RM 1767

HISTOLOGICAL TECHNIQUES

Manfred GABE

Laboratoire d'Évolution, Faculté des Sciences, Paris, France

HISTOLOGICAL TECHNIQUES

TRANSLATED BY

Robert E. BLACKITH

Department of Zoology, Trinity College, University of Dublin, Ireland

Aries KOVOOR

Laboratoire de Biologie de la différenciation cellulaire, Université de Paris VII, France.

MASSON
Paris New York Barcelone Milan

SPRINGER-VERLAG
New York Heidelberg Berlin

1976

MASSON S.A. 120 Bd Saint-Germain, Paris-6ᵉ
MASSON Inc. 111 West 57th Street, New York, N.Y.
TORAY MASSON Balmes 151, Barcelone 8
ETMI Via Settembrini 27, Milan
SPRINGER-VERLAG New York Heidelberg Berlin

Title of the French Edition:
TECHNIQUES HISTOLOGIQUES
© Masson et Cie, Paris, 1968

ISBN: 2-225-44154-5 Masson Paris
ISBN: 0-387-90162-0 Springer-Verlag New York Heidelberg Berlin
ISBN: 3-540-90162-0 Springer-Verlag Berlin Heidelberg New York

© *Masson, Paris, 1976. Copyright under the International Copyright Union. All rights are reserved. This book is protected by copyright. No part of it may be duplicated or reproduced in any manner without written permission from the publisher. Printed in Hungary.*

Dr. Manfred GABE died on the 12th September 1973. Before his death, he had updated the work for the English edition; publication was supervised by Dr. L. ARVY.

The fact that the translators had used widely different conventions for the spelling of technical words was not noticed until this work had been set up in type. Readers are asked to excuse what may appear to be irritating inconsistencies arising from this oversight, to correct which would have required very numerous changes in the proofs.

*
* *

Other works by DR. GABE *include:—*

Histochimie des polysaccharides chez les Invertébrés. *Hdb. der Histochemie* 1962, 2(I), 95 — 393, 133 Figs. Stuttgart, Gustav Fischer Verlag.

Neurosecretion. 1966, 872 pp., 586 Figs. Oxford, Pergamon Press.

Neurosécrétion. 1967, 1091 pp., 586 Figs. Paris, Gauthier-Villars.

Techniques histologiques. 1968, 1113 pp., Paris, Masson et Cie.

Polysaccharides in the Lower Vertebrates. *Hdb. der Histochemie* 1971, 2(3), 543 pp., 203 Figs. Stuttgart, Gustav Fischer Verlag.

TABLE OF CONTENTS

Foreword 1

Note concerning textual conventions 6

Introduction 7

    Histological research and diagnostic histology (9); Automatic, easy, difficult and capricious technique (10); Choice of a technique (11); Conclusion of technique (12).

PART ONE

GENERAL PRINCIPLES OF HISTOLOGICAL TECHNIQUE

CHAPTER 1. — *Vital examination* 15
    Removal of pieces 17
    Making preparations 17
    Examination under the light microscope 20
    Examination under the dark-field microscope 20
    Examination under the phase-contrast and interference microscope 21

CHAPTER 2. — *Vital Staining* 22
    Definition ....
    Objects, advantages and disadvantages 24
    Classification of vital stains 24
    Theories of vital staining 25
    General rules for applying vital stains 28

CHAPTER 3. — *Fixation* 30
    CLASSIFICATION AND MODE OF ACTION OF FIXATIVES 33
        Fixation by physical agents 33
            Fixation by heat (33); Fixation by drying at room temperature (34); Fixation by drying at low temperature (34); Fixation by freezing-substitution (41) ....
        Fixation by chemical agents 42
            Methanol, ethanol, acetone (44); Hydrochloric, nitric and sulfuric acids (45); Trichloracetic acid (45); Picric acid, Chloroplatinic acid (46); Mercuric chloride (47); Chromium trioxyde (48); Potassium dichromate (49);

Acetic acid (49); Formaldehyde (51); Other aldehydes (52); Osmium tetroxyde (54).

GENERAL REMARKS ON FIXATIVE MIXTURES 55
Fixative mixtures containing an "indifferent" salt 55
Mixtures containing several fixing agents 56
Period of fixation 59
Temperature of fixation 60

MODES OF FIXATION 61
Fixation with vapours 61
Fixation in liquids 61

CHOICE OF FIXATIVE 64

CHAPTER 4. — *Embedding and preparatory operations* 66

TERMINATION OF FIXATION 67
EMBEDDING IN PARAFFIN 68
Properties of the embedding medium 69
Procedure of paraffin embedding 69
  Dehydration (70); Impregnation with a solvent of paraffin (74); Penetration of paraffin into pieces (78); Moulding the block (80).
Choice of method for paraffin embedding and summary of operating procedure 83

EMBEDDING IN NITROCELLULOSE (CELLOIDIN, COLLODION) 85
Properties of the embedding mass 86
Procedure of embedding 88
  Imbedding in alcohol-celloidin (88); embedding in methanol-celloidin (89); embedding in glycerine-celloidin (89); embedding in pyridine-celloidin (90)

EMBEDDING IN GELATIN 90
Embedding in gelatin after Apathy 91
Embedding in gelatin after Heringa and Ten Berge 92
Embedding in gelatin after Baker 92
Embedding in gelatin after Pearse 93

OTHER METHODS OF EMBEDDING 93
The solid polyethylene-glycols 93
Steedman's ester-wax 94

DOUBLE EMBEDDING 94
Embedding in agar-paraffin 95
Embedding in celloidin-paraffin: the method of Apathy—the method of Pfuhl 96

CHAPTER 5. — *Cutting and sticking sections* 97

The razor 98
The razor-holder 102
The object-holder 103
The mechanism of advance 103
Choice of a microtome 103
Maintenance of the microtome 105
Cutting and handling paraffin sections 105
Preparing the block 105
Cutting sections 108
Handling and spreading sections 109
Cutting sections in paraffin-agar 116

    Cutting and handling celloidin and celloidin-paraffin sections 116
        Preparation of celloidin blocks to be cut under alcohol 117
        Preparation of celloiding blocks to be cut under terpineol 117
        Preparation of celloidin-paraffin blocks 118
        Cutting sections 118
        Sticking sections 118
    Cutting and handling gelatin sections 123
    Cutting and handling frozen sections 124
        Preparing blocks 125
        Cutting sections 125
        Handling and sticking sections 126

CHAPTER 6. — *Staining and mounting microscopical preparations* 128

    Definition and nomenclature 129
    General theory of staining and the classification of stains 131
    Theories of histological staining 134
        The chemical theory 134
        The concept of staining by inhibition and by precipitation 134
        Adsorption as a factor in the binding of stains 135
        Electrostatic adsorption as a mechanism of histological staining 135
        Theory of indirect staining 136
        The density of structures as a factor in histological staining 137
        The texture of tissue constituents and their penetration by stains 137
    General remarks on the practice of staining 138
        Choice of stains 138
        Preparation of solutions 139
        Glassware 140
        Deparaffining sections 141
        Collodioning sections 142
        Dissolving crystals of mercury 143
        Summary of operations preceding the staining of sections 143
    Mounting media miscible in water: Apathy's syrup; The glycerine gum;
    Laevulose syrup; Gelatinized glycerine 145
        Mounting media miscible with benzenic hydrocarbons 146
        Summary of different mounting procedures 149
        Luting the preparations 150
        Conservation of microscopical preparations 150

CHAPTER 7. — *The examination of histological preparations* 152

    The graphical representation of histological preparations 154
    The reconstruction of histological preparations 156
        Graphical reconstruction 158
        Plastic reconstruction 160
    The quantitative study of histological preparations 161
        The causes of error in measuring under the microscope 162
        Measuring lengths in the plane of the stage 163
        Measuring lengths along the optical axis of the microscope 163
        Measuring areas perpendicular to the optical axis of the microscope .. 164
        Procedures of linear integration to measure areas and relative volumes 165

APPENDIX. — *List of principal dye-stuffs used in histology* 168

    Anthraquinone (168)—Azins (168)—Azo-dyes (169)—Fluorochromes—Indulins—Natural dyes (170)—Nitro-dyes—Nitroso-dyes—Phenyl methanes (171)—Phthalocyanin— Pyrazolones—Quinolines—Thiazins (172) —Xanthenes (173)

Part Two

GENERAL METHODS

Chapter 8. — *Topographical fixation* 117

    The principal topographical fixatives 178
        Aqueous liquids 178
        Alcoholic liquids 185
    The practice of topographical fixation 187
        Choice of fixative 188
        Removal and fixation 189
        Stopping fixation and storing pieces 190
        Choice of embedding method 191

Chapter 9. — *Topographical staining* 192

    CLASSIFICATION OF TOPOGRAPHICAL STAINS 192
    NUCLEAR STAINING BY PROGRESSIVE HAEMATOXYLIN LAKES 194
        Aluminium lakes of haematein 195
        Progressive ferric lakes of haematein 197
        Progressive chromic lakes of haematein 199
    SELECTIVE STAINING OF COLLAGEN FIBRES 200
        Staining based on competition between two acidic dye-stuffs 200
            Haemalum-picro-indigocarmine (201); Ramon y Cajal's trichrome (202); Nuclear fast-red picro-indigocarmine (203); Van Giesons' method (204); Variants of Van Gieson's method (205); The method of Curtis (206); Variants of the method of Curtis (207); Gaussen's histo-polychrome (208); A. Prenant's triple stain (209);
            Advantages and disadvantages of methods based on competition between two acidic stains 209
        Staining that involves phosphomolybdic or phosphotungstic acid 211
            Original method of Mallory (212); Masson's trichrome (213); Gomori's trichrome (215); Variants of Gomori's trichrome (216); One-step trichrome: Gabe and Ms Martoja (217); Heidenhain's azan (219); Variants of the azan stain (223); Petersen's method (224).
            Advantages and disadvantages of methods involving phosphomolybdic or phosphotungstic acids 226
    STAINING BASED ON THE DEMONSTRATION OF CYTOPLASMIC TINCTORIAL AFFINITIES 227
        Nuclear staining with a haematoxylin lake followed by counter-staining with an acid dyestuff (227); Millot's triple staining (229); Safranin-light green (230); The Ehrlich-Biondi-Heidenhain method (231); Mann's technique (232); Dobell's variant (233); The Mann-Dominici method (233); Staining with azur eosinates (235)
        Advantages and disadvantages of the methods of this group 236
    BULK STAINING 237
        Coloration with the aluminium lake of gallamine blue (238); Staining with boracic carmine (239); Staining with Carmalum (239); Bulk staining with P. Mayer's haemalum (240); Staining with haematein IA of Apathy (240)

Chapter 10. — *Decalcifying and softening very hard tissues* 242

    DECALCIFYING 242
        Nitric acid—Sulfurous acid—Trichloracetic acid (244). Formic acid—

Chromic acid —Picric acid —Sodium ethylene-diamino-tetracetate (EDTA, versene)—Decalcifying by organic buffers (245)
Modifications of tinctorial affinities during decalcification and the choice of a decalcifying agent—Decalcifying pieces embedded in celloidin 246

SOFTENING CUTICULAR STRUCTURES AND KERATIN 247
Chlorine dioxide (248); Murrays' method (249)

PART THREE

HISTOCHEMICAL METHODS

CHAPTER 11. — *General introduction to the study of histochemical techniques*

DEFINITIONS 252
CURRENT PROGRESS IN HISTOCHEMICAL RESEARCH AND THE WAYS IN WHICH ITS TECHNIQUES MAY BE EMPLOYED 254
THE REQUIREMENTS EXACTED BY HISTOCHEMICAL INVESTIGATIONS 256
Chemical conditions 256
Morphological conditions 259
Histochemical fixation (259); Embedding (262); Sections cutting (263); Histochemical reactions (263)

CHAPTER 12. — *Histophysical methods* 226
ABSORPTION SPECTROPHOTOMETRY AND HISTOPHOTOMETRY 267
EMISSION HISTOSPECTROGRAPHY 271
FLUOROSCOPY AND FLUORESCENCE SPECTROGRAPHY 272
Apparatus 273
Fluoroscopy as a morphological technique 273
Primary fluorescence for histochemical identification 274
Secondary fluorescence following histochemical reactions 275
Immuno-histochemistry 276
Preparation of the antigen and antibodies; the conduct of immuno-histochemical reactions; labelling of antibodies with fluorochromes (276); preparations of sections and conduct of the reaction (277)

HISTORADIOGRAPHY 277
PHASE CONTRAST MICROSCOPY AND INTERFERENCE MICROSCOPY 279
MICROSCOPY IN POLARISED LIGHT 282
AUTORADIOGRAPHY 282

CHAPTER 13. — *Histochemical detection of mineral substances* 288
MICRO-INCINERATION 288
Fixation—Preparation and spreading of sections (289). Conduct of incineration (290). Mounting and examination of spodograms (291). Identification of mineral matter in spodograms (293).

DETECTION OF MINERAL ANIONS 292
Chlorides (293). Iodides and Thyroid iodine (294). Phosphorus (294). Sulphur (295). Arsenic (295). Silicon (296).

DETECTION OF MINERAL CATIONS 296
Sodium and Potassium 297
Calcium 298

Methods for staining with lakes 298
Chelation with sodium rhodizonate (300). Chelation with glyoxal bis (2-hydroxyanil) (301).
Substitution methods 303
Barium and strontium 307
Beryllium (glucinum): The azurine-solochrome method 308). The quinalizarin method (308). Staining with naphthochrome green B (308)
Magnesium 309
Zinc 309
Aluminium 311
Iron 311
The prussian blue reaction (312). Quincke's reaction (313). The Turnbull blue reaction (313)
Practical aspects of the histochemical study of iron 315
The choice of fixative (315). The chemical purity of reagents employed (315). The choice of techniques for detection (316)
Nickel and cobalt 317
Copper 317
Mercury 318
Silver 318
Gold 319
Bismuth and Lead 320

CHAPTER 14. — *Histochemical detection of properties common to several radicals and functional groups* 321

HISTOCHEMICAL DETECTION OF REDUCING COMPOUNDS 321
The ferric ferricyanide reaction: 322
Principles (322). Preparation of reagent (323). Practice of the reaction (323). Adam's method (324). Chèvremont and Frédéric's method (325). Interpretation of results (325).
The reduction of silver salts 325
Principles (326). Preparation of reagents (326). Fontana's solution (326). Silver hexamethylenetetramine (327). Silver piperazine (327). Ammoniacal silver carbonate (327).
Practice of the reaction: The classical argentaffin reaction of Masson (328). The silver hexamethylenetetramine reaction of Lillie and Burtner (328)
Interpretation of results (328)
The reduction of tetrazolium salts 329
Principles (329). Preparation of the reagent (331). Working technique (331).
Interpretation of results (331)

THE HISTOCHEMICAL STUDY OF ACIDOPHILIA 332
Working technique (333). Interpretation of results (333)

THE HISTOCHEMICAL STUDY OF BASOPHILIA 334
The physico-chemical factors influencing basophilia: 336
The action of fixative (336). The temperature (336). The effect of the concentration of dye (336). The type of stain used (337). The ionic strength of the dye solution (337). The pH of the staining bath (337)
The detection of basophilia for histochemical purposes: 339
Reagents (369). Working technique (340).
Estimation of the tissue zone containing proteins at isoelectric point 340
Reagents (340). Working technique (341)
The histochemical interpretation of basophilia in tissue 342

The histochemical study of metachromasia 343
  Metachromatic stains 344
  The mechanism of metachromasia 345
  The practical conduct of the metachromatic reaction 346
  Histochemical interpretation of the metachromatic reaction 348
    The sulphomucopolysaccharides (348). The mucopolysaccharides bearing carboxyl groups (348). The nucleic acids (348). The macromolecular metaphosphates (349). Certain lipids (349)
Other staining indicative of the presence of anions: 349
  Paraldehyde fuchsin 350
    The stain (350). Working technique (351). Histochemical interpretation (353)
  Paraldehyde thionine 354
  Phthalocyanins (alcian blue, alcian green, alcian yellow, astra blue) 354

Chapter 15. — *Histochemical detection of aldehydes and ketones* 357
  The Schiff reagent 358
    The preparation of Schiff's reagent 360
      Graumann's method (361). Coleman's method (361). Longley's method (361). Barger and De Lamater method (361). Preparation of Schiff's reagent equivalents (362). Method of use for Schiff's reagent and its equivalents (363). Histochemical interpretation (364)
  Alkaline silver complexes 365
  Benzidine and o-dianisidine 366
  Phenylhydrazine 367
  2-Hydroxy-3-naphthoic acid hydrazide 367
  p-Phenylenediamine 369
  Blocking reactions of the aldehyde groups: 370
    Aniline chlorhydrate. Hydroxylamine. Semicarbazide. Thiosemicarbazide. Phenylhydrazine. Sodium bisulphite
  The distinction between aldehydes and ketones 371

Chapter 16. — *Histochemical detection of phenols and naphthols* 372
  The azo-reaction 373
    The reagents (373). Lison's technique for the preparation of diazonium salts (377). Technique of Lillie and al. for the preparation of the diazo salt of safranine 0 (377). Technique of Lillie and Glenner for the preparation of the diazo salts of S acid (8-amino-naphthol-5 sulphonic acid) (377). Davis's technique for the diazotisation of pararosaniline (377). Coupling (378). Histochemical interpretation (380)
  The Indo-reaction 380
  The Gibbs reaction 381
  The argentaffin reaction 381
  The phaeochrome (chromaffin) reaction 382

Chapter 17. — *Histochemical detection of carbohydrates* 384
  Histochemical detection of glucose 384
  Histochemical detection of ascorbic acid 386
    Demonstration of ascorbic acid: in pieces of tissue, after freeze drying (387) and on cryostat section 387

HISTOCHEMICAL DETECTION OF POLYSACCHARIDES 388
   Classification of polysaccharides detectable by histochemical methods 389
   Techniques for the detection of polysaccharides 390
   Oxidative reactions: 391
      Periodic acid (391). Lead tetra-acetate (394). Sodium bismuthate (395). Manganese acetate (396). Phenyliodoso-acetate (396). Chromium trioxide (396). Potassium permanganate (397). The use of oxidative reactions in combination: periodic acid-Schiff reaction (398). PAS-haematoxylin-picro-indigocarmine (400). PAS-haematoxylin orange G (400). Allochrome method of Lillie (400). The method of Monné and Slautterback (401).
   Reagents and working technique 402
      The sodium bismuthate-Schiff (403). Methods with alkaline silver complex (403). Gomori's technique with silver-hexamethylenetetramine (403). Method of Arzac and Flores (404)
   Metachromatic reactions 405
   Sulfuric and phosphoric esterification 406
   Fixation of metallic ions 407
      Preparation of colloidal solutions of iron hydrate (408): Technique of Rinehart and Abul-Haj. Gomori's technique, Müller's technique and Mowry's technique 409
   Combination of the colloidal iron technique with the PAS-reaction 410
   Marker stainings 410
      Staining with: Best's carmine (411) and the phthalocyanines of the alcian blue group (412); Staining with alcian blue following Mowry's technique (413). Combination of the alcian blue stain with the PAS-reaction (413). Staining with alcian blue in saline solution (414). Staining with paraldehyde fuchsin (414). *Control tests* (415): Blocking the carbonyl groups (415). Inhibition of oxidation by lead tetra acetate (416). Decomposition of polysaccharides on sections (416): by amylase (416), sialidase (417), hyaluronidase (418). Chemical transformation of polysaccharides (418): by benzoylation (419), acetylation (419), reversible methylation (412).
   Histochemical identification of different kinds of polysaccharides 424
      Glycogen (424). Galactogen (428). Cellulose (429). Starch (420). Dextran (430). Neutral mucosubstances (430). Acid mucosubstances (434)
   The practice of histochemical tests for polysaccharides 439
      The fixation techniques (439). The embedding and cutting of the sections (440). The choice of diagnostic reaction and stains (440)

CHAPTER 18. — **Histochemical detection of fats and related compounds** 442

CLASSIFICATION OF FATS 443
PREPARATION OF THE TISSUES FOR A HISTOCHEMICAL STUDY OF LIPIDS 445
THE HISTOCHEMICAL DETECTION OF LIPIDS BY MEANS OF LYSOCHROMES 449
      By lysochromes in ethanol solution (451); by lysochromes in supersaturated isopropyl alcohol solution (452); by fluorescent lysochromes (453)
THE USE OF EXTRACTION TECHNIQUES IN THE HISTOCHEMICAL STUDY OF LIPIDS. 455
   Ciaccio's technique for selectively rendering insoluble the phospho-and sphingolipids 455
   Keilig's technique for the differential extraction of lipids 456
HISTOCHEMICAL REACTIONS AND STAINS PERMITTING THE IDENTIFICATION OF CERTAIN LIPIDS 457
   Optical anisotropy 457

Demonstration of the acid nature of lipids 459
   The Nile blue method (460). Tests for metachromasia (461). Staining with copper haematoxylin (462). Staining with phthalocyanins (463).
Demonstration of the unsaturated nature of lipids 464
   Reduction of osmium tetroxide (464). Addition reactions of the halogen (465). Oxidative reactions using peracids (467). Demonstration of peroxides formed during the oxidation of unsaturated lipids (465).
Demonstration of the complexes formed by lipids with chromium compounds 469
Demonstration of lipids bearing carbonyl groups 472
Demonstration of carbohydrate constituents of certain lipids 476
Demonstration of the sterol radical 477
HISTOCHEMICAL CHARACTERISTICS OF THE PRINCIPAL CATEGORIES OF LIPIDS 479
   Glycerides (480); Phosphatide esters (480); Plasmalogens (481); Sphingolipids (481); Steroids (481); Carotenoids (482); Chromolipoids (483); Ceroid pigment (486)- Lipofuscins (486); Haemofuscin (487)
DICHOTOMOUS KEYS FOR THE ANALYSIS OF LIPIDS 487

CHAPTER 19. — *The histochemical detection of amino-acids and proteins* 490

THE FIXATION OF PROTEINS 491
THE HISTOCHEMICAL REACTIONS OF PROTEINS AS SUCH 492
   THE HISTOCHEMICAL DETECTION OF THE α-AMINO-ACID GROUP 496
   Reactions depending on the formation of azomethines 496
   Reactions of condensation with dinitrofluorobenzene 497
   Reactions depending on oxidative deamination 499
   Blocking reactions for primary amine groups 502
   REACTIONS FOR THE SELECTIVE DETECTION OF CERTAIN AMINO-ACIDS 504
   Demonstration of the guanidyl radical and of arginine 504
   Demonstration of the imidazol group 507
   Demonstration of tyrosine 508
      Reactions of Millon-Baker (508) and Millon-Pollister-Ris (508); Danielli's coupled tetrazonium reaction (509); Morel and Sisley's reaction (511)
   Demonstration of indole groups and in particular of tryptophane 513
   Demonstration of thiol and disulphide groups 517
      Reactions for the histochemical detection of the thiol group (517); reactions based on the reducing capacity (518); methods based on the formation of mercaptides (519); techniques which depend on esterification of the thiol radical (520); methods based on the selective oxidation of disulphide linkages in cystine (523); Preparation of tissue for detection of protein-bound sulphydryls (526); Reduction of disulphide linkages to thiol groups (527): by alkaline sulphides, alkaline cyanides, sodium hydrosulphite, thioglycollic acid, thioglycerol (528), thiolacetic acid and dimercaptopropanol (529); Blocking reactions for thiol groups, by iodine, mercuric bichloride and ethylmaleilimide (529); sodium iodo-acetate or chloropicrin (530); The practice of the histochemical tests for protein-bound sulphydryls (530)
DEMONSTRATION OF ELECTROPOLAR FEATURES OF PROTEINS 531
   Tests for acidophilia as a method for the identification of proteins 532
   The evaluation of the zone of the isoelectric point in the histochemical study of proteins 533
THE IDENTIFICATION OF CERTAIN PROTEINS BY ENZYMATIC DIGESTION 534

Trypsine, chrymotrypsine, pepsine (535); collagenase (536); elastase 536).
THE IDENTIFICATION OF PROTEINS BY DIFFERENTIAL SOLUBILITY 536

CHAPTER 20. — *Histochemical detection of nucleoproteins and metalloproteins* 538
HISTOCHEMICAL DETECTION OF NUCLEOPROTEINS 538
Demonstration of nucleic acids through their ultraviolet absorption 539
Demonstration of nucleic acids through their basophilia 540
Chromic lake of gallocyanine (541); methyl green (543)
Demonstration of nucleic acids by staining with two basic dyes........ 545
Nucleal reactions 549
The nucleal reaction of Turchini and al. (549); The nucleal reaction of Feulgen and Rossenbeck (551); Other nucleal reactions (556); De Lamater's technique (557), Himes and Moriber's technique (558), Benson's technique (559)
Techniques for extraction of nucleic acids 560
Extraction with ribonuclease (561); Extraction with deoxyribonuclease (563); The general extraction of nucleic acids (564); Selective extraction of ribonucleic acid (564) *The preparation of the tissues for detection of nucleic acids* 565
HISTOCHEMICAL DETECTION OF METALLOPROTEINS 566
Histospectroscopy 567
Pseudo-peroxidase properties 567

CHAPTER 21. — *Histochemical detection of some products of protein metabolism* 571
COMPOUNDS ASSOCIATED WITH THE METABOLISM OF PHENYLALANINE AND TYROSINE 571
Fluoroscopic detection of biogenic monoamines 571
Histochemical detection of catecholamines 574
Simultaneous demonstration of adrenaline and noradrenaline (575); Selective demonstration of noradrenaline (577); The osmium-iodide technique of Champy and Coujard (579)
Histochemical detection of melanins 580
Methods for bleaching (581)
COMPOUNDS RELATED TO THE METABOLISM OF TRYPTOPHANE 584
COMPOUNDS RELATED TO THE METABOLISM OF HISTIDINE 586
COMPOUNDS RELATED TO THE METABOLISM OF HAEMOGLOBIN 587
Hemosiderins 588
Bile pigments 589
Porphyrins 591
WASTE-PRODUCTS OF PROTEIN METABOLISM 591
The histochemical detection of urea 591
Histochemical detection of purines 592

CHAPTER 22. — *The histochemical detection of the principal enzymes* 595
THE PREPARATION OF TISSUES INTENDED FOR HISTO-ENZYMOLOGICAL RESEARCH 597
THE GENERAL COURSE OF HISTO-ENZYMOLOGICAL REACTIONS 598
HISTOCHEMICAL DETECTION OF HYDROLASES 601
Phosphatases
Non-specific alkaline phosphomonoesterase 602
Techniques using sodium glycerophosphate (602); Techniques involving

naphthylphosphates (602); Preparation of tissue intended for the demonstration of non specific alkaline phosphomonoesterases (609)
Adenosine-triphosphatases 612
  Technique of Padykula and Herman (612); Technique of Wachstein and Meisel (613).
5-Nucleotidase (Adenosine 5-phosphatase) 614
  Gomori's technique (614); Wachstein and Meisel technique (614)
Non-specific acid phosphomonoesterase 615
  Gomori's technique using lead nitrate (616); Techniques using naphthol phosphates (617).
Phosphamidase 619
  Technique of Gomori (169); Meyer and Weinmann's technique (620)
Glucose-6-Phosphatase 620
  Chiquoine's technique (621); Wachstein and Meisel's technique (621)
Carboxylic esterases 622
Cholinesterases 622
  Coer's technique (624), Arvy's technique (625); The technique of Wachstein and al., (626)
Non-specific esterases 627
  Preparation of tissues (619); Techniques involving naphthylacetates (629); Techniques involving indoxyl acetates (631)
Lipases 632
Sulphatases 634
Glucosidases (glycosidases) 635
Carbonic anhydrase 636
Peptidases 637
Deoxyribonuclease 639

HISTOCHEMICAL DETECTION OF TRANSFERASES 640

HISTOCHEMICAL DETECTION OF OXIDO-REDUCTASES 643
  Oxidases 643
    Cytochrome-oxidase 643
    Tyrosinase and Dopa-oxidase 646
    Polyphenoloxidases 647
  Peroxidases 649
  Aerobic dehydrogenases 650
  Anaerobic dehydrogenases 652
    The succinic-dehydrogenase system 653
    The NAD-dehydrogenases-NAD diaphorase and NADP-dehydrogenase-NADP-diaphorases system 655
      Modern techniques for the detection of diaphorases (655); Modern techniques for the detection of NAD- and NADP-dehydrogenase (657)
  Δ^5-3-β-Hydroxysteroidodehydrogenase 659

APPENDIX 661
  Table of atomic weights (661); Formulae and molecular weights of the principal chemicals in the preparation of the buffer solutions (662); Preparation of normal solutions of hydrochloric acid; nitric acid and sulphuric acid from commercial concentrated acids (662); Buffers (663); Equivalents between Fahrenheit and centigrade thermometric scales (672); Number of drops to a gram of several usual reagents (673); Metric equivalents of the english (Imperial) system of measures of weight and capacity (674); Suggestions for a histochemical nomenclature of tissue carbohydrates (674); List of recommended material used in tests for the main compounds mentioned in the third part of this book (676)

Part four

THE METHODS OF GENERAL CYTOLOGY

CHAPTER 23. — *Introduction to the techniques of general cytology* 681

THE PROBLEM OF CYTOLOGICAL FIXATION 682
    Chromo-osmic solutions 684
    Chromic fluids without osmium tetroxide and acetic acid 686
    Fluids based on heavy metals other than chromium and osmium 687
    Chromo-acetic fluids 688
    Regressive staining with haematoxylin lakes 689
        Ferric lakes 690
        Heidenhain's technique and its variants 690
        Dobell-Hirschler haematoxylin 694
        Cupric lakes 695

CHAPTER 24. — *Techniques for studying the nucleus* 697

THE GENERAL STUDY OF NUCLEAR STRUCTURES 697
    Vital observation 697
    Vital stains 698
    Nuclear structures in smears 698
    Nuclear structures on sections 701

PREPARATIONS FOR THE STUDY OF CARYOTYPE 702

PREPARATIONS FOR STUDYING THE SEX CHROMATIN 704

MORPHOLOGICAL STUDY OF THE NUCLEOLUS 705

DEMONSTRATION OF INTRANUCLEAR INCLUSIONS DIFFERENT FROM THE NUCLEOLE 707

CHAPTER 25. — *Techniques for demonstrating the golgi apparatus* 709

    Osmic impregnation 710
    Silver impregnation 713
    Choice between osmic and silver impregnation 716
    Demonstration of the Golgi apparatus by staining or histochemical reactions 716

CHAPTER 26. — *Techniques for demonstrating the chondriome* 717

MITOCHONDRIAL FIXATIONS 719
PREPARATION OF PIECES FOR MITOCHONDRIAL STAINING 722
MITOCHONDRIAL STAINS 726
    Staining with acid fuchsin 726
        Dichromic techniques 728
        Polychromic techniques 729
        Rectifying errors of postchromatization on slides 733
        The significance of Altmann's stain 734
    Staining with crystal violet 734
        Benda's method 734
        Nassonov's method 735
        Rectifying of mitochondrial staining by crystal violet 737
    Regressive staining of the chondriosomes with the haematoxylin lakes 737
    Silver impregnation of the chondriome 739
        The tannin-silver variant of Del Rio Hortega 739
        Technique of Fernandez-Galiano 741
    Choice of mitochondrial techniques 741

TABLE OF CONTENTS

CHAPTER. 27 — **Techniques for demonstrating the ergastoplasm and related structures** 743

   Ergastoplasm and ergastoplasmic parasomes 744
   Techniques for demonstrating yolk nuclei 746

CHAPTER 28. — **Techniques for studying the centrosome and fibrillar differentiation of the cytoplasm** 747

   Techniques for demonstrating the centrosome 748
   Techniques for demonstrating tonofibrils 751
   Techniques for brush borders and striated borders 752
   Techniques for demonstrating cilia 753

CHAPTER 29. — **Techniques for demonstrating secretory granules** 754

   Topographical stains 755
   Cytological techniques 756
   Staining with neutral dyes 756
   Gomori's method and its variants 757
     Chromic haematoxylin phloxine (759); The Mann-Dominici stain after permanganate oxidation (760); the paraldehyde-fuchsin, Groat's haematoxylin and picro-indigocarmine stain (761)
   Method of Solcia, Vassallo and Capella: 761
     Staining with toluidine blue (763); Staining with astra blue (763); Staining with pseudo-isocyanin (764)
   Silver impregnation techniques 765
     Distinction between secretory granules and lysosomes 765

PART FIVE

HISTOLOGICAL EXAMINATION OF THE PRINCIPAL TISSUES AND ORGANS

CHAPTER 30. — **Techniques for isolation and maceration and the demonstration of cell boundary** 769

   Maceration techniques 770
   Demonstration of cell boundaries on spread membranes 772
   Demonstration of cell boundaries by bulk staining 773
   Demonstration of cell boundaries on paraffin wax sections 773

CHAPTER 31. — **Techniques for the histological study of the integument and of its outgrowths** 775

   The integument of vertebrates and its outgrowths 775
   Vital examination 775
   Preparations in toto 776
   Examination of sections 776
     Topographical study (776); Morphological details of the epidermal cells (776); Histochemical characteristics (779); Cutaneous blood vessels (780) Cutaneous nerves and tactile receptors (781); Skin and hair follicles (781); Horny excrescences: nails, horns (781); Cutaneous glands (782); Tissue blocks containing fragments of bone (782).
   The integument of Arthropods and of other animals having an epidermis covered with a cuticule 783

The integument of Molluscs and of other animals with a ciliated epidermis on which glandular cells are scattered 784

CHAPTER 32. — **Techniques of the histological study of blood and of haematopoietic organs** 786

Histological examination of the circulating blood 787
Blood sampling 787
Vital examination 788
Permanent preparations 788
Hematological stains 791
Enumeration of the free elements of the blood 794
  Enumeration of the erythrocytes of vertebrates (795); Enumeration of the nucleated elements in the blood of mammals (797); Enumeration of leucocytes and thrombocytes in the blood of Sauropsida and Anamniota (798); Enumeration of blood platelets of mammals (798); Enumeration of the blood cells of invertebrates (799); the leucocyte formula (799).
Histological examination of the haematopoietic organs 800
Techniques specially required for the study of haematopoietic organs ... 800
The histological examination of bone marrow 804
Histological examination of the spleen 805
Histological examination of the thymus 806
Histological examination of the lymph nodes and related structures (Tonsils, Peyer patches, in the intestine, etc.) 807
Histological examination of the haematopoietic organs of invertebrates 807

CHAPTER 33. — **Techniques of the histological study of the connective tissue** 809

The histological study of the ground substance 809
Histological study of the connective fibres 811
Collagen fibres 811
Reticulin fibres 812
  Selective impregnation of reticulin according to Del Rio Hortega (813); Silver impregnation according to Gomori (813); Silver impregnation according to Oliveira (815)
Elastic fibres 816
  Staining with orcein (817); Staining with resorcine-fuchsin (819); Staining with Gallego's ferric-fuchsin (820); Staining with paraldehyde-fuchsin (821)
Fibrin 821
Fibrinoid 824
Oxytalan fibres 824
The use of enzymatic preparations for the identification of connective fibres 824
Histological study of the connective cells 825

CHAPTER 34. — **Techniques for the histological study of cartilaginous, bony and dental tissues** 828

Selective staining of cartilage and of bone on whole mounts 829
Histological examination of cartilage 830
Techniques specially recommended for the study of chondrocytes 831
Techniques particularly recommended for a study of the ground substance 831
Techniques specially recommended for the study of fibrillar structures 833
Histological examination of bony tissue 834
Study of sections of bony tissue prepared by grinding and polishing 835
Study of bony tissue on sections taken from fixed material 838
Histological examination of dental tissue 843

Chapter 35. — Techniques for the histological study of muscles and tendons 846

Identification of muscle fibres as such 847
Demonstration of the structural details of striated muscle fibres 848
Demonstration of the structural details of smooth muscle fibres 851
Demonstration of the innervation of muscle fibres 851
Demonstration of the fibres of tendons 852

Chapter 36. — Techniques for the histological study of the circulatory apparatus 853

Techniques for the histological study of the heart 853
Techniques for the histological study of blood vessels 854
Methods of following the flow of blood in the tissues and organs 856
Techniques which depend on staining the normal content of blood vessels 857
Techniques depending on the selective staining of the vascular walls 858
Techniques of vascular injection 859

Chapter 37. — Techniques for the histological study of the digestive apparatus 864

Histological examination of the anterior part of the digestive tract 864
Histological examination of the stomach 865
Histological examination of the intestine 869
Gastro-intestinal endocrine cells of the vertebrates: 872
  Demonstration of all types of endocrine cells by staining with lead haematoxylin (873); Methods for selectively demonstrating endocrine cells using silver impregnation (873); Methods for the selective demonstration of enterochromaffine cells (875); Demonstration of the enterochromaffin-like cells or histamine-storing cells (877); Demonstration of gastrin cells (877)
Histological examination of the lymphoidal formations of the digestive tract of vertebrates 878
Demonstration of blood vessels and nerves of the gastric and intestinal walls 879
Histological examination of the salivary glands 879
Histological examination of the exocrine pancreas 882
Histological examination of the liver 883
Histological examination of the digestive glands of Invertebrates 887
The secretory cycle of the glandular formation of the digestive apparatus ... 889

Chapter 38. — Techniques for the histological study of the respiratory system 890

Histological examination of the respiratory tract of Tetrapods 890
Histological examination of the pulmonary tissue 891
Histological examination of the swim bladder 893
Histological examination of gills 893
Histological examination of trachea of Arthropods and related animals   894

Chapter 39. — Techniques for the histological study of the excretory system 897

Histological examination of the kidney of Vertebrates 897
Histological examination of the urinary tract of the Vertebrates 903
Histological examination of the excretory system of Invertebrates 903

Chapter 40. — Techniques for the histological study of the nervous system 906

NEUROHISTOLOGICAL TECHNIQUES 907
Techniques for the detection of Nissl bodies 807
Selective coloration of the ganglion cells and their prolongation 910
  Mac Conaill's stain with lead haematoxylin (910); vital staining with methylene blue (911)

TABLE OF CONTENTS

Selective metallic impregnations of the ganglion cells and of their prolongations 914
  Silver chromate impregnation after Golgi-Cajal (916); Bubenaite's impregnation with silver chromate (918); Cox's impregnation with mercury (918); Fox's impregnation with zinc-chromate-silver nitrate (919).
Techniques for neurofibrils 919
  Gold techniques for neurofibrils 920
  Techniques for neurofibrils derived from Bielschowsky's method 921
    Gross-Schultze (921); Tinel (923); Agduhr (925); Boeke (926)
  Nerve-fiber impregnations derived from the silver reduction method 926
    Ramon y Cajal's silver reduction technique (927); Foley's technique for impregnation (929); Favorsky's technique for bulk impregnation (930); Davenport's technique for impregnation of sections (930); Bodian's technique for impregnation of sections (931); Holmes's technique for impregnation on sections (933); Palmgren's technique for impregnation of sections (934); Schultze's technique for impregnation of frozen sections (937); Romane's technique for neurofibril impregnation (939); Samuel's technique for neurofibril impregnation (940); Fraser Rowell's technique for neurofibril impregnation (943).
The osmium-iodide technique for staining nerve-fibres and nerve endings 943
Myelin methods 944
Production of nerves treated with osmium tetroxide 945
Myelin methods derived from Weigert's method 945
Histochemical reactions and diagnostic stainings applicable to the detection of myelin sheaths 949
Marchi's method 950
Neuroglia techniques 952
Stains for the neuroglia 952
  Holzer's stain for neuroglia (952); Anderson's neuroglia stain (953); Staining of the neuroglia with Mallory's phosphotungstic haematoxylin (954)
Metallic impregnation of neuroglia 955
  Ramon y Cajal's gold-sublimate method (956); Gold sublimate method (957); Fourth tannin-silver variant of Del Rio Hortega (957); Del Rio Hortega technique for astrocytes (958); Technique of Del Rio Hortega for oligodendroglia (959); Del Rio Hortega technique for microglia and perivascular neuroglia (959), Penfield's technique for microglia and oligodendroglia (960).

TECHNIQUES FOR THE HISTOLOGICAL STUDY OF NEUROSECRETORY CELLS 961
Neurosecretory products which are acidophilic in spite of permanganic oxidation of the sections 964
Neurosecretory products which are basophilic after permanganic oxidation 964
Recommendations concerning histological techniques applied to the study of the nervous system 969

CHAPTER 41. — **Techniques for the histological study of sense organs** 973

Histological examination of the tactile corpuscules 973
Histological examination of the pituitary mucosa 974
Histological examination of taste buds 976
Histological examination of the visual apparatus 977
Vital examination of the vertebrate eye 977
Histological examination of the eye as a whole 978
Methods particularly recommended for the study of different parts of the visual apparatus 979
Histological examination of the stato- acoustic apparatus 983

CHAPTER 42. — *Techniques for the histological study of the endocrine glands* 986

TECHNIQUE FOR THE HISTOLOGICAL STUDY OF THE NEUROHAEMAL ORGANS ... 987
TECHNIQUES FOR THE HISTOLOGICAL STUDY OF ENDOCRINE GLANDS WITHOUT
ACCUMULATION OF PARTICULAR SUBSTANCES 989
TECHNIQUES FOR THE HISTOLOGICAL STUDY OF ENDOCRINE GLANDS WHICH
ACCUMULATE SECRETORY PRODUCTS 991
The distal lobe of the adenohypophysis 992
   Anatomical study 992
   Identification of cellular categories 993
      Staining (955); Histochemical reactions (998); Marker stains (1000)
   General histochemical and cytological techniques 1006
The intermediate lobe of adenohypophysis 1007
The endocrine pancreas 1007
   Techniques for the quantitative study of the endocrine pancreas 1007
   Techniques for identifying the different types of cell in the endocrine
   pancreas 1011
      Preparation of the material (1012); Techniques for the selective demonstration of B Cells (1013); Techniques for the selective demonstration of the A cells (1019); Techniques for the selective demonstration of D cells (1024); Staining sequences for demonstrating different types of cell in selected islets (1030); Techniques for demonstrating other types of cell (1030).
The adrenal gland 1031
   Techniques for the topographical study of the adrenal gland 1032
   Techniques specially recommended for the study of the interrenal tissue 1034
   Techniques particularly suitable for the study of the adrenal tissue ... 1036
Endocrine tissues of Vertebrate gonads 1038
   Interstitial tissue of the testes 1038
   Internal theca of the follicles 1039
   Corpora lutea 1040
Thyroid gland 1041
Epiphysis 1044
Histological study of hormonal target organs during histophysiological studies on the endocrine glands 1046

CHAPTER 43. — *Techniques for the histological study of the reproductive system* 1048

Histological examination of the male genital system 1048
Microscopic anatomy of the Vertebrate testes 1048
Microscopic anatomy of the Invertebrate testes 1049
The study of spermatogenesis 1050
The study of the excretory ducts for sperm and of the glands attached to the
  the male genital system of Vertebrates 1051
Study of the male genital tracts and of their auxiliary glands in Invertebrates 1053
Histological study of the female genital system 1054
Microscopic anatomy of the Vertebrate ovary 1054
Microscopic anatomy of the female gonads of Invertebrates 1056
Cytological and histochemical study of ovogenesis 1056
Histological study of the female genital tracts of Vertebrates 1057
Histological study of the female genital tracts of Invertebrates 1059

APPENDIX IX. — *The mass production of histological preparations for
              teaching purposes* 1061

By way of bibliography 1063

Index of subjects 1067

FOREWORD

> Ἐγὼ φωνὴ βοῶντος ἐν τῇ ἐρήμῳ
> JOHN, I, 23

A SURVEY OF THE PRINCIPAL WORKS on histological technique that have appeared since the end of the 19th century shows such a diversity of concept and directive ideas, in spite of the fundamental unity of subject, that the choice of the underlying orientation was perhaps the most difficult problem facing me when MM. Masson & Cie, requested me to write this book.

A classification of these works based on their particular orientation and carrying the excess inherent in all that is schematic would lead to the definition of three types of books.

Some are handbooks or treatises on "microscopy". They are tacitly limited to the biological applications of the microscope, all of which are reviewed, and include in the same volume the techniques of histology proper along with those of bacteriology, botany and embryology. Such a work, on the scale of an encyclopaedic treatise contributed by specialists from a number of disciplines and meant to be consulted as a dictionary, may have a certain value if it is really exhaustive and periodically revised. But it is no longer possible on the scale of a handbook. A single person, however gifted, cannot have acquired sufficient mastery over all the techniques of the above disciplines to be able to speak from personal experience. Several ideas are discussed at second hand in the type of work that I allude to and a knowing judge often detects omissions that are apparently insignificant but really essential.

Others, devoted to histological technique or to some of its aspects, are in fact doctrinal works on methodology rather than on techniques. They faithfully reflect, in fact too closely, the scientific antecedents of other authors. Thus, the histologist who studies a particular problem over a number of years naturally chooses and improves on the techniques that serve him best; and true to human nature he is inclined to forget that his choice is not always the ideal one for all cases.

Yet others, and not necessarily the lesser ones, are books of recipes, clearly not intended by their authors to be read from cover to cover. The techniques are described in all their minute detail conducive to a good preparation, but the unfortunate reader never grasps the reason for a particular acid or alkaline wash, for a mordant or for a certain type of differentiation and toning. The reactive mechanisms of the agents used in histology and the true implications of the various operations are as clear as in the recipes of Valentin Basile so that many a young worker is left with the impression that histological techniques form a mean task whose empiricism calls for no intellectual faculty other than that of memory and whose success is, in the last resort, governed by chance.

Nothing is more inexact. Hazard and intuition have certainly played a role in the invention of a number of techniques. The physico-chemical basis of several methods has not yet been elucidated, and the era of formulae, graphs or computerization in devising histological preparations is still remote. However most techniques can now be submitted to a rational analysis, with the difference that in many cases rigorous proof is replaced by personal experience. Though certain descriptive stainings cannot yet be interpreted with rigour, histochemical reactions are open to strict analysis since no step of the procedure results from the fantasy or superstition of the author.

A true grasp of histological technique thus calls for a certain amount of theoretical knowledge that should not be underestimated. It would be vain to expect a cytological preparation showing fundamental organelles from a person who does not have an exact knowledge of the organelles in question. An understanding of the chemical mechanism of histochemical reactions is a *sine qua non* for their success, and the choice of the exergue at the head of Part Three of this book is not merely a courteous gesture but stems from profound conviction. But it goes without saying that the relevant elements of theory have no place in a book devoted to technique. The need for a sufficiently solid acquaintance of chemistry should be emphasized from the very first pages of a book that includes histochemical techniques, but is no reason why the work should be burdened with matter that can be found in any good handbook.

In practice a histological preparation should not be a case of fishing in troubled waters. The choice of method is the first, and probably the most difficult, question to be resolved. Once the technique has been chosen it should be studied methodically. The significance of each operation should be perfectly clear at the time of its execution, and the practice of blindly following a book or technical notes is quite disastrous.

The above concepts guided me in writing this book. It is not a handbook of microscopy, and in fact the manipulation of the microscope is not described. Other and better qualified authors have treated this subject in works that I strongly recommend to the beginner and even to histologists who no longer consider themselves as beginners. The allied techniques of protistology, bacteriology, botany, embryology, micromanipulation and of tissue and organ culture have evidently been left aside. They were comprised in histology during the last century but have since been emancipated to constitute autonomous disciplines with their specialised literature.

Even in such context certain limitations have to be made. Thus, the study of some tissues calls for special methods that cannot be justifiably applied to any others; their methodological problems are so particular that these branches of histology are almost autonomous disciplines. One of these is neurohistology, the techniques of which will only be briefly discussed. Among the histochemical techniques, those used to detect enzymatic activity occupy a similar position, and like neurohistological techniques they also tend to form an independent discipline. Many excellent and recent books on histoenzymology amply justify a reduction of the space devoted to it here.

The actual technique of making histological preparations is certainly my immediate objective, but I have reserved due place to methodology. The theoretical basis of the various techniques and the underlying reasons for each of their steps are to my mind as important as the operating procedure itself. Contrary to an unfortunate and widespread prejudice a technique is amenable to a truly rational analysis, and it is precisely the capacity for such an analysis that distinguishes a scientific investigator from the clockwork that transfers pieces or sections from dish to dish. I have therefore found it impossible to follow the current practice of expurgating the main text of purely technical details and relegating the operating procedures to an Appendix. The vogue that I allude to is the fruit of a most regrettable evolution of the divorce between the "technicality of ideas" and plain technicality itself. This partition between technicians and thinkers is to be banished from histology. In spite of the ceaselessly growing mechanisation of modern life, histological research remains a handicraft that is incompatible with the assembly-line that produces consumer goods and not prototypes. In fact histology progresses by prototypes and not by mass—produced articles.

The success of a histological preparation depends to a large extent on the choice of the technique adopted, and it is just this choice that a great number of works on histological technique neglect to beyond reasonable limits. I have therefore laid much emphasis on it, but I must first draw the attention of the beginners to a fundamental point: a master-technique applicable to all cases and yielding equally satisfactory results does not exist. The ideal fixative amenable to all techniques, and the universal stain that shows up everything are yet to be invented and probably never will be. The history of the great discoveries that we owe to the giants of histology clearly shows that the choice of technique is a necessary, though not sufficient, condition for success. It is therefore important to facilitate this choice as far as possible.

It follows clearly from the above notions that histological methods should be classified according to the object to be studied. It thus leads to the abandon of the classical plan of all handbooks on histological technique which successively describe the examination of fresh tissue, fixation, embedding, cutting and staining. With the latter method a single chapter would have to include techniques that differ greatly in their principles and indications. It leads to numerous repetitions by the author or the incessant turning of pages by the reader. After giving much thought to the various possibilities I have adopted the following subdivisions while being quite conscious of what is arbitrary in them.

Part one is devoted to the general principles of histological technique. The theories of fixation and staining are considered in addition to the rules governing the operations common to most techniques such as embedding, section-cutting, and mounting.

Part two describes the so-called general methods, that is techniques of histological topography. The fixatives and stains used in preparing material for microscopical anatomy are described.

Part three provides the essential details of histochemical technique.

Techniques devoted to demonstrating the fundamental organelles common to all, or widespread in many, Metazoan cells are contained in *Part Four*.

Part Five includes the special techniques meant for the study of the principal organs and tissues. Certain procedures are described in connection with their application, which is quite particular; others already described elsewhere in the book are indicated when opportune.

I evidently do not have the folly of pretending to be complete and exhaustive. Certain omissions that strike the knowing reader, of which there are quite a few, result from gaps in my knowledge and my apologies are due to those whose work has escaped my attention. Other omissions are meant to be such and correspond to methods that do not have any particular advantage or which have given me only mediocre results. True objectivity is an ideal towards which one should strive but which is probably out of the reach of common mortals. Though trying to treat the subject as uniformly as possible I may have devoted too much to my personal preference. Thus it is certain that fervent adepts of fluoroscopy will be rightly astonished by the little attention I have paid to their favorite technique while those who fancy yet some other stain will reproach me for my disdain of procedures that serve them daily.

It is almost impossible to correctly describe a technique without having practised it a certain number of times. For this reason I have stopped respectfully before entering into the domain of electron microscopy of which my knowledge is both rudimentary and theoretical. It has also led me to omit certain methods of light microscopy of which I have no personal experience. These have either been mentioned summarily or described word for word from the original after indicating their source. Those techniques of which I have acquired experience are described as they have given me the best results and important modifications of the original procedure are duly noted.

My undertaking owes much to the authors of books and reviews cited at the end. It is based on more than a quarter of a century of reading, reflexion and especially of the daily practice of histological technique. It is addressed to those who in turn wish to experience the harsh joys of encountering a subject that is difficult but of inexhaustible wealth.

NOTE CONCERNING TEXTUAL CONVENTIONS

One of the conventions adopted in the text concerns the use of small type which differs from usual practice. In what follows, small type *does not denote passages of minor importance but rather signifies theoretical or doctrinal comments*. However, so many such notions need to be discussed that all those not directly implicated have been excluded so as not to unduly increase the volume of the work.

For the same reason certain repetitions have been omitted; thus, for instance, the absolute necessity of removing mercuric crystals before staining material has been emphasized in chapter 6, but is thereafter considered to be a well-acquired precept.

Notions given, even in small type, before or after the actual operating procedure are often useful or indispensable for properly executing techniques. As a whole the book has been planned to be read through rather than to be consulted from time to time.

Volumes are expressed as *milliliters* (ml) and *weights* as *grams* (g) or *milligrams* (mg). A practice which might seem to be too "medical" for some readers, but which avoids many possible errors, has led me to indicate the number of *drops* or reagents in certain formulas by *roman numerals*. An *aqueous solution* if not stated otherwise, implies that it is prepared in *distilled water*. The term *alcohol* by itself refers to *ethanol*, the term *ether* to *diethyl ether (ethyl oxide)* and *formalin* to the *commercial solution* that is 35–40% by weight. All *temperatures* are given in degrees centigrade. *96% alcohol* denotes the commercial product, which may, in fact, be 95 or 96%, and is uniformly adopted in all formulae; clearly, a difference of one degree in the level of alcohol does not modify the final results of the different techniques.

INTRODUCTION

> Judged by the quality of the prerations used as basis for many investigations, the importance of technical process is not fully appreciated. The value of the results obtained from any microscopical study is directly dependent upon the quality of the techniques employed in preparing the material.
>
> C. M. McClung (1929).

THE POSSIBILITIES AND LIMITS OF HISTOLOGICAL TECHNIQUE

As with all other techniques of research, histological technique is only a means and not an end by itself. It undoubtedly provides a certain aesthetic satisfaction in that a successful preparation is beautiful to view, but it would be an error to go into ecstasies before its multicoloured hues, however fascinating they may be, without seeking their significance. Its value lies in the amount of scientific information it yields. Impeccable technique is thus an indispensable prerequisite though it does not suffice by itself.

Nevertheless few young workers realise the profound truth of the words of Professor Mac Clung cited at the head of this chapter. It should besides be admitted that the organisation of higher education in most European countries hardly prepares the beginner with a healthy appreciation of techniques. It is often through a teacher of philosophy that the future scientist is introduced to the elements of scientific methodology in school.

At the University the Professor has barely the time to give a brief insight into the discipline, insisting only on the salient facts and their importance while leaving aside the hesitations, tentatives and errors that have always strewn the path of scientific truth. What is true for *ex cathedra* teaching is even more so for textbooks and popularization.

The young post-graduate embarking on a career of research has often been lulled for years on global attitudes. In nine cases out of ten he imagines that the primordial condition for success in scientific work is aptitude for philosophical generalization. Ready to juggle with fundamental ideas and edify grand hypotheses, our post-graduate would at the most design to perform an *experimentum crucis* but would reject indignantly as a basely material task the very idea of having to handle a microtome, pipette or precision balance. Those of our future scientists who turn towards histology dream of sitting before an excellent microscope and examining preparations that have been made, cleaned and labelled by technicians to finally produce a theory of the structure of living matter. In the absence of such "working" conditions our novices cut and stain samples carelessly, are satisfied with mediocre results and imagine that the exquisite drawings with which classical authors have illustrated their monographs have been adapted to the purpose.

Some readers may take the above lines to be facetious but it is unfortunately not so. A brief survey of novices in histology will show that hardly seven out of ten go beyond the stage of haematoxylin and eosin and the splendid stain that is iron-haematoxylin is gradually going out of use. The vogue for the so-called automatic procedures which tend to replace the classical regressive stains is sad testimony to this.

What is more serious is that apprentice histologists, and even those who are no longer apprentices, are not interested in technique. They do not show the slightest desire to improve their knowledge in this field to keep in touch with progress and to learn new ones. Those who frequent research laboratories where histological techniques are practised will find dozens of workers whose devotion to science can only be praised but whose methods are restricted to those learnt during their early work.

In fact the remarks of Professor Mac Clung have lost none of their pertinence. It is by the careful practice of technique that any scientific work should commence, whether it be histology or any other discipline. When a technique is well executed its results may be fully exploited and with luck new facts may be unearthed which finally are the best reward a worker can expect for they ensure the permanence of his work.

In spite of its importance the material part of histological technique is not all; it should be properly applied. As in all other techniques of research, those of histology have their recommendations and counter—recommendations which should be neglected on no account. When for instance the motor branches of the brachial plexus of the muscles of the upper limb of an adult mammal are to be studied the use of histological technique would only prove the lack of critical sense in the author of such an attempt. Conversely the anatomical study of a small Arthropod pertains to histology rather than to dissection. The most thorough histological study can only yield presumptions as to the functional significance of a gland associated with the digestive tract while physiological experimentation and biochemical analysis would furnish definite results. Conversely only a properly conducted histological examination can ensure the localization of a physiologically active principle in a particular category of cells in a complex organ. It is chemical analysis and not histochemistry that should be resorted to in studying variations in the level of liver glycogen under experimental conditions; but the detection of glycogen in the particular elements of a complex organ is on the contrary a matter of histochemistry.

The above examples, which may be multiplied *ad infinitum* clearly show that only a judicious application of histological techniques will allow the maximum benefit to be drawn from them.

HISTOLOGICAL RESEARCH AND DIAGNOSTIC HISTOLOGY

There is a great diversity of the context in which histological technique is practised so that a corresponding classification is inconvenient. However two large groups of histological methods may be distinguished; those intended for research and those applied to diagnostic purposes.

By histological research I mean work whose object is the investigation of a type of cell, tissue or organ that has not been studied before, the morphological examination of a hitherto unknown structure or the analysis of organelles, cells and tissues under novel physiological or pathological conditions. The aim of diagnostic histology, on the other hand, is to obtain precise information concerning cells, tissues or organs whose normal structure is well established. It is obvious that the general approach to the types of study is quite different.

Histological research cannot really be codified. In fact, many great discoveries have resulted from the invention of new techniques or from the first application of a technique, often fortuitous, to a given object. One advances into the realm of the unknown, not only with regard to the interpretation of the results but also in the preparation of the specimen, and even an experienced histologist can have surprises in store for him when he attacks a new material. Knowledge gained from previous research may permit at the most the formulation of some general rules and no technical manual will exempt one from the indispensable trial and error in the use of fixatives and stains with every new object.

Diagnostic histology is practised in an entirely different context. The normal state of the object in question, its behaviour to various histological reagents and the means of detecting particular modifications are all well known or at least should be known. Consequently the very first attempt should be successful. There is no occasion for the inevitable trial and error in choosing fixatives and stains demanded by a research problem since the investigator has at hand all the data that enable him to select the techniques best suited to the relevant diagnostic elements. Codification of techniques, impossible for research, is thus easy for diagnostic purposes.

In histological research one should never lose sight of the fact that the various manipulations are liable to seriously alter cellular structure. In fact every time that the study departs from the domain of microscopical anatomy to enter into that of cytology, the investigator should be literally obsessed with possibility of artefacts and all his efforts should be devoted to ensuring that they do not arise either by establishing a concordance of results obtained with different methods or by observations made on living material. It can be quite otherwise in diagnostic histology where artefacts often arise from well-defined technical conditions and are themselves criteria in diagnosis. The real structure *in vivo* of the nuclei of blood cells is of limited diagnostic significance since rigorously standardized conditions of fixation and staining yield constant figures for a given cell type that enable its identification. Thus "equivalent images" in the sense of Nissl are perfectly compatible with diagnostic histology.

The *primum movens* of histological research is the wish to enrich our knowledge of the structure of an organ, a tissue or a type of cell. Their authors therefore possess the mentality of histologists. However in diagnostic histology the author is not necessarily interested in structure as such and what he observes only serves, to his mind, as an indication of functional modification. Its value may be compared to that of a biochemical assay or an electrogram. In other words diagnostic histology may be practised by those who adopt histological techniques but who are not histologists and who do not feel the least attraction to morphological research in the strict sense of the term.

AUTOMATIC, EASY, DIFFICULT AND CAPRICIOUS TECHNIQUES

In the latter half of the 19th century a good histological preparation was quite an achievement and justly afforded its author occasion for rejoicing. At present, improved apparatus and highly perfected techniques have rendered such preparations commonplace. However, it remains a fact that terms such as automatic, easy or difficult, delicate and capricious, that are used to describe techniques, are often encountered and it should be made clear as to what they signify.

In fact no histological technique is really automatic and the experienced histologist will not be astonished when I maintain that even the notorious haemalum-eosin can have various degree of success. Quite a few techniques, none the less, tolerate considerable deviation before actual failure ensues. Certain procedures among the so-called topographic stains may be so standardized as to be entrusted to automatic programmation without the slightest inconvenience. Some fixatives, like that of Bouin, are easier to handle than others. It is obvious that easy and automatic techniques are recommended when the aim of the examination is purely diagnostic.

The term "difficult technique" should be confined to methods where the general procedure is well defined and the mechanism thoroughly understood but whose practice implies multiple manipulations that have to be rigorously followed. A good example is that of azan staining. Each well-analyzed step of this excellent technique has its particular purpose and a slight lack or excess in its execution bears on the final result so that a practised worker can obtain at will the desired colour in a predetermined structure. The experience of a worker shows especially in the handling of difficult techniques. Their frequent practice on widely differing material ensures one the requisite knack for success.

The methods considered to be capricious are quite different. They are often procedures whose true mechanism is yet unknown, so that the ideal conditions for success cannot be laid down, many of them depending on chance. A classical example is the silver chromate impregnation of nerve cells after Golgi. It is obviously advantageous to learn such methods, but any real progress can be made only from a detailed study of their mechanism. So many capricious techniques have become very easy the day that their mechanism was elucidated. I may recall as an example, the countless failures that marked all empirical attempts to apply Romanowsky's stain in contrast to the absolute safety of the Azur eosinate stains that have come to be established scientifically.

CHOICE OF A TECHNIQUE

The preceding paragraphs have emphasized the importance and difficulty of this choice, and only a few general rules will be given here.

The first consists in establishing a reasonable proposition between the technical efforts involved and the expected result. It would thus be absurd to employ cytological techniques to ascertain from serial sections whether a thyroidectomy or a hypophysectomy is complete; the most ordinary of topographical techniques would do. Similarly, topographical methods allow an appreciation of the functional state of the thyroid or of the mammalian female genital apparatus and they would suffice for a diagnostic histological examination of these organs. The histochemical detection of lipids is on the other hand an integral part of any histological examination, even diagnostic, of the adrenal cortex of the testicular interstitial cells. The histological study of most exocrine glands, of the digestive tract and of the excreting system draws heavily on the techniques of classical cytology and their absence from any work, even diagnostic, devoted to these organs is a serious handicap.

One should, besides, take into account the nature and the condition of the material and the various possibilities open at the time of choice. A very voluminous piece that cannot be cut because certain anatomical relations have to be maintained should not be submitted to poorly penetrating fixatives. All the methods of classical cytology are unacceptable whenever the material is not perfectly fresh. Warm stains and treatment at a high pH should be avoided as far as possible when sections are rich in bone cartilage or chitin, which render them liable to be detached especially when more than 5 μ in thickness. The recommended delay in the accomplishment of certain techniques should be strictly observed. Thus it is better to abandon a silver impregnation of the Golgi apparatus when one is not assured of being able to achieve all operations from fixation to reduction in the 48 hours that follow removal of the specimen.

Another point to be considered is that of risking the material with certain techniques. In fact, the occasion arises when a histologist has to work on samples from rare animals or on material issuing from unique or difficult experiments. The danger of losing material of this type should also be considered in the choice of technique. Under these circumstances the capricious methods are evidently to be excluded, and the investigator is left with the choice between easy and difficult techniques. Of the two possible solutions some workers avoid the slightest risk and adopt summary techniques that always succeed but which never lead to a profound study. Others avoid the risk by previous methodical practice of difficult techniques which yield rich results. The option between the two possibilities is a matter of temperament as much as it is one of competence.

CONCLUSION OF TECHNIQUE

That which is expected of a histological preparation is not the same in histological research and in diagnostic histology.

In histological research, or whenever one is dealing with very rare material, the end of technical effort is achieved with a perfect preparation as far as its perfection is humanly possible. The only preparations that may be kept and shown are those that are utterly irreproachable in every respect and not criticizable by a competent and unindulgent histologist. The interpretation of preparations is not to be included as part of the technique in histological research.

The quality of preparations is less exacting in diagnostic histology. It is enough if the morphological criteria that serve to define the functional state of the object in question appear clearly. There is no point in obtaining spectacular preparations. However the technical aspect of the study is not over after the preparations have been mounted. In fact the functional condition of most vertebrate tissues, particularly of Mammals, can be determined from exact criteria a knowledge of which is part of the technique as much as the methods of fixation and staining employed. In diagnostic histology the theoretical aspect does not begin with the observation and interpretation of the preparations but with the explanations of their particular characteristics.

PART ONE

GENERAL PRINCIPLES OF HISTOLOGICAL TECHNIQUE

Towards 1800 the Parisian anatomist Xavier Bichat propounded the notion of a tissue and thus laid the foundations of histology, a science devoted to the morphological study of tissues and their constitutive elements. However, at that time the optical instruments available to biologists were so unsatisfactory that the founder of histology scorned their use. Bichat in fact based the distinction into the 23 tissues, which according to him constituted the human body, on those characters that could be perceived on macroscopical examination.

The situation is quite different today. Progress in optics has led to spectacular improvements in both the lens and the microscope. The practice is now inseparably bound to the use of microscope and the essential technical problem is that of providing cells and tissues in a suitable condition for such examination.

In certain cases cells can be examined simply after mounting between slide and coverslip. There are in fact tissues that can be reduced to sufficiently thin blades, without undue traumatism, to be observed under the light microscope in the absence of any reagent. But such vital examination is of mainly doctrinal interest and is reinforced to great advantage in all cases by the study of fixed and stained preparations.

In cases other than those of free cells or very thin blades of tissues it is necessary to cut sections sufficiently thin to permit their observation under the microscope. The cutting of sections, an operation that is usually effected between fixation and staining, can bring into play several methods each of which requires a particular preparation of the object.

Freshly removed pieces, without fixation, can be cut into thin sections after hardening by freezing. This method which was laborious at the time of the classical freezing-microtome has now been greatly improved with the advent of the contrivance to cool the knife (Schultz—Brauns, 1928). Even further progress has been achieved by placing the microtome in a chamber that can be cooled to the desired temperature. With the help of the cryostat the cutting of uniformly thin sections of most vertebrate tissues has become a routine operation that is of considerable importance in histochemical technique.

Pieces fixed in an aqueous medium may be cut in a freezing-microtome without much difficulty, thus avoiding any intermediate operation between washing the fixed piece and cutting. Nevertheless embedding in agar or gelatin often facilitates the attainment of thin and regular sections.

In the great majority of cases sections are cut from pieces embedded in paraffin or a nitrocellulose (collodion, celloidin).

Each of these methods necessitates different preliminary operations. A great number of other embedding media also exist but none of them has so far attained the vogue of the above two fundamental methods.

Staining before microscopical examination can be effected on fresh objects or after fixation. In the latter case it can be done either before (bulk staining, *coloration en masse, Stückfärbung*) or after cutting into sections.

In any case a histological preparation is completed by mounting in a medium that is favorable for both microscopical observation as well as conservation of the stain.

CHAPTER 1

VITAL EXAMINATION

> Die neuere Entwicklung der Mikrotechnik wird im wesentlichen durch die alte, immer wieder zum Durchbruch kommende Erkenntnis bestimmt, dass Wesen und Dynamik mikroskopischer Strukturen niemals mit Sicherheit am fixierten Dauerpräparat abgelesen werden kann. Der Aufschwung auf diesem Gebiete in den letzten Jahrzehnten hat aber auch die altbekannten und vom Standpunkt der Strukturforschung grundsätzlichen Mängel der Bilder lebender Objekte in ihrer Gültigkeit für die gesamte histologische Formenwelt bestätigt.
>
> A. Zeiger (1938).

Examination in the fresh state is the oldest of histological techniques. It has led to great discoveries. The 19th—century histologists acquired their first exact notions of the structure of organs and tissues by the study of rapidly removed pieces that were teased and examined under the microscope after mounting between slide and coverslip. Even today vital examination remains a fundamental technique whose judicious use permits a quite extensive morphological study of living matter. However it is important to know its limits and drawbacks.

Some authors have the habit of considering vital examination as an easy method, but a look into their writings will show that they refer to the simple microscopical examination of fluids from an organism with a view to determining the presence of structured elements, especially parasites. It is obvious that the histologist attributes an entirely different connotation to the term "vital examination". The chief aim of the method, in his mind, is to study the elements of the living cell without submitting them to any physical or chemical agent that is likely to cause artefacts. In other words, vital examination presents all its advantages to the cytologist only when the object has been removed and examined under conditions that do not seriously alter its vitality. If out of distrust for chemical fixatives one seeks to study the fresh mammalian kidney by hand-sections, dissociation or even by cryostat-sections one is only replacing a particular cause of artefacts by another. Shock, anaerobic conditions, the brusque supression of metabolites and freezing can *a priori* give rise to artefacts as well as by fixation with chemical agents, and experience has shown that the fanatic of vital examination loses in the bargain. A similar criticism can be levelled at those who wishing to examine very thick objects submit them to a compression, albeit "micro" on the human scale. Vital staining practised under defective conditions is as devoid of interest as would be a study of the physiology and behaviour of normal Man made on the inmates of a German concentration camp.

Vital examination in its strict sense, that which indeed bears any real interest, is a method that should be confined to the study of certain favorable objects.

The ideal material consists of cells that are normally found free in a liquid intercellular medium. This is the case with blood cells and most Protists. The excellent results obtained from the vital study of these objects are too well known to be recalled here; and it goes without saying that such a study is an essential step in any protistological or hematological research.

Small and sufficiently transparent Metazoans lend themselves well to such study and one should never fail to resort to it when studying Rotifers, small worms, certain Arthropod, Mollusc and Echinoderm larvae.

Another relatively favorable case is that of cells which though not really free can be easily separated from each other. It usually suffices to carefully rupture the connective envelope of an Invertebrate gonad to isolate living gonocytes at the risk of only slight traumatism. Fragments of epithelium can often be detached from underlying tissue by means of gentle scraping and their vital examination can yield valuable information.

Certain organs of Molluscs, Arthropods and Vertebrates are sufficiently transparent for vital examination. The branchiae of Mussels, the wings of Insects, the tongue, interdigital membranes and lungs of the frog are classical objects known to every student. Certain tegumentary zones of Crustaceans, the mesenteron of small Mammals and the pancreas of rodents are exceptionally favourable objects that enable the use of the most powerful optical devices of the light microscope for their study. The vital examination of the anterior segment of the eye is common ophthalmological practice. The insertion of transparent windows or the construction of observation chambers to hold mobile organs while maintaining their vascular and nervous connections greatly enlarge the scope of vital examination.

It should however be remembered that only a few Vertebrate tissues are suitable for vital examination. In spite of great ingenuity and material facilities the limit of possibility is soon attained; and I can only cite the fairly recent work of Vonwiller (1948) as an example illustrating the disproportion between the means employed and the final results.

The greatest circumspection is called for when vital examination necessitates dissection, slicing or teasing with needles. One should never lose sight of the fact that only observation of the living cell is of relevant interest in the present context.

It should not be forgotten that during vital examination only structures with a different refractive index from that of the surrounding medium can be observed under the microscope. The existence of a structure cannot therefore be denied on the grounds that it is not visible during vital examination. Besides, vital examination unaccompanied by any added reagent limits the criteria of identification to their form, so that in this respect stained preparations are a far richer source of information.

As a whole vital examination is a long and laborious method except in the case of certain very favorable objects. If all goes well a whole morning of work would yield two or three sketches or a few photographs. One should not expect success at the very first attempt and the details of the structure sought after are not perceived right away. A previous knowledge of the object gained from permanent preparations is useful if not indispensable. In most cases vital examination is thus a confirmatory method that pertains to histological research rather than to diagnosis.

REMOVAL OF PIECES

The technique of vital examination differs widely according to the nature of the material. The four following schematic cases can be distinguished.

1° Examination of free cells or those easily freed.
2° Mounting sufficiently small and transparent objects *in toto*.
3° Mounting a tissue in a slide while maintaining its connection with the rest of the organism.
4° Possible examination only after dissection or teasing the tissue.

Removal. — In the vital examination of blood cells sampling consists of puncturing a vessel in species with closed circulatory systems and the body cavity in those with open circulation. The gonocytes of Polychaete annelids and the Sipunculids, animals whose germ cells develop in the coelom, may be obtained in the same manner. Protists and small Metazoans living in a liquid medium may be removed by pipetting if necessary under a dissecting microscope. When it is desired to enrich the medium in such cases, *cautious* centrifugation may be practised.

Tissues that form thin blades may be carefully removed from the rest of the organism and mounted on a slide. Where connection with the rest of the animal can be maintained the value of the examination is greatly enhanced. In such cases the anaesthetized animal is held on a superstage adapted to the organ to be studied. The preparation is usually mounted on a glass plate that covers the aperture of the superstage corresponding to that of the microscope stage itself.

When a tissue has to be removed by dissection it is essential to avoid all rough treatment and any loss of time. In this connection it should be remembered that such removal for histological study, especially vital examination, has nothing in common with the dissection practised by anatomists where tissues are stretched and torn out brutally.

Obviously there is no special problem in the case of tissue cultures which may be examined directly under the microscope.

MAKING PREPARATIONS

Apart from the case of superficial organs or those exposed without any practical removal which may be observed in reflected light, vital examination necessitates a microscopical preparation. Such preparations may be mounted on a slide, in a moist or oil chamber.

Observation medium. — The best observation medium is the liquid that normally bathes the objects to be examined, such as plasma or serum for blood cells and fresh, brackish or sea water for small aquatic animals. The use of physiological salines is advised only when it is really difficult to obtain the serum of the particular animal.

The simplest of the physiological salines is one of 0.9% sodium chloride for homoiotherms, 0.6% for poikilothermic Vertebrates and fresh water Invertebrates. Sea water is generally used for marine Invertebrates.

The only advantages of physiological salines are the simplicity of preparation and ease of sterilisation by boiling or autoclaving in sealed ampoules. On the other hand they have several disadvantages since these solutions satisfy only one of the requisites of a truly physiological solution, namely that of isotonicity. Hence physiological saline should be used only for short periods when no other medium is available and is perhaps best completely done away with if possible.

Ringer's solution is far better than physiological saline for examining the tissues of poikilothermic Vertebrates and terrestrial or fresh-water Invertebrates:

Distilled water	1000 ml
Sodium chloride	6.5 g
Potassium chloride	0.25 g
Sodium bicarbonate	0.20 g
Calcium chloride	0.50 g

It is preferable to dissolve the products in the above order to prevent precipitation.

Homoiothermic Vertebrate tissues may be examined in **Locke's solution:**

Distilled water	1000 ml
Sodium chloride	8.5 g
Potassium chloride	0.42 g
Sodium bicarbonate	0.20 g
Glucose	2.5 g
Calcium chloride	0.25 g

or **Tyrode's solution:**

Distilled water	1000 ml
Sodium chloride	8.0 g
Potassium chloride	0.20 g
Calcium chloride	0.20 g
Magnesium chloride	0.10 g
Sodium phosphate	0.05 g
Sodium bicarbonate	1.0 g

In the case of long term observations the above solutions may be sterilized by filtration.

Von Albertini (1951) particularly recommends, for the tissues of homoiotherms, a solution which he has named *tyrofusine K.A.* and which gives very satisfactory results under phase-contrast:

Sodium phosphate	0.05 g
Sodium bicarbonate	5.0 g
Sodium chloride	85.0 g
Potassium chloride	4.2 g
Calcium chloride	2.5 g
Magnesium chloride	0.05 g
Glucose	10.0 g
Distilled water	10 liters

In any case none of these solutions serves as well as the natural internal medium of the animal whose tissues are studied. This is so for media like the amniotic fluid, ascites fluid and the aqueous humour as well. These latter, which were much in favour with the older histologists, are certainly better than physiological saline but they are difficult to procure, especially under aseptic conditions of extraction and storage. In most cases it is much easier to remove a little blood of the same animal, add an anticoagulant and centrifuge it to get rid of structured elements.

Mounting. — Methods of mounting differ according to the material and the intended period of observation. Free cells that are to be observed only for a few minutes can be mounted directly on a slide without any further precaution. When the cells are very large or fragile artefacts due to the weight of the coverslip may be avoided by propping the coverslip up at its corners (with suitable broken fragments, hairs etc.). Drops of paraffin may be laid at the corners or the tips may be folded down by melting carefully in a very low Bunsen flame.

If the preparation is to be protected from evaporation, an important precaution for prolonged observation, it is best to make a vaseline chamber. A needle is fitted on to a syringe loaded with pure vaseline (perfumed vaselines might contain substances toxic for cells) and a circle is traced on a slide, at the centre of which the object is placed with a drop of the chosen medium; a coverslip is gently lowered and brought into contact with the vaseline. The preparation is thus enclosed in a chamber whose height can be adjusted up to a certain limit by slight pressure.

The hanging drop, where the coverslip carrying the object in its medium is inverted over the ring of a chamber of van Tieghem and Le Monnier or a hollow slide prevents both the drying and compression of cells, but only those elements touching the coverslip can be studied with objectives of short focal length.

The oil chamber of de Fontbrune is the best means to prevent drying and is evidently indicated for the prolonged study of isolated cells.

It is clear that any drop in temperature during the vital examination of the tissues of a homoiotherm should be carefully avoided. The old oven-microscopes, much appreciated by classical authors, have now been entirely supplanted by observation chambers mounted on heating stages specially meant for studying Mammalian spermatozoa but which can also be used for a variety of other objects.

EXAMINATION UNDER THE LIGHT-FIELD MICROSCOPE

The technique of examination against a light field is about the same for vital or for fixed and stained preparations. It is therefore enough to draw attention to some essential but often neglected precautions. In fact vital examination is, among all the biological applications of the microscope, the most exacting with respect to the adjustment of lighting (light source, condenser, field and aperture diaphragms) and the cleanliness of optical surfaces. It would not be too much to advise all beginners not to regret the time and effort spent in acquiring a solid knowledge of the functioning of an instrument which for them is going to be of daily use all along their career. The effort is particularly worth while for vital examination.

Vital examination must necessarily commence with an examination of the preparation under low magnification. It is only too frequent to see biologists begin by observing under an immersion objective. Such a procedure, which is always to be deplored, can be particularly wrong in vital examination. In fact a preliminary inspection under low power not only permits the rapid choice of interesting regions but also helps to avoid those that are not amenable to study under objectives of short focal length. Its omission can cause the immersion objective to fill the role of a compressor, crushing the preparation or even damaging its frontal lens.

Vital preparations generally afford much less topographical information than stained ones. It is therefore highly advantageous to first be acquainted with the structure of a tissue by an attentive study of permanent preparations before passing on to a vital examination. In all cases however vital preparations are temporary and a photograph or a sketch is necessary for every aspect that is deemed of interest.

EXAMINATION UNDER THE DARK-FIELD MICROSCOPE

Preparations destined for the dark-field microscope do not differ particularly from those described above except that the preparations should be of exacting thinness, slides and coverslip should conform to the thickness prescribed by the makers of the condenser used and the mounting medium should be perfectly clear.

EXAMINATION UNDER THE PHASE-CONTRAST AND INTERFERENTIAL MICROSCOPES

The introduction of the first phase-contrast microscopes led to an extraordinary craze among histologists for this method which by an admirably ingenious and simple optical artifice brought out details of structure that were difficult or impossible to observe under the usual conditions of the light-field microscope. The invention of the interferential microscope did not provoke the same enthusiasm since at the time of its appearance on the market most cytologists were held in suspence by the spectacular progress of the electron microscope.

In the field of the biology vital examination is the typical application of the phase-contrast and the interferential microscopes. In fact the study of membranes fixed smears or unstained sections is easier with such instruments. But staining or metal impregnation can bring out with maximum distinctness those structures that are difficult or impossible to detect when they are unstained. With living material it is otherwise. No physical or chemical agent can be used to modify contrast or refractive index, and it is here that the phase-contrast and interferential microscopes are invaluable.

Preparation and mounting call for no particular comment apart from the necessity of scrupulously following the indications of the manufacturers regarding the thickness of slides and coverslips. The actual techniques of examination are described in manuals of microscopy and will not be detailed here.

Looking back upon the twenty odd years since its arrival on the scene one can now judge the phase-contrast microscope calmly. Spectacular results have certainly been obtained with some chosen objects, but it should never be imagined that these microscopes are the universal panacea for the histologist. Many objects are inaccessible to these methods because of their thickness. With fixed material the advantage is at the most that of avoiding a particular stain or metal impregnation. In the whole field of histology it is vital examination that gains most by these methods and naturally the same precautions have to be observed in their interpretation. Thus while it is important to authenticate the existence of a given structure in a living cell its final identification is possible only after a series of stains and histochemical reactions which cannot at all be compensated by use of the phase-contrast microscope. As in all techniques of vital examination study under phase contrast is a method of control; it is of greatest value only when used in conjunction with classical and histological techniques. It can be of much doctrinal importance and give spectacular results when the object has been properly chosen with the optical possibilities of the method in mind, but it would be an error to make a routine technique out of it.

CHAPTER 2

VITAL STAINING

> Alles in allem kann gesagt werden, dass jede Vitalfärbung ein physiologisches Experiment ist.
>
> P. Vonwiller (1929).

Vital staining is a method whose theoretical impact goes well beyond that of a simple demonstration of structural details in tissues or cells. The considerable importance of this type of study was realised by investigators from the very first systematic efforts and several biological disciplines have gained from it.

In fact the understanding of the mechanism of vital staining and the interpretation of results call for physico-chemical and physiological notions to a much greater extent than in all other physiological techniques. Vital staining is by definition applied to living material whose infinite complexity has to be taken into closer consideration than in the case of staining celloidin or paraffin sections. It is by itself an experiment in cell physiology where every step should be carefully controlled and the results critically assayed. In other words, vital staining is not quite a routine method.

The origin of vital staining certainly lies in the effort to demonstrate cells and organelles more or less specifically by administering suitable stains to the living animal. But this is no longer so. Certain vital stains are used, as in the past, for purely morphological purposes, but the chief advantage is that it is a means of exploring cell and tissue permeability, phenomena related to the absorption, transport, accumulation and the excretion of substances artificially introduced into the internal milieu.

DEFINITION

In spite of numerous publications and much polemic, no satisfactory definition of vital staining has been reached.

Fischer (1910) has proposed that all staining of certain histological structures that can be effected without previous killing of the animal be designated as vital staining. This Viennese author does not commit himself as to the actual "vitality" of the structures that are stained and insists on the impossibility of rigorous definition since in any case the morphological criteria of "life" escape unequivocal definition. Möllendorff (1920, 1926) has confined the term to stains applied during the life of the animal; that is to vital staining which in his mind is opposed to supra-vital or post vital stains, applied to animals that have just been killed, and to the staining of fixed tissue. However the distinction between vital and post-mortem staining is not so absolute since he readily admits that certain stains administered to the living animal most certainly give rise to post-lethal phenomena at the cellular level. Vonwiller (1929/30) has favoured a broad definition of vital staining by applying it to all stains of organisms or parts of organisms obtained when the organisms or their parts are alive. Gicklhorn (1931) quite justly emphasizes the impossibility of a rigorous and absolute definition of the frontier between vital and post-mortem staining. His point of view may be illustrated by citing the following example:

"An isolated granule in a cell or the cell-sap of an adult plant cell is evidently not living in the sense generally adopted to characterize life, whether the particular structures take stain or not. However, if this granular or cell-sap is stained inside a living cell the entire cell is involved in the appearance, after a given time, of stain in the granule or cell-sap. This implies that attention should be paid to the origination of stain and not to the optical image, that is, the accumulation of stain. The image produced by vital staining can always be distinguished from post-mortem staining by taking into consideration the time—factor, by the presence or absence of stain in other organelles, cells or tissues etc. Instead of seeking a definition in the ordinary sense of the term, one should rather aim at specifying criteria that help to judge the vital nature of a stain..."

It thus seems legitimate to reserve the term "vital" to any staining applied to living elements. It is by adhering too literally to the first memoir of v. Möllendorff (1920) that Parat (1926) attempted to distinguish vital stains administered to the entire animal from post-vital stains acting on cells or tissues removal from the living organism. Nothing justifies such a distinction. In fact, v. Möllendorff himself insists on the fact that the staining of certain structures obtained under conditions regarded as "vital" for the whole organism can very well correspond to a post-mortem phenomenon at the cellular level. Inversely it is well known that the life of a cell does not necessarily cease as it is removed from an organism, and it can indeed continue indefinitely in a favorable milieu. It is quite out of the question to consider the staining of a fibroblast culture as post-vital under the pretext that the stain has been added to the medium and not injected into the donor chick embryo. The interpretation of certain authors according to whom vital staining occurs inside tissues in the absence of air whereas post-vital staining is aerobic is equally untenable. Certainly less oxygen is available in the vital staining of leucocytes under luted coverslips according to Sabin and Doan than in circulating blood.

It goes without saying that "vital", "supra-vital" and "post-vital" used by some haematologists to designate basic blue staining of reticulocytes on dry smears is but a regrettable misuse of language.

OBJECTS, ADVANTAGES AND DISADVANTAGES

It can be concluded from the above notions that vital staining is more than a histological technique in the ordinary sense of the term. Evidently the determination of the accumulation of a stain in certain structures can be a purely morphological indication, but in most cases vital staining is practised with physiological aspects in view. In spite of its considerable importance the latter orientation is outside the scope of this book and only vital stains meant for morphological study will be considered here.

From this point of view, the theoretical interest of vital staining corresponds to that of vital examination discussed in the preceding chapter. However vital staining has the advantage of providing a considerable better delineation of structure. In addition, the interpretation of these structures is not based only on shape and form, since the behaviour of organelles towards vital stains furnishes very valuable information concerning their nature. In that, vital staining is, in practice, an indispensable complement to vital examination, especially at the cellular level.

Some of the disadvantages of vital staining are the same as those of vital examination and the strict limitation to favorable objects is recommended in both cases. In addition, vital stains involve chemical compounds whose innocuity, far from being evident, should be shown in each case and for each object.

Vital staining is therefore, like vital examination, a method of research and not of diagnosis. Its practice demands much care and patience. A extensive theoretical knowledge and a profound acquaintance of the tissue to be examined are nearly indispensable; the interpretation of results calls for a maximum of critical sense. Vital staining is, in most cases, a difficult task that requires to be prepared thoroughly, and which does not always give the expected result at the first attempt.

The list of vital stains and the number of objects that can be stained are quite considerable. The technique of vital staining varies according to the object and the stain. The operating procedures adopted to some structures will be found in the particular chapters devoted to them. Thus, vital staining with neutral red, Janus green or methylene blue will be considered in the study of the cell in general; methylene blue staining of nerve fibres is described in the chapter on techniques for the nervous system; staining of bone with alizarin in the pages devoted to this tissue etc.

CLASSIFICATION OF VITAL STAINS

It is usual to distinguish between acidic and basic vital stains. However such a classification excludes the family of Sudans which can be considered to be vital stains of lipids since their administration by ingestion or injection into the living animal enable the staining of all structured lipid inclusions whose melting point is below the body temperature. Apart from these compounds which are generally grouped as "indifferent" stains, the principal vital stains may be classified as follows.

Acid stains. — **Alizarin.** — This oxyquinone is the oldest known of the vital stains. Its use was formerly confined to the staining of bone, but the findings of the school of Keller and particular the work of Gicklhorn (1930 to 1936) have shown that this stain can be put to much wider use.

Trypan blue, pyrrol blue and Congo red. — These three stains are tetrazocompounds and their use as vital stains dates from Goldman (1912). Trypan blue is used in most cases. They are chiefly indicated for demonstrating the histiocytes by vital fixation (athrocytosis), for the study of excretion and for examining lymphatic vessels.

Indian ink, lithium-carmin, ammonium carminate. — Though they are not stains in the proper sense of the term, they should be mentioned here as they are used in place of trypan blue to demonstrate histiocytes.

Basic stains. — **Methylene blue, toluidine blue and Methylene azure.** — These are thiazines of which methylene blue is most used especially for the classical demonstration of nerve cells introduced into histological technique by Ehrlich.

Neutral red and Janus green (diazine green). — These diazines are of considerable importance as vital stains. The former is considered as the best vital stain for the "vacuome" and has been widely used in both plant and animal cytology. The latter introduced by Michaelis (1900) is typical of the vital stains of the chondriome.

Cresyl violet is an oxazine recommended by some authors for the vital staining of the chondriome. Two other oxazines, namely Nile blue and brilliant cresyl blue have been used by botanists for the "vacuome".

Nigrosin is an induline that Vonwiller has suggested for certain nerve fibres.

Dahlia violet and **methyl violet** are triphenylmethanes that have been used for staining the chondriome.

THEORIES OF VITAL STAINING

The interpretation of vital staining and the explanation of its mechanisms are highly complex problems. The physico-chemical aspects of the vital staining of cells and organelles have yet to be understood, and it would be illusory, in the present state of the science, to anticipate a unified and unequivocal theory that allows an interpretation of all the results obtained with vital stains. The mechanisms involved in the entire phenomenon of the staining of diverse structures *in vivo* are certainly numerous and varied. Furthermore the mechanism of vital staining pertains more to cell physiology than to histological technique. Consequently the various theories that have been proposed are only briefly considered here; while the reviews of v. Möllendorff (1926), Zeiger (1938) and Baker (1958) provide an excellent documentary source for a more detailed study of this question.

a) The different stages of vital staining. — It is v. Möllendorff (1920, 1926) who deserves credit for having first pointed out the importance of studying vital staining as a function of time. He defined three successive stages in every vital staining, namely the absorption, the intracellular distribution and the selective accumulation of stain. There is nothing absolute about the limits of the three phenomena, but each one obeys different laws and is influenced by different conditions, so that it is highly important to clearly distinguish the three stages in every description of vital staining.

Gicklhorn (1931) has provided a very clear analysis of the above three stages. Penetration evidently depends on the permeability, whether normal or modified, of the particular cell, as well as its capacity to fix the stain in question. The distribution of stain involves specificity at the level of the cell, tissue or organ. As for the accumulation of stain, it depends on the structure and chemical composition of cells and tissues. Each theory of vital staining concerns more particularly one of the three stages.

b) The physico-chemical characteristics of solutions of vital stains. — As Zeiger (1938) justly remarks the old chemical classification of vital stains is evidently valuable, but from 1920 to 1935 evidence has accumulated in favour of v. Möllendorff's opinion that the chemical structure of stains is of lesser importance than the physico-chemical characteristics of the solution used. This is especially true for vital staining with acid stains. The chemical nature of the stain is only one of the several factors which as a whole determine the properties of the solution that is administrated to the animal. The size of particles, electric charges, pH, osmotic pressure, viscosity, dielectric constant of the medium, presence of colloids and several other factors influence the physico-chemical characteristics of a solution on which the final result of a vital staining evidently depends. It follows that a careful physico-chemical investigation is essential in all cases that go beyond a simple morphological demonstration of structure. The works of Keller and his school happily complete the older works of Schuleman and Evans, of Oswald and of v. Möllendorff. Nevertheless the biologist is often forced to define by himself the physico-chemical characteristics of the solutions used in his experiments. A description of the relevant methods will not be given here; Zeiger's (1938) monograph gives several references to classical work on this question.

c) Theories of penetration of vital stains into cells. — The oldest of the theories that seek to explain the penetration of vital stains into cells is the classical concept of the lipidic cytoplasmic membrane due to Overton. This point of view, although accepted by several authors in the beginning of the 20th century, is however open to criticism. In fact several basic vital stains are strictly insoluble in lipids and, inversely, several liposoluble stains do not penetrate into living cells. The concept of "physiological permeability" propounded by Höber to overcome this difficulty is only a manner of thinking rather than an experimental fact. On the whole modern research is hardly favourable to the idea according to which liposolubility is the chief factor determining the penetration of vital stains into cells.

According to the theory of ultra-filtration due to Küster (1911) and elaborated by Ruhland (1912) the cell membrane acts as an ultra-filter and the penetration of particles into the cells is determined by their degree of dispersion. This point of view is open to the serious criticism made by Höber, namely that liposoluble stains of large particle size succeed in penetrating into cells whereas particles of other compounds of undoubtedly smaller size do not. Experiments made on models and various Mammalian tissues have led authors like Collander (1928). Michaelis (1926) and Netter (1928) to the conclusion that the size of particles is not at all the essential factor controlling the penetration of vital stains into cells. On these grounds, and from his own findings, Gicklhorn observes that the theory of ultra-filtration has been neither confirmed nor invalidated formally.

The theory of reactivity, due to Bethe, attributes an essential role to cell acidity or basicity. Apart from stains of very large particle size the penetration of all other acidic or basic vital stains would depend on the corresponding acidic or basic reaction of the particular cell. In fact trials on blocks of gelatin have shown that this ampholyte can, according to the pH, fix either acidic or basic stains, but attempts at verification *in vivo* have given ambiguous results.

Indeed the opinion of Kedrowsky (1931), upheld by Zeiger (1938), according to which each of these theories envisages one of the factors of penetration while neglecting all others seems to retain all its aptness.

d) Theories of the accumulation of vital stains inside cells. — A diffuse staining of cells and tissues after the action of a vital stain was taken by older authors as a sure sign of alteration and even cell death. But recent work has shown on the contrary that certain diffuse stains by acidic or basic dyes are quite compatible with a vital phenomenon. Depending on technical conditions, especially the abundance of stain in the medium, such a diffuse stain may become attenuated with time and disappear or become granular after the specific staining of certain intracellular structures. Unambiguous experiments on animal and plant cells have shown the possibility of such diffuse vital staining by various stains, especially by chrysoidine and vesuvine.

However, the accumulation of stain in the granular form is by far the most frequent type of vital staining. Such accumulation follows quite different modalities with basic and acidic stains. Basic stains accumulate as a rule in pre-formations among the cell organelles or in the paraplasm. Acidic stains, on the other hand accumulate, in granules or vacuoles formed at the time of accumulation. In spite of some restrictions following recent work, this rule formulated by v. Möllendorff remains generally valid. As for the mechanism of accumulation it is one of flocculation according to v. Möllendorff, whereas Keller and his school evoke electrostatic phenomena in their explanation. For v. Möllendorff flocculation, depends on the level of acidic colloids in certain structures and occurs at the moment of fixation of basic vital stains on them. This precipitation, controlled by phenomena of electro-adsorption, may explain the rapidity with which certain organelles are revealed by basic vital stains.

Nirenstein, on the other hand, considers that the level of lipids in stainable structures plays an important rôle; staining being dependent on the reaction of the basic stain with the liposoluble acids contained in the lipidic component of the stained granules. However, as Rumjantzew, Kedrovsky and other authors have remarked the views of Nirenstein are difficult to reconcile with the absence of lipid that can be histochemically demonstrated in structures that stain intensely with basic vital stains.

The slow appearance of granular staining with acidic vital stains is related, according to v. Möllendorff, to the fact that flocculation occurs only when the local concentration of stain is high. The process is supposed to consist of a gradual enrichment in stain of newly formed "vacuoles" and the decrease in this dispersion culminates in flocculation. Electrolytes probably intervene in this decrease and surface phenomena also play a rôle in the appearance of this kind of granular staining which is a typical "vital" feature.

Seki's large-scale experimental research supports the views of v. Möllendorff. According to the Japanese author the essential condition for granular vital staining is the propensity of the stain to flocculate or its weak electric charge which facilitates adsorption. Neutral red, which flocculates with difficulty, especially stains liquid inclusions that contain lipids, a fact which is in agreement with the liposoluble nature of this compound. The vital staining of the chondriome by Janus green is due, according to Seki, to the easy flocculation of the stain and the density of structure of the chondriosomes. Contrary to v. Möllendorff, Seki considers that the accumulation of acidic stains is also dependent on the reciprocal flocculation of basic cell substrates and stains with a weak negative charge. This interpretation is based on the demonstration of basic substances in histiocytes and on the possibility of substituting one acid vital stain for another; which also indicates the presence of acidophilie substances precisely where vital stain accumulates.

The electrostatic hypothesis propounded by Keller requires that the distribution of vital stains in the organism follows chieflly the proportion of electric charges so that the charge of the stain used is the essential factor in vital staining; the staining should thus be interpreted according to the laws of electrostatics. Certain experimental data of Keller and of Gicklhorn support this, but the electrostatic theory cannot account for differing results given by stains having the same charge. Zeiger (1938) insists on the fact that such a point of view does not explain the most important of the vital stains.

This brief review of the principal classical theories shows that it is quite impossible to reduce all vital staining to a common denominator. In all probability each of the above concepts is valid, at least in part and for particular cases, but none of them can entirely account for all the phenomena that occur during vital staining. Remarkable progress has been made in the interpretation of certain vital stains, especially that of the chondriosomes by Janus green and that of nerve cells by methylene blue. In fact the recent findings to which I refer have been obtained on these structures.

GENERAL RULES FOR APPLYING VITAL STAINS

The method of applying vital stains varies in large measure according to the structure to be demonstrated and the function to be studied. The practical details concerning the use of vital stains in morphological technique are dealt with in connection with the principal structures that can be so stained. A few general rules only are compiled here to avoid repetition.

The use of acidic stains. — Certain stains can be administered orally as in the case of trypan blue. However, the results are satisfactory only with some Invertebrates. Injection of the stain into the internal milieu of the animal is thus the prefered method.

With Vertebrates, injection can be sub-cutaneous, intra-peritoneal or intra-venous. In every case "local" or "neighbourhood" staining is observed (connective tissue adjacent to the point of sub-cutaneous injection, omentum in intra-peritoneal injection, histiocytes of the liver, spleen and bone marrow after intra-venous injection). The specific accumulation of stain in certain tissues or organs is preceded by a stage when it is diffuse over the whole body of the animal. (*Allgemeinfärbung* of v. Möllendorff). The rapidity of appearance in a given organ evidently depends on the type of administration. Intra-venous injection leads to the most homogenous distribution of stain in the body of the animal and to its fastest accumulation in the organs. However, its major inconvenience is the toxicity of most solutions of vital stains which imposes a considerable reduction in the dose tolerated intra-venously.

Solutions to be injected should be freshly prepared. Most solutions of vital stains acquire upon aging (even when stored aseptically and at low temperature), a toxicity whose origin is still unknown but which is none the less real. A single injection gives the best results in some cases; others may require repeated injections at regular intervals.

The histological examination of cells and tissues stained with acid vital stains can be made on fresh or fixed preparations. Contrary to the basic stains, the accumulation of acidic vital stains can be maintained in place after applying a whole series of chemical fixatives. However such practice may lead to serious errors of interpretation on which v. Möllendorff insists and which are equally emphasized by Lison. The ideal operating procedure is therefore to examine both *in vivo* and in *situ* cells and tissues that contain accumulated acidic stains. This is easy for certain privileged objects (mesenteron, Frog's lungs, cornea) possible for another (Mouse kidneys, Ghiron, 1920) and impossible in the great majority of cases. It is here that dissociated preparations examined on a warm stage for tissues of Homoeiotherms and frozen sections of fresh material acquire all their importance.

The choice of fixative, later treatment and background staining mainly depend on the vital stain used and the tissue to be examined. They will be described in other chapters.

The use of basic stains. — The application and especially the technique of examination are very particular in the case of basic vital stains. In fact, conservation by chemical fixing is impossible in almost all cases, and hence it becomes necessary to follow *in vivo* all the phases of staining.

Certain stains such as Janus green are used only in local application. Others such as neutral red or methylene blue can be either applied locally, injected into the internal milieu or added to the surrounding medium.

The precautions to be observed in the preparation of acid vital stains are evidently valid for basic stains as well.

CHAPTER 3

FIXATION

> Das Fixations-Färbebild wird jedoch immer mit der Abtötung des lebenden Objektes erkauft und diese Tatsache liegt wie ein Verhängnis auf vielen Gebieten mikromorphologischer Forschung. Das Verfahren arbeitet auf dem bedenklichen Umwege über die Zelleiche und vieles, was es gerade im Bereich der Zelle zeigt, bedarf einer eingehenden Kritik, wenn daraus auf die Wirklichkeit des Lebens Bezug genommen werden soll.
>
> H. PETERSEN (1935).

To fix is to immobilize. The aim of histological fixation is to immobilize structures, while maintaining their morphology as far as possible, and to preserve them so that permanent preparations may be made.

As Baker (1958) has aptly remarked "fixation" and "preservation" are not synonymous.

In fact the rôle of a preservative liquid in histology is to prevent the cadaveric autolysis of tissues and cells, to conserve a specimen in a state that approaches as far as possible its morphology *in vivo* and to permit its observation under the microscope. Both the liquid of Ripert and Petit as well as Amman's lactophenol satisfy these requirements. Quite different properties are however demanded of a fixative liquid. It should not only conserve details of structures, but also render them amenable to subsequent operations. The immobilization of morphological details must be sufficient for the pieces to resist both section—cutting and its prior manipulation, without undue alteration. In most cases a given fixative liquid also forestalls a good staining by certain procedures.

The above distinction is not merely theoretical. In fact the preservative liquids mentioned above are not fixatives in the sense of histological technique since pieces immersed in them would undergo serious alteration if paraffin embedding were to be attempted. Conversely, several fixative liquids as such are not preservative and they should be applied within well—defined limits if extreme alteration of tissues and cells is to be avoided.

Is an ideal fixation that spares both the structure and chemical composition of living matter ever possible? One has every reason to doubt it. The infinitely labile and perpetually changing edifice of living cells must necessarily collapse under the action of fixatives however faithful. It is thus easy to see that fixation is one of the crucial problems of ultrastructural cytology and defective fixation heads the list of causes of failure in electron microscopy, the more so that this technique of morphological examination cannot be verified by comparing permanent preparations and living objects.

The outlook is less gloomy in histology with the light microscope. The histologist is concerned only with modifications that are sufficient to bring about a change of aspect that exceeds the lower resolving limit of the light microscope. Besides, cytology, as practised with the light microscope, has at its disposal the admirable means of verification against both permanent preparations as well as the living cell. It is thus possible to follow, step by step, the action of fixatives, embedding media and stains on favorable objects. Topographical histology, on the other hand, is almost free of the above problem. The safety of the methods of fixation, embedding, cutting and staining for microscopical anatomy have been verified so often that the histologist can operate in all tranquillity. This does not imply that the proper conservation of tissues is automatic and that alteration due to technical errors have been obviated by progress in histology. However most causes of artifacts are known and it is easy to appreciate the extent of damage and to limit it.

The importance of morphological modifications that stem from fixation should be envisaged both on the scale of microscopical anatomy and of cytology.

Careless fixation can create artifacts on the scale of the whole organ. When a small Arthropod is completely immersed in an alcoholic fixative the site of loosely attached organs in the body cavity may be seriously modified. The flow of liquid, unequal variations in volume during the dehydration of tissues, whose water content and consistency are not uniform, are sufficient cause for this type of artifact. It is obvious that these deceive only the superficial and incompetent observer.

The various tissues of an organ and the cells that constitute a tissue can exhibit, in stained sections, relations that do not correspond to reality. As examples I might recall the varying shrinkage caused by fixation, dehydration and especially paraffin embedding in the intestinal tunica of Vertebrates, the shrinkage of chondrocytes in the ground substance and the "empty" loculi that surround negligent preparations of pericaryons in Vertebrate nerve centres. A little critical sense is evidently enough to avoid such errors.

The true problem of artifacts arises at the cellular level. A faithful image cannot be distinguished from an artifact in cytology as it can be in microscopical anatomy. In fact intermediate cases range from a rigorously faithful image of structures to aspects wholly created by fixation and subsequent manipulations. The four classical eventualities as distinguished by Zeiger (1938) are as follows.

Faithful conservation, the eventual ideal of every cytologist, can be expected only when structures possess a certain amount of rigidity with solid bodies or irreversible inelastic gels preponderant. From the morphological point of view vital observation and that of fixed and stained preparations give strictly identical results in these cases.

Some structures become visible after fixation although this operation does not really create them. The rôle of fixation in this case is merely to render the refractive index of these structures different from that of the medium. These "masked" structures (Zeiger, 1938) invisible under the technical conditions of light field vital observation, need not necessarily undergo any morphological modification detectable under the light microscope. It may even be unfounded to use the term "artifact" for these structures whose number in any case is bound to diminish with progress in phase contrast and interferential microscopy.

Other structures, depending on the macromolecular architecture characteristic of living matter and without any real existence on the scale of the microscope, appear after fixation and, for that matter, cannot be considered as morphological entities. The relation between protoplasmic ultrastructure and these "latent" structures (Peterfi, 1929) is sufficiently close for different fixatives to produce comparable results. They may thus be considered as products of histological techniques and not as true artifacts.

The extreme case of this series is one where wholly new structures appear during histological manipulation, especially on fixation. Even these artifacts in the usual sense of histological terminology are not entirely independent of the ultrastructure of living matter, but the connection between them and the aspect of permanent preparations is more remote than in the preceding case so that their morphology varies considerably according to the particular fixative used.

The above notions have considerable bearing since fixation is the essential step of histological examination. In fact, a great many preparations can be completely destained if they are judged to be unsatisfactory and restained afresh. Faults in embedding and dehydration may be rectified up to a certain extent. Bad fixation, on the other hand, implies the irremediable loss of a piece. It is therefore important to know exactly the advantages of the different techniques of fixation, to choose the fixative according to the aim of research and not to strive after the impossible, that is an equally satisfactory conservation of all structural details and all chemical constituants by a single given fixative.

Anyone who has realized the importance of fixation in histological technique can only be surprised by the far too few methodical studies devoted to this essential operation. Most handbooks of microscopy and histological technique provide only details concerning the operating procedure of fixatives and the subsequent treatment of pieces. Certain authors emphasize the variety of factors that influence fixation by chemical agents and insist on the impossibility of an unambiguous interpretation of the phenomenon. Only recent manuals of histochemistry devote a few pages to the mode of action of fixatives. The general theoretical problems of fixation are reviewed only in the works of Fischer (1899), Mann (1902), Baker (1931), Zeiger (1938) and Baker (1958). This indifference of histologists to one of the crucial problems of their discipline finds its counterpart in the tenacity with which many of them cling to the use of a fixative devoid of advantages but sanctioned by custom or personal routine.

Histological fixation has thus been—and still is—given over to a certain amount of empiricism. While some authors persist in using outmoded fixative liquids, others have sought to multiply the various formulae beyond reasonable limits. Baker (1958) estimates the number of fixative mixtures based on formalin as more than 200. The catalogue of histological techniques compiled by Gray (1954) includes about 700 mixtures and it is likely that even the author of this admirably meticulous repertory considers the list as incomplete. In fact, on going over it one is struck by the absence of certain of the most frequently used fixatives. A really exhaustive index of fixatives proposed since the very beginnings of histology would require a methodical search of all zoological, histological and histopathological publications. It goes without saying that such a task is beyond the capacity of single individual; it is besides of no use whatever. Outside the domain of neurofibrillar impregnations, where several methods include special fixation by bulk impregnation, the histologist who has acquired the experience of about twenty fixatives can consider himself to be well armed.

The knowledge of hundreds of formulae that give equivalent results is useful only in a critical study of such methods.

The diversity of the mode of action of fixatives, the number of existing mixtures and the lack of information concerning the mechanism of fixation evidently do not permit a global account of this essential aspect of histological technique. The particular advantages, recommendations and operating procedures of the various methods of fixation will be found in the later parts of this book.

Only the general aspects of classification, mode of action, advantages and disadvantages of fixatives will be considered in this chapter.

CLASSIFICATION AND MODE OF ACTION OF FIXATIVES

It is now implicit in all methods that the essential problem of histological fixation is to denature proteins so that the morphology of the cell is altered as little as possible with due respect to the characteristics of its chemical constituents. It should be recalled once more that this is only an ideal approachable in a certain measure but vain to imagine as attainable.

The traditional classification of fixatives into physical and chemical agents still remains valid and will be adopted here.

FIXATION BY PHYSICAL AGENTS

It is usual to include under this term those methods involving the use of heat, drying at room temperature and drying at low temperature (freezing-drying, cryodesiccation). Techniques in which cooling of the object is followed by the use of a liquid fixative (freezing-substitution) may also be added to this list. Cooling by itself is not a means of fixation. It has the effect of stopping autolytic processes, which can be very useful, but this prevention of post-mortem modification evidently ceases on return to room temperature and hence it is indispensable to complete it with genuine fixation. It should be recalled that cryostat sections made on tissues that are merely cooled are really sections of fresh tissue; all the artifacts whose appearance has been prevented by suitable cooling will reappear upon warming if certain precautions are not observed.

1° *Fixation by heat*

This is one of the oldest methods of fixation and is based on the principle that proteins coagulate under the effect of heat. Even classical authors were conscious of the major drawbacks of this type of protein denaturation from the morphological point of view. One of the principal applications of fixation by heat, due to Ehrlich (1877) lies in the preparation of blood smears for staining with the well known triacid mixture. The author himself notes the "brutal" nature of the method and points out that the only purpose of its use is to avoid the interference of chemical agents during fixation; this type of fixation has been superseded by other methods and is cited here only as a reminder. The morphological results are disastrous even in the most favorable of cases where previously dried blood smears are exposed to the strictly time—controlled action of heat. The artifacts produced by the action of heat on larger pieces are even worse, and I strongly advise against the method which consists of commencing the fixation of small Arthropods by immersing them in water at 60°.

2° Fixation by drying at room temperature

Quick drying at room temperature is important in preparing blood smears for staining by the methods of morphological haematology. It can evidently be applied under the same conditions to smears of bone marrow and organ imprints. Apart from these cases, its applications are limited and it should be noted that it is not a true fixation. In fact the denaturation of proteins thus obtained does not extend up to their loss of solubility in water, so that drying should always be completed by another fixative at the time of staining. For example, during panoptic staining which is generally used in this case the methanol used to dissolve the methylene blue eosinate serves this purpose (May—Grünwald stain).

3° Fixation by drying at low temperature

In 1890 Altmann had the idea of applying this method to histology. It consists in drying tissues at low temperature and has led to several important applications. Its use in histology was proposed after a long period of neglect except for some isolated attempts by the school of Bentley. The early technical improvements due to Gersch (1932) resulted in a series of spectacular cytological results (Bensley and Gersch, 1933), but the widespread practice of cryodesiccation over the last twenty years is rather devoted to histochemical ends.

Freezing-drying is not a means of fixation in the proper sense of the term because it does not ensure any denaturation of the tissue proteins. Its simple principle is based on the elimination of water by sublimation from pieces that have been cooled to less than 0° and held in a vacuum whose pressure is less than 4.6 mm of mercury.

Its numerous industrial applications have led to considerable work on the physical principles and technical aspects of freezing-drying. The reviews of

Neumann (1958), Lison (1960) and Pearse (1960) give the essential facts concerning the rôle of cryodesiccation in histological technique.

Technically the practice of cryodesiccation in histology consists of three steps, namely, freezing, drying under vacuum and later treatment.

Freezing. — The aim of this operation is to render all the water in a piece solid as well as to stop immediately all vital phenomena. Experience has shown that quite low temperatures ($-50°$ to $-70°$) are necessary to stop all enzymatic reactions likely to occur in tissues, and physical considerations also plead in favour of extreme cooling. All authors agree that freezing is the critical step of the method. When well performed the results compare with those of the best chemical fixatives, whereas faulty freezing produces clumsy artifacts that render the piece worthless.

The principal artifact is the "reticulation" of tissues which is caused by the formation, during freezing, of ice crystals whose size exceeds the resolving power of the light microscope. Crystals measuring several microns can be formed by careless freezing. As Neumann (1958) remarks, the same phenomenon can occur while freezing fresh pieces on the stage of the ordinary freezing microtome, without the artifact appearing on histological examination since frozen sections are not dried but rehydrated shortly afterwards and the tissues swell to fill the cavities formed by ice crystals. In cryodesiccation the tissues are dried under vacuum and embedded in paraffin so that all the artifacts of reticulation are retained.

The size of ice crystals formed during freezing depends on the number of crystals seeded per unit time and the rate of crystallization. These two factors, apart from others beyond the control of the operator such as concentration, viscosity and the chemical nature of dissolved salts, vary according to the temperature. Crystals are larger when, at the time of their formation, the solid and liquid phases coexist for longer periods. The practical solution therefore consists in cooling the piece as rapidly as possible. In addition to above 80 cal/g, corresponding to the drop in temperature, a further 70 cal/g, representing the heat of crystallization, have to be absorbed. It is clear that this cannot be achieved instantaneously. Apart from the size of pieces, the factors that control the rate of cooling are the thermal conductivity inside tissues, conduction between the tissues and the cooling medium, the temperature gradient between the two and the thermal properties of the medium itself.

From the practical point of view the use of very small pieces is imperative; at least one dimension of the piece should under no condition exceed 1 mm; several authors even consider that satisfactory results cannot be obtained if it exceeds 0.1 mm. Direct cooling by liquid air, as used by Gersh (1932) has been abandoned because the advantage of a steep thermal gradient is entirely lost through poor conductivity. Following Scott (1933) all authors now use a liquid, with a very low melting point, cooled by liquid air or, better still, liquid nitrogen. n-pentane, isopentane, propane-isopentane mixtures, difluoromethane (freon) and ethyl alcohol are most frequently used.

Concentration changes during freezing should also be taken into account. In fact, the movement of water towards crystal seeds can carry along substances, modify osmotic conditions and change the concentration of the liquid phase. When the salt concentration increases beyond the eutectic point, the freezing point drops considerably and the period of coexistence between solid and liquid phases is prolonged with the consequent disadvantages described above.

Changes in volume of the piece are of little importance when histological examination is purely qualitative, or even when mensuration is intended. Neumann (1958) estimates a linear increase of about 2% following freeze-drying.

Sublimation of water. — This second step in cryodesiccation is aimed at eliminating water, a great part of which is contained as ice crystals in the interstitial spaces of tissues, while only a small fraction (residual moisture) is adsorbed on to the internal surfaces of the piece. During this process the boundary that separates the outer dehydrated parts from the inside that still contains ice is progressively displaced towards the centre. Escaping water molecules have consequently a longer distance to cover and dehydration is prolonged. The persistance of ice in the inner zones evidently necessitates the maintenance of a sufficiently low temperature throughout dehydration. Sublimation obviously ceases when the partial pressure of water vapour rises above the level of saturation, which varies according to the temperature (0.77 mm Hg at $-20°C$; $9.3 \cdot 10^{-2}$ mm Hg et $40°C$; $7.0 \cdot 10^{-3}$ mm Hg at $-60°C$). The rate of dehydration depends on the ratio between the pressure in the chamber and the saturation pressure corresponding to the temperature of the piece. Experience has shown that in practice it is best that the pressure be about a tenth of the saturation pressure of water vapour, that is, about $3 \cdot 10^{-3}$ mm Hg when desiccation is carried out at $-50°C$. Water molecules that are released from the tissue and fill the chamber may be removed in three ways, by direct pumping, by chemical or physical fixation on hygroscopic substances or by freezing on a special cold trap. The first of these appears to be the simplest, but its practical disadvantages are considerable. In fact the volume occupied by a given quantity of water vapour increases very rapidly as the pressure drops, and hence pumps are required to have a high efficiency. The usual mechanical pumps are inadequate since their efficiency drops at pressures lower than 10^{-2} mm of mercury. They have thus to be used in conjunction with a diffusion pump, which evidently entails a considerable increase in cost. However, the use of such low-temperature desiccators can be simpler than that of the devices based on the other two methods. Altmann adopted the solution of absorbing water vapour by hygroscopic substances; buth this practice has now been abandoned because of the major disadvantage caused by the progressive enriching of the absorbent with water, so that after a time the effect of the vacuum is directed to the absorbent rather than to the piece to be dehydrated. The third principle, that of holding water vapour in a cold-trap, has been adopted in most devices destined for histology. Extreme cooling of the trap is necessary since dehydration of the piece ceases when its vapour tension equals that of the trap. If the trap is not maintained at a sufficiently low temperature the last phase of the desiccation of histological samples, namely the removal of residual water, is considerably prolonged. It is therefore advisable to maintain the trap at a temperature that corresponds to a saturation tension ten times less than that of the piece being dehydrated. This implies cooling of the trap with liquid air or nitrogen.

Sometimes a combination of the principles discussed above may be involved in an apparatus. Thus a cold trap may serve to retain the large quantity of water eliminated during the first part of desiccation while a diffusion pump extracts residual moisture at the end. The cold trap is excluded from the circuit where the diffusion pump is brought into play. In addition, some recent models use a stream of dry gas, instead of a vacuum, to remove molecules of water. Among these, the apparatus of Kramer and Hill is remarkable for its simplicity and ease of operation.

Subsequent treatment of pieces. — Macroscopical examination does not show any shrinkage of dehydrated pieces with respect to the fresh state. Pieces are light, yellowish, more brittle than fresh tissues and very hygroscopic. Rehydration may attain up to 25% of dry weight in a few hours. Tissue proteins are dry but not denatured and for this reason cryodesiccation cannot be considered as a true fixation. However, as Neumann (1958) points out, freeze-drying greatly increases the resistance of proteins to heat. In any case, the absence of any real denaturation of tissue proteins and the danger of rapid rehydration closely determine the subsequent treatment of pieces.

Some authors have proposed that hand-sections be made on removing pieces from the desiccator. This procedure, and that of embedding pieces in nitrocellulose (collodion, celloidin), are however rarely followed. Paraffin embedding, which is widely practised, needs no intermediate step since the medium immediately penetrates the dehydrated tissue and proteins have moreover increased heat resistance following cryodesiccation. Such embedding may be effected in the desiccator itself with certain types of apparatus, while with others the pieces have to be transferred to a paraffin oven as rapidly as possible to prevent rehydration. The period required in warm paraffin is less than that after classical dehydration and, evidently, varies according to the nature of the pieces. No temperature precaution is necessary following the increased heat resistance of proteins after cryodesiccation.

Section-cutting presents no particular problem, but it should be remembered that since proteins have not been denatured contact with moisture while handling sections may lead to chemical modifications or even serious morphological alteration due to the dissolution of tissue constituents. Sections should therefore be spread avoiding contact with water, either dry or in a non-aqueous medium. If they are to be spread dry a short ribbon is preferable, one end of which is applied against a slightly warmed slide while the other is held at a short distance from the glass with forceps or a brush in the left hand. The sections are spread with another brush held in the right hand and the operation may be completed by exerting light pressure. Sections adhere better if the slide has been coated with a thin film of glycerin albumin as in the method of Apathy described for paraffin sections. When sections are spread on a non-aqueous liquid a Petri dish placed over a warm plate is used. When fully spread they may be retrieved on a slide coated with albumin. Spreading on mercury, as suggested by Danielli, is suitable for cytological research, but Neumann advises against its use in histochemistry, for which Mayersbach (1957) prefers mineral oil.

Dried sections may be dewaxed by benzenic hydrocarbons routinely used for paraffin sections, by petroleum ether or by isopentane. The solvent is in turn removed by drying. Such sections can be submitted to certain histochemical reactions; but in these cases, which are unavoidable especially when certain small molecules are to be detected, there is evidently a serious risk of not conserving structures. Most histophysical research (autoradiography, microradiography) can be performed on dry sections that have not been submitted to any denaturation. Mounting in glycerol or an aliphatic hydrocarbon (generally nonane) is the best choice for examination under phase contrast or in polarized light. In all other cases it is essential to denature proteins. It can be obtained by heating up to 15°C or by immersion in absolute or 96% ethanol. The optimal period for immersion varies, according to different authors, from 15 minutes to 12 hours.

Summary of operating procedure. — Cryodesiccation for histology consists of the following steps:

1° Cool the vacuum chamber to the temperature (usually $-30°C$ to $-50°$) using a mixture of dry ice in ethanol or acetone. Pour the required quantity of isopentane, propane or freon, chosen for cooling the piece, into a cylindrical brass vessel and place in it a small metal sieve attached to a long handle which will serve to mix the fluid as well as to extract the frozen piece.

2° Cool the hydrocarbon chosen for freezing with liquid nitrogen (avoid as far as possible liquid air which forms an explosive mixture with hydrocarbons) until it has a syrupy consistency.

3° Remove the piece to be examined as quickly as possible and cut it into slices of less then 1 mm (use if necessary the double-bladed razor devised for the purpose by Gersh) and fix the pieces of tissue on to very fine metal wires or, even better, on aluminium foil (Gersh).

4° Plunge the pieces into the cooled hydrocarbon and agitate taking care that they do not stick to the sides of the vessel or the handle of the sieve.

5° Transfer the pieces of tissue as quickly as possible to the desiccating chamber with a cold forceps and establish the vacuum; if the apparatus has a water-cooled trap it should be made to function following the manufacturer's instructions.

6° During desiccation the temperature of the chamber as well as of the trap should be checked. The end of the first phase (loss of ice-crystals) can be ascertained by weighing or by pressure readings in some types of apparatus. In others it has to be judged empirically. Cooling of the chamber may be stopped when only residual moisture remains in the pieces, and the last phase of desiccation completed at room temperature.

7° Embed in paraffin after desiccation. This may be done in the desiccation chamber itself in certain types of apparatus; otherwise pieces have to be quickly transferred to a paraffin oven.

8° Blocks are cut in the usual manner and sections spread dry or on a non-aqueous liquid. Dry, dewax, remove solvent by air-drying and treat section as indicated previously.

Advantages, recommendations and precautions. — The theoretical advantages of cryodesiccation are evident and largely explain the enthusiastic reception accorded to the method as soon as suitable instruments were available on the market. In fact, rapid freezing stops all enzymatic reactions in tissues and ensures against post-mortem autolysis. Desiccation in a solid medium also prevents any displacement of substances during the process. Furthermore, no chemical reagent is employed, so that the method of Altmann-Gersch appears *a priori* to be ideal for histochemical research.

In fact ideas have changed since the time when every histologist who did not have access to the means of cryodesiccation could not help feeling frustrated. Twenty years of intensive research in the field have brought out the limits and disadvantages of freezing-drying.

Some of the disadvantages of cryodesiccation were evident from the beginning, although they did not retain the interest of authors. One of the most important is the need to use only very small pieces, a drawback that was calmly accepted by the pioneers in view of the particular orientation of this work. They were primarily concerned with cytological and histological problems in homogenous Mammalian tissue whose microscopical anatomy was thoroughly well understood. There never arose any need to cryodesiccate objects whose anatomical connections had to be maintained and which could not be cut into 0.1 mm slices without serious alteration. In fact this is a real disadvantage, since it purely and simply prohibits cryodesiccation in most histological research on Invertebrates and renders the task complicated in the case of certain Vertebrate organs.

But this is not the worst disadvantage of cryodesiccation. While spectacular results have been obtained showing that the quality of preparations can attain that produced by the best chemical fixatives, such successes are neither automatic nor easy to achieve. Though the preservation of structures can be perfect when all goes well, serious damage may be caused, during freezing, by the formation of ice crystals that are larger than the resolving power of the light microscope. It is impossible to prevent such "reticulation" of pieces when the object exceeds 2 mm in its smallest dimension, and in other cases even when the limitation in size is duly observed. Lison (1960) notes that some tissues (liver, pancreas, Mammalian tegument) are well preserved by the Altmann–Gersch method, others (intestine, kidney) sufficiently well while yet others like the testicle, nervous tissue, bone marrow and lymph nodes of the same animal may be wholly unsatisfactory. The occurrence of a veritable zonation in voluminous pieces fixed by cryodesiccation has been known since Simpson (1941). In this instance a peripheral layer, where fixation is excellent, covers a badly damaged zone while the centre of the piece fares better, though less well than the periphery. From the morphological point of view cryodesiccation can yield results, in favorable cases, that compare with the best chemical fixations; but the procedure is less dependable and materially more expensive. The cytological results obtained by this method are of considerable doctrinal importance, but do not warrant its systematic substitution for chemical fixation. It becomes indispensable only when the effect of chemical fixatives on cell organelles has to be precisely established.

When cryodesiccation is indicated for histochemistry it is discussed in the relevant portions of this book. However, it should be remarked here that the majority of modern authors do not share the enthusiasm of its pioneers for whom cryodesiccation was destined to replace all methods of chemical fixation in histochemistry. Histochemists today do not deny the advantages of the method but believe that it should be confined to particular cases while in all others it is not in any way superior to procedures that are besides more rapid, cheaper and less delicate.

4° *Fixation by freezing—substitution*

This procedure, invented by Simpson (1941) and used by number of others (Lison, 1949; Blanck *et al.*, 1951; Adamstone, 1951; Woods and Pollister, 1955; Hancox 1957) has enjoyed a lesser vogue than freezing-drying. Its principle is closely related to that of cryodesiccation and, as Lison (1960) has observed, its advantages are but slightly less.

The first step of the method is the same as that of cryodesiccation; very small pieces are frozen with the same precautions. However, dehydration is based on quite a different principle. The frozen tissue is transferred to an organic solvent that has been cooled to between $-20°$ and $-50°$. An equilibrium is thus established between the solid phase, which is ice, and a liquid phase consisting of water and the organic solvent in proportions that vary according to the temperature. Equilibrium is attained at $-20°$ for water–ethanol mixtures containing about 30% of water. When the solvent is in considerable excess all the water may be extracted from a piece without the alcohol in the immediate neighbourhood dropping below 30%. The diffusion of water molecules into excess of solvent ensures gradual dehydration without a return of water in the tissue to a liquid state. However solid and liquid phases do coexist within the piece all through dehydration; and as Neumann (1958) has remarked, thawing in the physical sense takes place. Nevertheless, the retention in the piece of all substances that are insoluble in the phase that is in equilibrium (30% ethanol in this example) can be expected. Freed (1955) and Hancox (1957) have shown that tissue proteins are not denatured by freezing-substitution.

From the practical point of view the process is considerably simplified. The frozen tissue is merely placed in a large excess of the chosen exchange liquid cooled to about $-50°$. It is maintained until the complete disappearance of ice crystals which may be determined empirically. The temperature is then allowed to rise slowly to room temperature and the treatment of tissues is pursued in the usual manner.

It should however not be ignored that the fixation is really by chemical agents, though diffusion phenomena depending on the movement of water in the liquid phase are avoided. Simpson (1941) insists on this fact in his principal publication on the method. Lison (1949) further illustrates it when he advises replacing alcohol by Gendre's liquid without acetic acid when applying freezing-substitution for demonstrating glycogen. The coexistence of liquid and solid phases within the piece during dehydration implies the risk of shrinkage or swelling from the morphological point of view and the migration of substances from the chemical point of view.

Although it does not offer the theoretical guarantees of cryodesiccation, freezing-substitution provides very satisfactory morphological preparations.

Paraffin sections should be denatured, for which Hancock (1957) recommends spreading on 85% alcohol. This denaturation is evidently effected on return to room temperature when the exchange liquid is ethanol or any other protein denaturing agent, so that the situation is that of the usual chemical fixation. However, it is obvious that many of the chemical characteristics of tissue constituents can undergo important modification at this stage.

FIXATION BY CHEMICAL AGENTS

Of all the physical agents described previously, heat is the only one that ensures genuine fixation, that is, denaturation of the tissue proteins. With freezing-drying it is necessary to employ chemical agents that produce such denaturation. It is thus easy to appreciate the essential role of chemical fixatives in histological technique. The introduction to this chapter has furthermore emphasized the preponderance of empiricism in the practice of fixation.

The astonishing and surely excessive multiplicity of formulae adopted by classical authors for fixatives aptly illustrates a basic fact already observed, namely, that it is impossible to devise a universal fixative that can be used in all circumstances and which ensures reliable conservation of morphological details as well as all the chemical features of cells and organelles. A thorough acquaintance with the advantages and disadvantages of fixatives is therefore essential since the correct choice of one governs, in a large measure, the success of a histological preparation. This choice carries a certain scientific responsability and hence should not be left to the decision of a technician. The latter's role may be that of following instructions minutely, but the decision can be taken only by one who possesses all the elements that lead to a rational choice.

The indications and counter-indications of fixative mixtures depend largely on their constitutive fixing agents. Thus the properties of fixatives in relation to the methods for which they are particularly recommended will be treated in later chapters, while the present chapter will give the known essential facts concerning fixing agents.

Though the number of mixtures is considerable, the agents, that is, the active chemical compounds, are relatively few. Baker (1958) has compiled a list of 14 such fixing agents and a comparison with the numerous mixtures mentioned in certain handbooks of microscopy shows that only occasional compounds, devoid of any real interest in histological practice, have been ignored by this British cytologist.

Among the criteria for classifying fixing agents, that based on chemical structure adopted by certain authors is better dismissed. A logical criterion is the action of fixatives on proteins, since the denaturation of proteins is, as I have often remarked, the touchstone of histological fixation. A comparison of the classical work of Zeiger (1938) with more recent reviews

(Wolman, 1955; Zeiger 1957; Baker 1958; Pearse 1960) gives evidence of the considerable change that has occured over the last twenty years in the interpretation of the histological fixation of proteins. During Zeiger's time the dominant concern was to accord the phenomena of fixation with the physico-chemical concepts of colloids. Today the concept that protoplasm is a colloidal gel with micellar organization has been abandoned. Most authors agree that the basic structural element of living matter is made up of chains of structural proteins linked to each other and to carbohydrate, lipid and other molecules. These links evolve perpetually and some of their modifications have been analysed experimentally. Several molecules, some of which are proteinic (corpuscular or globular proteins) are found in these loose networks; the aqueous moiety of protoplasm may be linked to the polar groups of structural proteins, bound to other molecules or may be free.

During the denaturation of proteins, which is accompanied by a clearly apparent change in solubility, the structural protein chains are unfolded, new intermolecular bonds appear which render the whole somewhat more rigid and previously blocked groups become reactive while other active groups get blocked. As Wolman (1955) has rightly observed denaturation is not a uniformly constant phenomenon; different agents can produce denaturations that vary in the particular properties of the proteins involved. The effect of protein denaturation, during histological fixation, on the immobilization of other compounds on which the agent has no direct action should also be emphasized. In most cases such immobilization is enough to permit operations that precede section cutting. This only corroborates what has been often verified in practice, namely that fixatives which guarantee a good fixation of proteins have an advantage over all the so-called indifferent fixatives, except in cases where they are proscribed for precise chemical reasons.

Fixing agents can be classified according to their type of action (flocculation or coagulation) on ovalbumen into coagulants (methanol, ethanol, acetone, nitric acid, hydrochloric acid, trichloracetic acid, picric acid, chloroplatinic acid, chromium trioxyde, mercuric chloride) and non-coagulants (acetic acid, osmium tetroxyde, potassium dichromate, formaldehyde and other aldehydes).

Data other than those on the mode of action on tissue proteins should also be considered in a review, however brief, of fixing agents. Their action on carbohydrates and tissue lipids is evidently of interest. Furthermore, one should take into account their rate of penetration into the tissue, the consequent shrinkage or swelling of tissues, their hardening, the morphological modifications of organelles, their suitability for different modes of embedding and staining and, finally, the general appearance of the preparations obtained.

Some of the above information can be appreciated by objective criteria. The rate of penetration into tissues can be measured and expressed generally as mm per hour. An object may be easily measured before and after fixation to evaluate the degree of shrinkage or swelling. But the figures thus obtained are evidently valid only for a given object. For example, the careful investigations of v. Tellyesniczky (1926) have shown that the rate of hourly penetration of the same agent can vary up to thrice the value depending on whether it is measured in the liver, spleen, kidney or brain of the mouse. The same holds true for shrinkage or swelling. Hardening of tissues upon fixation does not seem to have been studied quantitatively, so that indications provided in various texts are necessarily subjective.

The other features enumerated above are likely to be even more subjectively appreciated by different authors and this should be remembered when considering the various fixing agents described below.

1° *Methanol, ethanol, acetone*

These three liquids are used in the pure form, apart from those cases where they are associated with other ingredients to constitute fixative mixtures. Fixation by methanol is almost exclusively reserved for treating blood smears. The other two have a certain role in histochemical research, especially in the preparation of tissues for some histo-enzymological reactions.

Their mode of action has been ill-understood by the great majority of classical authors, for whom dehydration was the chief mechanism involved. The unfortunate term "indifferent fixative" has been attributed again to ethanol in the work of Zeiger (1938) and certain more recent manuals of histological technique still perpetuate the error. In fact, the three compounds are non-additive coagulant fixatives, they do not enter into chemical bonds with the proteins they denature. Seki (1937) who was the first to break with the traditional explanation of histological fixation by methanol and ethanol, believes that the coagulation of proteins is due to a drop in the electrical charges of hydrated active groups and the lowering of the dielectric constant which enables protein molecules to approach each other. Recent authors add to this the probable extraction by these agents, of the lipid groups linked to protein molecules by their hydrophilic radicals which facilitates the formation of intermolecular bonds. The shift in the iso-electric point of tissue proteins is less during fixation by alcohol or acetone than when other fixatives are used. Nucleoproteins are not coagulated by these, although the same compounds precipitate nucleoproteins in solution. Carbohydrate components of tissue are not fixed in the true sense of the term although they are partially retained in place by the action on proteins. The extraction of lipids is more or less intense and varies according to their chemical nature and association with other compounds. The penetration of methanol into tissues does not seem to have been studied quantitatively and this lack is related to its use being almost exclusively confined to haematology. The penetration of ethanol is generally evaluated at 1 mm per hour in tests mostly effected on Mammalian liver. The tables published by v. Tellyesniczky do not carry any results on the penetration of acetone; experience has shown that it is slightly slower than ethanol. Shrinkage of tissues is great, hardening intense and the consequent penetration of paraffin quite mediocre. The non-additive nature of the three compounds renders any special washing unnecessary afterwards. All three are furthermore completely miscible with the intermediary solvents generally employed for paraffin embedding.

As for their effects on structures, Baker (1958) has reported a crude reticulation of the cytoplasm, the destruction of the chondriome and Golgi apparatus and the coalescence and more or less complete extraction of lipid inclusions. Several secretory granules are dissolved. In addition, the three liquids produce the well known phenomenon of withdrawal from the diffusion front. Many substances, and almost all organelles, are displaced in the cell following the direction of penetration of the fixative. The particular circumstances in which blood smears are fixed with methanol ensure against any artifact, but it occurs with all three fixatives of the group when fragments of tissue are concerned. This property is exhibited even in the action of certain fixative mixtures containing ethanol or acetone. The staining affinities of cell constituents that survive fixation undergo little modification; the basophily of nucleic acids is well retained, but their fixation is far from perfect; certain enzymatic activities are also quite acceptably conserved. All three agents leave calcified inclusions intact.

2° *Hydrochloric, nitric and sulfuric acids*

These three compounds are non-additive coagulant fixing agents. Their use in current histological practice is most limited. To the best of my knowledge only two fixative mixtures contain hydrochloric acid, namely that of Takahashi (1908) of which the other constituents are osmium tetroxyde and chromium trioxyde, and that of Meyer (1912) which contains ethanol, hydrochloric acid and mercuric chloride. Sulfuric acid is included in Kleineberg's (1879) solution and nitric acid in that of Gilson (1898) and that of Perenyi (1882). In all cases these mixtures are almost completely neglected now, and were used by their authors only for microscopical anatomy. With the result systematic tests have to be made afresh before the suitable data concerning these agents can be provided. Figures given by v. Tellyesniczky show a very rapid penetration of nitric acid into Mammalian tissues; at 2,5 mm per hour it is faster than that of any other fixing agent.

3° *Trichloracetic acid*

The action of this compound on tissue proteins differs from that of all other short-chain aliphatic acids; as opposed to them it is coagulant, although non-additive. Frequently used, both as a fixative and a decalcifying agent, trichloracetic acid does not seem to have been methodically studied especially in its mode of action on tissue proteins. It is known to have a fast rate of penetration (1 to 2 mm per hour according to the tissue). It does not seem to have any particular action on carbohydrates and lipids, apart from a non-specific effect due to its acidity. The latter property explains the dissolution of all inorganic inclusions, even quite stable ones, and especially those of calcified structures. The shrinkage of tissues thus fixed is slight and hardening moderate. They allow a good penetration of paraffin. Collagen fibers undergo marked swelling after trichloracetic acid fixation and washing. Hence it is necessary to remove all excess of fixative by directly transferring to strong alcohol or washing in an aqueous solution of sodium sulfate. With regard to the conservation of structures a slight reticulation of the cytoplasm is noted. Secretory granules and even chondriomes are conserved when the level of trichloracetic acid in the mixture does not exceed 5%. The tendency for withdrawal and the over-fixation of peripheral regions is weak. Most staining affinities are retained.

4° *Picric acid, Chloroplatinic acid*

The first of these two compounds is one of the most commonly used fixative agents, while the second appears in classical formulae and although neglected by several modern authors it does give admirable results. Both strongly precipitate alkaloids and are classed among the additive coagulants according to their action on tissue proteins. Little is known about the mechanism of fixation of proteins by chloroplatinic acid (the commercial name "platinum chloride", has an erroneous basis since the metal is present as the reactive complex $[PtCl_6]^{--}$). Classical authors have noted its poor penetration and v. Tellyesniczky (1926) goes to the extent of considering its capacity as a fixative to be practically nil. In fact, however, mixtures based on chloroplatinic acid are among the best fixative liquids for classical cytology, and from the morphological point of view they give results comparable to those obtained with osmic fixatives.

Data obtained with picric acid (2,4,6-trinitrophenol) are much more precise. Its action on proteins is now explained on the basis of the role of dipole inductors played by the 2,4,6-nitro groups and by the existence of several states of resonance of the molecule which create bonds between the molecules of fibrous proteins. Furthermore, the induction of polarity in the polarisable side chains of protein molecules cause other intermolecular linkages. It seems to have no action on tissue lipids. Neither is picric acid a fixative of carbohydrates; its advantages in conserving glycogen can be explained by its strong action on proteins. Penetration is somewhat slow (0.3 to 0.5 mm/hour, according to the object and the author). Shrinkage of tissues, which is great, can attain almost that caused by ethanol, though pieces are not at all hardened, and this is one of the chief advantages of picric acid as a fixative. It prepares well for paraffin embedding, but is clearly unsuitable before embedding in nitrocellulose (celloidin, collodion).

With regard to structures, a more or less fine reticulation of cytoplasm should be noted. Chondriosomes are not destroyed by picric acid alone, though they may undergo slight modification in form. The ergastoplasm and intranuclear structures are quite well conserved, but certain histochemical reactions and the staining of nucleic acids are poor. The natural acidophily of cytoplasmic structures is increased after fixation with picric acid.

It should be noted that in spite of the additive nature of the fixation, treatment with picric acid does not call for any particular subsequent measure. The usual preparation for embedding and staining is enough in most cases to eliminate any excess of picric acid. If necessary a rapid treatment with a saturated solution of lithium carbonate or ammonium acetate suffices to ensure elimination.

5° *Mercuric chloride*

This is an additive coagulant fixative frequently used in histological technique. Its action on proteins is well known. Fixation of this compound on tissue proteins involves three different mechanisms. The first of these is the classical formation of mercaptides with the SH-groups of cysteine. Furthermore, in an acidic medium mercuric chloride forms secondary bonds with the amino groups and primary bonds with the carbonyl groups of amino acids; in neutral or weakly alkaline media the secondary bonds with the amino groups predominate. When the pH is close to the isoelectric point of the protein fixation on amino groups is also an essential factor in the "addition" of mercuric chloride, though it is due to primary bonds.

There is no reason in favour of a direct action of mercuric chloride on tissue carbohydrate; the excellent fixation of certain mucins can be due to the coagulation of proteins. The action on tissue lipids is essentially that of a hydrolysis of the plasmalogen, discussed in the histochemistry of lipids. Triglycerides are not affected by mercuric chloride. Chemical data indicate the possibility of combination with phospholipids but its implications in histological technique do not seem to have been explored. Baker (1958) has noted signs that certain conjugated lipids are rendered insoluble by mercuric chloride, a phenomenon that is comparable to the well known action of cadmium salts.

Penetration of mercuric chloride into animal tissues is slower than that of ethanol or trichloracetic acid. The estimations of v. Tellyesniczky (1926) and Baker (1958) lie between 0.7 and 0.8 mm per hour. Fixation by itself causes only moderate shrinkage of tissues but this shrinkage becomes considerable during dehydration with ethanol. Similarly, tissues harden slightly during fixation and much more on dehydration. Subsequent embedding by all the usual procedures is good. After fixation with mercuric chloride, or other salts of mercury, black extracellular precipitates appear under light-field examination. Such precipitates should be removed before embedding or staining by treatment with a solution of iodine.

All cell organelles and nuclear structures are well conserved. Mercuric chloride is one of the best of fixative agents and in addition has the advantage of giving particularly bright tints with most classical stains. When used alone it does not help to conserve chromosomes in paraffin sections, but this drawback can be overcome if it is associated with other agents.

Fixation with mercuric chloride is not recommended for histochemical purposes when the case is evident from its chemical properties; several authors thus advise against its use for the histochemical detection of glycogen.

6° *Chromium trioxyde*

The common usage of calling this compound chromic acid in histological technique is doubly erroneous in that the aqueous solutions used by the histologist do not even contain chromic acid, H_2CrO_4, but dichromic acid H_2CrO_7. The commercial product, CrO_3, is in the form of highly soluble red crystals. Freshly dissolved solutions are preferred for certain histochemical uses; this precaution need not be observed when the solutions are to be included in fixatives.

As Baker (1958) has noted the mechanism of the action of chromium trioxyde is poorly understood. All the data provided by the intensive study of industrial tanning cannot be of avail to the histologist since the conditions of using the compound in both cases are entirely different. In any case, it is a powerful coagulant of proteins and probably additive in nature. As for the mechanism of coagulation, the strong acidity of chromium trioxyde solutions cannot be the only factor involved since the coagulation obtained goes as far as preventing subsequent digestion by proteolytic enzymes, which is not the case after coagulation by hydrochloric or nitric acid. Neither does reaction with the amino group of aminoacids seem probable since this should reduce the acidophily of fixed tissues, which is apparently not the case. The oxidative properties of the fixing agent cannot however be excluded from a role; from the chemical point of view reactions with the SH-group of cysteine, the phenyl of tyrosine, the indole of tryptophane and the imidazole of histidine are quite conceivable.

At any rate coagulative action on tissue proteins is very strong; nucleic acids are also precipitated. Its action on tissue lipids can be explained by its oxidative nature, that is, the oxidation of unsaturated fatty acids and the insolubilization of certain lipids similar to that caused by potassium dichromate. In the same way its action on carbohydrates is one of oxidation which can extend further than the conversion of alcohols to aldehydes and hence cause a possible loss of histochemically detectable groups. This agent is therefore not recommended before the histochemical investigation of glycogen.

Penetration into tissues is slightly more rapid than that of picric acid (an average of 1 mm per hour). Shrinkage and hardening of tissues are moderate.

Careful elimination of all excess fixative by prolonged washing in running water is essential before further treatment of pieces.

The fixation of chromosomes is of good quality, though cytoplasmic organelles are badly conserved. Chondriomes are destroyed, lipid inclusions coalesce and cytoplasmic reticulation often exceeds the resolving power of the microscope so that troublesome artifacts appear under the light microscope. The nuclear membrane is clearly demonstrated. Cytoplasmic acidophily increases after chromium trioxyde fixation; chromatin also shows some tendency towards acidophily when fixation in a solution containing chromium trioxyde is prolonged beyond the optimal time.

The chemical properties of chromium trioxyde, especially its oxidative properties, justify reserves as to its use in fixing for histochemical purposes about which Pearse (1960) is explicit.

7° *Potassium dichromate*

This is a non-coagulant fixative agent about whose additive nature opinion is divided among authors.

The mode of action of aqueous solutions of potassium dichromate on tissue proteins is not well known. From classical work (see Gustavson 1949 for a detailed account) it is known that hexavalent complexes of chromium can react with both the carboxyl as well as amino groups of amino-acids. According to Green (1953) the simple formation of chromic salts with the carbonyl groups is not enough to account for the stabilization of structures and he consequently envisages the primary reaction to be followed by the amino and hydroxyl groups in coordination resulting finally in the establishment of chromium-rich linkages between protein molecules.

Considerable progress in the understanding of the action of potassium dichromate on tissues at the histological level is due to Zirkle (1928, 1933) whose studies on *Zea mays* have led to a demonstration of the essential role of pH in fixation. This notion has been applied to animal cytology by the school of Baker (see especially Baker, 1958, Casselman 1955).

It turns out from these studies that acidic solutions of potassium dichromate contain the same ions as those of chromium trioxyde, though the corrsponding pH for equivalent levels of chromium is quite different. Thus a 2,5% solution of potassium dichromate has a pH of 4.05 while a solution of chromium trioxyde containing the same quantity of chromium has a pH of 0.85. At a given pH the ionic composition of the two solutions is identical but for the presence of the potassium cations and the corresponding anions of the added acid.

Experience has shown that below the pH range of 3.4 to 3.8 solutions of potassium dichromate have the same effect on tissue proteins as solutions of chromium trioxyde, that is, strong coagulation is observed. At a higher pH the result is quite different; proteins do not coagulate but slowly form a gel. Nucleoproteins are not insolubilized by solutions of potassium dichromate that have not been acidified. The insolubilization of certain lipids after prolonged treatment with solutions of potassium dichromate has been known since a long time and is the basis of Weigert's myelinic method. From the chemical point of view potassium dichromate can act on lipids either as an oxidizing agent, a polymerizing agent or as an additive fixative with the formation of chromic complexes. In acid solutions its action on tissue carbohydrates is comparable to that of chromium trioxyde; solutions whose pH exceeds 4 do not have any effect on the carbohydrates of animal tissues.

Penetration into tissues is quite rapid (1.33 mm per hour according to v. Tellyesniczky (1926) but, as Baker (1958) remarks, one may doubt whether it corresponds to a truly effective fixation of tissues. At the time of fixation tissues undergo slight swelling but very strong shrinkage is exhibited after the steps preceding embedding in paraffin. There is little hardening during fixation and moderate hardening after dehydration. Embedding in paraffin is not as good as that following fixation with chromium trioxyde.

When the pH of solutions exceeds 3.8 the conservation of chromatin is mediocre, chondriosomes are not destroyed but undergo modifications in shape, most secretory granules remain intact and the cytoplasm becomes granular. Acidic solutions have the same effect on organelles as solutions of chromium trioxyde.

Washing in running water is essential after potassium dichromate just as it is after chromium trioxyde.

The staining affinities of cell constituents are not much modified after fixation in potassium dichromate. The chemical properties of this compound do not allow its use as a routine fixative for histochemical studies, but it is indispensable for certain methods such as some of those for lipid detection and the pheo-chromic reaction.

8° *Acetic acid*

This too is a non-coagulant fixative whose non-additive nature is quite probable if not certain.

The mode of action of acetic acid on tissue proteins is still not precisely known. According to the classical observations of v. Tellyesniczky (1926) the proteins of the nucleus are well fixed by this agent, while those of the cytoplasm are on the contrary dissolved. More recent observations have confirmed this view since acetic acid precipitates nucleoproteins from solution while its effect on albumins and globulins is one of swelling. It can be held that fixation by acetic acid is limited to proteins whose isoelectric point is close to the pH of the solution employed and that the appearance of intermolecular bonds is due to the disappearance of water molecules surrounding the ionized groups of the protein molecule caused by the drop in electrical charge.

Acetic acid has no action on tissue lipids and carbohydrates other than that of dissolving some of them.

Penetration into tissue seems to be rapid but difficult to evaluate since it has no coagulative effect on the cytoplasm; v. Tellyesniczky estimates it to be 1.2 mm per hour. Its immediate effect on tissues is a conspicuous swelling followed by strong shrinkage during subsequent operations. Pieces do not harden after this fixation. It is convenient for the traditional procedures of embedding. No particular precaution need be taken with regard to the elimination of excess fixative since acetic acid is miscible in all proportions with the ethanol used for dehydration.

The nuclear membrane and nucleoli are well demonstrated while the conservation of interphase chromatin is mediocre. Chondriosomes are destroyed and the hyaloplasm loses its homogeneity. The usual staining affinities of the cell organelles do not undergo any particular modification.

9° *Formaldehyde*

The vogue for this well known non-coagulant additive agent need not be recalled here. It is obtained commercially as an aqueous solution (formol, formalin) containing 35 to 40% of its weight in formic aldehyde. All the figures indicated in the present work refer to this solution; the dilute formalin generally used as a fixative liquid (1 volume of formalin for 9 volumes of water) therefore contains about 4% of formaldehyde. The slight variations in the level of formaldehyde in commercial formalin do not appreciably affect the quality of histological fixation.

It has long been known that formaldehyde does not coagulate albumin but that it can perfectly stabilize gels of gelatin by insolubilizing them. Its action on tissue proteins has been studied in detail and is well known; histologists have been able to gain from knowledge acquired in the field of industrial tanning. The first step in its action is the formation of a methylol group ($-CH_2OH$) with an amine or other radical containing an atom of active hydrogen, which in turn gives rise to methylene chains that link the protein molecules. An appreciable number of functions can produce this type of reaction (amine, amide, peptide, imine, guanidine, indol, alcoholic hydroxyl, thiol, disulfide, carbonyl).

It does not exert any direct chemical action on tissue carbohydrates, but they are very well conserved after formaldehyde fixation because of the excellent insolubilization of cell proteins. As for lipids there are clear indications that prolonged fixation provokes chemical modification; however they are sufficiently well maintained in place to warrant the routine use of short formaldehyde fixation in the histochemistry of lipids.

Penetration into tissues is quite rapid and roughly corresponds to that of mercuric chloride. The slight swelling on fixation is followed by strong shrinkage during the steps that precede embedding. Hardening of pieces is considerable. In fact, among all the agents reviewed here only ethanol and acetone cause more hardening. Subsequent embedding in nitrocellulose (collodion, celloidin) is acceptable, while that in paraffin is one of the worst.

The conservation of cell structures is generally good. The cytoplasm acquires a granular structure after fixation in formalin; chondriosomes are most often well conserved. The nuclear membrane is clearly delineated and the karyolymph, like the cytoplasm, can show a granular aspect. Fixation of chromatin is better than that of the nucleolus.

No particular precaution need be observed in removing excess fixative before subsequent treatment of pieces.

The formalin fixation of pieces of Vertebrate organs often results in the appearance of brown or black extracellular precipitates, especially in zones that are rich in blood. This "formalin pigment" that arises from the reaction of formaldehyde with haematin may be easily removed by a rapid treatment of sections in a 1% solution of potassium hydroxide in 80° alcohol. According to Baker (1958) the same result may be obtained with an alcoholic solution of picric acid.

Most authors consider that fixation in formalin accentuates the basophily of all structures. However, several of these appreciations are based on the examination of paraffin sections, and in view of the mediocre results it is difficult to attribute that which is due to modifications in staining affinity and that due to poor embedding.

10° *Other aldehydes*

Electron microscopical research has resulted in the introduction in histological technique of certain aldehydes other than the first one of the aldehyde series. Among them are glutaraldehyde, hydroxyadipinic aldehyde and acrolein. Only the first of these will be considered here for its importance in applications for the light microscope. The chemical interpretation of the effect of the above aldehydes on tissue proteins is less certain than that of the action of formaldehyde since, in this case, the histologist cannot benefit from the experience of the tanning industry. However, from the quality of preparations observed under both the light and electron microscopes one has to admit that, as far as histological technique is concerned, the denaturation of proteins is perceptibly better than that produced by formaldehyde.

The conservation of the carbohydrate and lipid constituents of tissues in preparations for the light microscope have not yet been systematically studied.

The penetration of all the above aldehydes is slow; most authors agree that it is roughly equal to that of osmium tetroxyde. This is confirmed by the methodical investigations and well documented work of Reale and Luciano (1970). Contrary to formaldehyde the actual fixation occurs rapidly and a prolonged stay in the fixative is not justified. No particular precaution is to be observed in the subsequent treatment of pieces.

Modifications in the volume of pieces during fixation and afterwards do not seem to have been studied. The hardening of pieces is considerable and when these aldehydes are used without any adjuvant the subsequent embedding in paraffin is as mediocre as after osmium tetroxyde.

From the cytological point of view the cell organelles are remarkably well preserved. In this respect light microscope preparations fixed in glutaraldehyde recall the weak penetration and irregularities of fixation due to osmium tetroxyde. Impeccably fixed cells and coarse artifacts co-exist in the same section only a few dozen microns away. Weak penetration of these fixatives accounts for the very distinct zonation of pieces. Unpublished attempts, referred to in connection with mitochondrial fixation, show that the irregularity and poor penetration of glutaraldehyde can be attenuated by associating it with other fixative agents.

Systematic research on a wide basis will most surely lead to very interesting and useful fixative mixtures.

The importance of the fixations described here is equally great from the histochemical point of view. Certain derivatives of protein metabolism are conserved after fixation in glutaraldehyde much better than after formaldehyde. Thus, this fixation plays an important role in much modern research on 5-hydroxytryptamine. According to unpublished tests the conservation of glycogen is as good under the light microscope as under the electron microscope. All modern authors acknowledge the importance of these fixatives in histo-enzymological research. Evidently a certain inhibition of enzymatic activity in the peripheral zones of the block should be allowed for. Certain authors attribute this inhibition, at least partly, to impurities in commercial solutions of glutaraldehyde whose degree of purity varies considerably from one supplier to another. All authors agree that the activities of phosphatases and esterases are well conserved after fixation in glutaraldehyde. Some maintain that succinodehydrogenasic activity is conserved after fixation in hydroxyadipinic aldehyde while others report the total loss of it.

11° *Osmium tetroxyde*

This non-coagulant and additive fixative, familiar to cytologists since the latter half of the 19th century, has enjoyed a renewed interest with the advent of infrastructural cytology. Its qualities as a fixative of cytoplasmic structures have been well established but its mode of action is not yet known with certainty.

Most recent authors (Wolman 1955, Baker 1958, Pearse 1960) consider that its action on tissue proteins is in two steps. The first is that of the formation of an additive compound between osmium tetroxyde and a group carrying a double bond or two adjacent hydroxyls. A second similar reaction involving the oxygen atoms of the tetroxyde that remains free after the first reaction results in the establishment of intermolecular bonds. From the *in vitro* studies of Baker (1955) it is known that osmium tetroxyde reacts immediately with thiols and disuphides, rapidly with alcohol and ether, slowly with saturated hydrocarbons and not at all with their halogen derivatives. Reactivity with amines, aldehydes and ketones increases with chain length.

Osmium tetroxyde does not seem to react with tissue carbohydrates; its ability to fix glycogen follows from the good conservation of cytoplasmic proteins. With lipids the characteristic osmic blackening is due to reduction of osmium tetroxyde, a powerful oxidant, to the black dioxyde. This reaction is a consequence of the oxidation of the double bond of unsaturated lipids. Since these compounds are widely distributed in the lipid deposits of the Vertebrate organism it follows that treatment with osmium tetroxyde demonstrates several intracellular lipid inclusions. The insolubilization of these lipids is probably due to the formation of an additive compound.

Penetration into tissues is very slow. According to classical data, confirmed by Baker (1958), the rate does not exceed 0.5 mm in 12 hours and is even considerably slower afterwards. It is thus one of the least penetrating agents. Very slight swelling upon fixation is followed by moderate shrinkage during later steps. It is preferable to remove excess osmium tetroxyde by washing in running water before treating pieces with ethanol since contact with the latter produces progressive blackening. This fixation is suitably followed by celloidin embedding rather than paraffin, which is quite poor.

Cytoplasmic structures are remarkably well conserved after this fixation by itself. All authors agree that under favorable conditions it is osmium tetroxyde that ensures a fixation that is closest to the living state. But most of the qualities of osmic fixation are lost in paraffin sections. Comparative examination under the electron microscope shows that modifications occur at the time of embedding and sectioning.

From the histochemical point of view this fixation is only inapplicable when the particular chemical properties of osmium tetroxyde render it unsuitable.

Osmium tetroxyde is expensive and easily reduced; certain precautions should therefore be observed in preparing and handling solutions. Containers should be closed with rubber stoppers; cork or polythene stoppers are not suited, while costly and fragile ground-glass stoppers may be dispensed with. Osmium tetroxyde is usually supplied in ampoules of 0.5 g, and the simplest procedure is to clean the exterior of an ampoule and crush it in the required volume of distilled water. The presence of chromium trioxyde or potassium dichromate in the solution exerts a protective effect on osmium tetroxyde, but such chromo-osmic solutions are suitable only for certain histological uses; they are to be particularly avoided in the osmic impregnation of the Golgi apparatus.

GENERAL REMARKS ON FIXATIVE MIXTURES

In certain cases the fixing agents that have been reviewed here are used alone (the simple fixatives of early authors). Formalin, ethanol and methanol are thus used without the addition of any other compound.

In other cases the agent and the solvent are not the only constituents of the liquid used for fixation; these liquids represent the fixative mixtures (the compound fixatives of classical authors). The term has however been accepted differently. Certain authors, such as Baker, hold that only liquids containing several fixing agents should be considered as real fixative "mixtures" while those containing a single agent, the solvent and other compounds that are not themselves fixing agents remain simple fixatives. In fact it seems logical to use the term "fixative mixture" whenever the result produced is not due to the action of the agent alone. From such a point of view, therefore, one should include, in the group of fixative mixtures, those liquids that contain, in addition to the agent and the solvent, metallic salts which are not themselves fixing agents but whose presence improves the final result.

FIXATIVE MIXTURES CONTAINING AN "INDIFFERENT" SALT

The salts used as adjuvants in fixative mixtures are predominantly sodium sulfate and sodium chloride. The sulfate has been associated with potassium dichromate in the classic liquid of Müller from which those of Zenker, of Helly and of Maximow are derived. None of the authors who have used these liquids gives the slightest indication as to the mode of action of sodium sulfate, and some even consider its use to be a quite unnecessary measure. It is equally difficult to interpret the addition of sodium chloride to solutions of mercuric chloride used as histological fixatives. This practice, introduced by Heidenhain, is faithfully followed by all modern authors though no explanation for such an association has been provided. Similarly, the addition of various salts to solutions of formaldehyde has been proposed when using it both as a general histological or histochemical fixative. Some of the proposed additions have a solid chemical basis and should be considered as perfectly coherent. Such is the case with the formulae invented by Baker and designated as formaldehyde—calcium and formaldehyde—calcium—cadmium. As for the addition of sodium chloride that is so often proposed ("saline formalin") its reasons are not clear. In fact, the concern of the authors of these formulae, which is to obtain a fixative liquid more or less isotonic for the cells to be fixed, is quite pointless. From a series of studies, reviewed by Baker (1958), it turns out that osmotic factors are scarcely involved in determining the quality of fixation for light microscopy.

In spite of these theoretical doubts, however, certain additions of indifferent salts are not without their value. Very clear differences in the fixation of the stellar ganglion of *Sepia officinalis* have been reported by Young (1935) depending on whether distilled water or sea water is used as the solvent for picric acid, chromium trioxyde, osmium tetroxyde, potassium dichromate or formaldehyde. On the other hand he emphasizes that in the case of acetic acid or mercuric chloride the difference becomes insignificant.

Since there are very real difference in the quality of certain fixations depending on the presence or absence of "indifferent salts" it appears reasonable, in our present state of knowledge, to conform to the formulae proposed in each case. Even if doubts persist as to the efficacity of the addition, it is certainly quite innocuous. The modestly priced products and the negligible time taken for preparation are further arguments in favour of a pragmatic conservatism in this matter.

MIXTURES CONTAINING SEVERAL FIXING AGENTS

These "compound fixatives" form the great majority of liquids used in histological practice. Their number is considerable, and the excessive proliferation of formulae, some of which are practically identical to well known liquids, has been mentioned at the beginning of this chapter.

The chemical **compatibility** or rather **incompatibility**, of the fixing agents that constitute a mixture is, evidently, one of the primary features to be taken into consideration in appreciating a given fixative mixture. The mutual incompatibilities of the principal fixing agents are summarized in Table 1 after the data of Baker (1958). Some of the facts in the Table call for no comment. The incompatibility of ethanol and chromium trioxyde, a powerful oxidant, is evident; this is equally true for the incompatibility of ethanol with potassium dichromate and osmium tetroxyde. In other cases incompatibility is clear from the chemical point of view (e.g. formaldehyde and chromium trioxyde) but the histologist should overlook it. In fact, Sanfelice's liquid, which is justly considered as one of the best fixatives for general histology and karyology, contains both chromium trioxyde and formaldehyde in addition to acetic acid. Similarly though association of potassium dichromate and formaldehyde can be criticized from the chemical aspect, it forms the basis of some of the best fixatives of classical cytology such as the liquids of Orth, of Kopsch and of Regaud. Real incompatibility is thus less frequent than expected from a simple consideration of the chemical properties of the agents. This apparent contradiction may be easily explained if the conditions of application of certain supposedly "irrational" fixatives are taken into account. In practice, these mixtures are prepared freshly and their period of action is strictly limited. Very often the expected chemical reaction, to which the "irrational" nature of the mixture is attributed, is slow so that its qualities as a fixative are not affected. Such a change of quality, when it occurs, is often betrayed by an alteration in the colour of the mixture.

Besides strictly chemical incompatibility other difficulties arise, as in the case of potassium dichromate, from the mode of action on tissue proteins. The studies of Zirkle and of the school of Baker have shown that potassium dichromate exhibits all its qualities as a fixative of cytoplasmic organelles only when the pH of the mixture is above 3.8 or 4. Consequently, its conjoint use with a strong acid or chromium trioxyde deprives fixative mixtures containing potassium dichromate of most of their advantages. Thus, in spite of its vogue, Champy's liquid is better abandoned in favour of chromo-osmic fixatives that do not contain chromium trioxyde. Similarly, the presence of non-negligible quantities of acetic acid in Zenker's fluid easily explains the relative superiority of Helly's fixative where acetic acid is replaced by formaldehyde. Though the latter is thus rendered unstable and "irrational" it allows access to the qualities of potassium dichromate as a cytoplasmic fixative.

When fixative mixture are classified according to the *nature of the solvent* their frequency of use shows aqueous solutions to predominate over alcoholic liquids. The latter are favoured only in cases where the treatment of pieces in an aqueous medium is to be avoided for chemical reasons or when the objects are known to be poorly penetrated by aqueous solutions.

Another remarkable fact is the preponderance of *acid solutions*. The pH of a great majority of common histological fixatives lies between 0.5 and 5; among the routine mixtures Baker's formaldehyde-calcium is the only one that clearly has a pH above 7 (9.0 according to the estimation of Baker, 1958). Certain manuals of histological technique still claim that good fixation is impossible in alkaline or neutral fluids; though the considerable success of fixing in osmium tetroxyde dissolved in an alkaline buffer, as practised by Palade (1952) for

Table 1. — COMPATIBILITIES OF THE PRINCIPAL FIXATIVE AGENTS (partly from the data of BAKER, 1958). C = Chemical compatibility; I = Chemical incompatibility; PC = Partial compatibility (unstable mixtures to be prepared freshly).

	Methanol	Ethanol	Acetone	Trichloride acid	Picric acid	Chloroplatinic acid	Mercuric chloride	Chromium trioxyde	Potassium dichromate	Acetic acid	Formaldehyde	Osmium tetroxyde
Methanol	\	C	C	C	C	C	C	I	I	C	C	I
Ethanol	C	\	C	C	C	C	C	I	I	C	C	I
Acetone	C	C	\	C	C	C	C	I	I	C	C	I
Trichloracetic acid	C	C	C	\	C	C	C	C	C	C	C	C
Picric acid	C	C	C	C	\	C	C	C	C	C	C	C
Chloroplatinic acid	C	C	C	C	C	\	C	C	C	C	C	C
Mercuric chloride	C	C	C	C	C	C	\	C	C	C	C	C
Chromium trioxyde	I	I	I	C	C	C	C	\	C	C	PC	C
Potassium dichromate	I	I	I	C	C	C	C	C	\	C	PC	C
Acetic acid	C	C	C	C	C	C	C	C	C	\	C	C
Formaldehyde	C	C	C	C	C	C	C	PC	PC	C	\	I
Osmium tetroxyde	I	I	I	C	C	C	C	C	C	C	I	\

electron micrography, is enough to belie this assertion. Experience, however, shows that embedding in paraffin is especially good after fixation at a low pH.

Empiricism has been, in most cases, the guiding spirit in the formulation of the classical fixatives, and it is often quite impossible to understand, even *a posteriori*, the reason for certain associations. In other cases, however, the particular properties of fixing agents justify their association in a given mixture. Thus, when acetic acid is associated with a coagulating agent and formaldehyde (the latter being replaceable by osmium tetroxyde or chloroplatinic acid) excellent mixtures are obtained where the disadvantages of each agent are remedied by the others. A remarkable fact clearly noted by Baker (1958) is that the final shrinkage of tissues after fixation in these mixtures and paraffin embedding is definitely less than after fixation in each agent alone. The absence of acetic acid and powerful coagulants from mixtures meant for the detailed study of cytoplasmic structures is easily explained. However, it should be noted that the harmful action of acetic acid on the chondriome is not due to its acidity. A study by Casselman and Gordan (1955) has shown that the hepatic chondriome, which is always destroyed by acetic acid, is conserved by hydrochloric acid.

The penetration of the various agents of a mixture is of importance. There is, in fact, considerable difference in the rates of penetration, into a given tissue, of the common constituents of fixative mixtures. This may be easily verified by a careful examination of slices of tissue after a certain time. It explains the inequalities of fixation of a zone according to its distance from the surface of the piece. Thus the formaldehyde and the acetic acid of Bouin's fluid penetrate much more rapidly than the picric acid. Similarly, the difference in the penetration of acetic acid and potassium dichromate in v. Tellyesniczky's mixture is so great that one wonders whether such an association is really feasible. In fact, the centre of a piece of reasonable dimensions is attained by the potassium dichromate long after its cytoplasm has suffered the harmful action of acetic acid. In addition the advantages of a proper fixation of the cytoplasm by potassium dichromates are lost due to the presence of acetic acid in this liquid since the pH of the fixative drops well below 3.8. When a mixture contains agents with widely differing rates of penetration, autolysis is stopped by the fastest of these agents, but the quality of fixation expected of the association is obtained only in the region close to the surface where the differences in the period of contact with the various agents is not too great. This argues in favour of reducing the size of pieces to less than 3 mm in one dimension whenever it can be done without destroying anatomical connections or crushing the tissue.

PERIOD OF FIXATION

The *period of action* of fixative mixtures has usually been prescribed by their authors more or less strictly. In histological practice this is of small importance. Apart from formalin none of the usual fixatives conserves at the same time; hence it is necessary to stop fixation after a definite lapse of time. This lapse cannot be determined from the rate of penetration alone since the period required for the agents to exert their action on tissues varies. Thus, at the cellular level, fixation by osmium tetroxyde is practically instantaneous. Prolonging the period of contact makes sense only if further chemical reactions involving osmium tetroxyde and certain cell constituents are envisaged. Formaldehyde is quite the opposite since it is much more penetrating than osmium tetroxyde but its action on tissue proteins, which leads to fixation, is very much slower. Prolongation of contact with the agent after the cells have been reached, in this particular case, improves the final result. Differences in the "rate of fixation" are only one aspect of the problem. When a mixture is "irrational" in the chemical sense it is obvious that tissues should be removed before the chemical transformations, discussed in an earlier paragraph, set in and the composition of the liquid is extensively modified. In addition, the shrinkage and hardening of tissues caused by certain agents can only increase with longer periods of exposure; hence it is necessary to determine, by trial and error, the optimum period that is just sufficient for good fixation before excessive shrinkage or hardening occurs.

Actual fixation of tissues in the strict sense is not the only factor that has to be taken into consideration in estimating the period of action of fixative mixtures. In fact, the best possible preparation for the subsequent embedding of piece is also one of the objectives of fixation. Experience proves that this is not always obtained during the period that is sufficient for fixation. It is particularly true for fixatives based on formalin or acetic acid, especially that of Bouin. When pieces that are too bulky for the satisfactory fixation of the inner regions at the cellular level are maintained in the liquid for several days the final result in these regions is relatively improved, not because of better "fixation" but because it is a better prelude to embedding in paraffin.

This is probably a partial explanation of the striking differences in opinion as to the time of fixation that the reader will surely notice in many original articles in cytology and histology. Certain authors systematically prefer short fixation. From their personal orientation they often turn out to be cytologists working on smears who do not usually insist on the uniform conservation of all the structures of a piece. On the contrary others who are preoccupied with microscopical anatomy or topographical histology are partisans of long fixation. Truth evidently lies somewhere in between.

In practice it may be assumed that a fixation of about 12 hours is not likely to exceed the limit and cause damage. Baker (1958) admits this period but does not remark notable exceptions, some of which follow from purely chemical considerations and mostly involve fixation for histo-enzymological studies. Another very important exception is that of fixation in the liquid of Helly or of Maximow (without tetroxyde) which should be stopped after 6 hours at the latest by washing in running water if it is to be followed by certain stains. The same applies to all fixations before silver impregnation of the Golgi apparatus.

TEMPERATURE OF FIXATION

The practical importance of the temperature of fixation should not be ignored In most cases pieces for topographical study are fixed at room temperature. Warm fixation, suggested for objects that are difficult to penetrate or for animals that have to be spread out for fixing (worms, insect larvae), is not advisable for the conservation of structures; at the most it results in a bad coagulation of tissue proteins due to heat long before the fixative agents of the mixture have been able to act. Fixation in the cold is, on the contrary, quite a logical and coherent step since the low temperature (about 0°) considerably slows autolytic phenomena without affecting the rate of penetration of the fixative. Apart from histo-enzymological research, where cold fixation is almost compulsory, I would strongly advise it for all cytological fixation as well, except in cases where osmium tetroxyde is involved. In fact experience has shown that this agent fixes better at temperatures between 12 and 24° rather than at 0°.

MODES OF FIXATION

The modes of "fixation" by physical agents, described in the beginning of this chapter, follow well defined norms. Fixation by chemical agents is somewhat more "lax" in this respect, and their modes of application are reviewed below.

FIXATION WITH VAPOURS

Chemical fixing agents can act as vapours and this type of fixation plays an important role in studies on isolated cells. It is the protistologist who benefits more from fixation by vapours; other modifications of the method are useful to the haematologist. Osmium tetroxyde is the chief of such agents; examples of fixation by formaldehyde vapours are less frequent; iodine vapours, once favoured by classical authors, is almost completely neglected now.

FIXATION IN LIQUIDS

In the great majority of cases fixatives act on tissues in the *liquid phase*. In practice this may consist of *immersion*, of *injection into the body cavity* of an animal with an open circulatory system, or by *perfusion* of the liquid in an animal with a closed circulatory system. *Interstitial injection* of the fixative has been used in some cases, expecially when it is impossible to obtain slices of pieces that are too bulky to be fixed by simple immersion. It is however better to avoid this method as it distends and damages tissue.

1° Apart from considerations of the size of pieces and the temperature of the fixative, discussed in a preceding paragraph, *fixation by immersion* should take into account the dilution that follow the introduction of pieces which on the average contain 70 to 90% of water. It is therefore indispensable to envisage, whenever the cost of fixing agents does not forbid it, a large excess of liquid. All authors agree that its volume should be about 50 times that of the pieces, except in the case of osmic fixatives where 10 times would do.

Great care should be taken that the fixative attains the piece from all sides. I strongly advise against the practice of placing a piece in a vessel and then pouring the fixative over it. The best method is to first pour the fixative into a vessel in which some cotton or glass wool has been placed, according to the nature of the liquid, and then immersing the piece in it. It is only rarely necessary to suspend the piece by a thread in the centre of the liquid.

Pieces that are coated by a layer of coagulated blood or mucus fix badly; the layer should therefore be rapidly removed before immersion. Another essential precaution, often neglected, is to remove any contained gas by placing the recipient in which fixation is being carried out in the moderate vacuum of a filter-pump. Obviously the fixative should be renewed on returning to normal pressure. Vacuum should be applied repeatedly when pieces containing calcified inclusions are fixed with a liquid containing decalcifying agents.

If pieces cannot be easily wetted by aqueous liquids they may be immersed in absolute alcohol for a few seconds before plunging them into the fixative. By observing this simple precaution aqueous fixations generally give, in certain cases, results that are as satisfactory as those of alcoholic liquids.

Though direct sunlight obviously does no good to any fixation, keeping pieces in obscurity during fixation is really necessary only in very few cases. I suggest that pieces fixed in formalin or liquids containing osmium tetroxyde be sheltered from daylight in a cupboard.

The choice of the vessel in which fixation is carried out evidently depends on the chemical characteristics of the liquid used. Almost all modern authors prefer glassware. The vogue of vials with polythene caps is entirely justified; they need be avoided only for fixation in osmic liquids, when rubber-stoppered tubes are quite convenient. Cork is evidently unsuited, while ground—glass which is costly, fragile and difficult to clean is quite unnecessary. The cleaning of glassware does not call for any particular precaution; the usual sulfuric — acid — dichromate mixture, routine in chemical laboratories, followed through rinsing in running water is sufficient. A last rinse in distilled water is necessary only when the vessels are intended for osmic fixation. I strongly advise against the use of modern detergents which are really difficult to remove and also surface-active.

2° **Fixation by injection into the body cavity** is useful for fixing small animals *in toto*; it should be followed by immersion in the particular fixative.

3° **Fixation by perfusion** may at first appear to be the ideal procedure for animals with a closed circulatory system, especially the Vertebrates. However it has a certain number of practical disadvantages.

Theoretically the method has obvious advantages since the fixative is directly placed in contact with the cells to be fixed and this reduces the possibility of autolysis before fixation to a minimum. It is thus possible to fix correctly pieces that are far too bulky to be fixed by immersion. It is also the only means of fixing certain organs that are not easily accessible; the Mammalian internal ear is one such example. This procedure is also recommended when a truly faultless fixation of the brain is required in Mammals, even of moderate size (rabbit, cat).

Among its disadvantages the chief one is the need for apparatus that is much more complicated than in fixation by immersion. Furthermore, all the organs of an animal are evidently fixed by the same liquid unless one resorts to very complicated operations. In certain cases the cost of the liquid chosen should also be considered. As a rule this method is more relevant for histological research than for diagnosis.

The first step in fixation by perfusion consists of removing, as rapidly and completely as possible, all the blood from the particular vascular region. For this a cannula is inserted into the afferent blood vessel after deep anesthesia (perfusion of the whole body from the left ventricule or the aorta gives acceptable results only in animals smaller than the rabbit). The blood is displaced by an isotonic solution that contains no substance likely to react with the fixative, and which should be brought to body temprature for homoiothermic animals. It is advantageous to add a little amyl nitrite to this solution to provoke strong vasodilatation. A free flow of blood and the rinse may be ensured by opening a large vein or even better, the right auricle. As soon as the effluent from this opening contains no appreciable quantity of blood the fixative is rapidly injected taking care to avoid too much pressure and air bubbles which prevent access of the fixative to certain regions. It is obvious that metallic cannulae should not be used with fixatives containing mercuric chloride.

In general, large quantities of fixatives are required; classical authors, on the other hand, advise that the vessels be flushed before the injection of fixative with as little liquid as possible.

After perfusion the chosen organs are fixed by immersion in the particular liquid. The slicing of tissues is greatly facilitated by their modified consistency following perfusion with the fixative.

Apart from the disadvantages mentioned earlier fixation by perfusion can cause significant histological modification in the walls of vessels and oedematose reactions in the pericapillary regions of various organs. It is to reduce these reactions as far as possible, which occur during the flushing prior to injection, that authors advise one to diminish the quantity of rinsing solution.

Perfusion using a syringe can be performed only with animals of the size of mice or small frogs. In all other cases the rinsing solution and fixative are held in a flask with a lateral outlet and the pressure of injection regulated by varying the height of the flask above the animal.

CHOICE OF FIXATIVE

From the preceding discussion it follows that the choice of a fixative is one of the most important aspects of histological examination; its difficulty varies with the case. The choice of certain fixatives is laid down by the subsequent treatment of pieces. Thus, for the study of alkaline phosphomonoesterase activity in paraffin sections there is no other alternative but alcohol, acetone or perhaps Danielli's formalin-pyridine. Only the liquids of Ramon y Cajal, of da Fano and of Aoyama, which give almost equivalent results, render pieces suitable for proper silver impregnation of the Golgi apparatus. The use of Helly's or Maximow's liquids, of very similar composition, is almost compulsory in the study of Vertebrate haematopoietic organs to be stained by the panoptic method. In other cases dozens of fixative liquids can be used *a priori*. A review of the principal criteria of choice is thus called for; precise recommendations of particular techniques are given in the other chapters.

One of the factors that may be secondary in most cases but which can sometimes be the essential concern is the cost of fixative agents. Two of them, osmium tetroxyde and chloroplatinic acid, little used today, are really quite expensive. Even here the actual expense is not great when they are used for fixation by immersion of pieces meant for cytology. Financial considerations however become preponderant if fixation is by perfusion. The late Professor E. Scharrer once told me that a perfusion of the head of a foal, for a histological study of the brain, had cost him as much as 120 litres of Helly's liquid. Obviously even the head of a richly endowed laboratory cannot dream of a similar use of Altmann's or Champy's liquids.

Apart from such particular circumstances, only the final results of fixations weigh in the choice of a fixative mixture. This choice is difficult since it is very often a compromise. Even in those cases where the use of a fixative is imposed by chemical considerations, such as the conservation of certain enzymatic activities or certain inorganic or organic constituents of tissues, the feasibility of the operation is liable to discussion if the material happens to be out of the ordinary. Since no universal fixative exists the use of any one of the numerous formulae implies that certain stains or histochemical reactions have to be ruled out.

It is with mixtures based on formalin and acetic acid that one stands the greatest chance of properly fixing the bulkier pieces; but after such fixation a great number of cytological techniques cannot be envisaged. The use of chromo-osmic liquids, on the other hand, ensures excellent conservation of cytoplasmic structures in the well-fixed regions but precludes any study of microscopical anatomy.

Consequently the purpose of examining and the fate of the piece should be precisely known at the time of choosing the fixative, since very often the possibility or impossibility of applying certain stains follows from this choice. In addition to the data accumulated over a century of histological research there are the incertitudes that always reign when an object is studied by a given method for the first time. Thus, apart from the imperative precautions that follows from the action of fixatives on cell organelles or histochemically detectable compounds there exists no general rule that is valid for all cases. A necessary corollary to this is that the precautions and recommendations particular to the different formulae given elsewhere in this book will be discussed along with the methods of studying various structures.

The disproportionality between the large number of formulae described since the beginning of histological research and the relatively few mixtures that have entered into current practice is due partly to what Baker (1958) calls the "natural selection" against unsuitable liquids that are soon forgotten.

But such selection is not the only cause. Traditions, usages, routine and prejudices are involved to a degree not easily foreseen by one who is uninitiated in the discipline. There is indeed no other possible explanation for the furious obstinacy with which anatomo-pathologists fix all their pieces in dilute formalin, which, of all the usual fixatives, guarantees the worst imaginable embedding in paraffin.

The danger of definitely adopting a standard fixation is particularly great in comparative histology; in fact a liquid that admirably suits a given object can produce monstruous artifacts in another. The difficulties of fixation vary greatly according to the material and the histologist who specializes in Mammals can scarcely surmise the problems confronted in retaining the secretory products of the hypobranchial gland of a Gasteropod. The adaptation of the method of fixation to the given object is one of the essential prerequisites of success.

CHAPTER 4

EMBEDDING AND PREPARATORY OPERATIONS

> Manchem geübten Techniker wird dieser Aufsatz zu weitschweifig sein; er wird darin vieles finden, was ihm als selbstverständlich vorkommt. Doch habe ich in meiner... mikrotechnischen Praxis... die Erfahrung gemacht, dass in der Mikrotechnik nichts selbstverständlich ist. Im Gegenteil gilt hier der Satz: Es ist selbstverständlich, also muss es eigens gesagt werden. Dies zu meiner Entschuldigung!
>
> St. v. APATHY (1912/13).

The aims of the operations situated between the end of fixation and the cutting of sections are to remove the pieces from further action of the fixative, to prepare the tissues for penetration by the embedding mass and to ensure this penetration. Theoretical considerations in the description of these operations are quite scant and the methods of practice are far fewer than those of fixation or staining. It therefore appears justifiable and opportune to consider in this chapter both the general procedure as well as the practical method which is the same for most organs and tissues.

Only one of the operations discussed here is rigorously obligatory, namely the termination of fixation. In fact pieces, one of whose dimensions is very small (flat membranes, gills of Molluscs etc.) can be stained and mounted on a slide without embedding or cutting sections. Some stains and histochemical reactions can be applied in bulk before embedding and section-cutting. I shall therefore consider successively the termination of fixation and embedding by the three main procedures, namely in paraffin, celloidin and gelatin, along with their variants.

TERMINATION OF FIXATION

Most fixations are automatically stopped at the beginning of the operations that prepare for embedding. Thus, picric acid, acetic acid, formaldehyde and mercuric chloride are soluble in both water and alcohol, so that the desired result is obtained during dehydration or the aqueous rinsing before embedding in gelatin. Special washing in running water or frequent changes of it need be provided for only when the fixative contains chromium trioxyde, potassium dichromate, osmium tetroxyde or chloroplatinic acid. In these cases the complete elimination of all excess fixative is essential. Neglect of this rule irremediably compromises the fate of pieces because all four compounds react with the usual dehydrating agents and produce serious alterations in staining affinities as well as precipitates in tissues that are almost impossible to eliminate.

In washing one should take account of the fact that solutions of the fixative agents to be eliminated have a specific gravity that is higher than that of water. It is therefore important to use recipients with a wide base, to ensure that the pieces do not remain at the bottom and to evacuate water from below.

Excess fixative may be removed by washing in frequently renewed tap water in the vessel used for fixation. One is evidently slave to the operation, especially if some thirty or forty samples have to be thus attended to about twenty times a day. Its advantage however lies in the ease of verification. Thus incomplete washing after chromic fixation (osmium tetroxyde and chloroplatinic acid are rarely used without the addition of either chromium trioxyde or potassium dichromate) is betrayed by the yellow colour of the water, and further washing is consequently necessary.

Most histologists prefer washing in running water and several devices have been proposed for this purpose. It is besides quite easy to improvise one, allowing for the difference in specific gravity between water and fixative solutions. P. Masson recommends that pieces be wrapped in little bags of gauze or similar material and suspended midway in a tall jar in which the water is changed every one or two hours. Such a set-up may be easily adapted to running water by a choosing a jar with a lateral orifice near the bottom; a cork with an L-shaped tube is attached, the upper limb of which regulates the level of water in the jar. When placed under a tap it automatically ensures the evacuation of water by the bottom and the rapid elimination of fixative. When a large number of pieces are being manipulated they may be left in the bags during dehydration if sufficiently big vessels are used.

Fairchild tubes are round-bottomed, cylindrical recipients in porcelain whose walls are perforated. Pieces are inserted in this tube which is then closed with a cork that is sufficiently voluminous that it floats on the surface. Several different pieces or groups of pieces may thus be washed in a single jar if the relevant label written in soft pencil or India ink is enclosed in each tube. Fairchild tubes can be used for washing in running water as described above, and pieces may be kept in them during dehydration. Care should evidently be taken that the tubes are well corked; the result of negligence in this respect is quite obvious when a large number of different pieces are washed together.

Fairchild tubes may be replaced by glass tubes that are corked at one end and covered by a firmly tied muslin at the other. A constriction at one end or a bell-rimmed mouth have been described to ensure fastening of the muslin.

Metal baskets suspended in a recipient of water may also be used for washing. Automatic rinsing devices have also been specially designed for the histologist. Recent models process a number of pieces simultaneously with frequent and complete renewal of water, and their efficacity is greatly improved by constant agitation.

Most authors consider that washing in running water for 12 to 24 hours is enough to remove all the excess of chromic or osmic fixative. This period may be even reduced with the automatic devices. When pieces are washed in changes of water, the end of the operation is determined by observing that the last washings, in which the pieces have been left for two or three hours, remain colourless.

The removal of excess picric acid or mercuric chloride is ensured at the beginning of dehydration for embedding in paraffin or nitrocellulose. Some authors nevertheless advise that pieces fixed in high concentrations of picric acid be washed in 70% alcohol saturated with lithium carbonate or ammonium acetate. This step appears superfluous to me for the above cases, but is on the contrary very useful when small pieces have to be stained and mounted *in toto*, without embedding or cutting, since it shortens the period in alcohol. The black and very often extracellular crystals formed during fixation in liquids based on mercuric chloride can be removed by treatment with a 0.5% solution of iodine in alcohol. Here also the step which is followed by destaining in a 5% aqueous solution of sodium thiosulfate is useful only for pieces to be mounted *in toto*. Those that are to be embedded and sectioned are better freed of crystals by rapidly passing sections in Lugol's fluid.

EMBEDDING IN PARAFFIN

Embedding in paraffin, introduced into histological technique by Klebs (1869) remains even today the most frequently used method of embedding. None of the other suggested compounds has succeeded in replacing paraffin, which clearly illustrates its advantages.

It has to be admitted that only minor modifications in procedure have been made since the beginning and that most histologists practise it quite empirically. The scientific study of phenomena occurring during embedding has been very rarely attempted. General investigations on the physical characteristics of paraffin that bear an importance in histology are few; that of Piller (1953) is a rare example. The practical results of these studies are trivial and most often only confirm the empirical directives of classical authors.

PROPERTIES OF THE EMBEDDING MEDIUM

The commercial product sold as paraffin is a mixture of aliphatic hydrocarbons having the general formula C_nH_{2n+2}, where n is usually between 21 and 34. These fluctuations along with varying quantities of impurities of the olein group (C_nH_{2n}) account for the differences in commercial samples whose constitution is never rigorously defined. Even the paraffin that is sold for histological use is a mixture and its melting point is specified within a range of 2°. In most cases hot filtration of commercial paraffin is necessary before use in histology; this may effected with ordinary filter paper in an oven at a suitable temperature or in a funnel with a heating jacket.

Among the physical characteristics of the paraffin those that influence the quality of embedding and sectioning are principally the degree of *fissuration*, which betrays the presence of liquid impurities and air between crystals, *hardness*, *plasticity* and *viscosity*.

As regards the solubility of the product it may be recalled that paraffin is not miscible in either water, methanol, ethanol, propanol, glycerin, methyl benzoate, methyl salicylate or terpineol. On the contrary it is miscible with ether, aniline, gasoline, dioxan, butanol, chloroform, Cedarwood oil, bergamot oil, petroleum ether, carbon disulfide and benzenic hydrocarbons.

Evidently the general procedure of embedding depends on the above properties of solubility. Perfect penetration of the embedding medium into the piece requires, first of all, impeccable dehydration and, secondly, impregnation with a liquid that is miscible with paraffin. Only pieces submitted to freezing-drying may be properly impregnated with paraffin without resorting to any intermediate treatment.

PROCEDURE OF PARAFFIN EMBEDDING

The whole process of embedding thus consists of dehydrating the pieces, impregnating them with a solvent of paraffin, penetrating with paraffin and moulding the block. These four steps will be successively discussed.

1° Dehydration

Treatment with progressively increasing concentrations of ethanol is the traditional method of dehydration adopted to start the removal of water from pieces even when it is terminated with the help of some other substance. The concentrations and periods of treatment are diversely estimated by different authors. A comparison of their recommendations gives the impression that most precepts stem from routine rather than from reasoning or methodical trials. Apart from dehydration with ethanol, that using dioxan can play an important role in histological technique, but its advantages are counterbalanced by certain disadvantages which have led most European laboratories to renounce its use.

a) In the practice of **dehydration with ethanol** an elementary but often neglected fact should be remembered, namely that the specific gravity of water-ethanol mixtures is greater than that of pure ethanol. Consequently dehydration should be carried out in wide-bottomed vessels and the use of a large quantity of alcohol makes sense only if the tubes are often agitated or if the pieces are suspended at mid-height in the tube. In all other cases it is definitely preferable to pour only a sufficient quantity to cover the pieces with about one cm of alcohol, but to frequently renew it. When changing it should evidently be seen that the last drops of liquid at the bottom are emptied, as these are the richest in water. Progressive, as opposed to abrupt, dehydration and the number of stages to be followed have given rise to much discussion. Many authors advise a very progressive dehydration for cytological research, increasing the level of ethanol in steps of 10° at a time. The same authors accept dehydration to commence with 60% alcohol when pieces are meant for topographical histology. Others observe that weak alcohol is an excellent macerating agent, that the danger of dissociating *fixed* pieces is not at all increased by immersion in strong alcohol and that gradual dehydration is not any better than when it is rapid. Having followed from the very outset the counsel of P. Masson (1923) in histological technique, which consists in dehydrating pieces fixed in aqueous fixatives straightaway in 96% alcohol, I feel justified, after a quarter of a century of daily practice, in entirely confirming the views of this great French histopathologist. Methodical trials have convinced me that it is pointless to submit pieces intended for the techniques of light microscopy to progressive dehydration. It may perhaps be advantageous when the external shape of pieces rich in water has to be scrupulously maintained; and in fact several devices that enable the strength of alcohol to be gradually raised have been described for the purpose. But I am certain that a direct transfer into 96% alcohol of pieces that have been *properly* fixed in an aqueous liquid does not expose them to any risk. I therefore advise, without hesitation, the direct transfer from an aqueous fixative or a wash in water to 96% alcohol in all cases.

The time required to be spent in 96% alcohol evidently depends on the quantity of water to be removed from the tissues, and consequently on their dimensions. Equilibrium with the dehydrating medium is generally reached, in the cases of tissue slices not exceeding 5 mm in thickness, within a few hours and this period can be considerably reduced when the pieces are small. Frequent changes of alcohol and agitation of the medium also accelerate the process.

It is obvious that complete dehydration of the piece cannot be obtained with 96% alcohol alone. When benzenic hydrocarbons are used as intermediates between the dehydrating agent and paraffin, dehydration should be completed with absolute alcohol. Three changes of a few hours duration are sufficient in most cases, the second and third of which may be prolonged without harm to 12 hours; this often enables its convenient insertion in the daily program of the laboratory. I must remark here that the harmful action of a prolonged stay in absolute alcohol that is claimed for the results of classical mitochondrial stains is more of a legend. I can affirm from systematic studies that properly fixed and postchromatized chondriomes can easily withstand absolute alcohol for more than a week.

Many histologists substitute butanol in place of absolute ethanol; this is excellent practice, the more so that butanol is miscible with molten paraffin and the use of another intermediate is thus dispensed with. The practical procedure for its use is described under the impregnation of pieces with solvents of paraffin.

When pieces have been fixed in an alcoholic liquid, even the most timorous of cytologists admit starting dehydration at a strength of alcohol that is higher than that of the fixative (96% or absolute alcohol for the fixatives of Duboscq-Brazil and of Gendre, absolute alcohol for those of Clarke and of Carnoy).

The practical problems of using ethanol as a dehydrating agent are few. In most European countries both 95-96% and absolute alcohol are sold for scientific use free of tax, which is sufficient to render the recovery of used alcohol, as practised by classical authors, unnecessary. Apart from exceptional circumstances, the redistillation of used alcohol is thus no longer routine in histological laboratories. It is however advisable to store used alcohols; that of 96% can be used to clean glassware especially after stains that are more soluble in alcohol than in water. Absolute alcohol that has been once used can be used a second time for dehydration if it immediately follows 96% alcohol.

In most cases commercial absolute alcohol, which contains 1-2% water, may be used as such. Rigorously anhydrous alcohol is required only in particular cases; it is obtained by distillation over calcium. However, several precautions have to be observed in this operation, so that when a laboratory does not possess the special equipment or trained personnel it is preferable to pur-

Table 2. — Gay-Lussac's table for the dilution of alcohol
(after Langeron, 1949)

In ml of water to be added to 100 ml of the alcohol to be diluted.

Desired strength of alcohol	Strength of alcohol to be diluted								
	100	99	98	97	96	95	94	93	92
95	6.50	5.15	3.83	2.53	1.25				
90	13.25	11.83	10.43	9.07	7.73	6.41	5.10	3.80	2.54
85	20.54	19.05	17.58	16.15	14.73	13.33	11.96	10.59	9.24
80	28.59	27.01	25.47	23.95	22.45	20.95	19.49	18.04	16.61
75	37.58	35.90	34.28	32.67	31.08	29.52	27.97	26.43	24.94
70	47.75	45.98	44.25	42.54	40.85	39.18	37.53	35.89	34.27
65	59.37	57.49	55.63	53.81	52	50.22	48.45	46.70	44.85
60	72.82	70.80	68.80	66.85	64.92	63.	61.10	59.21	57.33
55	88.60	86.42	84.28	82.16	80.06	77.99	75.93	73.88	71.85
50	107.44	105.07	102.75	100.44	98.15	95.89	93.64	91.41	89.19
45	130.26	127.67	125.11	122.57	120.06	117.57	115.09	112.64	110.18
40	158.56	155.68	152.84	150.02	147.22	144.46	141.70	138.95	136.23
35	194.63	191.39	188.19	185.01	181.85	178.71	175.60	172.49	169.39
30	242.38	238.67	234.99	231.33	227.70	224.08	220.49	216.90	213.33
25	308.90	304.52	300.18	295.86	291.56	287.28	283.02	278.77	274.53
20	408.50	403.13	397.79	392.47	387.17	381.90	376.64	371.40	366.16
15	574.75	567.43	560.53	553.55	546.59	539.66	532.74	525.83	518.94
10	907.09	896.73	886.40	876.10	865.15	855.55	845.31	835.08	824.86

Desired strength of alcohol	Strength of alcohol to be diluted								
	90	85	80	75	70	65	60	55	50
85	6.56								
80	13.79	6.83							
75	21.89	14.48	7.20						
70	31.05	23.14	15.35	7.64					
65	41.53	33.03	24.66	16.37	8.15				
60	53.65	44.48	35.44	26.47	17.58	8.76			
55	67.87	57.90	48.07	38.32	28.63	19.02	9.47		
50	84.71	73.90	63.04	52.43	41.73	31.25	20.47	10.35	
45	105.34	93.30	81.38	69.54	57.78	46.09	34.46	22.90	11.41
40	130.80	117.34	104.01	90.76	77.58	64.48	51.43	38.46	25.55
35	163.28	148.01	132.88	117.83	102.84	87.93	73.08	58.31	43.59
30	206.22	188.57	171.05	153.61	136.04	118.94	101.71	84.54	67.45
25	266.12	245.15	224.30	203.61	182.83	162.21	141.65	121.16	100.73
20	355.80	329.84	304.01	278.26	252.58	226.98	201.43	175.96	150.55
15	505.27	471.00	436.85	402.81	368.83	334.91	301.07	267.29	233.64
10	804.50	753.65	702.89	652.21	601.06	551.60	500.50	450.19	399.85

chase the analytical reagent grade anhydrous ethanol that is available commercially. Treating alcohol with anhydrous copper sulfate to remove water, as advised by many histologists, is most often quite ineffective.

Apart from measuring the alcohol with an alcoholometer, the presence of water beyond the tolerable limit for routine use may be verified by the acetylene evolved when a pinch of calcium carbide is added to the alcohol or by the cloudiness formed when the alcohol is poured down the sides of a test-tube half full of benzene or toluene.

Though absolute alcohol is not as hygroscopic as it is reputed to be it is advisable to take certain precautions if excessive hydration is to be avoided. When delivered in large carboys or drums it is better to redistribute the contents into well-stoppered bottles of less than one liter. It is not advisable to keep absolute alcohol in wash-bottles when it is intended for dehydrating slides since the alcohol absorbs the humidity of the air that is introduced into the bottle every time it is used.

Dehydration with ethanol is often carried out in the vessel used for fixation. Transferring pieces held in Fairchild tubes, Caullery and Chapelier's tubes or metal baskets into large vessels where the same quantity of alcohol serves to dehydrate several lots of pieces is worthwhile only when the output of a laboratory is considerable. Similarly, it is worth acquiring an apparatus that automatically transfers pieces through a series of increasing concentrations of alcohol only when a really large number of pieces have to be processed. In all cases dehydration should always be terminated in fresh absolute alcohol that has not been used before.

b) Theoretically, **dehydration with dioxan** has undoubted advantages over that with ethanol. In fact dioxan (1.4-diethylene dioxyde) is miscible in all proportions with both water as well as molten paraffin. It is therefore the ideal intermediate between aqueous fixatives or washes and paraffin. This a however counterbalanced by severe disadvantages. One of them is the poor water tolerance of dioxan-paraffin mixtures; two phases are formed, the lower one containing dioxan and water while the upper consists of dioxan and paraffin. Furthermore, dioxan is quite expensive (it is about ten times costlier than the tax-free absolute alcohol usually granted to laboratories). It is also very toxic. Its absorption through the skin or its inhalation can cause grave hepato-nephritis than can lead to death from anuria. Careful precautions should therefore be observed during manipulation, some of which seriously complicate the task of the histologist. Thus all vapours should be captured as stipulated by the labour legislation governing industrial establishments, glassware should be stopped with ground-glass, contact with the liquid should be avoided, it should be poured only under a fume-hood and paraffin ovens should be airtight with means for evacuating gases. It is easy to see that most European laboratories do without the use of this substance.

Commercial dioxan is often hydrated. It is therefore advisable to pass pieces wrapped in muslin or in metal baskets through 3 or 4 vessels with quick lime at the bottom over which the dioxan is filled to about four-fifths of the vessel. The vessels should be well stoppered.

*c) **Isopropanol*** (isopropyl alcohol) has been proposed in place of ethanol for dehydrating pieces before paraffin-embedding. Its cost is moderate, it is less hygroscopic than ethanol and may be obtained on the market really anhydrous. But dehydration with it is definitely much slower than with ethanol. Those who favour it in histological technique advise its use after 96% ethanol, with three changes of isopropanol in each of which medium—sized pieces should be left for at least 24 hours.

d) Dehydration with ***aniline***, suggested by Allen, has the advantage of causing very little shrinkage of pieces, but the procedure for its use is quite complicated and few seem to have adopted it.

The passage through absolute alcohol of pieces that are to be embedded in paraffin using a benzenic hydrocarbon can be avoided by completing dehydration in phenolic mixtures of benzene, toluene or xylene (3 parts of the hydrocarbon to one part of phenol by weight). This old formula, due to Weigert, is an expedient that is now used only exceptionally. Similarly, replacing absolute alcohol by mixtures of 96% alcohol and benzene as suggested by Kisser (successive passages in 1/3, 1/1, 3/1, 7/100 by volume of 96% alcohol and benzene followed by pure benzene) is useful only when it is impossible to obtain absolute alcohol and when benzene must necessarily be the intermediate before paraffin embedding.

2° *Impregnation with a solvent of paraffin*

Of all the techniques of dehydration considered above, that using ethanol calls for the most rigorous elimination of traces of alcohol and a complete impregnation with the solvent of paraffin before the pieces are brought into contact with the latter. In fact ethanol is not miscible with paraffin so that the embedding mass will not penetrate into those regions of the piece where traces of alcohol remain. Serious shrinkage results and the consistency of the block is furthermore most unsuitable for sectioning. On the contrary passage through an intermediate medium is quite unnecessary when dehydration has been effected with dioxan or butanol. Both these compounds are miscible with liquid paraffin in all proportions, and hence can penetrate into interstitial spaces and even into cells to give satisfactory embedding.

Numerous intermediate liquids have been proposed, which only goes to show that none is quite free of disadvantages.

*a) **The benzenic hydrocarbons*** (benzene, toluene, xylene) are probably the most used but not the best of these intermediates. Their chief advantage is the speed of penetration. They produce a clearing of pieces which become translucid so that any persistence of opaque zones indicates the presence of badly dehydrated regions and calls for a renewed passage through absolute alcohol. These advantages are offset by the toxicity of the compounds and resulting consistency of the blocks. Most histologists ignore the serious disorders of the blood that can be caused by inhaling hydrocarbons of the benzene family. It is to be regretted that the precautionary measures stipulated by labour legislation (capture of vapours at their source, suitable ventilation, periodic medical examination of personnel) only too often remain a dead letter. Furthermore, the tendency of pieces to harden is greater with benzenic hydrocarbons than with other intermediates.

The methodical researches of Seki (1937) have shown that of the three hydrocarbons used as intermediates benzene has the most advantages. Being more volatile than toluene, and *a fortiori* than xylene, it is rapidly eliminated from pieces during penetration by paraffin. It hardens pieces the least of all the three compounds, and its cost is definitely cheaper than that of xylene which is still too widely used.

The procedure for using benzenic hydrocarbons to impregnate pieces is corollary to the fact that their specific gravity is greater than that of ethanol. Hence, as opposed to the recommendations concerning rehydration, narrow tall recipients should be used in this case. It is preferable to cover pieces with a considerable height of hydrocarbon and not to agitate them during impregnation. During renewal it serves no particular purpose to remove the last traces of hydrocarbon in contact with the pieces at the bottom. In most cases a satisfactory clearing of pieces, which is the test of good impregnation, is obtained in one or two hours with pieces of normal size. When pieces are too voluminous to be entirely cleared in two or three hours it is better to resort to some other intermediate between ethanol and paraffin since the hardening of pieces considerably increases with the time spent in the three hydrocarbons.

Benzene that has been once used may serve for the first of the two or three changes; it however goes without saying that impregnation should terminate with fresh benzene.

Used benzene may be saved for washing or deparaffining sections before staining. It is however better to use fresh benzene for mounting preparations. It is evidently not worth recuperating benzene and allied solvents by distillation as their toxicity and inflammability entail the observation of precautions that are too elaborate for most histological laboratories.

From a knowledge of the solubilities of alcohol, the benzenic hydrocarbons and paraffin it can be expected that success in embedding by the above method is closely dependant on perfect dehydration and complete elimination of the last traces of alcohol from the piece during impregnation. The importance of the clearing of pieces as an indication of proper impregnation has already been pointed out; however, the onset of transparency is difficult to appreciate when the tissues are dark to begin with, or when they have been fixed in mixtures containing potassium dichromate or osmium tetroxyde. In any case the removal of the last traces of water and alcohol can be ensured by the timely insertion between absolute alcohol and benzene of a few transfers in some other liquid that is miscible in both ethanol and benzene. Such procedures are described in most handbooks of histological technique as *mixed celloidin—paraffin embedding* since a little nitrocellulose is often added to the intermediate solvent. In fact, as Romeis (1948) correctly observes, it is not really mixed embedding since the quantity of nitrocellulose is hardly sufficient to modify the consistency of the piece when embedded. The first of these methods appears to be that of Millot (1926) which consists of transferring pieces after dehydration into a mixture of equal parts of alcohol and ether followed by a period in a 1% solution of collodion in the same mixture. This solution, which is a fivefold dilution of the solution of collodion obtained commercially, is left in contact with the pieces for 24 to 48 hours. They are then transferred to the benzenic hydrocarbon for clearing. From the composition of the intermediate liquid it is clear that the ethanol is hardly eliminated, so that the above procedure is now completely abandoned in favour of that of Peterfi (1929). According to this author dehydrated pieces are treated in methyl benzoate in which dry commercial celloidin has been dissolved to a concentration of 1%. At first, pieces float in this solution since the specific gravity of methyl benzoate is higher than that of ethanol; they gradually get clearer and drop to the bottom. Complete removal of alcohol is ensured by a second treatment in methyl benzoate. The whole operation takes about 24 hours for medium-sized pieces. It should be noted that pieces may be left in methyl benzoate almost indefinitely since there is not the slightest morphological alteration and the outcome of subsequent embedding is not in the least affected. Methyl benzoate is thus an excellent medium for storing dehydrated pieces. According to Turchini and collaborators (1951) it may be replaced by methly salicylate which is slightly cheaper.

From the practical point of view it is not sure whether the addition of 1% nitrocellulose to methyl benzoate is of any real use, though most authors follow the indications of Peterfi in this respect. Preparing this solution by mixing 4 volumes of methyl benzoate with one volume of a 5% commercial solution of collodion is bad practice, since the consequent addition of alcohol or ether, the usual solvents of collodion, diminishes the efficacy of the clearing medium with regard to the elimination of the last traces of alcohol from the pieces. It is by far preferable to dissolve 1% celloidin (an inflammable and explosive compound) directly in methyl benzoate. Complete dissolution takes quite a long time (one or two weeks, shaking the flask twice daily). The first treatment in this mixture should last about 12 hours, while the second may be prolonged indefinitely if the pieces are to be conserved in it, or it may last 12 hours if immediate embedding is desired.

After the second treatment pieces are briefly wiped with filter paper before immersion in benzene. Two changes of half an hour each in benzene suffice to remove all methyl benzoate before transferring pieces to molten paraffin.

The advantages of benzenic hydrocarbons as intermediates between alcohol and paraffin hence lie in their speed of impregnation and the possibility of visually appreciating its quality; among their disadvantages are the tendency of hardening and the incomplete elimination of alcohol. The latter, however, may be largely attenuated by adopting the methyl benzoate method of Peterfi, though it demands lengthier manipulation.

b) **The essence of Cedar,** not to be confounded with immersion oil, lends the most favorable consistency to pieces meant for the microtome. It causes the least alteration of structures and its complete elimination before embedding is of slight concern since, in fact, small quantities of essence remaining in the paraffin do not impair section cutting. In addition, the use of Cedar essence ensures against any risk of dissolving osmified lipids and the progress of impregnation may be followed visually from the clearing of pieces. But it is also one of the most expensive procedures for impregnation. Cedar essence is quite costly, each bath of which can serve only twice, and the paraffin used for penetration has to be very frequently changed. Thus, in spite of its qualities I am reluctant to recommend it for routine work; but I have no hesitation in maintaining that it should be preferred to all other intermediates for genuine cytological research.

The procedure for its use is the same as that for benzene, except that impregnation is less rapid; the first bath should last 12 hours and the second from 12 to 24 hours. Pieces that are not embedded immediately may be left for years in the second bath without undergoing the slightest alteration. Cork is preferable to polythene caps for closing vials as the plastic is attacked by Cedar essence.

c) **Chloroform,** whose merits have been described at length by Apathy (1912/13) also possesses the advantage of not hardening pieces and of rendering them favorable for sectioning; shrinkage during embedding is also less than with most other intermediates and its complete elimination is not as imperative as with the benzenic hydrocarbons or methyl benzoate (or salicylate). However, only rigorously anhydrous and alcohol-free chloroform is suitable for treating pieces intended for paraffin embedding. Such a pure grade product is costly and conserves poorly; it should especially be stored in darkness. This is probably one reason why its use is limited today. Furthermore, complete impregnation is not signified by any change in the appearance of pieces.

The operating procedure is simple. Narrow tall recipients are preferred, in which pieces issuing from alcohol float at first before falling gradually to the bottom. When this occurs the chloroform should be changed; complete impregnation is obtained in about 24 hours for medium-sized pieces.

d) Benzyl benzoate, preceded by a treatment of dehydrated pieces in creosote, *carbon disulfide* and decalin (naphthalene decahydride) are among the intermediate fluids that have been used episodically without being pursued any further.

e) An intermediate fluid is of no use whatever when dehydration has been carried out in butanol or dioxan. In the first case pieces leaving 96% alcohol are passed through three successive baths of butanol or isobutanol for an average of 24 hours in each of the first two, while the third may last for several months. In fact butanol, originally prescribed for embedding pieces rich in chitin, is an excellent intermediate and I urge its systematic use whenever histological examination is not called for with any urgence. Shrinkage and hardening of tissues is at a minimum. Butanol completes dehydration and serves as intermediate simultaneously; its cost, though higher than that of absolute alcohol, is not excessive; each bath may be used twice, the last one evidently fresh. Its two disadvantages are the long delay of impregnation (48 hours to 3 days) and embedding (at least 48 hours) and the absence of any modification in the appearance of pieces that indicates the quality of impregnation.

The procedure for using dioxan has been described in connection with dehydration. On leaving this liquid, pieces may go directly into paraffin.

3° The penetration of paraffin into pieces

This part of the procedure is aimed at obtaining an impregnation of pieces that is as complete as possible, so that when the blocks are moulded the cooling transforms the tissue that is originally heterogeneous in consistency and elasticity into a homogeneous mass whose different zones behave uniformly upon cutting.

From the melting point of paraffin it is clear that these operations require to be performed when it is warm. The time during which pieces may remain in the oven depends both on their consistency and the nature of the liquid used for impregnation. In fact, really complete penetration necessitates, first of all, a mixture of paraffin and the intermediate fluid that is as homogenous as possible, followed afterwards by the most extensive elimination of the latter. Obviously this second step is more rapidly achieved when the liquid chosen for impregnation is more volatile.

The use of a mixture of impregnating liquids (chloroform, Cedar essence, dioxan, butanol) with paraffin appears quite justified theoretically, but experience has shown that the improvement in the quality of blocks and sections is not worth the additional complication in operation. The same comment holds for the recommendation of certain authors to impregnate pieces first with a soft, low melting-point paraffin followed by the penetration of a harder one.

The two classical precautions concerning the period of exposure to warm paraffin and its temperature, obligingly reiterated in most handbooks of histological technique, appear quite fictitious to me.

Most authors advise that the time spent by pieces in the embedding oven be reduced to a minimum as far as possible, from a fear of excessive shrinkage and hardening or even alteration of certain cellular constituents. Such fears are quite unfounded, except when enzymatic activity has to be detected, since enzymes are inactivated during paraffin embedding to such an extent that even a short stay in the oven can be harmful. It is thus better to abandon this type of embedding whenever it is possible to do so in histo-enzymological work. In all other cases, however, prolonged stay in warm paraffin has no adverse effect. I feel all the more impelled to emphasize this point as renowned histologists often hold the contrary. Thus Hirsch and Bretschneider (1937) claim that mitochondria can be stained properly only if the pieces are kept in warm paraffin for not more than 90 minutes. Systematic trials have shown me that the form of the renal chondriomes of albino rats as well the affinity of chondriomes for Altmann's fuchsin or iron haematoxylin do not undergo the slightest modification after three weeks in paraffin at 60°, evidently on condition that all the operations preceding embedding have been scrupulously executed.

Similarly the temperature at which paraffin penetrates the pieces is not as important as supposed by certain authors. When a piece has been perfectly dehydrated and all trace of alcohol removed a rise in temperature to 65° or even 70° does not affect the morphology of tissues, though as can be easily imagined, inactivation of enzymes is accelerated.

Though many of my readers would be shocked by this point of view, I must say that it is based strictly on fact; I should besides be worried if my opinion were not to agree with that of acknowledged masters of histological technique like St. v. Apathy and P. Masson. Contrary to an idea that is both solidly established and quite erroneous, the "overdone" appearance of preparations does not signify an overlong stay in paraffin that is too warm but rather an insufficient penetration of the embedding mass, or, as in Massons' vivid terms, it is "underdone".

A precaution that is always useful and easy to observe with modern appliances, is to make the paraffin penetrate under vacuum. Some commercial ovens allow the use of low pressure. A high vacuum is not needed, and the use of a diffusion pump quite unnecessary. Any good filter pump would do to create a sufficiently low pressure in the oven to considerably hasten the elimination of volatile intermediate liquids. The usual precautions to prevent the backflow of water should obviously be taken.

The operating procedure for paraffin embedding depends largely on the particular liquid used as intermediate. The benzenic hydrocarbons, dioxan and chloroform, all volatile, are removed by evaporation. Consequently, paraffin treatment should be carried out in wide-mouthed, large vessels and the quantity of paraffin used is of less importance than an efficacious aeration of the oven. Theoretically, a single long bath in paraffin should suffice; in practice, however, it is better to use two successive ones, the first of which dissolves away certain constituents of the piece in addition to the intermediate liquid. The case of cedarwood oil is evidently quite different for it has to be removed by dissolving in paraffin and not by evaporation. Large quantities of paraffin have thus to be used for each bath and the same one should not be used more than thrice. The relatively high cost of cedarwood oil is thus aggravated by the consumption of much more paraffin than in other methods of embedding.

Butanol is also removed by evaporation, but its complete elimination requires a much longer stay than in the case of the benzenic hydrocarbons.

Apart from the nature of the intermediate liquid the consistency of pieces plays an important role in the penetration of paraffin. It is clear that a piece of lung is more rapidly penetrated than bone, cartilage or skin. The penetration of very small pieces with a rigid exterior (small Arthropods) occurs by capillarity and is slowed, the more so as molten paraffin is relatively viscous. The time required for good embedding can be safely evaluated only after some experience of the material. In all cases, apart from pieces meant for histo-enzymological study, it is better to exceed the limit rather than to be short of it. Slices of mammalian organs of less than 5 mm can be penetrated by paraffin in 3 hours if the intermediate is benzene, while 48 to 72 hours may be necessary with cedarwood oil or butanol.

4° Moulding the block

This last step of paraffin embedding is aimed at giving the piece and its surrounding paraffin the uniform consistency of solid paraffin. In spite of its apparent simplicity it calls for the observance of a series of precautions that are often neglected.

Most of these precautions may be foreseen by considering the physical properties of paraffin. In fact its manner of crystallization explains why the block should be cooled quite quickly but not brusquely and why one face of the block should be maintained in the liquid state for as long as possible. Slow cooling brings about the formation of large crystals in the central regions of the block, an irregular consistency and the appearance of fissures which harmfully affect the quality of sections. If cooling is too rapid the difference in shrinkage of the piece and the paraffin can result in their actual detachment from each other.

When the free face of the block solidifies before the deeper regions, where the pieces lie, remnants of the intermediate liquid and impurities are invariably trapped in contact with the piece resulting in fissuration and an irregular consistency.

Obviously paraffin used for making blocks should not be stored in proximity to the space set apart for the impregnation of pieces. Disregard for this rule leads to the paraffin of all blocks being saturated with the various volatile intermediates used in impregnation whose presence, even in small quantities, has disastrous consequences for the mechanical properties of the paraffin, and hence of sections. They become brittle, tear easily and their unequal consistency hinders proper spreading. Paraffin intended for blocks should therefore be stored, molten and filtered, in a chamber of the oven that does not communicate with the dishes in which the pieces are impregnated.

It is known from experience that blocks are of better quality if the paraffin used for embedding has been maintained liquid for a certain time. Apart from the sedimentation of impurities, possible in a liquid, the evaporation of volatile compounds can also contribute to this "improvement". According to certain classical authors paraffin heated to a higher temperature and then brought down to the melting point gives particularly good results; the recommendation seems to be unfounded and I consider its practice quite unnecessary

Widely differing receptacles can serve for moulding paraffin blocks. Apart from paper, folded as illustrated in Fig 1, and on which pieces may be labelled, plastic pharmaceutical capsules, coverslip boxes and similar containers are convenient. Leuckart bars are more suitable when a large number of pieces have to be embedded. They are L-shaped metal pieces whose shorter limb is usually of the width of a slide. When two of them are suitably juxtaposed on a metal or glass plate a mould is obtained, one dimension of which can be adjusted at will by sliding the bars. No particular precaution need be taken if the bottom is a metal plate, but if it is of glass lightly smearing with glycerol is often useful.

The operating procedure follows from the facts described above. When the mould is ready, paraffin for embedding, stored away from the impregnating baths, is poured into it. The piece is removed from the final impregnating bath with a pair of forceps lightly heated in a flame or with a warm spatula and placed in the mould in contact with the crust of solid paraffin that forms at the bottom. Warm forceps or needles are used to orient the piece; this also suffices to maintain a layer of liquid paraffin on the surface whose advantages have been pointed out. When the pieces are properly oriented the bottom and the sides of the mould are cooled by surrounding them with water. If the mould is a small box it is simpler to float it on the surface of a dish of tap water at about 15°; Leuckart bars are placed in Petri dishes in which water is poured taking care that its level does not exceed the height of the mould. The surface of the block

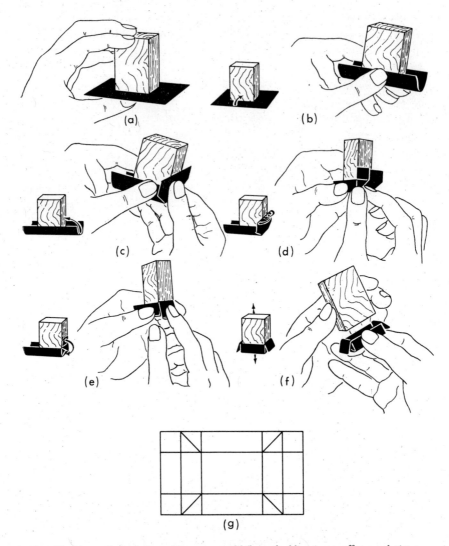

Fig. 1. — *Construction of a paper mould for embedding in paraffin or gelatin*
a—f: successive steps when the paper is folded with the help of a supporting object such as a box or a block of wood (after Gray 1954). *g*: Folds when no support is used.

is maintained liquid by the warm forceps until all the paraffin that surrounds the piece has solidified. It is only then that the surface of the block is cooled by blowing on it and the whole is plunged into water at 15°. Blocks moulded in paper, cardboard or plastic are removed at the time of cutting and hence can be labelled at the bottom or on the sides. When Leuckart bars are used the labels written in pencil or India ink are coated with paraffin and stuck into each block before it solidifies. This label is really made at the beginning and it accompanies the piece through all the liquid baths except osmic fixatives. Five to ten minutes in water at 15° are usually enough for the Leuckart bars to be detached easily, after which the block is put back into the same water.

Unless it is really urgent, blocks should not be cut on the very day that they are made. Several hours are needed for the complete solidification of the paraffin, and cutting a block whose centre has not attained its final consistency can result in internal displacement inside the piece.

Paraffin blocks may be stored at room temperature except when they are intended for histo-enzymology, in which case they are better kept in a refrigerator. Except for histo-enzymology again, conservation is excellent, and a collection of blocks is the surest reserve of a histologist. One should hence adopt a rigid convention as to the orientation of a piece in a block, since it is often difficult to discern it after solidification. A useful precaution is to wrap each block with its label in thin paper, just in case the label is detached accidentally. Engraving a serial number on each block appears less reliable to me since the numbers can be effaced when several blocks rub against each other in the same box.

CHOICE OF METHOD FOR PARAFFIN EMBEDDING AND SUMMARY OF OPERATING PROCEDURE

Apart from bases that may be analysed rationally, the choice that the histologist makes from among the different techniques of paraffin embedding that have been described evidently depends on personal factors such as the current practice of the laboratory or habits learnt early in his career. I advise the following procedures, depending on the particular type of work:

1° Dehydration in increasing concentrations of alcohol, impregnation in benzene and embedding in paraffin without any other intermediate liquid in cases when histological examination must be rapid or when a prolonged stay in warm paraffin is harmful (for enzymatic activity).

2° Dehydration in increasing alcohol, methyl benzoate, impregnation in benzene and paraffin embedding as routine procedure.

3° Dehydration in 96% alcohol and butanol, impregnation in the latter and paraffin embedding in all cases where hardening is expected and when histological examination is not really urgent.

4° Dehydration in increasing alcohol, impregnation in cedarwood oil and paraffin embedding for all pieces meant for cytological studies.

The different periods of treatment indicated below are only relative. They are valid for pieces of not more than 5 mm in one dimension and of ordinary consistency; they may be reduced for smaller or loose fragments and increased for voluminous or dense ones.

1° Paraffin embedding with benzene as the only intermediate

Proceeding from an aqueous fixative or washing in water.

1° 96% Alcohol.	3 baths of 2 hours each, the third may last up to 12 hours.
2° Absolute alcohol.	3 baths of one hour, the third may last for 12 hours.
3° Benzene.	3 baths of 30 to 45 minutes.
4° Paraffin.	2 baths of 1 to 2 hours at normal pressure or 15 to 20 minutes or 15 to 20 minutes in an oven under moderate vacuum.
5° Moulding	

Proceeding from an alcoholic fixative

The bath in 96% is unnecessary and dehydration may commence in absolute alcohol following the same times indicated above.

Proceeding from fixation in acetone for histo-enzymology

1° Acetone. 3 baths of 2 hours, the third can last for 12 hours.
2° 1 or 1,5% solution of nitrocellulose in acetone for 12 to 24 hours.
3° Benzene. 3 baths of 30 minutes.
4° Paraffin. 2 baths of 45 minutes at normal pressure or 15 minutes in an oven under moderate vacuum.
5° Moulding.

2° Paraffin embedding passing through methyl benzoate ("celloidin-paraffin").

Proceeding from an aqueous fixative or washing in water

1° 96% alcohol.	3 baths of 2 hours, the third can last for 12 hours.
2° Absolute alcohol.	3 baths of one hour, the third can last for 12 hours.
3° 1% dry celloidin dissolved in methyl	benzoate or salicylate 2 baths of 12 hours, the second can be prolonged almost indefinitely.
4° Rapid wiping in filter paper.	
5° Benzene.	2 baths of 30 minutes.
6° Paraffin.	2 baths of 1 to 2 hours at normal pressure, 15 to 20 minutes under moderate vacuum.
7° Moulding.	

Proceeding from an alcoholic fixative

As before the 96% alcohol bath is unnecessary and dehydration may commence in absolute alcohol without any modification of the above times.

3° Paraffin embedding passing through butanol

PROCEEDING FROM AN AQUEOUS FIXATIVE OR WASHING IN WATER

1° 96% alcohol. 3 baths of 2 hours, the third can last for 12 hours.
2° Butanol. 3 baths of 24 hours, the last can be prolonged almost indefinitely.
3° Paraffin. 2 baths of *at least* 24 hours at normal pressure, 1 to 3 hours under moderate vacuum.
4° Moulding.

PROCEEDING FROM AN ALCOHOLIC FIXATIVE

1° 96% alcohol. 2 baths of one hour, meant to dissolve any possible excess of fixative that is less soluble in butanol.
2° Butanol and paraffin treatment as in proceeding from an aqueous fixative.

4° Paraffin embedding passing through Cedarwood oil

PROCEEDING FROM AN AQUEOUS FIXATIVE OR WASHING IN WATER

1° 96% alcohol. 3 baths of 2 hours, the third can last for 12 hours.
2° Absolute alcohol. 3 baths of one hour, the third can last for 12 hours.
3° Cedarwood oil. 2 baths of 24 hours, the third can be prolonged almost indefinitely.
4° Very rapid wash (5 seconds) in benzene, meant to remove excess of cedarwood oil.
5° Paraffin. 3 baths of 12 to 24 hours, the paraffin of the first two should be changed often.
6° Moulding.

EMBEDDING IN NITROCELLULOSE

(CELLOIDIN, COLLODION)

The procedure for embedding in nitrocellulose, invented by Mathias Duval in 1879, enjoyed great vogue with certain classical histologists, but modern authors have a tendency to abandon it in favour of paraffin embedding. Truly enough, its former vogue was a bit exaggerated but its present neglect is indeed equally unwarranted. Both paraffin and celloidin (the terms nitrocellulose, celloidin and collodion are synonymously used by histologists) have their respective advantages and disadvantages, and the choice of one or the other should depend only on its suitability for a given study.

Paraffin embedding is by far the quicker of the two procedures; even with the slowest of the methods described in the preceding paragraphs a block can be obtained four or five times more rapidly than by celloidin embedding. Time is also saved during sectioning; cutting blocks into serial sections and sticking them on slides are much simpler and more rapid with paraffin. Even the storage of celloidin blocks calls for certain precautions that need not be observed with paraffin. Furthermore, the handling of paraffin has probably never caused any serious accident, while celloidin is highly inflammable when dissolved in the usual solvents and, when dry, the possibility of explosion is sufficiently real for more than one head of a laboratory to have banned its use.

Celloidin has however appreciable advantages. All the steps of embedding are carried out at room temperature and, consequently, there is no shrinkage of pieces which is otherwise almost impossible to avoid in paraffin embedding where a decrease of from 8% to 20% in the overall dimensions of a piece can be noted when compared to a completely dehydrated piece. Inequalities in the consistency of pieces can produce deformations that are quite undesirable in anatomical studies. With celloidin embedding the dimensions of a piece remain unchanged and the topographical relations of tissues are not modified.

Penetration by celloidin is closer than that by paraffin; with the result the cutting of sections from hard or very heterogenous tissues, quite impossible with paraffin, becomes possible with celloidin. Those fixations which prepare poorly for paraffin may be followed by celloidin embedding to give quite satisfactory preparations. The dimensions of pieces submitted to celloidin embedding can be considerably greater than when intended for paraffin embedding.

All this only shows the impossibility of a general choice; opting for one of the two procedures is a question to be answered according to the case in point. The exclusive adoption of celloidin embedding by great histologists like Maximow and Schaffer is an extreme attitude. On the other hand, to persist in embedding unhomogenous, shrinkable pieces with voluminous bone fragments, even though decalcified, is the other extreme. Truth, as in most cases, is the happy mean.

PROPERTIES OF THE EMBEDDING MASS

This mass is a mixture of mono and dinitrocellulose whose proportions vary according to the manufacturer. It is sold either as a solution in equal parts of absolute alcohol and ethyl ether or as a solid that is dry or moistened with a little alcohol. *Dry nitrocellulose is very explosive; when melted with alcohol or even in solution it remains highly inflammable.*

The use of celloidin for embedding is based on the property of its solution to solidify when brought into contact with certain reagents such as 70% alcohol or chloroform. The consistency of the gel that results evidently depends on the initial concentration of nitrocellulose; thus, sufficient hardness for making thin sections requires a fairly high concentration. However, as Apathy (1912/13) so properly emphasizes, solutions of nitrocellulose whose concentrations are high enough to give blocks that can be cut at less than 15μ remain liquid only if they are anhydrous. It is thus essential to ensure an impeccable dehydration of pieces. All substances used for embedding should be genuinely anhydrous and any absorption of atmospheric humidity should be prevented during operation. Apathy goes to the extent of advising that most steps of the method be carried out in desiccators over sulfuric acid.

The sheets of celloidin that used to be supplied in former times were always soaked in alcohol, and the first step in preparing solutions was to cut it into small pieces with a pair of scissors or to scrape it with a suitable kitchen utensil so that it could be dried at room temperature protected from dust. Today manufacturers supply for histological purposes celloidin that is finely ground and soaked in a specified quantity of alcohol. It is best to prepare solutions at the concentrations necessary for embedding as soon as the product is obtained and to dilute them as required, rather than to store the product as a solid. Its usual solvents are hygroscopic and it is recommended to store all solutions of celloidin in bottles with properly greased ground-glass stoppers. The mouth and the stoppers should always be carefully cleaned before restoppering.

All authors dissolve celloidin in a mixture of equal parts of absolute ethanol and ethyl ether, except Seki who prefers methanol. With this solvent penetration into pieces is improved and the time taken for impregnating with the embedding mass can be shortened, but the hardness of the block is considerably less and it is usually quite impossible to obtain sections of less than 10 μ.

In practice, therefore, the stock solution is prepared by dissolving dry celloidin at a concentration of 8% in a mixture of equal parts of absolute alcohol and ether or in methanol. Certain samples that are now available on the market are packed ready to be dissolved in the mixture. If the celloidin comes in sheets it should be fragmented, dried and covered with the required quantity of alcohol; the ether is added only on the next day. At first it swells considerably without actually dissolving; it is only after the addition of ether that it begins to dissolve and this may take up to several days. The 4% and 2% solutions used for impregnation are made from the 8% solution by diluting in the same alcohol-ether mixture.

It is important to check the anhydrous nature of the alcohol and ether while preparing solutions of celloidin. When celloidin embedding is not practised frequently it is more convenient to buy reagent grade anhydrous ether rather than to dehydrate it by treatment with calcium chloride, filtration and removal of the last traces of water with sodium metal.

A prerequisite of celloidin embedding is the impeccable dehydration of pieces. This is obtained, as for paraffin embedding, by increasing concentrations of ethyl alcohol. Dehydration by glycerine and by pyridine have also been proposed for celloidin embedding and the technique is described below. These two methods of dehydration shorten the time required to obtain blocks, but they are more expensive, especially the one using glycerine, than the classical method.

PROCEDURE OF EMBEDDING

The most often used method is the classical one involving dehydration in absolute alcohol and impregnation with celloidin dissolved in a mixture of ethanol and ether.

1° Embedding in alcohol-celloidin

Of all the variants of the method that of Apathy (1912/13) gives the best results and has been adopted by the great majority of modern authors.

Pieces that have been completely dehydrated in absolute alcohol are immersed in a mixture of equal parts of absolute alcohol and ether in which they are left from 4 to 8 hours depending on their size and consistency. They are then transferred to a 2% solution of celloidin in the same mixture where they remain for 2 to 4 days followed by another passage for the same length of time in a 4% solution. The last and longest bath in an 8% solution may be for one or two weeks and the same solution is used in moulding the blocks. For the actual moulding, the piece, immersed in a suitable receptacle containing the celloidin solution, is placed in a desiccator with sulfuric acid. The evaporation of the alcohol and ether is allowed to continue until the volume of the solution is reduced to half; which amounts to embedding in a solution of celloidin at 16%. Only perfectly anhydrous solutions become solid at this concentration, hence the imperative need to avoid any hydration during manipulation. Furthermore, care should be taken that the "thickening" of the embedding medium is brought about gradually and regularly so that the consistency of the block is uniform at the centre and the periphery. Apathy therefore recommends covering the receptacle that contains the piece with a lid from time to time. The original quantity of 8% solution should evidently be sufficient so that after the reduction of its volume to half the piece is still covered by a layer of at least 3 mm. If a solid crust is formed on the surface of the celloidin before the volume comes down to half it indicates that conditions have not been rigorously anhydrous and the desired thickening cannot be attained; such blocks can yield only relatively thick sections. The formation of air bubbles in the embedding mass during its thickening should be avoided; if it does happen a small quantity of the alcohol-ether mixture should be immediatly added and the receptacle covered until the bubbles rise to the surface when they may be pricked with a needle. The initial volume of the solution should be marked on the outside of the receptacle so that the reduction in volume may be duly appreciated. When the evaporation has attained the desired extent the receptacle is placed in a suitable dish containing a layer of about 1 cm of 70% alcohol at the bottom and covered. In a few hours a solid film will form on the surface of the thickened celloidin. When this occurs the receptacle containing the embedding mass may be filled with 70% alcohol and the hardening continued for 24 to 48 hours. The hardened block is then carefully extruded from the receptacle by detaching it from the walls with the help of a scalpel. It is trimmed and stored in 70% alcohol.

Hardening of the block in alcohol as described above further reduces its size from the time the celloidin attains 16%.

If it is desired to avoid this shrinkage, hardening may be effected in chloroform in the same manner, and the blocks stored in 70% alcohol as before.

2° Embedding in methanol-celloidin

This method, devised by Seki (1937), has an advantage over the classical one in that it enables a quicker and better penetration of the embedding medium into the pieces, but the blocks thus obtained are softer and more difficult to cut into thin sections. The solvent is anhydrous methanol and the solutions of celloidin have the same concentrations as those proposed by Apathy.

Absolute ethanol is replaced by anhydrous methanol in the dehydration of pieces and impregnation is carried out in 2%, 4% and 8% solutions of celloidin in anhydrous methanol. Seki recommends 24 hours, 2 days and 4 days of treatment in the three solutions for pieces of average size and consistency. Clearly, these treatments are to be prolonged for bigger and harder pieces. When impregnation is complete the piece is placed in 8% celloidin in methanol at the bottom of a suitable receptacle. The surface is then rendered into a gel by projecting a jet of steam for 20 or 30 seconds. The steam may be generated from boiling water in a flask carrying a stopper with a suitably bent tube. As soon as a film is formed the celloidin is covered with a mixture of three parts of chloroform to ten parts of 70% ethanol. Exposure to this mixture should last from 24 hours to 6 days and it is preferable to renew the mixture at least once. The block is then trimmed and stored in 70% ethanol. It is better to let it harden further for several days before cutting sections.

3° Embedding in glycerine-celloidin

This technique, described by Wolf (1939), is a considerable simplication of embedding in celloidin; its use really saves time, but not money (!!)

After washing in water, meant to remove excess fixative, the pieces are dehydrated in ordinary glycerine (density 1.23). It is advisable to use increasing concentrations of glycerine mixed with water if the risk of shrinkage is great (pieces with cavities). When impregnation with ordinary glycerine is complete the pieces are treated, in a well-stoppered flask, with anhydrous glycerine (density I, 26) for 6 to 12 hours. They are then directly transferred to an 8% solution of celloidin in alcohol-ether after rapidly wiping them in filter paper to remove excess glycerine that adheres to the surface. Each piece should be suspended with a string midway in the well stopped receptacle containing the solution of celloidin. A considerable excess of celloidin should be provided for (20 ml per piece of 3×6×6 mm).

Impregnation with celloidin is quite rapid and the glycerine drops to the bottom of the vessel; Wolf estimates 2 to 4 days for pieces of moderate size. The actual embedding is carried out as in Apathy's method for celloidin in alcohol.

4° *Embedding in pyridine-celloidin*

The advantage of this method described by Bauer (1941) also lies in the appreciable shortening of the time required for impregnation with celloidin. Its chief disadvantage is the danger of shrinkage which is undoubtedly greater than with any of the other techniques of embedding in nitrocellulose.

Pieces fixed in formalin are transferred directly from the fixative into a mixture of equal parts of pyridine (anhydrous analytical grade) and a 4% solution of celloidin in the alcohol-ether mixture. This bath is renewed once during the course of impregnation which should last from 2 to 4 days according to the size of the pieces. From there they are transferred to 8% celloidin for one or two days. Hardening and embedding in blocks is carried out according to Apathy in chloroform.

The methods of celloidin-paraffin embedding are described later under double embedding.

EMBEDDING IN GELATIN

Embedding in gelatin is aimed at two quite different objectives. Certain methods are meant to conserve impeccably very fragile ground substances and are of great use in the study of tissues and organisms with a high water content, such as most pelagic Prochordata or Molluscs.

They involve the use of strong alcohol and hence do not conserve lipids. Other methods with gelatin are meant to enable cutting sections without any dehydration and so avoid the use of lipid solvents. The second type of technique is more frequently used than the first. However, one of the first type of techniques, namely that of Apathy, will be described. Of the several techniques meant to conserve lipids based on the fundamental work of Gaskell, only two have been retained, that of Heringa and ten Berge (1923) and that of Baker (1941); the first allows the gelatin to be dissolved after sectioning while in the second the embedding mass is insolubilized before cutting.

EMBEDDING IN GELATIN AFTER APATHY

Apart from the perfect conservation of ground substances with a high water content this method avoids the shrinkage of pieces more than any of the other techniques of embedding. But in practice it is neither rapid nor particularly simple. The embedding mass is prepared by dissolving 50 g of good quality gelatin in 175 ml of water and 25 g. of glycerine. When fully dissolved the solution is filtered in an oven and maintained there, but in a desiccator with calcium chloride, until all the water is evaporated and a viscous mass is obtained "that can be barely stretched in threads" (Apathy). When such a consistency is attained the mass is cooled, cut into pieces and stored in a well stoppered bottle.

The operating procedure for fixed pieces, washed and treated in 96% alcohol is as follows:

1° The pieces are transferred gradually into a mixture of 5 volumes of water and 4 volumes of glycerine. This is effected, according to the suggestion of Apathy, by superposing in a tall cylinder layers of the water-glycerine mixture, distilled water, 35%, 70% and 90% alcohol. The pieces are placed in the 90% alcohol and allowed to drop by themselves to the bottom, which can take up to several days.

2° The water-glycerine bath is renewed three or four times to remove all traces of alcohol.

3° The pieces are placed in a mixture of equal parts of water-glycerine and gelatin in an oven at 40° for at least 24 hours. The gelatin is prepared by dissolving three parts of the embedding mass described above in 7 parts of hot water.

4° Pour the piece along with the embedding medium of water-glycerine-gelatin into a suitable mould placed in a desiccator with calcium chloride and leave the whole in an oven at 60° until the volume is reduced to half.

5° Remove the mould from the oven and allow it to cool. At this stage the block contains, apart from the piece, about one part of gelatin for three parts of glycerine and one of water.

6° Trim the block with a razor blade coated with paraffin oil taking care that at least one dimension does not exceed 5 mm. Pin the block on to the lower face of a cork so that it can be held immersed in a closed tube containing about 50 ml of absolute alcohol which serves to remove the glycerine. The bath of alcohol should be renewed daily; Apathy estimates 24 hours of this treatment for every mm of thickness of the block.

7° The cork, with the block pinned on, is used to close a receptacle containing terpineol in the same manner so that the piece covered with gelatin is immersed. As in the case of the absolute alcohol bath, 1mm of penetration should be expected in 24 hours. Change the terpineol once or twice during penetration. When the terpineol has completely penetrated into the block sections may be either made immediately in a microtome for celloidin or the dry blocks may be stored indefinitely in a well-stoppered vessel.

EMBEDDING IN GELATIN AFTER HERINGA AND TEN BERGE

This procedure, derived from the original technique of Gaskell, allows the preparation of blocks that are sufficiently consistant to be cut in a freezing microtome without having to submit pieces to the action of lipid solvents and without raising the embedding temperature beyond 37°. Furthermore, the embedding mass is not insolubilized and it may be extracted with hot water after the sections have been stuck. The embedding mass is a 20% solution of gelatin that is prepared by adding the required amount of good quality gelatin (commercial gelatin sold as a powder dissolves better than the sheets) to distilled water to which 1% thymol, or better still, phenol has been added. A solution of half this concentration is used to prepare the pieces for penetration. The operating procedure is much simpler than in the method of Apathy.

> Pieces have been fixed in formalin, all traces of which are removed by washing for 2 to 6 hours in running water.
> 1° Treat with a 10% solution of gelatin in an oven at 37% for 2 to 5 hours according to the size of the piece.
> 2° Transfer to the 20% solution of gelatin and maintain in the oven at 37% for 5 to 24 hours.
> 3° Pour into a suitable mould, cool in cold water and allow the block to solidify.

The block may be cut in a freezing microtome as soon as it is cooled or it may be stored for quite a short time in a well stoppered bottle in the refrigerator. Further treatment is described under the technique for frozen sections.

EMBEDDING IN GELATIN AFTER BAKER

This procedure, as the preceding one, is meant for pieces fixed in formalin and to be cut in the freezing microtome. It is the simplest of all and I recommend its use whenever the presence of the embedding mass on the slide causes no inconvenience. The embedding mass is 10% gelatin in distilled water to which an anti-microbial agent can be added. In fact good gelatin in powder dissolves at this concentration after about two hours in the paraffin oven, and hence I do not advise the preparation of a stock solution which always deteriorates in due course. The operating procedure is simpler than in the method of Heringa and ten Berge since penetration is effected directly in the embedding mass. The concentration of gelatin, which is lower by half, requires that the blocks be hardened by formalin, and this in turn insolubilizes the gelatin which hence cannot be removed from the sections.

Pieces are fixed in formalin and all traces of the latter removed by washing for 2 to 5 hours in running water.

1° Treat with 10% gelatin in an oven at 37° for 12 to 24 hours according to the size of the pieces.
2° Pour the embedding mass into a suitable mould and allow to cool.
3° Harden for at least 24 hours with 10% formalin or with formaldehyde-calcium.
4° Store in the same liquid or in Baker's formaldehyde calcium-cadmium if the pieces are meant for a histochemical study of phosphatids.

EMBEDDING IN GELATIN AFTER PEARSE

Pearse (1960) has described an adaptation of this method for histo-enzymology. It differs from the procedure of Baker in that the embedding mass is richer in gelatin (15 g of gelatin powder, 15 ml of glycerine, 70 ml of distilled water and a small crystal of thymol) and in the period of embedding and of hardening.

Small pieces are fixed for 10 to 16 hours in dilute formalin at 4°.
1° Wash in running water for 30 minutes.
2° Treat for one hour with the embedding mass in an oven at 37°.
3° Mould the block and cool rapidly.
4° Harden for one hour with a commercial solution of formaldehyde (35–40%).
5° Cut sections immediately and store them at 4°.

Pearse notes that hardening in pure formalin does not alter enzymatic activities if the piece itself is well within a few mm of the outer surface of the block. A mould of suitable dimensions should consequently be chosen.

OTHER METHODS OF EMBEDDING

Several embedding media have been proposed in place of those just described. Some of them differ from commercial paraffin only in that the mixture of hydrocarbons is chosen especially for the purpose and undivulged products have been added. This improves, the mechanical qualities of the medium, though no modifications in procedure are required. Others do not really deserve to be cited in histological technique; however, those that have appeared frequently in recent literature will be briefly mentioned.

The solid polyethylene-glycols (carbowax) would seem at first to offer enough advantages to dethrone paraffin as an embedding medium. They are compounds whose melting point is close to that of paraffin and of the same solid consistency so that sections may be cut by the usual procedures. In addition, when in the liquid state they are miscible with water in all proportions while as solids they are easily dissolved in water. This physical property implies that dehydration before embedding in carbowax is quite unnecessary. Pieces that have been fixed and washed of excess fixative are placed directly in the embedding mass in an oven at 55—60°. About 40 minutes of infiltration are necessary for each mm in the thickness of the block. A prolonged stay (4 days) in the oven does not cause serious alteration of the tissues. Moulding is as in the case of paraffin.

Most authors however seem to have abandoned embedding in carbowax after a few trials because of the difficulties in spreading sections, which will be discussed in the chapter devoted to this part of histological technique.

Steedman's ester-wax has been adapted mainly to avoid some of the disadvantages of paraffin, especially the lumping of thin sections associated with the crystalline structure of the embedding mass. It is a mixture consisting of 73% by weight of diethylene glycol distearate, 10% diethylene glycol monostearate, 4% ethyl cellulose, 5% stearic acid and 8% castor oil. The mixture can be prepared in the laboratory, though it is much simpler to buy it ready made from suppliers of material for microscopy in the form of bars having the consistency of paraffin.

The embedding mass is soluble in a great many substances, such as the benzenic hydrocarbons, generally used to clear pieces before embedding in paraffin, but in view of their tendency to harden pieces their use can be avoided. Steedman recommends the traditional method of increasing concentrations of alcohol for dehydration or, better still, the use of ethyl cellosolve (2-ethoxy ethanol). This substance is equally suitable for impregnation though dioxan, cedarwood oil and other intermediates can also be used.

The time of penetration is longer than that with paraffin; a cat's brain in a block measuring $34 \times 25 \times 10$ mm is penetrated only after 60 hours in the oven.

While moulding the blocks rapid cooling is desirable, but care should be taken to maintain a layer of liquid on the surface of the block as long as possible to avoid any infiltration of air into the immediate neighbourhood of the piece.

Recommendations for cutting and spreading sections are given in the following chapter.

DOUBLE EMBEDDING

Apart from techniques such as the one called mixed embedding with celloidin-paraffin, mentioned in a preceding paragraph, where the quantity of nitrocellulose used is not really sufficient to modify the consistency of the block, there are other methods of double embedding where the piece is truly embedded in two different masses. Of these, two will be described here, namely agar-paraffin embedding and the authentic double embedding in celloidin-paraffin as codified by Apathy (1912/13).

EMBEDDING IN AGAR-PARAFFIN

This technique, invented by Chatton (1923) greatly facilitates the embedding of objects that are too small to be oriented conveniently at the time of moulding the block. It also allows several small objects to be grouped and embedded in the same block. The method, as originally conceived, is actually one where the object is coated with agar followed by embedding it in paraffin rather than a real embedding in two masses.

The mass for coating is prepared by first soaking and then dissolving agar-agar at a concentration of 1.3% in boiling water. Formalin at 2.5% is added and the preparation can be stored for a certain time in the refrigerator.

The procedure is quite simple. The agar preparation is melted in a water-bath and is poured over a slide to give a cushion of about 2 to 3 mm in thickness. The objects to be embedded are laid on this cushion, if necessary while observing under a dissecting microscope, and covered with another layer of melted agar which is however not too hot. The block is trimmed after cooling and the plane of sectioning is conveniently oriented, but it is not detached from the slide until after a passage through 70% alcohol which ensures hardening of the agar and the beginning of dehydration. The remaining steps for embedding in paraffin are those that have been described earlier. Chatton remarks that a bath in warm toluene-paraffin facilitates the penetration of paraffin, though this precaution does not appear to me as particularly indispensable. There can be a certain advantage in lightly staining the block of agar with eosin or safranin to render its handling easier.

Authentic double embedding in agar-paraffin is recommended by Wigglesworth (1959) for cutting particularly thin sections (0.5 to 1 μ); the effect of the agar being to increase the elasticity of the block and to decrease its compression under the shock of the razor.

This method, applied by Wigglesworth to tissues fixed in Palade's osmium tetroxyde fixative bulk-stained with ethyl-gallate and washed, consists of a treatment for one hour in 5% agar in an oven at 60° followed by cooling, trimming of the block and dehydration in increasing concentrations of alcohol. Wigglesworth practises clearing in cellosolve and embedding in Steedman's ester-wax, but obviously embedding in paraffin is also possible.

It should also be noted that embedding in agar, in place of gelatin, has been suggested for freeze-sectioning.

EMBEDDING IN CELLOIDIN-PARAFFIN

Embedding in celloidin-paraffin, painstakingly codified by Apathy, can be of immense use when difficulty in the cutting of sections is expected from the nature of the pieces and when series of thin sections are nevertheless required. The method is therefore recommended when objects are very fragile and direct embedding in paraffin can cause troublesome shrinkage or when pieces are very hard and paraffin does not penetrate easily. Apart from the procedure described by Apathy, which gives remarkable results but which requires several operations, the simpler method of Pfuhl (1950) is also given here.

1° The method of Apathy commences by embedding in celloidin as described in the relevant paragraph of this chapter. If very thin sections are desired the procedure is followed up to the impregnation in 16% celloidin in a desiccator over sulfuric acid. If sections are to be of more than 10 μ it is on the contrary better to avoid concentrating the celloidin and the 8% solution is coagulated instead. In both cases, coagulation is effected by chloroform and not by alcohol. After coagulation the block is hardened by immersion in anhydrous chloroform for 24 hours. The last traces of water are removed by a 24 to 48 hour treatment in a "mixture of essential oils" devised for the purpose (by mixing in a brown bottle 4 parts, by *weight*, of chloroform, 2 parts of origanum oil, 4 parts of cedarwood oil, 1 part of absolute alcohol and 1 part of phenol.). The block should become entirely transparent and persistence of the slightest opacity indicates insufficient dehydration and calls for prolonged stay in the mixture. It is better to change this mixture once or twice during impregnation; dehydration of the mixture itself may be ensured by adding anhydrous sodium sulfate. When the block is quite clear the mixture, particularly the alcohol, is removed by several changes in benzene. The block is then transferred to warm paraffin and left in the oven for at least 24 hours, while doubling or even tripling this time is advantageous. Moulding the block is carried out as in ordinary paraffin embedding if impregnation has been effected in 8% celloidin. If the celloidin has been concentrated up to 16%, the block should be placed, on leaving the warm paraffin, between two slides and the whole is immersed in water with a weight on the upper slide.

2° The method of Pfuhl which is simpler and quicker, consists in bringing the pieces, as in celloidin embedding, up to a 4% solution. After several days in this solution, the pieces are wiped to remove excess celloidin, immersed in chloroform where they gradually fall to the bottom, cleared in phenolic benzene (1 part by weight of phenol for 10 parts of benzene) and embedded in paraffin. Moulding the block does not call for any particular precaution.

CHAPTER 5

CUTTING AND STICKING SECTIONS

> Das Mikrotom muss man meistern
> lernen wie ein Musikinstrument.
>
> L. J. Akkeringa (1929).

The cutting of sections is certainly the least esteemed of all the manipulations leading to a histological preparation. Turning the wheel of a microtome is a gesture of such seeming banality that every budding histologist dreams of the approaching day when a technician will relieve him of this basely tedious task; and inversely, every technician is supposed to know how to make sections.

But the facts are otherwise. To cut a block correctly into sections that will satisfy an exacting examiner is not an easy matter, neither is the operation codifiable. In spite of the great progress accomplished over a century, numerous imponderable factors remain that contribute to real success in making sections, and only long experience with the microtome can reduce the uncertainties of this aspect of histological technique to an acceptable minimum.

Contrary to a widespread prejudice, the way in which sections are made shows in the optical qualities of the final preparation almost as much as the fixation. Many artifacts imputed to fixation are really due to faulty sectioning. Apart from the clumsy faults that are evident even to a beginner, the inefficient handling of the microtome can produce alterations in structure of the final preparation that appear only under the microscope; ribbons that look well-made can be really quite unsuitable.

The indifference with which the cutting of sections and the corresponding instruments are held is to be emphatically deplored. The manufacturers of paraffin and celloidin microtomes have never made the effort that has been devoted, for instance, to improvement of the ultramicrotome. Very simple ameliorations that any experienced user could have suggested to the makers are sadly lacking even in the most modern instruments. The user, in turn, refuses to acquaint himself with an instrument that he uses daily, does not realise that it is one of high precision and, most often, makes no effort whatever to create the conditions which make the most out of it.

Fresh and fixed pieces, whether embedded or not, can be cut freehand; however, this technique, though still widely used in plant anatomy, is practised much less frequently in animal histology. Its execution is greatly facilitated by the use of a small hand microtome, most present day models of which are derived from Ranviers' microtome.

In most cases sections are made with automatic microtomes, where the advance of the block is ensured, before each passage of the razor, by a micrometer screw. The technical aspects of this mechanism and the devices of various makers will not be described here; they are usually described in the brochures that accompany each instrument. Only some general notions concerning the microtome will be discussed here before passing on to the actual methods of cutting sections.

GENERAL DESCRIPTION OF THE MICROTOME

The essential parts of a microtome are the razor which cuts the sections, the razor-holder which also permits orientation of the razor, the object-holder and finally the mechanism that controls the progressive advance of either the razor or the block.

THE RAZOR

Early histologists made their sections with ordinary razors which have long since been abandoned; this historical detail explains why the term "razor" has been retained by several authors; certain, however, prefer to use the name "knife".

Some of the qualities required of a good blade are well known and need not be dwelt upon further; they concern the quality of the steel used, case hardening and tempering. It is useful to remind oneself that the thickness of sections made with a given blade depends on the radius of curvature of the cutting edge, that is, on the size of the steel crystals at this edge. It is generally held that the thickness of sections cannot be less than the radius of curvature of the edge and obviously the edge wears more rapidly the smaller the radius. Furthermore, one should constantly keep in mind that only the outer "shell" of blades conforms to the standards of case-hardening and tempering mentionned above, so that too frequent and unwarranted honing is to be avoided.

The other characteristics of blades follow from their form. It is usual to distinguish, after their profile, biconcave blades (profile A of certain manufacturers), plano-concave blades (profile B or profile I) biplanar blades (profile C or profile II) and those that are biplanar and bevelled (profile D). Biconcave blades are used only for celloidin or gelatin sections, plano-concave and biplanar blades for paraffin and freeze-sections while bevelled biplanar ones are meant for plastic and other very hard material rarely used in light microscopy.

All blades carry ground facets, to facilitate maintenance, and this modifies the actual part of the blade that is involved in cutting from the rest of the blade. The profile of the razor and its orientation with respect to the plane of the section gives rise to the definition of the following angles (fig. 2):

— angle of the blade (α) which indicates the general thickness of the bevelling; in biplanar blades it is the width of the blade divided by its dorsal thickness.

— interior angle of the facets (β); most manufacturers adjust it to 45° which experience has shown to be the most suitable; angles higher than 45° cause deformation of sections and those much less than 45° render the bevelled edge too fragile and liable to be deformed by the pressure of the block.
— exterior angles of the facets (γ, δ), also called honing angles.
— clearance angle of the sections or slope (ε).
— angle of attack (η).

The angle of the blade is determined once and for all by the manufacturer; it cannot be modified by the user in the case of paraffin microtomes where the angle between the cutting edge of the blade and the direction of cutting (movement of the block or razor) is of 90°. This cutting angle, however, can and should be reduced for celloidin or gelatin blocks by tilting the razor with respect to the direction of cutting, which amounts to effectively lengthening the bevel and reducing the angle of the blade.

The interior angles, and consequently the exterior ones also, are defined by the first honing in the hands of the manufacturer, but they may be modified by subsequent honing. Care should obviously be taken that the bevel maintains its regularity and its shape. Most authors prefer symmetrical facets, but P. Masson advises the use of razors whose bevelling is asymmetrical, that is, one of the exterior angles of the facets is considerably more open than the other. This angle should be turned towards the block while cutting to obtain sections that are less compressed than with symmetrical facets.

The clearance angle (slope) and the angle of attack can be modified each time by inclining the razor and this adjustment is one of the important steps in preparing the microtome. Evidently the angle of attack should be greater than the slope (clearance angle of the sections), for the microtome is meant to function in the manner of a planer and this is in fact possible only when such a proportion is given to the two angles. If by error the angle of attack equals the clearance angle the facet of the razor only slides over the block polishing it. A further decrease in the angle of attack prevents the cutting edge from touching the block at all and the ridge between the facet and the face of the blade scrapes the block. Inversely, if the razor is inclined so as to form an excessive angle of attack, certain disadvantages are produced. Sections are deformed as cutting progresses, there is a risk of breaks and the vibration of the razor can produce an uneven thickness in the same section especially with large pieces. This should however not be confounded with alternating thick and thin sections in a ribbon, which are, on the contrary, due to an angle of attack that is too small.

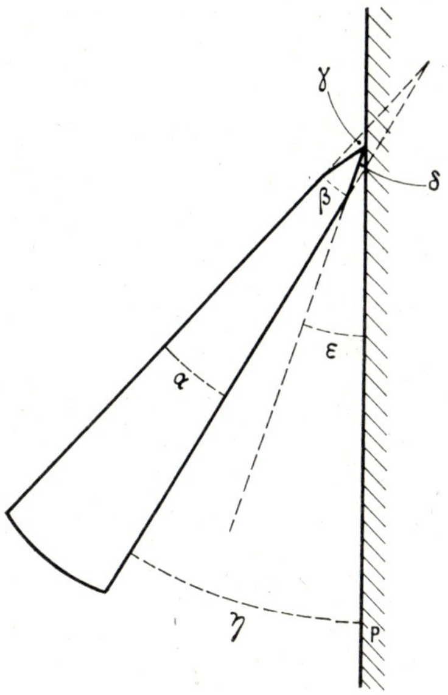

FIG. 2. — *Schematic drawing of the position of the razor on a Minot-type microtome.*

α angle of the blade; β interior angle of the facets; γ, δ exterior angles of the facets; ε clear- angle or slope; η angle of attack; P plane of the section.

It follows from the above facts that each of both the angle of attack and the clearance angle have to be adjusted to suit the consistency of the block. However, it is quite obviously impossible to vary these angles independently of each other in a given razor. The histologist who has to cut widely differing types of tissues is therefore advised to have at his disposal a series of razors whose facets have been ground at different angles so that the most suitable blade can be chosen for a particular block.

In practice, with the exterior angle of the facet at about 6 to 8°, the razor is oriented so that the angle of attack is close to the discharge angle of the sections in the case of hard blocks (paraffin, ester-wax, paraffin-celloidin of Apathy). On the contrary, the angle of attack should be definitely much greater than the slope with soft blocks (celloidin, gelatin). Evidently a certain amount of trial and error is necessary in most cases before obtaining the proper orientation of the razor for a block.

The most important measures to be taken for keeping a microtome razor in good condition are its maintenance in a perfectly clean state, its protection from dust, rust and contact of the cutting edge with any hard or metallic objects. It is to prevent such chipping that many manufacturers and histologists advise that sections be manipulated only with a brush. The cutting edge wears quite rapidly and periodical sharpening is an imperious necessity. Three different operations are actually included under the term sharpening. One is within the capability of every user of a microtome, then second requires either simple equipment and considerable skill or relatively costly equipment, while the third can be carried out only under factory conditions.

This third operation which is described only for the sake of information concerns the grinding of the facets when they are chipped to such an extent that the cutting edge cannot be remade by the ordinary means at one's disposal. On principle, careful and prolonged honing should do, but most histologists today do not possess the skill neither do they have the time to devote to such an operation, it is by far more convenient to get it done by the factory.

Routine *honing* (*affûtage, Schleifen*) and **stropping** (*polissage, Abziehen*) are however within the means of every user of a microtome. Only a good leather strop is required for stropping, and the practice of honing has been considerably simplified by the availability of mechanical sharpeners which, though expensive, are quite worth while in all laboratories where histological techniques are practised frequently.

Stropping is meant to give a finish to facets that have been honed, to remove the rough edge and to smooth the irregularities of the cutting edge with the help of a leather strop. The back of the blade is inserted into the special trough that is supplied with the razor for the purpose. The thickness of this trough determines the profile of the facets. One side of the leather is coated with a very fine abrasive paste (the red paste of most suppliers). The razor is held flat and passed to and fro, *backwards*, covering the whole surface of the leather and imparting a certain lateral movement; that is, at the beginning of the passage the left corner of the blade touches the operator's end of the leather, while at the end of the movement the right corner is at the opposite end of the leather. The leather may be fixed in a clamp or held between the operator's chest and a rigid object. At the end of each movement, the razor is rotated on its back and the other face of the blade is passed over the leather following exactly the inverse movement at the end of which another rotation places the razor in its starting position. All movements should be accomplished regularly and uniformly without exerting undue pressure on the blade. It is better to count the number of strokes so that the two facets are equally polished; usually about fifty would do for each face.

After stropping with the abrasive the razor is carefully cleaned to remove all traces of paste. A soft rag soaked in benzene or toluene will help, but no object other than the pulp of the finger should actually come into contact with the facets themselves. An oblique movement of the finger from one end of the blade to the other and from the back towards the cutting edge ensures against wounding oneself. All contacts between the finger-nails and the edge should be avoided.

After cleaning, further stropping on the uncoated side of the leather finishes the operation. It is at this stage that the facets acquire their final polish and the rough edge is removed. The procedure is identical to that with the abrasive and about fifty strokes may be given for each face. It should however be borne in mind that if the strokes on uncoated leather are too vigorous the cutting edge can get rounded and unsuitable for very thin sections.

Honing is necessary when the wear on the cutting edge and the irregularities of the facets cannot be rectified by stropping. Stropping is relatively harmless to the blade and can be resorted to frequently. Honing on the other hand causes a far from negligible wear of the outer "shell" that has been properly case-hardened and tempered and which is the really functional zone of the blade. Thus, frequent honing, even though perfectly done, decreases the longevity of the razor.

Using an abrasive paste of larger grain (black paste of some suppliers) than that recommended for the first stropping on leather is usually of no avail in correcting faults that are beyond a certain limit. Thus, honing on a special stone or a mechanical device has to be resorted to.

Honing stones are supplied by the manufacturers of microtome razors. The operation differs from that of stropping in that the blade, whose back is fixed in the trough which regulates the profile of the facets, is passed over the stone coated with oil or glycerine *cutting edge forwards*; in other respects the strokes are the same as in stropping. The whole face of the blade should come into contact with all the surface of the stone in the course of each stroke, and as before, the back is the axis of rotation before each return stroke. All movements should be regular and exerting pressure on the blade is unnecessary as its own weight is sufficient to ensure contact with the stone.

The stone can be replaced by a thick and perfectly plane glass sheet carrying the abrasive of larger grain; this is adopted in the mechanical devices for the purpose.

Honing may be checked under a microscope or dissecting lens; it can be terminated when all the irregularities of the cutting edge have disappeared and when the facets appear perfectly smooth and straight. Evidently, each time a blade is honed it should also be carefully stropped before it is used.

Honing by hand is a long operation even when done by a skilled manipulator. It only illustrates the real advantages of the mechanical instruments that automatically pass the razor over the glass laid with abrasive and turn it over at the proper time. A minimum of time is actually spent in the operation, probably less than that required to pack blades and dispatch them to a professional. Consequently, it is worth investing in such an instrument even when the number of razors in use in a laboratory does not guarantee a rapid return on the initial cost.

When the user himself cannot carry out the honing the choice of a qualified person is important. Ordinary establishments handling cutlery are not equipped for attending to microtome razors and their staff do not have the specialized experience; it is therefore best to entrust the work to the makers of the razors themselves.

Microtome blades have been replaced by safety razor blades, fixed in a special holder that has the form of the traditional microtome razor, by certain authors. It can give good results if suitable blades are chosen. In most cases, the interior angle of the facets of safety-razor blades is not suited for paraffin blocks since it is too acute; the cutting edge is severely compressed with each passage over the block and serious irregularities in the sections are caused.

The angle may, however, be modified by careful honing and verification under the microscope; the technique of this type of honing of blades meant for ultra-thin sections has been described in detail by Sjostrand (1953).

THE RAZOR-HOLDER

This varies considerably according to the type of the microtome. In those that are solely meant for paraffin sections, such as the rotary microtomes of the Minot type or rocking microtomes, the holder does not allow any variation in the angle of cutting; the cutting edge is always oriented perpendicularly to the direction in which the block advances. In microtomes with a horizontal chariot, which can be used for cutting paraffin as well as celloïdin or gelatin, this angle can be modified at will. All models allow a modification of the angle of attack, but this angle is calibrated only in few commercial instruments; a lack which clearly illustrates the indifference already mentioned towards one of the essential measures of histological technique. From a practical point of view, the user should pay attention to the distance separating the two arms of the holder because this span puts a limit to one of the dimensions of the blocks that the microtome can take, and moreover, the chances of the razor vibrating increase as they are further apart. The gaps between the clamps that hold the razor are also of practical importance as certain models take only razors that have a relatively narrow back.

THE OBJECT-HOLDER

According to the model the holder may take a small metallic stage on which the block is stuck or a similar piece of wood or synthetic resin. A ball-head or analogous mechanism allows the orientation of the block. A glaring drawback of most instruments should be noted here, namely the interdependance of the mechanism that fixes the stage carrying the block with that governing its orientation. This denial of elementary common sense has been manifested by many makers in an effort to reduce the cost of manufacture; it particularly complicates the task of the user who, in orienting the block, has to allow for the shift produced while tightening the nut to render the whole rigid.

THE MECHANISM OF ADVANCE

This mechanism is quite differently conceived according to the microtome. Models where the razor is fixed and the block mobile should be distinguished from those where the block is fixed and the razor is displaced during cutting. The first of these two conceptions is followed in rocking microtomes and those of the Minot type. The trajectory of the block over a single cutting cycle is an arc in rocking microtomes and a whole circle in the rotary ones. A micrometer screw governs the advance of the block at each passage before the razor, and the degree of advance can be controlled. Impulsion for movement is by traction on a chain in rocking microtomes or by rotation of a wheel as in microtomes of the Minot type. There also exist microtomes with fixed razors where the sledge holding the block is pushed by hand along a horizontal slide-bar.

In microtomes where the razor is mobile, it rotates around an axis corresponding to one of its extremities that is fixed while the other runs in a guide. This is so in freezing microtomes where each point on the cutting edge describes the arc of a circle at every stroke. In other models, the razor is held in a clamp and moves to and fro either by the rotation of a wheel or by hand; the piece held in the object-holder moves upward before the sweep of the razor either by a micrometer screw or by being displaced on an inclined plane.

The plane of cutting is thus vertical in microtomes of the Minot type, almost vertical in rocking microtomes and horizontal in all the others.

CHOICE OF A MICROTOME

Certain criteria in the choice of a microtome are dictated by the nature of the work. Rosking microtomes, for instance, can be used only for small blocks; they are not suitable for celloidin, celloidin-paraffin or gelatin sections. Frozen sections may, in the last resort, be made with these instruments, but such an expedient is rather avoided as far as possible. The Minot-type instruments are ideal for paraffin, especially when the pieces are not too big. The apparent inconvenience of the orthogonal disposition of the two guides controlling the sledge of the object-holder does not show in the quality of the sections for light microscopy. Sections are obtained in ribbons more easily and quickly than with other models. Theoretically, celloidin sections can be made with the help of special razor-holders which permit the desired inclination with respect to the direction of cutting; special stages of the object-holders also allow frozen-sections; but these two modifications of the Minot-type microtome are, however, expedients that are not quite recommendable. Microtomes with horizontal slide-bars and razor-holders that permit varying the cutting angle are the best adapted for celloidin, celloidin-paraffin and gelatin sections. They can also be used for paraffin sections and are even preferable to the Minot-type microtomes for large blocks. As for frozen sections, it is by far best to use the microtomes that are specially made for the purpose.

Other factors influencing the choice are the financial possibilities of the acquirer and his working habits; they cannot hence be codified. The qualities of the various commercial models cannot be discussed either; however, it is legitimate to briefly enumerate the technical points that should be considered when purchasing a microtome of the Minot type or one with horizontal slide-bars. Apart from the quality of the finish and the stability, which are necessary requisites of all instruments, the Minot-type ones should be chosen for the possibilities of giving a desired and measurable orientation to the razor, of adapting the instrument to blades of varying thickness, of spacing the clamps of the object-holder, of separate fixing and orientation of the object-holder, of a wide choice in the thickness of sections and for the stabilization of the sledge. This last characteristic depends on the ratio of the weights of the sledge and the wheel; good stabilization is indicated when the sledge and wheel can be maintained in equilibrium in any position whatever. In badly equilibrated microtomes the sledge drops when left in mid-course during cutting and more muscular effort is necessary. The above qualities are also required of microtomes with horizontal slide-bars; in addition, the stroke of the sledge should be sufficiently long, and models where the advance of the block between sections is not automatic are better avoided. In spite of their higher cost, microtomes with an accessory cuvette that serve for celloidin sections are preferable to others. The functional length of the micrometer screw and the range of possible thicknesses of sections are of as much importance as in the Minot-type instruments.

It is useful to recall here that *a microtome is an instrument of high precision and should not be entrusted to several hands*. This is of course a precept that many heads of laboratories are reluctant to follow, but none the less a very real one. Even a very skilled operator is at his best only with an instrument to which he is used and whose controls have not been distorted by the indiscriminate use of others. Laboratory administrations will not easily agree to buy as many microtomes with cuvettes as there are investigators; but I feel that every histologist deserves to have his own microtome, at least of the Minot type, that is, if the head of the laboratory is honestly concerned with the quality of work produced.

MAINTENANCE OF THE MICROTOME

Maintenance and care of this instrument varies according to the model; the instructions accompanying each instrument give precise indications as to the points to be greased and they should be followed closely. It is obvious that careful cleaning is necessary after each use; particular care should be taken that no dust or paraffin enters the guide or slide-bars. The instrument should obviously be left under a dust-cover when not in use, an elementary precaution but which needs to be often recalled. It is equally evident that the user has nothing to gain by taking to pieces the fixed parts of the instrument, especially the slide-bars; adjustment of the bearings calls for special tools and a certain experience lacking in the great majority of histologists, so that any attempt at odd repairs will only risk causing damage. Periodical inspection of microtomes that are constantly used is strongly recommended and this is better entrusted to the makers of the instrument.

Finally, I must recall a very obvious precaution, but those neglect has led to grave accidents, namely that the razor should never be left on the instrument when not in use.

CUTTING AND HANDLING PARAFFIN SECTIONS

Cutting blocks of paraffin in the Minot-type microtome is about the most usual method of making sections for study under the light microscope. Several steps can be distinguished in the whole operation such as the preparation of the block and mounting it on the stage of the microtome, the actual cutting and the subsequent handling of the sections, especially their spreading.

PREPARING THE BLOCK

The block of paraffin that has been cooled for more than 12 hours, except in urgent cases, is *trimmed* to remove as much paraffin as possible from the four sides that will border the sections. The cross-section is also thinned with a scalpel to bring the surface closer to the piece; it is however necessary to leave a certain thickness of paraffin on the basal side which will serve to stick the block on to the stage of the object-holder of the microtome. Attention should be paid to the length-by-width ratio of the future sections; in fact, if blocks are long and narrow they generally cut badly through a considerably greater risk of vibration. It is, besides, advisable to give a trapezoidal shape to the cross-section by slanting the lateral slides as it allows the boundary between sections to be easily distinguished on the ribbon. In any case, after fixation on the stage of Minot-type microtomes, the upper and lower edges of the block should be rigorously parallel if straight ribbons are to be obtained. The same rule applies to microtomes with a slide-bar; the edges of the block corresponding to the direction of cutting should be parallel. Clearly, the final trimming of the block, especially that of the parallel edges, can be done after it is fixed on the object-holder. There do exist devices for ensuring parallelism automatically which are however replaced to advantage by the skill of the operator.

Certain precautions have to be observed in trimming. If the removal of too much paraffin at a time is attempted, there is great risk of breaking or fissuring the block. The block should therefore be trimmed by removing shavings with a sharp scalpel. When several pieces are embedded in the same block and they are to be separated, the block should be cut with extreme care; a notch is made along the desired line and gradually deepened. Some authors advise the use of a warmed cutting-saw.

Blocks are stuck on to the object-holder with paraffin. A layer of paraffin is placed on the stage and made to melt by applying a heated spatula or pair of forceps, and the base of the block is held against it until it solidifies. The edges of the block in contact with the stage are similarly melted with the heated instrument to ensure better adhesion and the whole stage with the attacked block is immersed for a few instants in cold water. Some authors use a glass slide that has been heated in a bunsen flame. The warm slide is held over paraffin shavings lying on the stage; the block in turn is held over the warm slide with one hand and the slide is deftly withdrawn with the other. I strongly advise against the practice of warming the whole stage itself in a bunsen flame; it cannot be done with plastic stages but only with metallic ones and, besides, exposes the piece to considerable risk especially if the layer of paraffin separating it from the stage is not particularly thick.

The stage with the attached block is fixed in the clamp of the object-holder of the microtome and oriented to obtain the desired plane of sections. In fact, the particular orientation should be anticipated at the time of trimming and sticking the block, but minor adjustment may be made by suitably inclining the object-holder. It is useful to remember that the shape of pieces is not easily discernible through the layer of paraffin and the practice of orienting a piece inside the block with respect to a given side at the time of casting can be very helpful.

ING PARAFFIN SECTIONS 107

n excessively hardened during embedding
ual cutting of sections. It would be quite
or of this practice as it is casually referred
e great majority of handbooks on techni-
ose authors who do mention it apparently
eserves. It is however considerable since
ined especially when the piece contains
ch as decalcified bone, collagenous tissue,
retory products. This softening is quite
ck, that has been partially cut to expose a
hours to about 10 days. Baker (1941) has
txure of 34 parts of water, 54 parts of 96%
ifford (1950) has obtained good results on
e except that glycerine is replaced by acetic
ent to the water used for soaking has also
experience, the essential factor is that the
d the other ingredients referred to do not
ently, care should be taken that immersion
s complete, if necessary by ballasting it or
stuffing cotton to maintain ... to the bottom of the vessel during soaking.

Contrary to what one might think, penetration of water into tissues is quite rapid even when embedding is faultless. There is no risk of harm to the pieces especially if embedding is good and they are firmly lodged in the paraffin. The time required for soaking depends on the tissue and the quality of embedding. When pieces are very voluminous it is sometimes necessary to interrupt sectioning and submit them to renewed soaking.

The above procedure is to be avoided only in cases of very bad embedding when the impregnation of paraffin has been really insufficient. In all other cases, it seems best to apply it systematically. The omission of this operation, though it has been described in handbooks as long ago as the end of the 19th century, again illustrates the indifference of most authors towards purely technical problems.

After the block has been mounted on the microtome the razor is fixed and suitably oriented; during this step it is recommended to immobilize the sledge by means of the device intended for it in Minot-type microtomes. The choice of the particular orientation has been discussed under the general descripton of this instrument. It need only be recalled that good paraffin sections require that the angle of attack be slightly greater than the clearance angle of sections, for which 15 to 19° may be a rough average and further fine adjustment can be determined by trial.

The other characteristics of the razor are not at all to be ignored. Soft blocks should be cut with a plano-concave razor with the concave face turned towards the block; bi-planar razors are suitable for hard blocks. If a user has access to several razors, it is better to choose one with a large back, that is, with a wider blade angle, for the harder pieces. Often pieces that are really hard can be cut with a plano-concave razor if the plane face is turned towards the block.

CUTTING SECTIONS

The proper mechanical functioning of the microtome should be checked before actually cutting sections, but only after fixing the block in the object-holder so that it oscillates at a slight distance away from the edge of the razor when the wheel is rotated. This permits detecting any faulty movement or lack of greasing. The block is then brought up to the edge of the razor, the thickness of sections adjusted by the mechanism meant for the purpose and cutting may be commenced.

When the block has been neither soaked previously nor trimmed with a scalpel before being placed on the object-holder the first section consists only of the embedding paraffin. This should be taken advantage of to verify the absence of striations which indicate defects in the blade, to ensure a straight ribbon which is obtained only when the two faces parallel to the cutting edge are themselves parallel and, finally, to judge the ambient thermal conditions. The importance of thermal conditions is, besides, far from negligible. If the temperature of the room in which sections are cut is much colder than the melting point of the paraffin used, the sections curl and the ribbon is badly formed. If, on the contrary, the room is too warm the sections tend to pile up or are unduly pleated. It is only after the piece itself is exposed that the final orientation of the razor can be adjusted, the thickness of sections chosen according to the consistency of the block and a suitable speed of cutting adopted.

The proper rate of cutting is variously judged. Certain authors and makers of microtomes advise very slow cutting especially when pieces are hard. In fact, the choice of speed depends largely on the consistency of the block, ambient conditions, size of the block and the mechanical characteristics of the razor and the microtome. A simple experience will show that for a given setting with the same block the thickness of sections can vary according to the speed of cutting. It is therefore essential that a constant speed of cutting should be observed, especially in serial sections.

Another recommendation of manufacturers that should not be followed to the letter concerns the uniformity of the rotation imported to the wheel. By analogy with the functioning of slide-bar microtomes, where the movement of the clamp holding the razor should be as uniform as possible, makers generally advise the same uniformity for Minot-type instruments, also without any regard for the position of the object-holder in its course.

It should not be forgotten that in the Minot-type microtome, the actual cutting corresponds only to a small fraction of the turn of the wheel, in fact, to that fraction of a revolution when the whole mechanism consisting of wheel, sledge and object-holder is submitted to a braking effect. Turning the wheel as uniformly as possible is certainly no way of ensuring the desired effect, namely that of actually crossing the block at a perfectly uniform speed. It can be seen from experience that such uniformity is obtained much more easily by exerting a slight impulsion to the wheel just when the object-holder is at the height of its trajectory.

When all adjustments are correct and other conditions for sectioning are suitable the first section spreads itself on the blade while adhering by its upper edge to the cutting edge of the razor; the second section joins on to the first, and so on to form a ribbon. It is essential to cut paraffin blocks in ribbons even if it is meant to separate individual sections later on.

In practice, the ribbon is held and lightly drawn with the left hand, which greatly facilitates the unfolding of sections when spreading them. I strongly advise against the practice of allowing sections to accumulate on the other side of the blade away from the block; they risk jutting out and can be snatched back by the object-holder; they are also more likely to pile up if the ribbon is not stretched during cutting.

Adjustable ribbon-carriers are provided with certain models of microtomes; from experience, however, these conveyor belts are not so easy to manipulate and most users prefer to do without them.

The chief causes of trouble that one is likely to encounter while making paraffin sections in a Minot-type microtome and their possible remedies are given in Table 3.

HANDLING AND SPREADING SECTIONS

When the ribbon that is held in the left hand with a brush or any suitable instrument (glass rod, scalpel, mounted needle) has attained a certain length the rotation of the wheel with the right hand is stopped so that the object-holder is at its lowest position. The last section, whose upper edge remains attached to the edge of the razor, is very carefully detached by a light upward pull if necessary. This may be effected with a brush, but the use of the blade of a scalpel held in the right hand is more convenient. Any contact with the cutting edge of the razor should obviously be avoided. The ribbon, held at its ends by the two hands, is then laid on a flat and clean surface whose colour is chosen so that the sections are easily visible against it (light for osmified or chromated pieces and dark for faintly coloured pieces) and which permits cutting out stretches of the ribbon with a scalpel. Such ribbons can be stored for years if they are sheltered from heat and dust, but obviously such a stock is infinitely

Table 3. — Principal causes of trouble in cutting paraffin sections with a Minot-type microtome

Trouble	Cause	Remedy
Vibrated sections (alternating thick and thin zones *in the same section*)	Angle of attack too great	Straighten razor
Sections of different thickness that alternate more or less regularly	Angle of attack too small	Incline the razor a little more
	Badly fixed razor	Tighten the clamp of the razor-holder.
	Block badly fixed to the object-holder	Verify and, if necessary, remove block and stick it again.
	Defective micrometer screw	Revision of the instrument
Extremely folded sections	Blunt razor	Honing, or at least stropping
	Paraffin too soft for the particular thickness of sections.	Lower the room temperature; cool the block; if necessary, re-embed in paraffin with a higher melting point; if possible, cut thicker sections.
Sections crumple without however having a chalky appearance that is characteristic of poor embedding	Pieces are too hard	Reduce the thickness of sections; this is the ideal case where much is gained by soaking the cut block in water.
Sections are torn, break off, and have the chalky aspect due to bad impregnation of the embedding medium.	Incomplete elimination of the alcohol used for dehydration or poor impregnation	Try, but without undue expectations, returning through warm paraffin, the intermediate, and even back to absolute alcohol; in no case should it be soaked in water.
Section curl up on the blade and do not form ribbons.	Paraffin is too hard for the chosen thickness of sections and for the ambient temperature.	Reduce the thickness of sections; cut the first section slowly and with the help of a mounted needle or camel-hair brush spread it along the side of the razor; raise the temperature of both block and razor, which can often be done by blowing on to the zone of the razor that actually cuts the block.
Sections appear good but no ribbon is formed.	Paraffin is too cold for the chosen thickness and for the ambient temperature.	Proceed as above or increase the speed of cutting.

CUTTING AND HANDLING PARAFFIN SECTIONS

Table 3. continued

Trouble	Cause	Remedy
The sections of the piece detach from the paraffin ribbon.	Faulty impregnation of paraffin due to the consistency of the outer zone of the piece and to a low temperature of embedding.	Try a slower speed of cutting; apply collodion with a brush to the surface of the block before each section; re-embed; abandon the piece if a chalky appearance shows that the centre is also badly impregnated.
On the upward stroke the block carries along with it sections lying on the razor.	Electrostatic attraction.	Try to discharge the razor by lighting a Bunsen burner nearby or by bombarding with α particles (a sovereign remedy, if any, but expensive considering the cost of a generator).
	Clearance angle too small.	Incline razor.
	Paraffin debris accumulated on the lower edge of the block.	Free edges of debris constantly.
	Paraffin debris accumulated on the side of the razor turned towards the block.	Clean the razor.
Ribbon is curved.	Upper and lower edges of the block are not parallel.	Retrim block.
	Unequal sharpening of the the razor results in an asymmetrical compression of the block.	Shift razor, or trim the block to compensate (by decreasing the dimension of the edge corresponding to the convexity of the ribbon).
Ribbon is curved	The two screws of the clamp of the object-holder are not equally tightened.	Retighten screws or retrim block as before.
Striated ribbon	Defective sharpening of the razor.	Honing, or at least stropping.
	Debris on the side of the razor towards the block that causes striations.	Remove debris with the pulp of the finger.
	Presence of hard objects or particles in the piece.	Remove them with a needle if necessary.

more cumbersome than a collection of blocks. It is therefore advisable to cut blocks only when one disposes of enough time to continue the rest of the procedure.

Spreading paraffin sections can be done dry, on an inert liquid or combined with sticking by using a liquid containing substances that ensure the adherence of tissues to the slide.

Dry sticking has been mentioned in connection with the treatment of blocks obtained by freezing-drying. It is quite a laborious operation that gives acceptable results only when sections are not at all folded at the time of cutting. The slide may be coated with glycerine-albumine or just thoroughly cleaned; it may be gently warmed (to about 30 °C). A short piece of ribbon is cut out with a scalpel and one of its ends applied against the right edge of the slide while the other, held with a scalpel in the left hand is maintained at a short distance from the warm slide; any folds are straightened with the help of a brush in the right hand and the sections in the middle, which are generally the only ones that can be utilized, are laid down on the slide when perfectly unfolded. Adherence can be reinforced by covering them with cigarette paper and applying *mild* pressure with the finger or a rubber roller.

Spreading over an inert liquid (mercury or mineral oil) is easier. A Petri dish containing a suitable quantity of the liquid is placed on a hot-plate set to 35°–40°. When a stable temperature is attained it is enough to cut out a portion of ribbon and lay it over the warm liquid for the sections to spread by themselves. They may then be removed by gliding a slide coated with glycerine-albumine from underneath the ribbon. This is carried out by using a mounted needle held in the right hand to apply the left end of the ribbon to a slide held in the left hand and dipping at about 20° or 30°. The slide is then gradually withdrawn with the left hand and the ribbon lays itself on the slide over its whole length.

When the type of work does not call for either sticking dry or spreading over an inert liquid, both operations of spreading and sticking may be combined in one by using a solution that aids adherence to the slide. The most commonly employed of such solutions are glycerine-albumine, glycerine-water and Ruyter's fluid.

Sticking with glycerine-albumine was introduced into histological technique by P. Mayer (1883) who used a mixture of equal parts of the white of an egg and glycerine preserved by adding a little thymol, camphor or a 1% solution of sodium salicylate or formalin. After vigorous and repeated agitation the mixture should be filtered, which can be time consuming. It is often more convenient to buy ready made glycerine-albumine since most commercial preparations are quite satisfactory.

Undiluted glycerine-albumin smeared as a thin film on the surface of slides serves for sticking dry or after spreading on an indifferent liquid. In the case of sections spread over water various modifications of sticking with glycerine-albumen have been described. Two of them are particularly recommended, namely sticking with albuminous water and that using glycerine-albumin with 30% alcohol.

Sticking with albuminous water was first practised by the French cytologist Henneguy (1897), undoubtedly the reason why a great many histologists judge it proper to call it the Japanese method. Sections are spread over glycerine-albumin diluted 20 times with distilled water in the manner described below.

Sticking with glycerine-albumen after spreading over 30% alcohol, as introduced by Apathy, ensures better adherence of sections but is more complicated. Perfectly clean slides are coated with a thin film of glycerine-albumin and heated, albuminized face upward, over a flame or a hot-plate until fumes of acrolein are evolved. Such slides can be stored for months. At the time of use the albuminized face is covered with 30% alcohol on which the sections are spread.

Although practised in most histological laboratories, the various methods of sticking with glycerine-albumen are in fact inferior to sticking with gelatin. I advise its use only in cases where the presence of a layer of gelatin can cause difficulty in the subsequent treatment of sections, especially when silver impregnation or certain stains such as Mann's methyl-blue-eosin are intended.

Sticking with gelatin, whose authorship is difficult to ascertain, is the method of choice in most cases. Adherence of sections is quite satisfactory, the preparation of the reagent very simple, and most staining procedures and histochemical reactions are compatible with the procedure. A 0.1 or 0.2% solution of gelatin in distilled water is used. It dissolves very rapidly especially when warmed to about 50°. Gelatine solutions, as such, keep badly and most users advise that the quantity for a day's use be prepared freshly. In practice, however, it is possible to conserve it for a week by adding sufficient potassium dichromate to give it the yellow colour of a saturated solution of picric acid (that is, from three to five drops of a 3% solution of potassium dichromate for 20 ml of gelatine solution).

Sticking with Ruyter's fluid (1931) is especially advantageous with pieces rich in tissue that is difficult to spread (bone, cartilage). The mixture consists of 8 ml of distilled water, 2 ml of acetone, a drop of methyl benzoate and three drops of glycerine-albumen. It is most convenient for spreading paraffin-celloidin sections.

The procedure for sticking differs according to whether spreading has been effected on a slide or in a Petri dish. The first must be adopted with the method of Apathy, and is by far the most suitable for sticking serial sections. The second is advantageous for large sections, which explains why it is preferred by pathologists.

In any case slides used for sticking sections should be very clean and free of any trace of grease which will surely endanger the final result. If any detergent has been used for cleaning it should be thoroughly removed. The cleanliness of slides obtained commercially varies according to the supplier and it is difficult to prescribe a constant procedure. Dry wiping is enough in some cases; in others, washing in 5% acetic acid followed by thorough rinsing is called for. Sometimes slides arrive in a condition that requires treatment with a sulfuric-acid-dichromate mixture followed by extensive washing in water.

The clean slide is placed before the operator and its number or other suitable indication is scratched with a diamond on the side on which the sections are to be stuck. I recommend marking on the upper right corner as in the pagination of a book. The liquid used for spreading and sticking is pipetted on to this surface. It is not necesssary to layer this liquid over the whole surface of the slide if it is to receive only a single section or a small piece of ribbon, but in every case it should well extend beyond the edges of the paraffin. Any uneven spreading of the liquid indicates insufficient cleaning of the slide. The desired fragment of ribbon is cut off with a scalpel. The point of the scalpel, wetted with the liquid is then held under the ribbon and the ribbon placed on the slide. The shiny side of the ribbon that was facing the razor at the time of cutting is laid against the slide. Care should be taken that the dull side of the ribbon turned upwards is perfectly dry. The slide is then placed on a hot plate. The optimal temperature for the spreading of sections varies from 35 to 45° according to the sample of paraffin. The operator should keep control of the unfolding due to expansion of the paraffin and if necessary help with a mounted needle. Obviously the melting point of the paraffin should never be attained during spreading. When spreading is complete, the slide is taken by one end in the left hand while the section is held against the slide with the help of a needle or scalpel in the right hand. The slide is tilted to drain off the liquid used for spreading.

At this stage, the final position of the section on the slide is adjusted with the right hand. It is often necessary to return the slides to the hot plate for a few minutes to remove any folds produced during draining.

After cooling any liquid left is further drained off or mopped up and the slide is dried.

Spreading in Petri dishes is practised just as in treating sections that should not come into contact with water, except that mercury or mineral oil is replaced by the liquid chosen for spreading. The shiny side of the section should be in contact with the liquid. When fully spread the sections are taken out by slipping a slide underneath, drained or mopped up and dried. There exist water-baths with thermostats specially meant for the purpose. Most electric hot-plates are sufficiently big to hold a Petri dish of the required size; if necessary a Malassez plate can also be used. Evidently the electric plates are always preferable to the old gas plates.

The spreading of serial sections calls for further remarks concerning the disposition of ribbons and their alignment.

Ribbons may be placed in horizontal or vertical rows using the maximum available space on the slide. Expansion of the paraffin during spreading, in the direction in which sections were cut, should be allowed for. The strips of ribbon should contain the same number of sections in each row, and any missing sections should be denoted by a blank space.

Considerable time is gained during the exploration of preparations by aligning sections horizontally or vertically and it is essential to keep this in mind at the time of cutting to obtain ribbons that are as straight as possible. It is worth practising the transfer of ribbons from one slide to another by slipping a scalpel underneath the sections. Clearly, long series that cover the whole slide cannot be satisfactory if sections are very folded and have to be unfolded individually.

Another method of spreading that is very useful in histophysiological and histochemical research should also be mentioned. It consists of sticking single sections, cut out of a ribbon, on slides that are numbered consecutively so that sets of slides are obtained where all the different zones of the piece are represented in each set. Thus if 10 such sets are desired the first set will carry, in order, the 1st, 11th, 21st, 31st, etc..., while the second set will carry the 2nd, 12th, 22nd, 32nd, etc..., of the sections of the ribbon. If the sections are sufficiently thin two sections of the same cell can be studied by two different methods. Particular care should be taken in aligning sections since their position on the slide is the only means of identifying their individual order. It is often convenient to apply the liquid for spreading as stripes corresponding to the number of rows of sections. More liquid necessary for proper spreading may then be added after the sections have been placed. Any drying of sections while placing them in position on the slide should be avoided; paraffin sections once stuck without being unfolded are generally irretrievable.

Sections may be **drained** after spreading by placing them on a grooved board (Vigier's board) and allowing the liquid to flow off the slanted slides. Mopping can be more suitable in the case of thin sections. This may be done by laying a pad of blotting paper on a perfectly plane surface and inverting the slide carrying sections over it. The slide may then be quite firmly pressed downwards by its ends or even in the middle, but any lateral displacement should be carefully avoided. The operation gives the final touch to spreading and I disapprove of it only when sections exceed 15 μ in thickness, which is rarely so with paraffin embedding.

The *drying* of sections should closely follow draining and mopping. The practice of leaving sections at room temperature is quite simply disastrous, because the paraffin is never applied closely enough against the glass. In fact, at less than 30° paraffin is relatively stiff and air can easily penetrate between section and slide, so that examination of the lower side in oblique light will show shiny patches, a sure indication of later detachment during staining. As P. Masson has observed even drying at 37° does not guarantee against this. In fact, the temperature chosen should be close to the melting point of paraffin. I personally hold what might appear to be an outrageous affirmation to some adepts of histological technique, namely that melting the embedding mass, which can be a catastrophe when sections are not dry, is of no serious consequence at all when all the liquid used for spreading has been removed by draining or mopping. It is thus quite feasible to dry sections, that have been *perfectly* drained, in an oven at 58° or 60° and save considerably time thereby.

Clearly, the drying of sections meant for histo-enzymology should be affected at or near 0°. It obviously takes longer, and it can be useful to warm sections, just before deparaffining, to the temperature of melting paraffin for a few seconds. This operation, suggested by Gomori (1952) greatly facilitates deparaffining and improves adherence.

CUTTING SECTIONS IN PARAFFIN-AGAR

The general procedure is the same as for paraffin sections. It is however preferable to trim the block so that the agar is exposed along the lateral edges while a layer of paraffin is left on the sides corresponding to the plane of the razor. In this manner the ribbon will show alternate bands of paraffin and of agar more or less penetrated with paraffin; trimming can be facilitated by lightly staining the agar, during dehydration, with an alcoholic solution of eosin.

Ruyter's liquid is particularly suited for spreading agar-paraffin sections.

CUTTING AND HANDLING CELLOIDIN AND CELLOIDIN-PARAFFIN SECTIONS

The main differences between cutting sections in celloidin and in paraffin are in the orientation of the razor and in the impossibility of obtaining ribbons of sections with celloidin-paraffin.

Blocks of celloidin-paraffin hardened after soaking in 4%, or even 8%, celloidin may be cut, like paraffin blocks, in a Minot-type microtome at a cutting angle of 90°. However, blocks of celloidin-paraffin that have gone through a 16% solution of celloidin must be cut with a microtome sliding horizontally. In fact such an instrument is almost indispensable for blocks made entirely in celloidin and the substitution of a Minot-type microtome with a holder that allows inclination of the razor is only a poor last resource.

Preparation of a celloidin block differs according to whether it is to be cut under alcohol or terpineol. The two procedures will be described followed by that for celloidin-paraffin blocks.

PREPARATION OF CELLOIDIN BLOCKS TO BE CUT UNDER ALCOHOL

The block, stored under 70% alcohol, is stuck firmly by means of an 8% solution of celloidin, on to a piece of wood or on to the block-holder supplied for the purpose with certain models of microtomes.

The wood, cut into smooth blocks of suitable dimensions, is rid of its tannin by boiling in dilute sodium hydroxide, in water and finally by washing several times in alcohol. The surfaces of the wood and the block to be brought into contact with each other are lightly roughened with a needle or a file. A few drops of the celloidin solution are placed on the surface of the wood and the celloidin block is applied to it and held tightly for one or two minutes.

Excess celloidin is wiped off and the whole immersed for a few hours in 70% alcohol. Apathy (1912) rightly insists on the shape that should be given to celloidin blocks. The most convenient profile is that of a rectangular prism attached to the holder by one of its larger sides. The width of projected sections should be about twice their length. As for the position of the piece in the block, it is preferable that the blade actually cuts the piece in the block after traversing a short thickness of celloidin while it cuts a much larger thickness after the piece. One of the corners of the block may be trimmed cantwise to enable identification of the orientation of the sections. The block prepared in the above manner may then be fixed in the object-holder clamp of the microtome.

PREPARATION OF CELLOIDIN BLOCKS TO BE CUT UNDER TERPINEOL

The block that was stored under 70% alcohol is transferred to 90% alcohol and left for 24 hours. It is then treated with the mixture of essential oils described for embedding in celloidin-paraffin (see page 96). When fully cleared the block is transferred to anhydrous terpineol that is renewed twice or thrice to remove the last traces of alcohol. From this stage onwards the block can be stored either in terpineol, or dry, in a well-stoppered bottle. Sticking on to the wooden cube or holder is effected by means of a mixture of three parts of a thick solution (8% or better 16%) of celloidin and one part of clove oil. After sticking and air-drying for about ten minutes it is immersed for a few hours in anhydrous terpineol. The recommended shape to be given to the block is the same as that for cutting under alcohol.

PREPARATION OF CELLOIDIN-PARAFFIN BLOCKS

Celloidin-paraffin blocks hardened after 16% celloidin are the only ones that require the use of a sliding microtome. The dimensions of the block would have been already determined at the time of embedding in paraffin and it suffices to stick the block on to the wood or the holder of the microtome. Sticking is effected as in the case of paraffin blocks. It is possible to modify the shape and size of blocks at the time of sticking by trimming off in little shavings. Apathy (1912) recommends, for celloidin-paraffin and paraffin sections, the opposite configuration, namely that pieces should be disposed so that the embedding mass traversed by the razor before the piece is larger than the layer following the piece.

CUTTING SECTIONS

The use of horizontally sliding microtomes calls for certain precautions that need not to be observed with the Minot-type instruments, which explains the great vogue of the latter. In fact, the slideways of the razor holder, and in some cases of the object holder, should be thoroughly cleaned to remove all traces of dust and oil remaining from previous use. They should then be coated with a *thin* even layer of mineral oil. It is often best to use the oil supplied by the makers. The instrument should be made to run free a few times so that all mobile parts settle into perfectly smooth movement. After these preliminaries the piece is fixed in the clamp and the razor in its holder, suitably oriented not only in its angle of attack but also in its cutting angle which can be adjusted in this type of microtome.

The choice of the angle of attack depends on the same factors as in paraffin sections but making allowance for the embedding material. With paraffin sections, as with celloidin-paraffin and gelatin sections, this angle may be just superior to the clearance angle. It should, however, be much greater for celloidin sections, and even more so for softer embedding. If razors with different facet angles are available, small angles should be chosen for paraffin and larger ones for celloidin.

The choice of cutting angle, always at 90° in the case of Minot-type microtomes for paraffin, depends on the embedding mass, its consistency and the shape of the block. It should always be less than 45° except when celloidin-paraffin blocks have been hardened after treatment in a low concentration (4%) of celloidin, in which case they may be cut in a Minot-type instrument. Celloidin blocks, trimmed according to the recommendations of Apathy described earlier, are cut by orienting the razor parallel to the diagonal of the rectangle represented by the upper surface of the block. The cutting angle thus ranges from 20 to 40°. The same orientation is suitable for celloidin paraffin blocks (hardened after thick solutions of celloidin). With gelatin sections, however, the angle should be further halved (10 to 20°). It is clear that such an orientation of the razor's edge with respect to the direction of cutting prevents the formation of ribbons, which is besides rendered impossible by the consistency of these embedding masses other than celloidin-paraffin.

The actual cutting in these microtomes is effected by displacement of the razor either by rotation of a wheel or by hand. The movement is translated, according to the model, directly on the razor-holder or through a handle held in the right hand of the operator. The movement should always be *uniform and slow*. The sledge should always be made to run its whole course, whatever the dimensions of the piece, to avoid any irregular wear of the slideway. Evidently no vertical pressure at all should be exerted on the razor holder to avoid irregularities in the thickness of sections. This is a particularly important precaution to be taken in instruments where the razor-holder is pushed directly by hand.

In all cases, the right hand is used to move the razor, whether directly, by means of a handle or by a rotating wheel. A fine flat brush in the left hand serves to gently hold the section against the upper side of the razor without causing too many folds. Evidently this should not in any way influence the regularity of movement of the right hand.

The blade and brush should remain dry when paraffin sections are cut in this manner, with the cutting angle at 90° and the brush serving to hold the ribbon as when manipulating a Minot-type microtome. Thick sections of celloidin paraffin may also be cut without wetting the razor especially when blocks have been hardened after celloidin solutions of less than 8%. In all other cases it is preferable not to cut dry sections but to moisten both razor and brush with alcohol or terpineol.

1° *Cutting under alcohol*

This method is confined to celloidin blocks. The zones of the razor that do not come into contact with the block are thinly coated with vaseline while that which touches the block and on which the section spreads after cutting is constantly maintained under a layer of 70% alcohol. This concentration of ethanol does not soften the celloidin and the block keeps its consistency, but the subsequent spreading of sections with bergamot oil, as proposed by Apathy, is no longer possible. Evidently the block also should be moistened with alcohol.

Microtomes with an attached cuvette, where sections are cut submerged in 70% alcohol in which the razor moves, are obviously ideal for this type of work. If such an instrument is not available, the required moistening is effected by daubing the razor and the block with a brush dipped in 70% alcohol or by fixing a drop bottle just above the razor and adjusting its output suitably. Certain microtomes are provided with an accessory of this type.

The sections are kept in place during cutting by the brush held in the left hand. After detaching from the block each section is removed with the brush, if necessary after spreading it on the blade of the razor. In removing, the brush is first brought into contact with the edge of the section that is closer to the back of the razor and the sections detached from the blade by a movement of the brush that goes from the back towards the cutting edge. Sections may be kept in 70% alcohol and stored thus until staining, or they may be stuck on to slides.

2° Cutting under terpineol

Sections may be cut under terpineol from blocks of celloidin-paraffin (after thick solutions) from blocks of gelatin embedded according to the method of Apathy after dehydration and impregnation with terpineol or from blocks of celloidin. Celloidin blocks should be prepared as indicated earlier.

The technique does not differ from that for sections made under alcohol. Obviously, microtomes with attached cuvettes are not required and the terpineol is applied to the razor and the block with a brush while zones of the razor not involved are coated with vaseline. Excess terpineol that flows off the razor and block may be recovered, according to Apathy (1912) in a ring-shaped metal receptacle that surrounds the wooden block or holder and which fits to its dimensions.

Sections may be removed with a brush. Apathy recommends the use of a paper spatula inserted into a handle (that of the brush is quite suitable). The spatula is applied over the spread section which is removed by a movement directed from the back of the razor towards the cutting edge.

These sections are not stored in alcohol but kept, in the desired order, between sheets of cigarette paper moistened with terpineol. There is no danger of drying. Furthermore, a rapid inspection under the microscope, much easier than in the case of sections cut under alcohol, is possible before sticking them on the slides.

STICKING SECTIONS

The procedure for sticking differs greatly according to the embedding mass and the technique adopted for cutting.

Dry celloidin-paraffin sections are to be treated as paraffin sections and all the methods described for the purpose may be applied. I particularly recommend spreading in Ruyter's liquid on slides coated with albumin-glycerine.

For ***celloidin and celloidin-paraffin sections cut under terpineol*** sticking according to Apathy is the best procedure. After removal with a paper spatula the sections are arranged in order on cigarette paper moistened with terpineol. The necessary labelling may be written on a corner of the sheet. It is convenient to lay this sheet on a metal foil that is bent around the back of the razor so that sections can be received on the paper as they are cut. When the sheet (supporting paper) is filled with sections it is covered with a second sheet of cigarette paper (covering paper) which need not be moistened with terpineol but which leaves exposed an edge of about 3 or 4 millimeters of the supporting paper. Sections thus placed between sheets may be stored for a long time since the terpineol which impregnates them is not volatile. At the time of sticking the two sheets enclosing the sections are laid flat on a pad of blotting paper with the supporting paper uppermost. After careful and even pressing downwards the supporting paper may be removed with a forceps while the sections remain attached to the covering paper. The covering paper carrying the sections is next turned and laid over a slide thinly coated with albumin-glycerine and the sections transferred in turn to the slide where they lie with the same face upwards as at the time of cutting. The slide carrying the sections is then covered with a dry sheet of cigarette paper and over it, a second clean slide and the whole placed on a hot plate at about 60°. The covering slide is carefully pressed with the finger and the pressure maintained until the warmth can be felt, which is an indication that the albumin used for sticking has coagulated. The two slides are then transferred to a vessel containing a mixture of equal parts of absolute alcohol and chloroform and slanting them so that the slide carrying sections faces downwards. In a few minutes the covering slide and cigarette paper can be easily detached while the sections remain firmly stuck to the slide.

Sticking celloidin sections cut under alcohol presents great difficulties and quite a number of procedures have been described between 1890 and 1920. It is also because of these difficulties that most authors prefer staining celloidin sections without previous sticking, and mounting only stained sections on the slide. In practice, however, this method cannot be applied to staining techniques that require the embedding mass to be first dissolved away.

The most frequently used of the methods of sticking, generally called the Russian method, has been described by Rubaschkin (1907). It is used today in the manner formulated by Maximow (1909). The section, moistened with 70% alcohol, is unfolded on the razor and transferred by means of a spatula, with as little 70% alcohol as possible, on to a slide thinly coated with albumin-glycerine and flattened by careful and uniform pressure exerted across a pad of blotting paper. It is immediately covered with pure clove oil and after clearing (5 to 20 minutes) the slide is placed in a tube filled with 95% alcohol for about ten minutes. Dehydration is completed by two baths in absolute alcohol followed by a mixture of equal parts of alcohol and ether until the celloidin is dissolved. After returning to 70% alcohol it may be hydrated and stained. The method is evidently applicable to sections that have been stored for a long time in 70% alcohol.

Carazzi (1910) recommends arranging sections on a sheet of thin unglazed paper (toilet paper) moistened with 70% alcohol and transferring them to an albuminized slide and proceeding as in the method of Maximow.

The methods of Obregia (1890) and of Levi (1937) are particularly suited for sticking celloidin sections cut under alcohol that have to be disposed in a definite order (serial sections for example).

The principle of Obregia's method is to arrange sections on a glass sheet coated with a thin and even layer of sugar, covering them with celloidin and transferring them on to the resulting film of celloidin by dissolving the sugar in water. To prepare the sugar coating a solution of 150 g of powdered sugar-candy is made in 150 ml of boiling distilled water, and another one of 50 g of yellow dextrin in 50 ml of boiling distilled water. After cooling, 200 ml of 80% alcohol are added to the sugar-candy solution followed by the dextrin solution. The mixture is shaken and any impurities removed by decantation.

A few ml of this solution are poured on to a clean glass sheet and spread uniformly by tilting the sheet in all directions. Excess solution is drained off and the glass sheet dried in an oven at 37°. A number of such sheets may be prepared beforehand. The coating of sugar should be perfectly smooth and shiny.

Celloidin sections cut under alcohol are laid in order on strips of glazed paper and wetted with 70% alcohol. These strips may be kept in waiting, until cutting is over, by leaving them on a pad of filter paper soaked in 70% alcohol. When all strips are ready, they are placed in the desired order on the glass sheet with the sections against the layer of sugar. After covering the whole with filter paper the sections can be made to adhere to the sugar by exerting careful and uniform pressure ensuring that the sheet is placed on a perfectly plane surface. The strips of paper are removed cautiously, as in transferring, to leave the sections on the glass sheet. A 5% solution of celloidin is immediately laid over the sections and tilted as before to render the layer uniform. Drying until the celloidin solidifies produces a film of the desired consistency. The film is incised along three sides at a few mm from the edge and the sheet immersed into water, which dissolves the sugar. The film of celloidin easily detaches from the glass and remains fixed to it along the edge that was not incised. The series of sections can be stained using the glass sheet as support and the film need be cut out into fragments for mounting only at the time of clearing stained sections.

In the method of Levi, the celloidin sections are arranged on a slide taking care that their edges touch or overlap. They should be constantly moistened with 70% alcohol throughout the operation. When all the sections are disposed on the slide, they are covered with a pad of blotting paper and quite firmly, but evenly, pressed against the slide. The slide is immediately dipped in a tube containing a mixture of one part of absolute alcohol and four parts of ether for 20 seconds, at the most, before transferring to 70% alcohol where the celloidin coagulates. At the end of about 10 minutes the sections become joined to each other and firmly attached to the slide. The slide may then be hydrated and stained.

CUTTING AND HANDLING GELATIN SECTIONS

Gelatin blocks prepared according to the techniques of Heringa and ten Berge or of Baker are meant to be cut in a freezing microtome. Their treatment does not differ much from that of pieces which are not embedded and it will be discussed under the cutting of frozen sections. Only treatment of blocks made according to the technique of Apathy, dehydrated and impregnated with terpineol, will be described below.

Blocks are fixed with the gelatin used for embedding. A little quantity is applied to the wooden piece or object-holder and the block held pressed against it until the gelatin hardens. This sticking may be effected before impregnation with terpineol.

Cutting requires the use of a microtome with horizontal sliding. The cutting angle should be definitely less than that adopted for celloidin blocks (generally about 20°). The shape and the position of the piece are as in the case of celloidin blocks and cutting is similarly carried out under terpineol.

The *handling* and *sticking* of sections follow the practice recommended for celloidin sections cut under terpineol. Sections are stuck according to the technique of Apathy using two sheets of cigarette paper but care should be taken not to apply too much heat while coagulating the albumin-glycerin.

CUTTING AND HANDLING FROZEN SECTIONS

The cutting of frozen sections is an essential procedure with which every histologist should be familiar. While quite indispensable in some cases, where morphological or histological studies are intended as well as in the detection of enzymatic activity, it remains a very useful technique on several other occasions. Its role in neurohistological technique is to well known to be recalled here, and pathological diagnosis benefits much from it. Furthermore, many tissues that are difficult to cut after paraffin embedding are relatively well processed with a freezing microtome; it is thus with large bony pieces that are not fully demineralized and with pieces which are rich in cartilage. Even when the type and consistency of the pieces do not render frozen sections indispensable the time gained when compared to paraffin, and especially celloidin, sections can tempt the histologist to adopt this method of cutting sections.

Frozen sections can be made from fresh pieces or from fixed ones, whether they are embedded or not. Certain techniques of embedding in gelatin, described in the previous chapter, are specially meant for blocks to be cut with a freezing microtome. It should also be noted that the method can be applied to celloidin blocks that are not sufficiently hard to be cut in a microtome with a horizontal slide-way. According to some authors even pieces that are embedded in paraffin that is too soft may be cut in this way since the cooling causes it to harden.

The actual cutting of fresh pieces with a freezing microtome is not particularly difficult but the subsequent handling of sections is usually very laborious. Considerable progress has been achieved by techniques for cooling the razor and especially by placing the instrument in a chamber that can be cooled to the desired temperature. Since these methods are mainly applied in histochemistry they will be described in the chapter concerning histochemical fixation. Only sections made with the usual freezing microtome will be discussed here.

In theory, any microtome can be used to cut freezing sections, but in practice, the use of a Minot-type instrument, even when fitted with a special object-holder is better avoided. Microtomes with a horizontal slideway and with an object-holder that permits freezing the piece are more suitable, and of course the best solution is that of microtomes specially intended for the purpose.

In most cases the razor of a freezing microtome pivots around a vertical axis to which it is held by one of its ends while the other rests in a slideway or runs freely. Thus, during the to and fro movement controlled by hand each point of the cutting edge describes an arc. A micrometer screw ensures the upward progression of the object-holder before each sweep of the razor. The stage of the object-holder is hollow and pierced with a number of holes. Carbon dioxide arrives by a central tube. Certain models carry a second tube that sends a jet of carbon dioxide to cool the razor.

PREPARING BLOCKS

Pieces fixed in an aqueous medium may be cut after brief washing to remove the excess of fixative, while those fixed in alcohol or acetone should obviously be rehydrated before freezing. Gelatin blocks are treated as pieces that have not been embedded. There is no hard and fast rule about the shape of the blocks and in this respect more is tolerated that in any of the other techniques of cutting.

Fixing on to the stage of the object-holder is effected at the time of refrigeration by placing the piece, suitably oriented, on a large drop of water deposited on the stage and filling the central cavity with frost by the intermittent opening and closing of the tap that introduces carbon dioxide. Certain authors advise the use of a very dilute solution of gelatin instead of the drop of water in the case of gelatin blocks, but this precaution is not really necessary. Very small pieces that are difficult to position may be lodged in fragments of formalin-fixed mammalian liver. Covering the pieces with water which freezes during refrigeration is obviously pointless since such a support for sections is bound to disappear just when it is most useful, that is, during the transfer of cut sections into water.

The angle of attack of the razor should be slightly greater than the clearance angle. Many models of freezing microtomes do not provide any means to orient the razor in the clamp of the razor-holder. However, the necessary adjustement is easily made in adapting the hardness of the block to the given orientation of the razor by choosing the particular moment during the warming of frozen pieces to cut sections.

CUTTING SECTIONS

When the block adheres sufficiently to the stage it is covered with a plastic cup to avoid loss of carbon dioxide and the tap is opened by fits and starts until frost accumulates on the stage. The tap is then fully closed and one waits until the piece attains the suitable consistency for cutting.

This consistency depends on the nature of the tissue, the profile of the razor and the desired thickness of sections. As a rule the piece should be colder for thinner sections, for pieces rich in adipose tissue and for gelatin blocks.

In practice, one proceeds by trial and error. If the piece is too hard the sections break and fritter away when transferred into water. Conversely, soft pieces produce crushed sections which stick to each other on transferring. Clearly, an experienced worker is quicker than a novice in judging the moment when the consistency of a block is most propitious for the desired thickness of cutting. The choice of thickness depends not only on the type of work but also on the practical possibilities that are open and the consistency of the tissue. Subsequent treatments that the sections undergo should be taken into account when cutting. Even the histologist well trained in the use of a freezing microtome gains by not cutting sections too thin if the material is submitted to multiple reagents. Furthermore, some types of work require really thick sections and for this the freezing-microtome is ideal.

The behaviour of sections during cutting thus depends on the hardness of the block, that is, on its extent of cooling. If the block is too hard for a given orientation of the razor the sections break up and scatter. When slightly less hard they remain entire but still bounce off and may be recovered in a small dish of water held suitably in the left hand. When the block is allowed to warm further sections fold themselves somewhat and pile up on the upper side of the razor. They may be picked up, by running the pulp of the finger from the back of the razor towards the cutting edge, and plunged into water where they spread themselves out. It can be useful to add a small crystal of thymol to this water so that the change in surface tension facilitates unfolding of the sections. If serial sections are desired each section is removed individually before cutting the next one and set aside in a numbered dish or Petri dish.

Gelatin blocks prepared according to the technique of Heringa and ten Berge or that of Baker are cut like unembedded tissue. Satisfactory sections are generally obtained with further cooling than for unembedded tissue. Romeis (1948) advises freezing blocks, allowing them to thaw to room temperature and freezing them a second time before cutting sections. Sections are cut dry as in the case of unembedded tissue.

HANDLING AND STICKING SECTIONS

In most cases freezing sections are stained without sticking by transferring them from reagent to reagent contained in small dishes. Mounted needles, spatulas or glass rods drawn out and bent at the end are commonly used for transferring. Fishing out sections can be very tedious in deeply stained reagents. It is often convenient to use flat glass receptacles on a bright surface or to place a source of light underneath.

In any case sections have to be mounted on slides at some time or other. The most practical method is to place the section in a sufficiently large Petri dish containing water and to remove it on a clean slide thinly coated with albumin-glycerin. This slide, held in the left hand, is immersed into the water inclined at about 30° and the section carefully guided with a mounted needle held in the right hand. When the section is brought into contact with the slide the latter is carefully withdrawn from the water while holding a corner of the section in place with the needle.

Among the several methods of sticking freezing sections the best for cases where the embedding gelatin is not to be removed subsequently is that of Iwanoff (1936). Slides are coated with albumin-glycerin and dried for 24 hours in a paraffin oven. Sections are mounted on these slides in the way described above. The slide is laid flat on a perfectly level surface and covered with two strips of filter paper of suitable dimensions. A clean slide is laid over the filter paper and the sections made to adhere by applying careful and uniform pressure. The covering slide is removed and the area corresponding to the section soaked across the filter paper with a few drops of commercial formalin, if the sections are meant for detecting lipids, or absolute alcohol in other cases. The covering slide is relaid and careful pressure exerted a second time. After this it suffices to remove the covering slide, soak the filter-paper with drops of water and peel off the paper carefully, starting from one of the edges of the slide. The sections may then be treated without any further precaution.

Sections from blocks prepared according to Heringa and ten Berge should be stuck according to the procedure described by these authors. Slides are smeared with a 3% solution of gelatin followed by air drying and hardening in a 5% solution of sodium sulfate for two hours. Sections are placed on these slides, covered with strips of filter paper and then with another slide that is clean. Several such assemblies of slides carrying sections can be piled up on each other, held down with a small weight and left in an oven at 37° for about 10 minutes. After drying the whole assembly is immersed in warm water and held vertically. The filter paper detaches itself and the gelatin dissolves away, which can be followed by observing the slides by transparence. Prolonged stay in warm water can result in the sections detaching themselves as well.

Whatever the method of sticking adopted, frozen sections mounted on slides should be treated immediately afterwards. They run a serious risk of shrinkage if kept aside for more than a few hours. Unmounted sections can be stored in water for one or two days, adding a little formalin if necessary. In principle, this period of storage can be prolonged considerably by keeping sections under 10% formalin in well-stoppered bottles, but this manner of keeping material in reserve is of no practical interest.

CHAPTER 6

STAINING AND MOUNTING MICROSCOPICAL PREPARATIONS

> The method of staining, once having taken root in the animal histologist, grew and grew, till to be an histologist became practically synonymous with being a dyer, with this difference, that the professional dyer knew what he was about, while the histologist with few exceptions, did not know, nor does he to the present day.
>
> G. Mann (1902).

> On ne saurait donc trop répéter que les colorations ne sont pas toute l'histologie et que le premier devoir du micrographe n'est pas d'être un teinturier, mais de savoir regarder au microscope.
>
> M. Langeron (1949).

Although written at an interval of about half a century, the two quotations cited at the head of this chapter are still quite relevant. They stigmatize one of the erroneous attitudes of histologists when confronted with the problem of staining sections which results in an unbelievable crop of methods, modifications and variants that are really quite unnecessary. Paradoxically, the opposite excess is also widespread in the staining of sections, where largely outmoded methods enjoy a vogue that is almost impossible to understand and an unfortunately great number of histologists cling to them with a tenacity that is deserved of much better causes. This state of affairs can probably be explained by the established practice of a laboratory, habits learnt as a beginner and indifference towards what most biologists consider as a sort of "cookery" with no intellectual bearing. It however renders the task of compiling a work on histological technique arduous. From a rational point of view, the chaff is easily separated from the grain. Thus at present, there is no valid reason to maintain the fifteen odd formulae meant for the aluminium lake of haematin, and with a knowledge of two of them one is sufficiently well provided for against any eventuality. But the reader of any manual that claims to survey histological technique resorts to it not only for finding a formula that suits his own investigation, but also to be informed of a technique used elsewhere in the literature that he may be reading, and this is probably one of the reasons why many manuals carry an appreciable number of obsolete recipes.

The theory of the mechanism of staining has been the source of much vehement discussion; at present it seems impossible to single out a theory of staining. Even the very term "staining" is equivocal and its true significance subject to discussion.

The task of the histologist is equally difficult from the practical point of view. The chemical industry manufactures stains for histology more as a matter of prestige than as a source of profit. Several manufacturers do frankly admit to a wide variation in the level of the active principle from one batch to another of the samples of stains on sale. A most frightening synonymy further leads to all manner of misunderstanding and the qualities of a given stain, as stipulated by the user, cannot be expressed rigorously as in the case of a chemical compound. The present author is quite aware of the value of precisely indicating a particular mark of stain to be used with each method and indeed his first intention was to share with readers his personal experience gained from a quarter of a century of daily histological practice. However this cannot be achieved. In fact the direct sale of stains for histology by the manufacturer is more and more rare; important firms like Ciba, Bayer and Geigy have ceased to do so. At present most suppliers of stains for histology are only retailers, which considerably decreases the chances of stability from lot to lot, the quality of the products and, consequently, the reliability of the given specifications. Furthermore, "judging" the quality of a stain supplied by a commercial firm involves the methodical testing of several lots, and given in a published work it could have a wider bearing than warranted by the actual authority of the writer. The only ones who are really qualified for such an opinion are the various Commissions of standards such as those that function in the U.S.A., recognized officially and accepted by the chemical industry. Although no recommendations for or against any particular mark of stain will be given, the author insists on drawing the attention of histologists to the great importance of the quality of a dye-stuff in carrying out staining. Dye-stuffs should be systematically tested before being put into routine use, and for this it is very useful to keep a stock of "blank" slides carrying unstained sections and whose proper fixation has been verified on other sections off the same block.

DEFINITIONS AND NOMENCLATURE

As all authors observe, the staining of histological sections originated empirically and empiricism still plays an important role in its improvement. The aim of histological staining, in the wider sense of the term, is to overcome one of the principal drawbacks of examining fresh or fixed tissue, which is the lack of contrast between different structures when no other treatment has been applied. Staining, as practised for light microscopy, is thus meant to introduce artificially contrasts in amplitude between light rays that traverse the different parts of a preparation and to make them absorb different bands of the visible spectrum.

As taken in its widest sense, the term "staining" covers very different processes some of which are not really cases of staining. It seems proper to distinguish the following cases as Baker (1958) has done:

1° Injection of a coloured material into the natural cavities of the object; the typical example of this operation is injection into the circulatory system for morphological studies; it is not a stain in the strict sense although it renders the injected vessels coloured.

2° Fixation by athrocytary cells of coloured particles which are generally insoluble and do not stain; cells appear coloured in sections but their tint is not due to genuine staining.

3° Dissolving of a coloured substance that does not impart its colour in the structure to be stained; the general methods of detecting lipids are based on this principle; clearly such dissolving of a "lysochrome" (Baker) is not a case of true staining.

4° Absorption from a solution of a coloured compound that does not impart its stain; the staining of structures rich in proteins by Lugol's fluid is an example.

5° Formation *in situ* of a non-staining coloured compound of which the detection of iron is the best known example.

6° Formation *in situ* of a stain that is insoluble in the medium; the detection of polyphenols by the azoreaction is the best example.

7° Fixation by structures of a stain used in solution; this last is the only case of strict staining.

Thus, a distinction has to be made among three fundamental processes; the introduction into structures of coloured substances (some of which may be dye-stuffs on their own but which do not act in this capacity), coloured reactions where a coloured compound or stain is formed in the structure studied and, finally, staining which is based on the extraction by the structures of a stain from the medium.

The essential feature of the phenomenon of staining is this capacity to extract the stain from the medium which carries it, so that it can result in a diminution of the level of stain in the bath. Though such a definition applies equally well to the dyeing of textile fibres, the objectives of the two operations are quite different.

The dyeing industry aims at obtaining a hue that is as uniform as possible while the histologist's goal is a maximum of differential staining according to the structures. The chief common requirement of both industrial dyeing and histological staining is fastness, that is, the migration of stain from the bath and its stable fixation on to the stained structure and its resistance to light, acid, alkali, oxydation and reduction. They differ in that the type of resistance to handling, required of textile and leather goods, is of no importance to the histologist while the industrial dyer is little concerned with resistance to the attack of organic solvents such as alcohol and benzenic hydrocarbons.

The development of staining techniques has led to the creation of a certain number of terms that do not have their equivalent in industrial usage.

Thus, the term *bulk staining* (*stückfärbung* in German and *coloration en masse* in French) is used to describe the staining of pieces before they are cut into sections. The same terminology is extended to metal impregnation (*bulk impregnation*).

Section staining denotes methods applied after cutting, whether on sections that are stuck or not.

Instain mounting (*Einschlussfärbung*) the section or piece to be stained is mounted on a slide in the staining solution.

Direct staining (the substantive staining of German authors) does not require any particular preparation of the object before it takes stain from an aqueous or alcoholic solution. When the use of a mordant is necessary to obtain staining the term *indirect* or *mordant staining* (adjective staining of the Germans) is used.

In *progressive staining* the process is stopped when the structures take on the desired colour. In *regressive staining* the treatment is carried to well beyond this point, and the return process during which the final tint is obtained is called *differentiation*. The phenomenon of *toning* implies modification of a colour.

In *simple staining* only one dye-stuff is used, while several are involved in *compound staining* where they may act either *simultaneously* in the same bath or *successively* in different ones.

All stains in the strict sense of the term used in histological technique are organic compounds, most of them belonging to aromatic series. Their classification is hence based on their chemical constitution and in particular following the radicals that are directly responsible for their staining capacity. A brief account of present theories of staining is therefore necessary before going on to the classification of dyestuffs and the theory of histological staining.

GENERAL THEORY OF STAINING AND THE CLASSIFICATION OF STAINS

The chemistry of dyestuffs and the physical explanation of staining have made considerable progress since the fundamental work of Witt (1876). It cannot obviously be reviewed here. The work of Venkataraman (1952) contains a good number of purely chemical notions on the question, while those of Baker (1958) of Conn (1959) and of Harms (1965) are particularly intended for the histologist and they are an excellent introduction to a deeper study of the field.

It is well known that the absorption of light by a molecule produces a change in its energy that can be defined by the following formula:

$$\varepsilon_2 - \varepsilon_1 = h\gamma$$

where ε_1 and ε_2 are the energies before and after the absorption of light ("extinction") γ is the frequency of absorbed light and h is Planck's constant.

A compound appears coloured only if the difference $\varepsilon_2 - \varepsilon_1$ is such that the frequency of the light absorbed, or its wavelength, corresponds to a value that falls within the visible spectrum. In the case of saturated organic compounds absorption is in the short wavelength ultraviolet, while absorption in the near ultraviolet or the visible corresponds to the presence of radicals in the molecule which are called chromophores following the studies of Witt. Compounds that possess one or more chromophores used to be called chromogens but this term is rarely used now since the quite different sense attributed to it by industrial chemists leads to confusion.

Quite a large number of chromophore groups exist; Table 4 which is compiled from the data of Harms, carries the structural formulae for the chief chromophores found in stains used in histology.

Table 4. PRINCIPAL CHROMOPHORE GROUPS

anthraquinone	azine	azo-
azomethine	oxazine	triphenylmethane
cetimine	thiazine	xanthene
indamine	phthalocyanine	quinone

It should be noted that a compound bearing one or several chromophores can be coloured but the presence of such groups is not enough to make a stain of it. The absorption of certain chromophores such as the double and triple bond or the cetimine radical is in the ultraviolet as it is for the benzene ring; only the conjunction of these groups or another adjunctive function will displace the absorption towards the visible (bathochromatic shift). Furthermore, compounds carrying chromophores become stains only by the addition, to the molecule, of radicals called auxochromes.

Auxochromes do not act only by endowing a compound with a staining capacity; they often exert a marked bathochromatic effect. From the chemical point of view they are most often simple functions without double bonds, either polar or semi-polar. Hydroxyl, amino, carboxyl, cyanogenic and sulfonic radicals are the principal auxochromes.

Chemical radicals that are neither chromophores nor auxochromes can act by modifying the colour of a stain; examples of these are methyl, phenyl and several other functions.

Modern authors admit to a close relationship between the staining capacity of conjugated double bonds and their rapid change in molecular configuration (resonance) which plays on essential role in the absorption of electro-magnetic waves.

Double bonds due to mobile electrons are the cause of unsaturated radicals being chromophores since these radicals lie in a state that is intermediate between the two extremes of structure that are possible (mesomery).

The shift of maximal absorption towards longer wavelengths, due to chromophores, increases with the number of double bonds, that is, with the length of the chain of resonance between auxochrome groups.

The mere presence of a conjugated double bond implies a "resonance bond" only when the compound is unionized. Stains containing polar groups carry, in addition, a "resonance charge" which, according to present concepts, is essential for a chemical radical to play the role of an auxochrome. Auxochromes capable of donating electrons to a mesomeric system can thus be distinguished from others (anti-auxochromes) which, inversely, receive them. The introduction of sulfonic acid groups into a molecule clearly illustrates yet another type of ionization of a stain.

The classification of stains is first of all based on the nature of their auxochromes; it is on this that acidic stains are distinguished from basic stains, although the particular terms do not in any way implicate the pH of their solutions. Stains are said to be basic when the moiety of a molecule responsible for staining carries a positive charge and migrates towards the cathode during electrolysis like a metal ion; the anion of such a compound is of no importance as far as its staining capacity is concerned. On the other hand the functional moiety of an acidic stain carries a negative charge and migrates to the anode in electrolysis, while its cation does not directly affect staining. Basic stains are usually sold as chlorides or sulfates, while acidic stains are available as salts of sodium or calcium.

Amphoteric stains also exist but they are of minor importance in histological technique.

Neutral stains, however, are essential in histological technique. Introduced by Ehrlich in 1880, their principal characteristic is that both anion and cation are stains. They are usually prepared by mixing aqueous solutions of a basic and an acidic stain in suitable proportions. Neutral stains are often insoluble or sparsely soluble in water and they can hence be dissolved in an organic solvent (often ethanol or methanol) or in a solution of the acid stain from which they have been derived.

Another factor in the classification of stains is the chemical structure of the chromophores. The list given in the Appendix to this part of the book has been established on the basis of this factor along with the acidic or basic nature of the stain. Most of the compounds indicated by Conn (1959) figure in this list even though they may not be referred to elsewhere in the book so that the reader can identify a stain that appears in any other publication. A special effort has been made to group synonyms, but the author has no illusions of being either complete or infallible. The reader's attention is also drawn, in parts of the book that follow, to the annoying confusion that arises when ordering or choosing a given stain.

THEORIES OF HISTOLOGICAL STAINING

The histologist is mainly concerned with the mechanism by which structures take on stains, and this has given rise to interpretations that are as numerous as they are contradictory. Although dominated at first by purely chemical considerations the theory of histological staining was oriented during the first half of this century towards quite different concepts where physical factors were given much more importance than the chemical constitution of the stained structures. At present, this second period seems to be over; most authors admit that when based on solid experimental evidence there is no real opposition between chemical and physical theories of histological staining.

THE CHEMICAL THEORY

The interpretation, clearly enunciated by Ehrlich (1879, 1880, 1891) according to which the taking of stain by a structure is a chemical reaction, that is, the formation of a salt between the anion or cation of the stain and certain chemical functions of the structure, has had considerable impact on the evolution of histological research. It has given rise to some of the terms commonly used in the language of histologists. According to this, *basophil* structures are those that can fix basic stains (cationic) and hence possess acidic functions. *Acidophil* structures fix acidic stains (anionic) and consequently carry basic functions. A third type of tinctorial affinity, called *amphophily*, denotes structures that take both basic and acidic stains.

During the end of the 19th and the beginning of the 20th century, the chromatic analysis (*Farbenanalyse* of Ehrlich) of preparations was an important aspect of histological research and descriptions were based on the definition of the tinctorial affinities of various structures. I must note here that this method of studying tissues has brought about excellent achievements; when combined with a careful analysis of nuclear structures it provided morphological haematology with the basis of a rational classification of Vertebrate blood cells. There is indeed no chapter of histology which has not benefited greatly from a discerning application of chromatic analysis. However, it is none the less true that a certain excess has undeservedly brought discredit to chromatic analysis as witnessed by the violence with which those who reacted against such exaggeration detracted from the chemical theory of histological staining. The work of Unna is in this respect a characteristic example; the refinement and subtlety with which he practised chromatic analysis was clearly contrary to commonsense and was aimed at an end that was far beyond what could be reasonably hoped for at that time.

To-day, the chemical theory of histological staining, enhanced by modern advances in chemistry, retains all its relevance. Experiments with models afford quantitative confirmation and Harms (1965) quite justly emphasizes that it is not at all in disaccord with the electrostatic theory, that is, one of the most solidly based of the physical theories of staining.

THE CONCEPT OF STAINING BY IMBIBITION AND BY PRECIPITATION

Even though admitting to the notions of acidic and basic stains, V. Möllendorff (1923–1924) has been led to reject entirely those of basophily and acidiphily. This author goes to the extent of denying any relation between the chemical constitution of the stained structure and the final result of staining. According to him staining by imbibition *(Durchtränkungsfärbung)* is to be distinguished from staining by precipitation *(Niederschlagsfärbung)*. The first is characterized optically by its transparence and general luminosity; its colour corresponds exactly to that of the staining solution. As the term denotes, it is due to the penetration of the stain into all parts of the stained structure and the only factors that affect the final result are the texture of the tissues and the diffusion coefficient of the stain. According to V. Möllendorff both acidic and basic stains can give rise to this type of staining. Staining by precipitation is characterized optically by its granular and opaque appearance; its colour may often be quite different from that of the staining solution. It is caused by the precipitation of the stain and the particles resulting from this flocculation being fixed on to the acidic colloids that are found on the surface of the structures that take the stain. Thus, according to the ideas of V. Möllendorff, the factors affecting such staining are also purely physical; he also notes that only basic stains can bring about staining by precipitation.

In spite of the violent attacks from protagonists of the chemical theory (Unna 1923) the concepts of V. Möllendorff enjoyed a degree of popularity that appear surprising today. Most of his partisans seem to have forgotten, as Harms (1965 p. 1/52) has observed, that following one of the points asserted in the principal article where this theory is propounded the staining of chromatin in the nuclei represents the precipitation of basic stains on the surface of the nuclear scaffold. Zeiger (1930–1938) has already formulated serious reserves as to the basis of the theory of V. Möllendorff which is today only of historical interest.

ADSORPTION AS A FACTOR IN THE BINDING OF STAINS

Even at the time when the chemical theory of histological staining was almost universally admitted certain authors attributed an important role to surface phenomena in the binding of histological stains. This tendency was widespread when research on the physical chemistry of colloids underwent its well known development. Following Michaelis many histologists considered Van Der Waals forces as having an essential role in the phenomena of staining, while eschewing the idea of any real combination between the stain and its substrate. But this orientation did not bear much fruit and Michaelis himself proposed to take into account the electrochemical characteristics of stains and their substrate in studying the absorption of stains. This saw the beginning of the transition towards an electrostatical interpretation of histological staining, which of all the physical theories is in closest agreement with experimental data. It has already been mentioned that in fact it substantially agrees with the chemical theory.

ELECTROSTATIC ADSORPTION AS A MECHANISM IN HISTOLOGICAL STAINING

The experiments of Bethe (1905) showing the considerable influence of the pH of the staining solution on the result of staining with toluidine blue, point to the impossibility of explaining certain histological stainings by the interaction of Van Der Waals forces. In fact, the affinity of Mammalian tissues, fixed in alcohol, diminishes when the solution is acidified with sulfuric acid and increases when rendered alkaline with sodium hydroxide. It should be recalled here that adsorption due to Van der Waals forces cannot vary as a function of pH.

The findings of Bethe have largely contributed to the evolution of physical theories to explain histological staining. They form, in fact, the basis of the classical work of Pischinger (1926–1927) which affords an unequivocal interpretation of certain characteristics of proteins as substrates for histological staining. It turns out that acidic stains take on to protein structures when the pH of the staining solution is inferior to the isoelectric point of the tissue proteins; basic stains, on the other hand, bind when the pH is superior to this point. The basophily or acidophily of tissue proteins is thus explained by their amphoteric nature. Pischinger concludes that theoretically the essential factor for the basophily or acidophily of a structure is its electrostatic charge and he goes on to apply it in practice to determine the approximate isoelectric point of structures in a section of tissue by staining in solutions of a suitably chosen pH. In general, these findings explain why acidic stains take with a maximal intensity on to sections of tissue when they are used in acidified solutions and their selective preference for the more acidophilic structures increases when the staining solution is made alkaline. Inversely, basic stains are most intense and stain widely in an alkaline medium while they are selective in acid solutions.

As Harms (1965) has observed, electrostatic forces have the longest range (about 100 Å) as compared with what are called short-range forces, namely covalent bonds, hydrogen bonds and Van der Waals forces.

Thus a link has been established between the classical chemical theory of histological staining and the electrostatic theory. In fact the negative and positive charges of structures, of which one spoke towards 1940 to avoid using the terms basophily and acidophily, are ultimately a consequence of their chemical constitution. The balancing of charges, which according to the electrostatic theory is the basis of staining, corresponds quite exactly to what the chemist calls combination. It is thus quite justly that Harms (1965) adopts the opinion of Mann (1902) Liesegang (1924), and Vickerstaff (1950) according to which the physical and chemical phenomena that occur during histological staining are inseparably linked since they are only two different aspects of the same process.

THEORY OF INDIRECT STAINING

Staining by lakes, characterized by the use of a mordant in addition to the stain itself, has an important place in histological technique. These techniques may be applied in histology, as in the tanning industry, in three different ways. In certain cases the object to be stained is first treated with the mordant and later with the stain. They are examples of indirect staining in the strict sense and they may be carried out progressively or regressively; if regressive it involves differentiation. In other cases, the object is submitted directly to the action of the lake and staining is effected in a simple step. Finally, in the third type, rare in histological technique but frequent in industrial dyeing, the mordant acts after the stain.

The majority of stains used to prepare the lakes used in histological technique are amphoteric, while the lake itself is always basic. The practical advantages of staining by lakes are great since the stain, once obtained, is generally very intense and the lakes fixed to tissues are insoluble in most of the liquids used to treat preparations.

As Baker (1958) has noted, staining by lakes raises two problems from the theoretical point of view, namely, the mode of linkage between the stain and the mordant and the mode of binding of the mordant on to the stained structures.

Most mordants used in histological technique are salts of aluminium, iron, chromium or allied salts. Sulfates or alums (double sulfates) are generally used, but they may be replaced by other salts. The metals form complex ions in the solutions of mordants and they link to the stain by chelation, where the hydrogen atom of a hydroxyl of the staining molecule is replaced by the metal and a neighbouring electron-donor atom establishes a second bond with the metal. Experience shows that the addition of an acid to the lake in solution has a stabilizing effect but the actual mechanism of this stabilization, used for the first time by Ehrlich, is still obscure.

As to the fixation of the mordant to the structures to be stained, there is every reason to think that the phosphate radicals of nucleic acids and the carboxyls of amino acids play an essential role. This is particularly the conclusion drawn form a methodical investigation of Wigglesworth (1952) on the fixation of iron by animal tissues. It may be remarked here that deamination does not at all modify the distribution of metals provided by mordants, while methylation reduces it considerably.

In short, staining by lakes entails the formation of a complex between the stained structure, mordant and the stain.

The differentiation of regressive staining can be obtained either by the action of the mordant, by that of an acid or by oxydation. During differentiation by a mordant the distribution of stain between the tissue and the differentiating liquid can change because the latter is in great excess, so that structures may even be entirely destained when its quantity is sufficient and its action prolonged. Generally, certain structures remain stained while others would have yielded all stain to the differentiating medium depending on the quantity of lake accumulated and the strength of its linkage to structures.

However, the phenomena occurring during the differentiation of stains by certain lakes are more complex; the regressive iron-hematoxylin method is such an example since the final stain does not at all correspond to the affinity of structures for ferric ions.

In any case, this "balancing" of stain between the structures and the differentiating medium opens the possibility of devising lakes where the concentrations of stain and mordant in the solution are equilibrated to ensure the staining of certain structures while the background runs no risk of being overstained. Obviously such solutions are particularly advantageous for bulk staining.

The mechanism of differentiation by acids is more complicated since the lake-tissue bonds as well as the mordant-stain bonds are liable to be attacked. It is generally admitted that the hydrogen ions of the differentiating acid reconstitute ionized acid groups in the tissues when they come into contact with the mordant-stain complex. But, as Baker (1958) has remarked, these phenomena ought to be in fact more complex since the ultimate links between stained structures, metal and stain are not electrovalent. However, since differentiation, as practised by histologists, does not have its equivalent in the textile industry, progress in the techniques of dyeing is of no avail in resolving the difficulty of interpretation in this case.

Interpreting differentiation by oxidising agents is no less uncertain. Potassium permanganate and chromium trioxyde have been used as differentiators and it may appear at first sight that their effect consists in transforming the stain into a colourless compound; regions of heavy accumulation would then be conspicuous against a light background. Other compounds such as picric acid and potassium ferricyanide have also been used but their mechanism of action is unknown. It should not be forgotten that both picric acid and chromium trioxyde are acidic as well as oxidants so that the two properties may be involved in differentiation.

Apart from the above mordants, whose metal takes part in complexing with the stain, other substances that many histologists include among the mordants, but whose mode of action is probably different, should also be mentioned. They are compounds that serve either to render the stain insoluble and which do not play a role in the binding of stain, or that stabilize the staining and give it resistance to subsequent treatment. The most commonly used of such compounds are tannin, iodine, picric acid, mercuric chloride and mercuric iodide. Most efforts to explain the mechanism by which these compounds act have not lead to any definite conclusions. Some of these agents (mercuric chloride, mercuric iodide, ammonium molybdate) do contain metals which, however, do not seem to act as in the case of genuine mordants. Insolubilization by these agents is restricted to basic stains and both the hypotheses put forward admit either immediate precipitation as soon as they enter into solution or the formation of a true complex with the insolubilizing agent.

THE DENSITY OF STRUCTURES AS A FACTOR IN HISTOLOGICAL STAINING

Apart from the factors reviewed above the density of structures, in the physical sense, also influences staining. Thus the presence of a greater quantity of stainable matter results in more intense staining during the progressive method and slower extraction in the case of the regressive one. This is the explanation of the selective staining of elastic fibres by orcein, an amphoteric stain that has not the slightest chemical affinity for elastin.

THE TEXTURE OF TISSUE CONSTITUENTS AND THEIR PENETRATION BY STAINS

Leaving aside the actual phenomenon of staining, that is, the binding of stain to structures, the ease with which particles of stain penetrate into a structure also influences the final result. This fact, clearly enunciated by Ehrlich in 1879, is invoked to explain the results of staining histological preparations with mixtures of acidic stains such as in the detection of collagen fibres. Experimental proof in favour of this interpretation has been provided by Collin (1923–1924) v. Möllendorff and Tomita (1926) and Seki (1932). Mann's stain (a mixture of methyl blue and eosin) applied to gelatin smears gives a blue colour if the gelatin solution that is smeared is dilute and red if it is concentrated. More diffusible stains therefore penetrate into more compact structures, while less diffusible ones enter only when the texture is less dense.

Diffusion coefficients measured by Seki actually show them to be less for the usual stains of collagen fibres than for those of the cytoplasm. According to its association with other stains, a given stain can turn out to be the most or the least diffusible of the mixture used. Thus acid fuchsin, which is associated with aniline blue in Masson's trichromic method, stains the cytoplasm while in Van Gieson's method, where it acts with picric acid, it stains collagen fibres.

The conditions of penetration of a stain can be modified by various factors, one of which is the temperature of staining; this explains the staining of the chondriosomes with acid fuchsin in Altmann's technique.

Apart from histochemical methods where the final colour acquired by structures is the result of a chemical reaction, other factors as varied as chemical affinity, density and texture of structures are involved in determining staining. Great prudence is therefore required in any attempt at interpretation, especially when the intensity of staining has to be estimated.

GENERAL REMARKS ON THE PRACTICE OF STAINING

The procedures for carrying out histological staining are so numerous and diverse that only a few general comments will be made here. In fact, the staining of microscopical preparations is a long series of particular cases ranging from histochemical methods that can be standardized as rigorously as most methods of quantitative analysis to quite empirical methods influenced by factors that are still obscure. Only the general rules concerning the choice of stains, preparation of solutions, deparaffining and hydration of sections, that are common to most techniques, will be discussed here.

CHOICE OF STAINS

The difficulties mentioned in the introduction to this chapter show the importance of the choice of stains and the danger to which a histologist exposes himself if he does not look into the qualities of a dye-stuff when it enters into a preparation. Products on sale are practically never definite chemical compounds as such. Their level of impurities, as also their nature, can vary from one lot to another of the same manufacturer and even more so among retailers; precise analytical criteria, as applied to the verification of pure chemical compounds, cannot be defined for stains. Spectroscopy, chromatography and other microanalytical techniques of routine do not offer sufficient guarantee in the case of stains and the only reliable test is its actual use by a competent histologist in the staining for which it is intended. It should be emphasized that stains which are quite suitable for a given method can be of no use in another. Thus, the U.S. Commission of Standards for biological stains delivers its certificates of guarantee only with respect to a defined use for a stain and most suppliers state the use for which a stain is meant on the label.

Apart from the opinion of colleagues, the best way to choose stains is to try them systematically and build up a stock of products whose quality has been verified experimentally. Contrary to a somewhat pessimistic view of Lillie (1954) most stains keep well if they are kept in well-stoppered bottles way from sunlight and extremes of temperatures. Of the twenty odd samples of methyl green and pyronin that I have had the occasion to use none was as good as that given to me by my teacher of clinical haematology, the late Professor Ch. Aubertin; these stains were purchased in 1902!

I have already pointed out the usefulness of having at one's disposal a collection of slides carrying sections on which stains and methods of staining can be tried out.

PREPARATION OF SOLUTIONS

The solutions of stains used in histological technique are mostly aqueous or alcoholic; other solvents are mainly restricted to histochemical reactions.

The choice of glassware and the chemical purity of solvents and ingredients are not as exacting as in analytical chemistry. It is however better to use glass of good quality; hard glass or storage in paraffined glassware is necessary in certain cases. All glassware should be thoroughly rid of the slightest trace of synthetic detersives; it is in fact best to avoid their use entirely. It is generally unnecessary to weigh ingredients in a precision balance; a good simple one would do except in cases where very small quantities of stain are prepared. Similarly, a measuring cylinder suffices for liquid volumes.

The order in which the various products are dissolved is of no importance in certain cases while it can be essential in others. It is best to always follow the order as given in the formula.

Certain stains can be used as soon as they are prepared; others contain compounds that dissolve very slowly while yet others require a certain amount of "ripening".

The storage of solutions of stains can vary according to the case; apart from the nature of the products, the influence of the physical conditions reigning in the laboratory is far from negligible. There exist solutions that can be stored almost indefinitely while others have to be prepared afresh each time.

The most important of the consequences is that the practice of staining calls for real planning and that there is no question of following an impulse of the moment. A histologist worthy of his name should see that he has constituted a stock of solutions that require ripening, such as haematoxylin and safranin, well ahead of time.

The above remarks on the storage of solutions quite clearly hold only for those that are not in constant use. Thus the stablest of solutions can undergo a certain dilution every time a section is introduced since the latter is never perfectly dry; inversely, every lot of sections treated will remove a quantity of the active dye-stuff that enters into the staining reaction as well as a certain volume of solution carried over mechanically.

Consequently, the loss of stain from dishes or tubes in use is much more rapid than from storage bottles. Furthermore, in spite of rinsing between solutions, there is always the inevitable contamination with the previous one, so that frequent renewal becomes necessary.

Apart from these factors, the cost of various stains is of secondary importance in determining the quantity of solution to be prepared at a time, since really expensive stains for sections are rare. This is however not so for certain histochemical reactions. The quantity of staining solution to be prepared at a time finally depends on its expected utilization and its storage properties.

GLASSWARE

Bulk staining can be carried out, according to the time required, in well-stoppered tubes, in covered or open staining dishes of adequate size or in Petri dishes. They can also be used for staining free sections which are manipulated with spatulas, rods of synthetic resin or glass rods with a bent tip drawn out in a flame. Obviously, the size of the staining vessel should be such that the sections can be easily removed from the solution. Large vessels (such as Petri dishes) containing a sufficient layer of liquid, but not too high, are the most suitable.

Sections that are fixed to slides may be stained by laying them on parallel rods (S-shaped glass rods or bent rods joined with rubber tubing) that are placed over a dish and pouring the staining solution over them. The operation is usually called *staining on slides*. It cannot be practised when the staining solution or histochemical reagent is volatile or when it has to act for a long time. Staining on slides can be rendered obligatory by the cost of reagents which can be so expensive for certain histochemical reagents that the quantity of solution used should be reduced by tracing a circle of paraffin or vaseline around sections after deparaffining them or by fixing sections to coverslips and treating them in very small dishes. If the staining or histochemical reaction is to be carried out with warming or when the treatment is very prolonged, it is best to use a moist chamber that is easily improvised. A layer of filter paper well imbibed with the solvent is laid at the bottom of a Petri dish. Two short glass rods on the paper carry the slide covered with the stain or reagent and the whole covered with the lid of the Petri dish.

In most cases, slides are stained by immersion in solutions. A large number of receptacles have been devised for the purpose. Jolly's tubes (a single slide or two back to back) Borrel's cylinders (three slides or six back to back in pairs) or various other models with grooves are used according to the quantity of solution and the number of slides to be stained. A convenient method of holding slides during transfer is to insert them by one end between the helices of a suitably sized brass spring; the level of liquid in receptacles should then be such that it does not come into contact with the spring. Of the various grooved receptacles available, I advise the use of Coplin jars which hold 5 slides, or 10 back to back, and which require 50 ml of liquid to attain a sufficient level even when the slides are fully covered with sections. There also exist metal or glass holders that carry a varying number of slides and which serve to transfer them through a series of rectangular vessels containing the different solutions; such an operating method is particularly recommended for large numbers of slides that do not require checking under the microscope and which can undergo a certain delay before mounting. It is however better not to place slides back to back as residual liquid can be trapped between slides and washing between treatments necessitates dismantling the series, for otherwise considerable contamination of solutions will result.

DEPARAFFINING SECTIONS

But for very rare exceptions, paraffin sections stuck to slides should be freed of the embedding substance before they can be submitted to stains or histochemical reagents. The removal of paraffin is brought about by various substances of which the most commonly used ones are the benzenic hydrocarbons. As in the case of clearing pieces there is really no reason to prefer xylene in place of toluene or benzene. The time required for dissolving away the paraffin depends evidently on the quantity of solvent and the quantity of paraffin, that is, the thickness and number of sections, as well as the temperature. A few minutes suffice usually.

I must emphasize the need for a complete removal of paraffin before any further treatment of the sections; any irregularity in deparaffining leads to uneven staining and several stains and histochemical reagents do not penetrate well into sections that are incompletely deparaffined. As a result each slide should be passed through at least two baths of solvent and these baths should be renewed quite often.

Deparaffining with solvents other than the benzenic hydrocarbons is resorted to only exceptionally and these techniques will be referred to elsewhere in the relevant chapters of this book.

Sections from bulk-stained material can be mounted directly after deparaffining following procedures that will be described in a later paragraph. The same is possible with metal impregnations which do not require their colour to be toned. In all other cases deparaffining should be completed by the removal of the benzenic hydrocarbon used to dissolve the paraffin. In the great majority of cases, absolute alcohol is used for this. The practice of dipping slides, after deparaffining, into a bath of absolute alcohol is evidently unsuitable. The absolute alcohol should, instead, be dropped from a drop-bottle on to both sides of the slide inclined at about 30°. A few drops on each face are enough. In those very rare cases where sections should not be treated with alcohol, the benzenic hydrocarbon can be removed with acetone.

Most authors recommend that the treatment with absolute alcohol be followed by baths in decreasing concentrations of ethanol in water. I wish to formally insist that this is quite pointless. In fact, sections may be transferred directly from absolute alcohol into water without their structures undergoing the slightest damage. It is however useful to insert, between the absolute alcohol and water, a bath of a mixture of alcohol and formalin (9 volumes of 96° alcohol and 1 volume of commercial formalin) whose purpose is to completely tan the gelatin or the albumin used to stick sections. Obviously, sections passed through acetone after deparaffining do not undergo this treatment but are transferred directly into water.

It is at the time of deparaffining that two other procedures have to be carried out if necessary, namely, collodioning sections and the removal of crystals of corrosive sublimate that accumulate during fixation with a fluid containing mercury salts.

COLLODIONING SECTIONS

The aim of this operation is to coat the slide with a thin layer of nitrocellulose and thus ensure the adherence of sections. It is very useful when sections are thick or when they contain bony or cartilagenous tissue, much muscle or cuticular formations which give a tendency for sections to detach themselves easily. Collodion is not recommended only in a very small number of cases where certain compounds used in staining or histochemical reactions do not penetrate the film easily.

For collodioning to be efficacious it has to be carried out on slides that are entirely dehydrated and the film produced should be as thin as possible. The slightest trace of water between the film and the slide is enough for the film to be detached and to render the operation useless. A film that is too thick also tends to detach and can even carry away the sections with it if they have not been fixed well enough at the time of spreading.

Collodioning is carried out immediately after deparaffining. The best way to perform it is to dip the slides as they come out of the second bath in the benzenic hydrocarbon into a vessel (Borrel cylinder or other wide-mouthed bottle) containing a 0.1% solution of collodion in a mixture of equal parts of alcohol and ether (24.5 volume of absolute alcohol, 24.5 volume of ether, 1 volume of 5% commercial collodion). The slides are left for 2 minutes, then removed *slowly* so that all excess collodion drains off and held vertically until they are half-dried in air (which may be verified by observing slides in oblique light). As soon as this stage is attained they are plunged into the 96° alcohol-formalin mixture mentioned above which hardens the film of collodion and tans the albumin or gelatin used for sticking at the same time.

DISSOLVING CRYSTALS OF MERCURY

This operation is intended for sections made from pieces fixed in liquids containing mercury salts. It is also recommended for pieces that have been treated with iodine-alcohol during dehydration. Slides taken out of the alcohol-formalin mixture are rapidly rinsed in tap-water and dipped for about 30 seconds in Lugol's liquid (1 g of iodine, 2 g of potassium iodide, 100 ml of distilled water). They are then rapidly rinsed in water and placed in a bath of 5% sodium hyposulfite until the yellow colour after treatment with Lugol's liquid is bleached. Excess sodium hyposulfite is removed by thorough washing in tap-water before the sections are ready for staining.

Crystals of mercury are removed in the same manner from celloidin, gelatin and frozen sections, whether stuck to slides or free. Both celloidin and gelatin sections that are fixed to slides before staining are treated like paraffin sections. Celloidin and frozen sections that are free are passed through Lugol's liquid and sodium hyposulfite after hydration.

SUMMARY OF OPERATIONS PRECEDING THE STAINING OF SECTIONS

Apart from paraffin sections that should not be treated with alcohol, staining in other cases should be preceded by the following precedure:

1° **Paraffin sections**

Xylene, benzene or toluene   2 baths of about 2 minutes
Pour absolute alcohol on both sides of the slide or apply collodion.
96% alcohol-formalin   1 bath of 2 minutes
Tap-water   1 bath of 1 minute.
Removal of sublimate crystals if necessary
Running water   2 to 5 minutes.

2° Celloidin or gelatin sections fixed to slides

Tap-water	2 minutes or more
Removal of sublimate crystals if necessary.	
Running water	2 to 5 minutes.

3° Free celloidin or frozen sections

Tap-water	2 minutes or more
Removal of sublimate crystals if necessary	
Tap-water	3 to 4 baths of 1 minute.

MOUNTING MEDIA MISCIBLE IN WATER

All these media have the common advantage of not requiring the dehydration of sections. They are therefore suitable in all cases where it is desired to conserve stains or histochemical reactions that do not resist alcohol and the benzenic hydrocarbons that are intermediates between the dehydrating alcohol and the mounting medium immiscible with water. This advantage is counterbalanced by disadvantages that are far from negligible. Most media miscible in water do not acquire the consistency of other media and some of them show a tendency to crystallize. Hence it is necessary to lute the final preparation. Their refractive index is much lower than that of media that require dehydration, which is disadvantageous with stained sections. Many stains, especially the haematoxylin lakes and the basic blues of the thiazine group, are badly conserved in these media. Furthermore, it is difficult to remove air bubbles from media miscible in water since they show no tendency to disappear spontaneously as in certain media immiscible in water.

Certain media of this group are liquid and remain so. This is the case with glycerine which can be used pure, diluted with water if shrinkage of sections is expected, or saturated with cadmium chloride, chloral hydrate or zinc iodide if its refractive index is to be raised. The conservation of most stains in such media is quite mediocre and hence is rarely adopted for permanent preparations.

The technique of mounting in glycerine is very simple. After washing in water the slide is laid flat on a plane surface with sections turned upwards. Drops of glycerine, pure, diluted or containing the above metallic salts, are deposited on the sections. A drop of the same medium is laid on a suitable coverslip. This coverslip, with the drop downwards, is brought close enough to the slide so that the drop comes into contact with those on the section. When contact is established one edge of the coverslip is applied to the slide and the opposite edge lowered very slowly to allow all the air bubbles to escape. It is evidently better to correctly estimate the quantity of medium required so any overflow beyond the coverslip is avoided. If it does overflow, it should be immediately wiped off with strips of filter paper as any traces of it prevent luting the preparation.

Other mounting media are liquid at room temperature, but tend to more or less harden by evaporation of the solvent. These are the most commonly used ones.

Apathy's syrup (1892) is prepared by dissolving in a water-bath, 50 g of gum arabic (very pure and transparent pieces) and 50 g of cane sugar (uncandied) in 50 ml of distilled water. One ml of formalin or 0.5 g of thymol is added to check microbial growth. Impurities, if any, in the gum arabic are removed by decantation or even by centrifugation since the consistency of the medium does not permit filtration by the usual means. Most specialized suppliers sell Apathy's syrup ready for use. I advise the purchase of small-sized bottles as frequent opening clearly increases the chances of deterioration. The technique of mounting is the same as for glycerine. Preparations may be dried in an oven at 37° after mounting. The syrup hardens in 24 to 48 hours and the slides can then be luted.

The glycerine gum of Farrants (1880) is prepared by dissolving 30 g of very pure gum arabic in 30 ml of distilled water and adding 30 ml of glycerine after it is dissolved; 0.1 g of arsenic trioxide may be added to conserve the solution.

Laevulose syrup is prepared by dissolving 30 g of pure fructose in 20 ml of distilled water and allowing the solution to settle in an open bottle for 24 hours in an oven at 37°. The time taken for hardening is as in the case of Apathy's syrup. The basic blue stains and carmine are well conserved, while the haematoxylin lakes are not.

Some histologists prefer mounting media that are solid at room temperature; warm mounting is therefore required, but drying before luting must be at room temperature.

Gelatinized glycerine (Kaiser 1880) is prepared by soaking 7 g of pure gelatin for 2 hours in 42 ml of distilled water. 50 g of glycerine and 0.5 g of phenol are added afterwards and the mixture heated in a water-bath till it is dissolved. The solution is filtered over glass wool, preferably in a warm funnel. Preparations are mounted by depositing drops of warmed medium on the slide and coverslip or by melting small pieces of the solidified medium placed on the slide and coverslip and holding both on a hot plate. Solidification on cooling is quite rapid. This medium enjoys a certain vogue and many dealers supply it ready for use. I advise against its use since it is probably the one, of all the media discussed here, that destroys nuclear stains by haematoxylin lakes the most rapidly.

The gelatinized balsam of Heringa and ten Berge (1923) is much preferable to gelatinized glycerine but it is not available commercially and it is probably the need to prepare it oneself that has dissuaded most users. 20 g of fructose are dissolved in 15 ml of distilled water in a water-bath at 55°. After dissolving, 1.125 g of gelatin are added and left to soak.

Further heating at 50° is followed by adding 0.075 g of potassium alum and filtering when it is warm. Before use, 1 ml of this mass, which can be kept fluid in a well-stoppered bottle in an oven at 37°, is taken and 2 drops of commercial formalin are added. From this point onwards the medium should not be allowed to cool as it is difficult to return it to the liquid state. Mounting is carried out on a hot plate at about 35°. Solidification is rapid and slides can be luted after 24 hours of drying at room temperature.

Certain water-miscible mounting media, whose exact composition is not always indicated, are available on the market. Some of them give very good results. That sold under the trade name of *Karion F* or *Sorbitol F* is a solution of sorbitol and is particularly suitable for conserving sections stained with the basic blues or with pseudo-isocyanine.

MOUNTING MEDIA MISCIBLE WITH ALCOHOL

The mounting media of this group require the dehydration of preparations in alcohol going up to 80 or 95%. Their use is therefore indicated when it is desired to avoid the use of absolute alcohol and the benzenic hydrocarbons necessary for mounting in Canada balsam or equivalent synthetic resins.

The most frequently used mounting medium that is miscible with alcohol is euparal (Gilson 1906) a mixture of gum sandarac, Camsal, eucalyptol and paraldehyde in unspecified proportions; it is sold ready-made. Slides coming from 80% alcohol, or better 95% alcohol, are ready to be mounted. Mounting itself is carried out as in the case of media miscible with water. It dries very rapidly and luting is unnecessary. According to all authors the conservation of most stains and histochemical reactions is excellent. The chief advantage of mounting in euparal is that the dehydration of free celloidin sections in absolute alcohol is avoided, and it is essentially meant for this purpose. Edges of the coverslip should be cleaned immediately since any excess euparal is very difficult to remove once it has dried.

MOUNTING MEDIA MISCIBLE WITH BENZENIC HYDROCARBONS

These media, of which Canada balsam is typical, require not only complete dehydration of sections but also impregnation with a solvent of the mounting substance which is often a benzenic hydrocarbon.

In addition to Canada balsam, dammar and a large number of synthetic resins are supplied as solutions of varying thickness in benzenic hydrocarbons or other solvents miscible with them.

In fact Canada balsam should have long since disappeared from histological practice since dammar and especially the synthetic resins are far superior. Their chemical inertness ensures much better conservation of all stains and the practical procedure is the same as for Canada balsam. I must also add that synthetic resins do not show a tendency to turn yellowish with time as does Canada balsam and that their cost is not particularly high. In addition to a lack of information, the difficulties of procuring them is probably a reason why they are not so frequently used by the European worker.

As I have remarked earlier, mounting in these resins calls for an impeccable dehydration of sections. Apart from special cases (Pappenheim's panchrome and certain histochemical reactions) paraffin sections are dehydrated in ethanol. In all cases where the technique of staining does not include a final differentiation in an alcoholic medium, this dehydration can be carried out directly in absolute alcohol. The use of increasing concentrations of alcohol is one of the legends that has firmly taken root in the minds of users, but has no solid basis. I formally advise against the practice of dehydrating in tubes or dishes where slides are introduced in holders. Slides to be dehydrated should be handled one by one; if they have been stained back to back they should be separated to avoid carrying over trapped water into the benzenic hydrocarbon used for clearing. The slide should therefore be held in the left hand inclined at about 30° and absolute alcohol dropped from a drop-bottle on to both sides of the slide so as to remove all traces of excess stain, rinsing liquid and water. After dehydration the slide is immediately immersed into a Borrel tube or a dish containing clean benzene, toluene or xylene. Defective dehydration is betrayed by the appearance of milky streaks on the slide and a lack of complete transparency of the sections; if the quantity of water is great the cloudiness can spread to the benzenic hydrocarbon as well. It evidently calls for renewed dehydration and a change of the clearing bath. After clearing, the slide is transferred to a fresh bath of the same hydrocarbon to remove the last traces of alcohol. The clearing baths should be renewed frequently since one of the conditions for a good conservation of sections is the complete elimination of alcohol before mounting.

Actual mounting can be practised as with the other media described above, but experience has shown it to be advantageous if performed warm. The following procedure has given me excellent results.

A hot plate adjusted to about 50° is covered with the required number of coverslips. A drop of Canada balsam, or better, a chosen synthetic resin (Caedax, Depex, Lustrex, Lustron, etc...; see Lillie, 1954, for information on the chemical composition of these commercial products) is deposited on each coverslip. The slides are removed one by one from the last clearing bath and brought, face downwards, into contact with the drop of medium and as soon as contact is made it is turned over and laid on the plate. During this operation, the coverslip is carried up by the slide along with the drop of medium, if of course the surface of the plate is clean. The mounting medium now spreads quickly and uniformly. Slides may be dried without any further precaution at 45–50° for 24 to 48 hours. I however recommend a preliminary cleaning immediately after mounting to remove excess medium and air bubbles if any. For this, the slide is held at one end between the index and thumb of the left hand and *very mild* pressure exerted on the coverslip with the right index to squeeze out excess medium. Then while firmly holding the coverslip in place with the left thumb the slide is plunged into a tube containing benzene or toluene; the whole surface of the slide can then be cleaned with a soft lint-free rag held in the right hand, except the zone of the slide actually held in the fingers of the left hand. This too may be cleaned after shifting the point of contact of the fingers, but any slipping of the coverslip should be carefully avoided.

When the dehydration of stained sections with absolute alcohol is to be avoided acetone or phenolic benzene (10 g of phenol for 100 ml of benzene) can be used instead. Slides can go from water to acetone. With phenolic benzene it is better to start dehydration by 80% alcohol or to replace it by carefully blotting stained sections on a pad of filter-paper as described for the sticking of paraffin sections. Blotting can be useful even when sections are dehydrated in absolute alcohol; it should be practised whenever the stains used badly withstand treatment in weak alcohol.

Substituting terpineol for absolute alcohol is especially indicated in the case of staining free celloidin sections.

The availability of synthetic resins has rendered pointless the use of oxidized balsam, as described by P. Masson, to improve the conservation of sections. This method consisted of dipping slides carrying sections into a dilute solution of Canada balsam in toluene or benzene and allowing them to dry protected from dust after having wiped the slides all around the sections. Final mounting in thick balsam was done only later. But this procedure can still be useful in mounting sections covered with a thick and irregular layer of celloidin or slides carrying autoradiographs. The stay in dilute balsam should then last 5 to 10 minutes and the drying for 24 hours in a dust-free atmosphere.

When frozen sections or free celloidin sections are to be mounted in balsam or a synthetic resin they are spread on to slides in 80% alcohol. The slides are blotted and covered with 96% alcohol followed by phenolic benzene or terpineol. After complete clearing of sections they are mounted as described above.

SUMMARY OF DIFFERENT MOUNTING PROCEDURES

The chief indication for mounting in a water-miscible medium is the impossibility of dehydrating with alcohol. Media miscible in alcohol are indicated especially when sections cannot withstand absolute alcohol (free celloidin sections). In all other cases synthetic resins soluble in benzene hydrocarbons should be preferred.

1° *Paraffin sections fixed to slides and which can be dehydrated in alcohol.*—Wipe off the rinsing liquid used to terminate staining from around the sections and blot if necessary.

Drop absolute alcohol on to both sides of the slide till dehydration is complete (generally a very small quantity suffices).

Immerse immediately in two baths of benzene or toluene. The second clearing bath can be used for a long stay if necessary.

Prepare a suitable coverslip with a drop of mounting resin on a hot-plate.

Take the slide out of the second clearing bath, bring the slide carrying sections into contact with the drop of resin on the coverslip, turn it over and lay it on the hot-plate as soon as the coverslip adheres to the slide. Allow the resin to spread by itself.

Remove excess resin and air bubbles by carefully pressing with the pulp of the finger, clean the preparation while holding the coverslip firmly in place and dry in an oven at 45° or 50° for 24 to 48 hours.

2° *Paraffin sections to be dehydrated in acetone.* — Wipe and blot sections as before.

Dip the slide into two baths of acetone of two minutes each (acetone is too volatile to be used from a drop-bottle).

Clear in benzene and mount in balsam as before.

3° *Celloidin sections, gelatin sections according to Apathy or frozen sections that can be dehydrated in alcohol.* — Proceed as for paraffin sections but replace absolute alcohol with terpineol or phenolic benzene.

4° *Free celloidin sections.* — Spread sections on slides in 80% alcohol, cover with strips of filter paper and blot carefully.

Pour 96% alcohol immediately, leave for 2 to 3 minutes and drain off excess.

Pour toluene or phenolic benzene and leave for 2 to 3 minutes.

Repeat the treatment and leave until complete clearing.

Add pure benzene or toluene, renew it and drain off excess of clearing medium. Lay the required quantity of mounting resin over the section.

Cover immediately with a coverslip and lay the slide on a hot-plate to quicken spreading of the resin.

Clean and dry as for paraffin sections.

5° *Mounting celloidin sections in euparal.* — Proceed as above up to and including 96% alcohol.

Lay a suitable quantity of euparal on the sections.

Cover with a coverslip and place on a hot-plate for spreading.

Clean with a rag soaked in 96% alcohol and dry as for paraffin sections.

6° *Paraffin sections to be mounted in media miscible in water.* — Wipe off the last wash after staining from around the sections and blot them if necessary.

Lay drops of the chosen mounting medium on the sections.

Operate on a hot-plate for gelatinized glycerine or gelatinized balsam, in the cold for other media.

Place a drop of suitable size of the same medium on a coverslip.

Bring the drops on slide and coverslip into contact and gradually lower the coverslip.

After the medium is fully spread, clean with a rag soaked in water and dry.

7° *Free frozen sections to be mounted in a medium miscible with water*. — After the last wash following staining the sections are spread on slides in tap water or distilled water.

Clean around the sections and blot them carefully if necessary.

Cover immediately with a drop of mounting medium.

Lay a second drop of medium on the lower slide of a coverslip, bring the drops into contact and place the slide on a hot-plate to hasten spreading.

Clean the edges of the preparation without exerting any pressure on the coverslip and dry.

LUTING OF PREPARATIONS

This operation which is useful only after mounting in a water-miscible medium is meant to seal off the preparation and guarantee against any subsequent crystallization of the medium, a major drawback that can render the most satisfactory preparations of no use.

Several old lutes, the best known of which is that of Rondeau du Noyer, have given place to enamel paints and cellulose varnishes, like nail varnish, that are now available on the market and which I strongly recommend.

Perfect dryness of the edges of the coverslip and the adjacent zones of the slide is the chief condition for successful luting. The procedure itself is of the greatest simplicity; a layer of enamel paint or varnish is applied around the edge of the coverslip so that it covers the surrounding zone of the slide as well. Drying is very rapid.

CONSERVATION OF MICROSCOPICAL PREPARATIONS

Recent preparations should be stored flat; this can be done with grooved boxes as well if the whole box is maintained vertically. After a few weeks they may be stored in any position whatever. It is preferable not to pile up in boxes or drawers any preparations before six months.

A large number of filing systems have been devised for the histologist, from cardboard boxes with hollows for about twenty slides to large cabinets with trays for fresh preparations, drawers in a spiral for those a few weeks old and drawers of different sizes in which dry slides may be piled up. The classical grooved boxes have the advantage that preparations concerning particular investigations can be grouped in each one separately. The large cabinets are really useful only to store thousands of slides separately, each slide being denoted by a serial number.

In all cases microscopical preparations should be stored away from direct sunlight, it is indeed preferable to replace them in the dark after examination under the microscope. After each examination under immersion oil the slide should be carefully cleaned before putting it back into its box or drawer. That slides should be protected from dust is too evident to be insisted upon.

CHAPTER 7

THE EXAMINATION OF HISTOLOGICAL PREPARATIONS

> ...le passage que toute science naturelle doit accomplir un jour ou l'autre et qui indique la transformation d'une science dans l'enfance en une science adulte, à savoir le passage du qualitatif au quantitatif.
>
> L. Lison (1960).

Examination under the microscope is the goal of histological technique. It can never bear too much repetition that perfect preparations from the technical point of view are hopelessly useless if they are not exploited as they should be. But examination under a microscope is an art that is both difficult to learn and difficult to teach.

Some of these difficulties concern manipulating the instrument itself. Contrary to what one may expect, the number of biologists who regularly use a microscope and who are quite ignorant of its manipulation is quite great. Uncontested leaders in the field of microscopy whom I have asked for an estimate of the proportion of biologists really competent in handling a microscope have evaluated it at 3 to 5 per cent, depending on their leniency, and I do not take that as a whim. It must be admitted that this state of affairs can be explained, above all, by the indifference of users. Modern instruments do "show something" even if they are deliberately used under disastrous conditions of observation, and the number of people for whom that would do is unfortunately very great. This part of the technique of microscopical examination is easy to learn; a careful reading of any good work on microscopy is enough to acquaint oneself with the general principles; a little practical advice from a specialist then allows one to acquire the finer points. This aspect of microscopical examination is evidently not discussed here; far more competent authors than I have stated the rules concerning work with a microscope and it seems quite pointless for me to paraphrase their writings.

There remains the more difficult aspect of the problem, namely the technique of exploring histological preparations. As opposed to the general manipulation of the microscope this part of histological technique cannot really be described. It calls for an apprenticeship of several years even if the apprentice is full of enthusiasm. One should learn, often the hard way, to look at everything and see everything, and yet, without being lost in detail, to go straight to the goal while remaining alert for unexpected aspects, to jettison one's desires and not perceive in sections what one wishes to encounter. It seems to me that learning to examine under the micro-, scope can be compared to learning a musical instrument; leaving aside the talents of a pupil, the lessons of the best teacher are of no effect if the pupil does not bow down to the rigorous discipline of the scales. Such exercises do exist in microscopical examination and are not necessarily replaced by a piece of research assigned to the beginner. Even important investigations can include elementary operations from the histological point of view but which do not carry considerable formative value. Thus, long periods of work at estimating the height or the measurements of the thyroid epithelium of a mammal is no training for exploring preparations in depth, for analysing the relationship between organelles or for the mental reconstruction of a series of optical planes required of an experienced histologist. The future histologist should learn his scales in cases where, in spite of the intellectual profit, the task does not possess true formative value as we understand it here. It consists in making preparations of classical work in histology, without any hope of coming across a "discovery" but only for personal training, and to examine them thoroughly, to compare one's visual perceptions with the classical figures and, in short, to learn to see what was perceived by the great authors of modern histology. The method of analysing a preparation is not the same when the aim is microscopical anatomy, cytology or histochemistry. It is indeed worth acquiring a wide training in the different ways of examination, rather than to be caught unawares during one's career.

In most cases beginners find it difficult to spend the number of hours over a microscope necessary in the making of a histologist. Experience has shown that an "exhaustive" examination of a preparation does not exist; even a well trained observer disregards that which does not actually interest him when he examines a section. It is therefore never futile to examine sections that have already been explored dozens of times; there is always a considerable statistical chance of seeing something new.

The exploration of a histological preparation should always begin under the lowest magnification of the microscope; examination under a lens or even with the naked eye can be useful for large and heterogenous sections. In the case of homogeneous organs examination under low power will show technically defective regions or structural particularities; far from being a waste of time, it can gain time. Also reciprocally, every study of a preparation should extend up to the highest optical combination available to the histologist whenever the condition of the preparation permits it.

The examination in depth of a slice of tissue, represented by the section, is an essential step in the study. The observer should constantly manipulate the fine focussing, note the resulting changes in aspect and infer the respective relationships between tissues, cells and organelles. The possibility of examining slices of tissue of a certain thickness is one of the advantages of the light microscope over the electron microscope where spatial relations would often have to be deduced from photographs of serial sections, which is quite laborious.

The actual technical training of the future histologist should be accompanied by his theoretical development; it is only when one has learnt that certain structures exist that one acquires the habit of seeing them and analysing them.

The smooth mechanism of visual perception and mental integration that go to make a "reader of sections" is thus long and difficult to attain; no advice or teaching can spare the future histologist years of work.

Though the art of "reading out" a section cannot be codified, other operations which form an integral part of examining preparations, such as their graphical representation and their quantitative study, will be described here.

THE GRAPHICAL REPRESENTATION OF HISTOLOGICAL PREPARATIONS

Besides a precise description of his observations the histologist disposes of two modes of graphical representation to record his impressions, namely drawings and photomicrographs. Clearly, there is no question of describing the technique of drawing or that of taking photomicrographs here; these descriptions will be found in all good books on microscopy. Only a few indications concerning the photographic reproduction of preparations obtained by different techniques are given in connection with the description of these techniques. On the other hand, it seems opportune to discuss the indications and recommendations relevant to the two procedures here.

The number of factors that determine the choice between a photograph and a drawing to illustrate a publication in histology is quite great and they are sufficiently diverse for them to be discussed successively.

The educative value of drawing a histological preparation is certainly very great; only the real understanding of a preparation permits a good drawing of it. Older authors freely admitted, the relation in declaring that only drawing allowed one to really "take charge" of a histological preparation. Such an assertion is certainly exaggerated; observation need not have to be carried out with a pencil in hand for it to be reliable, and a training in visual memory can perfectly well replace the "rough sketches" with which many histologists fill voluminous files. The desire to prove the thoroughness of histological examination by giving a number of drawings should therefore not influence one's choice of illustration.

The objectivity of the photographic document has been greatly over-valued; it does exist to a certain extent, but one should not be blind to the fact that, pushed to an extreme, a photomicrograph does not necessarily constitute proof in the juridical sense. The illustration of a histophysiological study by photomicrographs showing evident histological modifications does not prove that the experimental conditions were really those mentioned in the legend; a spiteful critic can formulate the same doubt concerning drawings, tables or any other data. The so-called scientific investigator who is capable of faking a drawing can also perfectly well choose his photographic illustrations to suit his criteria or contrive to "adjust" his figures of experimental analyses. Obviously the gain from such procedure is nil and in the long run "natural" selection eliminates those who "work" in this manner. Nevertheless, objectivity in photomicrography should be considered in quite another meaning of the term.

In fact once the good faith of the author has been established, without which no scientific debate is possible, a drawing and a photograph result from different operations and have different aims. The aim of a drawing is to illustrate an interpretation, and to show the manner in which the author himself perceives and integrates the differences of form, colour and contrast in a preparation; the influence of the personal element is thus not only admitted but even desirable. A rigorously true drawing can be made from several preparations treated, if necessary, by different techniques; composite drawings of this type are often the most useful. But no one would go to the ridiculous extent if insisting that an author should faithfully reproduce all the imperfections of his preparation such as streaks, uneven thickness and defects in the sticking of sections. Similarly, the author of a drawing has the right to neglect what seems accessory to him in making place for what he considers essential, to exaggerate or attenuate the contrasts of a preparation, in short, to emphasize his view and interpretation of the preparation by the means at his disposal.

The aim of photomicrography is to reproduce, by procedures that can be easily standardized to exclude the personal factor, an optical slice of the section. The thickness of this slice varies inversely as the magnifying power of the optical system. All the conditions under which the photo is taken can be defined—indeed, they should be in the legend to the figure—so that any competent operator will obtain strictly comparable photographs of the same field at the same focus. The essential difference between drawing and photomicrography is that the element of personal interpretation which is impossible to avoid in drawing, can be eliminated in photomicrography.

A drawing, in short, illustrates the impressions gained by the author while examining a preparation; it is understood that other authors of equal competence, but different orientation, can arrive at an entirely different drawing of the same preparation. A photomicrograph, on the other hand, shows impartially what is found in an optical plane of the section and all equivalent objectives projecting on to the same film would show the same morphological details.

Leaving aside the norms of publication and the aptitudes of the histologist, it is therefore a drawing that should be preferred in every case where it is desired to interpret the results obtained by examining a number of preparations or different focal planes of the same one; a photomicrograph suffices if the objective representation of a single optical plane is enough to illustrate the ideas of the author. The intellectual preferences of the author, his conception and his conclusions appear as clearly through a drawing as through a description; while a photomicrograph can show very clearly what has been passed over in silence in the text, or even what has not been perceived at all during examination. With the result the execution of a drawing in histology implies a responsibility that cannot be entrusted to someone else; all the manipulations of photomicrography can, however, be carried out by a competent technician after the framing and the choice of optical plane have been ensured. A drawing tells nothing of the technical qualities of a preparation; a photomicrograph speaks of it eloquently, for only good preparations give acceptable photographs.

Apart from factors that are inherent in the procedures of graphical representation practical considerations are necessarily involved in the choice between a drawing and a photomicrograph. There are those for whom any aptitude at drawing will always remain a day-dream; the present author is one of them. The learning of photographic technique calls only for little effort and willingness. Even a competent histologist, well trained in drawing, will take as much time to draw a preparation ready to be photographed as he will to take about fifty photographs good enough to be printed.

The norms of publication have also to be considered. Certain journals are printed on such paper that the insertion of a photographic illustration only betrays a lack of common sense on the part of the author; schematic line drawings are the most suitable in these cases. In principle the technical conditions that are good enough for a wash drawing also allow publication of a photograph, but it must be remembered that contrast in a drawing is greater than in a photograph so that the satisfactory reproduction of a half-tone drawing may not be so for a photograph. In passing I might also point out that it is worth publishing colour plates or aquarelles only if the typographical conditions ensure really satisfactory reproduction.

The particular orientation of the work should also be considered. The balance between the two modes of reproduction can be in favour of a drawing in didactive work where the essential is purposely emphasized or even exaggerated; in publications meant for specialists, however, photographic reproductions can be preferred.

THE RECONSTRUCTION OF HISTOLOGICAL PREPARATIONS

The aim of reconstruction is to furnish a view of the object, that has been cut into sections, that is either two-dimensional in a plane different from that of cutting or three-dimensional. The first of these objectives can be attained by the techniques of graphical reconstruction and a certain amount of relief can be given by the expedients of drawing. But only a plastic reconstruction will enable a truly three-dimensional reproduction of an object rendered into sections or of its parts.

Reconstruction is long and laborious; it demands the perfect cutting of serial sections. The didactive value of a good plastic reconstruction is indeed considerable, but it entails such effort that specialists of this type of work recommend it only when none of the other procedures that could lead to the same result (dissection, separation by maceration, dissociation, clearing thick slices) can be applied.

When the need for reconstructing can be anticipated before fixation and the external shape of the piece is unusual it is better make a series of drawings or photographs from various angles before embedding. Special precautions should be taken while embedding, generally in paraffin, because guiding-marks should be noted which allow a rigorous superposition of the drawings or photographs of the various sections. Old authors used to embed, along with the piece and joined to it, a fragment of osmified nerve to serve as a guide-line in cutting sections.

However, since Born (1898) embedding in a special glass chamber is preferred. The bottom of the chamber has a number of parallel grooves with respect to which the object is oriented during embedding. When the block is removed from its mould it is seen to carry a series of ridges on one of its faces, and the object lies close to this face since it is embedded at the bottom of the chamber. If this side is painted with a varnish that is insoluble in the solvents to be used subsequently and covered with a second layer of paraffin, then sections cut perpendicularly to this face will carry a regularly indented line on one side as a guide. Clearly the block should also be very carefully oriented when it is fixed to the object holder of the microtome. Devices are also available on the market to make regular ridges parallel to one side of blocks that are made in ordinary moulds.

In many cases the object itself contains its own guiding points. They are enough for an approximate orientation of sections during reconstruction (vertebral column or the dorsal chord of embryos, trajectory of large vessels etc...). The orientation following external contours is never really precise enough. Only directional lines made in the manner described above really guarantee against any mispositioning of sections during reconstruction.

Obviously sections should be of a known thickness that is rigorously equal throughout and the orientation of the razor should not undergo the slightest change during cutting. Any loss of sections should be avoided. The greatest care should be taken in sticking and aligning sections on slides. The detachment of certain sections at the time of staining brings about so much inconvenience that they are better collodioned systematically even if they are not likely to undergo treatment with particularly drastic reagents.

Only a complete series of flawless, well attached sections can be counted upon for a correct reconstruction. In all cases where the material is not exceptionally rare it is preferable to recommence cutting rather than to spend the necessary time and effort over a reconstruction of doubtful quality.

The starting point of all reconstruction is a series of suitably enlarged drawings or photographs of the sections of the piece. Evidently the drawings need not be very elaborate, but their outlines should be very carefully traced; the guiding line is also drawn along with each section and each drawing should evidently be on a separate sheet of paper.

Experience has shown that it is better to reconstruct from photographs. Serial sections are photographed, preferably on 24×36 mm film, under strictly standardized optical conditions and then suitably enlarged. If sections are large and the desired linear enlargement does not exceed 15 diameters it is more convenient to prepare the series of photos directly with a photographic enlarger. The slides are placed in the film-holder of the enlarger, the enlargement adjusted for the whole series (using the largest section of the series) and either a slow fine-grained negative film is exposed if positives are desired or prints are directly made on suitably graded paper. The latter method, quicker and cheaper, is enough in most cases. Incidentally, this technique of low enlargement photography, recommended in several recent publications and whose authorship is difficult to establish, can be of great use in other types of work than reconstruction.

Before any reconstruction the serial sections are aligned along with their drawings or photographs and duly numbered. An as exact knowledge as possible of structures is evidently indispensable during actual reconstruction.

The indications and the techniques of the two methods of reconstruction are so different that they will be discussed separately.

GRAPHICAL RECONSTRUCTION

As mentioned earlier, this provides a two-dimensional image in a plane which is different from that in which the sections were cut. The expedients of drawing allow some techniques to introduce a certain impression of relief though it can never be a true three-dimensional representation in space from which measurements can be made. Furthermore, the best of the procedures of graphical reconstruction fail when the shape of the object attains a certain degree of complexity. Lison (1936) who has devised one of the most elaborate techniques of graphical reconstruction, has himself remarked that his method, as well as all others, do not work in cases like that of the urinary tubes of vertebrates, that is, where the need for reconstruction is really great. It is therefore dangerous to harbour any illusions about the range of graphical reconstruction; only plastic reconstruction can really replace dissection whenever the latter is impossible.

The projective reconstruction of His (1887) gives a two-dimensional image in a plane that is perpendicular to that of the sections. It is the oldest and the most frequently used of all the procedures of graphical reconstruction. It is relatively simple, especially when the block is ridged during embedding so that sections carry a guide-line. It may be carried out in the following steps.

1° Make the series of drawings or photographs preferably at an enlargement of 1000 times the thickness of sections; this allows the use of commercial metric graph paper.

2° Draw on one of the drawings or photographs, the line of projection that corresponds to the desired plane of reconstruction (if the series of sections is transverse the plane of reconstruction can be sagittal or frontal). Produce this line to meet the guide-line, or draw another straight line to join the line of projection with the guide-line.

3° Trace these lines on tracing paper and transpose them to all the other drawings or photographs of the series taking care that the guide-line is always carefully aligned to fall on that of each member of the series. Important points are best marked by piercing them with a fine needle.

4° Draw a vertical line on the graph paper. This corresponds to all the points of intersection between the guide line and the line of projection, or the line joining the two of the various members of the series.

5° Arrange the drawings or photographs in serial order and number the horizontal lines of the graph paper accordingly. Measure out, on each member of the series, the distance between the following two points: the first point which is the intersection between the line of projection and the contours of the particular organ to be reconstructed; the second point which is the intersection between the line of projection and the guide-line or the line joining the two. Plot points at these distances on the particular horizontal line of the graph paper that corresponds to the serial order of the drawing or photograph. A similar operation is carried out for the intersection of the line of projection with the outer contours of the object.

6° When all the points of all sections have been plotted on the graph paper those corresponding to the contours of the organ are joined as well as those corresponding to the outer contours of the piece. This will give the profile of the organ in the piece in the desired plane of projection.

In those cases where guiding marks have not been put in place at the time of embedding the lines of projection to be traced on drawings may be oriented with respect to the outer contours or the characteristic structures of the piece. Measurements are greatly facilitated with an exact drawing of the entire piece according to the plane of projection (a profile if the reconstruction is sagittal and a dorsal or ventral view if the reconstruction is frontal). A tracing of this view, correctly enlarged, is stuck on to the graph paper taking care that the planes of sectioning are rigorously parallel to the horizontal lines of the paper. Measurements can then be made with respect to the outer contours.

Obviously, all sections need not be drawn when the shape of the organ to be reconstructed is simple and when the block has been cut into this sections; only one out of three or four sections need be considered and this should evidently be taken into account in evaluating the thickness of the slices involved in reconstruction.

If the operation were to be repeated along successive parallel planes of the object an idea of its spatial configuration will be obtained. Incidentally I may recall that His used such reconstructions as the basis of his famous free-hand models of embryos. Such practice requires considerable artistic talent on the part of the operator which is rarely encountered among histologists. Besides, it remains only an approximation which, though excellent for teaching, is quite unsuitable for truly quantitative studies.

The technique of "*graphical isolation*" is derived from a superposition of drawings made on transparent paper or sheets of glass. The technique, improved and codified by Kastschenko (1886) and by Lebedkin (1926) has been frequently used by early authors. The object to be reconstructed is represented as hypsometric curves which can be transformed by shading into a view that is perpendicular to the plane of sectioning. It requires the presence of either very precise identifying points in the sections or guides that have been put in place at the time of embedding (ridges in Born's embedding chamber or several fragments of osmified nerve).

The operating procedure is relatively simple. The contours of the organ to be reconstructed are reproduced on a sheet of paper, starting with the section facing the viewer and taking care that the guide-marks are rigorously superposed in the drawings of successive sections. Contours hidden by those that have been already traced are not depicted. It can be helpful to use a different colour to trace sections at certain intervals (one in about every five or ten sections).

The various techniques of *graphical reconstruction in perspective* (Odhner (1910); Dubreuil (1921); Peter (1922); Lison (1936)) are derived from the technique of graphical isolation just described. They have the added advantage of providing a view of the object from any angle whatever. They are all based on the same principle. The object is supposed to be included in a parallelepiped whose two faces are parallel to the plane of cutting. In reconstruction this plane is rotated through an angle α. The different sections are drawn with an adjustment calculated from the angle α and with a lateral shift to show the sides which do not appear in the simple graphical isolation of Kastschenko. I shall not describe these procedures here for two reasons. In fact, as with all other methods of graphical reconstruction, a projected drawing becomes inoperative as soon as the structures get complex, that is, in just those cases where a reconstruction turns out to be really necessary. Furthermore, the works of Lison (1936) and Jorgensen (1971) describe clearly and precisely all the useful details needed to carry out this type of reconstruction.

PLASTIC RECONSTRUCTION

Plastic reconstruction can be particularly long and laborious, but it gives results that are far better than those of graphical reconstruction since it gives a three-dimensional model of the object; it has sufficient fidelity to permit measurements and its didactive value is considerable.

Since its invention by Born (1900) the procedure, whose principle is very simple, has undergone only modifications of detail that involve especially the raw material used for reconstruction.

The method consists of tracing drawings of serial sections on sheets or plates of the chosen material, cutting out the portions to be reconstructed and of superposing them after proper juxtaposition; the thickness of the plates evidently depends on the desired enlargement and the resulting model is a plastic reconstruction of the structure under study.

The practical procedure depends on the raw material used. Born used plates of wax, moulded by hand, which can give rise to a certain imprecision in their thickness and are fairly expensive. Instruments are available that aid in moulding and suppliers of products for histology furnished, until quite recently, plates of wax correctly calibrated for the purpose. Other materials have been suggested. Thus Wilson (1915) replaced bee's wax by a mixture of two parts of wax, four parts of paraffin and one part of pine resin. Sheets or plates of cardboard, wood and plaster have been used by certain authors. More recently reconstruction has been carried out with sheets of foam-plastic.

In all cases the drawings of the organs to be reconstructed and the guide-lines are traced or pasted on to the chosen material. They are then cut out along their contours, taking care to leave a strip that joins the organ to the guide-line, which is also cut out. They are immediately numbered and then duly reassembled by superposition. The whole is then consolidated with a warm iron in the case of wax sheets or with a suitable adhesive in the case of other material. The strip joining the different sections to the guide-line is removed afterwards.

The chief advantage of wax sheets is the ease with which they can be cut out and with which the desired thickness can be obtained. However, the thickness is of less importance than one imagines since it is often simpler to choose an enlargement in accordance with the thickness of the available sheets. Cutting out the contours is much more laborious and is the chief disadvantage of reconstructing with cardboard or plywood; a saw has to be used, while a scalpel is enough for wax-sheets. Sheets of foam-plastic are cut with a metal wire that is heated electrically and whose temperature is controlled by a rheostat so that the plastic is cut without adhering to the hot wire.

Large-sized reconstructions obviously require a metal framework. One can, besides, carry out a "negative" reconstruction and obtain the final model by casting in plaster.

In any case the techniques described above result in models whose surface consists of discontinuous steps. They should therefore be smoothed out by filling with mastic and by sand-papering before applying the final varnish.

THE QUANTITATIVE STUDY OF HISTOLOGICAL PREPARATIONS

The quantitative study of histological preparations is gaining importance in modern research and this can only rejoice histologists since it indicates, in accord with the exergue to this chapter, the maturation of their discipline.

This evolution is particularly evident in the case of histochemistry and it is in the corresponding part of this work that I allude to the techniques which often require costly instruments and delicate handling, and are consequently practised in somewhat specialized laboratories. However, even ordinary histological practice also offers a large scope for quantitative work. Thus in cases where classical authors spoke of large and small nuclei or of tall and flat cells numerical data would be preferred in modern histology. A simple visual estimation of the relative proportions of two tissues in a section or the relative abundance of several types of cells will only gain by support from such data. Consequently, every histologist should know how to obtain measurements of lengths and surfaces in his preparations.

He should furthermore be exactly aware of the causes of error in measuring under the microscope and of the limits implied in numerical data in order to avoid the two equally unreliable extremes, one being a simple vague and subjective description and the other the false precision of indiscriminate measuring.

THE CAUSES OF ERROR IN MEASURING UNDER THE MICROSCOPE

It is obvious that all the rules that govern quantitative work apply to the present case. The errors of distribution and sampling are not particularly different from those of other disciplines and hold for measuring under the microscope as well; similarly, the techniques for the statistical treatment of data are the same and hence will not be described here.

Certain errors, due to accident, will be considered but not at length; they result from the defective functioning of an instrument or the inexperience of the operator.

A systematic source of error, not to be disregarded, while measuring histological preparations, is due to the shrinkage of tissues following fixation, dehydration and especially embedding in paraffin. In most cases microscopical measurements are made on paraffin sections and the existence of shrinkage is implicit; it can vary significantly from tissue to tissue only when pieces are really heterogenous. It is however in measuring organs, segments of embryos or very small animals that allowance should be made for such error.

Other causes of error are inherent in the instrument and cannot be entirely eliminated.

1° The errors of distortion due to curvature of the field and the errors of overlapping, which appear when the object is larger than the field and necessitates partial measurements, are greatly reduced by the availability of eye-pieces and objectives that give plane fields. It is however prudent to carry out all measuring in the centre of the field to avoid as far as possible deformations due to a defective plane.

2° Mechanical errors due to the elastic deformation of the parts of the instrument whose manipulation is unavoidable and the hysteresis of components can, as Policard, Bessis and Locquin (1957) remark, be reduced by a reconsideration of the mechanical principles on which present-day microscopes are based.

3° Diffraction errors affect the accuracy with which the edge of the object coincides with the graduations of the measuring instrument. They are practically nil at low power but become appreciable at higher magnifications. In the latter case, it is generally admitted that precision is increased under phase contrast.

4° Errors of deformation and compression of contrasts occur when measurements are not made under the microscope but from photographs.

5° Systematic errors in planimetry or linear integration are also likely in measuring surfaces; error in the aperture of the objective and others due to the particular shape of certain objects have to be kept in mind in measuring volumes.

All the above possibilities imply that an error of at least 5% can be expected for linear measurements and this can easily attain 25% for surfaces or very small volumes. It is thus quite illusory to measure, to the nearest tenths of a micron, an object whose length is less than 10 μ.

MEASURING LENGTHS IN THE PLANE OF THE STAGE

This type of measuring is the most frequent. It is based in all cases on a comparison of the object with a standard, either coincidentally or by substitution.

Coincidental measuring is done either by superposing the edges of the object on a micrometer scale placed in the eye-piece or by superposing the virtual images of the object and of the micrometer scale. The scale, in both cases, should be calibrated by comparing with an objective micrometer, that is, a micrometer scale placed on the stage of a microscope and examined as one would a histological preparation. Most such micrometer scales are one or two millimeters long with sub-divisions of 100 and 10 μ. Evidently each graduation appears under high power as an opaque strip of a certain thickness, and hence it is necessary to adopt a convention, in measuring and calibrating, of considering either the middle of each band or a particular edge of each one. Eye-piece micrometers are usually graduated in arbitrary units. The number of graduations of the objective micrometer that correspond to a division of the eye-piece micrometer should therefore be estimated for a particular magnification of the microscope and the true measurement calculated from the ratio. Certain eye-piece micrometers (contrast micrometers) carry, instead of the graduation, a series of aligned squares that touch each other by their angles which facilitates appreciating the coincidence with the edges of the object to be measured. Precision of reading can be further increased by using an eye-piece micrometer worked by a drum. Its principle consists of running a mobile guide, visible in the plane of the microscope, along the length to be measured by rotating a drum and reading off the distance covered from the graduations of the drum. Policard and his collaborators (1957) however note that the increase in precision is counteracted by the risk of mechanical errors from the elastic deformation of the microscope tube.

In measuring by substitution the object and the standard are projected successively on to the same graduated scale. It is the method of measuring by coincidence that is used in most cases.

MEASURING LENGTHS ALONG THE OPTICAL AXIS OF THE MICROSCOPE

Measuring thickness under the microscope is much more difficult and uncertain than measuring lengths perpendicular to the optical axis. The old procedure of using a micrometer drum provides only a rough approximation. It consists of focussing on to the lower side of the section and noting the corresponding division of the drum. The fine adjustment is then worked to bring the upper side of the section into focus and the second reading of the drum is taken. The drum carried by the fine adjustment screw is calibrated by makers of all good quality microscopes so that the approximate thickness of the section may be calculated.

One of the inherent difficulties lies in the need to focus on the upper and lower sides of the section. Since the depth of focus of objectives is never equal to zero the determination of the two focal levels is liable to an error that cannot be reduced within certain limits. Furthermore, the indications on the drum are valid only when the path of light lies in a homogenous medium; errors due to refraction creep in as soon as light passes through heterogeneous layers, especially layers of air. Measuring thickness by the above method is thus probably one of the most inaccurate of all the measurements made under the microscope.

Much progress in the field is due to the use of the interference microscope. A description of the instrument and an explanation of the technique is outside both the scope of this book and the competence of its author. A recent review of Barer (in Pollister 1966) gives all the necessary details and carries an extensive bibliography.

MEASURING AREAS PERPENDICULAR TO THE OPTICAL AXIS OF THE MICROSCOPE

The need to measure areas in the plane of the preparation may arise under various circumstances during histological examination. In certain cases it is the prelude to an evaluation of the volume of an organelle having a geometrical shape. In others an attempts is made to deduce the respective proportions of two or more tissues in the constitution of an organ. Sometimes the evaluation of area is in itself the aim of measuring.

When the area to be measured has a simple geometrical shape the task of estimation is reduced to measuring several lengths and the procedures already indicated suffice. But errors of measuring can render such a direct evaluation illusory in cases where very small lengths have to be measured; the difficulties of accurately estimating the surface area and volume of spherical nucleoli affords such an example. Caspersson, Fredrikson and Thorsson (1953) have solved the problem by devising a microplanimeter that enables direct planimetry under the microscope. This instrument has given excellent results in the hands of Sandritter and Hübotter (1954) for measuring nucleoli in the Rat adrenal cortex.

The principle of the instrument is very simple. A suitable convergent lens is inserted in the light-path of the microscope between the objective and eye-piece; its displacement causes a virtual shifting of the image, which leads to the possibility of running a fixed point on the lens along the outlines of the structure to be measured. The lens is attached to the arm of a planimeter from which the area corresponding to the trajectory effected by the point can be read off in arbitrary units. The ratio between the real area and the planimeter readings depends on the distance between the mobile lens and the eye-piece, on the power of the lens and the magnification of the objective. The calibration of the instrument, whose practice has been described by Sandritter and Hübotter (1954) is based on the planimetry of known areas (cell counting chambers, nuclei whose surface area has been determined by another method etc...). In the case of nucleoli the apparent area can be measured with the planimeter, from which the radius is deduced and the volume calculated. According to Sandritter and Hübotter, the margin of error is from 4 to 8% for the measurements of nucleoli and less than 4% for larger surfaces.

The earliest procedure for estimating an area in the plane of the preparation consists in drawing it at a known magnification, cutting it out from the sheet of paper and weighing it. The relative areas of different tissues can be immediately obtained from the weights of papers cut out from corresponding zones. Absolute areas are determined by comparing with the weight of a reference square cut out from the same paper and whose sides are chosen according to the enlargement of the drawing. Apart from the number of causes of error inherent in the microscope, the drawing appliance, tracing and cutting, the uneveness of the paper used can lead to faulty results. It is therefore advisable to choose a paper that is as uniform as possible from the same ream and to calibrate by weighing several reference squares from different sheets. The deviation of weights among reference squares evidently gives an idea of the degree of confidence that can be placed in the system.

Several authors recommend the planimetry of surfaces instead of cutting and weighing the paper. Considerable time is saved and it is easy to repeat the measurements and increase their precision. If the absolute area is desired calibrating is done by the planimetry of reference squares traced as for cutting and weighing, that is, taking into account the magnification.

Evidently, planimetry can be done on photographs but it introduces a certain error caused by deformation of the photographic paper during processing and the compression of contrasts. Some authors prefer measuring projected images rather than drawings or photographs; planimeters have been specially adapted for this.

PROCEDURES OF LINEAR INTEGRATION TO MEASURE AREAS AND RELATIVE VOLUMES

One of the aims of measuring areas mentioned in the preceding paragraphs is the estimation of the relative volumes of two or more tissues that constitute an organ. The importance of this evaluation strikes the mind. Several techniques particularly suited to the quantitative study of certain organs have been devised by various authors. Some of these are described under the techniques specially adapted for the study of vertebrate organs. The principle of all these methods is quite simple; relative areas are measured, by drawing and cutting out or by planimetry, from a certain number of sections; relative volumes of tissues are deduced and their weights may be calculated after applying factors of correction in certain cases.

> These methods are in fact based on the principle formulated in about 1850 by Delesse concerning the quantitative study of rocks. According to this the ratio of volumes of different constituents is equal to that of the surface areas they occupy in a sufficiently large number of thin sections through the object.
> It was in 1898 that the possibility of much more rapid measuring than by drawing or planimetry, but sufficiently precise, was pointed out by Rosiwal. According to the method of this author, which represents the classical technique of linear integration, the measurements of lengths replace those of areas. The total surface to be explored is covered by a certain number of straight lines. The segments corresponding to each of the various constituents are added up and the ratio of these total lengths is used instead of that of areas to estimate relative volumes. The vogue for this procedure was considerable, especially in industry and in geology. Special stages and eye-pieces for such integration have been devised by makers of optical instruments, which allow these measurements to be made under the microscope. They usually consist of a series of about six screws that control micrometric rods which can move a guide along a straight path across the field of the microscope. At the start each screw is allotted to one particular constituent of the preparation. The field is scanned in straight lines by the guide and every time it crosses a particular constituent the operator makes it advance by working the corresponding screw. At the end the total trajectory covered by the guide in each constituent can be read off from graduated drums. The ratios of these lengths are used in place of the areas estimated by the older procedures.
> Though saving considerable time when compared to the direct measurement of area, the techniques of linear integration are not quite free from criticism. In fact the time taken to measure lengths is far from negligible and the high precision (it is possible to limit the error to below 1%) is itself quite redundant in view of the wide dispersion in sampling.

The techniques of linear integration, which are based on an estimation of lengths, tend to give place to procedures where the operator merely counts the number of fixed guide-points that fall within a given constituent in the plane of the image. These guide-points are usually carried on a suitably etched reticulum that is placed in the eye-piece.

Hennig (1958) goes back to Glagoleff (1943) to cite the first application of this principle. Its use in histological technique is due to Chalkley (1943) who operated with an eye-piece carrying, in the plane of the image, four bristles whose free ends served as guide-points; a fifth one has been proposed as a "control" on one of the constituents whose relative proportion in the section has been explored, but this precaution turns out to be unnecessary. Chalkley was able to arrive at a satisfactory approximation of the nucleo-cytoplasm ratio in the liver cell by counting the number of hits on the nuclei in a sufficiently large sample of fields. In the technique of Haug (1955) who proposes to call it the method of "scoring hits" (*Treffermethode*) the number of points in a field is raised to 101 by the use of intersecting points of an ordinary reticulum placed in the eye-piece. This author emphasizes the need to consider while counting only an optical plane and not a slice ot tissue. The optics of the microscope should therefore be chosen to reduce the depth of focus as far as is possible accounting for the accommodation of the observer, that is, partly as a function of his age. Obviously any modification of the focus should be avoided during the scanning of a given field. The ratio of the number of hits to the total number of points gives quite a precise idea of the share of each constituent in the composition of a tissue without, of course, giving the slightest indication as to the absolute number or mass.

From the writings of Hennig (1956, 1957, 1958) reducing the number of guide-points carried by the reticulum of the integrator eye-piece to 25 has certain practical advantages as illustrated by statistics. Such eye-pieces are commercially available and the accompanying detailed instructions, which need not be repeated here, include an abacus that enables calculating the error under different conditions of use.

These methods therefore appear at present to be the best ones to appreciate, approximately enough for a histologist, the proportions of the different constituents that compose a tissue or an organ.

The principle of counting points has been applied by Hennig (1957, 1958) to measure, in ground and polished sections or in histological preparations, the surface area of bodies of any shape whatever that go to constitute the objects examined. The integrator eye-piece carries equidistant straight lines of defined length. Exploration of the preparation is aimed at counting the intersections of these lines with the tissue constituent whose surface area is to be determined. From this data, and using a formula developed by Hennig, the area can be calculated to an approximation that is good enough for the biologist. This type of integrator eye-piece is also available on the market along with detailed instructions.

The techniques of counting cells are described in other portions of this book in connection with their chief practical applications.

Most stereometric operations described here (measuring areas and relative volumes, totalling points, classifying structures according to their size etc.) may be carried out by automatic electronic analysers. Considerable time is saved and their use is only likely to increase in the future. Eventual computerization should also be kept in mind when staining to give the relevant structures and points enough contrast against the background. However, the cost of equipment limits such work to specialized laboratories. Hennig and his collaborators (1970) have recently published a detailed account of the techniques and problems of stereometry.

APPENDIX

LIST OF PRINCIPAL DYE-STUFFS USED IN HISTOLOGY

The following list, which does not at all claim to be complete, has been compiled following recent publications (especially Conn, 1959; Harms, 1965). It is confined to dyes in the strict sense, and histochemical reagents are excluded. In addition to the most commonly used name and the chief synonyms, the acidic, basic or lysochromic character is also indicated. It should be noted that Y (*yellowish*), J (*jaunâtre*) and G (*gelblich*) are equivalent. The various dyes, excepting the fluorochromes and natural dyes, are grouped according to the chemical constitution of their chromophores. Figures within brackets indicate the serial numbers in the second edition of the *"Colour Index"*.

1° Anthraquinones.

Acid alizarin blue BB (58 610)	Anthracene blue SWX	acid
Alizarin-cyanin RR (58 550)		acid
Alizarin red S (58 005)	Sodium alizarin sulfonate	acid
Alizarin-viridin (62 555)		acid
Anthracene blue SWR (58 605)		acid
BZL Blue		lysochrome
nuclear Fast red		acid
Oil blue NA (61 555)		lysochrome
Purpurin (58 205)	Alizarin purpurin	acid

2° Azins.

Azocarmine B (50 090)		acid
Azocarmine G (50 085)	Azocarmine GX	acid
	Rosazine	
	Rosinduline GXF	
Magdala red (50 375 b)	Naphthalene red	basic
	Naphthylamine pink	
Neutral red (50 040)	Toluylene red	basic
Pheno-safranin (50 200)	Safranin B extra	basic
Safranin O	Safranin Y, A or G	basic
	Gossypimine	

3° Azo-dyes.

a) MONO-AZO DYES

Amaranth (16 185)	Azarubin	acid
	Naphthol red S	
	Fast red	
	Bordeaux SF	
	Victoria rubin O	
	Wool red	
Azophloxine GA (18 050)	Amidonaphthol red G	acid
Bordeaux red	Fast red B or BN	acid
	Cerasin R	
	Azo-Bordeaux	
Brilliant yellow S (13 085)	Curcumine	acid
Chromotrope 2R (16 570)	Fast fuchsin G	acid
	XL Carmoisine 6R	
	Acid phloxine GR	
Chrysoidin Y (11 270)	Brown salt R	basic
Crystal Ponceau 6R (16 250)	Ponceau 6R	acid
Fast yellow (13 015)	Acid yellow	acid
	Fast yellow FY, G, S	acid
Janus green B (11 045)	Diazin green S	basic
Metanil yellow (13065)	Yellow M	acid
	Acid yellow R	
	Tropaeolin G	
Oil brown D (12 020)	Fast brown	lysochrome
	Fast brown III	
	Sudan brown	
Oil yellow III (11 020)	Butter yellow	lysochrome
	Oil yellow D	
	Fast oil yellow B	
Orange G (16 230)	Orange GG, GPM	acid
Orange II (15 510)	Methyl orange	
	Gold orange	
	Acid orange II	
	Mandarin G	
Ponceau 2R (16 150)	Ponceau R, RG, G, 4R, etc	
	Xylidine ponceau 3RS (?)	
	Brilliant ponceau G	
Sorbine red (14 895)	Azofuchsin 3B	acid
	Eriorubine G	
	Azo rhodine 3G	
Sudan II (12 140)	Oil scarlet	lysochrome
	red B	
	Fast ponceau	
	Orange RR	
Thiazine Red R (14 780)	Chlorazol pink Y	acid
	Rosophenine 10B	

b) POLY-AZO DYES.

Benzopurpurin 4B (23 500)	Cotton red 4B	acid
	Diamin red 4B	
	Direct red 4B	
Biebrich scarlet (water soluble) (26 905)	Croceine scarlet	acid
	Scarlet B	
	Ponceau B	

APPENDIX

Bismarck brown Y (21 010)	Vesuvin Manchester brown Excelsior brown	basic
Blue black B (27 255)		acid
Brilliant purpurin R (23 510)		acid
Chlorazol black E (30 235)	Pontamine black E Direct black	acid
Congo red (22 120)	Cotton red B, C Direct red	acid
Diamine blue BB (22 610)	Direct blue 2B	acid
Evans blue		acid
Naphthol blue black (20 470)	Amido black B	acid
Oil red O (26 125)		lysochrome
Oil red 4B (26 105)		lysochrome
Ponceau S (27 195)		acid
Sudan black B (26 150)	Ceres black, Cerol black	lysochrome
Sudan III (26 100)	Sudan G Scarlet B, fat soluble Fast ponceau G Cerasin red	lysochrome
Sudan IV (26 105)	Scarlet red Oil red IV Fast ponceau R or LB	lysochrome
Trypan blue (23 850)	Benzo blue 3B Dianil blue H3G Congo blue 3B Niagara blue 3B	acid
Trypan red (22 850)		acid
Vital red (23 570)	Brilliant Congo red R Brilliant vital red	acid

4° Fluorochromes.

Acridine orange (46 005)		basic
Acridine yellow (46 025)		basic
Acriflavine (46 000)	Trypaflavine	basic
Auramine O (41 000)		basic
Berberine sulfate (75 160)		basic
Coriphosphine O (46 020)		basic
Geranine G (14 930)		acid
Primulin (49 000)		acid
Thioflavine S (49 010)		acid
Thioflavine T (49 005)		basic
Titan yellow G (19 504)	Thiazol yellow	acid

5° Indulins.

Indulin (50 405)		basic
Nigrosin (50 420)	Nigrosin W Indulin black	basic

6° Natural dyes.

Brazilin (brazilein) (75 280)		acid
Carmine (carminic acid) (75 470)		acid

LIST OF PRINCIPAL DYE-STUFFS USED IN HISTOLOGY

Chlorophyll (75 810)		lysochrome
Haematoxylin (haematein) (75 290)		acid
Indigo-carmine (73 015)		acid
Orcein		basic
Saffron (75 100)		?

7° Nitro dyes.

Aurantia (10 360)	Imperial yellow Dipicrylamine	acid
Martius yellow (10 315)	Manchester yellow Naphthol yellow	acid
Naphthol yellow S (10 316)		acid
Picric acid (10 305)		acid

8° Nitroso dyes (quinone oximes).

Naphthol green B (10 020)	Naphthol green Green PL Acid green O	acid
Naphthol green Y (10 000)	Fast printing green	acid

9° Oxazins.

Brilliant cresyl blue (51 010)	Cresyl blue 2RN	basic
Celestin blue B (51 050)	Coreine 2R	basic
Cresyl violet	Cresyl fast violet	basic
Gallamin blue (51 045)		basic
Gallocyanin (51 030)	Alizarin blue RBN	basic
New blue R (51 175)	Naphthol blue R Fast blue 3R Meldola's blue	basic
Nile blue sulfate (51 180)		basic

10° Phenyl methanes.

Acid fuchsin (42 685)	Fuchsin S, SN, SS, ST, SIII Acid magenta Acid rubin	acid
Acid violet (42 576)	Eriocyanin A	acid
Anilin blue WS (42 755)	China blue Soluble blue 3M Marine blue V Cotton blue Water blue	acid
Basic fuchsin (42 510)	Fuchsin RFN Magenta Basic rubin Anilin red	basic
Brilliant green (42 040)	Ethyl green Malachite green G Emerald green crystals Fast green JJO Diamond green G	basic

Crystal violet (42 555)	Violet C, G, 7B	basic
	Hexamethyl violet	
	Methyl violet 10B	
	Gentian violet	
Ethyl green (42 590)		basic
Ethyl violet (42 600)	Ethyl purple 6B	basic
Night blue (44 085)		basic
Parasosanilin (42 500)	Parasosanilin hydrochloride	basic
	Magenta O	
Patent blue V (42 051)	Alphazurine 2G	acid
	Patent blue VF	
	Pontacyl brilliant blue V	
Rosanilin	Magenta I	basic
Spirit blue (42 775)	Gentian blue 6B	basic
	Anilin blue, alcohol soluble	
	Light blue	
	Lyon blue	
	Paris blue	
Victoria blue B (44 045)		basic
Victoria blue R (44 040)		basic
Victoria blue 4R (42 563)		basic
Wool green S (56 205)	Lissamine green B, BS	acid
	Acid green S	
Xylene cyanol FF (43 537)	Cyanol FF	acid

11° Phthalocyanins.

Alcian blue (74 240)	Alcian blue 8GS, 8GN 150	basic
Alcian green		basic
Alcian yellow		basic
Astra blue		basic
Luxol fast blue	Methasol blue	basic

12° Pyrazolones.

Fast yellow (13 015)	Fast yellow GG	acid
	Tuchechtgelb	

13° Quinolines.

Cyanin	Quinoline blue	basic
Pinacyanol		basic

14° Thiazins.

Azure A (52 005)		basic
Azure B (52 010)		basic
Azure C		basic
Methylene blue (52 015)	Swiss blue	basic
Methylene violet (50 120)		basic
Thionin (52 000)	Lauth's violet	basic
Toluidine blue O (52 040)		basic

15° Xanthenes.

Acridine red 3B (45 000)		basic
Eosin B (45 400)		acid
Eosin Y (45 380)	Eosin J, G	acid
	Eosin, water soluble	
Erythrosin B (45 430)	Pyrosin B	acid
	Iodeosin B	
	Dianthine B	
Erythrosin Y (45 425)	Erythrosin J, G	acid
	Pyrosin J	
	Dianthine G	
	Iodeosin G	
Ethyl eosin (45 386)	Eosin, alcohol soluble	acid
Methyl eosin (45 385)	Eosin, alcohol soluble	acid
Phloxine B (45 410)	Phloxine	acid
	Cyanosine	
	Eosin 10B	
Pyronin B (45 010)		basic
Pyronin Y (45 005)	Pyronin J, G	basic
Violamine R	Acid violet 4R	acid

PART TWO

GENERAL METHODS

> La technique n'est rien; la manière de l'appliquer est tout.
>
> A. Branca (1924)

Few notions in histological technique are as blurred and imprecise as that of the so-called general methods. Almost all authors of handbooks on microscopy seem impelled to distinguish between "general methods" and "special methods" but carefully refrain from a clear definition of the two and always avoid stating the criteria on which their classification is based. In most cases it is the individual orientation of the author and not any objective criterion that decides the issue, and consulting such works in rendered all the more difficult.

The confusion of criteria adopted by various authors is most striking in the chapter on "general staining". Some feel obliged to follow a historical order and attribute an importance to staining with carmine that is quite unjustified by the present state of histological technique. Others confine the chapter to routine methods practised in their own laboratories which leads them to include true topographic staining, cytological technique and even histochemical reactions in the same group.

In fact, "general methods" can be defined according to the object studied and it seems to me that this term can cover all the techniques meant to study the topography of organs and tissues with microscopical anatomy as their basis.

Such a point of view is evidently not beyond criticism; thus at the level of bacteria and, *a fortiori*, of viruses, anatomy is confounded with ultrastructural cytology. Preparations made for cytological studies often provide for excellent anatomical descriptions and are even indispensable in some cases. Histochemical reactions have been included among general method and their usefulness in topographical examination is such that they have partially replaced the routine staining methods in many laboratories. Nevertheless, whenever the objective is a topographical preparation (*Ubersichtspräparate*) it may be considered in most cases as a valid example of a general method.

Consequently, preparations meant for topographical analysis are grouped in the following sections of this book. This classification is neither exclusive nor limiting and some of the techniques mentioned are useful and even indispensable for a true cytological study of animal tissues. Conversely, certain techniques that are not primarily topographical can turn out to be very useful general methods in many cases.

Vital examination and vital staining, when intended for topographical study, do not call for any special comment and will not be described again; it is however not so with fixation and subsequent operations.

CHAPTER 8

TOPOGRAPHICAL FIXATION

Keeping in mind the arbitrary classification adopted here, one may enumerate the properties that are required of a topographical fixative as follows.

Penetration should be rapid and uniform so that one can treat comparatively large pieces that may not be sliced because anatomical relations have to be retained. A minimum-*shrinkage* during fixation and subsequent operations is very desirable. The chosen fixative should show wide *tolerance for the period of fixation* so that it can be used in expeditions, at sea or on difficult terrain. The technique should lead to a *good preparation for embedding* and for *as many stainings as possible*. The delay required for *subsequent treatment* should not be too lengthy and, finally, the *cost of material* is important when large series of preparations are intended.

The above conditions are not equally exacting and depend on the type of study. They often imply that liquids meant for the Golgi apparatus, the chondriomes and certain caryological fixatives are to be excluded from the list of topographical fixatives since their properties of conservation are too doubtful and they demand a strict period of fixation. Apart from very special cases, fixatives based on chloroplatinic acid and osmium tetroxyde or those containing formalin and the salts of heavy metals intended for the silver impregnation of the Golgi apparatus are not to be considered as topographical fixatives. Mixtures based on formalin and potassium dichromate however do have some reason to be included; they are clearly more penetrating than osmic mixtures and the conservation of structures is usually excellent, but paraffin-embedding results in excessive shrinkage and all such mixtures call for strict periods of fixation. Ethyl alcohol and acetone should be avoided as topographical fixatives.

In spite of the above reservations the number of fixative liquids that can be used for topographical study is great and it would be pointless to enumerate them here. As Baker (1958) has remarked the number of fixative mixtures that have really emerged and deserve to be cited in histological technique is quite low; the advantages of other liquids are insignificant or none at all.

The exacting size of pieces and the complex equipment required evidently rule out freezing-drying as a topographical fixation; this is equally true for freeze-substitution. Cutting fresh sections in a cryostat, whether followed by fixation or not, is now current practice in some laboratories of pathological anatomy.

In fact, the limitations to the size of pieces should equally apply to this method and it appears to me that, as usually practised, it is difficult to consider it as a topographical technique that would satisfy an exacting histologist.

THE PRINCIPAL TOPOGRAPHICAL FIXATIVES

The fixative liquids reviewed here are divided according to the nature of the solvent which can be water or ethyl alcohol; the latter has a double function since it is at the same time a fixing agent. Each of these two groups is divided into sub-groups according to the common fixing agent.

AQUEOUS LIQUIDS

The great majority of liquids used in current practice consists of fixative mixtures having water as the solvent. They are prepared in distilled water; the use of double distilled water as in analytical chemistry is clearly unnecessary. Tap water is always used to prepare dilute solutions of formalin.

1° Formalin is still one of the rare simple fixatives that is still widely used without the addition of any other agent. Very often a commercial solution is diluted to give a level of formaldehyde that varies from 4 to 10% (that is, the commercial solution is diluted with 9 to 3 volumes of tap-water). The latter concentration is an upper limit that should not be exceeded and is better not even equalled.

The characteristics of formalin as a fixing avent have been described in the paragraph devoted to general comments on such agents. From the practical point of view it should be noted that the strength of the commercial solution varies from 30 to 40% by weight of formaldehyde according to the supplier and the lot. Experience has shown such variation to be troublesome only in very particular cases. The commercial solution should be stored in well-stoppered bottles away from light and at above 10° since polymerization into trioxymethylene takes place rapidly at low temperatures.

The commercial solution of formalin is always acid, the formic acid resulting from a Cannizzaro reaction. This acidity can be inconvenient in a number of cases; it can be surmounted by storing commercial solutions intended for cytological or histochemical fixatives in the presence of an excess of powdered calcium carbonate. The same precaution may be taken for dilute solutions also if they are prepared beforehand.

The practical advantages of dilute formalin solutions as topographical fixatives lie in their low cost, their ease of preparation, the considerable tolerance in the period of fixation since pieces may be left for years, the fairly rapid and uniform penetration and the good conservation of structured lipids. These are however countered by serious disadvantages. Thus, although formalin certainly penetrates rapidly, it fixes slowly; the denaturation of tissue proteins that is a prerequisite for the proper treatment of pieces takes much longer than with other fixing agents. It is *one of the poorest preparations for paraffin-embedding* as it is for most of the so-called topographical stains. Only a combination of indifference and slavery to routine can account for the considerable vogue among anatomopathologists for fixation in formalin without any adjuvant.

It should be noted that dilute solutions of formalin are excellent conserving fluids for storing pieces fixed in other mixtures. They are strongly recommended for this purpose after all fixations in aqueous media except where osmic mixtures have been used.

Many authors have sought to attenuate the disadvantages of formalin as a fixing agent by associating it with various adjuvants. Diluting the commercial solution with one of sodium chloride that is isotonic to the medium of the animal from which the pieces originate has been advised by several histologists. Fixation in such *saline formol* (Policard 1922) is reputed to be much better than in simple aqueous dilutions of the commercial product. The addition of magnesium sulfate or acetate at a concentration of about 2% has been suggested by Schiller (1930); that of calcium chloride proposed by Baker is especially indicated for the histochemical study of lipids. Fixation in formalin-pyridine has been practised in neuro-histology and for the conservation of certain enzymatic activities; it will be discussed in the relevant chapters of this book.

The practice of fixing in formalin, whether diluted alone or with an added adjuvant, is thus quite simple. Pieces, one of whose dimensions should be less than 1 cm if the tissue is homogenous, are immersed in a large quantity of fixative liquid and left in the dark for at least 24 hours if they are intended for topographical study. Lengthening this period is only advantageous and it may last up to several years. No particular washing after fixation is required if embedding is intended in paraffin or celloidin since all formaldehyde is completely removed by the alcohol during dehydration. A rapid wash in tap-water is recommended before cutting freeze-sections; this washing in water should be thorough in cases where the pieces are to be embedded in gelatin without previous dehydration.

Several staining techniques, especially those involving the basic blues of the thiazin group turn out badly after fixation in formalin and embedding in paraffin. No subsequent operation enables improving the preparation for embedding, but the result of staining can be influenced for the better by submitting fixed pieces, and in certain cases even sections attached to slides, to a second fixation in a liquid that serves better before the desired stain.

2° **Bouin's liquid**, the prototype of all fixatives based on picric acid, should be considered as one of the best topographical fixatives. Its composition is defined with slight differences in various works on histological technique. I advise the use of the original formula which consists of mixing 75 ml of a saturated aqueous solution of picric acid, 25 ml of commercial formalin and 5 ml of glacial acetic acid. Some authors reduce the quantity of formalin to 20 ml. Many histologists recommend increasing the level of picric acid by saturating it, not in water but in a water-formalin mixture of suitable proportions so that only acetic acid is added before use. Incidentally, the recommendation to add acetic acid only just before use is not at all imperative; I have often used Bouin's liquid prepared beforehand without ever having evidence of the slightest difference from fixation in freshly prepared mixtures.

Bouin's liquid penetrates rapidly and fixes uniformly. Shrinkage at the time of fixation is less than with most other good fixatives. The optimal period of fixation is of about 24 hours for slices of tissue whose thickness does not exceed 1 cm, though a delay of 3 or even 5 days does not irremediably compromise the final result. It is excellent as a prelude to paraffin embedding, and it is this quality that justifies prolongation of fixation to 2 or 3 days especially when pieces are voluminous. *Preparation for celloidin-embedding is, on the contrary, very mediocre* and the use of Bouin's liquid, as indeed all other fixatives based on picric acid, is clearly to be avoided for pieces that are to be cut in celloidin. Freeze-sections may be made after fixing in Bouin's liquid; even the *morphological* study of structured lipids is possible. Preparation for most topographical stainings is excellent and many histochemical reactions can be performed on material fixed in this manner; *nucleal reactions are, however, poor*. Chondriomes and the Golgi apparatus are not conserved; certain secretory products are destroyed by Bouin's liquid while others are very well retained in their place. Bouin's liquid decalcifies; this action is enough to permit cutting sections, without special decalcification, of small pieces that are not too calcified.

The practice of fixing in Bouin's liquid is most simple; it suffices to ensure that with compact pieces one of the dimensions does not exceed 1 cm. No particular washing is called for at the end of fixation; pieces meant for paraffin embedding may be transferred directly from the fixative to the dehydrating alcohol. The pointless rite of going through a series of increasing alcohol has been dealt with in the general comments on histological fixation; the method of removing, if necessary, any excess picric acid remaining in the pieces has also been described in the same chapter. *Prolonged washing in water should be avoided* since it causes swelling of collagenous tissue.

One of the numerous variants of Bouin's liquid proposed by Allen (his PFA 3 liquid) differs from the original formula by the addition of one gram of urea to 100 ml of fixative. According to Allen this addition allows the period of fixation to be prolonged indefinitely without harm to the pieces.

3° *Hollande's liquid* (1918) differs from that of Bouin in two respects, namely, the higher level of picric acid and the presence of copper acetate. It was the first difference, aimed at a better insolubilization of proteins, that was sought for when this fixative liquid was invented, but the copper acetate included to solubilize the picric acid also ensures a better preparation for certain stains. The fixative is prepared by dissolving 2,5 g of neutral copper acetate, if necessary after grinding in a mortar, in 100 ml of distilled water; 4 g. of picric acid are then added in small quantities (*dry picric acid should never be ground in a mortar as it is explosive*); when fully dissolved the solution is filtered and 10 ml of commercial formalin and 1 ml of glacial acetic acid are added. The liquid can be stored indefinitely.

The general properties of this fixative are not essentially different from those of Bouin's liquid, but certain subsequent stainings, especially those involving several acidic dyes, are improved. The size of pieces may be of that recommended for Bouin's liquid; the optimal period of fixation is generally considered to be of two or three days. Hollande recommends washing for 24 hours in several changes of tap-water before dehydration.

4° *Gérard's liquid* is the same as Hollande's fixative to which 10% of a saturated aqueous solution of mercuric chloride has been added. The latter fixing agent improves the preparation for certain stains and also helps to keep in place certain secretory products; while on the other hand it reduces the penetrating power of the liquid. One of the dimensions of the piece should not exceed 5 mm. The period of fixation and washing is the same as that recommended for Hollande's liquid; obviously the mercuric precipitate formed in the piece should be removed during dehydration or, even better, before staining the sections.

5° *Kleineberg's liquid,* based on picric and sulfuric acids, and *Mayer's liquid,* based on picric and nitric acids, should be mentioned in passing. They were often used by entomologists at the beginning of the 20th century but in fact, they are quite disadvantageous when compared to Bouin's liquid and their abandon by modern histologists seems quite well founded.

6° *Lang's liquid* is prepared by mixing 100 ml of a saturated aqueous solution of mercuric chloride (about 7%) with 5 to 10 ml of acetic acid. The period of fixation can vary from 1 to 6 hours according to the size of the pieces. They are then transferred to 70% alcohol which removes excess of fixative and commences dehydration. Since its penetration is quite good this liquid has been recommended by certain authors for glandular tissues and in general for pieces poor in collagen fibres. In fact, however, it has no real advantage over modern fixatives, based on mercuric chloride and its abandon seems justified to me.

7° **Liquids based on formalin and on mercuric chloride** are still widely used in English-speaking countries. A great number of such formulae have been proposed; the oldest of these is that of Bouin (1900) consisting of 190 ml of distilled water, 62,5 ml of commercial formalin and 11,25 g of mercuric chloride. In Heidenhain's mixture (1916) 4,5 g of mercuric chloride and 0,5 g of sodium chloride are dissolved in 80 ml of distilled water and 20 ml of formalin. Dawson and Friedgood (1938) suggest dissolving 9 g of mercuric chloride and 1,8 g of sodium chloride in 225 ml of distilled water and 25 ml of commercial formalin. A mixture of 80 to 90 volumes of an aqueous saturated solution of mercuric chloride with 20 to 10 volumes of formalin has also been used in certain cases.

From the practical point of view it should be remembered that in preparing these solutions the mercuric chloride dissolves slowly and that the formalin should be neutralized with calcium carbonate.

All these fixative liquids penetrate moderately, conserve most secretory products well and afford a satisfactory preparation for embedding in paraffin or celloidin. Shrinkage during paraffin embedding can be considerable, but the preparation for the usual stains is good. The period of fixation varies from 2 to 24 hours according to the size of pieces. The fixative is followed by 70 or 96% alcohol. Mercuric precipitates that are formed in sections should be removed before staining.

Although the above fixative liquids are fancied by many histologists they have no particular advantages and to my mind should be abandoned in favour of the four following liquids.

8° **Heidenhain's Susa** (1916) is prepared by dissolving 4.5 g of mercuric chloride, 0.5 g of sodium chloride and 3 g of trichloracetic acid in 80 ml of distilled water and 20 ml of commercial formalin; when fully dissolved 4 ml of acetic acid are added and the mixture may be stored indefinitely. This is an excellent topographical fixative that penetrates rapidly, fixes uniformly, prepares well for paraffin or celloidin embedding and ensures good retention of staining affinities. The period of fixation varies from 4 to 24 hours according to the size of pieces. One proceeds directly from the fixative to the dehydrating alcohol since any washing in water should be avoided especially when tissues are rich in collagen fibres. Its decalcifying action is even stronger than that of Bouin's liquid.

*9° **Halmi's liquid*** (1952) is Susa to which a tenth of an aqueous saturated solution of picric acid has been added. It is used in the same manner as Susa. The addition of picric acid greatly improves the preparation for subsequent staining and I am inclined to consider this fixative as the best of those containing picric acid. However, the presence of picric acid is obviously a bad prelude for embedding in celloidin.

*10° **Romei's liquid*** (1918) contains 25 parts of an aqueous saturated solution of mercuric chloride, 20 parts of an aqueous 5% solution of trichloracetic acid and 5 parts of commercial formalin. The procedure for use is the same as that for Susa and the results are equally good.

*11° **Stieve's liquid*** is prepared by mixing 76 ml of an aqueous saturated solution of mercuric chloride, 20 ml of formalin and 4 ml of glacial acetic acid. It is perhaps the most penetrating of the topographical fixatives. This was the fixative used by Stieve in his sadly notorious investigations on the histological modifications of the female genital apparatus following somatic and psychic trauma; entire ovaries and whole fragments of the uterine wall could be conserved for detailed histological examination.

Fixation lasts from 1 to 3 days and pieces are transferred directly into the dehydrating alcohol.

*12° **Sanfelice's liquid*** (1918) is the only one among the fixatives based on chromium trioxyde whose penetration is sufficiently rapid for it to be considered as a topographical fixative. It is prepared by mixing, *just before use*, 160 ml of a 1% solution of chromium trioxyde, 80 ml of commercial formalin and 10 ml of glacial acetic acid. Fixation lasts, according to the size of pieces, from 12 hours to a maximum of 24 hours *which should not be exceeded*. Excess fixative should be removed by thorough washing (for at least 24 hours) in running water or several changes of it.

Penetration is quite good, preparation for embedding in paraffin and celloidin excellent and shrinkage is slight although more than with fixatives lacking chromium. A good preparation for most usual stains and the remarkable conservation of nuclear structures go to make of Sanfelice's liquid an excellent fixative for studies in microscopical anatomy and caryology. Its practical disadvantages are that it should be always freshly prepared, that the period of fixation is rigorously limited and that thorough washing is required afterwards.

*13° **V. Tellyesniczky's liquid*** (1898) is a mixture of 100 ml of a 3% potassium dichromate solution and 5 ml of glacial acetic acid freshly prepared just before use. Pieces, one of whose dimensions should not exceed 1 cm, are fixed for 1 to 2 days and washed for 24 hours in running water.

Penetration is quite good, the risk of peripheral over-fixation slight and the interesting structures for topographical examination are uniformly conserved. It prepares well for paraffin and celloidin embedding while the chief topographical stains give good results after it.

As Baker (1951, 1958) justly observes, this liquid, as well as all others of the same sub-group, is irrational in that the pH of the solution is too low for the ionic equilibrium to approach that of a solution of chromium trioxyde. These factors, discussed in more detail in the general comments of fixation, exclude cytoplasmic fixation of a quality obtained with potassium dichromate solutions having a pH higher than 3.8. From a practical point of view it seems logical to substitute chromium trioxyde for potassium dichromate in this liquid.

In any case, however, the two following fixatives are clearly superior to that of v. Tellyesniczky.

14° Liquids based on potassium dichromate, formalin and acetic acid, used principally by German authors and grouped by them under the name of Kaformacet are as irrational as the preceding fixative, and the potassium dichromate that they contain should in all logic be replaced by chromium trioxyde. Their penetration is rapid, fixation uniform and the preparation for paraffin and celloidin embedding as well as for staining is good. A considerable number of formulae have been proposed by different authors, all of which give equivalent results. Only that of Romeis is given here. It consists of 85 ml of a 3% potassium dichromate solution, 10 ml of commercial formalin and 5 ml of glacial acetic acid; The mixture should be prepared *just before use*. One of the dimensions of the piece should be less than 1 cm and the period of fixation should be of 24 hours at the most. On leaving the fixative the pieces are treated with a 5% solution of sodium sulfate whose action is to prevent the collagenous tissue from swelling subsequently. Excess fixative is then removed by washing as usual in running water.

The results of such fixation are good but do not in any way improve on the quality obtained more conveniently with mixtures of potassium dichromate and formalin without acetic acid.

15° Zenker's liquid (1894) enjoys considerable vogue; many laboratories have adopted it as a routine fixative though this preference does not seem to be really justified. It is prepared by adding, just before use, 5 ml of acetic acid to 100 ml of a stock solution which may be made beforehand. The stock solution contains 5 g of mercuric chloride, 2.5 g of potassium dichromate and 1 g of sodium sulfate in 100 ml of water. One of the dimensions of the piece should be less than 1 cm. Fixation lasts 24 hours, followed by another 24 hours of washing in running water or in frequent changes of water.

Penetration of this fixative is quite good but pieces run a certain risk of peripheral over-fixation. The preparation for embedding in paraffin and in celloidin is excellent and so is the retention of staining affinity but shrinkage is more prevalent than with the majority of topographical fixatives that lack potassium dichromate.

The pH of this liquid is actually low enough to prevent it from displaying its qualities as a cytoplasmic fixative. The conservation of secretory granules is slightly better than with Bouin's liquid but clearly not as good as dichromate fixatives without acetic acid.

There is therefore no valid reason to accord Zenker's liquid the favour that it enjoys among many histologists.

It should be noted here that substituting formalin for acetic acid in this formula rectifies the irrationality of the mixture and yields fixatives that are among the best for cytology (liquids of Helly and of Maximow). But their penetrating power is insufficient and the shrinkage too great for them to be considered as topographical fixatives.

16° **Regaud's liquid** (1910) is a *freshly prepared* mixture of 4 volumes of a 3% aqueous solution of potassium dichromate with one volume of commercial formalin neutralized over calcium carbonate. A somewhat similar formula consisting of 4 volumes of a 3,5% potassium dichromate solution and 1 volume of neutralized formalin has been indicated by Kopsch (1896). Fixation lasts 24 hours and excess fixative is removed by washing in running water for 12 to 24 hours.

Its penetrating power is greater than that of Zenker's liquid but clearly less than that of Bouin's liquid. It affords good preparation for embedding in celloidin and in paraffin. Since its pH is higher that 4, it ensures an excellent conservation of cytoplasmic structures, especially secretory products.

Nuclear structures are also well fixed. The tendency to shrink is less than with Zenker's liquid but greater than with that of Bouin. Most stains and a large number of histochemical reactions give excellent results after this fixation. Its use is strongly recommended whenever pieces are not too voluminous and when the conservation of cytoplasmic structures in a perfect state is of importance for the study.

ALCOHOLIC LIQUIDS

It was recalled at the beginning of this chapter that ethyl alcohol does not possess all the properties required of a topographical fixative. It however enters into the composition of some frequently used fixative liquids whose common feature is that they do not ensure the conservation of structural lipids.

1° Clarke's liquid referred to in most publications under the name of Carnoy's liquid, first version or, abridged, Carnoy 1, is a mixture of 3 volumes of absolute alcohol and 1 volume of glacial acetic acid. The mixture is very penetrating; pieces less than 3 mm in thickness are fixed in about five hours. After fixation pieces are transferred directly into absolute alcohol. The preparation for embedding in paraffin and celloidin is excellent and shrinkage is moderate except when tissues are very rich in water. The general architecture of tissues is well conserved as are the nuclear structures, but structured lipids are dissolved and many secretory products are destroyed. It prepares well for the majority of stains, but methods such as Heidenhain's azan or Masson's trichrome give mediocre results.

2° Carnoy's liquid very similar to the preceding one, is prepared by mixing six volumes of absolute alcohol, three volume of chloroform and one volume of acetic acid. Many authors advise that it be prepared freshly each time, but it seems to me that it can be prepared beforehand on condition that it be stored away from light which hastens the decomposition of chloroform. The procedure for use and its results are the same as those of Clarke's liquid. After comparative tests with widely differing tissues I am inclined to consider this fixative as slightly better than that of Clarke, but the difference in value between the two is not very great.

3° Schaffer's liquid (1908) which is the prototype of mixtures of alcohol and formalin, contains two volumes of 80% alcohol and one volume of formalin (neutralized commercial solution). Fixation in this liquid lasts from 7 hours to 3 days depending on the size of pieces which are then transferred to the dehydrating alcohol.

Penetration is very rapid and homogeneous with little risk of peripheral over-fixation. Preparation for embedding in celloidin is excellent, while that for embedding in paraffin is much better than after fixation in formol or in alcohol singly. The tendency to shrink is as slight as that with Bouin's liquid and hardening of pieces is less than that with fixatives based on potassium dichromate. The preparation for topographical staining is good, but it should be observed that the conservation of secretory granules leaves much to be desired in certain cases.

4° Apathy's liquid is a solution of 4g of mercuric chloride and 0.5 g of sodium chloride in 100 ml of 50% alcohol. Pieces are fixed for 12 to 24 hours and then transferred to 70% alcohol.

This fixative is quite penetrating and ensures a good preparation for all types of embedding, while the tendency to shrink is not great. Most usual stains give good results.

5° **Schaudinn's liquid,** which is clearly not so advantageous as the above fixative, contains one volume of a saturated aqueous solution of mercuric chloride and two volumes of absolute alcohol. Schaudinn used this fixative with a warming (60–70°) for small objects that are difficult to penetrate such as Nematode eggs. The tendency to shrink is very strong and the conservation of cytoplasmic structures mediocre. In spite of its continued use by certain authors it does not really deserve to be retained for routine work.

6° **Brasil's liquid** (1904) formulated on the advice of Duboscq, is often referred to as Duboscq–Brasil liquid or alcoholic Bouin. It differs from the classical Bouin by the nature of its solvent. It contains 160 ml of 80% alcohol, 60 ml of commercial formalin, 15 ml of acetic acid and 1 g of picric acid. Contrary to a widely held prejudice, this liquid may be prepared beforehand; adding acetic acid to a stock solution containing all other components just before use does not give the slightest advantage.

This liquid penetrates to the same extent as Bouin's liquid and the preparation for paraffin embedding is equally good, while embedding in celloidin is evidently poor. Structures are generally not as well conserved as with Bouin's liquid and a large number of secretory products do not resist fixation. Obviously all structured lipids are destroyed. Preparation for staining is in general not as good as after Bouin's liquid.

Certain authors claim that fixation in Brasil's liquid can last much longer than in Bouin's liquid; I do not share this view. As in the case of the latter fixative a week is about the maximum that should not be exceeded and not even attained whenever possible. Pieces are transferred directly from the fixative to the dehydrating alcohol.

The vogue for this fixative is due, apart from a force of habit, to the delusion that penetration across cuticular structures is better because of the alcohol content of Brasil's liquid. In fact this argument cannot hold since it suffices to dip cuticular pieces very rapidly in alcohol to enable them to be wetted by all aqueous fixatives. From my personal experience Brasil's fixative is less advantageous than Bouin's liquid; it has no particular property to compensate for its drawbacks.

THE PRACTICE OF TOPOGRAPHICAL FIXATION

All the general considerations concerning the mode of operation and the choice of fixative described in an earlier chapter evidently apply to "topographical" fixation as well. However, certain problems particular to this type of fixation will be discussed below.

CHOICE OF FIXATIVE

The list of fixative mixtures given in the preceding paragraphs is much shorter than if it were a mere compilation and yet too long for it to contain only the really indispensable ones. They were chosen with a desire to avoid any bias and the need to mention fixatives whose advantages are doubtful which enjoy such a vogue that they have to be mentioned. Every histologist can, at some time or other, be led to treat at least part of his material under study by repeating exactly the work of a predecessor. In fact, the number of really efficacious topographical fixatives is much less than the number given earlier. According to the convention adopted in the introduction to this part of the book and from my personal experience, four types of fixation may be usefully retained for concomitant trials on an object of which one has not much previous experience. In the field of microscopical anatomy the differences in the final result obtained with Bouin's liquid on the one hand and the liquids of Hollande and of Gérard on the other hand are not significant enough to warrant preference for the latter two which are more complicated to prepare. Among the liquids based on mercuric chloride, but devoid of potassium dichromate, those of Romeis, of Halmi and Heidenhain's Susa give roughly equivalent results; I personally prefer that of Halmi. In the present context the liquid of Kopsch-Regaud seems to me the best of all fixatives based on potassium dichromate. Among the alcoholic liquids that of Carnoy satisfies best all requirements of a topographical fixative.

In short, I consider that the histologist who provides for fixation in the liquids of Bouin, Halmi, Regaud and of Carnoy in the case of material to be studied topographically for the first time reduces the chances of failure to a minimum and guards against unpleasant surprises at the time of examining preparations. It is quite rare that at least one of these four fixations fails to give satisfactory topographical preparations when correctly applied.

A personal experience of the material or the advice of an experienced colleague evidently permits the use of only one such fixative. Those who devote all their activity to the histology of Mammals have a tendency to forget that tissues of other animals react differently to fixatives. Thus Carnoy's fixative which gives excellent fixation with the tissues of insects and chilopods is clearly less suited for diplopods and arachnids. Fixation in formalin with any adjuvant is even more mediocre for tissues of Molluscs than for those of vertebrates.

Even though the chondriome and the Golgi apparatus are necessarily sacrificed in topographical fixation one should not neglect the possibility of practising certain histochemical reactions on part of the material. The choice of the above four fixatives provides for this in many respects.

In addition, provision should evidently made for fixing in dilute formalin, saline formaline or formaldehyde-calcium if the study of structured lipids is intended.

REMOVAL AND FIXATION

The speed of removing samples for topographical histology is evidently less exacting than for cytological or histochemical research; it is however better to do it rapidly. Certain invertebrate organs deteriorate at a really astonishing rate; good fixation of the branchial folioles of gastropods or the hypobranchial gland are obtained only if the object is plunged alive into the fixative. In general it may be admitted that pieces should find themselves in the fixative within 15 minutes after death, which does not necessarily coincide with that of the whole animal.

The indications concerning the size of pieces given earlier relate to compact organs. Obviously when large natural cavities are found in pieces into which the fixative has access the size of the piece can be increased. Similarly, organs with a loose texture can be cut into larger pieces than dense parenchyma. The type of tissue also has its influence; thus those elaborating proteolytic enzymes have evidently a tendency for greater autolysis than others.

In all cases it is important to bring about contact of the tissues to be fixed with the fixative as rapidly as possible. Pieces that are covered with a cuticle which is not easily wetted (teguments of most terrestrial arthropods) should be dipped for a few instants in alcohol before treating them with aqueous fixatives. It is essential that the surfaces of pieces should be cleaned of layers of blood or mucus as far as possible before placing in the fixative. Incising the tegument and cutting animals to be fixed *in toto* into suitable segments are useful precautions; this should be carried out progressively when the body of the animal is turgescent (dipteran larvae, opisthosoma of araneids etc...).

Injecting fixative into the general cavity can be of great use; it should be effected, in the case of fixatives containing mercuric chloride, with a drawn-out pipette and not with a metallic needle. Interstitial injection of fixative, which is also sometimes useful, should be carefully done as too much distension of tissues can seriously modify anatomical proportions; the same prudence should be observed while injecting fixative into hollow organs. Fixation by vascular perfusion can be advantageous in the case of animals with a closed circulatory system.

The volume of fixative into which pieces are immersed should be as large as possible. The relatively cheap cost of topographical fixatives removes any scruple in this matter and there is no reason not to use systematically a volume of fixative that is at least 50 times that of the pieces. Evidently the piece should be in contact with the fixative on all sides; it should never be placed first in an empty vessel and then covered with fixative, and many authors recommend a layer of cotton at the bottom. The precaution of suspending pieces midway in the fixative with a piece of string can be useful in some cases.

When pieces containing air are fixed it is strongly advisable to remove the air by gradually creating a moderate vacuum; I consider this operation as almost indispensable when fixing terrestrial arthropods. The vacuum obtained with a filter-pump is sufficient for the purpose. The fixative liquid should be renewed on returning to normal pressure. The fixation of pieces containing calcium salts in decalcifying liquids is also greatly improved by establishing a vacuum which removes the gas bubbles that are produced and which prevent the fixative from coming into even contact with certain zones of the piece.

The suitable periods of fixation have been indicated for each mixture. They are evidently a rough estimate and should be adjusted according to the size and the consistency of pieces. The nature of the fixative mixtures is also to be considered. Any delay of over 24 hours is harmful with fixatives based on potassium dichromate and formalin which are unstable liquids whose decomposition is besides denoted by a change in colour.

Past this delay pieces get very much hardened and shrink considerably during subsequent operations. Certain staining affinities are also irremediably altered. Exceeding the period of fixation with Carnoy's liquid also produces much hardening and shrinkage. In the case of fixatives based on picric acid exceeding the optimal period affects especially the staining affinity of certain tissue components and is less serious.

STOPPING FIXATION AND STORING PIECES

Of all the liquids described here, only those based on potassium dichromate necessitate the immediate removal of excess fixative by careful and prolonged washing in tap water. In all others cases transferring into dehydrating alcohol suffices.

Storing pieces in 70 or 96% alcohol when they are not to be treated immediately is a solidly established habit among histologists. It does not generally harm pieces that are fixed in liquids devoid of potassium dichromate; when they do contain dichromate the hardening caused can be troublesome while cutting sections. But storing in ethyl alcohol is far from being the most suitable expedient.

In all cases where dehydration can be carried out immediately it is best to store in methyl benzoate, with or without added celloidin, or in butanol. These liquids do not at all modify the consistency of pieces and they maintain staining affinities. Embedding can follow rapidly after two baths in benzene, when conservation is in methyl benzoate (or salicylate), or directly if conserved in butanol. These storage liquids, which are also suitable intermediates for paraffin embedding, show a much lesser tendency to evaporate than ethanol so that constant inspection of stored material is less important.

In cases where pieces fixed in an aqueous liquid cannot be dehydrated immediately, the best storage medium, in my opinion, is not alcohol but formalin diluted to 10% (4% of formaldehyde). The use of Baker's formula (1944) which is a mixture of 90 ml of water, 10 ml of formalin, 1 g of calcium chloride and 1 g of cadmium chloride, ensures very good conservation of lipid inclusions so that even histochemical studies may be carried out on them satisfactorily. The tendency to evaporate is less than with alcohol and dehydration can commence immediately on leaving the conserving solution without washing.

Obviously, storage in a conserving liquid is resorted to when circumstances do not permit otherwise; immediate embedding should be preferred whenever possible. In fact, it is in paraffin or celloidin that material fixed for histological study is best conserved.

CHOICE OF EMBEDDING METHOD

Pieces meant for demonstrating lipids are cut in a freezing microtome, if necessary, after embedding in gelatin following the technique of Baker or of Heringa and ten Berge. Others are embedded in celloidin or paraffin, the choice between the two depending on the habits of the operator, the practice of the laboratory, the type of material and the aim of the study. Generally, paraffin embedding permits serial sections rapidly and conveniently; it allows the regular and uniform cutting that is necessary for reconstruction; it is also the quicker of the two and the only one that enables cutting sections less than 5 μ. However, pieces should be quite small; certain tissues tend to harden considerably when going through warm paraffin, while shrinkage is greater than in celloidin.

The latter is therefore to be preferred for larger pieces or for those with an uneven consistency such as when they contain bone or cartilage.

CHAPTER 9

TOPOGRAPHICAL STAINING

The task of compiling all the technical details concerning topographical staining is rendered difficult for want of an exact definition of such methods and by the unbelievable multiplicity of modifications and variants of the fundamental procedures, many of which are really of no great use at all. Even when differences in detail between formulae derived from the same procedure are neglected, it has to be admitted that many methods give a more or less equivalent differentiation of structures, but for the colour, so that the choice among techniques becomes preponderantly subjective. A general review of topographical staining would therefore differ greatly in length according to whether it includes only really useful formulae or whether it covers the greatest possible number of procedures. Clearly, a complete inventory of all the techniques used in microscopical anatomy since the very beginnings of histological research would be only of limited interest. On the other hand, confining this chapter to those methods considered indispensable would have the disadvantage of excluding many that are frequently used and described so often in works that even those who do not actually practise them personally should be acquainted with them.

Topographical staining may be applied to sections or to pieces when the latter are intended for mounting *in toto* or eventual embedding and cutting into sections. Such "bulk staining" is described at the end of the chapter.

The general course of staining as well as the techniques of dewaxing and mounting have been described in the first part of this book. Only those techniques proper to staining are described below.

CLASSIFICATION OF TOPOGRAPHICAL STAINS

The impossibility of rigorously defining topographical staining evidently rules out any proper classification of these procedures. However, the simple enumeration of a certain number of techniques as they are given in many handbooks of microscopy and histological technique does not at all satisfy the mind. Some authors have solved the difficulty by classifying the methods according to the nature of the stains used; but it seems to me that a classification based on the final result obtained is more advantageous for the user.

The classification adopted here follows from a consideration of the factors that contribute to the "legibility" of a section stained by any topographical method. Apart from the quality of nuclear staining and the clearness of the preparation, the ease of identifying different structures and of distinguishing between organs and tissues depends on a good demonstration of fibrous structures, basement membranes and ground substance as well as the differential staining of the cytoplasm and secretory products. It therefore seems justifiable to me to distinguish, among the so-called topographical stains, those that ensure a selective staining of connective fibres, especially collagenous tissue, and those that function by revealing the tinctorial affinities of the cytoplasm and secretory products.

Such a classification has evidently nothing absolute about it since methods that satisfy both the above requirements do exist. However, the distinction between the two groups of stains is of practical interest since it orients the choice of the operator from the outset. In fact, the methods of the first or the second group are indicated according to whether fibrous structures or glandular parenchyma dominate the piece and are the prior concern of the investigator. Roughly speaking the demonstration of collagen is especially convenient for the anatomical study of animals whose bodies are rich in fibrous structures; they "render" better with vertebrates and molluscs than with arthropods. On the other hand, those of the second group should be preferred while examining pieces whose different tissues are interwoven without the insertion of any large bundles of connective fibres.

In any case, a very good demonstration of nuclear structures is essential for a satisfactory topographical preparation and for this reason staining by the progressive haematoxylin lakes holds a privileged place in histological technique. They are used alone or, very often, as nuclear stains in a combined technique. Their use is so frequent that one seems justified in devoting a special paragraph to them.

The following pages will therefore describe successively nuclear stains by haematoxylin lakes, selective staining of collagenous tissue and methods whose chief aim is to bring out the staining affinities of the cytoplasm or secretory products. The main bulk stains used in the topographical study of tissues and organs are treated at the end.

NUCLEAR STAINING BY PROGRESSIVE HAEMATOXYLIN LAKES

Haematoxylin is a compound extracted from the wood of *Haematoxylon campechianum* whose use for staining plant or animal fabrics (cotton, wool, etc.) was known to the peoples of Central America before the Spanish Conquest. Introduced afterwards into Europe, the extract of logwood (Campeachy) was used empirically in the textile industry. Its linear formula established by Chevreul (1810) is $C_{16}H_{14}O_6$. The fundamental work of Erdmann (1842) has shown that haematoxylin itself is not a stain but that it acquires the properties of one after oxydation to haematein, $C_{16}H_{12}O_6$. The loss of two atoms of hydrogen occurs without the addition of oxygen to the molecule. Its structural formula has been elucidated by Perkins and Robinson (1908); it indicates that the transformation of haematoxylin into hematein results, from the staining point of view, in the appearance of a quinonoid chromophore on the ring that carries the oxygen atom (carbon 9).

It is thus hematein and not hematoxylin that is the stain so widely used by histologists; but the misuse of the expression "hematoxylin staining" is so prevalent that it would be quite pointless to strive against it, and any attempt to replace it with the correct chemical terminology is likely to result only in misunderstanding.

Hematein is used in histological technique—as in industrial dyeing—only in the form of lakes; its structural formula clearly brings out the possibility of chelation with metals.

Suppliers of histological products sell both hematoxylin and hematein. Their qualities, especially of the latter, vary greatly according to the brand and the batch. One should therefore submit products of different origins to methodical trials and stock supplies of those of reliable quality. Hematoxylin comes in the form of yellowish crystals or a yellowish brown powder, while hematein appears as a brown powder. The former is quite soluble in water (1–2%) and very soluble in alcohol (more than 20%) while the latter is only very slightly soluble in both water or alcohol.

Among the several histological applications of hematoxylin some require the use of "ripened" solutions where the compound is oxidized into hematein. Every histologist worthy of the name should have at his disposal a stock of a 10% solution of hematoxylin in 96% alcohol that has ripened over at least six months. This solution keeps very well especially if care is taken to store it in bottles of glass out of which little alkali leaches. Desired dilutions in alcohol or water are made from such a stock solution according the formula required for the chosen technique.

The nuclear stainings with hematoxylin discussed here involve aluminium, ferric or chromic lakes that act progressively. The regressive techniques described elsewhere in this book evidently give admirable nuclear staining, but they are not really topographical methods and are therefore included among the cytological techniques.

ALUMINIUM LAKES OF HEMATEIN

These lakes, grouped by histologists under the term "*hemalum*", are prepared from potassium alum (the double sulfate of aluminium and potassium). They provide a convenient and excellent nuclear stain that ranges from blue to deep violet. Their specificity is sufficient to render any differentiation unnecessary, and I even strongly advise against any attempt at differentiation as the stain is not "bound" well enough to withstand the operation. Staining is generally very fast but does not resist the action of certain acid stains well enough. Progressive ferric lakes should be preferred for combined staining involving such acidic dyestuffs. Staining solutions keep well for several months.

*1° **Hansen's hemalum*** (1895), based on hematoxylin, has the advantage over other formulae of this type in that the lake shows excellent conservation. Hematoxylin is oxidized into hematein by the action of potassium permanganate. Other oxidants can in fact be used as well. Thus, Hansen (1926) has indicated the following quantities required to transform 1 g of hematoxylin into hematein:

Potassium permanganate	0.177 g
Potassium dichromate	0.276 g
Potassium chlorate	0.114 g
Potassium perchlorate	0.097 g
Potassium iodate	0.200 g
Potassium di-iodate	0.182 g
Sodium iodate	0.197 g

Baker and Jordan (1953) advise reducing these quantities if the staining solutions are to be kept for a very long time; only part of the hematoxylin is oxidized at first, which suffices for immediate use, while the rest gets oxidized gradually in air. Spreading oxidation over a period guarantees against a rapid alteration of the dyestuff.

Hansen's hemalum may be prepared as follows. 1 g of hematoxylin is dissolved in 10 ml of distilled water with heating. Another solution of 20 g of potassium alum in 200 ml of distilled water is also made with heating. A day later, the two solutions are mixed and 0.177 g of potassium permanganate (or 3 ml of a solution containing 1 g of potassium permanganate and 16 ml) of water are added. The mixture is boiled for one minute, cooled and filtered. The solution should be stored in a well-stoppered bottle.

2° **P. Masson's hemalum** is prepared directly with hematein and so does not require oxidation. 0.20 g of good quality hematein is added to 100 ml of a saturated aqueous solution of potassium alum (about 10%) and the mixture boiled for one to three minutes, cooled and filtered.

Both Hansen's and Masson's hemalum can be acetified with 2 ml of acetic acid per 100 ml of stain. Such a lowering of pH is recommended by certain authors to increase specificity as a nuclear stain. I am not entirely convinced of the usefulness of this measure; it could however lead to a better conservation of the solution.

3° **Method of using hemalum.** — The typical example of its use is in progressive nuclear staining; it gives good results after any of the fixations described in the previous chapter. Its use is however, not recommended after prolonged fixation in mixtures based on potassium dichromate, after post-chromatization and after fixation in liquids containing osmium tetroxyde or chloroplatinic acid. In using hemalum overstaining should be avoided by following, under the microscope, the progressive staining of the nuclei and stopping the process when the desired tint is obtained. Differentiation of very deep staining is possible by treating sections with either very dilute acetic acid (1 or 2%) or a 2% solution of potassium alum. Differentiation in alcohol-hydrochloric acid (99.5 ml of absolute alcohol and 0.5 ml of hydrochloric acid) so often recommended, seems to me the worst possible procedure since the action takes place in a matter of seconds, while the former two liquids act over several minutes and enable the process to be followed conveniently. In all cases, staining with hemalum, with or without differentiation should end with through washing (for several minutes) in running water. It is during this wash, aimed at removing the last traces of alum, that the nuclei take on their final tint. Proper washing is essential for the conservation of preparations.

Generally, staining with hemalum is practised as follows:

— Sections are dewaxed, collodioned when desired and hydrated after the removal of mercuric chloride crystals if any.

— Staining is checked by examination under the microscope after a rinse in tap water.

— Wash for 3 or 5 minutes in tap-water.

— Mount in balsam or carry out a further background stain.

In some cases it is preferable to use very dilute solutions of hemalum and lengthen the time of staining consequently. Solutions that have been diluted with 50 or 100 volumes of distilled water can stain in 4 to 24 hours. This kind of procedure is particularly suitable when the affinity of certain mucins for the aluminium lakes of hematoxylin is the basis of staining. The use of solutions diluted a tenfold is also recommended for staining frozen sections.

4° **Results of staining.** — The final result of staining with hemalum is essentially a blue or violet stain of nuclei, but other structures can also take stain. The ergastoplasm and calcic inclusions appear blue, while certain mucins stain very deeply. There are some secretory products that have a very strong affinity for the aluminium lakes of hematein; ground substances rich in acidic mucopolysaccharides also stain deeply. One should therefore not count on staining being limited to nuclei only; even the entire cytoplasm can take on a grey or bluish tint, especially when the staining solution is not very fresh, but in practice this is not really troublesome.

PROGRESSIVE FERRIC LAKES OF HEMATEIN

These lakes differ from hemalum in that they give a nuclear stain that shows greater resistance to acidic stains and differentiators. They are also more specific, which can be both an advantage or a disadvantage according to the circumstances. They should therefore be preferred to aluminium lakes whenever staining has to be restricted to the nuclei and when subsequent treatment involves powerful reagents. Three out of the several formulae that exist are retained here. That of Weigert seems to me quite outmoded by the other two and I personally never use it. However, so many histologists adopt it that I cannot avoid mentioning it. As for the two other ferric lakes included here, ferric trioxyhematein and Groat's hematoxylin, both give equivalent results on paraffin sections, but the first is dissolved in water and the second in 50% alcohol. Consequently, Groat's hematoxylin cannot be used as a background stain after stains or histochemical reagents which require treatment and mounting in an aqueous medium. The two lakes cannot therefore be used interchangeably.

1° **Weigert's iron hematoxylin** is prepared freshly before use by mixing equal parts of a 1% solution of hematoxylin in 96% alcohol (ripening is necessary, and a sufficient quantity should be prepared well in advance) and an acidic solution of ferric chloride (1.16 g of ferric chloride, 98 ml of distilled water and 1 ml of 25% hydrochloric acid). The hydrochloric acid of the required concentration for the latter solution is prepared by adding 50 ml of distilled water to 100 ml of the concentrated hydrochloric acid (d = 1.19) obtained commercially. Each of the two solutions may be stored for several years, but their mixture deteriorates in a few days, and hence should be prepared in small quantities as the need arises.

The operating procedure is quite simple and corresponds in all its details to that of hemalum. Highly selective staining of nuclei is obtained in about two minutes. The differentiation of overstained sections is possible; unlike in the case of aluminium lakes 0.1–0 5% hydrochloric acid in alcohol may be used for the purpose. Washing in water should be as thorough as in staining with hemalum.

*2° **Hansen's ferric trioxyhematein*** may be prepared beforehand as it can be stored for about three months. 10 g of iron alum and 1.4 g of ammonium sulfate are dissolved with slight warming, but not boiling, in 150 ml of distilled water. A second solution of 1.6 g of hematoxylin in 75 ml of distilled water is also made, warming if necessary to a little less than 100°. After cooling the solution of iron alum is poured into that of hematoxylin (and not the inverse), the mixture placed in a pyrex flask and brought to the boil for about 40 seconds. It should then be cooled rapidly to avoid too much oxydation. The stain is stored in a well stoppered pyrex or paraffined glass bottle; it should be filtered each time before use. Ferric trioxyhematein is used in the same manner as hemalum or Weigert's hematoxylin. The selectivity of nuclear staining may be increased by acidifying with 2–4 ml of 1% sulfuric acid per 8 ml of stain.

*3° **Groat's hematoxylin*** has greater practical advantages than the two other ferric lakes mentioned here, and I strongly recommend its use whenever operating in an aqueous medium can be dispensed with. According to Groat's formula (1948, 1949) 1 g of iron alum is dissolved in 50 ml of distilled water followed by the addition of 0.8 ml of sulfuric acid, 50 ml of 90 or 96% alcohol and, finally, 0.5 g of hematoxylin. Dissolution of the latter is facilitated by preparing the mixture of water, iron alum and sulfuric acid separately, and pouring into it the alcohol in which the hematoxylin has been dissolved. Filtration is not always necessary. When stored in well-stoppered bottles, the stain retains all its qualities for at least three months.

The operating procedure is the same as that for other ferric lakes. The need for thorough washing in water is particularly evident in the case of this lake which is dissolved in a very acidic medium. It is only during washing that nuclei take on the clearly black stain that is characteristic of this method.

Apart from the above qualities these three progressive ferric lakes of hematoxylin possess the advantage of staining celloidin and gelatin only very weakly. They are therefore particularly suitable for staining sections that have been embedded in such media or for tissue cultures that have been bulk-stained in their medium. The tint of the ergastoplasm, the ground substances rich in mucopolysaccharides and of mucins is definitely lighter than with hemalum. Furthermore, these ferric lakes give acceptable results in some cases where hemalum is quite without effect, that is, after prolonged fixation in a liquid based on potassium dichromate or after osmic fixation.

PROGRESSIVE CHROMIC LAKES OF HEMATEIN

The chromic lakes of hematoxylin play a far less important role than the aluminium or ferric lakes in the topographical staining practised by classical authors. This is rather due to a force of habit than to any eventual disadvantages of the chromic lakes, which, in fact, give excellent nuclear staining and are better suited than the aluminium or ferric lakes for bulk staining. Yet another reason for not disregarding these lakes is the vogue, as a stain for certain secretory products, of a particular chromic lake of hematoxylin described by Gomori (1939, 1941) and which largely corresponds to the chromic lakes of Hansen (1905) described below.

The investigations of Hansen have shown that hematein can produce several chromic lakes that differ according to the degree of oxydation of the dye molecule. As Harms (1965) has remarked, it is a case of hydrogen atoms being lost without a corresponding addition of oxygen to the molecule. Actually, the quantitative data available concerning the oxidative derivatives of hematoxylin are not precise enough for Hansen's results to be interpreted in chemical terms; however, in spite of their empiricism their practical advantages should not be neglected.

The chromic lake which can be particularly recommended as a nuclear stain is that designated by Hansen as chromic dioxyhematein. It is prepared in the following steps:

Dissolve 10 g of chrome alum in 250 ml of distilled water. Boil until the solution turns green, and allow to cool.

Dissolve 1 g of hematoxylin in 10–15 ml of distilled water with warming. Add this solution to the previous one. The hematoxylin may also be dissolved in the boiling solution of chrome alum.

After cooling add 0.5 g of sulfuric acid, that is, about 5 ml of a 10% solution of sulfuric acid. Add 0.55 g of potassium dichromate dissolved in 20 ml of distilled water. This should be added in small quantities with shaking.

Boil the mixture and maintain it for 2 or 4 minutes before cooling.

The solution may be used as soon as it is cooled. It can be stored in a well-stoppered bottle for several years. It should be filtered each time before use.

The operating procedure is similar to the other progressive lakes of hematoxylin. Good topographical staining usually requires 5 to 10 minutes, with practically no risk of overstaining even if prolonged to beyond an hour. The stain resists treatment with acids and the action of sunlight. Reducing the level of sulfuric acid in the above formula increases the intensity of cytoplasmic staining, which can be desirable in some cases and undesirable in others. Obviously, staining is terminated by thorough washing in tap water.

In practice, the choice among the various progressive lakes of hematoxylin depends largely on routine habits. Generally, ferric and chromic lakes are preferred to hemalum when a very selective and resistant staining of nuclei is desired. Hansen's ferric trioxyhematein and chromic dioxyhematein as well as Groat's hematoxylin are all equivalent in this respect. The last of these has the great advantage that it can be prepared without heating. It is unsuitable only in the case of sections that contain substances that cannot resist 50% alcohol.

SELECTIVE STAINING OF COLLAGEN FIBRES

A great many topographical stains are characterized by the striking appearance of collagenous tissue against the rest of the preparation. This result can be attained in many ways and the proliferation of techniques, often quite unjustified, has been particularly rampant in this group. The topographical value of such preparations is very great and the importance of certain procedures bears well beyond the range of microscopical anatomy. There exist some methods of demonstrating collagen fibres which do not yield preparations particularly suited for topographical study; they will be discussed in the chapter devoted to the techniques concerning connective tissue.

The classification of the selective stains for collagen fibres described here is simple. They are in fact based on two different mechanisms. Certain methods involve a competition between two acidic stains whose particle size and diffusion coefficients differ sufficiently. Others have the common feature of including the action of phosphomolybdic or phosphotungstic acid.

STAINING BASED ON COMPETITION BETWEEN TWO ACIDIC DYE-STUFFS

The principle of these methods has been described in the chapter devoted to general remarks on histological staining in connection with the role of diffusion in determining the colour of sections. It is quite simple and is based on a certain number of experimental data, especially those of Collin (1923, 1924), v. Möllendorff and Tomita (1926) and Seki (1932). When a section is treated, simultaneously or successively, with two acidic dye-stuffs whose diffusion coefficients differ sufficiently, the more diffusible of the two fixes itself on to the denser structures while the other is rather restricted to the looser structures. In spite of certain objections such a conception accounts for the phenomenon as a whole, and electron microscopical evidence confirms it especially in the interpretation of differences in the tinctorial affinities of certain secretory granules. The number of possible stain combinations is evidently very great; that of techniques is even greater since various nuclear stains may be applied before carrying out acid staining. Only the most useful of the several techniques will be described here. They may be grouped according to the particular dyestuffs. One of these is always picric acid, used as a saturated aqueous solution; the other can be indigocarmine, a natural dye which is the only case of an indigo derivative used in histological technique, acid fuchsin, ponceau, thiazine red, methyl blue, aniline blue or any of the acid blues among the poly-azo dyes.

1° *Hemalum-picro-indigocarmine*

This is the only method of the group that permits nuclear staining with hemalum, since exposure to the acid stain is very short and the browning of the nuclear stain that results does not appreciably affect examination of the preparation.

Reagents:

> Masson's or Hansen's hemalum;
> Picro-indigocarmine (0.4 g of indigocarmine is dissolved in 100 ml of aqueous saturated picric acid).

Operating procedure:

> Sections are dewaxed, collodioned if necessary, cleaned of mercuric precipitates and hydrated.
> Stain with hemalum so that the nuclei take on a deep shade.
> Wash for about 3 minutes in running water.
> Stain with picro-indigocarmine for 10 seconds in a dish or on slides.
> Dehydrate directly with absolute alcohol, clear in benzene or toluene and mount in balsam or a synthetic resin.

The action of the picric acid in picro-indigocarmine further brings out the staining of the nuclei. Since indigocarmine is very soluble in water, washing in the latter or in alcohol-water mixtures should be avoided afterwards; dehydration is therefore carried out in absolute alcohol with no other intermediate.

Results. — Collagen fibres are coloured blue; nuclei, the ergastoplasm and other cytoplasmic structures that show an affinity for hemalum are stained brown; the cytoplasm itself ranges from yellow to green. When the hemalum is of good quality, which mainly depends on the hematein used in preparing it, the blue stain of structures rich in mucopolysaccharides persists in spite of the action of picric acid. When properly mounted the preparations may be kept indefinitely. The clear-cut tints give by this method render its choice advantageous for anatomical analysis; photography is easy (slow panchromatic emulsion with a green filter if the fibres stained blue are to be subdued and an orange filter if the contrary is desired).

2° *Ramon y Cajal's trichrome*

This magnificient stain is disdained by too many histologists, probably because most descriptions of the operating procedure are quite imprecise and lead to frequent failure. In fact, success is easily ensured if the use of the alcoholic solution of basic fuchsin, advocated at the beginning of the century, is avoided. With the basic fuchsin that is now available on the market, a dilute phenolic solution (Ziehl) will almost certainly give a good stain.

Reagents:

> Ziehl's phenolic fuchsin (grind 1 g of basic fuchsin and 5 g of phenol with 10 ml of 96% alcohol in a mortar; add 90 ml of distilled water in small quantities; filter the solution, which may be kept for a long time).
> Picro-indigocarmine.
> Water acidified with acetic acid to 0.3–0.5%.

Operating procedure:

> Sections are dewaxed, collodioned and hydrated.
> Stain for 10 minutes at room temperature in the following mixture:
> > Ziehl's fuchsin .... 1 vol.
> > Distilled water .... 9 vol.
> > (this mixture keeps for 48 hours at the most, and hence should be prepared in small quantities);
> Rinse in tap-water and treat with water acidified with acetic acid until the excess of basic fuchsin has been extracted.
> Stain for 5 to 10 minutes with picro-indigocarmine.
> Treat for 20 to 30 seconds with acidified water.
> Differentiate on slides until all the excess of basic fuchsin has been extracted with absolute alcohol; those regions of the section that are poor in nuclei should take on a greyish blue tint.
> Clear in benzene or toluene and mount in balsam or a synthetic resin.

Results. — Nuclei are stained red as precisely as they are with iron-hematoxylin; the cytoplasm ranges from pink to yellow; structures rich in acid mucopolysaccharides (e. g. ground substance of cartilage) take a metachromatic violet tint with some samples of basic fuchsin; certain secretory granules stain red, while others stain yellow or blue. Collagen fibres appear a very pure blue; reticulin fibres are not stained at all while certain elastic fibres may take a red tint. This method is particularly suited for staining sections that contain structures coloured black either naturally or following silver impregnation or vital injection of India ink, etc... Preparations conserve very well. I advise the use of a green filter for photography if demonstration of collagen fibres can be neglected, and an orange filter otherwise.

Krause (1911) has devised a variant which differs from Ramon y Cajal's trichrome only in the nuclear stain, which is carried out in an aqueous-alcoholic solution of safranin (1 g of safranin is first dissolved in 100 ml of absolute alcohol and then 50 ml of distilled water are added; the solution keeps well). The times of staining are the same as for Ramon y Cajal's trichrome; metachromatic staining of structures rich in acid mucopolysaccharides is often more distinct, but nuclei are stained less brightly.

3° *Nuclear fast-red picro-indigocarmine*

This combination, which I have been using since about ten years, does not figure, as far as I am aware, in manuals of histological technique. It has the advantage of using, as a nuclear stain, the aluminium lake of an anthraquinone that is related to alizarin red S. This lake is insoluble in absolute alcohol and is not at all altered by picroindigocarmine. The tints that are obtained are less bright than with Ramon y Cajal's trichrome, but the method offers absolute security. It may be remarked here that the aluminium lake of nuclear fast red tends to replace more and more the preparations based on carmine that were formerly used to stain sections. Its introduction into histological technique is due to Domagk (1932).

Reagents:

> Aluminium lake of nuclear fast red (dissolve, with heating, 0.1 g of nuclear fast red —not to be confounded with fast red or fast red salt B—and 5 g of ammonium sulfate in 100 ml of distilled water, leave to settle for 24 hours, filter and add 1 ml of commercial formalin to prevent contamination; the solution keeps for two or three months).
> Picro-indigocarmine
> Water acidified with acetic acid to 0.3-0.5%.

Operating procedure:

> Sections are dewaxed, collodioned and hydrated.
> Stain for 2 to 4 minutes with the aluminium lake of nuclear fast red.
> Rinse in tap water.
> Stain for 5 minutes with picro-indigocarmine.
> Rinse in acidified water.
> Dehydrate in absolute alcohol, clear and mount in balsam or a synthetic resin.

Results. — Nuclei stain red, as precisely but lighter than after basic fuchsin. The cytoplasm stains pale pink, grey or yellow. Collagen fibres take the same colour as in Ramon y Cajal's trichrome. Structures rich in mucopolysaccharides and elastic fibres do not contrast against the rest. Photography may follow the recommendations given for Ramon y Cajal's trichrome.

4° *Van Gieson's method*

This method of staining, described in 1889, is based on the same principle as the previous ones. After nuclear staining with a hematoxylin lake the sections are treated with a mixture of an aqueous saturated solution of picric acid and a solution of acid fuchsin; the latter renders collagen fibres more or less intensely red and the cytoplasm yellow. Other red acid stains of the triphenyl-methane group or the azo group may be substituted for acid fuchsin.

Since the invention of this stain a large number of variants have been suggested that are particularly meant for paraffin, celloidin and frozen sections. Of these, Hansen's formula is the best when acid fuchsin is adopted as a stain for collagen fibres. The practice of staining nuclei with hemalum, common in certain laboratories of pathology, should be definitely avoided; it is not fast enough to resist the action of picric acid and the resulting brownish tint of the nuclei is very inconvenient for examining sections.

Reagents:

>   Weigert's hematoxylin, ferric trioxyhematein or Groat's hematoxylin.
>   Picrofuchsin (0.1 g of acid fuchsin in 100 ml of a saturated aqueous solution of picric acid).

Operating procedure:

>   Dewaxed sections are hydrated; collodioning is possible.
>   Stain nuclei intensely with a progressive ferric lake of hematoxylin.
>   Wash for 3 to 5 minutes in running water.
>   Stain, in dishes or on slides, for 5 to 10 seconds with picrofuchsin.
>   Dehydrate directly in absolute alcohol, clear and mount.

It is essential to avoid any washing in water after staining with picrofuchsin. When free celloidin sections have undergone this stain they may be briefly rinsed in picrofuchsin diluted twenty to thirtyfold in either distilled water or 1% acetic acid and blotted between sheets of filter paper before dehydrating in 96% alcohol. Paraffin sections and all sections fixed to slides may be treated directly in absolute alcohol.

Results. — The nuclei take on hematoxylin and appear black if the time of action of the picrofuchsin has been properly adjusted; the cytoplasm is yellow and the collagen fibres red, both contrasting sharply against the background. Basement membranes and ground substances rich in acid mucopolysaccharides can take a pink stain which facilitates their identification. Photomicrography with a green filter furnishes pictures that are particularly suited for microscopical anatomy. Disadvantages of the method lie in the pale colour of the cytoplasm which does not lend itself to a detailed analysis of structure, and a tendency for the stain of collagen fibres to fade. In fact, all stains with acid fuchsin keep badly, especially when the slides are of ordinary glass, since the fading is due to the alkali that leaches from the glass and not to the presence of picric acid as wrongly supposed by certain authors. This alteration, however, occurs over several years.

5° *Variants of van Gieson's method*

Those modifications of van Gieson's method that are described here concern mainly the substitution of other red stains for the acid fuchsin. The different types of ponceau and Biebrich scarlet may be used; they are dissolved in picric acid of the same concentration as for acid fuchsin. Collagen fibres are stained less brilliantly than with the latter dyestuff, but preparations made following the directions given below are conserved much better. The substitution of thiazin red for acid fuchsin was suggested for the first time by Heidenhain (1903) but his formula is clearly not as advantageous as that of Domagk (1933) in which the picrofuchsin is replaced by a mixture of 100 ml of a saturated aqueous solution of picric acid and 7.5 ml of a 1% aqueous solution of thiazin red. The action of this solution can be prolonged for several minutes; sections that have been thus treated resist washing in distilled water before dehydration. Collagen fibres stain as brilliantly as with picrofuchsin and the preparations may be conserved almost indefinitely.

If it is desired to avoid the use of a red dyestuff (vascular injection with a red mass or vital fixation with lithium carmine, etc.) one may follow the advice of Dubreuil (1904) which is to replace van Gieson's picrofuchsin with a mixture of 80 ml of a saturated aqueous solution of picric acid and 8 ml of a 1% aqueous solution of methyl blue or anilin blue. The operating procedure is the same as with picrofuchsin. The intense blue stain of collagen fibres alone differentiates these preparations from those obtained by van Gieson's method.

It should be observed that picrofuchsin is an excellent background stain for preparations that have been submitted to neurofibrillar impregnation; it is thus often used following the method of Bodian. It is also suitable after the ammonium silver carbonate impregnation of Del Rio Hortega which allows very good nuclear staining to be obtained with frozen sections and hence is useful in anatomo-pathological technique. It is applied to pieces fixed in formalin, the period of fixation for pieces of 5 mm thickness being two days at room temperature, 5 to 10 minutes at 60° and one minute with boiling.

Reagents:

Ammonium-silver carbonate (add 150 ml of a 5% aqueous solution of sodium carbonate to 50 ml of a 10% aqueous solution of silver nitrate; dissolve the resulting precipitate by adding ammonia slowly with agitation and dropwise at the end to avoid excess; after it is fully dissolved 550 ml of distilled water are added; the solution may be stored for several months in a cool place in the dark).
Commercial formalin diluted a hundredfold.
0.2% aqueous solution of gold chloride.
5% aqueous solution of sodium hyposulfite.
van Gieson's picrofuchsin.
Clearing mixture: 1 part of phenol, 1 part of beech creosote, 1 part of benzene, 8 parts of toluene or xylene (by weight).

Operating procedure:

Frozen sections are collected in distilled water;
Transfer, using glass rods, to the ammonium-silver carbonate solution heated to 45–50, for one or two minutes; the sections should take on a very pale yellow colour.
Transfer without washing to dilute formalin and gently agitate the sections; the yellow tint should intensify; if it remains greyish treatment in ammonium-silver carbonate should be reapplied for one minute.
Pass the sections rapidly through distilled water.
Tone in the solution of gold chloride for about 30 seconds.
Pass rapidly in the sodium hyposulfite solution.
Rinse in tap water.
Spread the sections on slides.
Treat for 5 seconds in van Gieson's picrofuchsin.
Remove excess stain in 96% alcohol and also commence dehydration in it.
Terminate dehydration and clear in the phenol-creosote-benzene mixture.
Carry through pure benzene and mount in balsam or a synthetic resin.

Results. — The quality of nuclear stain is equivalent to that of the ferric lakes of hematoxylin, the black stain being particularly intense; the cytoplasm and collagen fibres are stained as in the classical van Gieson's method. The procedure is valuable for its rapidity; an experienced operator will not take more than six minutes after cutting the sections for the preparation to be ready for examination under the microscope.

6° *The method of Curtis*

Credit for the use of naphthol black (blue black B) and related azo-dyes for the selective staining of collagen fibres should undoubtedly go to Curtis (1905), whose formula is based on the same principle as van Gieson's picrofuchsin, that is, association of an azo-dye with a saturated aqueous solution of picric acid. However, the formula of Heidenhain (1908) is more practical and I advise its use. It consists of staining nuclei with a red dye as a first step; Heidenhain used carmalum instead of the safranin suggested by Curtis; nuclear fast red or basic fuchsin can be used according to the procedure intended for Ramon y Cajal's trichrome. Sections are then treated with picronaphthol-black; no differentiation is necessary if nuclei have been stained with carmalum, which however I do not recommend, or with nuclear fast red; both basic fuchsin and safranin are automatically differentiated during dehydration.

Reagents:

>   Red nuclear stain (aluminium lake of nuclear fast red, safranin, dilute Ziehl's fuchsin etc...).
>   Heidenhain's picro-naphthol-black. (Dissolve 1 g of blue black B in 400 ml of a saturated aqueous solution of picric acid, add 80 ml of methanol and 320 ml of distilled water; Romeis (1948) advises diluting to half just before use). Heidenhain's solution and its dilutions keep very well.

Operating procedure:

>   Sections are dewaxed, collodioned if necessary and hydrated.
>   Stain nuclei by any one of the chosen methods.
>   Rinse in dilute acetic acid after staining with Ziehl's fuchsin or safranin, or in tap water after nuclear fast red.
>   Stain for 1 or 2 minutes in a pure solution, or 2 to 5 minutes in a dilute solution, of picro-naphthol-black (the optimum varies according to the particular commercial sample).
>   Rinse rapidly in dilute acetic acid (0.5%).
>   Dehydrate in absolute alcohol, taking care to extract all excess of red dye if the nuclei have been stained with Ziehl's fuchsin or with safranin.
>   Clear in benzene, mount in balsam or a synthetic resin.

Results. — Nuclei take on a stain that corresponds to that described for Ramon y Cajal's trichrome; cytoplasm that is very acidophilic appears yellow, while others range from pink to greenish-grey. Collagen fibres are blue-black and are brought out more clearly than by any of the other methods mentioned previously. Photomicrography with a green filter gives excellent results.

7° *Variants of the method of Curtis*

Certain modifications of this method, whose spectacular demonstration of collagenous tissue has been noted, are restricted to the substitution of related stains in place of blue black B; diamine blue BB, naphthol blue black (amido black 10 B) and trypan blue can be used instead of blue black B in the above formula. A more extensive modification, due to Lillie (1945), of the original formula is aimed at improving cytoplasmic stains. Nuclei are stained with a progressive ferric lake of hematoxylin, the cytoplasm with a mixture of acidic azo-dyes and collagen fibres with picro-naphthol-black B.

Reagents:

> Wiegert's hematoxylin, ferric trioxyhematein or Groat's hematoxylin.
> Catoplasmic stain: 0.6 g brilliant purpurin R, 0.4 g sorbine red, 1 ml acetic acid and distilled water to make 100 ml.
> Collagen stain: 50 to 100 ml of naphthol blue black B, 100 ml of saturated aqueous picric acid.

Operating procedure:

> Dilute acetic acid (1%).
> Sections are dewaxed, collodioned if necessary and hydrated.
> Stain nuclei with the progressive ferric lake of hematoxylin.
> Wash in tap water.
> Stain for five minutes in the purpurin- sorbine-red mixture.
> Rinse in tap water.
> Stain for one to five minutes in picro-blue.
> Wash for two minutes in dilute acetic acid.
> Dehydrate, clear and mount in balsam or a synthetic resin.

Results. — Nuclei are stained black, muscle fibres a clear brown, cytoplasm brown, pink or greenish, blood cells red, mucus pale blue and collagen fibres, basement membranes as well as reticulum fibres are a deep green; elastic fibres remain unstained.

8° *Gaussen's histo-polychrome*

This method, described in 1926, has been welcomed by histologists with incomprehensible indifference. In fact, it gives excellent results, its only drawback being the lack of strong contrast between the stain of the nuclei and the cytoplasm. Few topographical methods are as rapid and dependable. Gaussen's stain is based on the competition between three acidic stains, namely, ponceau, picric acid and anilin blue mixed in suitable proportions, while nuclear stain is ensured by basic fuchsin added to the three acidic stains. Excess fuchsin is removed by absolute alcohol during dehydration.

Reagents:

> 1 g "ponceau de xylidine", 100 ml distilled water and 1 ml acetic acid.
> 3 g of anilin blue in 100 ml of distilled water (dissolve with boiling and allow to cool). Add 2.5 ml of acetic acid and filter.
> Saturated alcoholic solution of picric acid.
> 0.5 g of basic fuchsin in 100 ml of 96% alcohol.

Operating procedure:

Sections are dewaxed, collodioned and hydrated.
Stain for 2 minutes in the following mixture:
    anilin blue solution .... 0.4 to 0.8 ml
    ponceau solution .... 1.2 to 0.8 ml
    picric acid solution 6   to 0.8 ml
    basic fuchsin solution 6   to 0.8 ml
    distilled water .... 11 to 0.8 ml
(The dyes are added to distilled water in the above order; alcoholic solutions are added in small quantities with agitation).
Drain slides and dehydrate directly in absolute alcohol (for about 10 seconds).
Clear and mount in balsam or a synthetic resin.

Results. — Nuclei stain red, cytoplasm greyish pink, collagenous tissue blue, fibroglia and certain elastic fibres red, blood cells yellow, and mucins and ground substances rich in mucopolysaccharides a bluish violet. The intensity of staining collagenous tissue and mucins can be adjusted by varying the level of anilin blue in the mixture within the limits indicated above.

Gaussen recommends the method to be practised in dishes; from my own experience it succeeds equally well on slides if the duration of each step is lengthened by a minute. Gaussen's description does not include any indication as to the conservation of solutions; clearly, stock solutions from which the mixture is prepared may be kept for several years, though in my opinion the staining mixture itself cannot be kept for more than 48 hours. Gaussen also observes that the staining mixture without anilin blue is a very good background stain for preparations that contain structures stained black.

9° A. Prenant's triple stain

The original formula of this stain is also based on the competition between two acidic stains for demonstrating collagen fibres, namely eosin and light green; but the mechanism of staining of the other tissue constituents is more complex. This method gives preparations that are admirably suited for topographical study, but its importance clearly extends beyond the limits of microscopical anatomy; it is in fact a cytological technique and is therefore discussed elsewhere in the relevant pages of this book.

ADVANTAGES AND DISADVANTAGES OF METHODS BASED ON COMPETITION BETWEEN TWO ACIDIC STAINS

Among the practical advantages of the techniques that have just been reviewed, their simplicity of execution should be remarked; none of them involves any differentiation that has to be carefully followed under the microscope, so that they are perfectly well suited to a large series of slides. Staining is of short duration in all cases and particularly in Gaussen's histo-polychrome. No aggressive reagents or stains are included which are likely to detach sections, and all operations can be carried out at room temperature, which is of considerable advantage with pieces rich in bone, cartilage or muscle.

The good demonstration of collagen fibres facilitates the analysis of sections of vertebrate and molluscan organs; among the arthropods these fibres are of lesser importance in the structure of organs, though the clear staining of basement membranes is of great value in examining sections.

The light cytoplasmic stain given by these methods, excepting Lillie's variant of the technique of Curtis, has certain advantages; it increases the clearness of structures in sections and permits its application to sections thicker than 10 μ. It also follows from the light cytoplasmic stain that with these techniques acceptable preparations may be obtained even from material that has not been quite well fixed. Experience shows that the very first artifacts of tissue autolysis are in fact cytoplasmic; if they are not very pronounced they do not distract especially when cytoplasmic staining is not intense.

However, in other respects the weak staining of the cytoplasm is the chief drawback of these techniques; apart from Lillie's variant of the method of Curtis, they render the cytoplasm yellow or pink, grey in some cases, which is not suitable for the detailed analysis of structures. Distinguishing the different secretory products and the study of the structural details of muscular fibres are hardly facilitated.

In cases other than the special study of fibrous structures of connective tissue, these techniques are adopted as topographical methods whenever a detailed analysis of cytoplasmic structures is not essential. They are very convenient in all cases where an abundant collagenous tissue lends good "structuration" to the stained preparation. The identification of different morphological types of nuclei is also easy, but all these methods are of little use when anatomical study is chiefly based on a distinction between different types of glandular cells or different cytoplasmic structures.

As for the choice among the different procedures of this group subjective factors are involved to a certain degree. In general, hemalum-picro-indigo-carmine and van Gieson's original method can be recommended for their rapidity; the choice between the two depends on whether a differential staining of ground substances rich in acid mucopolysaccharides is desired or not; such a differential stain is given by hemalum-picro-indicarmine and not by van Gieson's method; the latter however is very convenient for the photography of bundles of collagen fibres. The demonstration of nuclear structural details is better with the original formula of Ramon y Cajal's trichrome than with its variants based on safranin or nuclear fast red; but the latter variant offers absolute security while destaining of the nuclei during dehydration might occur if Ziehl's fuchsin has been used as a nuclear stain. The method of Curtis practised following Heidenhain's formula shows collagen fibres most clearly but it also gives the most uniform cytoplasmic stain. Impregnation with picro-fuchsin is a rapid diagnostic technique for frozen sections and its use may be confined to really urgent histological examination.

STAINING THAT INVOLVES PHOSPHOMOLYBDIC OR PHOSPHOTUNGSTIC ACID

All the methods of this group derive from that of Mallory (1900) which is based on the use of phosphomolybdic acid to confine stains like anilin blue, methyl blue or light green to collagen fibres only. Unfortunately, a great many descriptions of these procedures carry the term phosphomolybdic or phosphotungstic "mordanting". Baker (1958) quite rightly points out that the action of these acids is just the opposite of mordanting. They are, in fact, compounds that limit the action of certain selective stains of collagen fibres, for otherwise the stains take on too strongly. The studies of v. Möllendorff (1924) and of Seki (1936) have shown that there really is a "competition" between these acids and the particular dyes; this competition occurs only in loose structures which permit the diffusion of phosphomolybdic and phosphotungstic acids and in high molecular weight particles especially when hydrated.

Certain methods of this group consist in the successive action of a cytoplasmic stain, phosphomolybdic or phosphotungstic acid and a selective stain for collagen fibres; others involve mixtures containing one of these acids and one or more acidic stains. The former are regressive stains which can be followed under the microscope while the latter are generally applied as progressive stains. Gomori (1950) should be credited with having shown that the association of phosphomolybdic or phosphotungstic acid with the stain of collagen fibres, already suggested by Mallory in 1905, could be extended to cytoplasmic staining and hence to the possibility of two-step methods of fascinating simplicity.

This finding of Gomori quite naturally leads to the development of one-step methods which are based either on the association of a second stain meant for nuclei with the mixture of one of these acids and an acidic stain, or of abandoning the selective nuclear stain.

A considerable number of formulae have been proposed following the original work of Mallory which is based on limiting the stain of collagen fibres with phosphomolybdic or phosphotungstic acid. They have been adapted not only to paraffin and celloidin sections but also to smears. It is especially in the latter field that so many variants and modifications have been proposed that the objective reader might wonder whether they are all really useful. Even if one holds that many of the variants described here owe their existence to a desire for originality rather than to be useful one cannot leave them aside since every histologist should be acquainted with them even if he does not intend to use them personally.

1° *The original method of Mallory*

This method whose undoubted historical and doctrinal interest has been emphasized above is, however, typical of those procedures that are outmoded and should be abandoned. But it still has numerous adepts and it appears impossible for me to ignore it.

Reagents:

    Aqueous solution of acid fuchsin (0.5%).
    0.5 g anilin blue, 2 g Orange G, 1 g phosphomolybdic acid and 100 ml of distilled water.

Operating procedure:

    Sections are dewaxed, collodioned if necessary and hydrated.
    Stain for 5 minutes in the solution of acid fuchsin.
    Drain and blot if necessary, but do not wash in water.
    Stain for 10 to 20 minutes in the mixture of anilin blue, Orange G and phosphomolybdic acid.
    Rinse in 96% alcohol, dehydrate in absolute alcohol, clear and mount in balsam or a synthetic resin.

The above procedure was indicated by Mallory in 1905: that of 1900 included staining of the nuclei and cytoplasm with a 0.1% solution of acid fuchsin followed by treatment in a 1% solution of phosphomolybdic acid and then staining with the mixture of anilin blue and Orange G acidified with 2 g of oxalic acid per 100 ml of stain. A more recent formula of Mallory (1936) differs only in that phosphotungstic acid is used instead of phosphomolybdic acid at the same concentration.

Results. — Collagen fibres are stained an intense blue clear enough to satisfy the most exacting observer. In this respect the result is really spectacular; cartilage, the bone matrix and mucins are more or less a light blue; blood cells and the myelin sheath take a yellow stain, while fibrin, the nuclei and the cytoplasm are red.

The best results are obtained on paraffin sections of material fixed with a liquid based on mercuric chloride. The intensity of staining is such that sections which are somewhat thick become quite unrecognisable. Nuclear staining is quite mediocre and this is one of the principal disadvantages of the method; it justifies the substitution of other stains for acid fuchsin. Obviously, Mallory's method suits only paraffin sections.

Variants. — Cason (1950) has proposed a variant of Mallory's method which is based on an association of all the stains in the same solution; it is prepared by dissolving 1 g of phosphotungstic acid in 200 ml of distilled water followed by 2 g Orange G, 1 g of anilin blue and, finally, 3 g of acid fuchsin. Dewaxed and hydrated sections are stained for 5 minutes, dehydrated and mounted. This variant is open to the same criticism as the original formula; the very intense shades demand thin sections, while nuclear staining is quite mediocre. Cason's stain, as adapted by Mendelson (1951) for celloidin sections, has, on the contrary, a certain advantage. Staining with the mixture, whose composition has been given above, lasts for only *20 seconds* at the most; after rapid rinsing in distilled water the sections are treated, until destaining of the celloidin, with a mixture of 3 ml of anilin, 12 ml of chloroform and 85 ml of 96° alcohol. They are then rinsed in a mixture of 7 volumes of chloroform and 1 volume of 96% alcohol followed by a mixture of 3 volumes of xylene (toluene or benzene) and 1 volume of terpineol before clearing in a benzenic hydrocarbon and mounting in balsam or a synthetic resin.

2° *Masson's trichrome*

This trichrome is an important improvement on Mallory's method in that the nuclear stain is ensured by a ferric lake of hematoxylin, and, consequently, intracellular structures are much clearer in preparations, while all the advantages of anilin blue as a stain for collagen are retained. The original operating procedure of this technique includes staining nuclei with Regaud's hematoxylin followed by differentiation in alcoholic picric acid. The cytoplasm is then stained with acid fuchsin or ponceau; treatment with phosphomolybdic acid uncoats the collagen fibres which are then stained with anilin blue.

This method has enjoyed a considerable and well deserved vogue, but the original formula, whose principle has just been described, has undergone several modifications. The use of Regaud's hematoxylin to stain nuclei entails, in fact, a loss of time and is quite an unnecessary complication. It is surely one of the most precious among the cytological methods, and it should hence be described in the relevant chapters of this book, but the differentiation in alcoholic picric acid suggested by Masson deprives it of all its advantages and the results are not any better than with the progressive ferric lakes of hematoxylin. Thus, Weigert's hematoxylin, Hansen's ferric trioxyhematein and Groat's hematoxylin are excellent substitutes for the nuclear stain proposed by Masson. I must, however, remark that nuclear staining with hemalum, often practised as the first step in Masson's trichrome, is most unsuitable for the purpose; the aluminium lakes of hematein are not fast enough for this type of staining and in most cases the nuclei take on the acid cytoplasmic stain which completely masks the hemalum.

Other modifications of the original formula concern the stains of the cytoplasm and of the collagen fibres. Most authors tend to use solutions that are less concentrated than those of Masson, which is preferable since the final preparations are more transparent. Azophloxine and Biebrich's scarlet have been used instead of acid fuchsin and ponceau. As for staining collagen fibres many histologists prefer light green or fast green FCF to anilin blue; this also increases the transparency of preparations.

I recommend the procedure suggested by Goldner (1938) among the several variants of this stain.

Reagents:

Weigert's hematoxylin, Hansen's trioxyhematein or Groat's hematoxylin.
0.2 g of ponceau, 0.1 g of acid fuchsin.
300 ml of distilled water and 0.6 ml of acetic acid.
3 to 5 g of phosphomolybdic or phosphotungstic acid.
100 ml of distilled water, 2 g of orange G.
0.1 to 0.2 g of light green or fast green FCF, 100 ml of distilled water and 0.2 ml of acetic acid.
Dilute acetic acid (1%).

Operating procedure:

Sections are dewaxed, collodioned and hydrated.
Stain nuclei with a progressive ferric lake of hematoxylin (taking particular care to avoid any overstaining which can obscure the sections).
Wash in running water.
Stain for 5 minutes in the fuchsin-ponceau mixture.
Rinse in dilute acetic acid.
Treat for 5 minutes with Orange G and phosphomolybdic acid.
Rinse in dilute acetic acid.
Stain for 5 minutes with light green.
Rinse in dilute acetic acid.
Dehydrate in absolute alcohol, clear and mount.

Results. — Nuclei are stained a brownish-black; the cytoplasm can range from a bright red to greenish; blood cells appear yellow, while collagen fibres and structures rich in acid mucopolysaccharides take on a definite green stain. Photography of the latter shade requires the use of panchromatic emulsions and an orange or red filter.

The method gives excellent preparations for the study of cytoplasmic structures. The morphological details of muscle fibres appear very clearly and the precision of stain shown by collagenous and other fibrous structures leads to no hesitation at all in the interpretation of sections. Differentiation of the various types of secretory granules is also quite good. It should be emphasized that in practice Goldner's variant of Masson's trichrome gives very good results after aqueous fixatives; it is less successful after fixation in Clarke's liquid, Carnoy's liquid or alcohol. It is easily standardized and can be conveniently adopted for staining a large number of slides in series since they can be left for 10 to 30 minutes in the last dilute acetic acid rinse.

3° *Gomori's trichrome (1950)*

This trichrome is both a simplification of the staining technique and an important contribution to the methodology of the procedures derived from Masson's trichrome. The systematic trials of Gomori have shown that the acid arylmethanes usually employed in these techniques as stains for collagen fibres (anilin blue, methyl blue, light green, fast green and patent blue) can be mixed with the phosphomolybdic or phosphotungstic acid used to limit their action as well as with the sulfonated azo-dyes that generally serve to stain the cytoplasm (chromotrope 2R, azophloxine, ponceau, Biebrich's scarlet and amaranth); 1% acetic acid may be added to the mixture with advantage.

Certain factors that are likely to modify the equilibrium between the two stains have also been elucidated by Gomori. Phosphotungstic acid favors red dyes, while phosphomolybdic acid does so with blue and green ones. The addition of ethanol to staining solutions greatly reduces the binding of red dyes; they predominate in sections stained for a short period, while longer staining results in more green or blue. Pretreatment of sections with Bouin's liquid (2 to 5 minutes at 60°) followed by rinsing in water to remove excess of picric acid considerably intensifies red stains. Washing in tap water after staining, on the contrary, weakens these shades, while washing in 0.2% acetic acid renders sections more transparent without modifying the balance of stains.

Reagents:

0.6 g of chromotrope 2R; 0.3 g of light green or fast green FCF; 0.6 to 0.7 g of phosphotungstic acid, 100 ml of distilled water; 1 ml of acetic acid.
Weigert's hematoxylin, ferric trioxyhematein or Groat's hematoxylin.
Dilute acetic acid (0.2%).

Operating procedure:

Thin sections (less than 10 μ) are deparaffined, collodioned if necessary and hydrated.
Stain nuclei with a progressive ferric lake of hematoxylin, avoiding any overstaining.
Wash in tap water.
Stain for 5 to 20 minutes in the mixture of acid dyes.
Rinse rapidly in dilute acetic acid, dehydrate in absolute alcohol, clear and mount in balsam or a synthetic resin.

Results. — The stains taken by the different structures correspond to those given by the Masson-Goldner trichrome. The intensity of the stain is such that thick sections might be rendered obscure; for this reason Gomori advises sections of less than 10 μ.

Lillie (1954, p. 355) has proposed nuclear staining with an aluminium lake of hematoxylin before treating sections with the mixture of acid stains; this suggestion clearly extends beyond the idea of Gomori who does not specify, in the text, the particular hematoxylin lake intended as background stain. I have found, from personal experience, that the progressive ferric lakes are far superior to hemalum. The remarks concerning Masson's trichrome are also valid for that of Gomori.

4° *Variants of Gomori's trichrome*

Certain possible modifications of the operating procedure have been suggested by Gomori and it is not necessary to enlarge on them here since their effect on the final result of staining has been described above. In spite of all its qualities, Gomori's trichrome, however, has a disadvantage which it shares, besides, with all the other methods derived from Masson's trichrome. In spite of being carried out with the greatest care nuclear staining is not always pure; the red cytoplasmic stains of the azo group have an unfortunate tendency to superpose themselves on the black tint of ferric hematoxylin which very often results in nuclei that are stained a dark brown or even red. This minor defect, which is inherent in the method and probably due to the affinity of these dyes for the basic proteins associated with the nucleic acid, is obviously not reproduced in black-and-white photographs.

However, an attempt to obviate this seemed worth the while, and this was achieved by resorting to a red dye of the xanthene family, namely eosin, instead of the red sulfonated azo-dye for staining the cytoplasm (Gabe, 1954). This particular method was given as a variant of the triple stain of A. Prenant, which is indeed quite true with respect to the results since the preparations can hardly be distinguished from those provided by the classical method. But from the theoretical point of view there is a heresy and it calls for rectification. In fact, restriction of staining with light green is obtained not by the simple competition between acid dyes, as in the classical triple stain of A. Prenant, but by the introduction of phosphotungstic acid into the mixture of acid dyes. In practice it gives results that are superior to the other variants of Masson's trichrome in the brightness of preparations; nuclear staining is very pure and it is easy to discriminate between cytoplasmic structures. The intensity of the red stain is, however, less than in Masson's trichrome, which can be disadvantageous for the detailed study of muscle fibres or certain secretory products.

Reagents:

Progressive ferric lake of hematoxylin (Weigert, Hansen or Groat).
1 g of eosin Y, 0.2 g of light green or fast green FCF, 0.5 g of phosphotungstic acid, 100 ml of distilled water and 0.5 ml of acetic acid.

Operating procedure:

Sections are deparaffined, collodioned if necessary and hydrated.
Stain nuclei with the progressive ferric lake of hematoxylin.
Wash in running water.
Stain for 5 to 10 minutes with the mixture of acid stains.
Drain, dehydrate directly in absolute alcohol, clear and mount in balsam or a synthetic resin.

Results. — The nuclei take on a very pure black stain; the eosin shows no tendency to superpose itself on them. Cytoplasmic stain may range from red through grey to green. The erythrophilous and cyanophilous affinities of secretory granules appear very clearly. Mucins and all structures rich in acid mucopolysaccharides stain green, as do the collagen fibres. Elastic fibres remain unstained. Photography using a yellow-green filter and a slow panchromatic emulsion gives excellent results.

From the practical point of view it may be noted that the mixture of acid stains can be kept for several years. The only precaution to be taken in carrying out the operation, whose success is almost automatic, is to avoid any aqueous wash between the mixture of acid dyes and the dehydration in absolute alcohol. Holding slides in 1% acetic acid, an inevitable measure that is resorted to when making serial sections, is better avoided otherwise.

5° One-step trichrome (Gabe and Ms Martoja, 1957)

This is also based on the principle of Gomori's trichrome, but the hematoxylin lake is abandoned in favour of azorubine S in the mixture as a nuclear stain.

Reagents:

0.5 g of azorubine S (amaranth), 0.5 g of phosphomolybdic acid, 0.2 g fast green FCF, 100 ml of distilled water, 1 ml of acetic acid and saturated Martius yellow or 0.01 g of water-soluble naphthol yellow.
All the ingredients may be added and left to dissolve for one or two hours for the Martius yellow to attain saturation before filtering. Alternatively, the other ingredients may be added in the above order to a previously saturated solution of Martius yellow. If water-soluble naphthol yellow is used it is enough to add the ingredients in the given order, filtration being quite unnecessary.

Operating procedure:

Sections are deparaffined, collodioned if necessary and hydrated.
Stain for 10 minutes, in tubes or on slides, with the mixture indicated above.
Rinse in distilled water, dehydrate directly in absolute alcohol, clear and mount in balsam or a synthetic resin.
Neither water (distilled, or acidified with 0.5% acetic acid) nor absolute alcohol has any effect on the staining; they only remove the excess dye that has not bound to the structures.
The stain persists for up to 24 hours in any of the above three liquids without any notable change in the balance of colours. Stained slides of serial sections can therefore be easily left in them.

Results. — The azorubine S gives a red stain to the nuclei, the ergatoplasm and certain secretory granules. The cytoplasm may be stained pink, grey or green according to its affinity. Highly acidophilous structures are yellow, while fast green takes on to collagen fibres, all structures rich in acid mucopolysaccharides and certain secretory granules. The use of a green or orange filter according to the particular tinctorial affinity to be emphasized gives very clear photographs.

In addition this method affords a very satisfactory background stain after fuchsin-paraldehyde; technical details are given with the description of the latter technique.

Certain advantages of the above staining method are obvious, namely, the resistance to washing, the speed of execution and the wide range of colours obtained without any particular effort on the part of the operator. Furthermore, it should be noted that the mixture of dyes can be kept for several years and that the stain is effective not only after the usual fixatives but even with osmified pieces. In the latter case it is better to stain in the paraffin oven (54 to 60°) and to extend the period of treatment up to 45 minutes.

The products used to prepare the mixture of dyes should be chosen with great care; a rather annoying synonymy prevails in this domain. Azorubine S is, for instance, often sold as amaranth or fast red, and care should be taken not to confound it with fast red salt B (the diazo derivative of 5-nitro-anisidine) which is frequently used in histochemical technique. Fast green FCF should be unequivocally distinguished from malachite green, a basic dye of the triarylmethane group, often sold as fast green and which, unlike fast green FCF, is in the form of crystals. Some suppliers go as far as selling methyl green under the name of fast green. The synonymy in the group of naphthol yellow is no less complicated, and the quality of the dye-stuff used in preparing the trichrome should be systematically verified.

The two disadvantages of the method correspond to those that I should mention with respect to the azan technique. The one-step trichrome calls for a good quality of fixation whose defects become much more apparent than with any of the stains of the first group. Besides, as in the case of azan, nuclear staining is not very striking under low magnification when cells are rich in ribonucleoproteins or acidophil secretory products.

6° *Heidenhain's azan (1916)*

This, to my mind, is the most refined of the so-called general staining methods. It combines the advantages of anilin blue as a stain for collagen fibres with a nuclear stain that equals the regressive hematoxylin lakes and the nucleal reactions in their precision. Furthermore, few methods ensure such a differential staining of secretory granules. But, the azan technique (the term is an acronym derived from a contraction of azocarmine-anilin, which seems to be neglected by some authors who refer to "Azan's" stain) is not an automatic one and its great flexibility allows it to be adapted to all circumstances. As I have remarked in the Introduction, it is typical of a difficult technique each step of which requires to be carefully followed and really controlled. I consider that the way in which a histologist applies this method is a good measure of his technical talents.

Lillie (1952, 1954) feels that the flexibility and adaptability of the azan stain are drawbacks, since it follows that practice of the technique calls for those whom he describes as "the more skilled technicians". This aspect of the problem should on no account really deter the histologist, but other features of the procedure are, however, quite inconvenient. In fact, the stain is very exacting as to the quality of fixation, and one of its essential steps is carried out a 60° which exposes the sections to a real risk of being detached. The procedure is, in addition, quite long.

The essential difference between the azan technique and that of Mallory, its immediate precursor, lies in doing away with nuclear staining by acid fuchsin. Heidenhain uses instead the regressive staining of nuclei by azocarmine, an acid azin dye. Azocarmine B is the acid sodium salt of phenylrosindulin-trisulfonic acid, while azocarmine G is the disodium salt of phenylrosindulin disulfonic acid. As Harms (1965) has observed, the position of the sulfonic acid radical on the molecule of phenylrosindulin is not yet known. It has been shown that nuclear staining by azocarmine is not due to the presence of nucleic acids but to that of the associated basic proteins. Both types of azocarmine can be used for staining, but it is azocarmin G that gives the brightest tints and which better withstands differentiation as recommended by Heidenhain, that is, in anilinic alcohol. It should be applied with warming (1 hour in an oven at 60°) while azocarmin B may be used cold.

After differentiation in anilinic alcohol sections are treated with an aqueous solution of phosphotungstic acid, during which the extraction of dye continues.

It is at this stage that destaining of the collagen fibres also occurs. They may then be stained with a mixture of anilin blue and orange G, similar to that of Mallory; the fixation of these compounds on to structures depends on the way in which the previous operations have been carried out.

Reagents:

> Saturated aqueous solution of azocarmine G (from 0.05 to 0.1%) acidified with 1 to 2 ml of acetic acid for 100 ml of stain.
> Anilinic alcohol (100 ml of 70% alcohol, 1 ml of anilin).
> Acetic alcohol (100 ml of 96% alcohol, 1 ml of acetic acid).
> Aqueous solution of phosphotungstic acid (5%).
> Heidenhain's blue (dissolve, with warming, 0.5 g of anilin blue and 2 g of orange G in 100 ml of distilled water; leave to cool, add 8 ml of acetic acid and dilute before use with 2 or 3 volumes of distilled water).
> All solutions keep well.

Operating procedure:

> Dewax sections, collodion if necessary and hydrate.
> Stain for 1 hour in the solution of azocarmine warmed to 60°.
> Rinse in distilled water.
> Differentiate under the microscope with alcoholic anilin.
> Leave for 30 seconds to 1 minute in acetic alcohol.
> Rinse in distilled water.
> Treat for 30 to 60 minutes with the phosphotungstic acid.
> Rinse in distilled water.
> Treat for 30 to 60 minutes in the dilute solution of Heidenhain's blue.
> Rinse in distilled water, 96% alcohol or dehydrate directly in absolute alcohol, according to the case, clear and mount in balsam or a synthetic resin.

Results. — Nuclei take on a bright red tint and the precision of their staining is really remarkable. When differentiation has been properly carried out most cytoplasms are a magnificent yellow that is quite pleasing to the eye. Collagen fibres are a deep blue and more distinctly stained than by any of the other methods described here. Secretory products may range from an intense red to deep blue, passing through a series of pinks, yellows and violets. Structures rich in acid mucopolysaccharides stain a light blue and the ground substance of the bone red or yellow. Structural details of striated muscle fibres appear red, orange or yellow according to the way differentiation has been carried out. Elastic fibres remain unstained, while fibroglia often take on a pale red tint.

Technical comments. — The operating procedure described above does not strictly conform to that of Heidenhain and differs considerably from that indicated in certain manuals of histological technique. I therefore take the opportunity to comment on the successive steps.

Staining with azocarmine G should be effected as soon as sections are hydrated if any of the usual fixatives have been used. When pieces have spent a long time in an acid fixative, or when decalcification has been necessary, it is advisable to precede staining with a stay of section in anilinic alcohol as used for differentiation. Experience has shown that when sections are rendered alkaline in this manner the fixation of dye is greatly improved. Such an operation becomes indispensable when the azan technique is applied after any stain that requires differentiation in an acid medium (technique of Romeis for the hypophysis). It is rarely useful to prolong the stay in anilinic alcohol beyond 30 minutes; after this bath sections are briefly rinsed in distilled water and then stained. The concentration of azocarmine proposed here is far lower than that indicated by Heidenhain and half that given in most manuals of histological technique; it is equivalent to 60% saturation and any increase seems to me quite unnecessary.

The duration of staining suggested here (1 hour at 60°) has been seen from experience to be useful since a well-bound dye permits differentiation to be carried out conveniently. Even much longer periods can be adopted when the method is practised with certain pretreatments; one such variant is described for the histological examination of the endocrine pancreas.

Contrary to what is generally described in most technical manuals. I do not advise leaving slides in the staining bath for about 10 minutes after removal from the oven as indicated in certain formulae. In fact, azocarmine G is much less soluble in the cold, and the only effect of the slow cooling in the bath is a deposit of numerous microscopic crystals of azocarmine all over the surface of the slide. They would undoubtedly dissolve away during differentiation and subsequent steps, but are of apparently no use at all for the success of the operation. I therefore suggest removing slides from the stain as soon as the bath is taken out of the oven and rinsing them immediately in distilled water in which they may be left awaiting differentiation. Azocarmine staining is very sensitive to an alkaline medium; *all washes should therefore be carried out in distilled water.*

Differentiation is controlled under the microscope by removing the slide from the bath of anilinic alcohol and examining under low power. It is besides quite useful to survey the preparation rapidly before differentiation to judge the quality of staining which should be an intense and uniform red except for some structures that never take azocarmine. The concentration of anilin in the differentiator is much higher than that used by Heidenhain, while the level of alcohol is less; practice has shown, in fact, that more homogenous differentiation is obtained under these conditions. In this manner it takes about two or three minutes to go through a preparation, sometimes longer, rarely less. Nuclear staining and that of certain secretory products are fast enough to afford a sufficient margin of security for scrutinizing and controlling cytoplasmic destaining. It is the most critical step of the method and calls for much experience and dexterity. In fact, tints do not remain unchanged after differentiation in anilinic alcohol; the treatment with phosphotungstic acid extracts almost all the azocarmine retained by the collagen fibres, which indeed can be completely destained even without any differentiation in anilinic alcohol; dye that is fixed by muscular fibres is also partly extracted and even the shade of the cytoplasm can be "lowered" with respect to that which persists after differentiation in anilinic alcohol. Mild differentiation therefore favours blue and yellow ones. Nuclear staining generally remains as it is in the phosphotungstic acid, but excess differentiation results in the nuclear structures taking on anilin blue. Obviously insufficient differentiation is shown in the final preparation by the horribly smudged nuclei and should be avoided at all cost.

Differentiation is terminated immediately on plunging the slide into acetic alcohol. It is good practice to maintain the slide in it for at least 20 seconds; it may indeed be left for hours without the slightest harm; acetic alcohol is thus a convenient step for holding over the procedure if time does not permit its completion.

Treating sections with phosphotungstic acid very often requires 30 to 60 minutes but this may be adjusted to suite the differentiation of the azocarmine or the particular result that is desired. When the treatment with anilinic alcohol has been carried far enough for destaining the cytoplasm almost completely, there is no point in retaining slides for more than 30 minutes in phosphotungstic acid; 20 minutes whould suffice. If, however, a strong red tint persists in the cytoplasm after differentiation in anilinic alcohol treatment with phosphotungstic acid may be prolonged for three hours or more. Observation under the microscope easily shows when the action of phosphotungstic acid is completed; fully destained collagen fibres indicate that staining may be resumed with Heidenhain's blue after a brief rinsing in distilled water to remove excess phosphotungstic acid.

The period to be spent by sections in the dilute solution of Heidenhain's blue depends on the precedent differentiation and length of treatment with phosphotungstic acid; extensive differentiation in anilinic alcohol and a shortened stay in phosphotungstic acid call for a brief exposure to the mixture of anilin blue and orange G, while the converse also holds. It is, however, rare to exceed one hour in staining with Heidenhain's blue. The action of this stain depends on its age, blues predominating with freshly prepared solutions and old ones giving yellow shades.

The treatment of sections after staining with blue-orange is determined according to the precedent steps and the result that is desired. When the deepest possible stain of collagen fibres is required, when differentiation in anilinic alcohol has been extended and other steps shortened it is better to dehydrate directly in absolute alcohol, in which anilin blue is strictly insoluble. Washing in 96% alcohol renders preparations more transparent but slightly decreases the intensity of blue tints. Washing in distilled water should be resorted to only if one expects a too intense binding of anilin blue.

Contrary to a belief complacently admitted in certain works on histological technique, the conservation of slides is excellent. Preparations that I have made in 1946 still maintain all their brightness.

I have also had the privilege of examining in 1949 preparations made by the author of this method in 1920; their tints had not undergone the slightest modification over almost 30 years.

The reagents also keep very well; the same solution of acetified azocarmine G can serve for almost one year if it is stored at room temperature and well stoppered in between use; at 60° it loses its staining capacity in about ten days. The anilinic alcohol, acetified alcohol and phosphotungstic acid can be kept for years; they need to be renewed only when the red tint that they usually take becomes really intense. The solutions of Heidenhain's blue can be stored for about two years.

The rapid destaining of sections stained by azan is easily obtained by treating slides in an alkaline liquid; 1% ammonia or a saturated aqueous solution of lithium carbonate can bring this about in less than five minutes.

Clearly, this method is meant only for paraffin sections; collodioning is possible, and even recommended, but it is very important that the film of celloidin be sufficiently thin; in fact, the azocarmine does not penetrate at all beyond a certain thickness. In any case this method is to be envisaged only in rare cases for celloidin sections, even if they are fixed to slides and the embedding mass removed, since the intensity of shades is such that only thin sections (maximum: 10μ) give acceptable results.

Variants. — Certain modifications of the azan stain are specially adapted for studying the secretory products of certain glandular cells; they will be described among the techniques meant for the particular organs. Other variants are aimed at simplifying the method, particularly by avoiding staining with azocarmine G in an oven which is the chief cause of the detachment of sections. It should, however, be emphasized that none of the variants can match with the original method for the brightness of preparations.

On some variants azocarmine B is substituted for azocarmine G; the former is used as a saturated aqueous solution (about 0.1%) acetified, as in the case of azocarmine G, but in the cold. The resulting shades tend more towards the violet than with azocarmine G and the fixation on to structures is not as fast. Consequently, it is advisable to reduce the level of anilin in the differentiating solution and to increase its alcohol content; 0.1% anilin in 96% alcohol is quite suitable. Differentiation is more rapid than with azocarmine G. All other steps of the method remain unchanged.

Other methods, of much less value, consist in replacing the azocarmine with other red nuclear stains. They give results that do not differ appreciably from those of the original method with respect to collagen fibres, but evidently entail sacrificing the staining of certain cell organelles and secretory products with azocarmine. In the simplest of these variants the nuclei are stained with the aluminium lake of nuclear fast red followed by treatment with 5% phosphotungstic acid, rinsing in distilled water and finally staining with Heidenhain's blue. Nuclear staining is carried out in the manner described for Ramon y Cajal's trichrome; the phosphotungstic acid step may be reduced to 5 minutes and that of Heidenhain's blue to 5–10 minutes; rinsing in distilled water before dehydrating in absolute alcohol is often useful. The results correspond to those of the original method with respect to collagen fibres but they evidently do not provide the whole range of red, orange and yellow shades produced by it. Nuclear staining with Ziehl's fuchsin has also been suggested; it is effected as in Ramon and Cajal's trichrome with the rinse in dilute acetic acid followed by washing in distilled water before exposure to phosphotungstic acid; slides are held in this acid and in Heidenhain's blue for the same length of time as in the case of slides stained with nuclear fast red. Lastly, a very advantageous combination is that of first carrying out the nucleal reaction of Feulgen and Rossenbeck and then treating with phosphotungstic acid followed by staining with Heidenhain's blue. This method, proposed by Huber (1946), combines the advantages of the nucleal reaction with its precise demonstration of deoxyribonucleic acid and those of the azan stain for the background and for certain secretory products. The phosphotungstic acid may be allowed to act for 5 to 10 minutes, while for the blue I would strongly advise not to exceed 5 minutes to avoid any superposition of the blue and the red of the nucleal stain; in view of the brief treatment with the blue, slides are washed and dehydrated directly in absolute alcohol.

In fact, the original method with azocarmine G is superior to all the variants; it may be applied after all the usual fixations, and only post-chromatized or osmified pieces give mediocre results! For one who has any experience with Heidenhain's azan it is difficult to understand Geidies (1941) who ventures that the nuclear fast red variant, which he calls *azan novum*, is superior to the original formula; this author also neglects to draw the attention of his readers to the fact that the stain, of which he believes himself to be the inventor, was in fact already proposed by Domagk in 1933!

7° *Petersen's method (1924)*

In certain respects this is a modification of the azan technique since the staining of collagen fibres is effected as in Heidenhain's method; but the mechanism of nuclear staining is essentially different and has been the basis of two recent methods, of which one is particularly suitable for demonstrating elastic fibres and the other for certain secretory products. It is therefore fit to devote a special paragraph to Petersen's stain.

The nuclear stain used by Petersen is acid alizarin blue BB of the anthraquinone group (*not to be mistaken with alizarin blue S*); the aluminium lakes of this compound impart a diffuse violet shade to tissues; treatment with phosphungstic acid tones it to a red, and strips connective fibres and most of the cytoplasm entirely; muscular fibres remain stained.

Phosphomolybdic acid has the same "differentiating" effect but tones shades to blue. Clearly, phosphotungstic acid should be chosen if it is desired to stain collagen fibres with anilin blue.

Reagents:

> Aluminium lake of acid alizarin blue (boil 10 g. of aluminium sulfate and 0.5 g. of acid alizarin blue in 100 ml of water, maintain boiling for 5 to 10 minutes, cool, filter and readjust to 100 ml; it may be kept for at least six months.)
> 5% phosphotungstic acid in distilled water.
> Heidenhain's blue.

Operating procedure:

> Sections are dewaxed, collodioned if necessary and hydrated.
> Stain for 5 minutes at room temperature with the aluminium lake of acid alizarin blue.
> Rinse in distilled water.
> Treat with Heidenhain's blue for 30 minutes to one hour.
> Rinse rapidly in distilled water, dehydrate with absolute alcohol, clear and mount in balsam or a synthetic resin.

Results. — Nuclei stain red, the cytoplasm is pink, yellow or grey and muscular fibres generally retain their red, while collagen fibres and mucins stain as with azan.

As Romeis (1948) has remarked the result of Petersen's stain largely depends on the fixation used. Following formalin, Zenker's liquid or fixatives based on mercuric chloride but without picric or trichloracetic acids, sections are as beautiful as those given by azan, except that secretory products which otherwise fix azocarmine do not show up. If picric or trichloracetic acids have been used in fixation, the azan technique is definitely preferable to that of Petersen.

It is important not to prolong unduly the period of staining in the aluminium lake of acid alizarin blue if one wishes to avoid prolonging the treatment in phosphotungstic acid also for hours.

One of the great advantages of Petersen's method is that it may be applied to collodion sections that are not stuck to slides. In fact, the embedding mass is deeply stained with the aluminium lake of acid alizarin blue but it is completely destained in the phosphotungstic acid.

Obviously, sections can be stripped in phosphotungstic acid (5 or 10%

aqueous solution) and the collagen fibres stained green or red by any of the appropriate stains described previously.

Among the variants of Petersen's method, Kornhauser's "quad" should be noted; it includes staining with orcein in addition to a trichrome resembling that of Petersen and is specially meant to demonstrate elastic fibres. Another one is the tetrachrome of Herlant (1959) aimed at discriminating between the cell types of the distal lobe of the adenohypophysis. The two methods are described elsewhere in this work.

ADVANTAGES AND DISADVANTAGES OF METHODS INVOLVING PHOSPHOMOLYBDIC OR PHOSPHOTUNGSTIC ACIDS

The methods of this second group vary more than those of the first with respect to their difficulty of execution and the time taken for staining sections. Some of the procedures described here are quite rapid and do not require any real differentiation; the one-step trichrome is one such example. Others are relatively short and do not include any "critical" step that is likely to endanger the final result, but they require frequent renewal of reagents. Finally, there are those that are truly regressive stains whose practice implies assuming a certain responsibility and cannot be entrusted to the routine effort of a technician who remains indifferent to the intellectual side of the task.

Generally, all these methods give cytoplasmic stains that are deeper than those given by the first group.

This is advantageous in certain respects since the results can serve multiple purposes; they permit anatomical study as well as the analysis of certain secretory processes and even the description of certain cytological details. But the price of this deeper and more differentiated staining lies in the rigours attached to fixation and the quality of sections. Even a method that is technically as simple as the one-step trichrome requires good fixation and proper section for best results.

Because of deeper cytoplasmic staining all defects in sections are pitilessly exposed by the methods of the second group and this can influence the choice of technique for a given lot of slides.

A practical consequence is that techniques for collagen fibres involving phosphotungstic or phosphomolybdic acids are more fruitful than those based on picric acid. In the particular case of "topographical" staining, they have the advantage of serving several purposes and of imparting a wide range of shades to different structures. But one should not forget the strict requirements of the procedures which should be taken into account when confronted with material whose quality of fixation and of sections is doubtful. Most of the techniques described here are suitable for paraffin sections that do not exceed 10μ in thickness; only some may be practised on nitrocellulose (celloidin) sections not attached to slides; in a manner of speaking none of these techniques may be applied to frozen sections.

The choice among the different methods of this group is influenced by subjective factors as much as in the case of methods involving picric acid. The one-step trichrome, Gomori's trichrome and the latter's variant with eosin are recommendable for their ease of execution. The Masson-Goldner trichrome is particularly suitable for staining a large number of slides in series because it allows, as does the one-step trichrome, a prolonged delay before mounting stained slides. In my opinion the original method of Mallory is outmoded.

Among the various stains of the group described here the azan technique occupies a place of its own; the remarkable demonstration of collagen fibres renders it precious from the anatomical point of view, and the quality of staining certain secretory products further increases its value. But the difficulties of the method prevent it from being used routinely; it is typical of the stainings that should be carried out by the investigator himself constantly checking the preparations at every step and adapting the procedure to suit the particular aim of the study.

STAINING BASED ON THE DEMONSTRATION OF CYTOPLASMIC TINCTORIAL AFFINITIES

As I have pointed out in the introduction to this chapter, the "differentiating" property of certain stains discussed here, that favours topographical examination, is not due to the demonstration of connective fibres, especially collagen, but to the shades signifying the tinctorial affinities of the cytoplasm and secretory products.

Some of the methods described in the previous paragraph, especially the trichrome of Masson and its variants, that of Gomori, the one-step trichrome and the azan technique do fulfil this requirement as well. Conversely some of the methods described below show up collagen fibres very clearly. It is none the less true that the essential aims of the two groups of methods are different and the distinction between them seems to me quite well founded.

1° *Nuclear staining with a hematoxylin lake followed by counter-staining with an acid dyestuff*

These are the simplest methods of this group. Their prototype is one that has been outmoded since long ago and should have disappeared, but most authors seem to cling to it with a tenacity that is really hard to understand; it is the hemalum-eosin technique.

It may appear unnecessary to put this technique on trial once again. P. Masson (1923) has emphasized its sketchy nature at length in trying to convince his pathologist colleagues that resorting to a stain that makes guesswork of the distinction between different fibrous structures and ground substances, that does not bring out any tinctorial affinity, in short, that shows really nothing, amounts to voluntarily depriving oneself of much information easily obtained by other techniques as sure as the indiscriminate smearing of eosin over sections whose nuclei have been stained with hemalum. The late M. Langeron expounded the same point of view throughout all the editions of his *"Précis de microscopie"*.

But such authoritative opinion has not prevented the hemalum-eosin technique from pursuing a career far too brilliant for what it deserves. Neither can its fervent adepts be accused of choosing a facile solution, for several of the methods mentioned previously are easier than the hemalum-eosin. It is really due to an indifference for histological technique and the force of habit that this method owes a triumph as undoubted as it is undeserved.

The present author has had the good fortune to follow the advice of P. Masson and of M. Langeron from his earliest contacts with histological technique, and he has never had the occasion to regret it. He has no intention of describing here the hemalum-eosin stain, a technique that is as obsolete as the several formulae of nuclear staining with carmine which have been included complacently, but without any illusions, by several authors in their manuals of histological technique.

It probably suffices to note that sections which have undergone nuclear staining with a progressive lake of hematoxylin can be treated with an acid dyestuff for background staining (eosin, erythrosin, azophloxine, rubin S, bordeaux red, chromotrope 2 R, orange G, light green or fast green FCF). Contrary to the usual practice in many laboratories it is preferable to use dilute solutions of the above stains (0.05 to 0.1% in distilled water); acidification with one to three drops of acetic acid per 100 ml of stain solution is necessary in most cases. A quick wash in distilled water followed by dehydration in alcohol, clearing and mounting in balsam will show that the tinctorial affinities of the nuclei are quite different from those of the cytoplasm, while only very marked differences can be discerned from one cytoplasm to another. Fibrous structures can be identified only from their morphological characteristics. In the last analysis, a simple comparison with sections from the same block but stained according to modern techniques will probably suffice to dampen one's enthusiasm for the rather summary procedures described here.

2° *Millot's triple staining (1926)*

This excellent method should be recommended for its brightness of nuclear staining and the range of cytoplasmic tints. It is based on the competition between two acid stains; Martius yellow and acid fuchsin. As far as I know the mechanism of this differential staining has not been systematically studied, and its author himself has remained silent on the question. It seems likely that the distribution of the two stains among the various stained structures is determined by their extent of penetration depending on their diffusion coefficient which is definitely lower in the case of Martius yellow and not far from that of picric acid. Some of the technical details given below have been formulated after my own experience; Millot does not state the various concentrations used in the original publication.

Reagents:

> P. Masson's hemalum.
> Altmann's fuchsin (20 g of acid fuchsin in 100 ml of anilin water; see p. 728).
> Saturated solution (about 0.1%) of Martius yellow in 40% alcohol.

Operating procedure:

> Sections are dewaxed, collodioned and hydrated.
> Deep nuclear staining with hemalum.
> Wash in tap water.
> Stain for about 5 minutes, with Altmann's fuchsin at room temperature.
> Rinse in 40% alcohol until all excess acid fuchsin is removed.
> Stain with Martius yellow until sections take a general yellow shade.
> Dehydrate directly in absolute alcohol, clear and mount in balsam or, preferably, in a commercial synthetic resin.

Results. — The nuclei are stained bluish violet by the hemalum, subsequent steps of this method maintaining the shade better than most other acid counter-stains. Highly acidophilic cytoplasms stain yellow and others red. Secretory granules show very clearly. As a whole the shades are pleasing to the eye and sections are easy to examine since there is generally no superposition of colours at all. The principal drawback of the method noted by Millot (1926) namely the fading of the yellow colour can be completely avoided by mounting in a synthetic resin.

The progressive lakes of hematoxylin and chromic dioxyhematein can be used in place of hemalum as nuclear stains. However, from the aesthetic point of view, it is hemalum that provides the most beautiful contrasts. The method can be adopted after all the usual fixations; but it is evidently inapplicable after osmic fixation when the hemalum is poorly taken up by nuclei.

3° Safranin-light green

This stain, invented by Benda, enjoyed great vogue at a time when most histologists preferred osmic and chloroplatinic fixatives; indeed these fixatives greatly facilitate the staining of nuclear structures with safranin. At present the method is most often used in caryological research and its application to smears and squashes is described in the relevant chapter of this book. It has however another advantage, namely, that a nuclear stain of very good quality may be obtained in those cases where the use of regressive ferric hematoxylin is prevented by abundant acidophilic structures (e. g. vitelline platelets). The method is very valuable in this respect.

Benda's operating procedure includes staining with the water-alcohol solution of safranin suggested for Ramon y Cajal's trichrome (p. 202) for 24 hours and differentiating the stain with a 1% alcoholic solution of light green followed by dehydrating in absolute alcohol and mounting in balsam. It gives good results only with material fixed in a liquid containing osmium tetroxyde or chloroplatinic acid. The following operating procedure has always given me satisfaction after fixation by "topographical" liquids.

Reagents:

  Water-alcohol solution of safranin (fully dissolve 1 g of safranin in 100 ml of absolute alcohol before adding 50 ml of distilled water).
  Saturated aqueous picric acid.
  0.2% aqueous solution of light green or fast green FCF, acidified with 0.2 to 0.5 ml of acetic acid per 100 ml of stain solution.

Operating procedure:

  Sections are dewaxed, collodioned and hydrated.
  Stain with the safranin solution for 24 hours at room temperature.
  Rinse rapidly in tap water.
  Differentiate, if necessary under the microscope, with the saturated solution of picric acid until the cytoplasm is extensively destained.
  Stain for 30 seconds with the dilute aqueous solution of light green or fast green FCF
  Dehydrate directly in absolute alcohol, clear and mount in balsam or a synthetic resin

Results. — Nuclei, centrosomes and ciliary corpuscles take a red stain which shows up strikingly against the background of the preparation which is green, while the yellow of the picric acid used for differentiating is retained only by the most acidophilic structures.

A typical example for applying this method is the staining of sections rich in structures that take acid stains violently and which require proper demonstration of nuclei.

Much of its success depends on the quality of safranin used. It should be noted, besides, that irregularity in quality according to the manufacturer, or even according to the batch, is particularly prevalent in the case of this dye-stuff.

4° *The Ehrlich-Biondi-Heidenhain method*

This is the adaptation, for sections, of the well known triacid stain invented for blood smears. It gives very clear topographical preparations, but succeeds only after certain fixations. Frozen sections may thus be stained after all the usual fixations. Only fixative mixtures containing mercuric chloride without potassium dichromate or Carnoy's liquid are well suited before this stain may be applied to sections cut in celloidin (which should be dissolved away from slides before staining) or paraffin. Material fixed in Bouin's liquid may be stained by the Ehrlich-Biondi-Heidenhain method if the need arises, but nuclear tints are often dull.

The principle of the method is recalled under hematological methods. The dye-stuff is sold as a powder by certain suppliers of material for microscopy. If one desires to prepare it the procedure recommended by Krause (1911) is the best. It consists of grinding 3.4 g of methyl green, 4.2 g of acid fuchsin and 3.0 g of orange G in a mortar to obtain a homogenous mixture which is added to a pyrex flask containing 100 ml of distilled water. This stock solution is ready for use after 24 hours at 35–37°; it keeps very well. Commercial powders are usually dissolved, just before use, at a concentration of 0.2 to 0.5% (following the instructions of the manufacturer) in slightly acetified water.

Reagents:

Triacid of Ehrlich (stock solution or commercial powder).
Water acidified with 0.5% acetic acid.

Operating procedure:

Sections are dewaxed, collodioned if necessary (taking care that the collodion is sufficiently thin) and hydrated.

Stain, from 10 minutes to several hours, with the 0.2–0.5% solution of the commercial powder or the stock solution diluted twenty times; it is advisable to acetify the staining solution slightly by pouring it into a cylinder which has not been rinsed after it has been emptied of 1% acetic acid.

Rinse rapidly in 0.5% acetic acid.

Remove excess stain by holding sections in 70% alcohol until an overall red shade is obtained (except in zones rich in nuclei).

Dehydrate in absolute alcohol, clear and mount in balsam or, preferably, in a synthetic resin.

Results. — Chromatin, mucins and cartilage take a green or bluish stain. Certain secretory granules are violet, while nucleoli, centrosomes, the ground substance of the bone, collagen and elastic fibres and acidophilic secretory granules show a wide range of reds. Blood cells appear orange. The poor keeping qualities of preparations, frequently noted by classical authors, is due above all to the quality of slides which allow alkali to leach out into the medium, and to the reducing properties of balsam; the latter is evidently circumvented by using synthetic resins.

Proper differentiation gives very clear and transparent preparations so that the technique may be applied to relatively thick sections.

5° Manns's technique

This method involving methyl blue and eosin (Mann bi-acide of French authors) much used in certain cytological investigations and studies of secretory granules, gives very beautiful topographical preparations and can be practised after most usual fixations. It suits only paraffin sections, though careful collodioning is possible if the film of nitrocellulose is kept very thin.

Albumin is preferable to gelatin for sticking slides and any smudge should be avoided as it stains a deep blue or violet.

Mann's mixture contains 35 ml of an aqueous 1% solution of methyl blue (*not to be confused with methylene blue*) 45 ml of an aqueous 1% solution of eosin and 100 ml of distilled water. Success depends largely on the quality of dye-stuffs used, and commercial samples are far from being equivalent.

Suppliers sell the Mann mixture as a powder, which may be dissolved in distilled water. From my personal experience some of these powders give good results; I consider a 0.2% solution preferable to the 0.5% often recommended by the manufacturers.

Background staining, with this mixture, of sections submitted to nuclear staining with hemalum (the rapid Mann of some authors) seems devoid of interest to me. The true Mann stain can be carried out in two ways, by the original procedure or by Dobell's variant.

Reagents:

Mann stain (mixture prepared by the user or a 0.2% solution of the aqueous powder).
Alkaline alcohol (Ten drops of an alcoholic solution of sodium hydroxide are added to 60 ml of absolute alcohol just before use. The alcoholic solution of sodium hydroxide contains 0.33 ml of 30% caustic soda in 10 ml of absolute alcohol; this stock solution can be stored in a stoppered bottle).
Water acidified with four or five drops of acetic acid in 60 ml of distilled water.

Operating procedure:

Sections that are stuck with albumin are dewaxed, collodioned and hydrated.
Stain with the Mann mixture for 24 to 48 hours at room temperature.
Rinse in distilled water.
Dehydrate carefully with absolute alcohol; sections should be a deep bluish-violet.
Immerse slides into the alkaline alcohol and leave them until they are definitely red; this toning may need five minutes or more; if it is too long add a few drops of the stock solution of alkaline alcohol.
Dehydrate carefully in absolute alcohol ensuring that the last traces of alkali are removed.
Immerse slides in the acetified water and leave them for 2 to 3 minutes.
Dehydrate in absolute alcohol, clear and mount in balsam or a synthetic resin.

Results. — Chromatin of the nuclei stains a deep blue and the nucleoli are bright red; this is a criterion of good differentiation. The cytoplasm may be violet, blue or pink, while erythrophilous and cyanophilous secretory granules appear very clearly. Blood cells take a red stain, muscular fibres are red or pink and collagen fibres generally blue.

Experience has shown that the treatment with alkaline alcohol does not harm any structure if it is carried out in a strictly anhydrous medium; that is indeed the aim of the first dehydration in absolute alcohol, while the second dehydration is meant to remove the sodium hydroxide completely without using water.

Dobell's variant. — This modification of Mann's original formula simplifies the operating procedure considerably. Sections are stained with the Mann mixture, as described above, and then differentiated in a very dilute (0.01 to 0.02%) solution of Orange G in 70% alcohol. Differentiation usually takes from 5 to 10 minutes and may be followed under the microscope. After differentiation the slides are dehydrated directly in absolute alcohol, cleared and mounted.

In some cases the shades obtained with the original method of Mann are brighter than those given by Dobell's variant, but the relative simplicity of the latter renders it preferable to the original and even more so as differentiation may be controlled under the microscope.

6° *The Mann-Dominici method*

This method using eosin, Orange G and toluidine blue was intended by its inventors for the study of nerve cells (Mann, 1894) and for hematopoietic tissues (Dominici, 1905). In fact it is an excellent general method that provides very clear preparations and gives, in addition to very good nuclear staining, an excellent demonstration of basophilic cytoplasm, metachromatic compounds as well as erythrophilous granules. The operating procedure has been modified repeatedly and the formulae given in various manuals of histological techniques differ significantly from each other. The following procedure appears to me preferable to the others.

Reagents:

Erythrosin-orange (dissolve 0.2 g of yellowish erythrosin and 0.6 g of orange G in 100 ml of distilled water and acidify it with a drop of acetic acid.)
0.5% aqueous solution of toluidine blue.
Water, acidified with 0.2% acetic acid.

Operating procedure:

Sections are dewaxed, collodioned and hydrated.
Stain for 2 to 5 minutes in the erythrosin-orange solution.
Rinse briefly in distilled water.
Stain for 1 to 3 minutes in toluidine blue; the sections should take on a uniform blue shade.
Rinse briefly in distilled water.
Immerse slides in acetified water and leave them until the sections take on a reddish shade; part of the excess toluidine goes into solution.
Terminate differentiation by leaving slides in 96% alcohol until a definite blue tint reappears in the basophil zones of the sections.
Dehydrate in absolute alcohol, clear and mount.

Results. — The chromatin, nucleoli and basophil cytoplasm show a very intense blue; acidophil cytoplasm is pink or yellow and collagen fibres pink; elastic fibres often remain unstained. Mucins and ground substances rich in acid mucopolysaccharides take a purple colour while erythrophil secretory granules appear a bright pink.

The results of this beautiful staining depend very much on the fixation; that with formalin is by far the poorest preparation for the Mann-Dominici method which may even be completely abandoned if one disposes of only formalin-fixed material. Sections of material fixed in Zenker's liquid or that of Regaud should be treated according to the operating procedure indicated above.

When pieces are fixed in a liquid without potassium dichromate the final result is greatly improved if staining is preceded by slight oxidation. A stay of 5 to 10 minutes in Lugol's liquid, used for dissolving mercuric precipitates, followed by destaining in 5% sodium hyposulfite and washing for 2 or 3 minutes in running water can be adopted before staining slides with erythrosin-orange G.

When pieces have been fixed in a liquid without mercuric chloride, the required oxidation is obtained more rapidly by treating dewaxed and hydrated slides with a 0.25% solution of potassium permanganate in distilled water until sections show a very light tobacco tint (in about 10 to 20 secondes); they are then bleached with a 3.5% aqueous solution of sodium metabisulfite and washed for 2 minutes in running water before staining.

It should be noted here that the results of the Mann-Dominici method are greatly modified if sections undergo very strong oxidation before staining; with such a pretreatment the method becomes very valuable for studying certain secretory products (B-cell granules of the endocrine pancreas, hypothalamic neurosecretory product).

7° Staining with azur eosinates

This method, derived from that of Romanowsky, gives preparations of great beauty. It has been much used by Maximow's school, and most modern histologists reserve its use for hematopoietic organs where it is indispensable, but the procedure can really be adopted for much wider uses.

The various applications that necessitate differentiation of slides individually, especially the panoptic method of Pappenheim, are discussed under the techniques meant for hematopoietic tissues. A variant of the procedure, due to Lillie and Pasternack (1944) deserves to be consecrated as a general method since the regularity of stain is such that its authors suggest carrying it out with the automatic appliances that are available on the market. This improvement is obtained by staining in a buffered medium, with the pH modified to suit the particular fixation adopted.

Reagents:

0.1% solution of Azur A in distilled water.
0.1% solution of bluish eosin in distilled water.
0.1 M solution of citric acid (19.212 g/l if anhydrous or 21.014 g/l if crystalline) in distilled water.
0.1 M solution of disodium phosphate (14.198 g/l) in distilled water.

Operating procedure:

Sections are dewaxed, collodioned if necessary (ensuring the thinness of the film of nitrocellulose) and hydrated.
Stain for one hour in the following mixture:

Azur A solution	4 ml
Eosin solution	4 ml
Citric acid solution	1.2 ml
Disodium phosphate solution	0.8 ml
Acetone (pure)	5 ml
Distilled water	25 ml

Dehydrate in *acetone*, clear in a mixture of equal parts of acetone and benzene, toluene or xylene, follow with two baths of benzenic hydrocarbon and mount in a synthetic resin.

The solution of Azur A and eosin can be replaced with 0.5 ml of a commercial solution of azur eosinate (Giemsa stain, for instance). The quantities of citric acid and phosphate indicated in the above formula give a pH of 4.1; for material fixed in formalin it is better to lower the pH to 3.75 (1.3 ml of citric acid and 0.7 ml of phosphate) and raise it after Zenker's liquid to 4.5 (1.1 ml of citric acid and 0.9 ml of phosphate). The mixture should be prepared just before use, and it is best used only once. However, Lillie (1954) gives a formula meant for the dishes of automatic staining instruments and which can be used for up to a week. It consists of a mixture of 6 ml of 1% Azur A solution, 6 ml of 1% eosin solution, 21 ml of the citric acid solution, 14 ml of the disodium phosphate solution, 90 ml of acetone, and 585 ml of distilled water. The stock solutions of Azur A and of eosin, which are ten times more concentrated than in the first formula, can be replaced by 10 ml of the commercial solution (1%) of azur eosinate.

Results. — The preparations show a wide range of colours. Lillie describes them as follows: nuclei, the ergastoplasm, bacteria and rickettsiae are coloured blue, mast cells and granulations of basophil leucocytes blue-violet, calcium deposits deep blue, ground substance of the cartilage reddish violet, cytoplasm of living cells at the time of fixation light blue or violettish, necrotic cytoplasm deep pink, erythrophil secretory granules pink, pheochrome granules green (only after chrome fixation), keratin, amyloid, fibrin, muscle fibres and the thyroidal colloid pink, and blood cells orange. The general tendency of colours is to shift towards red when the pH is lowered and towards blue when it is raised.

I must particularly insist on the advantages of this method. The spectacular results of staining with the azur eosinates have been known for a long time, but the need for carefully differentiating each slide individually and the poor conservation when mounted in balsam have discouraged many histologists from using techniques which have however given their best in the hands of Maximow and of Pappenheim. With the availability of synthetic resins and the improvements formulated by Lillie staining with the azur eosinates can now be adopted as a general method and its wider use will surely be most profitable.

ADVANTAGES AND DISADVANTAGES OF THE METHODS OF THIS GROUP

None of the methods assembled in this paragraph is really difficult and all give satisfactory results if the stains used have been carefully chosen. The sketchy and unrefined practice of nuclear staining with a progressive lake of hematoxylin followed by background staining with a red acid dye has been emphasized earlier and it is desirable that such methods should be abandoned. Safranin-light-green is really recommendable only in particular cases (osmified material requiring very selective demonstration of nuclei in sections rich in acidophil structures). Millot's triple stain gives an excellent demonstration of nuclei and erythrophil secretory granules; results are less spectacular for discriminating between different ground substances and for staining cyanophil secretory granules. Mann's method and Dobell's variant of it give very clear preparations of fine distinction, their only real drawback being the quite long (48 hours) stay in the staining solution. The Mann-Diminici stain requires that slides be differentiated individually and is not suitable on a large scale, but it gives very valuable information on the distribution of ribonucleoproteins and metachromatic substances. Though the older formulae of staining by the azur eosinates require manipulating in an oven and individual supervision of slides Lillie's variant does away with these drawbacks and deserves to be adopted as routine practice in all laboratories of histology.

In fact, the various stains described here complement each other mutually and experience will soon show which one is best suited for each of the various particular cases.

BULK STAINING

Bulk staining or impregnation before section-cutting still plays an important role in neurohistology; all the methods of demonstrating the Golgi apparatus under the light microscope are based on silver or osmium impregnation of small pieces; certain histochemical reactions also call for treating entire pieces to be cut into sections later. But bulk staining in topographical histology has gradually diminished to a point where certain modern books on histological technique do not even mention it.

In fact, bulk staining is necessary for the topographical study of animal tissues in two quite different cases. The first arises when objects are small enough to be mounted *in toto* between slide and coverslip after staining and clearing. The other is when pieces are stained to be embedded in gelatin according Apathy's method, to avoid the slightest shrinkage.

Most of the staining techniques described in the preceding paragraphs can be applied to the first of these cases. It is clear that spread membranes or small flat animals can be attached to slides by the terpineol technique suggested by Apathy and thereafter manipulated like paraffin sections. Evidently, with such objects warm staining and too deep cytoplasmic stains should be avoided. It is imprudent to use a cytoplasmic stain for preparations that exceed 25 μ in thickness; nuclear staining generally suffices.

For this certain lakes of hematoxylin are very convenient; apart from them gallocyanim, whose use is described for the histochemical detection of nucleic acids, ensures a selective staining of nuclear structures; the aluminium lake of gallamin blue, used to give a blue nuclear stain in sections, has also been suggested for bulk staining. In addition to these sections, two carmine lakes, no longer adopted for sections, can be very useful for bulk staining; they are boracic carmine and carmalum. The progressive lakes of hematoxylin can also be used; Hansen's chromic dioxyhematein gives good results. Among the aluminium lakes, Mayer's acid hemalum, corresponding to the two formulae given in a previous paragraph for staining sections is even superior for bulk staining, while the results of staining with Apathy's hematein IA are particularly striking.

1° Staining with the aluminium lake of gallamin blue

This technique involves the aluminium lake of an oxazin which also gives very good nuclear staining in sections. Structures which are rich in acid mucopolysaccharides take a reddish-violet colour and the cytoplasm turns green if the staining solution is not quite fresh.

Reagents:

>Aluminium lake of gallamin blue (dissolve, with boiling, 0.5 g of gallamin blue an 5 g of aluminium chloride in 100 ml of distilled water, leave to cool and filter; dilute to half with a 5% solution of aluminium chloride before use).

Operating procedure:

>Quite small pieces, fixed in any one of the topographical fixatives described in the relevant chapter, are freed of excess fixative. Treatment with lithium-alcohol is necessary if fixation is based on picric acid. Crystals of mercuric chloride are removed with iodine-alcohol. However treatment with sodium hyposulfite is reserved until after sections are cut. One side of the pieces should be less than 0.5 cm.
>Stain for 24 to 48 hours in the diluted aluminium lake of gallamin blue. Ensure that the stain has penetrated up to the centre, if necessary by making incisions in the less important zones of the piece.
>Wash for 12 to 24 hours in distilled water.
>Dehydrate, embed in celloidin or paraffin, cut sections and treat them with sodium hyposulfite, if they have been submitted to iodine-alcohol, before mounting.

If gallamin blue is meant for staining sections the lake is prepared as described above but the aluminium chloride is replaced by sodium or potassium alum and the staining solution is not diluted. Staining lasts from 6 to 24 hours and there is no risk of smudging.

2° Staining with boracic carmine

Bulk staining is, in my opinion, the only instance of a carmine lake used as a general method which had wider applications formerly. The chief advantage of staining with these lakes and with those of carminic acid is that a balance between stain and mordant is easily obtained so that only basophil structures are stained and the cytoplasm shows no tendency at all to take the lake. This minimizes any difference in staining between the periphery and the centre of the piece, and also prevents overstaining of the cytoplasm. Boracic carmine is the most suitable for bulk staining, while other lakes based on carmine are used especially for sections and are, besides, better replaced by safranin, basic fuchsin or nuclear fast red.

Reagents:

Boracic carmine (Grind 2 to 3 g of carmine and 4 g of borax (sodium tetraborate) in a mortar and dissolve it with boiling in 100 ml of water. Cool, add 100 ml of 70% alcohol, leave to settle for a week and filter. It keeps well).

Alcohol hydrochloric acid (100 ml of 70% alcohol and 0.25 to 0.50 ml of hydrochloric acid of density 1.19).

Operating procedure:

Pieces, fixed preferably in a liquid containing mercuric chloride, are treated for 2 to 3 days in 70% alcohol.

Immerse in boracic carmine for 1 to 3 days; terminate staining when the dye has entirely penetrated the piece.

Leave for 1 to 3 days in alcohol-hydrochloric acid which is renewed several times; this solution which effects a genuine differentiation should be allowed to act until all excess of red dye is removed.

When the last renewal of alcohol-hydrochloric acid is found to remain colourless the pieces are washed for 1 to 2 days in 70% alcohol which is changed several times. Dehydrate and mount in *toto* or embed in celloidin, paraffin or gelatin according to Apathy.

Cut sections and mount.

3° Staining with Carmalum

P. Mayer's carmalum (1892) has the advantage, over lakes based on carmine, of being prepared from a well-defined chemical compound, carminic acid. Commercially available samples of carmine owe their staining capacity to the presence of this acid and are besides more or less contaminated with impurities. The only drawback of this formula is the relatively high cost of carminic acid.

Reagents:

Carmalum (dissolve 10 g of potassium alum in 100 ml of distilled water with heating; add 1 g of carminic acid and heat till it is fully dissolved; cool, filter and add 0.2 g of salicylic acid or 1 ml of commercial formalin to prevent microbial contamination.)
1% aqueous solution of potassium alum.

Operating procedure:

Pieces, preferably fixed in a liquid containing mercuric chloride, are treated as in bulk staining with boracic carmine.
Immerse in carmalum for 24 to 48 hours.
Treat for 12 to 24 hours with the solution of potassium alum, when nuclear staining will be seen to improve in purity.
Wash for 24 hours in several changes of tap-water.
Dehydrate and mount in *toto* or embed as in the case of boracic carmine.

4° Bulk staining with P. Mayer's hemalum (1891)

This progressive aluminium lake of hematoxylin, which gives, with sections, results that are equivalent to those of Hansen's or P. Masson's hemalums is superior to the latter for bulk staining. It gives very pure nuclear staining.

Reagents:

Mayer's acid hemalum (dissolve 1 g of hematoxylin in 100 ml of water with warming if necessary; after cooling add 0.2 g of sodium iodate and 50 g of potassium alum; dissolve by shaking and without warming; after dissolving add 50 g of chloral hydrate and 1 g of citric acid.
Store in a well-stoppered bottle.

Operating procedure:

Pieces, fixed in a usual liquid (avoid osmic fixation) are freed of excess fixative.
Stain for 24 to 48 hours with acid hemalum, ensuring that the piece has been fully penetrated.
Wash for 24 hours in distilled water to remove all excess of alum and citric acid.
Wash for 24 hours in several changes of tap water to tone the nuclei blue.
Dehydrate and mount in *toto* or embed in paraffin or celloidin.
Hemalum staining withstands embedding in gelatin poorly.

5° Staining with hematein I A of Apathy (1897)

This bulk staining is not only selective for nuclei, but also stains cilia, basement membranes and, in favorable cases, nerve fibres. It was used by Apathy in his description of the "primordial nerve filaments".

Reagents:

1% solution of hematoxylin in 70% alcohol, ripened for 2 to 3 months.

Mordant (9 g of potassium alum, 0.1 g of salicylic acid and 3 ml of acetic acid made up to 100 ml in distilled water). Mix 1 volume of the hematoxylin solution, 1 volume of the mordant and 1 volume of pure glycerine. The mixture can be kept for years.

Operating procedure:

Pieces, fixed in a liquid that permits staining with the aluminium lakes of hematoxylin, are freed of all excess fixative and dehydrated up to 90% alcohol.

Immerse for 1 to 7 days in the hematein 1A (the optimum period is determined by trial and error).

Wash for 24 hours in *absolutely pure* distilled water (double glass-distilled). The piece should be suspended by a thread in the washing vessel. The period of washing is the critical step of the method for demonstrating "primordial nerve fibrils".

Tone for 3 to 5 hours in tap-water.

Wash for 2 hours at the most in distilled water.

Dehydrate *quickly* in absolute alcohol, embed in paraffin celloidin or gelatin keeping pieces sheltered from direct sunlight.

Cut sections and mount.

Good neurofibrillar staining is quite difficult to obtain with this method and requires trials especially for the period of washing in distilled water, but demonstration of the nuclei and other structures mentioned above almost always succeeds.

It may be remarked here that the nucleal reaction of Feulgen and Rossenbeck can be carried out on pieces as bulk staining to give a selective demonstration of the nuclei that evidently surpasses all the other methods described above.

CHAPTER 10

DECALCIFYING AND SOFTENING VERY HARD TISSUES

It is clear that special operations should be effected before embedding calcified pieces, highly sclerotized cuticular structures or tissues which are rich in hard keratin, although the embedding itself and the cutting of sections in most cases can conform to the usual practice indicated in the first part of this book. Pieces containing silica would also be best softened before cutting, but, as far as I am aware, no technique for this exists. None of the works that I have had the possibility to consult refers to the use of hydrofluoric acid in histological technique, which, at least theoretically, appears to be suitable; in other words, a method that could facilitate the cutting of such material remains open for future research. In this chapter techniques for decalcifying and those for softening cuticular structures as well as keratin will be described.

DECALCIFYING

The aim of decalcifying is to dissolve the calcium salts in a piece, as it is, in most cases, the only means that permits cutting thin sections. All the classical methods of decalcifying involve inorganic or organic acids whose action results in the transformation of the insoluble calcium salts of tissues into soluble compounds. Another and much more recent method consists of dissolving calcium salts with the help of a chelating agent such as ethylene-diamino-tetra-acetic acid (EDTA, versene).

Decalcifying may be carried out simultaneously with fixation or following it. Early authors feared the destruction of certain structures by fixatives containing decalcifying agents, and for this reason recommended against the use of liquids containing an acid which was likely to attack calcium salts for the fixation of tissues rich in such salts. Their fears have turned out to be founded only in a few cases where the incrustation of calcium salts is very heavy with a proportional reduction of organic matter, of which dental enamel is the classical example. In other cases decalcifying fixatives do not expose pieces to any real risk.

Fixatives of this type include Bouin's fluid, Heidenhain's Susa, Halmi's liquid and the fixative of Romeis. The picric acid and acetic acid contents of the first of these liquids and the presence of trichloracetic acid in the others account for their decalcifying action which is sufficiently strong for small and not too calcified objects (limbs of the Mouse and Frog, ribs of the Rat) to be embedded in paraffin and cut without any further treatment. Even formalin exerts a clearly decalcifying action in the long run, which is due to the formation of formic acid. Carnoy's liquid does not decalcify since the eventual reaction between calcium salts and acetic acid does not yield products that are soluble in alcohol.

As a rule, decalcification can be carried out immediately after fixation if the fixative itself has decalcifying properties and it is merely a question of completing its action. In all other cases it is preferable to start by dehydrating up to 96% alcohol before submitting pieces to the decalcifying agent. Very fragile tissues may be embedded in gelatin, agar or celloidin before being decalcified.

The use of fixatives containing formalin is advantageous in all cases where decalcification is intended. In fact, one of the chief artefacts caused by decalcification with an acid is the swelling of collagen fibres on contact with water, and this risk is reduced to a great measure by fixation in formalin. Whenever the decalcifying liquid is not removed by washing in alcohol the aqueous wash should be preceded by a stay for 12 to 24 hours in a 5% aqueous solution of sodium or lithium sulfate.

It goes without saying that decalcification with a large quantity of the liquid is advised in all cases, and the daily renewal of the decalcifying bath is indispensable if pieces are big.

The process of decalcification is evidently more rapid in a moderate vacuum; that afforded by a filter pump suffices in most cases.

Various procedures have been suggested to verify whether decalcification is advanced enough to permit the cutting of sections. In cases where the calcium deposits are confined to the surface of pieces (as in the calciferous incrustations of cuticular formations) careful palpation is enough to ascertain the extent of softening obtained. When, however, the deposits of calcium salts are set deep in the tissue or when the piece is calcified through its entire thickness it may be necessary to verify whether section cutting has become possible by actually cutting a slice with a razor blade. It is better not to verify softening, as the early histologists did, by pressing or twisting the piece as it can cause serious artefacts. By far the most elegant means of checking complete decalcification is evidently to test for the absence of calcium in the last of the decalcifying baths. When decalcification has been effected with nitric or any other inorganic acid the simplest procedure is to withdraw about 5 ml of the last bath, neutralize it with ammonia until a methyl orange indicator turns yellow, and add 2 ml of a saturated aqueous solution of ammonium oxalate; if a precipitate of calcium oxalate appears within an hour it indicates that an appreciable quantity of calcium salts persists in the piece and further decalcification is called for. Examination in X rays has been proposed to verify the decalcification of bulky pieces (Goldhammer, 1929).

Tissues rich in calcium salts, even when completely decalcified, show an annoying tendency to harden considerably during paraffin embedding. Celloidin embedding may thus be resorted to, especially with large pieces. Frozen sections are also easier to obtain than paraffin sections even with incompletely decalcified tissues. With paraffin however, it is better to use butanol or cedar wood oil as the intermediate between the dehydrating alcohol and the embedding medium.

Numerous acids have been proposed for decalcification and their procedures for use have given rise to a great many formulae, not all of which are evidently useful. Only the more important ones are retained here.

1° Nitric acid. — Decalcification with nitric acid, adapted for histological technique towards the end of the 19th century, is considered by many authors as a method that best conserves the microscopical anatomy of tissues. It is, besides, very rapid. Schaffer (1902, 1926) advises the use of nitric acid diluted in distilled water, the most suitable concentration being 5 to 7.5%. It is better to use a large quantity of liquid with frequent agitation. When decalcification is over the pieces are treated for 24 hours with the 5% solution of sodium sulfate mentioned above and washed for 24 hours in running water before dehydration. Only formalin, among the various additives proposed, is useful; when 10% is added to the decalcifying bath it further guarantees against the subsequent swelling of collagen fibres.

2° Sulfurous acid. — Ziegler (1899) introduced decalcification with sulfurous acid into histological technique. Used as an aqueous saturated solution (about 5%) its action is based on the transformation of the insoluble tri-calcium phosphates into mono-calcium phosphate which is readily soluble in water. Decalcification is rapid and homogeneous, causing no serious alteration of structures, while the tendency for collagenous tissue to swell is weak enough for hardening in sodium sulfate to be dispensed with. Washing for 24 hours in running water usually follows decalcification.

3° Trichloroacetic acid. — Trichloroacetic acid, widely used as a 5% aqueous solution, is an excellent decalcifying agent whose rapid and uniform action conserves the fine structural details of cells to perhaps an even greater extent than the two previous liquids. However, the tendency for collagenous tissue to swell is even greater with this acid than with nitric or sulfurous acids, so that it is expedient to add 10% of commercial formalin to the decalcifying solution and to avoid any aqueous wash. Decalcified pieces are consequently transferred straight away to 96% alcohol which is renewed several times.

4° Formic acid. — Most modern authors stress the advantages of using a 5% aqueous solution of formic acid as a decalcifying agent. Structures are not affected, most tinctorial affinities are retained and the tendency of collagen fibres to swell is not very marked especially when Schmorl's formulae, consisting of adding 10% of commercial formalin to the decalcifying liquid, is adopted. Richmann and his collaborators have proposed a mixture of formic acid (100 ml) hydrochloric acid (80 ml) and water (820 ml); the decalcification obtained with this mixture is rapid and spares structures, but the use of an electrolytic bath to carry out the operation, as recommended by the authors, is quite unnecessary. As justly remarked by Lillie (1954) the effect of this bath merely amounts to raising the temperature.

5° Chromic acid and dichromates. — Decalcifying with these agents is particularly mild and requires a long time. Either a 1 to 2% of chromium trioxyde or an aqueous solution of potassium dichromate is used. Müller's liquid, whose formula is included among the cytological fixatives, can also be used. Structures are very well conserved, but decalcifying the femur of a rat, for instance, takes about a month. Pieces show a considerable tendency to harden when embedded in paraffin.

6° Picric acid. — Decalcifying with picric acid, used as a saturated aqueous solution, though slightly more rapid than with chromic acid or dichromates is, however, much slower than with the strong acids previously mentioned. It has the advantage of a good conservation of structures and tinctorial affinities.

7° Sodium ethylene-diamino-tetracetate (EDTA, versene). — This decalcifying agent, proposed by Dotti, Paparo and Clarke (1951) acts by chelation and has enjoyed great vogue. Its action is not very rapid, but structures are very well conserved. It should not be overlooked that other inorganic deposits are also dissolved, and hence, for instance, it cannot be used to decalcify pieces which are to be examined for structures carrying iron.

Either a 5.5% solution in 10% formalin or a 5% aqueous solution of the compound may be used. After decalcification, pieces may be washed in water or alcohol before embedding.

8° Decalcifying by organic buffers. — Citric acid or alkaline citrate buffers have been suggested as decalcifying agents in cases where certain enzymatic activities have to be conserved. Their methods of use are described under histochemical techniques.

9° **Decalcifying pieces embedded in celloidin.** — When pieces to be decalcified are very fragile, it can be useful, and even necessary, to embed them beforehand in a medium that allows the penetration of the aqueous solutions of the acids used for dissolving calcium deposits. Embedding in gelatin or in agar which can be adopted to this effect, does not call for any technical comment, but its relative inefficacity should be stressed. Celloidin is much better suited to this purpose, but special precautions should be observed. The following procedure, advised by Burket (in Mc Clung 1937) gives very satisfactory results.

The piece is embedded in 8% celloidin following the procedure described in the first part of this book. The block, hardened in chloroform, is trimmed so that only a thin layer of celloidin is left around the piece. The chloroform is displaced by isopropyl alcohol (which does not dissolve celloidin) and the block is passed through 80% ethanol, 60% ethanol and then into water. After soaking, it may be decalcified, hardened in 5% sodium sulfate and washed for 24 hours in running water. It is then dehydrated, terminating with Apathy's mixture of essences, and embedded in paraffin according to the usual technique if the cavities resulting from decalcification are not too large. If however, too many cavities have to be filled in dehydration is terminated in isopropyl alcohol and the block then immersed in a 6% solution of celloidin until the embedding mass penetrates fully. It may then be hardened in chloroform and cut in a microtome with a horizontal slideway or impregnated with chloroform and embedded in paraffin. Thorough dehydration is obviously an essential factor for success in this operation.

MODIFICATIONS OF TINCTORIAL AFFINITIES DURING DECALCIFICATION AND THE CHOICE OF A DECALCIFYING AGENT.

The decalcifying agents described above obviously do not restrain themselves to dissolving away the calcium salts that encrust tissues but also extract other chemical constituents of pieces. Apart from enzymatic activities, which unavoidably incur at least partial loss when tissues are decalcified, nucleic acids are also extracted whenever the action of an acid on tissues is prolonged to any extent. As a result tinctorial affinities are considerably modified, cytoplasmic basophily showing a strong tendency to be attenuated. Glycogen is hydrolysed during decalcification and its products go into solution.

Experience has shown that a greater part of the glycogen contained in pieces is lost and the extreme attenuation of all stains indicative of the presence of ribonucleic acid is inevitable when the size of pieces to be decalcified necessitates a somewhat prolonged stay in the decalcifying agents described above. Even nuclear staining is affected when decalcification lasts beyond a certain limit.

In general, many pieces can be cut after simple fixation in a decalcifying fixative without incurring any of the disadvantages mentioned above. If it is necessary to decalcify a piece that has already been fixed, trichloracetic or formic acid is best used when the calcareous incrustation is not too heavy; strong inorganic acids may be kept for samples very rich in bony tissue. The solutions of chromium trioxyde and potassium dichromate enable very mild decalcification, but their action is slow and consequently they would seem suitable for pieces meant for cytological study.

SOFTENING CUTICULAR STRUCTURES AND KERATIN

Cutting paraffin sections of highly sclerotised cuticular structures or pieces rich in keratin can set the histologist difficult technical problems. The consistency of these formations and the difference in hardness with respect to the embedding mass and the rest of the piece often involves serious difficulty in cutting, especially of serial sections.

In quite a few cases these difficulties may be overcome by taking particular care over the dehydration of pieces, their impregnation with a suitably chosen intermediate between the alcohol and paraffin and, finally, the embedding itself. In this respect it should be noted that butanol and cedar wood oil are better than all other methods of embedding when pieces show a tendency to harden. A prolonged stay in warm paraffin (several days or even weeks) also ensures satisfactory penetration where hastening otherwise leads to failure. Finally, softening pieces before cutting greatly facilitates matters.

None of the methods for softening with chemical agents can lead to cytological preparations. Several secretory products are destroyed during softening, not to mention the chondriomes and the Golgi apparatus which are always sacrificed. Many chemical constituents are extracted by these procedures, some of which resort to very powerful oxydants. In other words, only topographical study remains possible when the consistency of the material really requires the application of any of these methods.

The choice of fixative is important; Carnoy's liquid is admirably suited to the fixation of Arthropod organs, while that of Clarke can also be very useful. Two other fixatives should be noted here; although they do not possess the qualities of the mixtures described for topographical fixation they are reputed to soften Arthropod cuticles and their penetrating power is very great.

Gilson's liquid contains 20 g of mercuric chloride, 100 ml of 60% alcohol, 880 ml of distilled water, 15 ml of nitric acid (d = 1.45) and 4 ml of glacial acetic acid. Pieces are fixed for 1 to 6 hours, washed in 96% alcohol, dehydrated and embedded in paraffin.

Henning's liquid (1900) is prepared by mixing 8 ml of concentrated nitric acid (d = 1.45) 8 ml of a 0.5% aqueous solution of chromium trioxyde, 12 ml of a saturated solution of mercuric chloride in absolute alcohol, 6 ml of a saturated aqueous solution of picric acid and 21 ml of absolute alcohol. Fixation lasts, according to the size of the pieces, from 12 to 24 hours; it is followed by washing in 96% alcohol, dehydration and embedding.

From their composition it can be understood that these fixative mixtures cannot leave unharmed the fragile organelles of the cell; even several secretory products are destroyed but anatomical conservation is quite good and topographical study is perfectly feasible.

The chief chemical agents that can soften cuticular structures and keratin in fixed pieces are chlorine dioxide and a mixture of chloral hydrate and phenol.

1° *Chlorine dioxide*

Chlorine dioxide, a yellow toxic gas, is generally used as a solution in acetic acid; it is the classical diaphanol of Schulze (1922) and is available from suppliers of products for microscopy. It is a powerful oxydant and can bleach melanin pigments. The softening action on cuticular formations and on keratin is rapid and strong, but many structures are destroyed and the tendency for pieces to swell is quite marked.

Pieces meant for diaphanol should be dehydrated up to 96% alcohol and then submitted to a bath in alcohol at 65% before immersing in a commercial solution of diaphanol for a period depending on the nature of the object. Solutions which have lost their colour are no longer active and should be renewed. It is recommended to incise pieces so that the gas that accumulates within during softening can escape. Softened (and also depigmented) pieces are washed in 65% alcohol, dehydrated and embedded.

Drahn (1926) advises using chlorine dioxide dissolved in sulfuric or nitric acid. This author prepares an aqueous saturated solution of the gas and mixes, just before use, 10 volumes of the solution with one of concentrated sulfuric or nitric acid. Treatment with the softening agent is carried out as in the method of Schulze. When the desired result is obtained, washing is effected for 24 hours in a mixture of equal parts of a 2.5% aqueous solution of sodium hyposulfite and a 5% aqueous solution of sodium nitrate. This is followed by washing in running water, dehydration in alcohol and embedding.

Softening is more or less rapid according to the nature of the object. The softening liquid should be renewed during the course of the operation as soon as it loses its colour or becomes cloudy. Drahn (1926) reports having obtained serial sections in paraffin of the hoof of a newborn foal with this technique.

Embedding in celloidin before softening is possible when pieces are fragile. Moller (1933) recommends the following technique.

Pieces, which have been embedded in celloidin and hardened in chloroform or alcohol, are brought to 60% alcohol. Blocks are trimmed so as to leave a thickness of not more than 1 mm of celloidin around the piece. Softening and washing are carried out as described above. The block is then dehydrated up to 96% alcohol renewed several times, treated with Apathy's mixture of essences until complete clearing, impregnated with benzene and embedded in paraffin.

Apart from its action on pieces, which is unavoidable and due to the chemical nature of the softening agent, a practical drawback of Drahn's method is that one has to prepare the aqueous solution of chlorine dioxide. This is a dangerous operation because of the toxicity of the product and the explosive properties of the reagents. The two techniques described here are the least risky. However, the histologist who lacks equipment or experience is strongly advised to seek the services of a competent and helpful chemist for preparing the chlorine dioxide.

Moller's method (1933) consists in laying 220 ml of distilled water in a jar of 1000 ml capacity. A beaker containing 12 ml of distilled water is then placed in the jar and 44 ml of concentrated sulfuric acid are added to the beaker in small quantities while observing the usual precautions.

After complete cooling of the solution of sulfuric acid 12 g of potassium chlorate (*never ground, as it is explosive*) are added to the beaker. The jar is hermetically closed (sealing the lid with vaseline) and left to rest for 24 to 36 hours protected from sunlight in a fume-cupboard or a well ventilated room. After this the beaker is removed and the water in the jar, which is saturated with chlorine dioxide, is poured into a brown, glass-stoppered bottle and stored in the cold.

Drahn's method (1926) is more rapid but carries greater risks; it consists in mixing, with all the prudence necessary, 150 g of ground oxalic acid and 40 g of potassium chlorate in a round-bottomed flask, adding 30 ml of distilled water and warming to 60° in a water-bath. The chlorine dioxide evolved is collected by bubbling into 500 ml of distilled water in a receiving flask held in ice.

2° *Murray's method (1937)*

This method has been applied, as far as I know, only to Arthropod tissues. It involves a mixture of equal parts by weight of chloral hydrate and phenol. The mixture melts towards 55–60° and remains liquid at room temperature. Pieces which have been fixed in any of the usual liquids are immersed into it at room temperature, after having been dehydrated and treated with a mixture of equal parts of absolute alcohol, chloroform and acetic acid, the whole saturated with mercuric chloride. A stay of 12 hours in this "dehydrating fixative" of Murray is enough to precede the action of the mixture of chloral hydrate and phenol, which can last from 24 hours to a week. After softening, pieces are washed in several baths of xylene and embedded in paraffin.

On the whole, its softening action is less powerful than that of chlorine dioxide, but structural alterations are less. The chief drawback of the procedure is its irregularity. Murray's technique, as I have personally practised it, has given me both excellent results and complete failures indiscriminately without my ever having been able to elucidate the reasons for the latter.

PART THREE

HISTOCHEMICAL METHODS

> There is no Histochemistry without Chemistry and no understanding of the methods without knowledge of their chemical background.
>
> A. G. E. Pearse (1953)

CHAPTER 11

GENERAL INTRODUCTION TO THE STUDY OF HISTOCHEMICAL TECHNIQUES

Even those biologists who have turned their backs on morphological research, and who proclaim in and out of season the weaknesses of its outdated techniques, are rather hesitant to set themselves up as detractors of histochemistry. This latter subject, at the present time, is the most flourishing branch of histological research and the one which the majority of histologists regard as central to their professional preoccupations; its results are enthusiastically received not only in the major histological journals but also in specialised publications restricted to research with a histochemical orientation.

The first attempt to elucidate the chemical constitution of the structures revealed under the microscope, by the earliest histological techniques, is to be found in the works of Raspail (see, in particular, 1830). From this date onwards, histochemistry has undergone a development which we may divide legitimately into three periods.

The first period, dating from the origins to about 1900, was full of promise; preoccupations of a chemical nature were very much in the minds of the nineteenth century histologists but the importance of their views concerning the structures which they described is necessarily restricted by virtue of the limited chemical background of that era. From a technical point of view it would be unjust not to recall that some methods which were developed well before 1900 have triumphantly survived the test of time and are still used as routine procedures; such is the case with the demonstration of the presence of glycogen using iodine (Claude Bernard, 1849), with the detection of ferric iron using Prussian blue (Perls, 1867) and with the blackening of certain lipids under the action of osmium tetroxide (Schultze and Rudneff, 1865).

The interest taken by histologists in the kind of work we are discussing here diminished at the very moment when biochemical studies began to develop rapidly; this fact appears to be paradoxical but it is indeed easy to explain in reality. Starting with the last decades of the 19th century, morphologists left histochemistry on one side and restricted themselves to the description of structures whose study had become possible because of progress in microscopy. The explanation of this transitory divorce between these two orientations in all probability rests on their progressive complication which made it impossible for most individuals to acquire the background knowledge needed for a synthesis; we should not forget that the narrow specialisation in a single sector of one science, nowadays regarded as a necessity, was not permitted at that time.

The period between 1900 and 1936, from a histochemical point of view, only rarely brought to light facts of outstanding interest, the most spectacular of which were probably the invention of the nucleal reaction of Feulgen and Rossenbeck (1924) and microincineration (Liesegang, 1910; Policard, 1924); there are a number of reviews (A. Prenant, 1909; Parat, 1927; Patzelt, 1929; Romeis, 1930) which collect together the new knowledge acquired during the first quarter of the 20th century.

The real turning point in the evolution of histochemistry took place in 1936, the date on which Lison's book entitled "Histochimie animale" appeared. It was this work that transformed a heteroclite collection of recipes into a scientific discipline. Lison united in a coherent body of knowledge all the data available prior to 1936; moreover, he rigorously codified the requirements of histochemical research; in fact, this author's book marks the renaissance of histochemistry. It is but rarely that one finds critical reviews which have had a comparable influence on the development of their respective disciplines.

Beginning in 1936, publications became more and more numerous, eventually reaching the impressive development characteristic of modern histochemistry. The two last editions of Lison's book (1953, 1960), the works of Gomori (1952), Pearse (1953, 1960, 1968), Lillie (1954, 1965), the Treatise on Histochemistry (Handbuch der Histochemie) which is currently being edited by W. Graumann and K. Neumann, the books and papers devoted to certain aspects of histochemistry, in particular to histoenzymology, are eloquent testimony to the progress accomplished in thirty years.

This development has led to modifications in the sense in which certain terms are used even though their meaning once appeared to be clearly established; new names have been created, not all of which were happily chosen; it is thus necessary to define the usage which is employed, in this part of the present work, for the terms in question.

DEFINITIONS

Up to 1938, the term "histochemistry" was scarcely capable of leading to confusion and everyone understood by it a branch of histological research whose objective was represented by the need to obtain histological preparations, capable of giving information on the chemical composition of tissues and their constituents, using methods analysable in chemical terms. The first source of misunderstandings appeared as a result of the spectacular progress accomplished under Linderström-Lang's influence by the chemical analysis of ever smaller quantities of animal tissues. The cryostat which was the fruit of this great Danish biochemist's imagination did in fact enable us to obtain, without difficulty, frozen sections of fresh tissue, so that it became possible to compare the results of the chemical analysis of one section with the morphological data obtained by microscopical investigation of the adjacent section. This close comparison of morphological and biochemical data has been exceedingly fruitful. A further step in the same direction was accomplished by the widespread development of techniques for fractionating the cellular constituents by differential centrifugation, techniques initiated by the great morphologist R. R. Bensley (Bensley and Hoerr, 1934). To an ever increasing extent, the authors of the biochemical studies, to which I have alluded, describe their results as being histochemical because their analyses do in fact deal with tissues, cells or cellular organelles.

Some workers have tried to remove this potential double meaning by introducing the term "cytochemistry" whose significance corresponded to that of "histochemistry" as used by authors prior to 1938. This new word was intended to indicate that the chemical considerations did in fact relate to knowledge at the cellular level, examination under the microscope being taken for granted. Lison (1953, 1960) tried to avoid this double meaning by suggesting a distinction between histochemistry *in situ*, without preliminary isolation of the tissues, cells or organelles which form the objective of the work, and histochemistry *extra situm* with which histochemistry *in situ* was contrasted. Histochemistry *extra situm* begins with the isolation and separation of tissues using techniques which vary a great deal according to the material studied, but the general objective of which is the same as the objective of those who study intact organs.

In fact, the two solutions adopted lay themselves open to criticism. Histochemistry *extra situm* in Lison's sense does indeed include the whole of analytical biochemistry applied to metazoan tissue. Those reactions which are called "cytochemical" are of great use in the study of intercellular material and of secretory products exuded from the cells which secreted them, and it is in no way indispensable to use a microscope in order to carry out chemical studies on isolated cells. Apart from those instances where samples of strictly equivalent cells are easy to obtain in quantities such that their study by common analytical procedures poses no problems, there exist cells of a size so great that any difficulty of this kind disappears. I might recall in this respect that the yolk of an unfertilised ostrich egg represents a single cell, but a cell whose introduction into the cartridge of Kumagawa's apparatus of a size normally used in laboratories would be rather difficult. It is, thus, evident that the term "cytochemistry" does not sufficiently call to mind the methodological peculiarities of the kind of work which it purports to designate.

This nomenclatorial difficulty would never have existed if the authors had been wise enough to admit that the root "histo-" of the term "histochemistry" did not necessarily bear upon the fact that the work related to tissues, but that it could also quite well indicate that the work in question devolved on histological preparations. The term histochemistry, when taken in this accepted sense, which was conceded by Gomori (1952) and by Pearse (1953, 1960, 1968), is preferable to that of topochemistry, proposed by Voss (1952). "Topochemical" results of the greatest interest can be obtained using Linderström-Lang's technique, but this is in no way histochemistry because the morphological results on the one hand and the chemical results on the other are obtained by the examination of different sections however close they may be one to another. The essential characteristic of the work of a histochemist is precisely the convergence of chemical and morphological techniques applied to the same section; when correctly practised, histochemistry remains within the framework of histology and should not become chemistry applied to sections.

It is, then, the classical meaning of the term "histochemistry" which is adopted in the following pages.

CURRENT PROGRESS IN HISTOCHEMICAL RESEARCH AND THE WAYS IN WHICH ITS TECHNIQUES MAY BE EMPLOYED

Prior to the spread of histochemistry as a discipline, the techniques which the older writers grouped together under the name of microchemical methods were put into effect by them simultaneously with staining reactions; tests for histochemically detectable compounds were usually inspired by desire to obtain information capable of clarifying a diagnosis in pathological anatomy or a histophysiological interpretation; the identification of compounds detectable in a structure was only rarely the moving spirit of a piece of research. The development of histochemical research has led to a profound change and the work of modern authors can be grouped into one of three, essentially different, orientations.

Some authors—and by no means the least—are principally interested in the methodology of histochemical research, their basic preoccupation being the development of methods which already exist and the initiation of new procedures capable of increasing the number of chemical substances or enzymatic activities detectable on sections, as well as to improve the reliability of these techniques. There exist people who would like to reduce histochemistry to its methodological aspects and for whom the application of an already standardized technique no longer falls within the purview of histochemistry. This way of looking at things is obviously excessive; no chemist would be so pretentious as to reduce his discipline solely to analytical techniques. It is nevertheless true that the amount of effort which needs to be invested in the development of techniques has been such that during the last thirty years those who hold the patently incorrect view, which I have just commented on, have some psychological excuses.

Other histochemists have the self-imposed task of studying the distribution, in various organs and tissues, of compounds, groups or enzymatic activity whose demonstration no longer poses various technical problems. Such workers, specialised in the application of a limited number of methods, produce inventories of great value; from the very fact of the specialisation implied by the orientation I have just mentioned, those who undertake this kind of work run a considerable risk of failing, themselves, to exploit all the discoveries that histochemistry owes to their efforts.

Lastly, other scientific workers call into play histochemical techniques during research which is not specially aimed at developing methods for the demonstration of compounds or functions; the distribution of these compounds in the tissues under investigation is not the object of the work; the objective is indeed descriptive or histophysiological, histochemical techniques being employed either to facilitate the identification of certain structures or to obtain information about the functional significance of tissues or cells or again to provide the elements of a histophysiological diagnosis. Scientists who work in this way are perhaps users of histochemical techniques rather than histochemists, but their orientation is no less valuable than that of the others since the technique represents a means to an end but not an end in itself.

Histochemical techniques can, therefore, be applied in widely diverse circumstances, each particular case being, in general, capable of being subsumed under one of the three orientations mentioned above.

It is the first of the orientations in question that requires the greatest chemical erudition or the closest contacts with competent chemists. To be successful, anyone who seeks to develop a new technique needs in addition to consider the choice of suitable material available in large amounts and, as far as is possible, already well known from the analytical chemical standpoint. The results obtained in what is, properly speaking, the histochemical part of the work may often be verified by tests on models, the compounds whose demonstration is sought being deposited on glass slides, where necessary after wrapping or dissolution in gelatin or agar, and then fixed and treated as if they were sections. For some compounds such tests are carried out on strips of filter paper impregnated with the substance that one is seeking to reveal. Such work should be undertaken, to the greatest possible extent, using substances closely related to that being tested for, in order to define the extent of the specificity of the reaction put forward; it is also very useful to know, at least approximately, how sensitive the reaction may be.

Those who study the distribution of a compound or of a functional group in diverse material may allow themselves to be guided either by the precepts of analytical biochemistry or by those of histophysiology; in fact, experience shows that close links exist between the functional significance of a particular type of cell or tissue on the one hand and its histochemical characteristics on the other. There are, moreover, some circumstances in which a methodical inventory is rendered necessary, all the tissues and organs of any given animal being subjected to tests for the particular compounds studied. This kind of work, which to some workers may seem of little consequence, has already led to important discoveries.

It is the third of the orientations discussed which to some extent represents a link between the methodology of histochemistry and morphological research. To adopt it the research worker needs to have cultivated a more extensive knowledge of histochemistry than is required for the two other orientations and he will also need to call into play a wider variety of histochemical techniques. The appropriateness of tests for such and such a chemical substance arises during investigations which have no histochemical preoccupations to begin with; the relevance of such tests may be suggested during the examination of preparations stained by so-called general histological techniques or by various cytological methods. As a result of all this the last of the three orientations mentioned is the least favourable to a high degree of specialisation but it does afford the most extensive experience with histochemical techniques.

Lastly, we may remark that histochemical techniques can be used for staining purposes by scientists who are quite indifferent to the histochemical aspect of their results. The histophysiologist who uses the periodic acid Schiff method to obtain a clear demonstration of the thyroid colloid may be totally uninterested in the chemical reactions which result in this colloid becoming intensely stained, and anyone who, in the course of a caryological study, adopts the nucleal reaction of Feulgen and Rossenbeck as a method for demonstrating the existence of chromatin is not necessarily preoccupied by the chemical consequences of the hydrolysis, using hydrochloric acid, of deoxyribonucleic acid. It would be a serious injustice to hold such a usage of histochemical techniques in disdain; their ultimate objective is to further our body of knowledge, whatever may be the intellectual reasons for their application.

THE REQUIREMENTS EXACTED BY HISTOCHEMICAL INVESTIGATIONS

Thirty years of intensive research have confirmed the opinions expressed by Lison (1936) setting out the special requirements needed for the work of a histochemist. It is therefore useful for us to reconsider here the key ideas of a text which has lost none of its topicality.

> The special conditions of a histochemist's work require him to adjust himself to all sorts of requirements, some of which are morphological and others chemical.

CHEMICAL CONDITIONS

Three *requirements of a chemical nature* need to be set out during a critical appreciation of a histochemical reaction; it should be specific, sensitive and reliable.

1° So far as **specificity** is concerned, the range of histochemical reactions runs the gamut, from reactions which are truly specific for a particular chemical compound or ion on the one hand, to techniques whose positive result on the other hand represents, at best, a presumption in favour of the existence of a particular category of chemical substances in the stained structures. Tests for ferric iron using Prussian blue and the nucleal reaction of Feulgen and Rossenbeck are examples of the first situation and, where a positive result is obtained, is the equivalent of a chemical analysis. The second extreme situation is illustrated by cytoplasmic basophilia obtained under good technical circumstances; it should lead us to suspect the existence of electronegative groups in the basophilic structures but a whole series of supplementary tests should be called into play before such basophilia could be related to any particular group of compounds.

Most reactions intended to demonstrate the presence of organic compounds detect not chemical substances but functional groups; supplementary tests and control reactions allow us, in certain cases, to go beyond this and to identify the compound which bears the reactive group, but, in what is unfortunately a large number of cases, what is implicated is not a single chemical compound but a whole category of compounds.

The reactive groups disclosed by a certain number of histochemical reactions may either be intrinsic to the compounds studied or appear in them as a consequence of various pretreatments it is these latter groups which then determine the specificity of the histochemical reaction A large number of organic compounds can be detected as a result of the appearance of the aldehyde group following treatments which differ according to the circumstances; any of the reactions used for the detection of these compounds thus results in the demonstration of primary carbonyl groups. In the same way, the azoreaction can be used, not only for the detection of polyphenolic compounds existing spontaneously in the tissues under investigation, but also to enable us to discern groupings of this kind introduced into the molecules which we have to detect by means of various procedures.

A theoretical analysis based uniquely on chemical considerations may well render us highly sceptical as to the value of a far from negligible number of histochemical reactions, but all the foreseeable sources of error are far from being realised under the working conditions actually met with. In this way one of the metals most easily detected in the free condition, namely calcium, is discerned histochemically by means of techniques the most commonly used of which do, in fact, only detect anions with which the calcium is combined in the insoluble deposits met with in animal tissue, namely the phosphates and carbonates. The chemist could never allow himself to be satisfied with the results of von Kossa's or Stoelzner's reactions; the histochemist knows, from the results of chemical analyses, that the solidified accumulations of phosphates and carbonates in animal tissue virtually always correspond to salts of calcium and, hence, that so far as animal histochemistry is concerned the methods in question are valid. The number of compounds theoretically detectable by the periodic acid Schiff method is such that, merely by taking into consideration the various possible outcomes, we should be led to abandon any attempt at an interpretation of a positive result; in fact, so far as the majority of cases are concerned, it is possible to circumscribe the problem by using analytical biochemical data. Lison (1960) quite rightly emphasizes the difference between the theoretical specificity of a histochemical reaction and its effective specificity (the actual specificity in Lison's terminology).

Classically we follow Lison (1936) in distinguishing direct and indirect histochemical reactions. The first are characterised by the fact that the substance for which we are looking forms a reaction product with the reagent, a reaction product which is immediately identifiable through its colour, its crystalline form or other physical properties. A non specific "adsorption" of the reagent by other constituents of the tissues or cells is in no way disadvantageous in the case of a direct reaction since the positive result stems not from the presence of the reagent in the preparation but from its action on the substance we seek to detect. It is quite otherwise in the case of indirect reactions the first stage of which is generally the fixation of the reagent on the structure to be analysed, a fixation which involves a chemical reaction, certain chemical characteristics of the aforesaid reagent being secondarily put to good use to obtain a colour reaction. The unspecific adsorption of the reagent on structures which do not contain the substance we wish to detect may then introduce serious sources of error. Other disadvantages of the indirect methods will be discussed in relation to the morphological circumstances under which histochemical analyses may be undertaken.

From the point of view of their chemical specificity, some histochemical techniques can thus be said to be of equivalent value to an *in vitro* chemical analysis; others characterise the presence, in the structures under investigation, of a chemical function or of a reactive grouping; yet others afford presumptions in favour of the existence of certain groups of compounds even though the analytical techniques at our disposal do not as yet permit us to go beyond that finding.

Alongside the histochemical reactions in the strict sense of the term, may be classified those procedures which give us a clue to the presence in some structure or other of a chemical compound or function, even though the colour conferred on the structures in question cannot be unequivocally interpreted. Methods of this kind have most appropriately been described by Lison (1953) as diagnostic (marker) stains; it is rather to be regretted that Lison has abandoned this idea in the third edition of his book; the term does indeed appear there (1960, p. 47) but no use is made of it in the general body of the book and the fact that it has been abandoned leads Lison to consider that paraldehyde-fuchsin, for example, is a "reagent" (1960, 44), a proposition which is patently inaccurate. The number of marker stains is rather large and their diagnostic value varies according to circumstances. It may not be unhelpful to recall that even the so-called general histological techniques provide the experienced worker with clues which may enable him to choose those histochemical techniques which will be most rewarding. Without at this point mentioning basophilia or metachromotropia (metachromasia) the evidence of which is unequivocal, a very strong acidophilia leads one to suspect that basic proteins are abundant, whereas a clear affinity for aniline blue and light green implicates the presence of mucopolysaccharides; a particular greenish tint after staining with toluidine blue argues in favour of the presence of metals such as calcium or iron in the coloured structures. None of these dyestuffs' affinities represents a real argument in favour of the effective occurrence of this or that chemical compound but a knowledge of them may save the experimenter both time and energy by aiding him to choose the appropriate histochemical techniques to be used.

2° The problem of the ***sensitivity*** of reactions, the importance of which does not need to be stressed, arises in a different way for the chemist and for the histochemist. Within rather wide limits the chemist can in fact vary not only the total amount of the material on which he is working but also its concentration in the medium in which the reaction is taking place. In the case of those colorimetric reactions which, from this standpoint, represent that part of a chemist's work most closely related to the conditions with which the histochemist has to contend, it is virtually always possible to concentrate the solution for colorimetric analysis and to choose the thickness of the spectrophotometric container for the liquid in the light of the intensity of the colour. This is not true in the case of the histochemist who by definition works *in situ* and who can only vary one of the parameters, namely the thickness of the sections subjected to histochemical reactions. The augmentation of this thickness may be useful in cases where the compounds are diffusely distributed in the cytoplasm; it is known that histochemical tests for proteins using various reactions which have proved their worth in analytical chemistry only give positive results when carried out using thick sections; in the same way, the histochemical detection of protein-bound sulphydryls using the sodium nitroprussate method gives good results when carried out on thick tissue slices, whereas it becomes quite inoperative on thin sections such as are generally used for histochemical examination. However, the histochemist cannot have recourse to this manoeuvre in any instance where the compounds to be detected are concentrated in the form of granules since the reactivity of the granules requires individual consideration. We should, moreover, appreciate that such an accumulation in granular form may in certain instances favour the histochemist. Lison (1960, p. 54) remarks that the Prussian blue method allows us to detect 2.5×10^{-7} µg of iron if such a quantity was to be concentrated in a granule of 1 µg diameter. Naturally, the same quantity of iron could not be detected if it was diffusely distributed in a sufficiently extensive cytoplasm. It is, then, the local concentration of the substance to be detected and not its total amount which matters to the histochemist, the idea of the relative sensitivity (the *Empfindlichkeitsgrenze* of German authors) of the reactions being much more important for him than that of the theoretical maximal sensitivity *(Erfassungsgrenze)*. The classical studies of the development of deoxyribonucleic acid in oocytes provide cogent evidence for the importance of this idea.

We must admit that, in general, the histochemical reactions that we have at our disposal are sensitive; nevertheless we lack numerical data which would permit of a rigorous evaluation of this sensitivity.

3° The condition of *reliability* makes itself felt for histochemical reactions in the same way as it does for biochemical techniques. A true histochemical reaction requires the rigorous standardization of the experimental conditions; the composition of the reagents, the durations of their action and the physical circumstances (temperature etc...) must be defined with the same precision as if we were conducting a quantitative analysis. From the practical point of view it is evidently preferable to use "robust" methods, which will work under suboptimal conditions, rather than those which make very strict demands but this advice ceases to be of the foremost importance as soon as the conditions for the success of the more demanding techniques are strictly defined. The conditions for the preparation of histochemical reagents differ from those which have been described for the preparation of stains; in fact, histochemical techniques use compounds which are rigorously defined from the chemical point of view so that the user can assure himself of the degree of their purity, verify the composition supplied by the manufacturer and complain vigorously if there is any departure from this composition. Apart from certain substrates for histoenzymological studies the purchase of the reagents will not bite too deeply into the budgets of laboratories where histochemical research is undertaken, since rather small amounts of these substances are used. This represents yet another argument for the exclusive adoption of rigorously pure substances certified for analytical purposes in histochemical work.

MORPHOLOGICAL CONDITIONS

No less strict are the *morphological conditions* of histochemical work. In order to come within the definition of histochemistry a technique must respect the integrity of the tissue and ensure that the substance under investigation remains in position. At the outset these requirements will remove from the histochemical aegis a certain number of chemical reactions, which involve either the passage into solution of the product to be detected or the use of drastic treatments which destroy the structures. Such desiderata, moreover, will determine the progress of the entire range of operations from the dissection of the tissue blocks to the mounting of the preparations. It is, obviously, during fixation that the most difficult problems arise but the operations which succeed fixation are by no means excluded from the considerations with which we are now dealing and they need to be discussed.

1° Histochemical fixation

This serves not only the objectives of any histochemical examination but also the need to preserve the compounds under investigation as faithfully as possible. Some of the requirements of histochemical fixation are obvious and they are mentioned only for the record. Thus we may say that fixation should neither destroy nor introduce to the tissue blocks the compound or compounds for which we are testing. The use of fixatives liable to dissolve the salts of calcium is obviously contraindicated when it is proposed to test for these compounds and there can be no question of fixing, in Zenker's fluid or in Heidenhain's Susa, material upon which histochemical tests for mercury are to be practised. Highly oxidising fixatives, especially those with a potassium bichromate base, are not particularly desirable in work which involves the study of the action of various oxidising agents on carbohydrates, and a considerable amount of depolymerisation of deoxyribonucleic acid during fixation by Bouin's fluid renders this latter fixative unsuitable as a preparation for nuclear reactions. It is in the domain of histo-enzymology that the requirements involved in the preservation of the compounds under investigation most seriously influence the choice of fixative agents and mixtures.

But the requirements of histochemical fixation go still further; the compounds under investigation should not only be maintained unaltered from the chemical point of view, it is also necessary to secure their immobilisation in a position as close as possible to that which they occupied in the living state. This imperative rule which allows of no exceptions prevents us from considering as histochemical a large number of methods which, from the chemical standpoint alone, are quite satisfactory. The difficulties with which the investigator meets, moreover, are highly variable according to the compound in question; there are several cases that require discussion.

When we are dealing with insoluble compounds which exist in the living cell, in the free condition, the only imperative precaution for us to take during fixation prior to histochemical investigation consists of not dissolving such compounds; the chosen fixative should not, moreover, impair the chemical characteristics which provide a basis for the reactions which will subsequently be employed. It is in this particularly favourable case that we should restrain ourselves from giving way to the temptation of choosing the simplest fixative and instead choose that which best conserves the tissues in general. This is a classical requirement expounded at length by A. Prenant (1909) and confirmed by the whole course of modern histochemisty; leaving aside cases of chemical incompatability, the best histochemical fixatives are those which ensure the best morphological preservation of the tissues and cells.

Other compounds which are soluble in fixatives, dehydrating agents or in the intermediates used during embedding can in fact be kept in place because they form part of a macromolecular structure whose preservation *in situ* is ensured by fixation in the histological sense of the term. A degree of "immobilisation" which is sufficient to withstand all subsequent treatments is to some extent due to their being "wrapped up" by intermolecular linkages created during fixation. It is to this mechanism and not to precipitation by the fixatives that the preservation of glycogen is due under the working conditions of the histochemist, which explains the mediocre results obtained by the older authors using alcoholic fixatives, since alcohol is a poor preservative of structures and an unsatisfactory agent for denaturing proteins. It is easy to understand that the quality of the in *situ* preservation which occurs during fixation may depend not only on the chemical constitution of the substance which it is desired to detect but also on the nature of the macromolecular structures in which it is caught up. Experience shows that the difficulties met with in preserving glycogen in place vary a great deal from one tissue to another, and that even structures as stable as are the ferruginous inclusions can be either well or poorly preserved. Criteria determining the choice of fixatives which are satisfactory from a morphological point of view, as expounded above, are just as valid in cases where the compounds are incorporated in macromolecules. In such cases, also, good histological fixatives give better results than do others except in cases of chemical incompatability.

The most unfavourable circumstances relate to the occurrence of soluble compounds which do not form a part of macromolecular structures whose immobilisation by the fixative does in fact represent a precipitation. As Lison (1936, 1953, 1960) has quite rightly commented, the difficulty does not reside in the development of precipitating agents but in applying them so as to meet the histochemical requirements. When the substance to be detected is of low molecular weight, diffusible and mobile, its movements are always more rapid than those of the reagent; even perfusion of the vascular system with the precipitating reagent or the immediate immersion in the reagent of sections prepared on a freezing microtome, will not secure a precipitation which corresponds in all respects to the "topography" of the compound in the living tissue. Purely physical phenomena such as the periodical precipitation in the form of Liesegang's rings still further complicate the result; the first precipitates play the part of seeds for crystallisation and precipitation is not instantaneous so that the end result, however irreproachable from a chemical standpoint, is devoid of any "topochemical" value. It is the xanthydrol test for urea, a technique which from the chemical point of view is rigorous, which exemplifies the special requirements of histochemical work; when this method is applied to animal tissues the crystalline rosettes of dixanthylurea which are obtained are of a size clearly greater than that of the cells and their distribution bears no relation to the cellular topography. The risks of error entrained by these methods, we may conclude, are such that it is perhaps better not to use them at all in the present state of our knowledge.

The choice of a histochemical fixative must then be made in the light of chemical and morphological needs, the two types of requirement converging in certain cases whereas they are contradictory in others. The older tendency, preferentially to employ so-called indifferent fixatives, has fortunately been abandoned, partially because modern research has destroyed the myth of the "indifference" of the fixatives in question of which ethanol is the type. In those cases, which are fortunately fairly numerous, where chemical incompatability does not forbid their use, recourse to good topographical and cytological fixatives is mandatory even when the essential objective of the work is histochemical in nature, but cases do exist where the use of good histological fixatives is prevented by the need to preserve the chemical properties of which use will be made for the detection reactions and the scientist may be lead deliberately to sacrifice the morphological conditions of the work by choosing a method of fixation which he knows to be defective. It is in the domain of histoenzymology that the need to do without satisfactory fixation of the tissues is often imposed by the requirement that the enzymatic activity should be preserved.

It is particularly with an eye on histochemical practice that freeze-drying and freeze-substitution have been proposed; these procedures were described in the first part of this work as part of a general discussion on histological fixation. The advantages and disadvantages, of the methods in question were discussed from a morphological standpoint. It is appropriate to recollect that freeze-drying does not constitute a fixation in the proper sense of the term and that the denaturation of the proteins, which should occur prior to the treatment of the sections is to be taken into account as a source of chemical changes and even of the displacement of substances. When freeze-substitution is practised using an indifferent fluid the tissue proteins do not undergo denaturation and the situation is the same as occurs during freeze-drying; if the technique is practised using alcohol or acetone it is obviously necessary to take into account the action of these chemical substances on the tissues. The practical remarks formulated for these methods, regarded as histological fixations, are also valid for histochemistry; magnificent successes have been obtained through their use but putting them into effect necessitates numerous precautions and implies limitations of the size of the tissue blocks which seriously limit their use.

The practice of frozen sections taken from fresh tissue was justifiably considered as a very laborious process so long as histologists did have at their disposal only the classical freezing microtome. The first progress in this respect, which is due to Schultz-Brauns (1931), has already been mentioned in relation to the technique for section cutting; it consisted of adding a tube allowing one to refrigerate the razor blade to the ordinary freezing microtome; under such conditions the sections take on a parchment-like consistency remaining stuck to the upper face of the razor blade and strongly adhering to the carrying slide brought into contact with this face. In this way the principal difficulty met with in handling unfixed frozen sections is bypassed, this difficulty being the very laborious unfolding of the sections. Of the improvements subsequent to this method the most important was the invention of the cryostat (Linderström-Lang and Mogesen, 1938), a refrigerated container at a temperature lower than —15° in which the microtome was placed and within which all the operations of cutting and sticking the sections to slides take place. Numerous commercial models include important technical advances over the prototype of the Danish authors but the principle of the method remains the same. The tissue blocks are rapidly chilled to a low temperature, stuck on the object carrier of the microtome, as during the preparation of frozen sections of fixed tissue, and then cut using a rocking microtome or one of the Minot type, placed in the refrigerated container. A suitably calibrated plastic plate, which can be tilted towards the exterior, keeps the section against the upper face of the razor blade and prevents it from rolling up. The sections can be removed with a paint brush or by applying a carrier slide, kept at laboratory temperatures, against the razor blade; adhesion is immediate and firm if the tissue is fresh whereas sections taken from fixed tissue will obviously not adhere to the slide since the tissue proteins already denatured during fixation do not act as an adhesive.

Sections so obtained from fresh tissue may either be fixed by a short immersion in a chosen fixative or even by exposure to the vapours of a fixative or else treated without fixation.

Naturally, the principle of the method is most attractive but its practical inconveniences should in no way be forgotten. The cutting of the sections certainly presents no technical difficulty, at least in so far as we have to deal with homogeneous tissue and it is easier to obtain serial sections than with a freezing microtome of the current type. However, all the sources of artefacts enumerated in relation to the first stage of freeze-drying also exist for work in the cryostat and are still further aggravated because most users of the apparatus do not take the minute precautions concerning the size of the tissue blocks and the speed with which they are refrigerated, precautions which are second nature to partisans of freeze-drying. Thus, a large number of cryostat users can tempt themselves with freezing, in carbondioxide snow, tissue blocks whose size would not allow of satisfactory treatment even if they were thrown into isopentane chilled to the temperature of liquid nitrogen. The result is that many preparations and photographic records taken from material so treated show artefacts which would be considered inadmissible if the work were intended for microscopical anatomy but which are accepted because of the orientation of the studies in question.

In fact, the requirements of histochemical fixation are still more rigorous than those of histological fixation in general; to the need for an impeccable preservation of the structures must be added an obligation to change the chemical composition of the tissue constituents as little as possible and not to introduce any factor likely to impede the reactions to which the tissue block will be subjected and to avoid, with all possible care, movement of the substance during the preparation of the sections. Those methods which seem most satisfactory from a chemical point of view do not necessarily represent a universal panacea; it is essential to have recourse to freeze drying or to a cryostat in certain cases but one should not make a habit of it. As in any other branch of histological research, the ill-thought out and routine application of a technique, however indispensable it may be in certain cases, leads to the Tarpeian rock rather than to the Capitol.

In this context we may mention that work done during the last five years has shown how many disadvantages stem from freezing the tissue-blocks, prior to histochemical studies at the cellular level, even when all possible precautions are taken.

Such authors as Novikoff et al. (1966), Seligman et al. (1967), Karnovsky (1967), Rutenburg et al. (1969) and Fahimi (1969) stress that the preservation of the general morphology of the tissues and cells as well as the localisation of chemical compounds and enzymes are much superior on sections of unfrozen tissue. There are two kinds of equipment designed for this kind of section.

One of these depends on the same principal as the cutters used for making tissue slices intended for respirometric work. The tissue fragment is cut dry, into a series of slices kept adherent to one another by a drop of agar gel, placed on one side of the fragment prior to sectioning. The relatively thick sections are then separated under a liquid and generally used for histo-enzymological reactions, followed by embedding and ultrathin section-cutting for electron microscopy.

In the other kind of apparatus, the blade is vibrated at low frequencies along its length, in the plane of the section. The sections are cut one by one, under liquid, and collected as needed.

A comparative study by Smith (1970) has shown that the first of these instruments is preferable when a piece of tissue needs to be cut rapidly into thick sections of equal size, but that the second gives much better results when thin, regular, sections are required, or, alternatively, when thin and thick sections are desired.

In a very recent investigation, Hökfelt and Ljungdahl (1972) emphasise the advantages of uch sections for work on the fluoroscopy of biogenic amines.

2° *Embedding*

Embedding and the manoeuvres which prepare for it do not, in a large number of cases, require modification because the tissue blocks will be submitted to histochemical reactions Generally speaking, embedding in celloidin plays a much less important role in histochemical technique than does embedding in paraffin wax. Dehydration can be practised in the way indicated in the first part of this work except in cases where the compounds to be detected would be changed by ethyl alcohol. In such cases we use chemically pure acetone: three baths of a total duration of 24 hours will suffice, all the more so because this treatment is generally allotted to tissue blocks fixed in acetone; benzene serves as the intermediary.

A substantial reduction of the time spent in hot paraffin wax is required only in investigations of enzymatic activity, the nature of the material preventing one from practising the reactions on frozen sections. It is in the case to which I have just alluded that the use of a vacuum embedding oven is particularly desirable.

3° *Sections cutting*

The preparation of sections for histochemical purposes is carried out in the usual way; I might recall that sections which are too fine are not advantageous when there is a need to detect certain compounds. The spreading of the sections does not, in general, require special precautions, some exceptions being noted in the following chapters. This in no way signifies that displacements and losses of material are impossible during the manoeuvres in question; the reality of the artefacts to which I have alluded might be illustrated with examples but it is generally possible to insure against such incidents by choosing the liquid fixative with this in mind.

Frozen sections play a greater role in histochemical technique than in most other branches of histology; it is upon this technique that the histochemical study of lipids rests, practically exclusively, and it is the method of choice for the histochemical detection of enzymatic activities.

4° *Histochemical reactions*

Histochemical reactions, the chemical conditions for the validity of which have been discussed above, need to be discussed from the standpoint of their morphological exactitude taking into account not only their action on tissues in general but that on the structures within which the chemical compounds are to be detected.

In an earlier section we mentioned that methods which use too drastic reagents cannot be considered as histochemical reactions. However, experience shows that animal tissues, when correctly fixed, embedded and sectioned in paraffin wax, withstand astonishingly well the action of strong and relatively concentrated acids and alkalis provided that we take various elementary precautions, the principal one of which consists of allowing these substances to act in an anhydrous medium in all cases where the chemical conditions of the reaction in question permit. Very vigorous oxidising agents are equally well withstood by the sections.

As for the action on the structures which are the object of the histochemical reaction, the passage into solution of the compound to be detected, as I have remarked, renders the method in question unworthy of the adjective histochemical. In fact, the essential problem which arises during the appreciation of histochemical reactions from the point of view with which we are now considering them is their localising value within the organelle or, at least, within the cell. From this point of view histochemistry offers us all intermediary stages between compounds which are effectively fixed and detectable without any additional manoeuvre because of certain of their characteristics, on the one hand, and on the other hand those whose detection requires complicated manipulations and a prolonged sequence of reactions.

Obviously it is the first set of circumstances which is most advantageous for the histochemist. The localisation of melanin granules poses no special technical problem; it suffices that the fixation was correct and the sections cut in a suitable way for the natural colour of the granulations to provide a rigorously exact intra-cellular localisation. In the same way, ultra-violet absorption spectrography provides an excellent localisation of nucleic acids as does microradiography for heavy metals; the waste pigments designated under the name of lipofuscins may be localised because of their natural colour and a few supplementary tests will suffice to verify, not the accuracy of the localisation, but that of the chemical interpretation.

In other cases the compound sought does not become detectable unless a chemical reaction can be found in which it effectively participates; of necessity when it is rendered insoluble by histological fixation the product of the reaction is also insolubilised. This is the case with the nucleal reaction of Feulgen and Rossenbeck and with the detection of glycogen using the periodic acid Schiff-reaction. Diffusion artefacts are rare in the case of these methods; they may occur through partial solubilisation of the compound to be detected during the reaction but, generally speaking, inexact localisations stem more from a diffusion of the substances at the time of fixation or during the other manoeuvres prior to the reaction, than from a displacement during the course of the reaction.

It is quite otherwise when the histochemical detection of a compound depends on putting into effect a chemical reaction in which the compound in question does not directly participate. Even if the fixation is irreproachable from a histochemical point of view, which indicates that the molecules are truly immobilised, the products of the reaction can undergo displacement such that the test loses all its value. Tests for reducing groups using the ferric ferricyanide method, most techniques which depend on the reduction of a silver salt and all methods for detecting enzymatic activity are suspect for this cause of error. It happens in this way that the product of the colour reaction, which remains in solution, becomes fixed on structures which do not contain the substance to be detected and are held there by mechanisms which have no relationship to the histochemical reaction which has been practised; we then have to deal, in Lison's phrase, with a false positive reaction. On other occasions the compound formed during the reaction remains in solution and leads to false negative results. This risk of error is obviously all the slighter when the reaction leading to the formation of the coloured substance is faster, when the solubility of the compound is slighter and when its affinity for the substrate where the compound which has brought about the reaction is situated is greater. In particular, we have in this way a rationale for the great effort undertaken by certain histochemists to synthesise diazonium salts which will give rise to coloured azodyestuffs with as slight a solubility as possible.

To these sources of error we must add those which, in the case of indirect reactions, stem from an unspecific adsorption of certain reagents and also those sources of error which may entrain the chemical transformation during the reaction of the materials used. The danger of unspecific adsorption of the reagent is particularly great in the case of methods which employ the salts of heavy metals (iron, silver etc...). In this respect it is highly significant that the authors of histochemical reactions, involving the use of a silver salt, formally insist on the absolute necessity to limit its action to the optimum time and to follow the progress of the reaction under the microscope in all cases where the reaction is applied to sections. All the argentaffin reactions, when the periods for which the tissue is kept in the reagent are exceeded, become techniques for demonstrating argyrophilia, a property common to a large number of structures and wholly devoid of chemical significance. As for the errors which may stem from a chemical transformation of the reagent, events which are possible in the nucleal reaction of Feulgen and Rossenbeck or, in a rather more general way, in any of the methods which make use of the Schiff reagent, provide typical examples. This reagent, which is leuco-pararosaniline-C-sulphone-N-sulphinic acid, can regain its colour either by chemical combination with aldehydes and the formation of a coloured compound chemically distinct from pararosaniline chlorhydrate (basic fuchsin), which was used initially for its preparation, or through a lowering of the sulphurous acid content (evaporation of SO_2, elevation of the pH by another mechanism) and true regeneration of the basic fuchsin. The second event may occur when the slides are treated with Schiff's reagent without taking certain precautions, so that the unwise manipulator may obtain, in addition to the desired histochemical reaction, an undesired and undesirable stain using basic fuchsin.

The histochemist should then be aware of errors of omission and commission. The first may be due to losses during the manipulations preparatory to the reaction (fixation, embedding, cutting and spreading of the sections, drying) whether we have to deal with the passage of the compound to be detected into solution or with its chemical transformation; they may equally occur during the reaction itself, the reaction product passing into solution instead of becoming fixed on the structures containing the reactive substance. As for errors of commission, leading to false localisations, they may reflect the displacement of the reactive compound during the manipulations preparatory to the reaction, a displacement of the coloured product at the time of the reaction, an unspecific adsorption or a chemical transformation of certain reagents. The best guarantee against the sources of error consists of the confrontation of results obtained using techniques which, if possible, should depend on different principles; it may also be very helpful to take biochemical information into account.

We may add that from the practical point of view the preparations obtained using histochemical reactions are often ephemeral and that the necessity of examining, drawing and photographing them immediately is generally more vital than in the so-called general methods or in the case of cytological techniques.

CHAPTER 12

HISTOPHYSICAL METHODS

It is customary to collect together under the generic term "histophysical methods" those procedures which give information about the chemical constitution of tissues and cells using histological preparations but involving physical techniques. Such methods are numerous and varied; their importance will no doubt increase steadily and they are among the first methods enabling us to obtain quantitative data. In the present state of our knowledge, the importance of these methods of investigation and the easy with which they can be brought into play vary a great deal according to circumstances. Some of the techniques in question—and among these the most valuable—involve the use of apparatus which is both costly and highly complicated; moreover, they require on the user's part a technical ability as a physicist rarely met with amongst histochemists. Other techniques are less difficult to handle and the equipment needed for their use does not represent a substantial investment; their value cannot be illustrated by such clear cut examples as those available for methods falling into the first group. Still more procedures can be used with the normal equipment of a histological laboratory and form a part of the technical resources of any histochemist worthy of the name.

In the first group we can include ultraviolet spectrography, electron probe microanalysis, and historadiography, techniques which have had enormous success to their credit but which are not available to all laboratories. Only teams of workers specially trained in this kind of work and provided with ample funds and equipment can ensure that such methods give the maximum returns. It seems to me indispensable to give a brief survey of the fundamental principles and the main recommendations of such techniques but the description of the apparatus and an account of their use would not only exceed the scope of this book but also the capabilities of its author.

Histophotometry using visible light has been greeted with enthusiasm and the publications devoted to it are to be counted in hundreds; it seems likely that it will have less scope for development than will ultraviolet spectrography and most commercial histophotometers are not provided with the various gadgets required for working in the ultraviolet spectrum. Most of the results obtained using such procedures deal with the nuclear constituents and it is the caryological applications which have given rise to the greatest number of methodological studies involving histophotometric techniques.

Emission histospectrography, one of the most elegant methods from the chemical point of view, leaves a lot to be desired when it comes to localisation at the cellular level or even at that of the tissue; its applications are rather rare and require special equipment which occurs only in the form of prototypes and in a few laboratories at that.

The histochemical applications of fluoroscopy are less demanding from the point of view of equipment than are the methods just mentioned, at least so long as the experimenter does not go beyond visual observation of the fluorescence; fluorescence histospectrography, which is a very useful complement to fluoroscopy in the strict sense of the term, obviously requires the use of a spectrograph.

The histochemical applications of phase contrast microscopy (determination of the refractive index of cells so that their water content may be calculated) and interference microscopy (measurement of dry matter content) require no equipment other than the apparatus just mentioned; their use seems to hold promise.

The use of the polarising microscope entered into modern histochemical practice a number of years ago; the study of lipids and of certain mineral substances benefits greatly from it and many other uses of this instrument are mentioned in the following chapters. Autoradiography also constitutes one of the means of investigation open to the histochemist and needs to be discussed here.

The manuals of histochemical technique differ greatly in the amount of space devoted to histophysical methods; although summarily mentioned by Gomori (1952), Lillie (1954) and Pearse (1960) these techniques are described in a more detailed way by Lison (1960). However this may be, the entry into the literature of histophysical techniques is easy. The first volume of the Treatise on Histochemistry published by Graumann and Neumann (1958), some of the proceedings of the first International Congress of Histochemistry (1960) and the reviews published under the direction of Oster and Pollister (1966) represent rich sources of documentation; specially qualified authors have devoted monographs to several of the histophysical techniques.

ABSORPTION SPECTROPHOTOMETRY AND HISTOPHOTOMETRY

These two methods have in common the application of the general principles of photometry to histological preparations; their objectives differ in certain respects. Absorption spectrophotometry involves the measurement of light transmission at several wave lengths, the values obtained allowing us at the same time to trace the absorption curve to obtain information about the nature of the substance studied as well as the evaluation of its concentration in the medium examined. In the case of histophotometry the measurements are only taken at one or two suitably chosen wavelengths, the object of the experimenter being to obtain quantitative information concerning compounds whose nature is known to him. These methods which were introduced into histological technique by Caspersson (1936) have been much in fashion; their earliest applications, dealing with the measurement of ultraviolet absorption and requiring complicated apparatus, have played an essential part in the evolution of our knowledge of cell biology; the work of Caspersson and his students does in fact represent the starting point of work on the biochemistry of nucleic acids, work whose development is too well known to require mention here. The first application of the method in the visible spectrum is due to Pollister and co-workers (1949); numerous monographs published since that date are mainly concerned with nuclear constituents, in particular deoxyribonucleic acid. Infra-red absorption spectrophotometry has also been adapted to histochemical ends but the results are much more fragmentary and less promising (see Lison, 1960; Lecomte, 1963).

The general principles of absorption spectrophotometry obviously apply to histochemical usage. A flux of incident light (I_0) passes through the structure under examination; a fraction I of this light is transmitted. The transmission T is defined by the formula

$$T = \frac{I}{I_0} = e^{-k.c.l}$$

where k is a constant which for a given wavelength is characteristic of the substance to be determined, c the molar concentration, l the thickness traversed. The extinction E is defined by the formula

$$\boxed{E = \log \frac{1}{T} = K.c.l}$$

K being a constant for the substance studied and the wavelength chosen for the measurement (the molecular extinction coefficient). This, the Bouger-Lambert-Beer law, allows us easily to calculate the total amount of the substance to be determined in cases where the object is spherical or has plane-parallel faces. This quantity q is given for objects with plane-parallel faces by the formula $q = v.c$, where v is the volume, and hence

$$q = \frac{E.v}{K.l} \quad \text{or} \quad q = \frac{E.s}{K}$$

s being the surface area of the measured structure.

In cases where the object is spherical with radius r, the extinction (optical density) is measured along an axis passing through the centre, the formula becoming

$$q = \frac{4}{3}\pi r^3.c, \quad \text{that is, } c \text{ being equal to} \quad \frac{E}{K.2r}, \quad \frac{2.E.\pi.r^2}{3.E} = \frac{2.E.s}{3.K}$$

In most histophotometric research, the measurements are made in arbitrary units, the real quantity being supposedly multiplied by a factor which is constant for the series of measurements; thus we multiply the optical density by the measured surface

$$q = E.s$$

Histophotometric measurements in the visible spectrum most often have the objective of comparing the concentrations of two structures in any given compound; such measurements in relative terms are much simpler, the relative concentrations C_1 and C_2 and the total relative contents for the areas s_1 and s_2 being given by the following formulae starting from the extinctions E_1 and E_2 and the thicknesses of l_1 and l_2

$$\frac{C_1}{C_2} = \frac{E_1.l_2}{E_2.l_1} \quad \text{and} \quad \frac{q_1}{q_2} = \frac{E_1.s_1}{E_2.s_2}$$

The practical problem thus reduces to the measurement of light transmission, under the conditions of microscopic examination, over a very small surface area which is exactly known, and with very low light intensities. This measurement involves a single wavelength in histophotometry and a whole series of wavelengths in absorption microspectrophotometry.

The essential equipment for histophotometry is, therefore, the microscope and the light source, the screen and the photoelectric cell, and lastly the electron multiplier. The image of the histological preparation is projected on the screen, the zone which it is required to measure being placed, by manipulation of the microscope carriage, so as to coincide with the diaphragm interposed between the screen and the photoelectric cell. The measurement gives transmitted light; a further measure involving an area of the preparation which does not contain the structures studied but which is as close as possible to that which has just been measured (the blank measurement) allows us to evaluate the incident light. These two values enable us to calculate the transmission, the logarithm of the reciprocal of which is the extinction (optical density). The different pieces of commercial equipment vary in details of their technical construction as well as in the greater or lesser ease with which the surface area can be measured; this may be carried out by photography or by sketching, when the image is projected onto the screen behind which is the photoelectric cell. Monochromatism of the light is ensured either by interference screens, the logical situation of which is just in front of the photoelectric cell, or by illuminating the preparation using a monochromator.

Obviously the material requirements are much greater when absorption microspectrophotometry is carried out in the ultraviolet. The microscope must be provided with a quartz lens system or one in which the light is reflected, the light source is represented by a mercury vapour arc, a cadmium electrode arc, or a xenon lamp. The use of a prism monochromator is practically indispensable, filters being of use only with light sources emitting at fixed wavelengths. Special gadgets must be incorporated for focusing when working with quartz optical systems; this focusing can be carried out using visible light with objectives consisting of mirrors. Measurements are carried out either by photographic procedures or directly. We should add to this that each measurement of absorption should be supplemented for each wavelength by a "blank" measurement when the objective of the work is to determine the absorption curve, so that it is necessary to have a highly developed mechanical arrangement enabling one to shuttle freely between the object and the reference zone. In certain equipment (Barer and co-workers, Mellors and co-workers) which use reflection optical systems the image of the object is projected on to the slit of a spectrograph so that each point corresponding to the vertical band entering the apparatus is spread out in a horizontal straight line; a single photographic record thus gives information over the whole range of wavelengths, analysis being carried out by means of a control photograph which is a projection on the lower part of the slit of the spectrograph of a rotating sector.

It is easy to understand why the conditions in which histophotometric measurements may validly be made have given rise to a large number of publications. Some of these conditions relate to the equipment (monochromatic light, illumination regulated according to the nature of the equipment, in conformity with Köhler's principle or to that of the critical illumination, an achromatic and aplanetic condenser with a reduced numerical aperture, an objective with a high numerical aperture); yet others deal with the measuring instrument which should be sensitive, reliable and stable. The microscopic field illuminated should be of very small dimensions; this piece of information which derives from applying the Schwarzschild-Villiger effect to microspectrophotometry was neglected by constructors of histophotometric equipment until the investigations of Naora (1952); as a result errors on the high side, which may be substantial, are to be suspected in the course of the measurements because internal reflection increases the measured light intensity in excess of that transmitted by the object. The Japanese author provided a palliative for this disadvantage of other histophotometric equipment by replacing the microscope condenser by a microscope working upside down which reduces to 1–5 μ the illuminated field. The refractive index of the mounting medium should be equal to that of the material under investigation and the dimensions of the object under study should be at least twice as large as the wavelength of the light used; non-specific absorption through reflection or refraction can be substantially diminished by conducting the measurement through the central parts of the object. Such an error, through non-specific absorption, needs particularly to be taken into account when the measurements are carried out in the ultraviolet.

To these sources of error we have to add the distributional error (l'erreur de distribution of French authors, Inhomogenitätsfehler of German authors). Unlike the situation found in chemical work, the distribution of the compound to be measured in the field traversed by the incident light is not homogeneous, so that deviations from the Lambert-Beer law represent "one of the most serious problems of histophotometry" (Lison, 1960, p. 85). The seriousness of this kind of error is very unequally appreciated; on the whole, authors who have specialised in this subject stress the seriousness of the situation but some think that the real error is a good deal less than that theoretically possible.

The correction of this distributional error has been attempted in various ways; one of the solutions consists of exploring the area which is being measured with a large number of point source measurements, calculating the optical density for each measurement and summing over the whole, such operations being possible with scanning and integrating equipment. Caspersson and his colleagues (1951) and Deeley (1955) have developed equipment which meet these requirements but which is of great complexity. Integration of microdensitometer measurements on photographic records has also been used. A simpler solution is to conduct photometry at two wavelengths as suggested by Ornstein (1952) and by Patau (1952). The procedure involves making two measurements of transmission on the same object at wavelengths chosen so that the molecular extinction coefficients are in the ratio 2/1; from such data the mean optical density can be calculated so as to eliminate the distributional error; tables have been drawn up for this purpose (Patau, 1952; Mendelsohn, 1957). However, the method cannot be applied when the illumination of the field being assessed is not completely homogeneous or when the staining is too intense; in any event the choice of the wavelengths to be used requires a preliminary investigation or the experimental determination of the absorption curve of the substance under investigation.

It is appropriate to mention, in addition, that the sources of error discussed above relate to the measurement itself but do not take into account the techniques which precede it. When we take into account all the manipulations from dissection to the stage at which crude numbers are available, the sources of error are even greater especially in relation to histophotometry in the visible spectrum. Ultraviolet absorption microspectrography is in this respect at a considerable advantage; a large number of compounds, such as the nucleic acids, certain proteins, and the lipids are directly accessible to the measurements provided that they are preserved during the handling preparatory to examination. The same is unfortunately not true of histophotometry in the visible spectrum. Apart from those rather rare cases where the compounds to be estimated have a sufficiently intense natural colour to be measured in itself, histophotometry amounts to the estimation of the results of stains or colour reactions; the existence of a strictly defined relationship between the amount of a reactive or stainable substance on the one hand and the intensity of the stain obtained on the other is by no means self evident and has to be demonstrated anew in each instance in which the method is applied. This preliminary but indispensable information has only been acquired to date in a small number of cases (the nucleal reaction of Feulgen and Rossenbeck, staining with gallocyanine, and the DDD reaction in particular).

From the theoretical standpoint the introduction of quantitative methods into practical, histochemistry, that is to say the replacement of subjective estimation by expression in numbers is psychologically satisfying but we should in no way lose sight of the current limitations of the possibilities of histophotometry in the visible spectrum. Lison (1960, p. 60) states in relation to the histophotometer that "this instrument is for the microscopist what the colorimeter or the spectrophotometer is in the biochemical laboratory", but this enthusiastic assertion is contradicted by the rest of the text; in fact, on p. 92 of the same work the reader is told that "the conditions for histophotometric measurement are very different from those of normal spectrophotometric measurement"..., because "in the latter absorption is measured over a band of parallel light crossing a homogeneous object"..., whereas "in histophotometric measurement, the absorption is measured on the image formed by a complicated optical system of an optically non homogeneous object illuminated by a convergent ray of light". Moreover, Lison admits that "attempts to make histophotometric measurements in absolute values cannot be considered satisfactory"..., but that "relative measurements by means of which we seek to compare biological objects with one another are generally valid". To all appearances, the conclusion of the chapter devoted by Lison to histophotometry in the visible spectrum is a far cry from the paeon of praise represented by the introduction to the same chapter.

In fact, the remark made by Pearse (1960, p. 763) has preserved all its topicality; the degree of specialisation of practitioners of histophotometry in the execution of measurements on nuclei treated with the reaction of Feulgen and Rossenbeck is certainly not accidental. It is in the caryological field that proponents of the technique not only choose the material for their personal investigations but also that for the demonstration of the success which the method has to its credit.

By way of conclusion it seems legitimate to consider that ultraviolet absorption microspectrography, a method which has tremendous successes to its credit, necessitates a high degree of specialisation in the laboratory and in the scientific workers involved in this kind of research because of the complexity of the equipment and the technical knowledge required for its deployment. Interesting results have been obtained through the use of histophotometry in the visible spectrum concerning the deoxyribonucleic acid content of the nucleus but most of the apparatus designed for this method seems to be specially adapted to this purpose alone, so that the technique in question is very far from occupying a place in histochemical work comparable with that held by spectrophotometry in the activity of the chemist.

EMISSION HISTOSPECTROGRAPHY

This is a method whose rigorous specificity from the chemical standpoint and whose inadequacies so far as histological localisation is concerned were mentioned in the introduction to this chapter. As used by Gerlach (1931, 1933) and by Policard and Morel (1932, 1933) it consists of throwing a high frequency spark between a conducting plate on which the section has been spread and a very small electrode whose point of contact with the section has previously been adjusted. The spectrogram of this spark contains, in addition to lines corresponding to the electrode and those corresponding to air, lines characteristic of the chemical elements present in the part of the section which has been destroyed by the passage of the spark.

The great sensitivity of the method and its rigorous specificity from the chemical standpoint is recognised; obviously, only the chemical elements can be identified, an examination of the spectrograms giving no information about the nature of the chemical combinations in which they are engaged.

From the histological standpoint, the localising value is not great; the amount of tissue destroyed by the high frequency spark corresponds to 0.1 mm^3, a limit below which it seems difficult to get; thick sections must be used and the localisation obtained is rough and ready.

FLUOROSCOPY AND FLUORESCENCE SPECTROGRAPHY

The earliest applications of fluoroscopy in histochemistry did indeed antedate the widespread development of morphological fluoroscopy. In fact, this method was applied as early as 1909 to trace porphyrins in the blood and tissues of various invertebrates (R. Dubois, Stuebel); the same compounds were also detected in 1924 in a variety of mammalian tissues (Derrien and Turchini), whereas the great development of fluoroscopy as a method for histological examination began with the work of Haitinger (1930, 1934).

Fluoroscopy depends on the fact that certain compounds are capable of emitting some part of the radiant energy that they absorb in the form of radiation of a wavelength higher than that of the radiation received (Stokes' law). When irradiated with ultraviolet light these compounds give out visible light, whose colour and spectrum are to some extent characteristic of the class of substances and even of the particular chemical compound under investigation. This is what we should call primary fluorescence, a property which has been exploited from the earliest histochemical investigations.

Moreover, fluorescent compounds can be attached to substances devoid of *primary fluorescence*, such fixation resulting in the appearance of *secondary fluorescence*. In such instances there may be a well defined chemical reaction and the techniques which allow us to obtain it are then true histochemical methods. In other circumstances, the fixation of the fluorochrome on the substrate we wish to detect is secured by means of an immunological reaction of the antigen-antibody type, such methods being designated by the name of immuno-histochemical techniques. Lastly, there are numerous ways of staining with fluorochromes whose chemical mechanism is as poorly known as that of a large number of stains used in microscopy with visible light. The morphological value of the procedures falling into this latter group may be substantial and they are of great service in bacteriology; their application to the study of animal and plant tissue is closely associated with the German-speaking countries, whereas English-speaking histologists neglect the purely morphological applications of fluoroscopy.

APPARATUS

The equipment necessary for fluoroscopic examination includes a source of ultraviolet light, heat filters, filters intended to remove the visible part of the light coming from the source, a microscope and a filter intended to suppress ultraviolet light which has traversed the preparation.

In most cases long wave ultraviolet light is used (3.000–4.000 Å units); a powerful source of the light is much to be desired, most equipment includes either carbon arcs or, more particularly, mercury vapour lamps. Filters of nickel oxide glass serve to eliminate the visible part of the spectrum emitted by the light source; a heat filter filled with an approximately 10% solution of copper sulphate (4 to 20% according to the author) or glass heat filters serve as a complement to the nickel filters. By contrast with an old preconceived idea, the use of quartz condensers is unnecessary since condensers made of ordinary glass, such as modern microscopes are equipped with, are sufficiently permeable to long wave ultraviolet light; in some cases the results are improved by using a condenser made of glass permeable to ultraviolet light. Only one requirement has to be mentioned, so far as the microscope optics are concerned, and that is the absence of lenses made out of fluorescent material (beware of objects containing fluorine, or apochromats). The filter which protects the eye is generally placed in the diaphragm of the eyepiece.

We need hardly add that it is essential for the mounting medium not to be fluorescent; Canada balsam is unsuitable for fluoroscopic research and some immersion oils cannot be used either. The classical research workers used glycerine for mounting preparations intended for this sort of work; currently, synthetic resins and immersion oils which are not fluorescent are commercially available.

In cases where the experimenter desires to go further than simple visual observation, possibly with photographic reproduction in black and white or in colour, the equipment may be supplemented with a spectrograph provided with a photographic chamber. The first equipment of this kind was described by Lehmann (1913); it was developed by Borst and Königsdörfer (1929), Euler and his colleagues (1935), De Lerma and Moncharmont (1942), Sjöstrand (1946), Seeds and Wilkins (1950), and Mellors (1950). Spectra which characterise the preparations, and control spectra which provide an estimate of the energy distribution in the rays of the light which forms the spectrum are photographed on the same plate, and the density in the various regions is measured using the microphotometer which allows us to trace curves corresponding to the fluorescence spectra.

FLUOROSCOPY AS A MORPHOLOGICAL TECHNIQUE

In addition to bacteriological applications which do not require description here, the fluoroscopy of objects treated with a variety of fluorochromes has been widely used in animal and plant histology. The reviews of Haitinger (1934,

1938), Haitinger and Hamperl (1933), Bukatsch (1941), Gottschewski (1954), Mellors (1953), Peters, and the work of Strugger (1949) summarise the rich literature on this subject.

From the strictly morphological point of view, the interest of fluoroscopic techniques resides in the rapidity with which we can obtain the preparations and in the fact that the stains which are used are virtually non-toxic, so that there is a wide possibility of applying them in the living condition. It is nevertheless true that such techniques show no structures which cannot be detected by other means; the equipment needed for the examination of the preparations is more complex and more costly than simple microscopy in visible light; special precautions have to be taken when mounting the preparations; the latter often keep rather poorly. From the optical point of view, it is essential not to lose sight of the fact that the definition at high magnifications is distinctly less good than when transmitted light is used and that the special conditions for fluoroscopic examination scarcely assist a topographical study of the preparations. The selectivity of the fluorescence is a great advantage during work on pathogenic organisms, blood parasites, etc..., since the attention of the observer is immediately attracted during the rapid exploration of the slides. Acridine yellow, rivanol, and trypaflavine are widely used by bacteriologists and anatomopathologists. Other fluorochromes allow us to demonstrate the nuclei very selectively; acridine orange which, according to certain authors, is a fluorochrome highly diagnostic for nucleic acids, coriphosphine 0, and berberine sulphate are often used for this purpose. Aurophosphine allows us to show up mucus clearly, geranine confers a red fluorescence on myelin, neutral fats appearing blue; collagen appears white, and muscle blue, when thiazol yellow is used; this latter fluorescence is also obtained with primulin; thioflavin confers a blue fluorescence on cartilage whereas leucocytes show up yellow; more dilute solutions of the same dyestuff give a deep blue secondary fluorescence to adipose tissue. The studies and general reviews mentioned above include many technical details; a list of the major fluorochromes is given by Harms (1965).

PRIMARY FLUORESCENCE
FOR HISTOCHEMICAL IDENTIFICATION

This histochemical application of fluoroscopy is the oldest of all. It allows us to localise vitamin A through its primary green fluorescence, vitamin B_2 also giving a green fluorescence, as well as thiochrome whose primary fluorescence is blue, oxidative derivatives of lipids of the chromolipoid group which are characterised by a brownisch yellow fluorescence, carotenoids whose fluorescence is green, and porphyrins which show up red. Tissue proteins show up as bluish-white, this fluorescence being due to aromatic amino-acids (phenylalanine, tyrosine, tryptophane). The primary fluorescence of pterins has been widely used for their localisation in tissue.

SECONDARY FLUORESCENCE
FOLLOWING HISTOCHEMICAL REACTIONS

Some of the techniques to be dealt with here involve the solution of a fluorescent lysochrome in free lipids; their mechanism is the same as is that of general stains for lipids but the sensitivity of the method is very great. The blue fluorescence after treatment of the sections with 3,4-benzpyrene has been put to good use by Graffi and Maas (1938); Berg (1951) has made great play with the advantages of this method. Anthracene and chrysene have been suggested for the same purpose. The fluoroscopic detection of testosterone after treatment with sulphuric acid was obtained by Burkl (1954).

The fluoroscopic examination of frozen sections of the adrenal gland fixed in formalin allows us to locate precisely those cells which contain noradrenalin; it is only these cells which, under such experimental conditions, give a very intense white fluorescence (Eränkö, 1955). Modern techniques for the localisation of monoamines (Chapter 21) depend on fluoroscopic examination.

IMMUNO-HISTOCHEMISTRY

Immuno-histochemical techniques which were introduced into histochemical practice following the work of Coons and his colleagues are of great elegance and the highest sensitivity, but their conduct involves substantial practical difficulties some of which are not concerned with the histological part, strictly speaking, of the operations. In most cases, the final stage of the operation is the fluoroscopic examination and this is the reason why immuno-histochemistry is mentioned in this paragraph. In other cases, the detection of antibodies is ensured by labelling, using a radioactive tracer, the technique then terminating with an autoradiographic study.

The principle of the method is admirable in its simplicity and ingenuity. Antibodies are obtained by the usual immunological techniques (injection of an antigen into a suitably chosen mammal, generally speaking the rabbit, and sampling to disclose the appearance of antibodies in the blood, followed by purification when the blood content appears to be sufficient when evaluated by classical techniques). Once purified, the antibodies are labelled using a fluorochrome (in the original work fluorescein isocyanate was used). The tissue sections are brought into contact with the labelled antibodies, washed, mounted in glycerine and examined under a fluorescence microscope. The fluorescence of fluorescein isocyanate only appears at the sites of the antigen corresponding to the antibodies used.

Nevertheless, the practical conduct of the method in question is much less simple than its theory; the difficulties being mainly of an immunological nature. The essential stages of the working technique are briefly mentioned below; numerous supplementary details are to be found in the reviews of Mayersbach (1958, 1966), a reading of which will provide an excellent introduction to a deeper study of immuno-histochemical techniques.

1° Preparation of the antigen and antibodies. — This part of the work is obviously of an immunological nature; it consists of the production of precipitins in the body fluids of an animal, precipitins which are later to be labelled using a fluorescent substance. The purification of the antigen represents one of the main difficulties of immuno-histochemical technique because it is the stage which determines the success of the work and because cross-reactions in the immunological sense are liable to occur with the greatest ease if the antigen is not rigorously homogeneous. The extraordinary sensitivity of immunological reactions still further increases this requirement of an absolute purity of the antigen.

Once the antiserum has been obtained it is not generally used as it is; the globulins, which are the antibodies, are precipitated by the addition of a half-saturated solution of ammonium sulphate before being coupled with the fluorescent compound.

On the whole, this part of the work is so far removed from histochemical techniques, and empirically based decisions are so numerous, that the advice of a competent immunologist is most earnestly recommended.

2° The conduct of immuno-histochemical reactions. — The simplest way to detect the antigens present in sections was sketched when we summarised the principle of the method. The antiserum labelled with a fluorescent substance is brought into contact with the sections, the latter then being examined under a fluorescence microscope. When we have to detect antibodies firmly fixed to the structures of cells, the sections are treated, as a first stage, with unlabelled antigen which is fixed; washing removes the fraction of the antigen which is simply adsorbed on the tissues and the section is then treated with labelled antibody which fixes the antigen attached to the sessile intra-cellular antibody. This "sandwich" method may also be used for the detection of antigens; an antibody which corresponds to them and which is unlabelled is fixed on them as a first stage, the fixed antibody being demonstrated by means of an anti-antibody which is labelled with a fluorochrome. This indirect method for detecting antigens can be useful when we need to increase the sensitivity or the specificity of the reaction because it allows us to reduce the sources of error through cross-reactions. A combination of *in vivo* and *in vitro* methods is due to Mellors and his colleagues (1953) with a view to detecting the sites at which antibodies are formed. Here is the principle: Rabbits are sensitised to the rat kidney and chicks to the rabbit globulins. The anti-kidney serum of the rat is injected into rats which are then autopsied; sections of the various organs are treated with the rabbit anti-γ-globulins serum previously labelled with a fluorochrome in order to detect the sites where the antigen antibody complex is formed.

3° Labelling of antibodies with fluorochromes. — The earliest immuno-histochemical investigations were carried out by coupling antibodies with fluorescein isocyanate, an unstable compound which has to be prepared immediately prior to use; the synthesis which uses resorcinol and nitrophthalic acid was devised by Coons and Kaplan (1950); it is rather lengthy and requires the use of phosgene, a compound well known for the dangers which attend its manipulation, so that special equipment and trained personnel are required. We might add that these difficulties have been considered as being among the principal obstacles to the widespread adoption of immuno-histochemical techniques. Currently, other fluorochromes can be used in place of fluorescein isocyanate. Clayton (1954) and Mayersbach (1958) have suggested the chloride of 1-dimethylaminonaphthalene-5-sulphonic acid which is a stable substance, easy to prepare by methylating 1-naphthylamino-5-sulphonic acid followed by treatment with phosphorus pentachloride. The process is not dangerous and requires no complicated equipment; moreover, its practice has been rendered unnecessary as the chloride is available commercially in a form which is ready for use. More recently lissamine-rhodamine-sulphonyl chloride, rhodamine B isocyanate and the isocyanates of rhodamine B and of fluorescein have been suggested.

In any event, coupling the globulins with the fluorochrome generally presents no difficulties; it takes place in an alkaline medium and at low temperatures, the time taken varying according to the circumstances. The reagent so obtained should be purified by dialysis and by adsorption of non-specific antibodies; in general practice the material is passed through an organ powder (especially powdered liver), this powder being subsequently removed by centrifugation. Not all unspecific reactivity can be eliminated by this treatment so that the results need to be interpreted critically.

4° Preparation of the sections and conduct of the reaction. — In most cases, it is essential to have recourse to freeze-drying or to working with sections of fresh tissue cut on a cryostat in order to avoid any modification of the antigenic properties under investigation; the denaturation of the tissue proteins can be undertaken with alcohol or acetone. A short fixation in alcohol, acetone or formalin is possible in some cases; even embedding in paraffin wax may preserve some antigens.

The sections are washed carefully before treatment with the labelled antiserum; further washing eliminates the excess of the latter. Mounting can be carried out in glycerine, in glycerine-treated physiological saline or in a non fluorescent synthetic resin, after dehydration with alcohol and clearing in a benzenoid hydrocarbon. The fluoroscopic examination itself requires no particular precautions.

Evidently, the essential histochemical information provided by this method is the localisation of proteins. Excellent results have been obtained, in spite of the methodological difficulties, in the detection of certain adenohypophysial hormones, insulin, and glucagon some enzymes and various proteins. We know from immunological research, upon which it would be inappropriate to expatiate here, that certain carbohydrates can also give rise to the formation of antibodies, a fact which obviously enlarges the framework of reference of immunohistochemical techniques.

HISTORADIOGRAPHY

The use of X-rays as a histological technique, and more particularly in histochemistry, runs up against grave practical difficulties but the theoretical advantages, which include a wavelength notably less than that of visible light, and the existence of strictly defined relationships between the absorption and the atomic number of the elements present in the structures traversed accounts for the efforts made to promote their histochemical use. The proceedings of a colloqium held in 1956, published by Cosslet, Engström and Pattee, the reviews of Neumann (1958) and Engström (*in* Oster and Pollister, 1966) provide a rich literature on the subject of this technique; only the essential features are mentioned here.

In theory three ways of applying X-rays for the study of histological preparations can be conceived, these include the use of X-ray microscopes, whose development has not yet gone beyond the experimental stage, contact microradiography which consists of preparing a radiograph of the histological preparation and examining it under the microscope, and lastly projection microradiography which affords an enlarged radiograph of the preparation. This latter method runs up against the serious practical difficulty of obtaining point sources of X-rays; most of the important findings of historadiography are associated with contact microradiography.

This method which was suggested by Goby (1913) was applied to the study of plant tissue by Dauvilliers (1930) and to animal tissue by Lamarque and Turchini (1938). The full development of contact microradiography is due to Engström and his colleagues.

Only very soft rays ($\lambda = 1-10$ Å units) emitted under low potentials can be used for microradiographic purposes; the emitting tubes should be constructed accordingly and most of the sources of supply used in laboratories which conduct microradiography also represent experimental prototypes. The apparatus developed by Van Den Broek (1957) is nevertheless commercially available. Certain workers use extremely soft rays (20, even 30 or 50 Å) which necessitates the taking of photographs under high vacuum. We can easily see how demanding will be the requirements as to grain and sensitivity of the emulsions used for the photography; Neumann's general review includes an indication of the emulsions which are commercially available and which allow the examination of microradiographs at linear enlargements of as much as 800 diameters.

Some applications of historadiography are qualitative; this method does indeed allow us easily to localise elements with a high atomic number because absorption increases very rapidly with atomic number; obviously the method provides no indication of the compounds into which the elements detected may be combined. Among the most important results obtained in this way we may cite the localisation of calcium in bony tissue and that of iodine in the thyroid gland.

Other applications are quantitative. A very ingenious technique for determining the total dry maas developed by Engström and Lindström (1950) depends on the fact that most of the elements making up animal tissue have low atomic numbers (less than 30), so that they are roughly equal in their absorption of X-rays with a wavelength around 10 Å; this absorption is therefore practically proportional to the density of the cell structure. In this particular case, the application of the Lambert-Beer law gives the formula

$$I = I_0 \cdot e^{-\frac{\mu}{\varrho} m}$$

where I is the intensity of the transmitted radiation, I_0 that of the incident radiation, e is the base of naperian logarithms, μ the density of the tissue traversed (in grams per cm^3), ϱ the distance travelled within the tissue (in cm^{-1}) and m the mass of the tissue traversed (in g:cm^2)

In practical terms, the microradiograph of the tissue under examination and the reference photograph representing a scale made up of nitrocellulose layers of known thickness are taken on the same plate, the two images being examined by means of a microdensitometer comparable with that used for the assessment of ultraviolet photomicrographs. The ratio $\frac{\mu}{\varrho}$ (the mass absorption coefficient) for a certain number of wavelengths and various elements has been measured by Lindström (1955); the data of this author and the methodological studies of Engström and Lindström (1950) show that the error does not exceed 5%; correction factors for hydrogen and for tissues whose elementary composition is very different from that of nitrocellulose taken as the reference system may also be introduced into the calculations. It is appropriate to remark that the determinations of dry mass by this method give results which agree to a most satisfactory extent with those of interference microscopy.

Brattgaard and Hyden (1952) have combined this measure of dry mass with the extraction of various tissue constituents so that it is possible to estimate on a microscale lipids, ribonucleic acid, etc... The studies of Stich and McIntyre (1958) on the proteins of the mitotic apparatus should also be mentioned here.

Historadiography at various wavelengths also allows us to identify certain chemical elements through the discontinuities of the absorption curve corresponding to sharp variations in the mass absorption coefficient. Such absorption spectrophotometry may even give quantitative information, the concentration of the element influencing the height of the discontinuity on the absorption curve. It is the discontinuity K which corresponds to variations of energy in the internal electron shell of the atom studied which are generally used for measurement. Important results have been obtained in this way during work on osteogenesis, on the deposition of calcium in atheromatous arteries, on the production of sulphur during epidermal keratinisation and on the phosphorus content of the sea urchin egg.

Electron probe microanalysis. — Galle (1964) was responsible for applying che analytical procedure developed by Castaing (1952) for crystallographic and hem ical research to the working conditions of the histologist. The method seems to show considerable promise at least so far as chemical elements with atomic numbers greater than 10 are concerned.

The principle of the method is simple. A very narrow electron beam (of the order of 1 micron) is thrown by a series of electromagnetic lenses on to a point of the sample under analysis. The X-rays produced under the impact of the electrons are directed towards equipment for spectrographic analysis, allowing us to identify the nature of the atoms entering into the composition of the "sampled" point. Scanning the preparation gives the distribution of the chosen element in the section with relatively high resolution (about one micron). This distribution can be explored quickly under the optical system of the equipment and a detailed morphological study of a neighbouring section greatly assists in providing points of reference.

The chemical specificity of the procedure is rigorous and its sensitivity is very great; localisation on the electron microscope scale is possible. Nevertheless it is evident that atoms and not chemical compounds are detected; this limitation is common to electron probe microanalysis and to contact microradiography.

PHASE CONTRAST MICROSCOPY AND INTERFERENCE MICROSCOPY

The biological applications of phase contrast and interference microscopy have given rise to numerous publications; the description of the equipment in question and an account of their use would exceed the scope of this work; the two instruments are summarily mentioned here only because they allow us to measure the refractive index of the objects studied from which we can make interesting deductions about the dry mass of the cell constituents. The interference microscope also represents a way of measuring the thickness of sections.

Only the basic principles of the methods of measurement which have just been mentioned are very succinctly described in this section. The recent general review of Barer (in Oster and Pollister, 1966) provides all the necessary details of the detailed literature on phase contrast and interference microscopy.

In the case of the phase contrast microscope the phase difference between the object and the medium which is associated with differences in the optical path, that is to say of refractive indices, is made visible by the interference of the direct image with images difracted laterally. This difference of optical path is a function of the thickness of the object, as well as of the difference in the refractive indices of the object and the medium

$$\varphi = (n_0 - n_m)t$$

where φ is the phase shift, n_0 and n_m the refractive indices, and t the thickness of the object. There is, moreover, a simple relationship between the refractive index of a solution and its concentration, a relationship given by the formula

$$C = \frac{n_s - n_m}{\alpha}$$

C being the concentration, n_s and n_m the refractive indices of the solution and pure solvent (medium), α a constant representing the increase in the refractive index for an augmentation of 1% of the concentration (specific refractive increment).

Experience shows that the value of the specific refractive increment is about 0.00180 for most protoplasmic constituents; knowing the index of refraction of water (1.333), it is possible, by measuring the refractive index of a cell, to calculate the concentration of total solids to within limits of about 5% and to deduce from this the water content. This measure of the refractive index using a phase contrast microscope (with positive contrast objectives) depends on the fact that the object under examination appears darker than the mounting medium if its refractive index is higher than that of the medium and lighter if it is lower; when the indices are equal the object becomes invisible. Following the investigations of Barer and Joseph (1955), most authors use the commercially available fraction V of ox serum-albumin solutions as a mounting medium for different refractive indices. This medium, which is non-toxic, does not penetrate into the interior of the cells and thus permits correct measurements on living objects. Between concentrations of 0 ($n = 1.333$) and 55% ($n = 1.430$), the refractive index increases linearly and follows the relationship

$$C = \frac{n - 1.333}{0.00182}$$

Obviously this method which depends on the measure of phase differences existing between interfaces cannot be used for the measurement of the refractive index of structures situated within the cells; only those parts of the cytoplasm which are in contact with a mounting medium lend themselves to measurement.

Measurement of the phase shift under the interference microscope, in conjunction with a knowledge of the area under exploration and that of the specific refractive increment of the compound under investigation, allows us to calculate the dry matter in a particularly elegant way. Experience has in fact shown that solutions of proteins do obey the relationship between the concentration and the refractive indices set out above. A cell can be considered as being primarily a solution of proteins. The value of the phase shift can then be found by combining the formulae (1) and (2) in the form

$$\varphi = \alpha . C . t$$

where C obviously represents the ratio of the protein content of a cell to its cellular volume, multiplied by 100. If we suppose that the structure examined has plane-parallel faces the volume is represented by the product $S.t$, where t is the thickness explored, and S the surface area. We deduce

$$\varphi = 100 . \alpha . t . \frac{m}{S.t} = 100 . \alpha . \frac{m}{S}, \quad \text{whence} \quad m = \frac{\varphi . S}{100 \alpha}$$

m being the content of proteins expressed in grams per cell.

As Barer (1955) has commented, this calculation eliminates the need for a measure of the thickness t, a measure whose uncertainty has been mentioned several times. Knowledge of the specific refractive increment is obviously required; as I remarked above, the use of an average value of 0.00182 introduces an error less than 10%.

When the measurement is made on heterogeneous objects the difficulties are the same as in histophotometric or microspectrophotometric measurements; scanning and integrating equipment enables us to reduce the distribution of errors through the use of a large number of point measurements and has been developed by several teams of workers.

Naturally the measure of phase shift in two media with different refractive indexes allows us to calculate the thickness of the object under examination (Barer, 1953); other interferometric methods which allow us to evaluate the thickness of the preparations depend on counting the interference fringes when the preparation is illuminated in a particular way (Richards, 1947; Mellors and co-workers, 1953).

MICROSCOPY IN POLARISED LIGHT

In histochemical research the polarising microscope plays a much smaller part than it does in the study of the ultramicroscopic structure of the protoplasm; it is nevertheless true that certain histochemical techniques involve the exploration of the preparations using polarised light so that a polarising microscope or polarising filters form part of the normal equipment of any histochemical laboratory.

Generally speaking, only intrinsic birefringence (crystalline) is sought during histochemical investigations; most often such methods merely require us to observe optical anisotropy; at the most, in certain cases, we need to determine the sign of the spherocrystals. In consequence, from the practical point of view, the purchase of a large polarising microscope is generally of no service because it is sufficient to possess polarising filters and a first order wedge of red gypsum.

The techniques for preparing the material and mounting the preparations call for no special comment apart from the need to avoid the action of those chemical substances which abolish birefringence (phenol) in any instance where the investigator thinks it might be interesting to examine the preparations under polarised light.

The principal applications of the polarising microscope which are discussed ni this part of the work involve the histochemical study of purines and their derivatives, the distinction between the various mineralogical forms of calcium, the histochemical analysis of lipids, and the demonstration of crystalline material or of spheroliths resulting from various reactions; suggestions for studies to be carried out under polarised light and the main results are mentioned in the corresponding chapters.

AUTORADIOGRAPHY

The demonstration of radioactive elements on histological preparations dates back to Lacassagne and Lattes (1924) who detected, in this way, polonium introduced experimentally into the body of the rabbit. Autoradiographic techniques developed rapidly with the use of radioactive tracers in biological research; currently, it is used under a wide range of circumstances; numerous and excellent reviews have been devoted to it. It is a histochemical method to the extent that localisation can be obtained on the tissue, cell or even organelle scale by examining histological preparations. Nevertheless, the procedure detects chemical elements without, of itself, providing the slightest information about the chemical compounds of which they may form a part; only supplementary tests, especially extractions, can provide clues of this nature. Moreover, we always have to deal with compounds which do not exist spontaneously in the tissues examined but which have been introduced experimentally.

The localising value of autoradiographic methods may be great; it is appropriate to mention that localisation on the organelle scale can be obtained, provided that certain precautions are taken, on electron micrographs. The sensitivity of the technique is great though not as great as that of the procedures which involve counting. So far as its specificity is concerned, the only sources of error which need to be considered are artefacts associated with the background of the photographic emulsion, electrocapillary phenomena, mechanical accidents during the treatment of the preparations, the reduction of silver halides by certain tissue constituents (protein-bound sulphydryls in particular), and lastly changes in the properties of the emulsion by the chemical substances used for treatment of the tissue or of the sections.

The main interest of autoradiography does not lie within the domain of histochemistry. The incorporation into the structures under investigation of an element which forms part of a compound the presence of which is shown by other techniques does indeed represent information of great value, but information concerning the movements of the compound within the organism into which it has been introduced, its fixation by tissues, cells or organelles, the rate at which it is eliminated are data of the greatest value from the point of view of the histophysiologist and of cell biology in general. We should add to this that labelling certain cells by means of a radioactive tracer often gives decisive information about their length of life, their movements within the tissue and other features of their development.

A large part of the operations which lead to autoradiography does not need description here; in effect, what is properly the radiobiological part of the work does not fall within the framework of histochemical research. We need only take into account techniques which are, strictly speaking, histological. It is nevertheless useful to mention that satisfactory autoradiographs are generally only obtained with radio-isotopes whose half-life is at least several hours and that the α and β rays lend themselves to detection on photographic emulsions of the same kind as are used in this sort of work.

Fixation for autoradiographic purposes is obviously subject to all the requirements of histological fixation in general; losses during this first stage of the histological process should be avoided so that the choice of fixative is to some extent determined by the nature of the chemical combinations in which the tracer to be detected is combined. It is possible to use sections of fresh tissue, cut in a cryostat, freeze-dried sections, freeze-substituted sections, frozen sections after formalin fixation, paraffin wax sections, celloidin sections, and smears.

The conditions for the success of work carried out on sections are the high quality of the sections and the care expended during their spreading; collodion treatment is cordially recommended by certain authors, with the obvious exception of cases where the radioactive tracer has been incorporated into lipids. This precaution, which is particularly useful when emulsion coating techniques are used, is replaced by some workers with a gelatin skin which is painted on prior to the sticking of the sections and is intended to aid the adherence of the emulsion to the glass. To do this the slides are plunged into a 0.5% gelatin solution and then dried in a position protected from dust.

Autoradiography itself can be carried out in various ways. It is customary to distinguish procedures which involve contact, mounting, coating and stripping emulsions.

In *contact procedures,* which are the simplest but which do not permit of very precise localisation of the tracer, the sections are simply spread out on sections, the latter being kept in contact with the emulsion for the whole exposure period. Dewaxing and staining can take place after developing once the slides bearing the sections and the emulsion have been separated; in cases where the sections have been dewaxed prior to exposure collodion treatment followed by drying in air is virtually imperative.

The techniques of *autoradiography by mounting* consist of spreading the sections, dry or under water, on a photographic emulsion; the section thus remains in contact with the latter during exposure and throughout the photographic and histological treatments. In consequence the serious problems of collecting the sections which arise during the contact procedures no longer obtain; however, the stains have to be chosen in the light of the risk of staining the photographic emulsion and a densitometric analysis of the autoradiographs is rendered impossible and histological treatments on the one hand and photographic treatments on the other may mutually interfere.

The sensitivity of the method can be increased by mounting "in a sandwich", the section being mounted on the photographic emulsion and brought into contact with a second layer of the same emulsion; after exposure, one of the emulsions can be developed independently of the section and used for densitometric studies, the other being treated as in the procedure involving mounting, and serving to collect the sections.

Techniques involving *coating methods* (*coulage de l'émulsion* of French speaking authors) use emulsions which can be liquified by warming to 37°. The dewaxed and collodion treated sections (the layer of collodion reduces the risk of chemical fogging) stained or not according to the circumstances, are covered with emulsion in the dark at 37° (a hot-plate, or water bath), the emulsion being spread out using a paint brush or, better still, a calibrated spreader. Some stains should be applied prior to exposure, others afterwards. During the mounting of the preparations we need to remember that the emulsion is present; concentrated solutions of Canada balsam or of commercial synthetic resins penetrate poorly across the emulsion and dehydration and clearing are thus rendered rather difficult. Clearing can be assisted either by treating the sections, which have been dehydrated in absolute alcohol, with beech creosote and then with the benzenoid hydrocarbon chosen for clearing; the use of mixtures of cedar-wood oil and of benzene or toluene is also advantageous. As for the mounting strictly speaking, it is often useful to keep the slides in a thin solution of Canada balsam or of the chosen synthetic resin to allow them to dry and only to mount in thick balsam after this.

The main disadvantage of the method is the difficulty of obtaining rigorously homogeneous layers of constant thickness which is an indispensable condition for densitometric study; apart from quantitative work, it is the method of choice.

It may be helpful in certain cases to detach the entirety of the preparation, the collodion layer and the emulsion, after exposure and development and to turn it upside down on another slide so that the preparation is exposed on the side opposite to the slide; this is the technique of *coating with inversion*, the preparation only being staining histologically after the development of the autoradiograph.

Stripping film techniques (*techniques a l'émulsion détachable* of French-speaking authors) consist of covering the dewaxed and collodion treated section, whether stained or not, with a layer of emulsion prepared on the spot and offered up on a support from which it is easily detached. Spreading is carried out on a water bath at 20°, drying taking place at laboratory temperatures. Certain types of support can be penetrated with the usual stains so that the sections can be stained either before or after the setting in place of the emulsion. The advantages of the method are the high resolution and the uniformity of the emulsion whose very homogeneous thickness facilitates quantitative study; but the sensitivity of the emulsions so presented is often weak and there are risks that it may become detached during the work.

Some precautions are common to all methods, namely the need to conduct the manipulations preceding exposure and the treatment of the exposed emulsions in light which does not affect them, varying according to the types of emulsion. It is highly advisable to choose the technique in the light of the work to be carried out on the autoradiographs; coating methods allow the sections to be most easily recovered because the preparation and the emulsion become one body from the moment in which the latter is applied to the sections; contact methods and stripping film techniques give more homogeneous layers which are better suited for the quantitative analysis of autoradiographs.

The characteristics of the emulsions vary a good deal according to the supplier and the category. Specialist works disclose a rich literature on this topic. On the whole, emulsions of the radiological type are still used when the activity of the preparations is very weak; they are in fact quite sensitive but their grain is too large to allow a detailed study of the autoradiographs. Nuclear emulsions which are available in the form of pourable gels or as detachable films are better suited for work at high magnifications.

The technique for development and fixing depends on the emulsion used; the recommendations of the supplier should be strictly adhered to.

Apart from contact procedures in which the histological preparation and the photographic emulsion are separated temporarily or definitively after exposure, it is impossible to avoid the action of either developers or photographic fixatives on the stained sections, or indeed that of the histological stains on the photographic emulsion. Certain precautions need to be taken in this respect.

The systematic investigations of Leblond and his colleagues have shown that most histological stains, as customarily used, react rather poorly to treatment with photographic developers and fixatives when they take part in coating methods. The colour of the aluminium lakes of haematoxylin becomes weakened, eosin is to some extent extracted from the sections; with Masson's trichrome destaining is almost complete; light green, fast green, and celestin blue do not withstand photographic developers; the results of the nucleal reaction of Feulgen and Rossenbeck are not affected and those of the PAS reaction also stand up to this treatment well as do the stains produced by alcian blue and those afforded by carmine or the aluminium lake of nuclear fast red.

It is, moreover, important to avoid staining prior to development and fixing in cases where the materials to be used may sensitise the photographic emulsion; this is the case with all the basic blue dyes of the thiazine group which can only be used after development and fixing of the autoradiographs, where necessary by inverting the sections.

It is obviously impracticable to give recommendations here dealing with the duration of exposure; this may vary from a few hours to several months. The nature of the radioactive material to be demonstrated, the extent to which it occurs in the structures, the thickness of the sections and the nature of the emulsion are all variables which affect the duration. In general, substances which produce high-energy radiation are unsuitable because diffusion images interfere with any attempt at localisation at the level of the organelle; the low-energy radiation emitted by tritium makes it the ideal tracer for autoradiographic work.

The practice of exposing at low temperatures is indispensable when working with unfixed sections; it is advisable in all instances; the slides which are placed in contact with the emulsion or are covered by it are, therefore, to be placed in receptacles which shelter them from light, which are hermetically sealed, and which are kept in a refrigerator for the time needed for exposure.

The examination of autoradiographs under the microscope calls for no particular comment. A quantitative study can be carried out either by densitometry of photographic pictures or photometry of projected images or by counting traces or grains. The counting of traces is easy when they are caused by α particles which give short and straight trajectories; it is more difficult in the case of β particles, especially if the background fogging is even slightly noticeable. In any case, traces parallel to the optical axis of the microscope are difficult to identify. In the view of the specialists most confidence can be placed in the quantitative technique involving grain counting when considering the analysis of autoradiographs.

CHAPTER 13

HISTOCHEMICAL DETECTION OF MINERAL SUBSTANCES

Methods for revealing certain mineral substances in histological preparations occur among the first histochemical techniques invented in the second half of the nineteenth century, and yet, the detection of mineral substances represents one of the least advanced sections of histochemistry. It is not a lack of analytical reactions capable of being adapted to the work of the histochemist that is the main reason for this, but rather, the near impossibility of preserving the mineral compounds in their original position under conditions compatible with histochemical work; and it is the study of these mineral compounds that would be of most interest from the histophysiological and physiological points of view. This fragmentary state of the possibilities open to the research worker is necessarily reflected in the appropriate chapters of all histochemical manuals and treatises.

The present chapter is divided into three parts of which the first is concerned with discovering the total mineral matter content by micro-incineration and the two others deal with the histochemical detection of mineral anions and cations.

MICRO-INCINERATION

Micro-incineration (histospodography) consists of the mineralisation of a histological preparation by heat, in such a way as to obtain, as it were, the "mineral skeleton" of the tissues, that is the ash remaining in place and outlining the topography of the histological structures. The result of this operation is known as an ash-pattern (*spodogramme, Aschenbild*).

The discovery of the method goes back to Raspail (1833), who applied it to the study of plant cells; other nineteenth century authors also made use of it but the first methodical research into the morphological validity of the method was that by Liesegang (1910) whose results were received with indifference by most of the histologists of that epoch. In fact, micro-incineration has acquired the right to be cited as a histochemical technique thanks to the research done by Policard (1921, 1924, 1933 and 1934), whose publications mark the beginning of an important series of notes, memoirs and other writings concerned with the method. The general reviews by Tschopp (1929), Scott (1933) and Policard and Okkels (1932) summarise what was learnt prior to 1930. Among more recent sources of information should be mentioned those of Gersh (1941), Richards (1956), Hintsche (1956) and Kruszynski (1966).

The purpose of histospodography is to obtain as exact an image as possible of the mineral matter at the level of resolution of the light microscope; it does not provide any details about the chemical structure in which are to be found the compounds revealed before the sections were incinerated, and only certain chemical elements can be identified with certainty unless the procedure is combined with other techniques, notably that of histospectrographic emission; but with such techniques histospodography loses its value as a method for localisation. Thus spodograms provide an exact topographic representation of the distribution of *total* mineral matter in the body of the sections. One should not forget that this representation is not absolutely complete since certain substances can be entirely or partially lost during mineralisation; such is the case with sulphur and even alkaline salts can be lost if the incineration is carried out at too high a temperature.

The technique of micro-incineration is simple. The different stages can be argued over as much from the point of view of the preservation of the structures as from the chemical validity.

*1° **Fixation*** must be carried out in such a way as to avoid the introduction of any mineral compounds, a requirement that prevents the usage of the group of fixative liquids with heavy metal salts as their base and also of all the mineral salts recommended as adjuvants (sodium sulphate or chloride etc...). The extraction of any mineral compounds must also be avoided. It was with micro-incineration in mind that Schultz-Brauns (1931) perfected the technique for cutting frozen sections of fresh tissue. Sections obtained in this way, or cut on the cryostat, may be used but experience has proved that fixed and embedded material withstands mineralisation much better and shows less distortion. Freeze drying and freeze substitution using any suitable liquid is even better because any denaturing of the tissue proteins is useless. Among chemical fixatives absolute alcohol was recommended by Scott (1933), but the results that he himself obtained with a mixture of 9 volumes of absolute alcohol and 1 volume of commercial formalin were much better. Even Bouin's liquid can be used, more especially when the worker is looking for certain mineral substances, in particular iron; it is of course necessary to take into consideration the decalcifying action of this latter fixative.

*2° **Preparation and spreading of the sections.*** — the procedure preparatory to embedding the sections should be carried out in the usual way. Only rarely is it necessary to embed in celloidin or in gelatin using Apathy's technique; in the exceptional case where sections embedded in celloidin have to be mineralised, it is imperative, first, to dissolve the embedded mass since its sudden combustion during micro-incineration will lead to actual displacement of the sections. In most cases one uses paraffin wax embedded sections. The amount of celloidin present in sections taken from blocks embedded, using the method of Peterfi, with methyl-benzoate celloidin is too small to be a nuisance during the incineration.

It is advisable to cut thin sections (3 to 5 μ, at the most 10 μ). If one wishes to know the precise distribution of the ashes, it is better to avoid spreading out the sections in water and to replace this liquid with paraffin oil. Glycerin, albumen and gelatin (particularly if it is bichromated) can cause errors if used to excess. Slides used for spreading out must be carefully washed and freed from dust; slides of hard glass (green) should be chosen.

It is not, of course, necessary to dewax the slides. When dealing with frozen sections which are rich in fats it is sometimes advisable to dissolve the fats in a mixture of ether and chloroform, remembering that this treatment, which Tschopp (1929) recommended should be maintained for two to five hours, can result in removal of mineral substances.

3° Conduct of the incineration. — The equipment which came to hand, such as was used by some classical authors, are now only of historical interest since the apparatus invented by Policard (1924), Schultz-Brauns (1931) and Scott (1933) is provided by industry. Policard's apparatus is the simplest and the cheapest. It consists of a quartz tube built to contain one standard slide supported by a quartz slide and with a resistance providing heating for the tube, which is lagged on the outside with asbestos; there is a second resistance for regulating the temperature. In the apparatus designed by Schultz-Brauns the temperature can be read continuously by means of a thermo-electric couple and air or nitrogen can be passed through the tube by a simple mechanism. Scott's apparatus has a much longer quartz tube than the preceding ones and, in addition, has a mechanism which automatically moves the slide from one end of the tube into the centre, where the temperature is highest, and then on to the other end of the tube. New slides can be added while the incineration is in progress and this continuity of the work can save much time.

During mineralisation, the first critical point is reached when the temperature gets up to about 70°C; at this temperature the collagen fibres contract and this is one of the principal causes of the distortion of spodograms when compared with sections. It is important to raise the temperature slowly in order to diminish this contraction; most authors recommend that one should allow at least 10 minutes to reach the temperature mentioned above.

Carbonisation of all the organic substances occurs at about 150°C; stopping the operation at this stage leaves an *anthracogram* which gives a surprisingly true representation of the tissue structure. Fine drops of tar may appear at this stage and their confluence, favoured by too rapid heating, represents a new source of artefacts.

The temperature at which this carbonisation is produced varies with the different structures and certain authors have attempted to put this fact to profitable use in the morphological analysis of anthracograms. But Hintsche (1956) pointed out that this carbonisation depended not only on the chemical composition of the tissue constituents but also on their abundance; thus carbonisation is slower for collagen fibres clustered into bundles than for similar fibres that are isolated.

As the temperature rises, the combustion of organic matter continues steadily and can be made more even by bathing the slide in a current of gas; air and oxygen were once recommended for this but now workers use nitrogen instead. The gas can be used from the beginning of the micro-incineration or when the temperature has reached 500°C; one thus obtains a spodogram in which the contractions and the artefacts produced by the confluence of the tar droplets are largely suppressed. It should be borne in mind that this current of gas can facilitate the evaporation of alkaline salts.

The maximum temperature to be aimed at and the time for which the sections should be kept at this temperature are assessed very diversely by different authors. Some advise heating to 630°C and leaving the sections there for 10 minutes; others prescribe lower temperatures (500–550°C) for a duration of about 40 minutes. This latter method seems the one best adapted for the preservation of alkaline salts, which are volatile above 600°C.

The slides should, of course, be cooled gradually; this is achieved in Scott's micro-incineration oven by moving the slides towards the cold end of the quartz tube, and in other forms of the apparatus by the gradual reduction of the intensity of the current supplying the resistance used for heating. At least one hour should be allowed for bringing the slides back to room temperature and they should not be removed from the quartz tube until this has cooled to the ambient temperature.

4° **Mounting and examination of the spodograms.** — Spodograms are fragile and hygroscopic, it is therefore essential to mount them under a coverslip immediately the slides are completely cooled; one can also make a preliminary check to see if the incineration is complete and that no trace of carbon remains.

Spodograms should be mounted dry, a coverslip of adequate size should be laid on top and sealed with paraffin wax or some other wax. It is advisable to apply varnish away from the edge of the coverslip. The various mounting media recommended by some classical authors should not be used.

Spodograms can, of course, be microscopically examined using a light background, this method being particularly useful when one is looking for coloured ashes; however the best method is to use oblique light or a dark background with a cardioid condenser. The early workers did their drawings on black pasteboard or on smoked bristol board, but this has now been superceded by photomicrography.

The granular appearance of spodograms is inevitable even when the technical conditions are irreproachable; Policard (1942) showed that this was due to the conflict between the thermal contraction of the tissue constituents and their adherence to the slide. When the spodograms have been correctly prepared this granular appearance should not mask the structures and even the nucleoli should be readily identifiable.

Hintsche's (1956) careful investigations have shown that the examination and photomicrography of spodograms using phase contrast offers some advantages over the use simply of a dark background, so that it is helpful to use both methods of study.

Spodograms that have been correctly mounted will keep almost indefinitely.

5° *Identification of mineral matter in spodograms*. — The chemical identification of the substances present in spodograms can be taken quite a long way provided the worker is able to use such techniques as histospectrography or electron diffraction. If this is not possible, one element, iron, is easy to identify through the colour of its ashes. In fact, no matter in what chemical combination this element occurs in the tissues, it appears in the form of the oxide Fe_2O_3 and can be immediately identified from its red colour. All the other ash is white.

It should be recognised that most attempts to analyse the ashes by chemical or physical methods give rather unsatisfactory results. Fluoroscopy, examination with polarised light and tests for solubility can give interesting indications but no generalisations can be made; with any of the microchemical reactions that have been recommended for use on spodograms, the histochemical character of the method is lost since precise localisation becomes impossible once a reagent has been added, even if the operator uses very fine pipettes and a micromanipulator. The general reviews by Horning (1951), Hintsche (1956) and Scott (1966) contain much technical and bibliographic information on this subject.

DETECTION OF MINERAL ANIONS

The difficulty of maintaining the position of mineral compounds during fixation, as already indicated in the introduction to this chapter, is more acutely felt when dealing with the histochemical detection of anions; there is no really satisfactory procedure, so that even though Lison devoted 14 pages of the third edition of his book (1960) to a theoretical discussion of the methods in question, none occurred in the list of particularly useful operative methods.

CHLORIDES

There is considerable interest in a reliable histochemical method for detecting the ion Cl^- and one can understand why so many and such diverse attempts have been made to this end, all based on the principle that chloride ions are precipitated by silver salts. The practice of the earlier authors was to immerse thin slices in 2% silver nitrate solution acidified with nitric acid at the rate of 3 ml to 100 ml of reagent. Excess silver nitrate was removed by washing and the silver chloride reduced, in the tissue pieces, by a solution of hydroquinone. These treated pieces can be embedded in paraffin wax, cut into sections and examined with or without a background stain; frozen sections can also be used. This is really the procedure used by Leschke (1914) for the detection of chlorides in the kidney.

The specificity of the method was greatly improved by Lison's work (1936); he precipitated the chlorides with silver nitrate using pieces of fresh material but carried out the reduction on sectioned material, resulting in an easier and more complete removal of silver nitrate. The liquid used for precipitation and fixation (2 g silver nitrate, 3 ml nitric acid, 100 ml distilled water, 100 ml formalin) is introduced into the tissues by vascular perfusion, after first washing out the blood system with isotonic glucose serum to which is added, when necessary, a small quantity of a vasodilator (amyl nitrite). The tissue pieces are then lifted up and left in the reagent used for the perfusion for 2 to 4 hours; they are treated for 12 hours with a 2% silver nitrate solution, to which 10% formalin has been added, dehydrated with alcohol and embedded in paraffin wax. The sections are dewaxed, washed in 3% nitric acid, which should be renewed several times, and then hydrated. All these operations shoud be carried out away from direct light. Having washed the sections in distilled water they are reduced by a mixture of equal parts of 15% potassium carbonate solution and a metol-hydroquinone developing agent (4 g metol, 8 g hydroquinone 10 g sodium sulphite, 1 g potassium bromide, 1000 ml distilled water). Each of the two liquids keeps well but the mixture should be made immediately before use. This reduction is carried out in full light and takes about 5 minutes. The sections are then washed; the background can be stained with a nuclear red before the section is dehydrated and mounted in Canada balsam. Lison himself noted the very weak penetrating power of the liquid used to precipitate the chloride ions and emphasised the need for a critical examination of the preparations, since the precipitation could assume a banded appearance (Liesegang rings).

In Gersh's method (1937) the sections are prepared by freeze-drying and then embedded in paraffin wax and spread out dry, a technique that considerably reduces the artefacts caused by displacement of the chloride ion during fixation. After dewaxing and air drying, the non-denatured sections are treated with an alcoholic solution of silver nitrate (0.1 to 2 g silver nitrate and 100 ml 95% alcohol); the sections are washed in 0.5% nitric acid and then reduced by light or by a photographic developer.

We should note here a technique developed by Komnick (1962) and specially designed to reveal chloride ions on electron micrographs. Komnick fixed very small tissue pieces in 1% osmium tetroxide solution to which was added 0.2 to 0.8 g of silver acetate or 0.3 to 1 g of silver lactate. The pH was adjusted to 7.2 to 7.4 using a M/100 solution of borax. The instructions given next by Komnick follow the requirements of electron microscopy (washing, dehydration, differentiation with uranyl acetate or phospho-tungstic acid, embedding in Vestopal) and have no particular histochemical interest, but the first stages in the method could provide a useful basis for perfecting a technique of use with the light microscope.

As Lison (1960) remarked, all these methods lay themselves open to criticism; their manipulation demands a great deal of care and the interpretation of the preparations requires much caution; in fact, it is not possible, at the moment, to recommend a single method for the detection of chloride ions which combines reliability, chemical specificity and correct morphological localisation of the ions.

IODIDES

Precipitating iodides *in situ* in the tissues is so difficult that it is advisable not to use the older methods employing lead nitrate, thallium acetate or silver nitrate; even when working with sections taken from material that has been freeze dried and embedded in paraffin wax, the results are only mediocre and the detection of these compounds using light histochemical methods (Gersh and Stieglitz, 1933 and Lison, 1960) should also be abandoned.

THYROID IODINE

The iodised compounds involved in the synthesis of thyroid hormones, in particular thyreoglobulin, can be detected by historadiography, electron probe microanalysis, by autoradiography after first administring radio-active iodine (^{131}J) or by absorption spectrography in ultra-violet light; in fact thyreoglobulin has a very characteristic absorption spectrum in ultraviolet light, with a first maximum at about 2800 Å corresponding to aromatic amino-acids (phenylalanine, especially tyrosine and tryptophane) and a second maximum, situated between 3200 and 3300 Å, which is linked to the presence of the thyroid hormones themselves (thyroxine, di-iodotyrosine, etc...). Extraction with an acid causes this absorption band to disappear. Gersh and Caspersson (1940) and Gersh and Baker (1943) have derived from this a method for the quantitative study of the thyroid hormones of the rat, using sections from tissue that has been freeze-dried and the technique of microspectrographic absorption in ultraviolet light.

PHOSPHORUS

This element occurs in various forms in the tissues. Classically one distinguishes ionic phosphorus, which can be demonstrated directly and masked phosphorus which occurs in organic combinations.

Ionic phosphorus, occurring in mineral combinations, is nearly always represented by calcium phosphate; the method for detecting this compound is given in connection with the salts of this metal. Soluble phosphates are rare so that the question of their detection hardly ever poses a problem except during experimental work; suffice it to say here that one of the recommended methods depends on its precipitation by 0.5% uranyl nitrate followed by detection of the precipitated uranyl phosphate with a potassium ferrocyanide giving potassium uraniferrocyanide which has a red colour (technique of Leschke, 1914). Winter and Smith (1922) suggested that the precipitation should be performed with ammonium molybdate solution acidified with nitric acid, the precipitate being transformed by potassium ferrocyanide into molybdenum blue. These two methods, although chemically correct, do not maintain the morphological conditions of a histochemical reaction and so are only of historical interest.

The techniques proposed for the detection of masked phosphorus also have faults. Everything rests on the principle of an acid "demasking" combined with precipitation by means of ammonium molybdate. The earliest of these methods, which was developed by Lilienfeld and Monti (1892), consists of the detection of the ammonium phosphomolybdate, formed during the precipitation, by conversion into molybdenum blue oxide after first reducing with pyrogallol. Other reducing agents have been suggested, such as tin chloride (Polacci, 1894), phenylhydrazine (Macallum, 1907) and benzidine (Serra and Queiros Lopez, 1945).

All present day histochemists agree that these methods should be rejected; Gomori (1952) and Lison (1960) emphasised that the relative solubility and slow formation of ammonium phospho-molybdate are sufficient to allow considerable displacements to take place during precipitation; the solubility of molybdenum blue represents a further source of artefacts.

SULPHUR

Among the numerous mineral combinations containing sulphur only the sulphates are of histochemical interest; their detection meets with the same difficulties as did the detection of the soluble compounds described in the preceeding paragraphs.

One method of detection proposed by Macallum (1912) consists of treating frozen sections taken from fresh material with a dilute solution of lead acetate; sulphates present in the tissues are precipitated as lead sulphate which is insoluble in dilute nitric acid; washing with the latter removes all other lead salt precipitates from the sections and the sulphate left behind is converted into the dark brown lead sulphide by means of a dilute aqueous solution of ammonium sulphide. This method can be applied to non-denatured sections taken from material that has been freeze dried; the results must, of course, be interpreted with great caution.

ARSENIC

The problem of histochemical research on this element only arises in the work of the histopathologist; the therapeutic importance of arsenical derivatives explains the considerable number of publications devoted to the detection of arsenical compounds in sections, but it should be recognised that none of the suggested techniques are sufficiently reliable for one to advise their use.

Methods using hydrogen sulphide were introduced by Justus (1905); the procedure is to treat tissue pieces that have been in formalin with a saturated aqueous solution of hydrogen sulphide. However these methods are very insensitive and Tannenholz and Muir (1933) have shown that the yellow granules that are revealed in the cells are not arsenic sulphide. In Castel's (1936) method the pieces are treated with copper sulphate solution which results in the arsenites in the tissues being precipitated as copper arsenite; this method gives positive results with fatty acids, phosphates, carbonates and numerous proteins. The silver methods advocated by Schumacher (1928) for the detection of arsenobenzenes are, in fact, argentaffin reactions which reveal the phenolic nucleus and not the arsenic.

SILICON

The problem of detecting, in sectioned material, the silica and hydrated silicates which are found in the lungs of people suffering from silicosis, is encountered principally during histopathological research into this disease. In addition to histospectrographic detection one can use the technique of micro-incineration followed by examination under polarised light when only the silica crystals will retain their birefringence. Another method that has been suggested is to destroy the tissues with warm perchloric acid and then to look for the silica crystals. This method is of course more microchemical than histochemical since it does not enable one to find the actual position of the substance in the cell and the same is true for the technique of emission histospectography used by Gerlach (1933) and by Policard (1933).

DETECTION OF MINERAL CATIONS

The histochemical detection of metals has various aspects depending on which cation one is looking for. Some of the recommended reactions are so good that one can have great confidence in the sensitivity of the recognition and the exactness of the localisation of the metals so identified. Other procedures use group reactions rather than methods for specific identification; they can be very useful when the nature of the cation under investigation is known and the object of the work is to discover its position at the cellular level or tissue level. Other methods should be rejected as lacking in chemical or morphological validity.

The actual importance of the procedures to be discussed here varies from case to case; some belong to the group of histochemical reactions that every histologist has to use regularly, others are only used occasionally and others are only used in exceptional circumstances since they detect metals not normally present in the organism but which have been introduced for experimental purposes.

In addition to the truly histochemical reactions, which are reviewed below, histospectrographic emission and, more especially, historadiography and electron probe microanalysis, are extremely valuable for ensuring the correct identification of a cation present in sectioned material.

SODIUM

It is generally considered that it is impossible to detect this alkaline metal under the working conditions of the histochemist. However it should be noted that Komnick (1962) and Nolte (1966), using electron microscopy, obtained a precipitate of sodium antimonate which could perhaps serve as the basis for a technique which could be used with the light microscope. Komnick, whose technique was used by Nolte, fixed the material in the cold for about 2 hours with a 2% solution of potassium antimonate in distilled water (warmed to dissolve) to which 1 g of osmium tetroxide per 100 ml is added after the solution has cooled. The pH is adjusted to 7.2 to 7.4 with N:100 acetic acid. Electron micrographs show amorphous precipitates which, according to the diffractograms are definitely those of sodium antimonate.

POTASSIUM

Among the three techniques suggested for the histochemical detection of potassium, that of Carere-Comes (1937) should be discarded since it consists of staining with aurantia. The method of Jacoby and Keuscher (1937) which produces a chloroplatinate precipitate does not appear to have been used since its publication and complementary research would be needed before its value could be ascertained. Macallum's (1905) technique based on precipitation with sodium cobalt hexanitrite has been strongly criticised by some authors but modifications introduced by Gersh (1938) and Crout and Jennings (1957) have overcome some of the difficulties inherent in the older variants of the method. Crout and Jennings method is given below:

> Sections 10 μ thick from freeze dried material which has not been denatured;
> Dewax in two lots of petroleum ether, spread out the sections on slides in the second bath of petroleum ether, wipe and leave to dry in the air;
> Treat with cobaltinitrite reagent for 15 minutes at the temperature of melting ice;
> Blot dry, wash in two baths of iced distilled water (for about 15 seconds);
> Dehydrate in absolute alcohol, clear and then mount in a synthetic resin.

The reagent is prepared by adding a mixture of 50 ml of a 50% solution of cobalt nitrite and 12.5 ml of acetic acid to 210 ml of a 66% aqueous solution of sodium nitrite; the nitrous fumes given off are removed by bubbling through water (1 to 2 hours). The reagent produced can be kept in ice for a limited time; it should be filtered before use.

If potassium is present it shows up as numerous yellow or brown granules; the chemical specificity of the method seems to be good but the validity of the localisation is less certain, even with freeze-dried material; obviously the uncertainties are even greater with the earlier variants of the method, using small pieces of material or frozen sections of fresh material.

CALCIUM

The detection of calcium holds an important place among histochemical techniques and much work has been concerned with this topic. An excellent general picture of the methods in question is given by the work of McGee Russel (1958) as well as by the manuals and treatises on histochemistry; McGee Russel's work gives explanations for the misunderstandings and contradictions which are so readily found when reading the literature prior to this date.

Calcium occurs in three forms in Metazoan organisms, firstly a soluble ionic form, attempts to precipitate which *in situ* gave results that do not enable this to be included as a histochemical method, secondly an insoluble ionic form which can be detected histochemically and finally a masked form which can only be detected by histophysical methods such as historadiography and microincineration. Only the insoluble ionic form will be discussed here.

The many reactions for revealing calcium in histological sections can be classified, according to the principle on which they are based, into methods for staining with lakes, methods for the substitution of other metals, methods for the conversion into coloured substances and methods for crystallisation. The conversion methods have no practical advantage over the other techniques or over crystallisation and since they are microchemical rather than histochemical hey are left out of the discussion.

1° *Methods for staining with lakes*

Among the stains whose lakes can be used to show up deposits of ionic calcium in the organism, two should be remembered, namely haematoxylin and gallamine blue. Haematoxylin will only form the calcium lakes, which are stained intensely blue, if the pH of the reagent is greater than 9 (McGee Russel, 1958); a 5% solution of haematoxylin in ammonia water stains the calciferous inclusions a very intense blue but since the preparations are unstable the method is of no practical interest. Gallamine blue, an oxazine close to gallocyanin, is used in the form of aluminium or ferric lakes as a nuclear stain; the work of

McGee Russel explains the contradictory results which pervade the literature dealing with the histochemical detection of calcium. In fact the stain, used as an aqueous solution, forms a soluble lake with the calcium and it is this lake that stains the bony matrix; although valuable as a morphological method this is not a histochemical method.

The anthraquinone group of stains is, on the other hand, of interest among histochemical reagents for calcium. Alizarin, sodium alizarin-sulphonate (alizarin red S), purpurin, quinalizarin and nuclear fast red (sodium aminoanthraquinone sulphonate) have been recommended for this purpose. The most advantageous of these stains are sodium alizarin-sulphonate and purpurin while quinalizarin can be useful in certain cases.

McGee Russel recommends the following technique for staining with sodium alizarin-sulphonate.

> Dewaxed sections, treated with collodion where appropriate and hydrated (do no leave too long in the water);
> Stain on slides for 30 seconds to 5 minutes, checking under a microscope, with a 2% aqueous solution of the stain at a pH adjusted to about 4.3 using dilute ammonia water;
> Throw away the excess reagent, wipe with tissue paper or rinse very rapidly with distilled water;
> Dehydrate with acetone, clear, mount in Canada balsam or in a synthetic resin.

The sites of calcium accumulation are covered and surrounded by a dense, red-orange, birefringent precipitate; the background stain is fairly pale to avoid any uncertainties when the preparations are examined.

Purpurin, used in an alcoholic solution by the early workers, can be used in the same way as sodium alizarin-sulphate, in a 2% aqueous solution provided the pH is raised to 8.5 by the addition of ammonia water. This solution is used in an identical way to that which has just been described; the preparations are, however, less stable and the intense stain given with purpurin makes it very difficult to regulate under the microscope. Nevertheless the purpurin technique is useful when one needs to work in an alkaline medium.

Staining with quinalizarin is of interest because, according to McGee Russel it stains not only the phosphates and carbonates but also calcium oxalate. It is used in a concentrated solution of potassium hydroxide (0.2 to 0.5 g of stain in 3 ml of 15% potassium hydroxide). Dewaxed sections treated with collodion where necessary, are covered with this reagent for 5 seconds to 3 minutes, drained, rinsed with water and the examined under water. The intense blue or purple stain of the calciferous inclusions does not last very well when mounted in Canada balsam.

It should be remembered that quinalizarin also gives blue lakes with beryllium and magnesium (Broda, 1936).

Methods for the detection of calcium deposits with lakes of anthraquinone are generally fairly specific in the chemical sense; they are not very sensitive and clear positive results are only obtained for rather high local concentrations of calcium salts. A comparison between McGee Russel's results and those of earlier authors leads one to believe that the pH of the staining solution is very important and it is possible that the optimum pH varies with different tissues; indeed, McGee Russel, who tried out the methods on calcium inclusions of invertebrates (the digestive gland of *Helix* and of *Carcinus*, and the left colleterial gland of *Periplaneta*) recommended that the pH of the solution of alizarin red S should be adjusted to 4.1–4.3, whereas Dahl (1952) working on the ossification sites in mammals obtained the best results with a pH of 6.3 to 6.5.

Other chelating agents have been suggested for the demonstration of calciferous deposits. Treatment with a solution of murexide (ammonium purpurate) gives the calcium inclusions a very stable red stain; naphthochrome green B or G stains the calcium deposits a brownish red when fixed in alcohol or formalin and green when fixed in corrosive sublimate and Pearse (1960) believes that this stain provides a good routine method for their detection. Very often the calcium inclusions are stained blue by cupric phthalocyanins dissolved either in water (alcian blue and durazol blue 8G) or in alcohol (Luxol fast blue and Methasol fast blue 2G).

2° Chelation with sodium rhodizonate

It merits a separate section. It was introduced into chemical analysis by Feigl (1924) for the detection of the alkaline earth metals barium and strontium with which it forms red chelated compounds; this method has been used by Waterhouse (1950) for the detection of these two metals in the tissues of insects. However, Gomori (1952) commented that the calcium deposits also take up an ochre stain when treated with sodium rhodizonate and this was confirmed by Molnar (1952). From *in vitro* tests it appears that it is only the oxide and hydroxide of calcium that give an ochre stain with sodium rhodizonate; Waterhouse maintains that only those calcium salts that satisfy spectroscopic standards of purity are not stained under the technical conditions of the sodium rhodizonate method.

Systematic tests carried out by McGee Russel have shown that some calciferous inclusions can be effectively revealed by sodium rhodizonate; as with all the other chelation methods the rhodizonate method does not reveal deposits of calcium oxalate. McGee Russel also notes some structures which do not stain under the technical conditions described here; these structures are the Swammerdam glands of the frog and the calciferous grains of the connective tissue of the freshwater mussel. The calciferous grains of the connective tissue of the snail, however, stain a clear red.

McGee Russel deduced that the positive results described above for the sodium rhodizonate method were probably caused by contamination with barium or strontium; nevertheless McGee Russel also pointed out the advantages of this method especially the very intense colour of the inclusions, the fact that no diffusion occurs and there is no background stain so that the sodium rhodizonate method can be of very real service and, in addition, the preparations are very stable. The technique is also very simple to perform; the dewaxed sections, treated with collodion if necessary, are left for about one hour in a saturated aqueous solution of sodium rhodizonate then washed in distilled water, dehydrated, cleared and then mounted in Canada balsam or a synthetic resin.

3° Chelation with glyoxal bis (2-hydroxyanyl)

It also merits a special mention since it gives excellent results.

The principle of the method is relatively simple. Glyoxal bis (2-hydroxyanyl), which was synthesised by Bayer (1957), gives chelation complexes with a whole series of metals (copper, uranium, nickel and cobalt, and manganese and zinc). Goldstein and Stark-Mayer showed (1958) that alkaline solutions of glyoxal bis (2-hydroxyanyl) give complexes with the alkaline earth metals and that the reaction can be made specific for calcium by the addition of sodium carbonate and potassium cyanide; the first of these additives decolourises the precipitate formed with barium and strontium while the second additive prevents chelation with cadmium, copper, cobalt and nickel.

Kashiwa and his collaborators (1963, 1964 and 1966) introduced the procedure into histochemical technique. The working technique varies according to whether one is looking for soluble ionic calcium, insoluble calcium or labile calcium.

a) Tests for soluble ionic calcium.

Reagents:

A 0.4% solution of glyoxal bis (2-hydroxyanyl) in absolute alcohol;
5% NaOH in deionised water;
90% alcohol saturated with sodium carbonate and potassium cyanide;
A 0.08% solution of fast green FCF in 95% alcohol.

Working technique:

Paraffin wax sections taken from pieces of tissue that have been freeze-dried, spread out without being denature or dewaxed;
Cover the sections with a mixture, freshly prepared, of 3 ml of an alcoholic solution of glyoxal bis (2-hydroxyanyl) and 0.3 ml of soda solution, leave for 3 minutes;

Rinse in 70% alcohol;
Treat for 15 minutes with an alcoholic solution of sodium carbonate-potassium cyanide;
Rinse in two baths of 95% alcohol;
Stain for 3 minutes in an alcoholic solution of fast green FCF;
Rinse in 3 baths of 95% alcohol;
Dehydrate in absolute alcohol, clear in a benzenoid hydrocarbon, mount in a commercial synthetic resin.

The presence of soluble ionic calcium is revealed as an intense granular red stain.

b) Tests for insoluble calcium salts (Kashiwa and House, 1964).

The search for soluble calcium salts using Kashiwa and Atkinson's (1963) technique constantly gives negative results. This technique has just been described. The hypothesis that the negative result is caused by working in an alcoholic medium led the authors to carry out a series of tests on models or on sections of tissue containing calciferous deposits. The hypothesis was confirmed and the following modifications to the method were proposed.

Reagents:

3.4% caustic soda in 75% alcohol;
90% alcohol saturated with sodium carbonate and potassium cyanide;
95% alcohol containing 0.1% fast green FCF and methylene blue.

Working technique:

Paraffin wax sections taken from tissue blocks that have been freeze—dried or freeze—substituted, these should be stuck to the slides dry, not denatured and not dewaxed;
Cover the sections with 2 ml of caustic soda solution in which 0.1 g of glyoxal bis(2-hydroxyanyl) is dissolved at the moment of use, and leave to act for 5 minutes;
Rinse in 70% alcohol and then in two baths of 95% alcohol;
Treat for 15 minutes with alcohol saturated with sodium carbonate and potassium cyanide;
Rinse in 3 baths of 95% alcohol;
Stain the background with a mixture of fast green and methylene blue;
Rinse in 3 baths of 95% alcohol;
Dehydrate in absolute alcohol, clear in a benzenoid hydrocarbon and mount in a synthetic resin.

As in the preceeding method, a positive result shows up as an intense, red, granular stain; the insoluble calcium salts react strongly.

c) Tests for labile calcium (Kashiwa, 1966)

The method is based on the precipitation of calcium salts *in situ* by rendering them insoluble; this is achieved by immersing pieces of fresh tissue in an alcoholic solution of glyoxal bis(2-hydroxyanyl). The other steps in the sequence are executed after paraffin wax sections have been cut.

Reagents:

> 3.4% caustic soda in 75% alcohol;
> 90% alcohol saturated with sodium carbonate and potassium cyanide;
> 50% alcohol containing 0.1% methylene blue.

Working technique:

> Immerse small pieces of tissue in the alcoholic soda solution, in which is dissolved, immediately prior to use, 0.1 g of glyoxal bis(2-hydroxyanyl) per 2 ml; leave in this solution for about 16 hours;
> Dehydrate in absolute alcohol, clear and embed in paraffin;
> Spread out the sections dry and treat them without dewaxing;
> Immerse for 15 minutes in alcohol saturated with sodium carbonate and potassium cyanide;
> Rinse in two baths of 95% alcohol;
> Stain the background for 1 to 3 minutes with an alcoholic solution of methylene blue;
> Rinse in two baths of 95% alcohol;
> Dehydrate in absolute alcohol, clear in a benzenoid hydrocarbon and mount in a synthetic resin.

Under these technical conditions the labile calcium is precipitated in the form of an intense red granular complex, but any insoluble calcium present in the pieces of tissue is not revealed. It may, however be stained by the variant of the method described previously, after the sections have been spread out.

4° Substitution methods

They are based on the replacement of calcium by other cations; thus the compound under investigation no longer forms part of the coloured molecule that one sees under the microscope. These are, therefore, indirect methods and are open to all the theoretical criticisms described in Chapter 10. As I remarked when speaking of the conditions under which histochemical methods are valid, all the so called calcium reactions relying on a substitution in fact reveal the phosphate and carbonate anions to which the calcium is associated in the deposits that one finds within animal tissues. These techniques cannot be used in plant histochemistry since magnesium phosphate deposits are common in plant tissue.

All the methods make use of the difference between the solubility constants of the calcium salts being studied and the solubility constants of the reagents. In the presence of silver nitrate, or ferric chloride the calcium of the phosphates, carbonates, oxalates and sulphates passes into solution in the form of the nitrate and the cation carried by the reagent is substituted for it. It is this cation that is revealed in the second stage of the process. Among the numerous techniques that are theoretically possible, about ten have been recommended by von Kossà (1901), Stoelzner (1905) and Roehl (1905). In fact the only ones of any practical interest are von Kossà's silver nitrate method and Stoelzner's cobalt nitrate method; they are mainly used not only for the detection of insoluble calcium salts occurring normally in sections, but also for detecting those that are precipitated within the tissues during tests for alkaline glycerophosphatases.

The reaction of von Kossà consists of immersing the slides in silver nitrate solution which transforms the silver phosphates and carbonates, which were deposited during the substitution described above, into black metallic silver by reduction either with light or with a photographic developer. It is this second form of the method, introduced into histological technique by Gomori, that is the best since it results in a clearer, well delimited, stain. The technique consists of the following stages.

Dewaxed sections, treated with collodion if necessary, (a thin coating) and hydrated;
Treat for 5 to 30 minutes in the dark with a 2–5% solution of silver nitrate in distilled water;
Rinse carefully, several times, in distilled water;
Treat for 2 minutes in daylight with an 0.5% aqueous solution of hydroquinone;
Rinse in distilled water;
Treat for 30 seconds to 1 minute with a 5% solution of sodium hyposulphite (thiosulphate);
Wash carefully in tap water, stain the background where appropriate, dehydrate, clear, and mount in Canada balsam or a synthetic resin.

The structures containing insoluble calcium salts show up in black and the background is very uniform if the reduction is performed with a photographic developer; if, on the other hand, the reduction is obtained by exposing the sections, which have been treated with silver nitrate and rinsed, to daylight or to ultraviolet light the background stains yellow and the borders of the structures stained in black also stain yellow and this can be a nuisance when making a detailed study of the preparations. This possibility mitigates against background staining; the most advantageous methods for staining the background are those using nuclear red stains; Ramon y Cajal's trichrome, the aluminium lake of nuclear fast red and safranine give good results.

One large source of error in the method is that deposits of uric acid and of urates react exactly like the calcium salts and stain in the same way. The distinction is, however, easy; treatment of short duration with a solution of dilute nitric acid or hydrochloric acid (0.2 to 0.5%) completely dissolves the calciferous deposits without altering the deposits of uric acid or urates; conversely, treatment with an aqueous solution of lithium carbonate, even if diluted, dissolves the uric concretions without modifying the calciferous deposits. Copper, mercury and lead also react positively under the technical conditions of von Kossà's method; *in vitro*, the reaction is given by phosphates and carbonates of barium and strontium.

This is not, therefore, a histochemical method in the strict sense of the term and certainly not a reaction of the calcium ion but is a process whose value in discovering the site of calcium is such that it has played an important role in the majority of histophysiological research concerned with calcification.

In Stoelzner's method using cobalt nitrate, the sections are treated with an aqueous solution of salt and the cobalt phosphates and carbonates resulting from the substitution are converted into cobalt sulphide and show up in black. This latter form of the method is at the most a reaction given by a group; many other metals given black sulphides with this technique. Experiments have shown that the concentration of the cobalt nitrate solution can vary within fairly wide limits without having the least effect on the result of the reaction; the sulphate and chloride of this metal can be substituted for the nitrate. The technique used by most authors consists of the following stages.

Dewaxed sections, treated with collodion if necessary, and hydrated;
Treat for 2 to 5 minutes with a 2–5% aqueous solution of cobalt nitrate;
Wash carefully in distilled water which should be changed several times;
Immerse in a dilute solution (1 ml of 20% commercial solution in 60 ml) of ammonium sulphide; leave the sections in for 1 to 2 minutes;
Wash in running water, stain the background if necessary, dehydrate, clear and mount.

The calciferous inclusions stain an intense black, which is homogeneous in the case of phosphates; with carbonates the black stain can be heterogeneous as some areas apparently do not react (McGee Russel, 1958). The importance of the background stain depends on the nature of the tissue and the care given to the washing process. Among background stains the techniques given in von Kossà's method are also suitable for the method of Stoelzner.

Apart from the indirect nature of Stoelzner's method criticism can also be levelled at the specificity of the method chosen to show up the result of the substitution. Chemically, the demonstration of insoluble cobalt salts, by converting them into the sulphide, contains many sources of error; the most important, because of the frequency with which it occurs, is the detection, by treating with ammonium sulphide, of all the ferruginous inclusions present in the tissues (reaction of Quincke). The confusion which results between calciferous and ferruginous inclusions can be avoided by using a method described in connection with the histochemical detection of iron. But other inclusions containing black metallic sulphides (copper, lead, mercury and nickel) cannot be identified as easily as can the sulphide of iron.

Besides this problem, linked to the nature of the reaction for detecting the cation substituted for calcium, other errors can arise from the adsorption of the cobalt contained in the reagent or even from the chemical reactions in which it plays a part. Adsorption by the tissue proteins explains the intensity of the background stain especially when the sections are not washed with enough care between the action of the cobalt salt and that of ammonium sulphide. The cysteic groups, which may occur in the sections, and, more particularly, the sulphuric acid groups of the sulphomucopolysaccharides which are so frequent in the sites of osteogenesis and, in a general way, in the organic matrix of all metallic inclusions in the animal cell, retain the cobalt by a chemical mechanism which is probably identical to that of the fixation of iron in Hale's method and its variants. It follows from this that the histochemical detection of the phosphates and carbonates of calcium by the method using cobalt salts is also a means of demonstrating electronegative groups; the histochemical reactions based on this principle have in fact been suggested.

This second source of error explains the long known and often wrongly interpreted fact that a positive result with Stoelzner's method in the sites of ossification persists after the complete decalcification of the sections with a dilute mineral acid. This fact was noted by Schuscik (1920) and Lison (1960) considered it to be a sufficient argument to contest any connection between a positive result with the method, on the one hand, and the presence of phosphates or carbonates of calcium on the other; this result would indicate, according to Lison, solely the affinities of the ground substance of the calcified tissues. Of course this way of looking at things is manifestly inexact; Stoelzner's method for rendering visible the calcium phosphate precipitated at the site of alkaline glycerophosphatase activity in the absence of any ground substance rich in mucopolysaccharides or mucoproteins is sufficient to render null and void the assertion to which I have just referred. Schuscik's observation is nevertheless exact; the sites of osteogenesis are characterised by the presence of phosphates and carbonates of calcium as well as acid mucopolysaccharides; each of these histochemical characters is enough to give positive results with Stoelzner's method, hence the persistence of the black stain after decalcification. However, the phosphates and carbonates of calcium not associated with mucopolysaccharides can also give the reaction and in this case the stain disappears after decalcification.

The results are obtained more rapidly with the method of Stoelzner than with that of von Kossà; the reagents cost less and the optical quality of the localisation of the substance being studied is superior, especially when the study has to be done using high magnifications. There is reason therefore to consider this as a method for rendering substances visible which is useful for routine work but in which a positive result has to be confirmed by other methods.

5° *Use of histochemical tests for calcium*

The opportunity to carry out histochemical research on the insoluble calcium salts occurs in rather diverse circumstances. The optical quality of the preparations, particularly the precision of the staining reaction, is the most important characteristic when one is concerned with the position of sodium salts which are already known to be present in the tissue under study; the chemical significance of the procedure becomes, by contrast, the chief preoccupation when one is trying to discover whether or not calcium is present in structures whose composition is not known. It should be mentioned in this respect that only the microchemical techniques, namely the gypsum reaction on sections or spodogrammes, (Schuejeninoff, 1897; Policard, 1924) are genuinely specific for calcium.

Some calcified tissues are very hard and the need for decalcification before sections can be cut means that the procedures that have just been discussed cannot be used. One method enabling sections to be cut of bone that has not been decalcified (Bloom and Bloom, 1940) is described in connection with the techniques for the study of bony tissue. In the other cases, it is important to avoid using acid liquids as fixatives, or fixatives which contain heavy metals as these can act as mordants (chromium, mercury). Frozen sections, celloidin, sections or paraffin wax sections can be used in most of the methods mentioned here; except in very special cases paraffin wax sections should be used.

It should not be forgotten that calciferous inclusions present in the digestive system and connective tissue of invertebrates are so labile that in order to preserve them fixation must be carried out with absolute alcohol or a mixture of absolute alcohol (6 volumes) and chloroform (4 volumes) as recommended by A. Prenant. In other cases formalin alcohol gives good results; many authors use Schaffer's formula, given in the section on topographic fixation; McGee Russel (1957) prefers a mixture of equal parts of absolute alcohol and commercial formalin, neutralised before use. The other steps preparatory to treating the sections with the different stains and reagents call for no special comment.

BARIUM AND STRONTIUM

Techniques for demonstrating the presence of alkaline earth metals have, in fact, been considered when dealing with the detection of calcium. Indeed, von Kossà's method gives, *in vitro*, positive results with the phosphates or carbonates of both barium and strontium, but, in the organism, these salts are always mixed with the corresponding calcium salts so that verification on sections is virtually impossible. The sodium rhodizonate technique, described in the preceeding section, stains inclusions containing one of the two alkaline earth metals an intense red; complementary tests enable the distinction to be made between barium and strontium. In fact barium rhodizonate is very soluble in potassium chromate solutions, resulting in decolouration, whereas strontium rhodizonate withstands this treatment, but can be rapidly decolourised by dilute mineral acids which do not affect barium rhodizonate.

BERYLLIUM (GLUCINIUM)

One only looks for this metal in animal tissues during experiments in which it has been administered. The authors of the techniques for detecting beryllium give no special requirements for fixation of the pieces of tissue; frozen sections or paraffin wax sections taken from material that has been in formalin are satisfactory in this respect. Three methods have been put forward, none of which is really specific for beryllium.

1° The azurine-solochrome method (solochrome azurine I.C.I.) uses dewaxed and hydrated sections; these are stained for 30 minutes with a 2% solution of the stain in 2% soda, then washed in distilled water, dehydrated cleared and mounted. The deposits of beryllium and of calcium show up black veering towards a brownish red when the stained sections are treated with an acid; Pearse (1960) pointed out that the possible presence of aluminium deposits could not be a source of error since they would be dissolved by the alkaline stain bath. As for the calcium deposits, they could be eliminated before staining by treating the sections with a dilute mineral acid.

2° The quinalizarin method, already mentioned in connection with the histochemical detection of calcium, is recommended by Pearse (1960) with a slightly different working technique from that given by McGee Russel for the detection of calcium. Frozen sections or paraffin wax sections which have been dewaxed and hydrated, are treated for 3 to 5 minutes with a 0.2% solution of quinalizarin in 4% soda. The sections are then washed carefully in distilled water and mounted either in a medium miscible with water or, after dehydration and clearing, in a synthetic resin. The deposits of beryllium and calcium stain an intense purple; complementary reactions are necessary to distinguish between these two substances.

3° Staining with naphthochrome green B (Denz, 1949) detects deposits of aluminium, calcium and beryllium. Frozen sections from material treated with formalin or paraffin wax sections cut from pieces of tissue that have been fixed in formalin, alcohol or formalin-alcohol can be used. In order to detect beryllium, the sections are stained for 30 minutes at 37° in a 0.2% solution of the stain in a M/10 Sörensen's buffer at a pH of 5 (?), then washed in water, differentiated, if need be, in absolute alcohol, cleared and mounted.

The formula given here is taken from the original memoir and it is probable that it contains a substantial error which prevents it from being correctly used; indeed, Sörensen's tables do not enable one to make up a mixture of phosphates with the desired pH; this error was also noted by Lillie (1954). By extrapolation one can recommend, approximately, the addition of one ml of a M/10 solution of disodium phosphate to 49 ml of a solution of monopotassium phosphate at the same concentration.

MAGNESIUM

Detection of this metal is primarily of importance in plant histochemistry. Apart from the quinalizarin technique, already mentioned, in which the magnesium deposits take on a blue stain which is resistant to the action of bromine in the presence of soda whereas the beryllium stain is destroyed under these conditions, there are two other methods which can be used.

Magnesium is stained an intense red by a mixture, prepared immediately before use, of equal parts of 0.2% solutions of Titan yellow and 2N soda; the material should be stained for an hour, then washed in distilled water, dehydrated, cleared and mounted in a synthetic resin. Although the stain is intense the preparations fade in 24 hours.

An intense blue stain, which is stable after dehydration and mounting in a synthetic resin, is obtained by treating the sections for an hour at 60° with a 1% solution of p-nitrobenzene-azo-1-naphthol (magneson) in 5% soda; the stained sections should be washed in dilute soda then dehydrated immediately.

ZINC

This metal is an essential constituent of insulin and of carbonic anhydrase; the prostate, the islets of Langerhans and the blood granulocytes are the principal sites in which it occurs in the mammalian organism; zinc is a specific activator of a number of enzymes. All these facts serve to explain the interest given to the histochemical detection of zinc.

The oldest of the suggested methods, that of Mendel and Bradley (1905) has been used for tests for zinc in the digestive gland of molluscs. Paraffin wax sections, taken from material which has been fixed in alcohol, are treated for 15 minutes at 50° with a 10% solution of sodium nitroprusside; washing removes all excess reagent (15 minutes in running water). A coverslip is then placed on the sections and a drop of concentrated potassium sulphate solution is introduced between the slide and the coverslip. If zinc is present an intense purple stain is produced. The preparations do not keep and this is probably the chief reason why the method has been abandoned by present-day histochemists.

The method of Okamoto using diphenylthiocarbazone (dithizone), is more in fashion. The Japanese author's working technique has been modified by Mager, McNary and Gibson (1953); it is this variant that gives the most satisfactory results. It can be used on paraffin wax sections taken from freeze-dried material or on sections taken from fresh pieces of material and cut with the freezing microtome. The preparation of the reagent involves the use of a mixture of salts designed to prevent the formation of stained complexes with metals other than zinc.

Reagents:

> solution of dithizone (10 mg dithizone, 100 ml chemically pure acetone) kept in the cold and the dark;
> mixture of salts (dissolve 55 g of sodium hyposulphite (thiosulphate), 9 g of sodium acetate and 1 g of potassium cyanide in 100 ml of distilled water, place in a separating funnel and extract with several portions of a solution of dithizone in carbon tetrachloride, until a clear green stain appears in the carbon tetrachloride layer; the purpose of this operation is to extract any traces of zinc which might be found in the products being used);
> 20% solution of the double tartrate of sodium and potassium; normal acetic acid.

Working technique:

> Sections from freeze dried tissue, cut on a freezing microtome or, if unavoidable, frozen sections or paraffin wax sections from material fixed in the cold with absolute alcohol;
> Dry the sections;
> Treat the dried sections for 5 to 10 minutes with a mixture prepared immediately before use as follows; add 18 ml of distilled water to 24 ml of dithizone solution, adjust the pH to 3.7 with normal acetic acid then add to this 5.8 ml of the mixture of salts and 0.2 ml of the solution of the double tartrate of sodium and potassium: do not keep or use more than once;
> Rinse with chloroform and drain;
> Rinse rapidly in distilled water and mount in a medium miscible with water.

Results. — The zinc is revealed in the form of red or purple stained granules or even in the form of a diffuse red stain.

A more recent method relying on the use of o-{2-α-(2-hydroxy-5-sulphophenylazo)-benzylidene} hydrazino benzoic acid (zincon of analytical chemistry) only seems to have been used on the blood and the hematopoietic organs (Arvy, 1959) and on the prostate (Rixon and Whitfield, 1959). The process is recommended for the simplicity of its technique, its apparent sensitivity and because it does not seem to give rise to any diffusion artefacts. The zincon dissolves at a concentration of 0.05 to 0.5 g in N/50 soda; it is advisable to dissolve the required quantity in 2 ml of N/1 soda and then make up to 100 ml with distilled water.

Blood smears can be treated after simple desiccation; fixation with 10% formalin is recommended when using frozen sections. The sections or smears are treated with the stock solution, the preparation of which is given above, and this should be diluted to a quarter or a fifth with Sörensen's buffer at a pH of 8.05 (5 ml of M/15 monopotassium phosphate and 95 ml of M/15 disodium phosphate) or with Clark and Lubs's buffer at a pH greater than 8.

A blue stain, of greater or lesser depth, appears very rapidly in the leucocyte granules in frozen sections of haematopoietic organs; in smears that have not been fixed, the stain tends towards a red colour. Pretreatment of the material with a chelating agent for zinc inhibits the reaction.

ALUMINIUM

The histochemical detection of aluminium is only used for experimental or anatomo-pathological research work. Most authors prefer the method of Irwin (in Lillie, 1954).

The reagent used is prepared by dissolving, at a concentration of 2%, the sodium or ammonium salt of aurinetricarboxylic acid, in a buffer of pH 5.2, containing 3.8 volumes of 5M ammonium acetate (385.3 g/l) and 1 volume of 6N hydrochloric acid (500 ml/l of concentrated hydrochloric acid).

Sections taken from material fixed in formalin or alcohol, and cut on a freezing microtome or after paraffin embedding, are treated for 5 minutes at 75° with the reagent prepared as above. They are then rinsed in cold distilled water, differentiated for 3 to 5 seconds in a mixture of 3.6 volumes of the buffer used in the preparation of the reagent, and 10 volumes of 1.6 M ammonium carbonate; a further rinse in distilled water may be followed by background staining with a saturated aqueous solution of picric acid or with a very dilute (0.01%) solution of methylene blue. The sections are then dehydrated, cleared and mounted in Canada balsam or in a synthetic resin.

If aluminium is present it appears as an intense red stain.

In addition it should be remembered that some of the methods given for the detection of the salts of calcium, beryllium and magnesium, will also show the presence of aluminium; when treated with a solution of 3,5,5,2′,4′-pentahydroxyflavanol (morin) the aluminium deposits become a very intense fluorescent green, but since other metallic deposits also become fluorescent, it may be necessary to study the fluorescent spectrum to make certain of the identification of the metal.

IRON

Tests for iron constitute one of the most important sections in mineral cation histochemistry; certain iron-bearing compounds are easily detectable by methods known for over a century and the biological importance of bodies containing iron is considerable.

It is classical to recall that two forms of iron occur in animal tissues; one, the ionic form, can be tested for using procedures which have a high chemical specificity whereas the other, the masked form, can only be detected, in certain cases, after the sections are treated with dilute acid or ammonium sulphide; this unmasking fails in a large number of cases, and the presence of iron in the constituents of the cells can then only be detected by micro-incineration of by histophysical methods. Apart from the latter, it is the study of spodograms that provides the most complete "topochemical" pictures of the distribution of iron; the metal appears in the form of the sesqui-oxide Fe_2O_3, which is immediately recognisable from its red colour.

Among the many histochemical reactions put forward for the identification of ionic iron, three have proved their worth and are described here; they are the Prussian blue method (Perls, 1867), the Turnbull blue method (Tirmann, 1898, Schmelzer, 1933) and the ammonium sulphide method (Quincke in Mayer, 1850).

1° The prussian blue reaction is rigorously specific for the Fe^{+++} ion; it only detects ferric compounds, which are almost the only ones to occur in the ionic state in vertebrates. Among the numerous variations in this method two should be retained in histochemical practice, namely those of Lison (1936) and of Gomori (1952).

In Lison's technique, frozen sections, paraffin wax sections or smears, which, where appropriate, have been dewaxed, treated with collodion and hydrated, are treated with a mixture of equal parts of a fresh 2% solution of potassium ferrocyanide and dilute hydrochloric acid (2 ml of commercial concentrated hydrochloric acid and 98 ml of distilled water). The reaction is generally completed in 10 minutes; Lison recommended that the reaction should be continued for 30 minutes, in which case it would seem prudent to renew the reagent after 15 minutes. Careful washing in distilled water removes excess reagent. Among the background stains, the best contrasts are given by nuclear stains using basic fuchsin, safranin or the aluminium lake of fast nuclear red, followed by staining of the cytoplasm with a saturated aqueous solution of picric acid (5 to 10 seconds). The sections are then dehydrated, cleared and mounted in a commercial synthetic resin; the blue stain of the ferruginous inclusions does not keep well in Canada balsam, but is very stable in synthetic resins.

The technique of Gomori takes into account the unequal penetration into the tissues of hydrochloric acid on the one hand and potassium ferrocyanide on the other; it would seem logical to get the ferrocyanide to react first so that the section is completely penetrated by it before the hydrochloric acid reaches it. According to Gomori, the sections are, therefore, treated for 5 minutes with a 5% solution of freshly prepared potassium ferrocyanide; then, while shaking carefully, $\frac{1}{2}$ the volume of 10% hydrochloric acid reagent is added; starting from this moment the action of the reagent lasts for 10 to 20 minutes. The rest of the method follows the instructions that have just been given.

The two variants of the Prussian blue method are applicable to celloidin sections provided that the sections are stuck to the slides and the celloidin dissolved before starting the treatment.

2° *Quincke's reaction* leaves much to be desired with regard to its chemical specificity, since it shows up the iron in the form of ferrous sulphide which is black and is indistinguishable, without complementary reactions, from the sulphides of nickel, cobalt, copper and mercury. This method should only be used when one wishes to confer a black stain on inclusions whose ferruginous character is already known and as a method preparatory to the Turnbull blue reaction.

It can be used on frozen sections, paraffin wax sections, and celloidin sections, when the celloidin has been dissolved and on smears. The sections are treated for 10 minutes to 1 hour with a dilute solutions of ammonium sulphide (1 volume of a fresh, 20% commercial solution which should be a clear yellow and 5 to 10 volumes of distilled water). The ferruginous inclusions rapidly take up a black stain and usually it is not necessary to prolong the action of the ammonium sulphide beyond 10 minutes. The sections are removed from the reagent and washed in tap water; the same background stains may be used as for the Prussian blue reaction.

3° *The Turnbull blue reaction*, which is rigorously specific for the Fe^{++} ion, has two stages. The aim of the first stage is to reduce, to the ferrous state, the ferric compounds which are in the majority in the vertebrate organism and in most invertebrates. The reduction is brought about by Quincke's reaction, but this time using a 20% commercial solution of ammonium sulphide. It is important to use only fresh solutions with clear yellow colour; the time taken for the solution to act is about 30 minutes. The ferrous sulphide is then converted into Turnbull blue by shaking the sections, which have been carefully washed in running water, in a freshly prepared mixture of a fresh 2% solution of potassium ferricyanide in distilled water and 2% hydrochloric acid. Next the sections are washed with great care in running water, the background is stained as in the previous methods and the preparations are cleared, dehydrated and mounted in a commercial synthetic resin. The ferruginous inclusions show up in blue.

Undoubtedly, this reaction has some serious disadvantages from the morphological standpoint; indeed, the shape of the ferruginous inclusions, which is in no way altered by the action of ammonium sulphide, is frequently modified by the action of potassium ferricyanide in an acid medium. When the ferruginous inclusions are not very abundant, their morphology generally remains unchanged, but the deposits, although of little importance, give rise to the appearance of vacuolisation and of "burgeoning" which can cause serious obfuscation of the sections. It is, nonetheless, true that this method must be retained among those still in use in spite of recommendations to the contrary given by authors of the competence of Lillie (1948), Gomori (1952) and Lison (1960).

Those who uphold the usefulness of the method of Tirmann and Schmelzer base their support mainly on results obtained with mammalian tissue, where the ionic iron is in the ferric state so that the Prussian blue reaction ensures complete detection of the iron without the morphological disadvantages of the Turnbull blue reaction; however, a comparison between the results given by the two reactions in certain invertebrate tissues, particularly those of molluscs, suffices to show immediately that the quantity of iron revealed by the Turnbull blue method is far greater than that revealed by the Prussian blue reaction. This difference may be due partly to the presence of ferrous iron, which is not detected by the potassium ferrocyanide reaction, and partly to the unmasking which occurs during the Quincke reaction, the first stage in the Turnbull blue method. According to my personal experience, the two methods are equivalent when testing for iron in mammalian organs but the Tirmann and Schmelzer method assures a much more complete detection of ionic iron than the Perls method, when one is using sections taken from poikilothermic vertebrates or from invertebrates.

The Turnbull blue method, carried out without first reducing the slides with ammonium sulphide, assures the detection of ferrous iron; inclusions or deposits of bivalent iron have not, to my knowledge been found in mammalian organisms.

The unmasking of "masked" iron has been attempted many times, and for the most part at the beginning of the 20th century. In fact the operation is only possible in certain cases. The methods most commonly used are those of Macallum; in one method the sections are treated with a commercial solution of ammonium sulphide, working at a temperature of 50° if necessary and continuing the action of the reagent for one week; in the other method, on the contrary, the sections are treated at laboratory temperature with a mixture of 96 volumes of 90% alcohol and 4 volumes of concentrated sulphuric acid. The optimum time for the reaction has to be determined by trial and error. In both the methods the sections are washed at the end of the unmasking and then treated by the methods used for the detection of ionic iron; obviously only the Turnbull blue reaction is applicable after unmasking with ammonium sulphide.

The real value of these techniques is debatable; the number of compounds in which the iron escapes, *in vitro*, from any unmasking by the reagents being used is rather large; their efficacity, under the working conditions of the histochemist, depends on the circumstances and a negative result does not in any way affirm the absence of masked iron; I note here, as an example, that the iron of haemoglobin escapes any unmasking.

Only micro-incineration ensures the complete detection of the iron present in sections and is therefore the method of choice in all cases where one wishes to study the total iron content.

The other techniques for the histochemical detection of iron have no practical advantages over those just described; any description of them would lengthen the text unnecessarily.

4° *Practical aspects of the histochemical study of iron.* — It is important to take note here of several causes of error.

The **choice of fixative** has been a frequent subject of discussion. The earlier preference for the so-called indifferent fixatives, especially for ethanol, has no justification; it has been shown, overwhelmingly, that bad morphological fixation goes, in the case we are dealing with here, hand in hand with a far from insignificant loss in iron and displacement within the tissues. I note, only as a reminder, the disastrous procedure used by Tartakowsky (1903) who fixed the material with a mixture of 95 parts of 70% alcohol and 5 parts of a commercial solution of ammonium sulphide; poor fixation with the weak alcohol added to the fatal effect of the alkalinity caused by the introduction of ammonium sulphide was such that one can have no confidence in the localisation of the iron so obtained. Many present-day authors strongly advise the use of dilute formalin as fixative (1 vol of the commercial solution to 9 of water) or saline formalin or Baker's formaldehyde-calcium. Bouin's liquid also gives good results and fear of losses because of its acidity seem to me to be unnecessary; I prefer it to formalin because it gives a better histological fixation. When carrying out histochemical tests for iron it is important to avoid all fixatives that might introduce heavy metals into the pieces of tissue; thus all fixatives with a base of corrosive sublimate, or those containing potassium bichromate or chromium trioxide, as well as the liquids of Hollande and Gérard, should not be used.

The **chemical purity of the reagents employed** is one of the essential elements for success in critical research work. Quite a number of the constituents of the tissues are strongly siderophilic; the nuclei and those secretory products which are rich in acid mucopolysaccharides are the most striking examples. The smallest trace of iron in any of the chemical products used during the research work can lead to errors. I can remember, on this subject, sterile discussions as to the presence or absence of iron in the nuclei arising from results which were in fact caused by the adsorption, onto the nuclear structures, of iron from the reagents. The risk of such adsorption must always be recognised when doing research on pieces of tissue that are particularly rich in iron; minute quantities, at the limit of resolution by chemical analysis, can be the origin of positive results with the reactions for detection and it is always to be feared that the deposits of iron may be partly dissolved during the technical manipulations.

As to the **choice of techniques for the detection,** the methods described previously supplement on another mutually. The reaction of Perls reveals the trivalent ionic iron, the Turnbull blue reaction reveals the bivalent ionic iron, the reactions of Quincke and of Tirmann and Schmelzer reveal all the ionic iron and micro-incineration reveals the total iron content (ionic and masked).

It should be recalled that an important role is played by the organic substrate, rich in acid mucopolysaccharides, in the composition of deposits of iron and of other metals within the metazoan organism; the methods for demonstrating these compounds can provide a useful complementary tool for research work on metallic inclusions (Gedigk and Strauss, 1953, 1954 and Gedigk and Pioch, 1956).

Ferritin, the principal form of iron deposited in mammals, and haemosiderin, representing surplus iron, cannot be detected histochemically by reactions for ionic iron; the protein part of the ferritin molecule (apoferritin) can be detected by a microchemical method based on the formation of yellow crystals after treatment with cadmium sulphate solution (Granick, 1946), but this technique does not necessarily give the position of the substance at the cellular level.

The demonstration of iron and other heavy metals in organs where they are very poorly represented has been attempted by Timm and his collaborators by applying the principle of physical development, following Liesegang. The metals are precipitated as sulphides and the ultramicroscopic grains which are formed act as seeds around which the silver is deposited in quantities sufficient to be visible under the light microscope.

The precipitation of heavy metals as sulphides can be achieved either by treating pieces of tissue of small size, with fixatives saturated with hydrogen sulphide, or by treating sections of fresh tissue, cut on a freezing microtome or with a razor, with gaseous hydrogen sulphide. The original method based, as it is, on the action of alcohol saturated with hydrogen sulphide, is of course open to all the criticisms levelled at fixation with alcohol. Recent modifications introduced by the Falkmer school (see particularly Pihl, 1968), namely the use of glutaraldehyde saturated with hydrogen sulphide, counteract, in part, this disadvantage.

For the physical development, Pihl and Falkmer (1967) recommend a mixture of 30 g of gum arabic, 0.43 g of citric acid, 0.17 g of quinol and 10 g of saccharose made up to 100 ml with distilled water; when dissolved the mixture should be left to stand for several days. Just before use, 0.09 ml of a 10% solution of silver nitrate is added to 10 ml of this solution; this mixture will not keep, whereas the colloidal solution of gum arabic can be kept, in the cold, for several weeks. The physical development itself takes place at laboratory temperatures and in the dark.

After careful rinsing, the sections can be given a background stain before they are mounted in the normal way.

A black precipitate shows the presence of heavy metals.

The method is very sensitive but does not enable the heavy metals to be distinguished from one another and its ability to show the position of the metal at the cellular level is questionable.

NICKEL AND COBALT

These two metals occur in such small quantities in the normal organism that their detection by histochemical means is only used for experimental purposes. According to Voigt and his collaborators, none of the methods suggested by the chemists give acceptable results on sectioned material. Only Timm's method shows the position of the metal, but it, of course, does not identify the metal so that it is essential to compare it with sections from a control animal which has not been given the metal in question.

COPPER

The occurrence of this metal, in small quantities in the liver of vertebrates and its part in the composition of the respiratory pigments of many invertebrates explain the interest taken in its histochemical detection. The older methods, such as precipitation as a sulphide, which is non-specific, and detection using haematoxylin, which gives a blue lake with copper salts, should be abandoned in favour of more sensitive methods, in particular those used by Okamoto and Utamura (1938).

Detection by means of rubeanhydric acid (rubeanic, dithioxamide) can be used on fresh tissue pieces and on frozen sections or paraffin wax sections. The latter, once dewaxed, are exposed to hydrochloric acid vapour for 15 minutes, then washed in water, the object being to unmask the copper. The remainder of the treatment is identical for both tissue pieces and sections.

> Immerse for 10 minutes in a 0.1% solution of dithioxamide in 70% alcohol;
> Add 200 mg of chemically pure sodium acetate, shake, then leave to act for 24 to 48 hours;
> Place in 70% alcohol for 60 to 90 minutes.

After this last stage in the method, the sections are dehydrated in absolute alcohol, cleared and mounted in Canada balsam or in a synthetic resin, the tissue pieces are dehydrated in absolute alcohol, impregnated with chloroform and embedded in paraffin wax. The sections cut from these blocks are dewaxed and mounted without a background stain.

A greenish black stain indicates the presence of copper. No systematic study seems to have been made on the effect of different fixatives on the result of the reaction; all authors have used paraffin wax sections of formalin-treated material.

The technique using p-dimethylaminobenzylidene-rhodanine should be carried out in the same way as that for silver and is described in the section on that metal. The presence of copper is revealed as a violet red stain.

In the diphenylcarbazide technique the sections are treated for 10 to 20 minutes with a mixture of 10 ml of a 1% solution of diphenylcarbazide in absolute alcohol and 100 ml of distilled water; the sections are then rinsed in distilled water and the slides should be examined under water. The presence of copper is indicated by a violet-red unstable precipitate.

MERCURY

The histochemical study of mercury is only used in experimental work. The older methods were based on the formation of the black sulphide HgS. Liquid fixatives with a base of hydrogen sulphide or other sulphides should, of course, not be used. Cambar (1940) suggested using formalin or a mixture of alcohol, formalin and acetic acid as a fixative. Paraffin wax sections are first dewaxed and hydrated and then treated with a mixture of 40 ml of 96% alcohol, 60 ml of distilled water and 50 ml of hydrochloric acid through which is passed, bubble by bubble, hydrogen sulphide throughout the whole of the 6 hours that the sections should remain in the liquid. The excess reagent is removed by careful washing first in 70% alcohol and then in water; the sections are mounted in Canada balsam, with or without a background stain. Mercury appears in the form of black grains.

In Lombardo's (1906) method, pieces of tissue fixed in dilute formalin, alcohol or Carnoy's liquid, then washed in distilled water, are treated for 12 to 24 hours with a 25% solution of tin chloride in a mixture of 25 g of concentrated hydrochloric acid in 75 ml of water; this treatment reduces the mercury salts to black metallic mercury. The tissue pieces are then given a long wash in distilled water, embedded in paraffin, cut into sections and mounted in Canada balsam with the background lightly stained if necessary. The mercury appears in the form of black grains.

The diphenylcarbazide and diphenylcarbazone reactions used by Brandino (1927) are severely criticised by most modern authors; the instability of the reagents explains the non-specific stains and the risk of error being caused by excess reagent.

SILVER

Histochemical identification of silver is only useful for research into spontaneous or experimentally induced silver poisoning. The black or brown deposits, characteristic of this condition, contain metallic silver bound to a substrate in which the proteins and mucopolysaccharides can be detected by histochemical methods. The older techniques for identification depended on staining the particles by treating with Farmer's photographic reducer (1 g of potassium ferricyanide, 20 g of sodium hyposulphite and 100 ml of distilled water) or with Lugol's solution and then bleaching with sodium hyposulphite; as a result, the black stain disappears in an interval of time that does not affect the melanins (1 to 2 hours).

The method of Okamoto using rubeanhydric acid (dithioxamide) gives excellent results; Gedigk and Pioch (1956) recommend this method with some modifications differing slightly from those given in connection with the histochemical reactions of copper. Paraffin wax sections from formalin treated material are dewaxed, hydrated and then treated for 10 to 20 minutes with chlorine water. Washing in water eliminates excess reagent. The sections should then be kept for 2 to 5 hours at 37° in a closed vessel containing a solution made up of 3 ml of 1% ammonia water, 3 ml of a 0.1% solution of dithioxamide in absolute alcohol and 94 ml of distilled water. The background can be stained with hemalum. The presence of silver is shown by an intense brown stain.

The p-dimethylaminobenzylidine-rhodanine reaction, carried out as for the detection of copper, also stains silver deposits red but diffusion artefacts are rather common. In this method the sections are treated for 24 to 48 hours at 37° with a mixture of 3 to 5 ml of a saturated solution of this compound in absolute alcohol and 1 to 3 ml of N/1 nitric acid and sufficient water to make up the volume to 100 ml; the background can be stained with hemalum.

GOLD

As with silver, the only time one looks for gold in animal tissues is after it has been introduced experimentally, therapeutically or accidentally.

The classical method of Christeller involves treating paraffin wax sections taken from formalin- or alcohol-fixed material for 36 hours at 56° with a mixture of 10 volumes of 5% tin chloride solution and one volume of concentrated hydrochloric acid. The sections are then washed and the background stained with a nuclear red or green stain; they can then be mounted in Canada balsam. A stain varying from brown to black indicates the presence of gold. Gérard and Cordier noted that diffusion artefacts were a possibility.

A very simple method introduced by Elftman and Elftman (1954) consists of treating the sections in an oven at 37° for 1 to 3 days with 3 volume hydrogen peroxide. Under these conditions all the black pigments, whose presence could make interpretation difficult, are decolourised and only the deposits of gold show up in red, purple, blue or black.

BISMUTH

The rather widespread therapeutic use of bismuth compounds and their use in experimental research work on metallic deposits explains the interest shown in the histochemical detection of bismuth in animal tissues. All authors use the Christeller-Komaya method (Komaya, 1925; Christeller, 1926).

Frozen or paraffin wax sections from formalin—fixed material are treated for 5 to 10 minutes with the reagent of Léger, then rinsed in dilute nitric acid (2 drops of 25% nitric acid for every 10 ml of distilled water), wiped with blotting paper, dehydrated in benzene-phenol, cleared in benzene and mounted in Canada balsam or a synthetic resin.

Léger's reagent, which must be prepared immediately before use, is a mixture of equal parts of an aqueous solution of quinine sulphate (1 g of quinine sulphate, 50 ml distilled water and 10 drops of 25% nitric acid) and a 4% solution of potassium iodide in distilled water.

This method stains the bismuth deposits a very characteristic yellow or orange.

It should also be noted that bismuth salts stain an intense black in the presence of hydrogen sulphide or alkaline sulphides.

LEAD

As with the metals just described, the histochemical detection of lead is only used during histopathological or experimental work.

The classical authors made use of the fact that deposits of lead can be converted, by the action of chromates or bichromates, into yellow lead chromate. Some simply fixed the material in a liquid with a potassium bichromate base and then embedded in paraffin wax and stained the background. Others treated paraffin wax sections taken from formalin-fixed material with a 3% solution of potassium chromate or bichromate acidified with several drops of acetic acid. The formation of the insoluble chromate of lead is completed in three days; the sections can then be washed and mounted after the background has been lightly stained with toluidine blue.

Molnar (1952) and Gedigk and Pioch (1956) used the sodium rhodizonate method. Sections taken from formalin-fixed material are treated for 40 minutes at laboratory temperature with a 0.5% solution of this compound in distilled water; the background can be stained with haemalum. The deposits of lead take on a dark brown stain.

CHAPTER 14

HISTOCHEMICAL DETECTION OF PROPERTIES COMMON TO SEVERAL RADICALS AND FUNCTIONAL GROUPS

Following Lison's (1960) excellent example, the present chapter collects together the marker stains and histochemical reactions common to a certain number of radicals and functional groups. None of these characters is specific to any given compound, but if we also take into consideration other histochemical features and data derived from analytical biochemistry we can arrive at a strong presumption in favour of the presence of a chemical substance, and even of its identification. The converse is also true; if we take into account one of the characters mentioned here we strengthen substantially the interpretation of the results obtained from the use of other marker stains or histochemical reactions.

Some of the methods noted above depend on electron transfer in the course of oxidation-reduction reactions. From the standpoint of the histochemist, the detection of the reducing capacity of certain structures is much more important than is that of the oxidising capacity. If we leave aside enzyme activities, since this is discussed in another chapter, the peroxides contained in certain lipids alone correspond to this second category, and their detection is described in relation to lipid histochemistry. On the other hand, the tests for reducing properties play an essential part in modern practical histochemistry.

Other procedures discussed in this chapter provide information about the electro-polarity of compounds contained in the structures under investigation; such information relates to tests for acidophilia and basophilia, metachromotropy (metachromasia) and a number of related marker stains.

HISTOCHEMICAL DETECTION OF REDUCING COMPOUNDS

The number of reducing compounds which may occur in material falling into the purview of animal histochemistry is quite large. All or some of the reactions discussed in this section are given by mono- and polyphenols, pyrroles and indoles, certain carbohydrates (ascorbic acid and hexoses), melanins, uric acid and its derivatives, unsaturated lipids and their derivatives formed by oxidation, as well as compounds bearing carbonyl groups. We should add to this list the fact that there are histochemical reactions which depend on the artificial introduction, into the compounds we need to detect, of reducing groups; such methods should evidently be discussed together with the compounds in question, and only methods of demonstrating reducing compounds will be dealt with here.

Techniques for the histochemical demonstration of reducing compounds depend on the reduction of ferric ferricyanide, silver salts, or of tetrazolium salts.

THE FERRIC FERRICYANIDE REACTION

This is a method introduced into histological technique by Golodetz and Unna (1909) to reveal 'sites of reduction'. The working technique has several times been modified (Schmorl, 1934; Chèvrement and Frédéric, 1943; Adams, 1956). This latest among the investigations mentioned above includes a rational analysis of the mechanism of the reaction.

Principles. — We know from *in vitro* studies (Adams, 1956) that ferric ferricyanide $Fe^{+++}[Fe^{+++}(CN)_6]$, prepared by mixing a solution of potassium ferricyanide and a ferric salt (chloride or sulphate) immediately prior to use, may react in three distinct ways in the presence of a reducing agent.

With weak reducing agents a green precipitate is formed (Prussian green) which in all probability corresponds to ferroso-ferric ferricyanide $Fe_4^{+++}F_3^{++}[(CN)_6]_6$, identified chemically by Lange (1937).

With stronger reducing agents Prussian blue, or ferric ferrocyanide $Fe_4^{+++}[Fe^{++}(CN)_6]_3$ is formed.

With very vigorous reducing agents, a white precipitate of ferric ferrocyanide $Fe^{+++}[Fe^{++}(CN)_6]$ is formed.

This last reaction only takes place with particularly strong reducing agents such as are not met with in animal tissue; only the first two possibilities need to be considered when the method is used in histochemistry. Experience shows that the two ways of reacting do indeed exist, the action of ferric ferricyanide on sections of tissue resulting either in the appearance of a green stain revealing the presence of weak reducing agents, or by that of a blue stain, disclosing stronger reducing agents. It cannot be too strongly emphasised that solutions of ferric ferricyanide undergo spontaneous reduction to Prussian green, this change being accelerated by strong sunlight or by a rise in temperature; from the practical aspect, it is thus imperative to use only solutions prepared just before they are needed, and to renew the reagent whenever the treatment is prolonged beyond a dozen or so minutes.

Preparation of the reagent. — In practical work, the reagent for the ferric ferricyanide reaction is, therefore, prepared by mixing a solution of potassium ferricyanide and one of ferric sulphate (in Chèvremont and Frédéric's method) or of ferric chloride (in all other variations) immediately before use. The rapidity with which these compounds dissolve, and the far from negligeable risk of deterioration in the solution of potassium ferricyanide, leads me to recommend that the two solutions which have to be mixed should themselves be prepared just prior to use. There are disparate opinions as to the proportions of the two solutions required, as is shown in Table 5.

Table 5. — Composition of the reagents recommended for the ferric ferricyanide technique

Authors	Potassium ferricyanide		Ferric salt		Iron/ferricyanide ratio
	Conc.	ml	Conc.	ml	
Golodetz and Unna	1%	50	1%	50	2/1
Schmorl	—	—	—	—	—
Chèvremont and Frédéric	0.1%	25	1%	75	50/1
Lillie	1%	10	1%	75	15/1
Adams	1%	10	1%	30	7/1

Gomori (1952) considers that the concentrations of ferric salt and of potassium ferricyanide are not critical. And yet, experience shows that the sensitivity of the reaction is greater when the iron/ferricyanide ratio is lower, but the lowering of the ratio increases the liability of among other things a scarcely specific, and hard to interpret, green colour in the sections. For such reasons we can understand that Chèvremont and Frédéric's formula results in preparations whose background staining is slighter than with any other variant of the ferric ferricyanide reaction, but that obtaining positive results with this variant necessitates a duration of action such that the reagent requires to be renewed twice during the process.

From my own experience, the formulae due to Adams and to Lillie give equivalent results, if we take into account the durations of treatment recommended in the two cases (5 minutes for Adams' formula, 10 minutes for that of Lillie).

Practice of the reaction. — The considerations set out above show that the various versions of the ferric ferricyanide technique are not equivalent. In fact, the methods due to Adams and to Lillie, which are of relatively short duration, disclose the sites of relatively vigorous reducing agents, compounds whose reducing capacity is weaker giving rise to a background stain which is pale green; Chèvremont and Frédéric's method, the sensitivity of the reagent being much less, but partly compensated for by the much longer duration of action, only shows up the sites of vigorous reducing agents; with the older method of Golodetz and Unna, the background stain is quite intense despite the short period for which the reagent is allowed to act, and of all the methods this is the one which least lends itself to interpretation of the green background stain, since that may be caused by the presence of weakly reducing groups as well as by an unspecific adsorption of ferroso-ferric ferricyanide (Prussian green). For this reason it seems to me legitimate to counsel against the use of this technique, and to restrict our discussion to Adams' method and that of Chèvremont and Frédéric.

It hardly needs saying that preparations obtained with the ferric ferricyanide reaction may be treated subsequently with various background stains; in most instances, nuclear staining in red gives the best contrasts; basic fuchsin, azocarmine, nuclear fast red, and safranine are the most widely used among background stains. So far as the mounting of the preparations is concerned, it is appropriate to stress the benefits accruing from a replacement of Canada balsam by synthetic resins, since the latter preserve Prussian blue much better.

a) **Adams' method.**—The working technique recommended by this author is suitable for paraffin wax sections, dewaxed, treated where appropriate with collodion, and hydrated.

> Treat for 5 minutes at laboratory temperatures with a mixture of one volume of ferricyanide solution and three volumes of ferric chloride solution, both at 1% concentration; the mixture should be prepared within the 5 minutes preceding its use, and I would advise the experimenter to prepare the constituent solutions just before they are required;
> Wash carefully with three baths of distilled water, the total duration of the washing being some 10 minutes.
> Where appropriate, stain the background using the aluminium lake of nuclear fast red (p. 203) safranine (p. 203) or basic fuchsin (p. 202); it does not seem to me desirable to use azocarmine as a background stain;
> Rinse rapidly in distilled water, dehydrate in absolute alcohol, clear and mount in a synthetic resin.

b) **Chèvremont and Frédéric's method.**—According to its authors, this method can be applied to frozen sections or to paraffin wax sections; only the duration of the treatment varies according to the nature of the material.

> Treat frozen section for about 10 minutes, paraffin wax ones which have been brought into water for three times 10 minutes, with the reagent prepared by mixing 25 ml of 0.1% potassium ferricyanide solution with 75 ml of a 1% solution of ferric sulphate; it is generally necessary to filter the reagent and it does not keep for more than 10 minutes; all contact with metallic instruments must be avoided, as well as the action of too bright a light;
> Wash for a long time in running water, stain the background and mount as above.

Interpretation of the results. — The presence of vigorous reducing agents is disclosed by the appearence of a blue colour; a green colour is of rather more delicate interpretative value, as it may be due to the presence of weakly reducing groups or to non-specific adsorption of Prussian green. It may prove useful to examine the sections under water, before the background has been stained, the better to appreciate any subsequent changes associated with that process.

In vitro trials and the conduct of the reaction on sections shows that results which are more or less strongly positive are obtained with thiol, mono- and polyphenol, pyrrole and indole groups; moreover, oxidative derivatives of lipids of the lipofuscin type stain green or blue; with ascorbic acid, the formation of Prussian green can be obtained *in vitro*, but the preservation of this acid is naturally uncertain under the experimental conditions described above. Reducing carbohydrates and aldehydes do not give the ferric ferricyanide reaction.

THE REDUCTION OF SILVER SALTS

The methods falling into this group, which have been known for a long time, depend on the reduction of a silver salt, with deposition of metallic silver, in contact with the sections; it is, therefore, the reducing agents present in the sections which are revealed.

Lison (1936, 1952, 1960) quite rightly emphasises the wrong use of language in respect of the histochemical use of silver salts. The histochemical reactions which involve these compounds bear no relation to the silver impregnations of general histological technique, where the fixation of a silver salt on the structures (argyrophilia) is revealed by the experimenter's introduction of a reducing agent. In the case of the procedures we wish to collect together under the name suggested by Cordier (1927), the argentaffin reaction, no reducing agent is added to the medium by the experimenter, as the whole object of the procedure is to detect groups endowed with this capacity in the structures under investigation. In consequence, the positive results obtained with the argentaffin reaction have a definite histochemical significance, whereas the demonstration of argyrophilia has none. The term "argentophilia" used by some recent authors should be formally proscribed; its barbarous mixed Greco-Latin derivation adds to the disquiet associated with its imprecise meaning.

Among the silver salts which can be used for the detection of reducing compounds, the nitrate is used, in practice, only for demonstrating the presence of ascorbic acid; the ways in which it is used are indicated in relation to the histochemical detection of this compound. The complex silver salts (argentamine, silver hexamethylenetetramine etc...) have a much wider range of uses as they allow us to demonstrate the presence of an appreciable number of reducing compounds (ortho- and parapolyphenols, aldehydes, uric acid and urates, ascorbic acid, reducing sugars, 5-hydroxytryptamine). It is appropriate to emphasise an important difference between the behaviour of certain reducing agents towards ferric ferricyanide, on the one hand, and towards complex silver salts on the other. So it is that aldehydes do not reduce ferric ferricyanide, but give the argentaffin reaction strongly, whereas the thiols, which are very vigorous reducing agents towards ferric ferricyanide, do not give the argentaffin reaction.

Principles. — The methods which involve silver diamine hydroxide and silver methenamine (hexamethylenetetramine) depend on the same principle. In the presence of a reducing compound, these complex silver salts are reduced, with the deposition of metallic silver in places where the reducing groups are situated. The preparations so obtained can be mounted and examined as they are; it is often desirable to tone them with gold and to stain the background. One of the peculiarities basic to all argentaffin reactions is the absence of any strictly defined end-point; when the action of the reagent is prolonged beyond an optimum which varies with the preparative technique and the temperature at which the reaction is carried out, sundry phenomena involving reduction, having no histochemical significance, result in a most annoying darkening of the preparations; in addition to the argentaffin reaction sections whose passage through the reagent has been unduly prolonged are characterised by a more or less intense blackening of argyrophilic structures, or even by haphazard precipitation of silver, unrelated to the structure of the given tissue. This peculiarity of argentaffin reactions is associated with the relative instability of silver complexes; it necessitates a close watch on the preparations during the course of the reaction.

Preparation of the reagents. — Among the numerous formulae for ammoniacal silver complexes, that of Fontana is used in the great majority of instances for the practical conduct of the argentaffin reaction. The silver hexamethylenetetramine methods (Gomori, 1948; Lillie and Burtner, 1949) are coming into ever wider use; they have the advantage of lower cost-benefit ratios for the reagent which acts more rapidly and keeps better than does Fontana's solution. Formulae based on ammoniacal silver carbonate or silver piperazine (Arzac and Flores, 1949) have also been put forward. Bryan (1964) recommends an ammoniacal silver complex obtained by adding ammonia to a 2% solution of silver nitrate until the precipitate redissolves.

a) **Fontana's solution.**—Add commerical ammonia to a 5% aqueous solution of silver nitrate until the precipitate redissolves; it is imperative not to overshoot the mark, so that the last additions should be made drop by drop, stirring each time. Once the precipitate has redissolved, add, drop by drop, the silver nitrate solution until a *persistent* cloudiness remains; remove the precipitate by settling and decantation. This "reverse titration" improves the sensitivity of the reagent which should not smell of ammonia.

We may recall that all the ammoniacal silver complexes are unstable, and that their decomposition results in *explosive compounds*, probably representing silver nitride:

$$Ag(NH_3)_2OH \rightarrow AgNH_2 + NH_3 + H_2O; \quad 3\,AgNH_2 \rightarrow Ag_3N + 2\,NH_3;$$

$$Ag_3N \rightarrow 3\,Ag + \tfrac{1}{2}\,N_2$$

This conversion into the nitride, involving an intermediate stage of silver amide, is rather slow and occurs in alkaline media; it is, then, strictly necessary to prevent the throwing away of solutions of ammoniacal silver complexes or their simple neglect, at laboratory temperatures; serious accidents caused by the failure to observe this rule have been reported.

b) **Silver hexamethylenetetramine.**—To 100 ml of a 3% aqueous solution of hexamethylenetetramine add 5 ml of 5% aqueous solution of silver nitrate; stir until the precipitate redissolves. This reagent can be kept in the cold and darkness for several months.

c) **Silver piperazine.**—Add 1 ml of a 10% aqueous solution of silver nitrate to 100 ml of a 0.5% aqueous solution of piperazine; stir until the precipitate redissolves; the keeping qualities are the same as for silver hexamethylenetetramine.

d) **Ammoniacal silver carbonate.**—To 16 ml of a saturated aqueous solution of lithium carbonate add 4 ml of a 10% aqueous solution of silver nitrate; redissolve the greater part of the precipitate by the prudent addition of ammonia, until a persistent turbidity is allowed to remain; make up to 100 ml with the saturated aqueous solution of lithium carbonate; this reagent may be kept in an ice-box.

In practice, the formulae of Arzac and Flores are no better than is silver hexamethylenetetramine; contrary to Lison's (1960, p. 726) opinions, the latter gives results as satisfactory as those obtained using Fontana's solution and has the advantages mentioned above over that preparation. It is, therefore, the one that I would recommend for practical use.

Practice of the reaction. — For all practical purposes, the argentaffin reaction is applied to paraffin wax sections, to smears, or to squash preparations; the older applications to tissue blocks have been abandoned. The slides may be treated with collodion and most authors explicitly advise that this step should be carried out. The duration of action of the silver complex and the temperature at which it acts vary according to circumstances.

a) **The classical argentaffin reaction** (Masson, 1923):

> Paraffin wax sections, dewaxed, hydrated;
> Wash with great care (1 to 2 hours) in distilled water several times renewed;
> Treat with Fontana's solution for 24 to 36 hours in darkness in a well-stoppered flask. The reaction takes place at laboratory temperatures;
> Rinse carefully in distilled water;
> Tone with gold chloride (0.1% aqueous solution) for 5 minutes;
> Rinse in distilled water;
> Treat with a 5% aqueous solution of sodium thiosulphate for 1 minute;
> Rinse at length (5 minutes) in tap water;
> Stain the background with Ramon y Cajal's trichrome, nuclear fast red-picro-indigo-carmine or safranine-picro-indogocarmine;
> Dehydrate, clear, mount in Canada balsam or in a synthetic resin.

b) **The silver hexamethylenetetramine reaction** (Lillie and Burtner's (1949) technique):

> Paraffin wax sections, dewaxed treated with collodion and hydrated;
> Treat for 10 minutes with Lugol's fluid (Potassium iodide 2 g, iodine 1 g, distilled water 100 ml);
> Bleach with a 5% aqueous solution of sodium thiosulphate;
> Wash for 10 minutes in running water;
> Rinse in two baths of distilled water;
> Treat in an oven at 60° in well-covered receptacles (Borrel or Coplin jars, staining-baths) with the mixture
> > silver hexamethylenetetramine solution .... 30 ml
> > borate buffer, pH 7.8 (1.24% solution of boric acid, 16 ml, 1.9% solution of sodium tetraborate decahydrate 4 ml) ..... 8 ml
>
> The duration of action is optimal at 30 to 60 minutes if the solution has been previously warmed to 60°, and at about three hours if the sections are steeped in it at laboratory temperatures and then moved to the oven.
> Rinse in distilled water;
> Tone with gold and stain the background and mount as in Masson's technique.

Interpretation of the results. — The presence of reducing compounds is revealed by an intense black stain. In conformity with what has been said above, it is mainly ortho- and parapolyphenols which are detected by the argentaffin reaction, together with uric acid and the urates, melanins, and aldehydes. *It gives negative results with thiols.* The optical qualities of the preparations are remarkable but in interpreting them we need to take into account the difficulty of deciding exactly on the optimal duration of action of the silver complex. Indeed, too short a duration results in errors of omission; when the action of the reagent is too prolonged, errors by excess may be induced because of the onset of some degree of argyrophilia of no histochemical significance. Should one, in fact, overshoot the mark the first sign is a blackening of the collagen fibres and such a result should be enough to act as a warning sign for the alert investigator. Naturally, nothing of histochemical value can be deduced once the nuclei, the muscle fibres, and the secretory granules can be seen, and, *a fortiori*, when precipitates of silver are seen in the sections.

THE REDUCTION OF TETRAZOLIUM SALTS

The tetrazolium salts are compounds which are soluble and but slightly coloured in the oxidised condition, but insoluble and strongly coloured in the reduced condition (formazans). Their principal use in histochemistry is for demonstrating dehydrogenases, diaphorases and endogenic reductases in histo-enzymology. Apart from this use, tetrazolium salts are much less used by histochemists than are silver complexes or ferric ferricyanide; one reason for this is probably the relatively high cost of the compounds in question, but the need to work in an alkaline medium and the lack of true chemical specificity are partly responsible for the relative lack of interest shown by investigators so far as these methods are concerned.

Principles. — As their name suggests, compounds of this group are characterised by heterocyclic rings with 4 nitrogen atoms and one carbon atom. They were known to chemists at the end of the 19th century, and have been used in biology since 1940. Jambor's work (1960) gives a very full account of chemical investigations prior to that date. The main salts of tetrazolium used in histochemistry are listed in Table 6. Some of the compounds have only a single tetrazolium nucleus; others contain two, linked by a radical attached to the atoms of nitrogen bearing the number 3 in each ring (N-N-ditetrazoles); tetrazoles the two rings of which are linked by carbon atoms (C-C-ditetrazoles) also exist. Reduction to formazan accompanies the opening of the ring; it gives rise to compounds which are brightly coloured and much less soluble in water than are the corresponding tetrazolium salts. The formazans vary in colour from red to violet, through a fairly deep blue.

Besides the factors such as the sensitivity of the reaction, the stability of the colour obtained, its intensity, and the insolubility of the formazan, the choice of the salts used in histochemistry has been primarily dictated by the need to end up with precipitates as finely divided as possible, so as to be able to do better than provide an approximate localisation of the enzymatic activity or substance which is the objective of the work. Those which seem to be most satisfactory from this standpoint are nitro tetrazolium blue, nitroneotetrazolium, and methyl thiazolyltetrazolium.

Table 6. — THE PRINCIPAL TETRAZOLIUM SALTS USED IN HISTOCHEMISTRY.
(after BURSTONE, 1963)

Chemical name	Common name and abbreviation	Molecular weight
a) 2, 3, 5-triphenyltetrazolium chloride	triphenyltetrazolium (TTC)	334.81
b) 2-(p-iodophenyl) -3-(p-nitrophenyl) -5-phenyltetrazolium chloride	iodonitrotetrazolium (INT)	541.18
c) 3-(4, 5-dimethylthiazol-2)-2, 5-diphenyltetrazolium bromide	methylthiazoltetrazolium (MTT)	414.35
d) (4,4−'diphenylene) bis-2-(3, 5-diphenyl)-tetrazolium chloride	neotetrazolium (NT)	703.65
e) 3, 3'-dianisol-bis-4, 4'-(3, 4)-diphenyltetrazolium chloride	blue tetrazolium (BT)	727.67
f) 2, 2'-di-paranitrophenyl-5, 5'-diphenyl-(3, 3'-dimethoxy-4, 4'-diphenylene) ditetrazolium chloride	nitrotetrazolium blue (nitro-BT)	871.72

Tests for reducing compounds in sections taken from fixed tissue, when carried out using tetrazolium salts, are always undertaken in an alkaline medium. The reaction occurs at 60° in the presence of an alkaline cyanide; the formazans produced by the reduction of the tetrazolium salt are soluble in alcohol and in benzenoid hydrocarbons, so that it is essential to mount them in a water-miscible medium.

As Lison (1960) has commented, the earliest of the techniques to be put forward, which comprised treatment of the sections with solutions whose pH was greater than 10 and which necessitated a period in an oven, have been practically abandoned. Today, it is Gomori's (1956) method which is the most used. This also involves the use of an oven at 60° but the pH of the reagent is only 8.5 to 8.8.

Preparation of the reagent. — Gomori's technique, the only one we give here, uses neotetrazolium, but tetrazolium blue or nitrotetrazolium blue can also be used. The reagent is prepared at the time of use by mixing the following materials *in the order indicated*

```
distilled water .......................................... 15 ml
sodium cyanide ......................................... 1 g
borate buffer of pH 8.8 ............................. 20 ml
N/I acetic acid .......................................... 15 ml
0.5% solution of neotetrazolium in absolute alcohol ...... 5 ml
```

The reagent, when prepared in this way, keeps for a certain length of time away from bright light and heat. It may be reused two or three times provided that it is carefully filtered. But the intensity of the stain so obtained diminished rapidly enough. In any event, there is no great advantage in preparing large quantities of the mixture.

Working technique. — So far as I am aware, the technique has only been applied to paraffin wax sections, dewaxed, treated with collodion, and hydrated.

Treat for one to two hours at 60°, with the alkaline tetrazolium solution;
Rinse in distilled water;
Stain the nuclei with haemalum (optional);
Wash for five minutes in running water;
Mount in a medium miscible with water.

Interpretation of the results. — The presence of reducing compounds is shown by a more or less intense purple colour. Generally speaking, there is strong contrast between the stained structures and the remainder, so that the optical qualities of the preparation are good. In my opinion, nuclear staining with haemalum serves no useful purpose and I would even advise against it, because it decreases the contrast.

In considering the histochemical significance of the results obtained, we need to bear in mind that the number of reducing agents capable of reacting under the experimental conditions defined above is quite large. Pearse's (1953, 1954) technique, which is disadvantagous from a morphological point of view because of the very high pH of the reagent, shows up protein-bound sulphydrils, lipofuscins and other compounds derived from the oxidation of lipids, myelin, certain mucins, and the polyphenolic compounds of the enterochromaffin cells of the intestine. Under the experimental conditions of Gomori's method, a positive result constitutes valuable evidence of the occurrence of protein-bound sulphydrils, but it is necessary to back this up with other means for the detection of these compounds before we can indeed affirm that thiosulphide groups are present. The value of the method as a reaction for protein-bound sulphydrils is discussed in relation to the demonstration of these compounds by histochemical means.

THE HISTOCHEMICAL STUDY OF ACIDOPHILIA

The identification of 'acidophilic' structures, that is to say those taking up acid (anionic) dyestuffs, has formed part of histological practice for almost a century, yet we cannot offer a rigorous definition of this stain affinity. On the contrary, in the language of histochemists the term 'acidophilic' has a precise meaning; it applies exclusively to the tissue proteins and indicates that anionic stains have become fixed on the basic radicals of the proteins, from a solution whose pH is low.

> The use of a solution whose pH is distinctly lower than that at which the ratio of ionised to unionised carboxyl groups of the proteins is equal to unity (often designated by the symbol pK) induces the carboxyl groups to become non-ionised, whereas the basic groups of the protein molecules become ionised. As a consequence, the proteins in question fix anions in numbers corresponding to those of the basic ionised groups.
>
> Experience fully confirms the predictions of the theory, showing that the number of anions fixed does not depend on the nature of the latter, but does correspond to the number of basic groups as indicated by chemical analysis. The same is true during the fixation of mineral acids by proteins. Numerous *in vitro* studies involving wool and other easily manipulatable proteins leave no doubt in this respect (see Vickerstaff, 1950, for a bibliography).

From the histochemical standpoint it follows that staining with an anionic stain at a sufficiently low pH should, in principle, allow us to evaluate the total number of basic groups present in the structure under investigation; this is the quantity which Lison (1960) proposed to designate as 'total acidophilia'.

Lison (1960) quite correctly mentions that priority for the histochemical application of the principle just discussed goes back to Hyden (1943); that author attempted to evaluate highly basic proteins, during a general study of nucleic acids in nerve cells, using as a stain ponceau 2R in a strongly acid medium. Fast green (fast green FCF, in order that it should not be confused with basic dyes sold under the same commercial name) has been suggested by Schrader and Leuchtenberger (1950) and by Bryan (1951) for the selective demonstration of accumulations of basic proteins. These authors used a solution of the stain in water acidified to pH 1.2. With the same objective, Deitch (1955) proposed that naphthol yellow S be used. It is the working technique of this latter author which seems to be the most satisfactory.

Working technique:

Paraffin wax sections, dewaxed, treated with collodion and hydrated;
Stain for 15 minutes at laboratory temperatures, with a 1% solution of naphtho yellow S in 1% acetic acid;
Transfer the sections to 1% acetic acid, leave them in it for 15 to 24 hours to extract the excess of the dye;
Blot with tissue paper;
Dehydrate with tertiary butyl alcohol;
Clear in a benzenoid hydrocarbon, mount in Canada balsam or in a commercial synthetic resin.

All contact between the sections and tap or distilled water should be avoided once they have left the stain-bath; similarly, dehydration with ethyl alchol may extract the stain and must, in consequence, be avoided.

Interpretation of the results. — We know from the very detailed experiments of Deitch that the method gives every satisfaction as to its fidelity; the time spent by the slides in the acetic acid is not critical and the same comment could be made for the duration of staining. Experiments on models of known chemical composition, moreover, show that acetylation or deamination decreases the intensity of the stain in a fashion predictable from a knowledge of the relative number of amine or other basic groups (guanidyl, imidazol) of the protein being studied.

The main disadvantage of Deitch's method was well brought out by Lison (1960); the stain was chosen because of its absorption maximum in the visible spectrum (435 μ), which is sufficiently displaced from that of the product of the nucleal reaction of Feulgen and Rossenbeck to avoid any interference between the absorption curves during comparative studies; in consequence, the preparations are mediocre from the optical standpoint, when Deitch's reaction is used without any other stain. We may also, as did Lison (1960 p. 327), enquire whether the pH of the solution is sufficiently low.

However that may be, the accumulation of substances rich in basic groups entrains a yellow colour in the structures in question.

Following Deitch's investigations, staining with naphthol yellow S has been introduced into sundry combined techniques, mainly those intended to reveal various carbohydrates by histochemical means (Himes and Moriber, 1956, Benson, 1966). Such procedures are discussed in relation to the histochemical study of nucleic acids.

THE HISTOCHEMICAL STUDY OF BASOPHILIA

The remarks concerning the different accepted meanings of the term 'acidophilia", according to whether the framework of reference is general histology or histochemistry, hold good for basophilia. We might even say that wrong uses of language are commoner in the second case; the nomenclature of the types of cell to be found in the distal lobe of the adenohypophysis is an example.

In conformity with Ehrlich's classical conception (1877), the basophilia of a structure is due, in the first place, to the presence of groups likely to undergo linkage, with a coloured cation, through a primary valency. However, other factors may intervene to increase or decrease this basophilia. The occurrence of cationic groups in the stained structure patently decreases its affinity for a cationic stain; any factors capable of reducing the ionisation of the electronegative groups of the stained substratum have the same effect; steric inhibitions, also, may reduce the basophilia of a given structure and this dyestuff affinity cannot, evidently, be manifested if the staining cations do not penetrate into the structure in which the groups with which they might combine are situated. Conversely, van der Waals forces, covalent bonds, and the aggregation of the dye into particles all increase the basophilia of the stained structure. From this fact, we can see that the quantity of basic stain fixed by a structure does not necessarily accord with the stoichiometric proportions expected if we were dealing with salt formation through primary valencies. The importance of this question for the generality of quantitative studies carried out by means of basic stains accounts for the large number of experimental investigations; as did Lison (1960), we have to admit that one of two possibilities may come to pass, the amount of stain fixed being stoichiometric in some instances and not so in others.

The principal chemical groups capable of fixing coloured cations, which need to be taken into account under the working conditions of the histochemist, are the sulphate radicals of acid mucopolysaccharides, the phosphate radicals of nucleic acids, the carboxyl radical of proteins, certain carbohydrates, uric acid, and the oxy-acid (keto-acid) radicals of the oxidation derivatives of lipids.

Naturally, basophilia does not show up unless the balance of electrostatic charges is favourable for anions; this observation is particularly important in the case of amphoteric substances such as proteins.

The physico-chemical factors which play a part in the fixation of basic dyes by the tissues have long been studied; Zeiger's (1938) work summarises the classical investigations; Singer's reviews (1952, 1954) give more recent data. The salient features of what is known should be recalled here, but it is germane to emphasise, in the first place, the elements of a histochemical definition of basophilia.

To have histochemical significance, basophilia must be observed under strictly defined conditions.

Following Lison (1960, p. 277) in this respect, I should say that only the use of basic dyestuffs allows us to observe basophilia. Those who find this remark trite might change their opinion if they read the works of some histologists, and by no means the least among them, who classify the structures studied into acidophilic and basiphilic according to the results of stains such as Heidenhain's azan or Mann's method using methyl blue—eosin, procedures which involve no basic dyestuff. The hoary absurdity by which adenohypophyseal cells are classified as acidophilic or basophilic according to whether they take up eosin or aniline blue has already been mentioned. In too many instances, basophilia in structures is judged by staining with haemalum; it may not be unhelpful to recall that the progressive lakes of haematoxylin possess certain attributes of basic dyes, but that they do not become fixed on the tissue by salt formation.

Only progressive stains can be discussed here, because we are looking for that basophilia which has histochemical significance. Very different factors, which vary from case to case and are little known, intervene during differentiation, so that it is essential not to use regressive stains.

Naturally, we should avoid allowing two basic dyestuffs to compete in instances where the basophilia of the structures needs to be interpreted in histochemical terms; even the results of staining with methyl green—pyronine need control experiments in order to be unequivocal. In my opinion, background stains with acid natures, intended to improve the optical qualities of the preparations, should also be handled with circumspection and the results so obtained should be verified, in difficult cases, through the examination of slides which have not undergone such background staining.

As Lison (1960) has commented, absolute basophilia in the sense of Ehrlich, which is manifested with all basic dyes and whatever the conditions under which they are applied, is a rare phenomenon. In most cases, histologists record relative basophilia which may be considerably modified by pretreatments of the tissue or by treatments applied after the stain, in the strict sense of the term.

In fact, the influence of pretreatments on the dyestuff affinities which go to make up the acidophilia and basophilia of structures may be considerable. Fixation does not only act to maintain certain elements of the tissue in position, whereas others are dissolved; the acidophilia and basophilia of the tissue constituents and cell constituents depends to a material extent on the choice of fixatives and the length of time for which they have acted. The way in which the main fixatives maintain dyestuff affinities was mentioned in the first part of this work. It is appropriate, moreover, to mention that the pretreatments to which the sections may be subjected may also modify, in all respects, the dyestuff affinities of any given structure, so that the statement that there is acidophilia or basophilia in a cell constituent takes on a meaning only if the experimental conditions are explicitly stated. In this connection I might recollect that sufficiently lengthy postchromatisation of tissue blocks, such as is practised for the demonstration of chondriome using Altmann's fuchsin or iron haematoxylin, results in the attenuation, or even the disappearance, of basophilia in structures such as the chromatin, nucleoli, and ergastoplasm. Conversely, structures devoid of affinity for basic dyes after certain fixatives have been used may become frankly basiphilic after others. The treatment of sections with a strongly oxidising agent prior to staining confers strong basophilia on many cell constituents and tissue components; the methods for selective staining of certain secretory products depend on this principle. It happens that the number of structures endowed with absolute acidophilia and refractory to basic dyestuffs under any experimental conditions is quite small. The two examples cited by Lison (1960, p. 278) namely the elastic fibres and granulations of eosinophilic leucocytes in Man, can be discounted because permanganate oxidation in an acid medium causes a strong basophilia to appear in both cases. Among the secretory products, that of the A cells of the endocrine pancreas and that of certain cells of the distal lobe of the adenohypophysis represent good examples of absolute acidophilia.

No less important in judging basophilia is the pretreatment to which the sections are subjected after removal from the basic stain. Some background stains can cause the colour obtained to change; treatments with dilute acids or alkalis, such as appear in certain formulae for staining, may abolish or augment the stain. Evidently, dehydration with ethyl alcohol may almost completely extract basic dyes fixed by certain materials, so that it is helpful to look at the sections whilst they are leaving the staining bath, an examination which should be preceded by a brief rinse in distilled water or in a buffer of pH identical with that of the stain. Most modern authors advise one not to use ethyl alcohol in difficult cases but to employ tertiary butyl alcohol which does no damage to the great majority of basic stains. The stained sections' after rinsing, are blotted with tissue paper and treated with two baths of tertiary butyl alcohol; the dehydration is generally complete in about 30 seconds and the sections may be cleared in a benzenoid hydrocarbon. A certain number of basic dyes do not tolerate Canada balsam well, and for their mounting it is useful to use a synthetic resin.

THE PHYSICO-CHEMICAL FACTORS INFLUENCING BASOPHILIA

We know from the survey given above that basophilia is one kind of affinity for dyestuffs; the action of a basic stain on the constituents of tissues and cells cannot be referred to any chemical reaction. The essential factor influencing the uptake of a basic stain by certain structures is, indeed, a simple phenomenon of electropolarity namely, salt formation on acidic groups by a coloured cation, but the intensity of the stain produced depends on many factors and other mechanisms may lead to the uptake of the stain. Modern treatises on histochemistry and the general reviews of Singer (1952, 1954) include many interesting facts, drawn not only from practical histochemistry, but also from experiments with models and experience in the dyestuffs industry. Naturally, only the essential data can be dealt with here.

1° The action of the fixative is known to influence basophilia and has been so since the beginnings of histochemical research; several observable features are mentioned above. We know from the experiments of Singer and Morrison (1948), undertaken with films of fibrin, that the dyestuff affinities of the unfixed model are as weak as are those of tissue proteins in the fresh condition; a clear increase in affinity for all stains resulted from fixation by physical or chemical means. This general effect may be the consequence of physical factors such as spatial rearrangements leading to a greater accessibility of the groups likely to fix the stain.

Molecular rearrangement may also facilitate the penetration of the stain within the network formed by the protein molecules. However, the nature of the fixative is relevant in that it determines the sense in which this increased affinity takes place, and also determines its importance. In this way formalin fixatives favour an affinity for basic dyes; fixing by the salts of heavy metals favours the uptake of acid dyes. Evidently, modifications of the chemical nature of the proteins are responsible for the secondary effect of the fixative.

Ferry and his colleagues (1947) emphasise the great sensitivity of the fibrin they chose as their model towards heat fixation; slight differences in the thermal treatment employed could be detected by a study of the uptake of dyes.

From the practical point of view, the classical results reviewed by Zeiger (1938), together with more modern data, illustrate how lacking in foundation was the old belief in an 'indifferent fixative'. No technique of fixation preserves the dyestuff affinities of the proteins in a condition which corresponds to that found in the living cell, and if ethyl alcohol has been considered by some authors as being, in this respect, the most reliable fixative such an interpretation is simply due to the fact that its action is intermediate between that of formalin and those of the heavy metal salts.

2° The temperature at which the staining takes place does not seem to have held the attention of histologists interested in the affinity for basic dyestuffs. In the vast majority of cases staining by basic dyes is carried out at laboratory temperatures and histological publications are very poor in published data on the effect of the temperature of staining on basophilia. There is, however, a rich literature on this topic from the dyestuffs industry. Vickerstaff's (1950) work summarises what is known and underlines the factors making up this temperature effect; these include modification of the freedom with which the stain diffuses, a change in the affinity of the reactive groups forming part of the stained protein—dyestuff complex, and, lastly, chemical transformations of the stained proteins. The theoretical interest of such data is obvious, but their practical bearing, for the histologist, is rather slight.

3° The effect of the concentration of dye on the total amount fixed by the tissue and cell structures is well known to histologists; it finds expression in the equilibrium between dyes which was examined empirically during the development of combined stains. The quantitative work of Singer and Morrison (1948), using films of fibrin, shows that the total amount of stain fixed by the model increases with the concentration, this finding being as valid for basic as for acidic stains. The limiting factor in deciding the amount so fixed is the 'saturation' of the reactive groups by coloured ions whose uptake would involve electrostatic forces; moreover, the coloured ions already fixed may exert steric or electrostatic hindrance on the other ions of the stain, and thus reduce the extent of their penetration into the structures. It may be useful to recall that changes in the fixation of various dyes as a function of the concentration have been interpreted by Előd (1933) in terms of the Donnan equilibrium.

4° *The type of stain used* plays an essential part in the result of the staining process, and this fact has dominated histological practice since the first attempts selectively to demonstrate certain tissue or cell structures. As Singer (1952) has quite rightly commented, instances of specific or exclusive affinity of proteins for dyes are rare, rather does the affinity vary according to the nature of the dyes used, some being fixed in greater amounts than others. The evaluation of the amount of stain fixed by any given protein as a function of the pH of the staining bath may give rise to curves whose appearance is quite different. To explain such differences, the influence of links other than those of primary valences between the ions of the stain and the stained structure are generally invoked; covalencies and hydrogen bonds may play an important part. Other authors (see, in particular, Steinhardt, 1942) take into account the degree of dissociation of the combination between the protein and the ionised dyestuff. Moreover, experience in the dyestuffs industry shows that the affinity increases with molecular weight and with the introduction into the molecule of the dye of new polar groups. Naturally, the number and nature of the reactive groups of the dye molecule also play a part.

5° *The ionic strength of the dye solution* has clear effects on the amount fixed by proteins of cations or anions. Generally speaking, the fixation of ions diminishes with increasing ionic strength of the dye solution. In conformity with the old explanation given by Előd (1933) one of the reasons for this phenomenon resides in changes of the equilibrium between the dye remaining in the medium and that in the protein itself; in conformity with Donnan's theory, the effective concentration of dyestuff ions, that is to say that concentration which is to be found in the structure to be stained, varies inversely with the ionic strength of the dye solution.

On the other hand, the hypothesis of competition between the dyestuff ions and the other ions to be found in the solution cannot be rejected. Furthermore, ionised salts suppress the electrostatic forces of the proteins, so that the attraction for anionic stains below the isoelectric point, and for cationic ones above it, diminishes, (Neale, 1946, 1947). In agreement with the remarks made by Michaelis (1947), the presence of salts in the solution favours the aggregation of the dye into particles of colloidal size, thus reducing their penetration within the structures whose staining is sought.

6° *The pH of the staining bath* is one of the vital factors in staining, and is a factor whose importance was intuitively seized upon by histologists at the end of the 19th century; the empirical formulae put forward at that time for the regulation of basic or acid stains included, in the majority of instances, accentuators or moderators of the stain. Mann (1902) stresses the fact that those compounds which accentuate basic dyestuffs are alkaline (sodium or potassium hydroxydes, sodium borate, sodium bicarbonate, soap, pyridine), those which favour the uptake of acid stains being themselves acid (phenol, acetic acid, sulphuric and oxalic acids, etc. . . .).

The first systematic study of ways of modifying the staining of tissue sections by changing the acidity of the stain solution are due to Bethe (1905) who used solutions of toluidine blue of constant concentration but to which suitably chosen amounts of acetic acid or of soda had been added. These experiments showed that alkalinity favoured the stain, which became diffuse once a certain level of alkalinity had been reached, whereas acidity restricted the uptake of the stain by certain structures and weakened the intensity of the stain. Such data were interpreted by Michaelis (1920) in the light of the data available at that time concerning the amphoteric nature of proteins; Thomas and Kelly (1922), Stearn and Stearn (1924 to 1928) and

Robbins (1923 to 1926) confirm these findings in the fields of animal histology, bacteriology, and botany.

In 1926 Pischinger suggested that staining with acid and basic dyes in buffered solutions of increasing pH values could be used for the determination of the isoelectric point of the tissue elements. A quantitative study of the fixation of stains by gelatin and ovalbumin shows that basic stains are not fixed below a pH corresponding to the isoelectric point; at higher pH values, the amount of stain fixed by the models increases regularly; conversely, acid stains are only taken up by proteins when the pH of the solution is lower than the isoelectric point. Applicatons to sections of mammalian tissue give results of the same order.

Numerous investigations serve to confirm Pischinger's views in their generality. In addition to publications which relate to the strictly histochemical applications of the method, we might in particular mention experiments with fibrin films (Singer and Morrison, 1948; Singer, 1952) which permits of a convenient and quantitative investigation of the influence of the pH of the dye solution on the uptake of acid and basic stains. Such experiments show that the pH of the solution is not the only factor to influence the fixation of stains, but that it can be considered as playing the principal role in the phenomenon.

This action of the pH is easy to interpret if we take into account the amphoteric nature of the tissue proteins. In fact, dissociation of the acid groups takes place when the pH of the solution is above the isoelectric point, so that it becomes possible to satisfy them by salt formation with cationic stains (basophilia); conversely, it is the basic groups which are ionised at pH values lower than the isoelectric point; a salt formation with anionic stains (acidophilia) can take place at the isoelectric point, the dissociation of the two kinds of groups is minimal, so that any clear affinity for acid or basic stains is absent. Naturally, a compound which carries strongly acid groups will remain basophilic even at very low pH values, and the presence of very strong basic groups will confer an acidophilia on the structures which will persist despite a relatively high pH of the staining solution.

Objectively, the practical application of Pischinger's method cannot be considered as a measurement in the sense which a physicist would give to the term. Amongst the reserves we may feel constrained to admit, some relate to the preparation of the tissue blocks and sections, others to the technique of evaluation itself.

Obviously, Pischinger's method is practically always applied to fixed tissue and the dénaturation of the proteins which is the principal phenomenon in histological fixation inevitably has its effects on the isoelectric point of these compounds. Pischinger's opinion, which was still reiterated by Zeiger (1938), that fixing in ethyl alcohol had no effect on the isoelectric point of the proteins, cannot now be substantiated, every form of fixation modifies the isoelectric point, but the shift resulting from the use of any given fixative occurs in a well-defined sense, and even its magnitude varies a little from one experiment to another. Naturally enough, the shift in question can take place in the same sense in respect of several tissue proteins, or in mutually opposed senses.

As for our reservations about the method of evaluation itself we need to consider the multiplicity of factors which condition the uptake of the acidic or basic stain by the proteins of the tissue. Certain physico-chemical factors other than pH of the stain-bath have been dealt with in the preceding sections; their very existence persuades us of the polyfactorial nature of the phenomenon. Indeed, experience shows that Pischinger's method, when compared with electrocatophoresis, shows substantial deviations when the two methods are applied to purified proteins. Levene (1940) considers these differences to be some two units, but the more recent work of Singer and Morrison (1948), in which films of fibrin were used, discloses much smaller deviations of approximately half a unit. As Singer (1952) has remarked, the deviation between the results of the two methods varies with the stain used

In consequence, Pischinger's method cannot be considered as a "measure of the isoelectric point" of the tissue proteins. The terms "isoelectric zone" (Stearn, 1933) or "isoelectric band" (Naylor, 1926) are more suitable. This terminology has the advantage over that of Lison (1960, pp. 327-333) who spoke of an "estimate purporting to be the isoelectric point", of being more euphonious and of indicating the sense of the restriction we wish to formulate.

THE DETECTION OF BASOPHILIA FOR HISTOCHEMICAL PURPOSES

The reserves formulated in the preceding sections show how impossible it is to deduce the basophilic nature of a cell or tissue constiuent, in the course of a histochemical investigation, from the results of a topological stain which uses both a basic dye and an acid dye. It is proper to take into account the conditions under which fixation was done, to avoid any pretreatment of the sections liable to induce the appearance of a basophilia which did not previously exist, unless, of course, such an event constitutes one of the objectives of the work, and to choose appropriately the conditions for the staining process itself.

In the majority of cases, in order to demonstrate basophilia, we use thiazine dyes (azur A, B, C, methylene blue, toluidine blue, thionine). Toluidine blue is the most widely used. All these stains give rise to the phenomenon of metachromasia, in such a way that their use under the conditions discussed above is confounded with the practice of the metachromatic reaction. The use of a rather dilute solution (0.1 to 0.5%) is advised by the majority of authors. An essential choice concerns the pH of the solution; some of the basophilic compounds we need to consider in animal histology show this dyestuff affinity even at the lowest pH values of the stain bath (sulpho-mucopolysaccharides, nucleic acids, derivatives of oxidised lipids); in other instances, a clearcut basophilia appears only at pH values near 4 (uric acid, the carboxyl groups of proteins and of certain carbohydrates). We should, obviously, choose a pH under 5, a value which is close to the isoelectric point of most tissue proteins, so as to obtain sufficiently selective stains. Most authors advise one to work at a pH of 4.6 or 4.2; the second of these values seems to me to be the better one.

The staining process itself is followed by a rapid rinse in a buffer of the same pH as that of the stain bath; the preparation is then examined as a temporary measure. When mounting is preceded by dehydration in ethanol, it is most helpful to pass the stained sections through a 5% solution of ammonium molybdate, as this compound has the property of rendering dyes of the thiazine group insoluble, and of increasing their resistance to extraction by ethyl alcohol. Careful washing should obviously be employed to remove the excess of ammonium molybdate, which is insoluble in alcohol.

Reagents:

a solution 0.2% of toluidine blue, or of another thiazine, in Walpole's buffer. pH 4.2 (1.2% acetic acid, 73 ml: 2.7% solution of sodium acetate trihydrate, 23 ml);
a 5% solution of ammonium molybdate in distilled water;

Working technique:

> dewaxed sections, treated with collodion where appropriate, and hydrated (the method is applicable to frozen sections and to celloidin sections, adhering to slides and freed from the embedding medium);
> Stain with a solution of toluidine blue at pH 4.2 for 5 minutes;
> rinse rapidly in the buffer;
> examine under the microscope, covering with a coverslip should the high power be required;
> treat for 5 minutes with the ammonium molybdate solution;
> wash for three to five minutes in running water;
> dehydrate in absolute alcohol, clear in a benzenoid hydrocarbon, mount in a synthetic resin or, if necessary, in Canada balsam.

When dehydration is undertaken using tertiary butyl alcohol, it is pointless to pass the sections through ammonium molybdate; the sections should then be blotted with tissue paper, treated with two baths of tertiary butyl alcohol, (20 seconds in each bath), then cleared and mounted.

The presence of basophilic substances is shown by a blue colour (orthochromatic), a violet one (β-metachromasia) or a reddish purple one (γ-metachromasia).

LOCALISATION OF THE TISSUE ZONE CONTAINING PROTEINS AT THE ISOELECTRIC POINT

Various procedures which have been put forward differ from the original one of Pischinger in details (choice of buffers, concentration of the stains, durations of staining). Methylene blue is the most widely adopted of the basic stains; as for the acid stain, some authors employ cyanol, but most prefer crystal ponceau. The working technique recommended here follows Lipp's procedure (1954).

Reagents:

> stock solution of methylene blue (dissolve 0.13 g of Analar methylene blue in 100 ml of boiled distilled water);
> stock solution of crystal ponceau (dissolve 0.18 g of crystal ponceau in 100 ml of boiled distilled water;
> Michaelis' sodium veronal—acetate buffer (p. 000); it is advisable to choose a range of pH values between 2 and 7, increasing the values by 0.25 units per slide;
> a 5% solution of ammonium molybdate.

Working technique:

> paraffin wax sections, floating on distilled water, dewaxed, treated with collodion where appropriate, and hydrated;
> stain the slide carrier bearing the serial sections with neighbouring ones close to one another, duly labelled, by the mixture
>
> > stock solution of methylene blue $\}$ equal parts
> > buffers
> >
> > *or*
> >
> > stock solution of crystal ponceau $\}$ equal parts
> > buffers
> >
> > for 10 minutes
>
> rinse rapidly with the mixture
>
> > buffer of pH equal to that of the stain bath $\}$ equal parts
> > distilled boiled water
>
> treat the stained slides with methylene blue using the ammonium molybdate solution applied for 10 minutes; follow this treatment by washing for 2 to 5 minutes in distilled water, renewed;
> Blot, dehydrate in absolute alcohol, clear, and mount in a synthetic resin or, if need be, in Canada balsam.

Slides stained with crystal ponceau should be dehydrated and mounted after the rinse, as the stain is insoluble in ethyl alcohol. When dehydration is carried out using tertiary butyl alcohol, no useful purpose is served by passing the slides through ammonium molybdate solution and the slides stained with methylene blue should also be mounted after rinsing and a rapid wiping with tissue paper.

The method is applicable to frozen sections; these should be treated with the stain solution for about 5 minutes, rinsed in buffers diluted with equal volumes of distilled water, freshly boiled, and then mounted in a medium miscible with water. It should be emphasised that such mounting is rapidly deleterious to the preservation of methylene blue stains, so that the preparations should soon be examined. The results depend, as has been mentioned above, on the quality of the fixation. Absolute alcohol is now almost abandoned; most workers use formalin-treated alcohol (Schaeffer's formula), formalin itself, Bouin's fluid, or Zenker's fluid (for short periods of action).

The working technique recommended by Singer and his colleagues (Dempsey and Singer, 1946; Dempsey, Wislocki and Singer, 1946; Singer and Wislocki, 1948) differs from that of Pischinger in using more dilute stain solutions and longer staining periods (24 hours at constant temperatures) so as to be sure of realising the equilibrium adsorption of the stain.

The examination of the preparations allows us to judge the intensity of the staining of the structures under investigation, whether by methylene blue or crystal ponceau, taking into account the pH of the stain bath. A greatly strengthened uptake of acid dyestuffs at low pH values, and of basic dyestuffs at high pH values, is evident from macroscopic inspection of the slides. The intensity of the stain obtained can be judged by reference to a subjective scale, by reference to graded colour charts, by using an ocular comparison, or even by histophotometry. Obviously, the last method is the most precise, but it requires work on sections whose thickness is rigorously controlled, and this degree of equality may be hard to attain using frozen sections.

In any event, the pH zone corresponding to the disappearance of the affinity for crystalline ponceau, and the appearance of that for methylene blue, is, subject to the reservations we formulated above, the approximate site of the isoelectric point of the amphoteric constituents of the tissue. Structures containing strongly acid groups retain their basophilia at pH values at the bottom of the range indicated above, and the converse is true for structures containing free, and strongly ionised, basic groups.

THE HISTOCHEMICAL INTERPRETATION OF BASOPHILIA IN TISSUE

Provided that it is observed under conditions compatible with histochemical interpretation, that is to say without any prolonged fixing in an oxidising medium, without any special pretreatment of the sections, and following progressive staining with a dyestuff of the thionine group operating at a pH lower than the isoelectric point of common tissue proteins, basophilia represents definite evidence for the presence of a certain number of compounds in the stained structures. The principal among these compounds are polysaccharides bearing acid groups, nucleic acids, certain compounds derived from the oxidation of lipids, and, lastly, uric acid and its derivatives. Supplementary tests, which have been set out in this work wherever we have discussed the histochemical detection of the compounds just listed, enable us to confirm their presence. Moreover, the nature of the basophilia affords clues as to their nature.

Among the polysaccharides with an acid group, the sulphomucopolysaccharides are characterised by a very strong metachromatic basophilia which still shows up even at pH values so low that all other basophilic tissue constituents stain either feebly or not at all. The basophilia of carbohydrates which carry solely the carboxyl radical is slighter; it does not become clearly apparent until pH values close to 4 are approached, and the metachromasia is often less pronounced.

The nucleic acids are characterised by a clear basophilia even at pH values less than 3; whether the stain obtained in structures containing these substances is orthochromatic or metachromatic has given rise to numerous discussions; the essential facts are summarised in the section dealing with metachromasia.

The compounds derived from the oxidation of lipids, in particular the chromolipids, are characterised by a clear basophilia at pH values between 2.5 and

3, and this is orthochromatic; in most instances, the stain obtained with basic dyes stands up well to extraction with dilute acid, such acid resistance being a distinctive feature which is useful in practical work.

Uric acid and its derivatives do not become basophilic except at pH values around 4; the basophilia is orthochromatic and the identification of the compounds responsible for it may be less easy than in other cases.

Summarising the facts just enunciated, basophilia, in all cases, discloses the presence of anionic groups (the phosphoric acid of nucleic acids, the sulphate or carboxyl of mucopolysaccharides, the keto-acid of chromolipids, the carboxyl of uric acid, and urates).

A large number of marker stains and histochemical reactions depend on the conversion of a radical of the molecule to be detected into an acid group, or upon fixing an acid group, borne by the reagent, to the molecule which we need to detect. Such procedures are dealt with in relation to the compounds whose detection they permit.

THE HISTOCHEMICAL STUDY OF METACHROMASIA

In conformity with the definition given by Ehrlich (1877) metachromasia consists of a state of affairs in which the stain obtained in certain structures is to some extent distinct in colour from that of the dye solution. The compounds present in the sections, which may give rise to this shift in colour, are designated by the name of chromotropes, the dyes which undergo the shift bear the name of metachromatic stains. The term metachromotropy is often employed by modern authors in place of metachromasia.

The phenomenon which has just been defined was discovered simultaneously, in 1875, by Ranvier, Cornil, Jürgens and Heschl in relation to an example which has been little studied since then, namely, the metachromatic stain of the amyloid substance after treatment of the sections with dahlia violet, and crystal violet, compounds which belong to the triphenylmethane group. Ehrlich (1877) reported the first instances of metachromatic staining using thiazine, and put forward the terms orthochromatic and metachromatic stains.

From that time onwards, our knowledge of metachromasia evolved in two periods, the first of which was characterised by the progressively growing interest, leading research workers to become physico-chemically oriented; the names of Michaelis and Holmes emerge from the substantial number of publications with this orientation. During the same period histologists, on the contrary, used metachromatic stains for purely morphological purposes and seemed indifferent to their chemical significance.

The second period of development of our knowledge of metachromasia, which was histochemical in the proper sense of the term, opened with the researches of Lison (1933 to 1935) Taking up methodically the survey of a large number of basic stains, Lison defined the chemical conditions required of a stain in order to give rise to the phenomenon of metachromasia. Tests *in vitro* and on sections led to the discovery of the nature of the main group of chromotropic substances in the vertebrate body, namely, the sulphomucopolysaccharides.

Very many studies have confirmed the essential findings of Lison; moreover, theoretical investigations on the phenomenon of metachromasia greatly enriched our knowledge of the mechanisms involved and of the significance of metachromasia arising after the use of basic dyes. The totality of our knowledge is considerable; even to summarise it would exceed the scope of this work, and would, indeed, be futile since most works on histochemistry devote long sections to developing this question and there are excellent general reviews, notably those of Kramer and Windrum (1955), Kelly (1956), Schubert and Hamerman (1956), Bergeron and Singer (1958), Vitry (1958), and Romhany (1963) which greatly facilitate a search of the literature. Only the essential theoretical ideas are, therefore, summarily set out here prior to the description of the methods for studying metachromasia and for interpreting the results so obtained.

METACHROMATIC STAINS

The phenomenon of metachromasia may take place either when acid or basic stains are applied, but only the latter needs to be dealt with here, within the framework of histochemical techniques.

Basic stains capable of showing the metachromatic phenomenon are numerous and varied; to follow Kelly's (1956) system, the belong to one of several groups according to their chromophores, (azines, oxazines, thiazines, xanthenes, azodyes, quinoleines, triphenylmethanes). In practice, it is the stains of the thiazine group that are used in the great majority of cases and most of the physico-chemical studies of the mechanism of metachromasia have dealt with stains of this group. The auxochrome is, in all cases, the free or substituted amine group. The anion of the stain (chloride, acetate, sulphate etc...) seems to play no part in it.

We know from Lison's investigations (1935) that quite closely related substances, from a chemical point of view, may have essentially different properties so far as metachromasia is concerned. The study of a large number of basic stains led Lison to put forward the following rules:

— to be metachromatic, a stain should have at least one unsubstituted amine group;
— to be metachromatic, a stain should be capable of being transformed into an imine base different in colour from the staining salt.

The first of these two rules has been verified in every case; as for the second, it would lead us to exclude methylene blue from the list of metachromatic stains, since it gives an ammonium base and not an imine base. *In vitro* experiments and histochemical usage in respect of this latter stain have given such a large number of contradictory opinions that it may be useful to mention the essential grounds for the debate, all the more so because methylene blue is so prominent in histochemical technology.

The histological application of methylene blue for tests of metachromasia leads to results which seem to confirm the rule enunciated by Lison; in fact, most authors emphasise the slight practical value of the results obtained and do not recommend its use; some say that it is a non-metachromatic stain (Gomori, 1951; Lillie, 1951); others grant its metachromatic nature, but recognise the lack of clarity of the colour shift, and, furthermore, the practical disadvantages of its use (Singer and his colleagues, 1951; Wislocki and Singer, 1950). We should stress that the results just outlined are valuable in as much as the authors quoted have sought to use samples of the stain which were, as far as could be ascertained, pure. Patently, even the usage of the term 'metachromasia' implies that the result has been obtained with the aid of a stain of unimpeachable purity. The staining of certain structures by an impurity of the sample used, an impurity not evident on visual examination of the solution, was called allochromasia by Michaelis (1903).

Nevertheless, *in vitro* studies conducted with all possible care show that the absorption spectral curve of methylene blue, to which a chromotropic substance has been added, has a maximum displaced towards the longer waves, a phenomenon which characterises metachromatic stains (Schubert and Hamerman, 1956; Bergeron and Singer, 1958, Romhany, 1963). Thus, from the point of view of *in vitro* work, we may legitimately consider methylene blue as a metachromatic stain, and this finding is all the more interesting because this thiazine is much easier to synthesize and to purify than any of the others. The disagreement which appears, as between the spectrophotometric data on the one hand and the results of practical histology on the other, is easily explicable; it so happens that the deviation between the orthochromatic and metachromatic colours is much less marked for methylene blue (665 for the orthochromatic, 570 for the metachromatic, i. e. a shift of 95 mμ) than for toluidine blue or azur A (from 630 to 480 mμ).

The practical corollary of these observations is the slight interest attaching to methylene blue as a stain for eliciting metachromasia on sections. The excellent results obtained with certain commercial samples is simply accounted for, in terms of contamination by other thiazines, in particular by azur A, B, or C (di-, tri-, or mono-methylthionine). Whilst we are on this subject, it seems useful to recollect the empirical formulae put forward by Unna (1891 and numerous later publications) with the aim of increasing the metachromatic stain produced by methylene blue. Polychrome methylene blue and blue polychrome (a term whose usual French translation "bleu polychrome" is an error sanctioned by use) are, in fact, solutions of methylene blue and of methylene and toluidine blues, warmed with potassium carbonate so that azur and methylene violet are formed.

If the number of stains capable of showing up the presence of chromotropic substances is, therefore, rather large, only toluidine blue and azur A, which are chemically closely related, can specifically be recommended for histochemical use; thionine may also be of service in this respect; the other stains are used only quite occasionally by modern authors.

THE MECHANISM OF METACHROMASIA

Most investigations concerning the physico-chemical mechanism of metachromasia take account of results obtained with solutions of metachromatic dyes; such working conditions are obviously much more favourable to quantitative study than are the stains of histological preparations. We can only sketch these different conceptions of the problem in the most summary way in this work; the reviews cited at the beginning of this section provide a rich introduction to the literature on this subject.

The older ideas of Michaelis (1910) and of Holmes (1924 to 1928) who considered that there was a close relationship between metachromasia in the histologist's sense on the one hand, and the behaviour of metachromatic stains in solution on the other, have been confirmed, by Lison (1933 to 1935) and all modern authors following him.

A spectrophotometric study shows that solutions of metachromatic stains do not follow the Lambert-Beer law, and that the colour changes considerably with the concentration, whereas this law is respected, within certain limits, when the liquid phase is non-aqueous (ethyl alcohol, acetic acid, etc. ...). Moreover, Lison's investigations (1935) showed that it was possible to produce the colour shift of metachromasia *in vitro*, by the addition of chromotropic substances some of which are active at astonishingly low concentrations. Such action is not stoichiometric and many factors (temperature, saline concentration of the medium, etc. ...) act jointly with the chromotropic substance.

Among the various explanations for the phenomenon of metachromasia in solution, the older theories regarding selective adsorption of the free base of the stain were founded exclusively on the examination of sections (Hansen, Pappenheim) or on the existence of several tautomeric forms of the stain; these explanations are no longer considered valid. The polymerisation theory, developed by Michaelis (1944), and by Michaelis and Granick (1945) was once fashionable. On this theory, the monomeric form corresponds to the orthochromatic colour, the dimeric form to what histochemists call β-metachromasia and the trimeric form to the histologists' γ-metachromasia. It is relevant to mention that these symbols do not have the same significance as the Greek letters used to designate the bands of the absorption spectrum of metachromatic stains, but that it happens to be expedient to retain their use in the language of histochemists (Pearse, 1960).

As Lison (1960) has remarked, the polymerisation theory rests on indirect arguments alone, and explains inadequately certain features of the phenomenon, in particular the abolition of metachromasia in solution by the addition of salts, which is a modification which ought to favour the aggregation of the particles of the stain. Similarly, the polymerisation theory cannot account for the suppression of metachromasia by the heat treatment of histological preparations.

A more recent interpretation proposed by Bergeron and Singer (1958) involves the concept of mesomerism. These authors comment that the methylene blue, which was used by them during work on metachromasia in solution and on metachromatic staining of fibrin films or histological sections, exists in three resonance hybrid forms, and that changes in the distribution of the charges in these hybrids may lie at the origin of metachromasia.

The explanation of metachromatic staining of certain structures in histological preparations must evidently take into account the data concerning metachromasia in solution. The fixation of anions of the stain on the structures is determined in the first place by the presence of anionic groups. It is to Lison's (1933 to 1935) investigations that we owe the first unequivocal demonstration of the strongly acid nature of groups which fix cationic stains under the conditions of the metachromatic reaction. As for the appearance of the metachromatic colour, most modern authors are in agreement that the essential factor is a certain density of acid groups on the stained structure. In this way hyaluronic acid, whose carboxyl groups are separated by intervals of some 10 Å, does not give rise to the metachromatic phenomenon in solution and its demonstration on sections by means of the metachromatic reaction has given rise to discussions full of contradictions. A weak metachromasia exists in the case of pectic acid, whose carboxyl groups are separated by some 5 Å; this metachromasia is very strong in the case of the mucopolysaccharides, in which the sulphate groups are separated by distances less than 4 Å. Since a local concentration of cations of the stain is obtained in this way, water molecules are immobilised between these cations and, because of their dipole nature, play an important role in the interactions between auxochrome groups terminal to the cations of the stain.

It is appropriate to recall the results of recent experiments by Kisser (1969) which might have the effect of throwing our interpretation of metachromasia back into the melting pot. This author reports that the addition of soda or of other strong alkalis to a solution of toluidine blue induces the same metachromasia as does that of a pentosan-polysulphoester. A spectroscopic study of the solutions shows that the absorption maximum undergoes the same displacement in both instances. Kisser agrees that the stain, when in alkaline media, represents a base in Brönstedt's definition, whereas when in acid media it represents an acid. In either case, the presence of mesomeric ions accounts for the colour, and the metachromasia, which is caused by the appearance of quinonoid structures, may be evidence either of the occurrence of anionic radicals, or of that of strong cationic radicals. It hardly needs to be added that further work along these lines would be highly desirable.

The recent work of Romhany (1963) illustrates the importance of the orientation of the stain cations on metachromatic structural elements. Studies of several subjects revealed to this author that a close parallel existed between the metachromasia itself, and the dichroism and metachromatic birefringence of the structures, giving rise to the hypothesis that the metachromatic reaction demonstrates an inframicroscopic anisotropy of the structures which are stained.

From the practical point of view, the analysis of the metachromatic phenomenon leads us to regard it as evidence of great value demonstrating the presence of terminal electronegative groups in the stained structures; these groups are capable of reacting and are distributed in such a manner that their density exceeds a certain threshold value.

THE PRACTICAL CONDUCT OF THE METACHROMATIC REACTION

Theoretical considerations obviously influence the working technique to choose for research on metachromatic compounds in histological preparations.

The importance attaching to the choice of stain goes without saying; most authors use toluidine blue; the azurs of methylene, notably azur A and thionine, are also used in current work. Among the other substances employed, we may mention methylene blue, crystal violet, pinacyanol, safranin, methyl violet, celestin blue, vesuvine (Bismark brown), cresyl violet and gallocyanine. In fact, these stains have no practical advantage over toluidine blue; nevertheless, they enter into numerous formulations for stains and it is, in consequence, useful to recall that the fact that a metachromatic stain has been obtained during the application of the procedures in question may well reorient the investigation.

Divergent opinions exist as to the concentrations of stain to be used; recent publications contain all intermediate values between very dilute solutions (0.01%) and relatively concentrated ones (0.5%). The duration of staining should be all the longer if the stain solution is weak. As for the pH of this solution, most authors adopt phosphate or acetate buffers whose pH values lie between 3 and 5.

Much importance attaches to the treatment to which the sections are subjected after staining in the strict sense of the term. The theoretical data allow us to understand the action of dehydration by ethanol on certain metachromatic structures and it is indispensible to examine, in all cases, the sections as they emerge from the stain bath, in case there is any subsequent modification of the staining during dehydration or mounting. Some authors advise one to mount all such preparations in media miscible with water, but thiazine stains keep very poorly under these conditions. The effect of alcoholic dehydration on the metachromatic stain of certain structures has been erected into a criterion for the differentiation between 'true' metachromasia and 'false' metachromasia. In any event, this effect should be taken into account during the interpretation of the preparations (Sylven, 1941, 1945; Kelly, 1956; Pearse, 1960).

The standard working technique recommended for tests involving basophilia (p. 339) is entirely suitable for routine work on the metachromatic reaction. Subsequent adjustments may be required for detailed studies (modification of the pH of the stain bath, reduction of the concentration of toluidine blue).

Compounds of the pseudo-isocyanine group were, at one time after 1957, fashionable as metachromatic stains. These compounds are interesting from the theoretical standpoint because the mechanism of their metachromasia has been carefully investigated and brought to light by Scheibe and his colleagues (see, in particular, Scheibe, 1937, 1938; Zimmermann and Scheibe, 1956; Schauer and Scheibe, 1958). This metachromasia depends on a reversible polymerisation of the molecule of the stain, a polymerisation which is detected by the appearance of a highly characteristic and very narrow absorption band, at 573 mμ, as well as by a yellow fluorescence.

From a practical point of view, we may mention that this metachromasia is not particularly helpful from the optical aspect, when the preparations are examined in white light, but that it becomes of the greatest clarity when monochromatic light, of the wavelength required, is employed, or when the work is pursued under the fluorescence microscope. Among the practical applications, the most important ones concern not the detection of mucins, but that of anionic groups which appear in secretory products (the beta-granules of the endocrine pancreas, the neurosecretory product of the hypothalamus) after energetic oxidation. These applications are discussed in the last part of this book.

HISTOCHEMICAL INTERPRETATION OF THE METACHROMATIC REACTION

If we observe a metachromatic stain under well defined experimental conditions (the use of a sufficiently dilute solution of a pure dye, a pH sufficiently low in that solution, adequate preservation of the stain after mounting) in certain structures, we can be sure of the presence of anionic groups set rather closely to one another. It may be diagnostic of a fair number of compounds; the distinction between the various chemical substances which might be responsible depends partly on other reactions or marker stains, which are not considered here, and on the characteristics of the metachromasia obtained.

The **sulphomucopolysaccharides** were the earliest known among the chromotropic compounds (Lison, 1935; Jorpes and Bergström, 1937). Their presence in sections is disclosed by a strong red or purple metachromasia (called γ-metachromasia) which is evident even if the pH of the solution of the dye is very low. The metachromatic stain withstands the dehydration by ethyl alcohol, and such alcohol resistance has been considered by some workers as being a criterion for the infallible identification of true metachromasia. In fact, the action of alcohol on stained sections is complicated, because not only may it suppress the metachromasia, but also it may extract the dye, so that a measure of prudence is appropriate in interpreting this action. Moreover, the metachromasia caused by sulphomucopolysaccharides occurs if a small amount of 0.001 N uranyl or barium nitrate is added to the stain, but it disappears if the concentration of these salts attains O.1N.

Mucopolysaccharides bearing carboxyl groups give a weak metachromasia which is violet in colour (called β-metachromasia); this does not usually withstand dehydration by alcohol and does not appear if the pH of the stain bath is below 3.4. The addition of a small amount of uranyl or barium nitrate (0.001 N) suppresses the metachromasia due to these compounds.

Nucleic acids were considered for a long time not to be chromotropes. In fact, their phosphoric radicals may lie behind a metachromasia whose expression may be most complicated (Lison and Mutsaars, 1948; Flax and Hilmes, 1952) and whose practical importance is slight.

Macromolecular metaphosphates whose degree of condensation is greater than 8 (Ebel and Müller, 1958) give rise to the metachromatic phenomenon; the typical example is that of the volutine granules in yeasts (Wiame, 1946). This metachromasia is strong and shows up even if the pH of the stain bath is less than 3.4; it also withstands dehydration by alcohol well; it does not appear when the staining solution contains 0.001N uranyl nitrate but can be obtained in the presence of the same molarity of barium nitrate.

Certain **lipids** are metachromatic; this characteristic is only found in frozen sections and the characteristic stain usually only appears after a rather prolonged duration of staining. The metachromasia in question does not withstand dehydration by alcohol and obviously is not to be seen if the lipids have previously been extracted from the sections. According to circumstances, it may be caused by sulphate or phosphate radicals.

OTHER STAINS INDICATIVE OF THE PRESENCE OF ANIONS

It seems appropriate to bring together at this point a certain number of stains brought into use in the last few years, the results of using which to some extent relate to those obtained from tests for metachromasia or basophilia. All the methods in question are indicative of the presence of anionic radicals in the stained structures, whether these exist spontaneously or are caused to appear by appropriate pretreatments. The results given by the stains in question can almost always be reproduced by the use of one of the classical basic stains, but the selectivity with which stained structures can be demonstrated is often greater and easier to obtain. This amounts to saying that the stains to be discussed have some of the properties of the classical basic stains, but differ from them in other ways. The range of action of the stains with which we are concerned here is too extensive for any positive reaction to be attributed to the presence of any given compound, or even a family of chemical compounds; it is only by taking into consideration the experimental conditions under which the affinity for dyes has been observed, and by resorting to supplementary histochemical reactions and marker stains that the results we are discussing can be interpreted in chemical terms.

The prototype of stains in this group is paraldehyde-fuchsin; it is, indeed, the ony one mentioned by Lison (1960) in this connection. Nevertheless, other stains require mention here. Paraldehyde-thionine (Paget, 1959) has all the staining properties of paraldehyde-fuchsin; in addition, some phthalocyanins (alcian blue, alcian green, alcian yellow) have special properties which lead us to include, at this point, a discussion of their use in histological technique.

PARALDEHYDE-FUCHSIN

Since its discovery by Gomori (1950) paraldehyde-fuchsin has been used by many authors, either for purely morphological purposes, or with a histochemical orientation. The publications of Halmi and Davis (1953), Scott (1953), Scott and Clayton (1953), Gastaldi (1954), Bangle (1954, 1956), Braun-Falco (1955, 1956), Landing, Hall and West (1956) and Konecny and Pliczka (1958) are directed towards the histochemical interpretation of the results obtained by this technique.

The stain

In the original method of Gomori (1950) the stain was prepared by adding 1 ml of concentrated hydrochloric acid and 1 ml of paraldehyde to 100 ml of a solution 0.5% of basic fuchsin in 70% alcohol. Under these conditions, we observe a progressive colour shift from red to violet; after two or three days, the staining properties of the basic fuchsin have quite disappeared, and the new material proves to be endowed with a strong affinity for a whole range of structures, in particular elastic fibres and acid mucopolysaccharides. Suitably chosen pretreatments allow us to stain certain secretory products with perfect selectivity, notably those which acquire a more or less marked basophilia subsequent to these pretreatments. Nevertheless this stain only keeps the entire range of its properties as a dye for a relatively short period (about 8 days).

The chemical reactions which take place during the preparation of Gomori's version of paraldehyde-fuchsin have been worked out by Bangle (1954). According to this author, each molecule of paraldehyde, in the presence of the hydrochloric acid acting as a catalyst, gives three molecules of acetaldehyde, capable of reacting with the amine groups of pararosaniline chlorhydrate (basic fuchsin) to form Schiff bases (azomethines). The compounds so formed are related, as their formulae indicate, to dyestuffs of the methyl violet family, the last term in the series characterised by the substitution of all the amine groups of the pararosaniline molecule being crystal violet (hexamethylated violet). This transformation is progressive; the substitution of three amine groups of the pararosaniline molecule causes that substance to lose its properties as a cationic dye, which explains its poor keeping qualities as a stain.

$$(CH_3 CHO)_3 \xrightarrow{HCl} 3\ CH_3 CHO$$

Paraldehyde → Acetaldehyde

Pararosaniline + 2 CH_3 CHO ⟶

Paraldehyde-fuchsin + 2 H_2O

These chemical data serve as an *a posteriori* justification for the way of separating out pure, stable, samples of paraldehyde-fuchsin which was first suggested on an empirical basis (Gabe, 1953). The procedure in question puts to good use the insolubility of paraldehyde-fuchsin in water, and consists of extracting the stain, as and when it is formed, from the substances which give rise to it (hydrochloric acid, paraldehyde). This objective is attained by conducting the preparation not in 70% alcohol but in distilled water; the three substances which are to react are soluble in water, but the product of their reaction, which is insoluble, is precipitated. In this way we can eliminate the last stage of the reaction, which is the substitution of the third amine radical of the pararosaniline, rendering the product unsuitable for the purposes considered here.

The working technique is of the simplest: 100 ml of a 0.5% aqueous solution of basic fuchsin are added to 1 ml concentrated hydrochloric acid and 1 ml of paraldehyde. The mixture is left to stand at laboratory temperatures and the progress of the reaction followed by capillary analysis, by dropping a drop of the liquid on a sheet of filter paper; the paraldehyde-fuchsin forms the central stain, surrounded by a red ring which corresponds to the as yet unreacted basic fuchsin. When the ring has almost entirely disappeared or when its extent and its colour do not change, the reaction is arrested by filtration, the precipitate being freed from the excess of paraldehyde and hydrochloric acid by washing with distilled water, followed by drying in an oven at 60°. It can be preserved in the dry state or dissolved in 70% alcohol. Its stability is great; the first samples so prepared (December 1952) have kept to this day (November 1967) all their staining capacity.

Experiments carried out since then have shown how advantageous it is to prepare paraldehyde-fuchsin from chemically pure pararosaniline and not from a commercial sample of basic fuchsin, which almost never consists of pure pararosaniline chlorhydrate. The only modification that needs to be added to the working technique described above is to double the amount of hydrochloric acid so as to ensure that the pararosaniline is transformed into the chlorhydrate. The sequence, then, is to dissolve 1 g of chemically pure pararosaniline (a substance insoluble in distilled water) in 200 ml of 2% hydrochloric acid, adding 2 ml of paraldehyde. The reaction is generally complete in 48 hours, and its yield is excellent, 1 g of pararosaniline giving about 1 g of dry paraldehydefuchsin.

About 0.5% serves to saturate 70% alcohol, which acts as the stock solution; I advise working with a 0.125% solution obtained by diluting the saturated stock solution with three parts of 70% alcohol. or by dissolving directly 0.125 g of the stain in 100 ml of 70% alcohol. Experience shows that paraldehyde-fuchsin dissolves rather slowly and that the solution does not give full value unless the amount of stain mentioned above is indeed dissolved. It is, therefore, desirable to prepare the solution at least 24 hours prior to use.

Another method of preparing pure paraldehyde-fuchsin in a stable powdered form depends on the extraction of the stain as it is formed by chloroform (Rosa, 1953). A solution of paraldehyde-fuchsin, prepared according to Gomori's formula, matures for 4 days, and is then extracted in a separating funnel with chloroform; the stain passes into this latter liquid and can be obtained in the dry state by evaporation. Less convenient than the procedure described earlier, Rosa's technique is also lower in yield and runs the risk of carrying down the impurities from the basic fuchsin, which serves as starting material, through the chloroform phase.

Working technique

Histologists who use the Gomori's version of paraldehyde-fuchsin have to keep an eye on its maturation; this source of worry disappears when purified paraldehyde-fuchsin is used. Experience shows that the stain should be allowed to act in an acid medium; such a situation is, *ipso facto*, realised in the first of the two situations outlined above, because of the hydrochloric acid present in the liquid phase in which the paraldehyde-fuchsin has been prepared; when the stain is prepared from powdered paraldehyde-fuchsin, it is advisable to add 1 ml of acetic acid to 100 ml of 0.125% solution in 70% alcohol. This acetified solution keeps very well.

The duration of staining with paraldehyde-fuchsin is short; it is rarely desirable to prolong the passage of the sections through the stain bath beyond five minutes. Some authors follow the staining with washing in 96% alcohol. I prefer to treat the sections for 10 to 20 seconds with 96% alcohol to which 0.5% hydrochloric acid has been added, and this particularly when the paraldehyde-fuchsin is used mainly for primarily morphological purposes. Extraction of the stain adsorbed is the more nearly complete, the background is better cleared, and systematic studies have shown that even 24 hours in the acidified alcohol does not extract the stain from structures for which is has a genuine affinity. I would, therefore, advise that staining by paraldehyde-fuchsin should be carried out in the following manner:

> Paraffin wax sections, dewaxed, treated with collodion where appropriate (taking care to ensure that the nitrocellulose coating remains thin enough) and hydrated, having undergone, in suitable cases, an appropriate pretreatment;
> Stain for 3 to 5 minutes on slides or in dishes, with the 0.125% solution of paraldehyde-fuchsin containing 1% acetic acid;
> Rinse rapidly in tap water, to remove the excess stain;
> Treat for 10 to 20 seconds with 96% alcohol to which 0.5% concentrated hydrochloric acid has been added;
> Wash in tap water;
> Stain the background, or dehydrate, clear, mount in Canada balsam or in a synthetic resin;
> A positive result is shown by an intense purple stain.

Histochemical interpretation

The number of structures which are spontaneously endowed with an affinity for paraldehyde—fuchsin, or are likely to acquire such an affinity after sundry pretreatments, is quite high. The principal morphological uses for the stain in question are reviewed in other chapters of this work; only the histochemical significance of the method is dealt with at this point.

Only one affinity for paraldehyde—fuchsin has so far failed to receive satisfactory interpretation, namely the case of the elastic fibres; the various ideas put forward on this topic are discussed in relation to techniques for the demonstration of elastic tissue.

In all other instances, experimental investigations have produced unequivocal conclusions; a spontaneous affinity for paraldehyde—fuchsin discloses the presence, in the stained structures, of anionic groups, and any pretreatments capable of inducing them to appear in the constituents of cells or tissues confers on the *structures* in which they appear an affinity of the same kind.

The *investigations* carried out in some detail by Scott and Clayton (1953), Braun–Falco (1955, 1956), and Konecny and Pliczka (1958) show that the groups which may give rise to an affinity for paraldehyde—fuchsin include aldehydes, carboxyls, and acidic groups with a sulphur base (sulphuric, sulphonic, sulphinic). In this way the strong affinity of the sulphomucopolysaccharides for this stain, which is manifest with no pretreatment, and is paralleled by the metachromatic reaction, is easily explained. Similarly, we can also understand that pretreatments likely to cause aldehyde groups to appear may result in the case of paraldehyde—fuchsin treatments, in preparations comparable with those which are given by the Schiff reagent.

It is in the same sense that we should interpret the intense staining of nuclei after hydrochloric acid hydrolysis (Konecny and Pliczka, 1958) and that of PAS—positive (PAS = periodic acid—Schiff) after oxidation with this acid followed by staining with paraldehyde—fuchsin (Scott and Clayton, 1953). On the other hand, oxidative reactions capable of transforming cysteine into cysteic (alanine β-sulphonic) acid results in a clear affinity for paraldehyde-fuchsin in all the structures which are rich in protein-bound sulphydrils.

In practice, the main interest of paraldehyde—fuchsin staining lies in its morphological implications, but the results are quite often capable of interpretation in chemical terms, and disclose the presence of anionic groups in the structures under investigation.

PARALDEHYDE—THIONINE

Paraldehyde—thionine has more recently been developed (Paget, 1959) than paraldehyde—fuchsin, and seems to have been used so far purely for morphological purposes. Paget (1959) nevertheless mentions trials which show that this new stain behaves like paraldehyde—fuchsin from a histochemical point of view. We can draw a parallel between the process of obtaining a stain from thionine, which is a thiazine, having properties comparable with those of paraldehyde—fuchsin, which is derived from triphenylmethane, and the possibility of preparing reagents of the Schiff type from triphenylmethanes and thiazines.

The technique for preparing paraldehyde—thionine is based on that for paraldehyde—fuchsin (the original formula of Gomori). 91.5 ml of 70% ethanol are mixed with 0.5 g of thionine, 7.5 ml of paraldehyde, and 1 ml of concentrated hydrochloric acid. The time taken for maturation, *in a well-stoppered bottle*, is from three to four days, and the solution can be used for about two weeks.

The working technique corresponds exactly to that for paraldehyde—fuchsin, with the exception that the duration of staining is longer (at least ten minutes). Once the sections have been stained, they are rinsed in tap water and mounted after dehydration and background staining.

In fact this stain seems to have only one advantage over paraldehyde—fuchsin, namely, a lesser tendency to stain the background in preparations which have been treated with chromium. Against this morphological advantage one has to offset some serious disadvantages, the difficulty which often arises of obtaining sufficiently pure samples of thionine, the need to allow it to mature, and its poor keeping qualities. The few data of a strictly chemical nature that we have in relation to paraldehyde—thionine, as compared with paraldehyde—fuchsin, is yet another disadvantage, especially when the stain is used for mainly histochemical purposes.

PHTHALOCYANINS
(alcian blue, alcian green, alcian yellow, astra blue)

Since their introduction into histological technique in order to stain mucins (Steedman, 1950) the phthalocyanins of the alcian blue group, stains whose composition has only partially been disclosed, have received a number of histochemical applications the principal one of which is the demonstration of acid mucopolysaccharides. Their use, however, is not limited to the detection of these compounds; we know from a whole series of investigations that alcian blue and other stains listed at the head of this section can be substituted for paraldehyde—fuchsin for certain of the purposes discussed here.

We know from recent publications (see, in particular, Scott and coworkers, 1964; Quintarelli and coworkers, 1964) that alcian blue represents, in reality a family of stains, six compounds having been sold by the chemical industry under this name; the differences in the constitutional formula are not fully known. In any event, they are basic stains and the same holds good for alcian yellow and alcian green, substances which are even less well known from the chemical standpoint than is alcian blue. The investigations to which I have alluded prove that alcian blue combines with tissue poly-anions by a simple electrostatic mechanism.

From the practical standpoint, some of the properties of alcian blue are highly advantageous for the histochemist. The inconstancy and mediocrity with which nuclei are stained can be explained (Scott, 1967, 1968, 1970) by the almost complete absence of affinity for nucleic acids, an absence which distinguishes the stains of this family from most other basic stains. There seems to be virtually no affinity for the carbonyl groups present in the sections, and even the affinity for carboxyls is not particularly marked. This affinity, on the contrary, becomes quite strong in the case of sulphur-containing acid groups (sulphuric, sulphonic, sulphinic) and it is their presence which is to be inferred, in the first instance, when any stain, however slight, is obtained with substances of this group.

Moreover, phthalocyanins such as alcian blue, or astra blue which is its German equivalent, alcian green and alcian yellow are primarily used for the detection of sulphomucopolysaccharides as well as for the demonstration of cysteic acid and other strong sulphur-containing acids, formed in the sections following vigorous oxidation. We may add that the high solubility of alcian blue in saline solutions renders it highly advantageous for the identification of polyanions by the technique which invokes critical electrolyte concentrations (Scott and Dorling, 1965).

Nevertheless, other characteristics of alcian blue are highly disadvantageous; principally, we should mention the inconsistency of the quality of commercial samples, which was very clearly shown by Mowry (1963) and by Scott (1972) and by many other users of this stain. Moreover, the obstinacy with which the manufacturers refuse to disclose the structural formula is a serious handicap in attempting to interpret the results obtained by the histochemist on a chemical basis.

We can add to this that commercial samples often contain an abundance of impurities added as 'diluents'. One of these diluents has recently been identified (Scott, 1972) as being boric acid; commercial samples studied by this author contained at least 20% by weight of this material.

A relatively simple technique for the elimination of this important and harmful impurity, developed by Scott (1972), is much to be commended for all histochemical uses of this dyestuff. It consists of mixing, with vigorous stirring by a magnetic stirrer, of one volume of 2 to 5% aqueous solution of alcian blue 8GX together with five to ten volumes of acetone. The dyestuff is precipitated and settles rapidly from the colourless liquid which it is easy to decant; the greater part of the boric acid remains in solution. The precipitate is washed in ether and dried; it keeps unaltered for several months.

The way in which phthalocyanins of the alcian blue group can be used for the detection of acid mucosubstances is described in chapter 17, their use in the course of the histochemical investigation of lipids and proteins is described in chapters 18 and 19; other stains with a phthalocyanin base are discussed in the last part of this book.

CHAPTER 15

HISTOCHEMICAL DETECTION OF ALDEHYDES AND KETONES

The histochemical detection of organic compounds depends, in most cases, not on the identification of chemical substances but on the detection of functional groups, which may exist in a chemically active state in the compounds for which the investigator is looking, or may be shown up as a result of appropriate pretreatments. This state of affairs could not very well pass unnoticed by a reviewer of Lison's sagacity; the third edition of his book thus includes two chapters devoted to the detection of aliphatic and aromatic functions. It would have been tempting to have followed his example, were it not that if we adopted such a plan it would inevitably lead to much repetition of material in the chapters dealing with the demonstration of the various groups of organic compounds; such repetition would be acceptable in a book whose theoretical approach to histochemical problems outweighed its emphasis on practical work, but it would not be acceptable in the present work.

It is, therefore, impossible to adopt an arrangement similar to that of Lison (1960), all the more so because the working technique for conducting the various reactions is not given here in the form of technical appendices, as it is in many recent works. It is no less true that two self-contained chapters need to be devoted to the detection of carbonyl groups by one set of chemical reactions and of the phenols and naphthols by another set.

In fact, these reactions emerge unchallenged from the plethora of procedures utilised for the demonstration of organic compounds; they represent the up shot of a very large number of suggested methods and are thoroughly reliable not only so far as their execution is concerned but in respect of the various possible control reactions. It is fundamental to modern histochemical technology that we should be able to show up aldehyde groups in an organic compound which we wish to detect, or to attach a naphthyl radical to it, and I would even go so far as to say that the two procedures in question are the very stuff of our discipline.

Free aldehyde and ketone groups, directly accessible to histochemical detection, are rare within animal tissues, but the numerous reactions which allow us to demonstrate such diverse compounds depend on the appearance of aldehyde groups in the molecule under investigation; the site of this aldehyde group is then revealed, during a further stage of the process, by techniques discussed in this chapter.

Among the many colour reactions of the carbonyl group which could, in principle, be of service in histochemistry, we need to discuss the Schiff reagent and its equivalents, the alkaline silver complexes, benzidine and *o*-dianisidine, phenylhydrazines and paraphenylenediamine. At the outset it should be stressed that the practical importance of the first of these reactions far exceeds that of all the others together.

THE SCHIFF REAGENT

Since its invention by H. Schiff (1867) the reagent which bears his name has been the subject of a substantial number of publications, which were exclusively chemical in orientation up to 1924, the date at which the studies of R. Feulgen and his colleagues ensured that they would be cited, as of right, in works on histochemical technique. At the present time, it is one of the most widely used techniques available to the histochemist, and the number of those who use it for purely morphological purposes increases daily. Recent general reviews (see, in particular, Kasten, 1960) serve to introduce the reader to the rich documentation on this topic, and only its essential features will be mentioned here.

The histological use of the Schiff reagent depends on the transformation of basic fuchsin under the influence of sulphur dioxide, into a colorless compound whose composition has been elucidated (Wieland and Scheuing, 1921); one molecule of sulphurous acid becomes attached to the central carbon atom of the pararosaniline molecule, giving as the reaction product pararosaniline leucosulphuric acid which is colorless and does not give a colour reaction with aldehydes; at a later stage of the reaction, another molecule of sulphurous acid reacts with one of the amine groups of the pararosaniline molecule, and thus, by the addition of SO_2 gives rise to N-sulphinic-pararosaniline leucosulphonic acid, representing the Schiff reagent In the presence of aldehydes, one molecule of the reagent condenses with two molecules of aldehyde and a molecular rearrangement transforms the compound into a coloured substance whose colour is due to the presence of a quinone chromophore. In fact, recent studies (see Kasten, 1960, for a detailed account of these reactions) show that during the Schiff reaction with acetaldehyde, at least two coloured substances are formed, differing in their absorption spectra; this observation is of no great consequence for qualitative analyses, since we have to deal with substances which are chemically very closely related to one another and are almost impossible to distinguish by simple visual examination, but obviously it has to be take into account in quantitative work.

The chemical findings thus permit us to make use of the term "regeneration of the colour of the Schiff reagent" which a number of authors has deprecated; nevertheless, the reappearance of this colour is patently not due to the 'regeneration' of the basic fuchsin, the new colour owing its existence to another chromophore, and this second way of expressing the phenomenon should be deleted from the vocabulary of histochemists. The regeneration of the basic fuchsin may, indeed, occur when the Schiff reagent is subjected to certain treatments, in particular when it is made alkaline or when the sulphur dioxide which is present in excess is driven off. Naturally, the phenomenon in question has no relationship with the reaction which enables us to carry out the histochemical Schiff reaction, and it represents a technical source of error which we would do well to beware of.

I—III = transformation of the pararosaniline chlorhydrate molecule during the preparation of Schiff's reagent; IV—VI = reaction of the latter with two molecules of aldehyde; note the quinone chromophore of the coloured compound formed (VI).

The employment in histochemical techniques of reagents equivalent to Schiff but prepared from other dyestuffs is a relatively recent development. Osterberg (1948), DeLamater (1951) and DeLamater and his colleagues (1955) make use of thionine-based preparations or those of azur A, treated with sulphur dioxide, and they obtain results equivalent to those obtained with the Schiff reagent. We know from the methodological studies of Kasten (1956, 1959) that numerous dyestuffs belonging to a variety of chemical categories may be used to prepare reagents capable of taking the place of that of Schiff. The chemical data relating to the reagents in question are less precise than those which concern the Schiff reagent, their practical interest, however, is no less great. It so happens that the colour given by some of these reagents may be even more advantageous from the optical standpoint than is that of the Schiff reagent, particularly when we need to carry out well-defined background staining. On the other hand, a study of the absorption spectra leads us to concede that the colour reactions in question are more advantageous in qualitative investigations. Moreover, the early work of Van Dujn (1956) and of Himes and Moriber (1956) illustrates the possibility of using mixtures into which two coloured reagents for aldehydes play a part, such reagents being intended to reveal the presence of carbonyl groups which appear successively after appropriate pretreatments. The number of technical possibilities offered by these new equivalents of Schiff's reagent is thus rather large; the most important ones are collected together in Table 7, based on the data of Kasten (1956, 1959).

The preparation of Schiff's reagent

The considerable number of formulae put forward for the preparation of Schiff's reagent is a symptom, of the greatest cogency, reflecting the difficulties which abound during work intended to produce a reagent which is at once sufficiently sensitive and sufficiently stable. Some of these difficulties stem from the poor quality of the commercial samples of basic fuchsin which serve as a starting point. Moreover, many authors have attempted to make use of a variety of sources of sulphur dioxide; the amounts of, respectively, basic fuchsin and sulphur dioxide, have also undergone a large number of modifications. Some formulae include a treatment of the reagent with active charcoal, because it adsorb simpurities which do not destain under the influence of sulphur dioxide.

In practice, the most rational solution is to prepare Schiff's reagent from pure pararosanaline, a chemical compound which has been placed on the market by good suppliers of requirements for microscopy; simple examination with the naked eye allows us to see if impurities are too abundant (a red or violet hue) and insolubility in distilled water is a second readily applicable means of guaranteeing purity. In addition to Graumann's formula, which I prefer to any other, several ways of preparing Schiff's reagent starting from basic fuchsin are mentioned below.

Graumann's method. — Dissolve 0.5 g of pure pararosaniline in 15 ml of normal hydrochloric acid (80 ml of concentrated hydrochloric acid, d = 1.19, in sufficient distilled water to make up to 1 l); dissolve 0.5 g sodium bisulphite in 85 ml distilled water; mix the two solutions, allow to stand for 24 h at laboratory temperatures. At the end of this period, if the pararosaniline used is of good quality, the reagent has taken on a rather pale yellow tint and decolorisation by charcoal is thus unnecessary. Should it be necessary, it is possible to add 0.3 g charcoal, followed by filtration after vigourous shaking for 15 to 30 s; the filtrate is usually pale pink and decolorises completely in a few hours.

Coleman's method. — Dissolve 1 g of basic fuchsin in 200 ml water; the dye is placed in cold distilled water, previously brought to boiling point, which it is often advisable to maintain for one or two minutes; allow to cool, filter after complete chilling, as this precaution helps to eliminate certain impurities; add 2 g of dry sodium or potassium bisulphite and 10 ml of Normal hydrochloric acid; allow to stand for 24 h in a well-stoppered flask. With very good samples of basic fuchsin, the colour of the reagent is yellow at the end of this lapse of time, decolouration by charcoal being unnecessary. Such decolouration may be carried out as for Graumann's method.

Longley's method. — Dissolve 0.5 g sodium metabisulphite or potassium metabisulphite in 100 ml of 0.15 N hydrochloric acid; add 0.5 g of basic fuchsin; stir, allow to stand for several hours at laboratory temperatures; add 0.3 g of activated charcoal, stir for two minutes, and filter through Whatman No. 2 paper.

Barger and DeLamater's method. — Add 0.25 ml of thionyl chloride to a solution of 0.25% basic fuchsin in distilled water. Allow to stand in a well-stoppered flask until it has lost its colour.

In any event, once the reagent has been prepared it should be kept in a well-stoppered flask. Generally, it is advisable to keep it away from light and in the cold, these precautions tending to slow down the loss of sulphur dioxide which constitutes the essential factor in the deterioration of Schiff's reagent.

The time for which the reagent will keep has been very diversely estimated by different authors and Kasten (1960) considers that the divergent estimates are partly associated with differences in the preparative techniques. It should be emphasised that the deterioration of the reagent does not necessarily lead to the appearance of a pink tinge, but if it does appear the reagent should at once be thrown away. The systematic use of Schiff's reagent prepared less than one month previously, as advised by Lison (1960, p. 166) seem to me to be excessive; it is best to test the reagent by means of one of the reactions for which it is suitable, using slides whose subsequent appearance is well known, before using the reagent on material which is new or difficult.

Preparation of Schiff's reagent equivalents

The preparation of these reagents depends on the same principle as does that of Schiff's reagent. A 1% solution (for dyestuffs of the acridine group) or 0.5% (for dyestuffs belonging to the other groups appearing in Table 7) is either saturated with gaseous sulphur dioxide or has several drops (0.10 to 0.25 ml) of thionyl chloride added to it. It is also possible to prepare the dyestuff solution, not in distilled water, but in a mixture of 5 ml of Normal hydrochloric acid, 5 ml of 5% sodium or potassium metabisulphite, and 90 ml of distilled water. Some decolourisation takes place only with solutions of acid fuchsin,

Table 7. — THE MAIN DYESTUFFS OF PRACTICAL IMPORTANCE WHICH YIELD EQUIVALENTS OF THE SCHIFF REAGENT
(after KASTEN, 1957, 1960)

Colour Index Number	Common name	Family	Reaction colour	Fluorescence
46 025	acridine orange	acridine	greenish-yellow	+
46 000	acriflavine	—	yellow	+
46 035	phosphine 5G	—	yellow	+
46 045	phosphine GN	—	yellow	+
50 040	neutral red	azine	brown	0
50 200	phenosafranine	—	red	0
50 240	safranine 0	—	red	0
11 320	chrysoidine R	azo	orange	0
21 010	Bismark brown R	—	brown	0
51 010	brilliant cresyl blue	oxazine	blue	0
41 000	auramine 0	phenyl-methane	yellow	+
42 535	methyl violet	—	violet	0
42 555	crystal violet	—	bluish-violet	0
42 685	acid fuchsin	—	red	0
52 000	thionine	thiazine	blue	0
52 005	azur A	—	blue-green	0
52 015	methylene blue	—	blue-green	0
52 040	toluidine blue	—	blue-green	0
45 010	pyronine B	xanthine	red	+
45 210	rhodamine 3GO	—	red	+

azur A and C, crystal violet, gentian violet, methylene blue, and thionine; it is never, so to speak, quite complete. Certain dyestuffs become partially precipitated during preparation; in such cases, the precipitate is removed by filtration.

On the whole, reagents prepared in this way keep less well than does that of Schiff; the keeping time has been estimated, for azur $A-SO_2$, at several weeks provided that before use on each occasion, several drops of a 5% or 10% solution of sodium or potassium metabisulphite are added (Himes and Moriber, 1956).

Method of use for Schiff's reagent and its equivalents

As I commented at the beginning of this section, tests for free carbonyl groups play only a limited role in animal histochemistry, but *their absence from sections should be verified whenever Schiff's reagent or one of its equivalents is used to detect aldehyde groups which appear in the tissues consequent upon an appropriate pretreatment.* Sections which have undergone this pretreatment, and control sections, are steeped in Schiff's reagent or in one of its equivalents for a period which depends on the method adopted; it is imperative to work in a closed recipient, to avoid the loss of SO_2 during the reaction, a possibility whose consequences have been set out above. At the end of the period in the reagent, the excess reagent must be removed, and this manoeuvre has given rise to some debate. In fact, simple washing in tap water results in raising the pH so as to entrain a regeneration of the basic dyestuff used for the preparation of the reagent, so that there is a possibility of error in that structures which are merely basophilic, but devoid of carbonyl groups, may become stained.

It was to avoid this source of error that Feulgen and his colleagues advised, from their earliest major publication, that excess Schiff's reagent should be removed by washing in sulphur dioxide water. Most authors have scrupulously followed this rule and washing with a dilute solution of sodium or potassium metabisulphite, whether or not it is acidified with hydrochloric acid, forms an integral part of many formulae. It so happens that this dogma seems less tenuous than it once did; the generalisation of the periodic acid-Schiff reaction as a routine method has shown that the essential element in the treatment of the sections when they are taken out of the Schiff's reagent is the elimination with all possible rapidity of the reagent, a result which may be attained, when using paraffin wax sections, by very vigorous washing in a sufficient amount of distilled water, without passing the sections through sulphur dioxide water. The same result is more difficult to ensure when the reaction is carried out with frozen sections, and, *a fortiori*, when it is undertaken on tissue blocks. It is, then, my considered opinion that the traditional passage through three baths of sodium metabisulphite solution, to which, where appropriate, a few drops of Normal hydrochloric acid have been added, is not indispensable when the work involves paraffin wax sections, and that it may be kept for cases which present special difficulty. Such washing, however, is essential when working with frozen sections or with blocks of tissue.

Experience shows that sections treated with Schiff's reagent, or with one of its equivalents, do not attain their definitive stain until they have been washed for several minutes in tap water, the chemical significance of this phenomenon being as yet unknown.

In any case, the colour reactions so obtained lend themselves to quite diverse background staining. As I remarked above, pretreatments intended to cause aldehyde groups to appear in diverse types of chemical structure, pretreatments followed by the action of reagents giving rise to different colours, may be carried out successively on one and the same section. Most of these combination stains call for a nuclear stain and the periodic acid-Schiff reaction; they are dealt with in the following chapters.

The general course of the reactions discussed here is, therefore, as follows:

Paraffin wax sections, frozen sections or tissue block material, having, where appropriate, undergone the appropriate pretreatments;

Treat with Schiff's reagent or one of its equivalents at the same time as control blocks, or sections, for which the pretreatment has been omitted, in a closed receptacle for a period varying between 5 min and 1 h 30 min or even longer (especially for tissue blocks);

Where appropriate, wash in several baths of a solution of sodium or potassium metabisulphite (1% concentration) to which several drops of N hydrochloric acid may or may not have been added;

Careful washing (for at least 10 min for paraffin wax sections, several hours for tissue blocks) in running tap water or frequently renewed water;

Where appropriate, stain the background or apply any other histochemical reaction to the sections; Dehydration, clearing and mounting for sections in paraffin way, mounting in a medium miscible with water for frozen sections, embedding or cutting on a freezing microtome for tissue blocks.

Histochemical interpretation

A positive result of the reaction involves the appearance, in structures containing primary carbonyl groups, of a colour varying between red and violet when the Schiff reagent is used; the stains obtained with its equivalents are shown in Table 7 so far as the nucleal reaction is concerned; other aldehydes may, with these reagents, give distinctly different colours. In any case, the criterion of success for this reaction is the absence of staining when the pretreatment has been omitted, or, in the case of tests for free aldehydes, when the sections have previously been subjected to a blocking reaction involving the carbonyl groups using one of the methods discussed in a following section.

In vitro investigations show that the Schiff reagent is not rigorously specific for aldehydes. Certain ketones, some unsaturated compounds such as oleic acid (Lison, 1932; Chu, 1950) and some acetyl derivatives may give a positive reaction; moreover, sundry oxidising agents may regenerate the colour of the Schiff reagent by regeneration of the pararosaniline chlorhydrate. Such sources of error do not interfere much in work on tissue sections. Under the experimental conditions of animal histochemistry, a positive result of the reaction carries with it virtual certainty that aldehyde groups are present in the stained structures.

When we are dealing with primary carbonyl groups which appear after pretreatment of the sections, comparison with control sections for which the pretreatment has been omitted greatly strengthens this interpretation. Among such treatments, we may mention at this point hydrolysis using hydrochloric acid, the first stage of the Feulgen and Rossenbeck nucleal reaction, the treatment of frozen sections with mercuric chloride, which forms the basis of the plasmal reaction of Feulgen and Voit, various types of oxidation (periodic acid, chromic acid, potassium permanganate) intended to convert glycols into aldehydes, performic or peracetic oxidation which causes carbonyl and acid groups to become detectable, in protein-bound sulphydrils and unsaturated lipids, oxidative deamination using alloxan or ninhydrin, and lastly treatment with ultraviolet light which enables us to detect carbonyl groups in certain unsaturated lipids.

ALKALINE SILVER COMPLEXES

The demonstration of primary carbonyl groups by means of alkaline silver complexes depends on their reducing capacity, which is a property that they have in common with the aldehydes and a large number of other compounds. From the chemical point of view, histochemical reactions which depend on the reduction of an alkaline silver complex are much less informative than those in which a colour reaction is obtained by means of the Schiff reagent or one of its equivalents. We have to add to this theoretical restriction the practical limitations of the argentaffin reaction which have already been mentioned in connection with work on tests for reducing compounds undertaken by these means; these limitations are the relatively high cost of the reagents, the difficulty of standardising the preparation of some of them, their instability, and, most of all, the problem of ensuring a clear distinction between the achievement of a true argentaffin reaction and the early stages of a non-specific precipitation which is quite without histochemical significance.

It is nevertheless true that the optical properties of the preparations which the argentaffin reaction provides will, in certain instances, justify its use in testing for the aldehyde groups, when these are made manifest in sections after various pretreatments. It is particularly in the domain of carbohydrate histochemistry that silver complexes have a certain part to play. Nucleal reactions depending on acid hydrolysis followed by the argentaffin reaction have been put forward by a certain number of authors but the practical value of these methods seems somewhat restricted. Lastly, we should remember that the argentaffin reaction plays an important part in the detection of polyphenols, and this application is discussed in another section of the present work.

In any case, with the exception of the pretreatment of the sections, the working technique corresponds to that set out in relation to the detection of reducing capacity. Comparison with control sections which have not undergone the pretreatment is even more useful than in the case where the detection of aldehyde groups is performed with the Schiff reagent.

In this context I might recall that another technique for testing for reducing compounds, namely the ferric ferricyanide reaction, is quite unsuitable for the demonstration of aldehyde groups; weakly positive or dubious results are obtained in some instances, and entirely negative results in others, so that the practical value of the ferric ferricyanide method in testing for carbonyl groups is nil.

BENZIDINE AND O-DIANISIDINE

The use of aromatic amines for the demonstration of carbonyl groups depends on a condensation reaction with the aldehydes, giving rise to the formation of aldimines the monomeric form of which is very unstable, so that trimerisation ensues (Van Eck, 1923). The compounds so formed are strongly coloured.

So far as I am aware, the reaction whose principle has just been sketched has only been used to demonstrate carbonyl groups which appear in carbohydrates after oxidation with periodic acid and lead tetra-acetate (Glegg, Clermont and Leblond, 1952) or with sodium bismuthate (Lhotka, 1952). These authors used a 1% solution of the selected amine in pure acetic acid; *o*-dianisidine, which is very light and highly irritating to the respiratory tract, should be used with due precautions. The reaction takes place in the warm, and results in a brown stain in places where primary carbonyl groups are to be found, the stain being almost as intense as it is after the Schiff reagent has been used.

The working technique is as follows:

> Paraffin wax sections, dewaxed, treated with collodion and hydrated, having undergone the appropriate pretreatment;
> Treat for 45 min at 50 °C with the solution
> pure acetic acid .... 100 ml
> benzidine or *o*-anisidine .... 1 g
> Rinse rapidly in acetic acid;
> Wash in distilled water (5 to 10 minutes);
> Stain the background and mount as after the use of Schiff reagent.

According to the observations of Glegg and his colleagues, the results obtained with some mammalian tissues correspond closely, with the single exception of lens fibres, to those obtained with the Schiff reagent after the same pretreatment.

The practical value of the technique which has just been described does not seem to be great, but its theoretical value cannot be doubted.

PHENYLHYDRAZINES

The condensation of phenylhydrazine with aldehydes and ketones, which has long been known from the chemical point of view, gives rise to coloured phenylhydrazones, and has been used in histochemistry in the hope of obtaining a selective demonstration of the carbonyl group of ketosteroids. This histochemical application of phenylhydrazines has, at present, only historical interest, but the tests in question lie behind work which shows that it is possible to employ substituted phenylhydrazines (in particular 2,4-dinitrophenylhydrazine) instead of the Schiff reagent for the detection of aldehyde groups.

This is the principle of Albert and Leblond's method (1944) for the detection of acetalphosphatides and of that put forward by Monné and Slautterback (1951) to discriminate between carbohydrates which can be oxidised by periodic acid; following this oxidation, the Swedish authors used treatment with 2,4-dinitrophenylhydrazine followed by the Schiff reagent. Under these conditions, some of the carbohydrates oxidised by periodic acid take on a red colour, others a yellow one. We know from the work of Danielli (1949) that substituted phenylhydrazines can replace the Schiff reagent in nucleal reactions; stains which are particularly advantageous because of their intensity are obtained with an azobenzene-phenylhydrazinesulphonic acid.

The stain obtained by condensing phenylhydrazines with aldehydes is often rather pale; Seligman, Gofstein and Rutenburg (1949) advise that these phenylhydrazines should be coupled with the diazo salt of *o*-dianisidine, with the form ation of a purple diformazan. The reaction takes place in the presence of pyridine. Pearse (1953, 1960) mentions a very clear demonstration of certain structures rich in carbohydrates when subjected to periodic oxidation and then to the above reaction, but he comments that the results are often different from those given by the Schiff reaction.

In practice only the methods of Albert and Leblond (1944) and Monné and Slautterback (1951) are in current use. These two techniques are described in relation to the histochemical detection of lipids and carbohydrates.

THE 2-HYDROXY-3-NAPHTHOIC ACID HYDRAZIDE

The principle of this method does not differ from that of the reactions involving phenylhydrazine and the aldehydes. The 2-hydroxy-3-naphthoic acid hydrazide, in fact, gives condensation products with primary or secondary carbonyl groups whose colour is no more intense than that given by the reaction of Albert and Leblond. Nevertheless, as Camber (1949) and Ashbel and Seligman (1949) have demonstrated, coupling of the product of this first reaction with the diazo-salt of *o*-dianisidine results in the formation of a coloured azo-dye which is intensely violet, so that preparations can be obtained which are, optically speaking, particularly advantageous. This reaction has been successfully applied to the study of certain lipids and can replace the action of Schiff's reagent in the nucleal reaction. The working technique is as follows.

(1) = 2-hydroxy-3-naphthoic acid hydrazide; (2) = product of its condensation with a compound bearing a primary carbonyl group; (3) = diazo-salt of o-dianisidine; (4) = the azo-dystuff which results from coupling.

Frozen or paraffin wax sections, the latter brought into water;
Use of the chosen pretreatment;
Treat for 1 to 3 hours at 60 °C with the solution
  2-hydroxy-3-naphthoic acid hydrazide .... 0.1 g
  50% alcohol .... 45 ml
  Acetic acid .... 5 ml
the hydrazide being dissolved by warming to 70°.
and stirring vigorously;
Wash in three baths of the ethanol-acetic acid mixture;
Wash in three baths of 50% alcohol;
Wash in distilled water;
Treat for 2 to 5 minutes with the mixture, prepared immediately prior to use,
  0.1 M Sörensen buffer, pH 7.2 to 7.5 .... 30 ml
  absolute alcohol .... 30 ml
  diazo-salt of o-dianisidine .... 50 mg
Wash carefully in tap water;
Mount the frozen sections in a medium miscible with water, the paraffin wax ones in a synthetic resin, dehydrating rapidly and avoiding any excessive length of time spent in the benzenoid hydrocarbon used as a clearing agent.

P-PHENYLENEDIAMINE

Woker (1914) discovered that there was a substantial acceleration of the oxidation of *p*-phenylenediamine by aldehydes in the presence of hydrogen peroxide; a technique used by Scarselli (1956, 1961) makes use of this discovery. The reaction leads to the condensation of three molecules of the diamine and the formation of a blue-violet compound which is insoluble in water. In the first version of Scarselli's method there was the inconvenience arising from the need to examine the preparations after they had been mounted in water, and from their poor keeping qualities, but these have been removed from the second version of the method because the colour is stabilised by means of a solution of gold chloride. In this way permanent preparations can be obtained, which may be hydrated and cleared by means of benzenoid hydrocarbons. The technique we give here represents the latest version of Scarselli's method, in which the peroxidase properties of aldehydes are put to good use.

Reagents:

A 1% solution of paraphenylenediamine in distilled water which has been boiled; keep in a well-stoppered flask away from the light;
1.5 volume hydrogen peroxide;
1% solution of gold chloride in distilled water.

Working technique:

Paraffin wax sections, dewaxed and brought into water, which have undergone the pretreatments intended to reveal the aldehyde groups;
Treat for 15 minutes, away from the light, with the mixture
    solution of *p*-phenylene-diamine   } equal parts
    hydrogen peroxide
Wash carefully in distilled water, several times renewed;
Treat for 5 minutes with the gold chloride solution;
Wash in distilled water;
Dehydrate, clear, and mount in Canada balsam or in a synthetic resin.

Structures which contain aldehyde groups take on a colour which varies from bluish-violet to black. After periodic oxidation, the results are comparable with those given by the Schiff reagent, but the stain is more selective and Scarselli (1961) stresses the greater sensitivity of the method. The reaction is wholly suppressed by blocking the aldehyde groups; ketones do not react under the experimental conditions defined above.

A technique which is quite distinct in principle involves the condensation of dimethylparaphenylenediamine and has been put forward by Spicer and Jarrels (1961) to distinguish between neutral and acid mucopolysaccharides; this method is discussed in relation to the histochemistry of the carbohydrates.

BLOCKING REACTIONS OF THE ALDEHYDE GROUPS

Blocking reactions for the carbonyl groups represent an important means of verifying the effectiveness of the methods discussed above; the histochemist should make use of them to obviate any interference between the free aldehyde groups in the sections and any which may appear as a results of the pretreatments which have been applied, or, perhaps, to verify the positive result of the reactions listed in this section to ensure that they do, indeed, reveal the presence of aldehydes.

The number of blocking reactions used since the pioneer work of Feulgen and Voit (1924) is quite considerable. Sodium bisulphite, alkaline cyanides, phenylhydrazine and its derivatives, dimethylcyclohexanedione (dimedon), semicarbazide and thiosemicarbazide, sulphanilic acid, aniline and aniline chloride have been used by various workers. All these compounds act by giving condensation products with aldehydes; these are coloured in the case of phenylhydrazine and its derivatives so that the use of these compounds for blocking serves at the same time as a means of demonstrating carbonyl groups.

Lillie (1954) suggests that, in practice, the following compounds should be made use of.

Aniline chlorhydrate.—Add 8 ml of concentrated hydrochloric acid to 9 ml of aniline; stir and make up to 100 ml with distilled water. Treat the sections with this reagent for from 1 to 3 hours at laboratory temperatures.

Hydroxylamine.—Dissolve 10 g hydroxylamine chlorhydrate and 20 g crystalline sodium acetate in 40 ml distilled water. Treat the sections for 1 to 3 hours at laboratory temperatures.

Semicarbazide.—Dissolve 2 g of semicarbazide chlorhydrate and 5 g crystalline sodium acetate in 40 ml distilled water. Treat the sections for 2 to 3 hours at 60° C.

Thiosemicarbazide.—Dissolve 4 g thiosemicarbazide in 40 ml distilled water; add 2 ml acetic acid. The duration of action should be the same as for the semicarbazide solution.

Phenylhydrazine.—Mix 5 ml phenylhydrazine and 10 ml acetic acid; make up to 50 ml with distilled water; treat the tissue blocks for 2 to 3 hours at 60°.

Sodium bisulphite.—Treat the sections for 2 to 8 hours at laboratory temperatures with a 0.1 N solution of sodium bisulphite in water.

THE DISTINCTION BETWEEN ALDEHYDES AND KETONES

As Lison (1960, p. 170) has quite rightly commented, none of the reactions mentioned above permits of a distinction between primary carbonyls (aldehydes) and secondary ones (ketones) under circumstances which do not elicit some degree of theoretical misgivings.

The repercussions of this state of affairs on histochemical practice are, nevertheless, minor ones. It so happens that free carbonyls, whether aldehydes or ketones, are rare in animal tissue, at least under the circumstances in which the histochemist studies them. The considerable interest which attaches to the histochemical detection of carbonyls stems from the fact that a large number of compounds become accessible to histochemical detection because pretreatments have rendered the functional group in question demonstrable. We need hardly add that the chemical mechanism of these pretreatments, which is readily analysable, and has indeed been analysed, *in vitro*, relieves us of any doubts as to the primary or secondary nature of the carbonyl groups which are revealed.

The single practical example in which the distinction to which I have alluded becomes genuinely important is that where attempts are made to identify ketosteroids histochemically by showing up their carbonyl group, whether or not this is done in association with other reactions. This question has been raised in connection with the histochemical detection of steroids; at the present moment it is appropriate to mention that recent work has overwhelmingly demonstrated the impossibility of detecting ketosteroids histochemically.

CHAPTER 16

HISTOCHEMICAL DETECTION OF PHENOLS AND NAPHTHOLS

The techniques considered here are applied on the one hand to studies of natural phenolic compounds, preserved in sections of animal tissue, and on the other hand to the demonstration of naphtholic compounds introduced artificially into bodies we wish to show up.

Unlike the case of the carboxy-groups, histochemical tests for free phenolic compounds in the course of studies on animal tissue present a far from negligible interest. An essential amino acid, tyrosine, can be detected because of its phenolic nucleus (Millon's reaction, the azo-reaction); the demonstration of sympathomimetic catecholamines and of related substances, such as the promelamines, depends on the presence of a diphenol group in these compounds. It is also true that the detection of naphthols artificially attached to molecules which exist in the sections, or which are precipitated there by enzymatic activity which we wish to detect, represents by far the most important of the practical applications of the various techniques which are considered in this chapter.

The reactions to be passed under review here are of quite unequal importance. Millon's reaction, already mentioned, serves uniquely to detect tyrosine and related amino acids; it rests on the formation of a mercuric complex of nitrosophenol in the presence of a mercuric salt and of nitrous acid and its description is to be found in the chapter devoted to the histochemical detection of proteins. The indoreaction (Lison, 1930) and Gibbs' reaction (1926) are but little utilised and only their theoretical interest justifies the summary mention of them which is made below. The osmium-iodide reaction of Champy (1913) is still debateable from the point of view of its chemical specificity. The pheochrome reaction (chromaffin) and the argentaffin reaction are widely used for the detection of ortho- and paradiphenols, but it is the azo-reaction (a term distinctly preferable to that of the diazo-reaction, diazonium reaction or azo-coupling reaction of certain anglo-saxon authors) which represents the essential technique for the histochemical detection of the groups considered in this chapter.

THE AZO-REACTION

It is Cordier and Lison (1930), and Lison (1930, 1931) to whom we owe the introduction into histochemical practice of a reaction based upon the condensation of diazonium salts with the phenols, resulting in the formation of azo-dyes.

The salts of diazonium, which have been known to chemists since the initial studies of Griess (1860), have given rise to many investigations, some of which are of purely chemical orientation and have no immediate bearing on histochemistry whereas others, concerning the application of the reaction which has just been mentioned (coupling) in industrial dying, bring out ideas which may have direct interest for histochemical practice. The work of Zollinger (1961) represents a full statement of our present knowledge in this field, and basic information concerning the histochemical use of diazonium salts can be found in the book by Burstone (1963).

The reagents

We know that the diazonium salts, which are prepared by allowing sodium nitrite to react with an aromatic amine or with its salt in the presence of hydrochloric acid, are unstable; their preservation in solution can only be assured in the cold and for a rather short length of time. Industrially, the stabilisation of diazonium salts in the dry condition is obtained either by associating them with various metallic salts (zinc, calcium, etc...) or by combining them with naphthol-sulphonic or naphthalene-β-sulphonic acids. It is in this stable form that the products in question are used, by coupling them with naphtholates, in industrial dyeing practice. In the pure state diazonium salts are explosive; samples for histology, which are sold commercially, contain a variable proportion of inert diluent; the diazonium salt content of products intended for microscopy does not generally exceed 20%.

The number of diazonium salts currently used by histologists is large; the table of the names proposed by the editors of the "Journal of Histochemistry and Cytochemistry" (1959) sets out 28 compounds, the list arranged by Burstone (1963) includes 52 and the number of such substances used experimentally or regularly by histochemists has probably increased further since that date. The most important among the amines corresponding to the diazonium salts used in histochemical practice are set out in Table 8, where the names proposed in order to standardize the nomenclature, by the editorial board of the journal noted above, are also to be found.

In principle, all the diazonium salts give rise to the formation of an azo-dye, by linkage with a phenolic or naphtholic compound; they should therefore be interchangeable so far as their histochemical use is concerned. In fact, several factors intervene to render the use of certain substances impracticable and to encourage the use of others.

Table 8. — NOMENCLATURE OF DIAZONIUM SALTS CURRENTLY USED IN HISTOCHEMISTRY
(after LILLIE, 1959)

The following table gives the common name, adopted after comparison of all the synonyms, and stating the latter, as expressed in the "Journal of Histochemistry and Cytochemistry", and includes the numbers indicated in the second edition of the "Colour Index". The amines corresponding to the diazonium salt are also given; the term 'salt' is understood in the common name.

N°	Name of amine	Proposed common name	Synonyms
37245	4, 4'-diaminodiphenylamine	Fast Black B	Black BS salt
37190	2, 5-dimethoxyaniline coupled with the diazo salt of *p*-nitroaniline	Fast Black K	Black NK salt
37235	*o*-dianisidine	Fast Blue B	Blue BNS salt; dianisidine blue; diazo blue B; Fast blue BN; naphthanile blue B
37175	4'-amino-2' 5'-diethosy-benzanilide	Fast Blue BB	Blue BB, 2Bs, NBB; fast diazoblue BB; fast blue 2B, EB, BBN
37155	4'-amino-2' 5'-methoxy-benzanilide	Fast Blue RR	blue RR; diazo blue RR; fast diazo blue NRR, RR
37255	B'-*p*-methoxy phenyl-*p*-phenyldiamine	Fast Blue VB	blue V, B, CB, NS, NSV; fast blue NB, BL; variamine blue BD; variamine blue B, BD, NB
27135	2-nitro-*p*-anisidine	Fast Bordeaux GP	Bordeaux GP; bordeaux Ciba IV; fast bordeaux GDN; GPN, GPS NGP 3NA
37020	3, 5-dichloro-*p*-phenylene-diamine	Fast Brown RR	brown RR
37200	4-methyl-*m*-anisidine coupled with the diazo salt of 2-chloro-4-nitroaniline	Fast Brown V	fast brown VA
37160	4'-amino-5'-chloro-*o*-benzanisidine	Fast Corinth LB	corinth LB; fast diazo corinth LB
37195	2, 5-dimethoxyaniline coupled with the diazo salt of 2, 6,-dichloro-4-nitroaniline	Fast Dark Blue R	navy blue RN
37210	*p*-toluidine coupled with the diazo salt of *o*-toluidine	Fast Garnet GBC	garnet GBC; bordeaux II
37015	*m*-toluidine coupled with the diazo salt of m-toluidine	Fast Garnet GC	fast garnet AC, GCD; fast diazo garnet GC
37025	*o*-nitroaniline	Fast Orange GR	fast orange GR salt
37275	1-aminoanthraquinone	Fast Red AL	fast diazo red AL; red naphthanil diazo AL
37125	4-nitro-*o*-anisidine	Fast Red B	fast red 5NA BN, E; red V, B, BS; fast diazo red B

N°	Name of amine	Proposed common name	Synonyms
37035	*p*-nitroaniline	Fast Red GG	nitroazol CF; red nitrosamine; red paranitraniline; red para; red GG, 2GS; fast red 2G, 2J
37110	2-nitro-*p*-toluidine	Fast Red GL	fast diazo red GL; diazo red G; fast red G, JL, 3NT; red G, GL; red VII
37040	4-chloro-2-nitroaniline	Fast Red 3GL	fast diazo red 3GL; diazo red 3G; fast red 2NC, 3JL; fast red 3G salt; red 3G, NBGL, 3GK F; salt red VI
37150	N' N'-diethyl-4-methoxy-metanilamide	Fast Red ITR	fast red ITRN; red ITR fast brentamine LTR
37120	B-chloro-*o*-anisidine	Fast Red RC	brown V, III; diazo red RC; fast red 4CA, RCN, RS; red RC, RCS
37100	4-nitro-*o*-toluidine	Fast Red RL	fast red NRL, 5NT; red RL; red base X; fast ponceau L; fast ponceau naphthosol L
37085	4-chloro-*o*-toluidine	Fast Red TR	fast diazo red TR; red fast red 5CT; TRN; salt red IX; red TA, TR, TRS
	5-chloro-*o*-toluidine-4-benzanilide	Fast Red Violet LB	red violet LB
37010	2, 5-dichloroaniline	Fast Scarlet GG	fast scarlet GGS, GGN 2J, DS; scarlet A, GG, 2G, I; fast diazo scarlet GG
37130	5-nitro-*o*-anisidine	Fast Scarlet R	fast scarlet 4NA, RC, RN; brown salt D, IV; scarlet NSR, R, RB, RC, RS, III
37165	4'-amino-6'methyl-*m*-benzanisidine	Fast Violet B	fast diazo violet B; fast violet BN; violet B, BN
37265	α-naphthylamine	α-naphthylamine	1-naphthylamine

The first element in this choice is the colour of the azo-dye-stuff obtained after coupling; experience shows that complicating the molecule of the amine which enters into the constitution of the diazonium salt has a deepening effect (bathochrome effect) of a quite distinct nature, so that there is a more intense staining of reactive structures and an improvement in the optical quality of the preparations.

Moreover, certain of these compounds only carry a single diazonium group (mono-diazo compounds), whereas others have two of them (bi-diazo compounds). These latter can give rise to a double coupling so that we obtain deeper and more intense stains, an eventuality which in certain cases may be highly advantageous. On other occasions the possibility of this double coupling, more or less complete, results in polychromatic preparations whose histological interpretation is less easy than that of slides treated with a mono-coupling reagent.

One of the essential factors, in choosing a diazonium salt to use in order to detect naphthols deposited in sections during a histo-enzymological reaction, is the property which in the dye-stuffs industry goes under the name of fastness. By this term is understood the affinity of dyes for the cellulose fibres or the firmness of their fixation on these fibres. In the language of histochemists, the same term serves to designate the affinity of the coloured reaction products for the structures which are shown up or the insoluble nature of the products of the staining reaction. Artefacts due to diffusion are evidently all the less when the fastness is very great.

Some strictly chemical factors also determine the choice before the histochemist. The stability of aqueous solutions, the speed of coupling and the pH requirements in order to obtain optimum coupling are not identical for all diazonium salts; at pH values greater than 9 most of these compounds are very unstable so that there is serious danger of decomposition with the formation of the corresponding phenol. This latter substance can give a coloured azo-dye with the diazonium salt present in the medium and can become attached to certain structures which may lead to overestimating the results obtained from the reaction.

The fineness of the particle size of the dye should also be taken into consideration; it varies for any given diazonium salt according to the substrate with which it is coupled and for any given reaction according to the way in which the tissue were fixed.

It is perhaps unnecessary to make a point of the practical elements which guide this choice, such as the facility with which any particular diazonium salt can be obtained in a stable form or, on the contrary, the need to prepare it as required.

The practical upshot of this discussion is that the histochemical worker will find it in his own interest to respect as far as possible the choice of diazonium salts made by the authors of the formulae put forward in the different cases.

In spite of the large number of stable diazonium salts, which are placed on the market by firms supplying products for microscopy, salts which are prepared as required have not lost their interest. It is in fact agreed that the results obtained when test for a natural phenolic compound are carried out using a diazonium salt prepared at the time of use are often better. It is therefore useful to set out the principal formulae, especially the general preparative techniques, as they have been codified by Lison (1931), together with certain recent formulae.

a) **Lison's technique for the preparation of diazonium salts as required.**—The amine to be diazotised is dissolved or suspended in 50 ml of distilled water; concentrated hydrochloric acid (density = 1.19) is added, the amounts required being shown in Table 9. This mixture is chilled at the temperature of melting ice. Once chilling is complete, an equally chilled solution of 5% sodium nitrite in distilled water is added in amounts indicated in Table 9, with appropriate stirring. The mixture is kept in a refrigerator for about 15 minutes; it keeps for from 24 to 48 hours.

Table 9. — Preparation of diazonium salts

Diazotised amine	Amine (g)	Quantity of hydrochloric acid (ml)	Sodium nitrite solution (ml)
Sulphanilic acid	0.20	4	3
Metaphenyl diamine	0.20	8	6
Napthylamine	0.15	4	2
Naphthoic acid	0.15	4	2
Benzidine	0.20	8	5
o-dianisidine	0.15	8	5
Benzidine-disulphonic acid	0.25	8	5
Dianisidine-sulphonic acid	0.12	8	5

b) **Technique of Lillie and collaborators (1953) for the preparation of the diazo salt of safranin O.**—Two stable stock solutions are prepared and chilled to about 4°C. The first is obtained by dissolving 3.6 g of safranin O in 60 ml of distilled water and adding 30 ml of normal hydrochloric acid, the second by dissolving 6.9 g of sodium nitrite in 100 ml of distilled water.

For the diazotisation, 4.5 ml of the solution of safranin are added to 0.5 ml of the sodium nitrite solution. The mixture, which instantly becomes blue, should be left for 15 minutes at the temperature of melting ice. This mixture keeps poorly and is diluted 40 times immediately prior to use, hence the small quantities which appear in the formula.

c) **Technique of Lillie and Glenner (1957) for the preparation of the diazo salt of S acid (8-amino-naphthol-5 sulphonic acid).**—240 mg of S acid are dissolved in 6 ml of distilled water; three ml of normal hydrochloric acid are added, the mixture then being chilled to 4°. After chilling, 1 ml of the 6.9% solution of sodium nitrite in distilled water is added. Diazotisation is obtained after a lapse of 15 minutes at 4°.

d) **Davis's technique (1959) for the diazotisation of pararosaniline.** — 1 g of pararosaniline chlorhydrate (basic fuchsin) is dissolved in 25 ml of 2N hydrochloric acid; this solution is kept at laboratory temperatures. 1 g of sodium nitrite is dissolved in 25 ml of distilled water and also kept at laboratory temperatures. The "hexazonium" salt (the molecule of pararosaniline contains three primary amine groups) is obtained by mixing at laboratory temperatures 4 drops of the solution of basic fuchsin and 4 drops of the solution of sodium nitrite in a small tube which is shaken for 30 seconds. After being rendered alkaline with 0.6 ml of N soda, the liquid is used at once.

Coupling

The chemical reaction which goes under this name only takes place in alkaline media. It can be represented in a general way by the equation

$$C_6H_5-N\!=\!N-Cl + C_6H_5-OH \rightarrow HCl + C_6H_5-N\!=\!N-C_6H_4-OH.$$

The product of the reaction contains the azo-chromophore; its colour varies a great deal according to the structure of the radicals represented here schematically by benzene rings.

In histochemical practice, coupling may be carried out with the stable diazonium salt of commerce or with solutions of these salts prepared immediately prior to use.

The stable commercially available diazonium salts can be used as they are in tests for natural phenolic compounds or for naphthols deposited in the first stages of the reaction through enzymic action (so called post coupling methods). However, when these salts are added in the course of the incubation intended for a histo-enzymological study, their preliminary purification can be useful in order to eliminate the metals which are added as stabilisers; certain of these metals can in fact have a very marked inhibiting action on the aminopeptidases and on certain oxidases as well as on other enzymes. Pearse (1960) advocates the removal of aluminium sulphate which is present in many commercial preparations of diazonium salts by the addition of a small quantity of saturated aqueous solution of purpurin, followed by filtration; Burstone (1958, 1963) prefers to add to the solution exchange resins for anions and cations.

The pH value of the medium in which the coupling is to take place should be above 7, but it is strongly advisable not to increase it to above 8.5, since the diazonium salts are very unstable at pH values reaching or exceeding 9. The optimum pH for each coupling reaction is produced in the case of the stable diazonium salts commercially available, by dissolving them in a buffer of the appropriate pH value, as indicated in relation to each method. The solutions of the diazonium salts prepared immediately prior to use can be diluted with a buffer or rendered alkaline by means of a solution of sodium carbonate chilled to 4°C according to the circumstances; when carbon dioxide is no longer given off and the colour of the solution turns to a pale yellow the required pH value is reached; it can also be checked using indicator papers. It may be mentioned at this point that some techniques (in particular tests for indol groupings using Glenner and Lillie's 1957 technique) involve coupling in an acid medium.

Once rendered alkaline, the solutions of diazonium salts are very unstable; from the practical point of view, it is thus essential only to prepare the amount strictly necessary for the practice of the reaction, to throw away any reagent prepared longer than fifteen minutes and to carry out even the coupling reaction in the cold (about 4°C) in all cases where its duration exceeds five minutes and where the contrary has not been expressly recommended in the instructions for use of the corresponding reaction.

In certain cases, the azo dyes so formed are insoluble in alcohol and in benzenoid hydrocarbons, which allows one to mount the preparations in Canada balsam or in the commercially available synthetic resins, but this is not always the case. The precautions which stem from this situation are indicated in relation to the various methods dealt with.

The diverse ways in which coupling to diazonium salts can take place prevent us from giving any standard working technique; what are, properly speaking, working methods are therefore suggested at the points where we deal with the demonstration of compounds which can be detected by the azo reaction.

It is appropriate to comment that bis-diazo-compounds can participate in a double coupling in widely varying circumstances. In certain cases, the double coupling is spontaneous, the two diazo-groups reacting with two phenol or

Table 10. — Coupling rate and solution stability of the principal diazonium salts used in histochemistry
(after Burstone, 1963)

Common name	Coupling rate	Solution stability
Fast Black B(salt)	Slow	Poor
Fast Blue B (salt)	Very slow	Good
Fast Blue BB (salt)	Slow	Good
Fast Blue VB (salt)	Very slow	Good
Fast Bordeaux GP (salt)	Rapid	Fair
Fast Corinth V (salt)	Fairly rapid	Very good
Fast Garnet GBC (salt)	Very rapid	Fair
Fast Red B (salt)	Very rapid	Very good
Fast Red GG (salt)	Very rapid	Good
Fast Red GL (salt)	Rapid	Fair
Fast Red LTR (salt)	Fairly rapid	Good
Fast Red RC (salt)	Rapid	Very good
Fast Red RL (salt)	Very rapid	Good
Fast Red TR (salt)	Rapid	Very good
Fast Scarlet G (salt)	Very rapid	Fair
Fast Scarlet GG (salt)	Very rapid	Very good
Fast Scarlet R (salt)	Very rapid	Fair
Fast Violet B (salt)	Slow	Good

naphthol groups of the preparation (as in the reaction of Barrnett and Seligman with DDD, followed by coupling with the diazo salt of ortho-dianisidine); in other cases, the double coupling is deliberately provoked by the manipulator who treats the preparation in which the coupling has taken place with a suitably chosen solution of a naphthol. This double coupling, which has been used since 1931 by Lison, increases the depth of colour and increases its intensity (as in the coupled tetrazonium reaction of Danielli).

The practical advantages (stability of the solutions, speed of coupling) of the principal salts of diazonium used in histochemical practice are indicated in Table 10.

Histochemical interpretation

We know from the studies of Lison (1931) and of all those who have followed him that the azo reaction is given by all phenolic compounds containing a non-substituted hydroxyl group, provided that at least one of the *ortho* or *para* positions with respect to the hydroxyl group are also free. Among the other substances that are of some consequence in animal histochemistry, only the indol and imidazol groups also give the azo-reaction. Stemming from this the azo-reaction may represent a method for the histochemical detection of histidine, this problem having been discussed in relation to the histochemistry of the proteins. The behaviour of indolic compounds, especially tryptophane, has also given rise to discussions which are mentioned in the same context.

Leaving aside errors by excess or omission related to poor working techniques, the azo-reaction can therefore be considered as being specific and reliable.

THE INDO-REACTION

This also is a method, developed by Lison (1931), whose practical importance is not great so that most modern authors neglect it; it is mentioned here summarily because of its theoretical interest.

The principle of the method rests on the formation of indo-anilines from a phenol and a paradiamine, in the presence of an oxidising agent; the mixture of a phenol and a para-aminophenol, under similar conditions, gives rise to indo-phenols. Both types of reaction product contain the quinone-imine chromophore; they give blue or green colourations.

The reaction is carried out by flooding the slide which bears the sections under investigation with a 1% solution of dimethylparaphenylenediamine or of para-aminophenol and adding, with a pipette, a 1% aqueous solution of potassium bichromate. The reaction is over in a few minutes; background staining in red can be practised and mounting in Canada balsam, or, better, in a commercial synthetic resin, is then possible. A positive result betrays structures which are rich in phenolic groups by a blue or green stain.

The indo-reaction only succeeds in a certain number of cases, even when the greatest possible care is taken to use freshly prepared reagents; it is not to be advised as a working tool.

THE GIBBS REACTION

In principle, this method, whose practical interest is also slight, resembles the indo-reaction. The condensation of a phenol with 2,6-dichloroquinone-chloro-imide gives rise to the appearance of a deep blue or black precipitate, corresponding to the formation of a stain of the quinone-imine group.

Gomori (1952) advocates the practice of Gibbs' reaction by treating dewaxed and hydrated sections with a solution containing 20 mg of 2,6-dichloroquinone-chloro-imide for each 20 ml of Michaelis's buffer containing sodium acetate-sodium veronal at pH 9; to get the material into solution often necessitates warming to about 70°. The optimal duration of action for the reagent is from 10 to 15 minutes. On being taken out, the sections are washed in running water for several minutes; the nuclei may be stained with neutral red (a 1% aqueous solution applied for 3 minutes). The slides are then dehydrated, cleared in a benzenoid hydrocarbon and mounted in a commercial synthetic resin. A positive result shows up as a black stain.

THE ARGENTAFFIN REACTION

Unlike the reactions which have just been reviewed the argentaffin reaction in no case permits one to detect phenols or naphthols as such; in fact a positive result is due to the existence, in the structures which are being demonstrated, of reducing compounds sufficiently vigorous to induce the precipitation of metallic silver from alkaline complexes of silver (silver-diamine, silver-hexamethylene-tetramine, etc....) without the intervention of reducing agents added by the experimenter. It is mentioned in this chapter solely because the most widespread of the natural reducing compounds which the histochemist meets with in animal tissues are the thiols and phenolic compounds.

All phenols do not reduce alkaline silver complexes; the argentaffin reaction is only positive with diphenols or polyphenols in the *ortho* or *para* positions. In addition, positive results can be obtained with aminophenols and polyamines satisfying the same stereochemical criteria. Lison (1931) makes the timely comment that positive results can be counted on with all members of the series of aromatic developers given by Lumière and Seyewetz.

Since the period when Cordier (1927), Cordier and Lison (1930), Gérard, Cordier and Lison (1930), and Lison (1931) undertook the first rational analysis of the methods for the histochemical demonstration of the phenol group many other applications have been found for the argentaffin reaction, in particular those relating to the detection of aldehyde groups which appear as the result of a pre-treatment and this observation underlines still further the very wide range of the procedure in question. Merely to obtain a positive result from the argentaffin reaction does not, then, in any case prove the existence of phenolic compounds in the structures which are stained black, but simply that of reducing substances.

That the argentaffin reaction keeps its place among the techniques for the histochemical demonstration of the phenols is due, as I have remarked above, to the fact that most naturally occurring reducing compounds present in sections of animal tissues are ortho-or paradiphenols; it is also due to the optical qualities of the preparations resulting from the reduction of alkaline silver complexes.

The working technique for the argentaffin reaction, when practised in order to detect phenolic compounds, differs in no way from that which has been set out in relation to the detection of carboxy-groups, since it is, in both cases, the reducing capacity which is being tested; as in the case of tests for aldehydes, methods using silver-hexamethylene-tetramine seem to me preferable to those using Fontana's liquid. The same technical precautions should be observed in both cases.

THE PHEOCHROME (CHROMAFFIN) REACTION

In use since the time of Henle (1865) the reaction designated by Kohn (1898) under the name "chromaffin" reaction has long been considered as resulting in the deposition of chromic compounds; the yellow or brown colour ensuing when this method is positive can in fact be so interpreted. We know from the studies of Gérard, Cordier and Lison (1930) that the colour mentioned above is due to the compounds which react and not to the reagent. It therefore seems logical to me to adopt, in order to describe the method in question, the term "pheochrome" proposed by Poll (1905, 1906) for that category of cells in the adrenal gland that it shows up selectively.

We know from tests made *in vitro* that the brown colour induced by the action of solutions of potassium bichromate can be obtained with polyphenols, aminophenols or polyamines, so long as these functional groups are placed in the *ortho-* or *para-*positions (Verne, 1922). The same browning can be obtained *in vitro* and on tissue sections using solutions of potassium iodate, which shows that the colour obtained is independent of the precipitation of chromic compounds (Gérard, Cordier and Lison, 1930). The conclusions of these authors have been verified by modern workers. In effect, chemical, historadiographic and autoradiographic studies do indeed show the presence of chromium in sections of the medullo-adrenal treated by the pheochrome reaction (Coupland, 1954), but the metal stays there even if one decolourises the sections by oxidising them with bromine water. The practice of the reaction with potassium iodate also results in the incorporation of iodine which does not take part in the staining.

One of the conclusions in the work of Gérard and his collaborators (1930) retains its full validity; the pheochrome reaction demonstrates the presence not of any reducing compound but of aromatic compounds corresponding to the series of developers listed by Lumière and Seyewetz; these compounds also give the argentaffin reaction.

As for the mechanism of the yellow or brown stain which results from a positive pheochrome reaction, modern authors agree that the first stage is represented by the formation of quinones or of quinone-imines which when turned into cyclic compounds followed by condensation result in compounds of the melanin type.

The pheochrome reaction may in principle be carried out either on pieces of tissue or on sections; it is the first of these two possibilities which in practice is the more important. Most authors start with a fixative employing a potassium bichromate base, containing neither acids nor other heavy metals; that is to say that the fixatives of Regaud, of Kopsch or of Orth are quite suitable. Fixation is followed by treatment for several days (5 on an average) with a 3%

aqueous solution of potassium bichromate at laboratory temperatures. The pieces of tissue are then washed in running water so as to eliminate all excess of potassium bichromate; the dehydration and embedding in paraffin wax take place in the usual manner. The sections can be mounted without background staining or may on the other hand be subjected to various stains and histochemical reactions intended to increase the contrasts. These methods are set out in Chapter 21 in relation to techniques for studying the adrenal gland, together with certain recent improvements in the histochemical detection of sympathomimetic catecholamines.

In conformity with the observations of Gérard and his collaborators, the pheochrome reaction can be carried out by fixing pieces of tissue in a mixture of 10 ml of formalin and 90 ml of water, in which 5 g of potassium iodate has been dissolved. The use of this liquid is particularly indicated in cases where it is necessary to avoid errors of interpretation resulting from the vigorous adsorption, by certain cells, of chromium salts. The classical example of this "pseudo-reaction" is represented by certain cells of the hypobranchial gland of the stenoglossan gastropods. Naturally, fixation should be completed by keeping the pieces of tissue in a 5% solution of potassium iodate, a stage which it is not generally useful to prolong beyond 3 days. The pieces of tissue are then washed, dehydrated and embedded as in the method using potassium bichromate.

The pheochrome reaction on sections is carried out by treating the slides for several hours with a 3% aqueous solution of potassium bichromate and then washing in tap water to the point where all excess of the bichromate has been removed.

Lastly, we may mention that the older reactions put forward in order to demonstrate the presence of adrenalin in the medullo-adrenal (the reaction of Vulpian using ferric chloride, that of Virchow, using iodine, and that of Grynfeltt and of Mulon using osmium tetroxide) are now substantially out of date and have only an historical interest.

CHAPTER 17

HISTOCHEMICAL DETECTION OF CARBOHYDRATES

The role of carbohydrates in the chemical constitution of animal tissues explains the importance of those methods which permit their detection on sections. On the whole, the histochemistry of the carbohydrates offers the investigator a considerable number of possibilities so far as the detection of many of the polysaccharides is concerned; the histochemical demonstration of monosaccharides on the other hand is at its very beginning. Only one method for the detection of glucose has been taken into consideration by recent authors; that is the method of Okamoto and his collaborators, but these trials have been carried out on only a few mammalian tissues (Müller, 1955, 1957, 1959) and further studies are greatly to be desired. With the methods for the detection of monosaccharides we may legitimately include those for ascorbic acid (vitamin C) since this is a derivative of L-glucofuranose.

HISTOCHEMICAL DETECTION OF GLUCOSE

As Müller (1957) has remarked, none of the staining reactions used in analytical chemistry for the detection of monosaccharides in general and of glucose in particular can be adapted to the working conditions of the histochemist.

The method of Okamoto, Kadota and Aoyama (1948) involves the *in situ* precipitation of tissue glucose through the immersion of very small pieces in methyl alcohol saturated with barium hydrate. Afterwards these pieces are embedded in paraffin wax, taking great care that they do not come into contact with water; the sections should be spread out dry; they are treated with an alcoholic solution of silver nitrate, washed in 96% alcohol, reduced by means of an alcoholic solution of formalin and then hydrated, washed and mounted. The presence of glucose at the moment of fixation is revealed by a black precipitate which is related to the replacement by silver of barium precipitated in the form of its glucose complex.

The working technique involves the following stages.

The slices of tissue which should be as thin as possible should be fixed for 24 hours at 4°C in methyl alcohol saturated with barium hydrate;
Dehydrate in three baths of absolute alcohol;
Embed in paraffin wax, passing the material through methyl benzoate (or salicylate) and benzene;
Cut the sections 10 μ thick, spreading the sections out dry;
Dewax and take into absolute alcohol;
Treat for 30 minutes in full illumination, with the following mixture
absolute alcohol .... 90 ml
20% aqueous solution of silver nitrate .... 5 ml
In appropriate instances, wash in absolute or 96% alcohol (at least 3 baths of 1 minute duration each) and reduce by means of the following solution
absolute alcohol .... 90 ml
commercial formalin .... 10 ml
Hydrate the sections;
Treat for 30 seconds with a 5% solution of sodium thiosulphate (hyposulphite);
Wash carefully in tap water, staining the background where appropriate with the aluminium lake of solid nuclear red;
Dehydrate, clear and mount in Canada balsam or in a synthetic resin.

We know from trials on models, carried out by Müller (1955) that only fixation with methanol saturated with barium hydrate allows one to obtain positive results. These disappear entirely if the sections, prior to treatment with silver nitrate, are washed with distilled water. Reduction by means of formalin is useful only if the sections scarcely become black when illuminated.

The same working technique should evidently result in the demonstration of lactose which also gives a precipitate which is insoluble in alcohol when treated with barium hydrate; nevertheless, to my knowledge, lactose has not yet been sought for in animal tissues by means of this technique.

We need hardly add that the method of Okamoto and his collaborators (1948) can be made the subject of numerous theoretical objections. In fact, any attempt at the immobilisation *in situ* of a molecule as small and as mobile as that of glucose might, *a priori*, appear doomed to failure. Moreover, the technique by which it is demonstrated rests on the histochemical detection of barium and corresponds very closely to a reaction of von Kossà in an alcoholic medium; we would then expect a positive reaction of all alkaline earth phosphates and the carbonates which are present in the sections prior to fixation or after treatment with methyl alcohol saturated with barium hydroxide. Müller (1957) has moreover noted a diffuse yellow colour of the keratinised structures which evidently tells us nothing relevant to the presence of glucose. We should then, in all cases, use as a control a slide which has been subjected to washing with distilled water prior to the treatment with an alcoholic solution of silver nitrate; only the silver precipitates which are completely suppressed by this washing can be considered as evidence of the presence of glucose; the precision with which this method localises substances may not be very great and it would be foolish to try to draw, from this kind of preparation, deductions about intracellular distribution of glucose or of lactose.

Moreover, work done by Müller (1955, 1957) shows that the sensitivity of the method is not very great; in fact this author obtained negative results in the kidney of the mouse even where tests for glucose-6-phosphatase, using the method of Chiquoine (1953), gave strongly positive results; indications corresponding to those of glucose-6-phosphatase have on the contrary been obtained in the liver of the mouse, and the study of intestinal absorption of glucose in the duodenum and the jejunum have been undertaken by means of this procedure. Positive results moreover have been obtained in the kidney by freeze-substitution (Müller 1959).

THE HISTOCHEMICAL DETECTION OF ASCORBIC ACID

The demonstration of ascorbic acid in slices of animal tissues did in fact precede the chemical identification of the antiscorbutic vitamin; it was in 1928 that Szent-Györgyi noticed the rapid darkening of slices of the adrenal gland when treated with a solution of silver nitrate, this reduction taking place even in darkness.

All the techniques for the histochemical demonstration of ascorbic acid rest on this observation of Szent-Györgyi. The methods of Bourne (1933), Giroud and Leblond (1934), Sosa (1948), Bacchus (1950), Eränkő (1954) differ from one another only in the details of the working technique.

The principle of the histochemical detecton of ascorbic acid by silver nitrate rests on the fact that reducing compounds which are sufficiently vigorous to act in an acid medium are rare in the animal body. Treatment with a solution of silver nitrate, acidified with 1% acetic acid, should obviously be carried out in darkness. The excess reagent may be removed either by treating the material with a dilute solution of thiosulphate (hyposulphite) of sodium, or in causing this reagent to act after the sections have been prepared; we need hardly add that all the manipulations would have to be carried out in the second case away from sunlight.

Experience shows that the treatment of pieces of tissue with the solution of sodium thiosulphate may be the cause of precipitates representing a serious source of error through over-treatment. For this reason Sosa (1948) has advised washing the pieces of tissue in a solution of sodium sulphite before treating them with thiosulphate.

The greatest obstacle to a convincing histochemical demonstration of ascorbic acid is the small size of the molecule and hence the ease with which it diffuses; it is thus essential that the reagent should penetrate rapidly in contact with the cells. The earliest workers sought to ensure this result by injecting the reagent using vascular perfusion, after washing the blood vessels with an isotonic solution of fructose; the same washing was advised in those cases where slices of tissue were immersed in the reagent. Such washing has been abandoned by modern authors. The demonstration of ascorbic acid in sections of tissue treated by freeze drying (Jensen and Kavaljian, 1956) or sectioned in a cryostat (Eränkő, 1954) represent a notable advance on the older methods.

1° Demonstration of ascorbic acid in pieces of tissue:

Immerse the pieces of tissue, which should be *freshly dissected and very small*, in the following solution
- silver nitrate .... 10 g
- distilled water .... 100 ml
- acetic acid .... 1 ml

for one hour in darkness;
Wash with great care in several baths of distilled water, dehydrate and embed in relative darkness, cutting the sections away from direct sunlight;
Or, (Sosa, 1948); wash for 1 hour with a solution of 10% sodium sulphite, the solution being several times renewed;
Treat for 1 hour with a 10% solution of sodium thiosulphate;
Bring the pieces into the light, wash in distilled water several times renewed, dehydrate, embed in paraffin wax and section without special precautions;
Mount the dewaxed sections or stain the background using safranin, basic fuchsin, or nuclear fast red etc.

2° Demonstration of ascorbic acid after freeze drying:

Treat the paraffin sections, about 10 μ thick, without dewaxing and denaturization, but after they have been stuck to the slide and dried, for about 10 hours, with an acidified 3% aqueous solution of silver nitrate;
Wash in 96% alcohol renewed several times;
Dehydrate in absolute alcohol, dewax, clear in a benzenoid hydrocarbon and mount in a commercial syntetic resin.

The preparations thus obtained should be kept in darkness; they blacken with age.

3° Demonstration of ascorbic acid on cryostat sections:

Cut the material into sections of 20 μ or more;
Float the sections for a period of 10 seconds to several minutes, on the surface of the following reagent:
- 96% alcohol .... 9 ml
- acetic acid .... 1 ml
- a 20% aqueous solution of silver nitrate .... 10 ml

Wash in 5% acetic acid;
Rinse rapidly in distilled water;
Mount in a medium miscible with water.

The chemical specificity of this method and its topochemical value in localising substances have given rise to much debate.

From the point of view of the chemical specificity the first idea which springs to mind is the partial nature of this demonstration which only shows up ascorbic acid and not dehydroascorbic acid with which it is in equilibrium in the tissues. Attempts have been made at the reduction of this latter acid by treating the pieces of tissue with hydrogen sulphide for 10 to 15 minutes, and then removing the gas by evacuation or else by placing sections, coming from pieces of tissue treated by freeze drying, and not dewaxed in a current of the same gas which is then driven out by a current of nitrogen; these methods seem not to have given very encouraging results.

Even with this reservation, the method is not out of critics; it demonstrates the presence of ascorbic acid solely by means of one of its reactions, that is to say its reducing power. Even though it is true that by carrying out the reaction in an acid medium one can eliminate interference from substances which have a feeble reducing power, more vigorous reducing agents may simulate the presence of ascorbic acid. Grains of melanin, the secretory product of the enterochromaffin cells, and adrenochrome under the technical conditions of the silver nitrate method behave like ascorbic acid. Deposits of phosphate are also shown up in the form of black precipitates. As Pearse (1960) has commented, some of the classic intracellular sites of ascorbic acid, namely the chondriome, the Golgi body and the cytoplasmic granules of the macrophages (lysosomes?), are known for their richness in phospholipids, compounds which are capable of reducing the salts of silver even in an acid medium.

It is, then, difficult to consider the reduction of silver nitrate in an acid medium as being a reaction specific to ascorbic acid; only a comparison with sections treated so as to show up, by other methods, the main compounds which themselves may give rise to this reaction allow us to conclude with a certain degree of confidence that ascorbic acid is present in tissues which have reduced the silver nitrate.

No less cogent are those objections which call into question the strictness of the localisation especially on the scale of the intracellular organelles, when using the silver nitrate technique.

A measure of prudence in the interpretation of the results may be induced just by considering the granular nature of the deposits of silver, since this localisation scarcely corresponds to the great solubility and easy diffusion of ascorbic acid. Moreover, studies by Deane and Morse (1948) and Sosa (1948) show that the appearance of these deposits varies considerably with the technique of fixation. *In vitro* trials prove that deposits of silver obtained by allowing a solution of silver nitrate to react with ascorbic acid have a strong tendency to concentrate at interfaces (Bourne, 1944). Wolf-Heidegger and Waldmann (1942) established a parallel between the physico-chemical phenomena which take place during the histochemical demonstration of ascorbic acid on the one hand, and the photographic techniques of "physical development" on the other hand. Voigt (1952) has expressed similar views.

It is, then, impossible in the present state of our knowledge to be sure that the intracellular localisations of ascorbic acid, such as were described in work published prior to 1940, are valid. The 'golgian' or 'mitochondrial' localisation of this compound might represent an artifact of fixation. Lison (1960) considers that localisation on the tissue scale is valid when the technical conditions are right and when the absence of other vigorous reducing agents has been verified.

HISTOCHEMICAL DETECTION OF POLYSACCHARIDES

The most important part of the histochemistry of the carbohydrates is the demonstration of polysaccharides in animal tissues. Some of the techniques used for this purpose are very old, others being much more recent. The number of reactions and colour tests brought into play during the last twenty years is such that only the main ones can be outlined here. In addition to the manuals of histochemistry which we have already noted many times, there are reviews by Hale (1957), Gabe (1958), Vitry (1958), McManus (1961), and Curran (1964) which contribute greatly towards a survey of the literature on the subject of the histochemistry of the polysaccharides.

A. — CLASSIFICATION OF POLYSACCHARIDES DETECTABLE BY HISTOCHEMICAL METHODS

In conformity with universally accepted practice those polysaccharides which are relevant to animal histochemistry have been classified following K. Meyer (1938, 1945) into simple polysaccharides, neutral and acid mucopolysaccharides which may be either simple or complex, mucoproteins, glycoproteins and glycolipids.

Simple polysaccharides (polyholosides in chemical nomenclature) are characterised by the fact that their hydrolysis furnishes only monosaccharides; these are then true "hydrates of carbon". Glycogen, galactogen, cellulose, and tunicine, together with starch, belong to this category.

The *neutral mucopolysaccharides*, which are generally associated with proteins in animal tissue, contain hexosamine groups in addition to monosaccharides. The simplest among them is chitin which consists solely of acetylglucosamine. Other neutral mucopolysaccharides contain in addition galactose, glucose, or other monosaccharides.

Acid mucopolysaccharides contain either acetylhexosamine and glucuronic acid (hyaluronic acid), or the same amine and pyruvic acid (the sialic acids), or in other cases, sulphuric acid (chondroitin and mucoitin-sulphates).

The *mucoproteins* are characterised by forming a stable chemical compound with the peptides, a chemical analysis of which shows the presence of more than 4% of nitrogen.

In the *glycoproteins* the union of the carbohydrate part of the molecule with the peptides is also quite stable, but the content of nitrogen is less than 4%. We need hardly add that the distinction between these two types of compounds is purely arbitrary.

In the *glycolipids*, chemical analysis shows the presence of a monosaccharide (glucose or galactose) a sphingosine and a fatty acid. These are the cerebrosides (phrenasin and kerasin).

B. — TECHNIQUES FOR THE DETECTION OF POLYSACCHARIDES

The numerous procedures for detecting polysaccharides in sections of animal tissue can be classified in several categories, the most important of which is that of the oxidative reaction. The metachromatic reaction, already mentioned, as well as the extent of the relative basophilia, which has also been dealt with in Chapter 13, are extremely useful in the study of these compounds. Moreover, sulphuric esterification, the fixation of metal ions and a certain number of diagnostic colour tests need to be covered here. Among the control reactions, the most important are reversible acetylation, reversible methylation and various enzymatic digestions. These techniques should evidently be summarised before discussion of the problems raised by the identification of the various kinds of polysaccharides.

OXIDATIVE REACTIONS

The most spectacular elements of the recent progress made in the histochemical study of carbohydrates are due to the oxidative reactions. Each of these methods comprises three stages, the first of which is the oxidation of carbohydrates present in the section which is being studied; the second stage consists of the detection of carbonyls which appear as a result of oxidation, and the third stage is represented by the various control reactions. These latter allow one to verify that the colour reaction obtained is indeed indicative of the aldehyde groups formed during the oxidation and, to a certain extent, that these aldehyde groups do indeed come from the oxidation of a carbohydrate; the nature of this latter, or at least whether it belongs to one of the groups enumerated in the preceding paragraph, can also be clarified.

The second stage of these reactions, that is to say the way in which we detect the carbonyls which have appeared as a result of oxidation, has been mentioned in Chapter 13. It is appropriate therefore to review the oxidising agents and the practice of the oxidative reactions in the histochemical detection of poly saccharides, the controls being treated in another part of this chapter. It is chromic oxidation (Bauer, 1933) which represents the earliest but not the best among the procedures that we have to consider; its chemical mechanism is little known and the same remark could be made in relation to permanganate oxidation (Casella, 1942). Periodate oxidation (Hotchkiss, 1948; Lillie, 1947; McManus, 1946) and that using lead tetra-acetate (Crippa, 1951) and sodium bismuthate (Lhotka, 1952) are, on the contrary, the direct derivatives of techniques widely used in chemical studies on the carbohydrates, so that their mechanism is well known. The latter is also well known in the case of oxidation by manganese acetates (Lhotka, 1952) and by aryl-iodoso-acetates (Lhotka, 1954), procedures whose practical importance is slight and which are mentioned here for the record.

a) Periodic acid

Periodate oxidation, which was discovered by Malaprade (1928, 1934) and studied from a chemical point of view by numerous authors, included among whom are Fleury and Lange (1933), Nicolet and Shinn (1939), Jackson (1941) and Fuson (1950), has become an essential tool in the study of polysaccharides. In an acid medium, at a pH around 2, it results in the formation of two primary carbonyl groups from the following radicals; 1,2-glycol, 1,2-amino-alcohol, 1,2-alkylamino-alcohol, 1,2-hydroxy-ketone (α-ketol); the carbon chain is broken between the two carbon atoms which carry the oxidised groups; in the case of polysaccharides the pyran or furan rings are thus opened, but the macromolecular skeleton undergoes no alteration. The process of oxidation which takes place at the temperature of the laboratory is quite rapid; under the conditions of temperature, of concentration of periodic acid and of the duration of action which is customary in histochemical usage, the oxidation does not go further than the aldehyde stage. It is evident that these properties are outstandingly advantageous to the histochemist. Lastly, we may recall that the substitution of 1,2 groups, especially their esterification, results in a loss of the capacity for periodic oxidation.

It follows from these facts that the formation of primary carbonyl groups following periodic oxidation is in no way the prerogative of the carbohydrates. Among the amino-acids, serine, threonine and hydroxylysine are oxidised (Nicolet and Shinn, 1939, 1944), this reaction having been applied to the quantitative estimation of the substances in question. Their demonstration on sections should therefore be possible and indeed it has been shown by the studies of Glegg, Clermont and Leblond (1952) that this particular occurrence can take place when serine or threonine occur in a terminal position in the protein molecule, hydroxylysine being capable of reaction whatever its position in the molecule. Hale's memoir (1957) includes an extensive literature survey dealing with those proteins which can be oxidised by periodic acid. Lipids, on the other hand, especially the phospholipids (sphingosine, cephaline, cardiolipine and phosphoinositides) can be oxidised by periodic acid with the liberation of aldehyde groups. The same remark may be made for the ceroid pigment, for certain fuscines, for adrenalin and noradrenalin (Lillie, 1950), the oxidation of the two latter compounds acting on the hydroxymethylamine grouping. It follows therefore that the pheochrome reaction, taking place on the catechol grouping, remains unaffected. Moreover, the chemical formula of ascorbic acid, of corticosterone and of dehydrocorticosterone should make us consider the possibility of periodic oxidation of these three substances.

It stems from all this that the list of substances capable of undergoing periodic oxidation with the appearance in the molecule of primary carbonyl groupings is a long one, and that the idea of a true chemical specificity of this method for the polysaccharides (Hotchkiss, 1948) can no longer be maintained. Table 11, which is taken from Hale (1957), includes the main compounds in which the histochemist may be interested and which may be detected by periodic oxidation followed by the demonstration of aldehydes.

Table 11. — Substances detectable by the periodic acid-Schiff method
(after Hale, 1957)

Polysaccharides	Glycogen Galactogen Starch Cellulose and tunicin Dextran
Neutral Mucopolysaccharides	Chitin (non-incrusted) Gastric mucus
Acid Mucopolysaccharides	Mucin Hyaluronic acid Heparin (mono- and bisulphate)
Mucoproteins	Thyroglobulin Thyrotropic hormone Gonadotropins Mucoids of the sub-maxillary gland Polysaccharides of the crystalline capsule
Glycoproteins	Gelatin Ovalbumin Serum albumin Collagen Reticulin
Glycolipids and lipids	Cerebrosides Sphingomyelin Cardiolipin Cephalin Ceroid pigment Lipofuscins
Sundry	Adrenalin Noradrenalin Corticosterone Dehydrocorticosterone Ascorbic acid

There is another restriction preventing us from affirming the true specificity of periodic oxidation for carbohydrates, that is to say the fact that authentic polysaccharides do not posses this capacity. The esterification of hydroxyl groups carried on carbon atoms 2 and 3 of the pyran or furan rings results in a loss of the capacity for oxidation; we can understand in this way that chondroitin-sulphuric acid and heparin trisulphuric acid do not give the reaction. Moreover, the β-glycol groups cannot be oxidised, so that polysaccharides whose glycoside linkage is borne on carbon atom 3 do not react.

Considering only the theoretical aspects, the omens are scarcely propitious so far as the specificity of periodic oxidation is concerned in the histochemical detection of carbohydrates. Things look a great deal brighter however so far as the effective specificity of the method is concerned (the actual specificity in the sense of Lison, 1960). In fact, the studies of the school of Leblond (see in particular Glegg and his collaborators, 1952; Leblond and collaborators, 1957) show that the positive results obtained on sections in paraffin wax can be related, with a high degree of probability, to polysaccharides or to the carbohydrate part of the molecules of glycoproteins in the broad sense of the term.

Table 12. — METHODS OF UTILIZATION PERIODIC ACID after LILLIE, 1954)

Author	Source of periodic acid	Concentration (%)	Molarity	pH	Solvent
MCMANUS (1946)	H_5IO_6	0,5	0,022	2,1	Distilled water
LILLIE (1947)	Na_4IO_5	1	0,036	1,6	0,5% HNO_3
HOTCHKISS (1948)	H_5IO_6	0,8	0,035	2,5	Na acetate in distilled water
HOTCHKISS (1948)	*id.*	*id.*	*id.*	2 4	Na acetate in 70% alcohol
LILLIE (1949)	KIO_4	0,8	0,055	1,9	0,3% HNO_3
LILLIE (1950)	—	0,69	0,030	1,9	*id.*
MOWRY (1952)	H_5IO_6	1	0,044	id.	90% alcohol

The practical methods by which periodic oxidation is used are summarised in Table 12, taken from Lillie (1954). The examination of these methods shows that the majority of investigators work in an aqueous medium. The concentrations of periodic acid can vary within rather wide limits without in any way influencing the result; according to Lhotka (1952) concentrations varying from 0.25 to 2.5% allow one to obtain rigorously equivalent preparations and errors attributable to an excess of the reagent need only be feared for concentrations of periodic acid higher than 6%. The duration of action of aqueous solutions has been estimated by the majority of investigators at 5 to 10 minutes; it is notably longer for alcoholic solutions (2 hours according to Mowry, 1952). The oxidation of *cis*-glycols seems to be more rapid than that of *trans*-glycols. In practice, periodic oxidation carried out at the temperature of the laboratory, with solutions whose concentration does not exceed 1%, incurs no risk of loss because the aldehyde stage of the oxidation of the glycols has been exceeded. The chemical industry now provides us with the dihydrate of periodic acid, which only needs to be dissolved in distilled water; formulae which make use of an alkaline periodate have thus lost much of their practical import. Solutions of periodic acid keep well but naturally become exhausted with use. It is generally considered that 100 cc of a 1% solution of periodic acid allow one to treat about 70 slides.

b) Lead tetra-acetate

This oxidation of glycols has been known to chemists since Criegee (1930) and was introduced into histochemical technique by Crippa (1951). The studies of Heidt, Gladding and Purves (1945) and Karrer (1948) have clarified the mechanism. This mechanism differs from that of periodic oxidation; in the first stage the glycol group forms an unstable cyclic compound with lead tetra-acetate, two molecules of acetic acid being liberated; in the second stage this compound undergoes a rupture of the link between the two carbon atoms bearing hydroxyl groups, with the formation of two aldehyde groups and the liberation of one molecule of lead di-acetate.

$$\begin{array}{c} R \\ | \\ H-C-OH \\ | \\ H-C-OH \\ | \\ R \end{array} + Pb(OCOCH_3)_4 \rightarrow$$

$$\begin{array}{c} R \\ | \\ H-C-O \\ | \diagdown \\ Pb(OCOCH_3)_2 + 2\ CH_3COOH \rightarrow \\ | \diagup \\ H-C-O \\ | \\ R \end{array}$$

$$\begin{array}{c} R \\ | \\ H-C=O \\ + Pb(OCOCH_3)_2 \\ H-C=O \\ | \\ R \end{array}$$

In addition to the *vic*-glycol groups (*vic* = *vicinus*, a neighbour) lead tetra-acetate oxidises amino-alcohol groups, but with the formation of a single carbonyl group, whereas their periodic oxidation causes two such groups to appear. The 1-hydroxy-2-ketonic groups and the hydroxy-aldehyde groups oxidised by periodic acid are not oxidised by lead tetra-acetate; conversely, the 1-carboxy-2-hydroxy groups (α-hydroxy-acids) which are not oxidised by periodic acid are so by lead tetra-acetate.

We know from the work of Glegg, Clermont and Leblond (1952) that the histochemical specificity of oxidation using lead tetra-acetate conforms with what one might predict from the chemical data. The periodic oxidation and that using lead tetra-acetate give comparable results in the case of carbohydrates but the optimal conditions of this second oxidation are much more strict than those of periodic oxidation, and so the margin of tolerance is much less.

As for the amino-acids, only hydroxylysine is oxidised, serine and threonine do not react, so that the range of action is narrower with the lead tetra-acetate method, resulting in a lighter background colour to the preparations. The oxidation of lipids by lead tetra-acetate seems not to have been explored so far as its repercussions on histochemical practice are concerned.

Table 13. — METHODS OF UTILIZATION LEAD TETRA-ACETATE
(after LIPP, 1955)

Author	Concentration	Solvent	Reaction time at 20°C
CRIPPA (1951)	1%	Acetic acid	30–60 minutes
SHIMIZU and KUMAMOTO (1952)	1%	Acetic acid 30 Na acetate 70 sat. sol.	10 minutes
LHOTKA	saturated	Acetic acid + 0,5M K acetate	2–3 minutes
GLEGG *et al.* (1952)	1%	Acetic acid	4 hours
JORDAN and MCMANUS (1952)	0,9%	50% acetic acid +25% Na acetate	?
HASHIM and ACRA (1953)	0,17N 0,23N	Acetic acid 50% Benzene 50 Acetic acid 50	5 minutes 5 minutes
GRAUMANN (1953)	0,5%	8N Acetic acid	15 minutes

The methods by which lead tetra-acetate are used are summarised in Table 13, as set out by Lipp (1955). All investigators agree in emphasizing the variability of the results according to the concentration, the duration of action, the temperature and the nature of the solvent. It is Graumann's variant (1953) which gives the best results, without in any way suppressing the practical inconvenience of oxidation using lead tetra-acetate, that is to say, the poor stability of the solutions *which must be prepared immediately before use and used only once,* the ease with which lead tetra-acetate decomposes, even in the solid condition (it should be kept in darkness in a hermetically sealed container and if possible under vacuum), and lastly the toxicity of the substance which is, moreover, very irritating to the skin.

c) *Sodium bismuthate*

We know from the work of Rigby (1949, 1950) that sodium bismuthate is capable of oxidising polysaccharides by means of a chemical reaction close to that which has just been described in relation to lead tetra-acetate; in the first stage, there is the formation of a cyclic compound, which by rupture of the carbon chain between the two carbon atoms which bear hydroxyl groups gives a molecule carrying two aldehyde groups; in addition, bismuth peroxide is liberated. A reaction of the same kind gives rise to the formation of aldehydes from α-hydroxy acids.

Lhotka (1952), to whom we owe the introduction of this oxidation into histochemical practice, emphasizes the theoretical advantages of the method, which seems to be highly specific for carbohydrates and which carries no risk of exceeding the aldehyde stage during oxidation of alcohol groups.

From the practical point of view, Lhotka suggests oxidising by means of a 1% solution of sodium bismuthate in 20% orthophosphoric acid. This solution should be prepared immediately before use and its optimal duration of action on the sections is 20 minutes at laboratory temperatures.

The theoretical interest of the method is undoubted but it seems not to have been studied methodically by histochemists, so that we cannot discuss the degree of effective specificity and the practical advantages.

d) *Manganese acetates*

The oxidation of carbohydrates by tri- and tetra-acetates of manganese, discovered by Zonis and collaborators (1950), takes place with the formation of alcoholates during the first stage, the decomposition of which during the second stage results in the appearance of aldehyde groups on the two carbon atoms bearing hydroxyl radicals, a rupture of the carbon chain and the liberation of manganese bi-acetate. The degree of specificity of this method is not known.

Lhotka (1953) has proposed that this method be applied in histochemistry, practising the oxidation by means of saturated solutions of tri- or tetra-acetate of manganese in glacial acetic acid, the optimal duration varying between 30 and 60 minutes at 60°C. The practical interest of this method seems slight.

e) *Phenyliodoso-acetate*

As with the preceding oxidation, that with aryliodoso acetates, introduced into organic chemistry by Criegee and Beucker (1939), has been applied in histochemistry by Lhotka (1954), who suggests the use of a 0.02 N solution of phenyliodoso-acetate in glacial acetic acid. The carbonyl groups formed from the two hydroxyls can be shown up by the Schiff reaction. The histochemical specificity seems not to have been studied and the practical advantages of this method, of which I have no experience, seem slight to me.

f) *Chromium trioxide*

The "Polysaccharidreaktion" of Bauer (1933), which was taken up by Bignardi (1935), without formal proof, as being an oxidative reaction of the carbohydrates, represents the oldest among the methods belonging to this group. The oxidation of carbohydrates by solutions of chromium trioxide does not seem to have been methodically studied by chemists, so that what we know of this matter stems almost exclusively from the work of histochemists, amongst whom it is appropriate to mention, primarily, Lillie (1951) and Mayersbach (1954). We know from their publications that chromic oxidation on the one hand and periodic oxidation on the other hand give results the general outlines of which are equivalent, which supports the hypothesis according to which the primary carbonyl groups which appear as a result of chemical oxidation occupy in the molecule of the oxidised carbohydrate the same position as those whose appearance is brought about by periodic oxidation, but notable differences exist between these two methods and all the differences are unfavourable to the Bauer reaction. In practice, oxidation by solutions of chromium trioxide very readily exceeds the aldehyde stage so that carboxyl groups appear and there is a loss of carbonyl groups which may result in a considerable weakening and even the disappearance of the staining reaction which takes place during the second stage of this method. This attenuation occurs when sections which have been subject to a preliminary oxidation with periodic acid undergo chromic oxidation in the second stage. At any given moment in the treatment with solutions of chromium trioxide some of the oxidisable hydroxyl groups have not been oxidised whereas others have already been transformed into carboxyls, so that the stage relevant to the reaction has been passed. The practical corollary is the need to adjust the duration of action of the solution of chromium trioxide with the greatest possible care, feeling one's way in stages which should be reconsidered in every new case. A second inconvenience is represented by the depolymerisation of carbohydrate macro-molecules during treatment with the oxidising solution, so that there is a possibility of loss and a danger of the diffusion of the oxidative product; treatment of the sections with collodion, which is optional in the case of periodic oxidation, is absolutely essential in that of chromic oxidation.

These inconveniences are not counter-balanced by any real advantage. The lack of chemical data prevents any closely argued discussion of the theoretical degree of specificity of the Bauer reaction and the histochemical data, which according to the authors of a dozen years ago were divergent, have now become concordant. To an ever increasing extent, the greater "selectivity" of the demonstration of certain structures rich in carbohydrates by the Bauer reaction is attributed not to a greater specificity but to losses during oxidation. Even Lison (1953, p. 312) who considered that the Bauer reaction was more specific for polysaccharides than that of the PAS reaction because it did not give positive results in certain structures, such as the collagen fibres (!), admits in the last edition of his work (1960, p. 401) that the Bauer reaction had been completely supplanted by that using periodic acid-Schiff (PAS).

It is then solely for the record that we comment on the way in which the Bauer reaction works. Dewaxed and collodion treated sections are subjected to the action of a freshly prepared 1–4% solution of chromic anhydride for a period which has to be determined by trial and error; the oxidation takes place at laboratory temperatures; it requires 30 to 75 minutes with the 4% solution and about 12 hours with the 1% solution. The sections are then washed in distilled water and subjected to tests for carbonyl groups.

We may recollect at this point that chromic oxidation confers a basophilic metachromasia on structures rich in polysaccharides. This phenomenon, which was discovered by Bignardi (1939), is particularly clear when oxidation proceeds beyond the optimum time for tests involving aldehyde groups. Whereas Clara (1940) suggested the liberation of masked sulphuric esters by chromic oxidation, modern authors, together with Bignardi (1940) and Lison (1953), consider that the metachromatic basophilia in question simply reflects the transformation of the hydroxyl groups of the carbohydrates into carboxyl groups, oxidation not being stopped at the carbonyl stage.

g) *Potassium permanganate*

As in the case of chromic oxidation, that using potassium permanganate does not rest on sound chemical foundations; it was introduced by Casella (1942) who suggested from the beginning of his work that the appearance of aldehyde groups could well be due to an oxidation of carbohydrates; in consequence, this Italian author suggested that this technique and the Bauer reaction should be considered together. The observations of Lillie (1951) confirmed Casella's point of view; as in the case of chromic oxidation, potassium permanganate oxidation can go beyond the transformation of hydroxyls into carbonyls; a metachromatic basophilia can appear after permanganate oxidation as it does after chromic oxidation. Thus, all the comments made in relation to the Bauer reaction can be applied to that of Casella. It is not possible to discuss the degree of specificity of the method in the light of chemical data and this method which includes the treatment of the sections with a 1% aqueous solution of potassium permanganate, the optimum time of action being about 20 minutes, is for all practical purposes no longer used by modern authors.

It is apparent from a review of the different oxidising agents that their effects are not strictly comparable; the principal differences are set out in Table 14.

Table 14. — NUMBER OF ALDEHYDE GROUPS FORMED BY THE OXIDATION OF THE RADICALS CONSIDERED HERE
(after GABE, 1958)

Radical	Periodic acid	Lead tetra-acetate	Na bismuthate	Mg acetate	Chromic acid	$KMnO_4$
1, 2-glycol	2	2	2	2	2(?)	2(?)
1-hydroxy 2-amino	2	1	0	0	?	?
1-hydroxy 2-alkylamino	2	1	0	0	?	?
1-hydroxy 2-keto	2	0	0	0	?	?
1-hydroxy 2-carboxy	0	1	1	?	?	?
Double bond	0	0	0	0	?	2

h) The combined use of oxidative reactions

The combination of various oxidative techniques, which have been reviewed above, with the different reactions of carbonyl groups, discussed in Chapter 13 of this work, potentially gives rise to a rather large number of theoretically possible reactions, but we need hardly add that only a few among the combinations in question have any real practical interest. Thus we shall only deal here with the periodic acid-Schiff reaction, that using lead tetra-acetate-Schiff, or that using sodium bismuthate-Schiff, as well as those involving periodic acid or chromic acid and silver complexes.

The periodic acid-Schiff reaction (PAS) is by far the most important of the techniques we have to deal with in this section. Its practical advantages have turned it into a universally used general method; cytology, microscopic anatomy and anatamo-pathological practice have greatly benefited from its use. I might note in passing that the adoption of the abbreviation PAS in a text prepared in any other language than English shows a deplorably sheeplike conformity.

Tables 12 and 15 set out the principal variations which have been put forward; two points deserve summary discussion, these are the reducing rinse, proposed by Hotchkiss (1948), at the end of the periodic oxidation, and the bath in sulphurous water at the end of the Schiff reagent action.

Table 15. — VARIATIONS IN THE PERIODIC ACID-SCHIFF REACTION after GABE, 1958)

	HOTCHKISS	MCMANUS	LILLIE	MOWRY	PEARSE
Oxidation time (minutes)	5	5	10	120	5
Reducing bath	+	0	0	0	+
Length of time in Schiff's reagent	10–45	15	10	30	20
Sulphurous acid wash	+	+	+	+	0

Most modern authors agree that the reducing rinse is useless; the liquid used by Hotchkiss (1948) (potassium iodide 1 g; sodium thiosulphate 1 g; distilled water 20 ml; absolute ethyl alcohol 30 ml; 2 N hydrochloric acid 0.5 ml) in fact acts as a blocking agent for the aldehydes; it has been at the present time abundantly demonstrated that washing in running water for from 2 to 5 minutes is sufficient to remove from the slides all traces of periodic acid.

So far as washing in sulphurous water is concerned, the comments we have made in relation to the use of the Schiff reagent for the detection of aldehydes in general are particularly relevant in the case of the PAS reaction. When the work is carried out on paraffin wax sections this washing in sulphurous water is quite useless, vigorous washing in distilled water sufficing to eliminate any artefact due to the staining of fuchsinophil structures. In the case of frozen sections, to which the PAS reaction may be applied in the same way as to wax sections, the washing cannot be carried out as quickly, and it may be useful to pass the sections through 2 or 3 baths of a dilute solution of an alkaline metabisulphite, whether or not this has been acidified.

Various background stains can be used after the PAS reaction; among the nuclear stains, haemalum, which is often used by anatomical pathologists, should be avoided, the progressive ferric lakes of haematoxylin giving much clearer preparations. When a particularly clear demonstration of acidophil cytoplasm not giving the reaction is required, it is best to use the formula suggested by Herlant (1950) for staining the adenohypophysis; the allochrome method of Lillie (1954) gives the most strongly polychrome preparations.

PAS-haematoxylin-picro-indigocarmine :

> Dewaxed sections, treated with collodion if appropriate, and hydrated;
> Treat for 5 minutes with a 0.5% solution of periodic acid in distilled water;
> Wash for two minutes in running water;
> Treat for 15 minutes in a closed receptacle with the Schiff reagent;
> Wash very vigorously in distilled water;
> Wash in running water for at least 5 minutes;
> Stain the nuclei with Groat's haematoxylin (p. 198);
> Wash for 2 minutes in running water;
> Treat for 10 to 20 seconds with picro-indigocarmine (p. 201);
> Dehydrate in absolute alcohol, clear in a benzenoid hydrocarbon, mount in Canada balsam or in a synthetic resin.

The PAS positive material is stained red or violet, the nuclei are stained black, and the acidophil cytoplasm in a clear yellow; the collagen fibres become a violet colour, resulting from the predominance of indigo-carmine during the background staining by PAS.

PAS-haematoxylin-orange G:

> Dewaxed sections, treated with collodion where appropriate, and hydrated;
> Use the PAS reaction and the nuclear staining as set out above;
> Replace the passage through picro-indigocarmine by a bath of about 1 minute in the mixture
>
> | | |
> |---|---|
> | distilled water | 100 ml |
> | phosphomolybdic acid | 1 g |
> | orange G | 2 g |
>
> Rinse in distilled water;
> Dehydrate in absolute alcohol, clear and mount in Canada balsam or in a synthetic resin.

The colouration of the PAS positive structures and of the nuclei is the same as in the preceding paragraph. The yellow of the acidophil cytoplasm is much clearer, the collagen fibres preserving the colour which the PAS reaction confers on them.

Allochrome method of Lillie:

> Dewaxed sections, treated with collodion where appropriate, and hydrated;
> Use the PAS reaction and the nuclear stain as above (Groat's haematoxylin gives results which can in all cases be compared with those using Weigert's haematoxylin, as advocated by Lillie);

After washing in running water, treat the sections for 6 minutes with the mixture-
aqueous saturated picric acid
    solution .... 100 ml
    methyl blue or water soluble aniline blue .... 0.4 g
Rinse twice with 96% alcohol, dehydrate in absolute alcohol, clear in a benzenoid hydrocarbon, and mount in a synthetic resin.

The nuclei are stained black or grey, the cytoplasm in grey or greenish-grey, the reticulin fibres in blue or red, the basement membranes are stained purple, the fibrin red, and the bony matrix in greyish-orange, the cartilage takes up a purple colour, the collagen fibres go pink, yellowish-grey or blue. The other PAS positive structures retain their reddish-purple appearance.

The PAS technique can be combined with various other histochemical reactions, particularly where it is required to detect simultaneously the various kinds of carbohydrates and of nucleic acids and carbohydrates jointly, etc... We consider such techniques in relation to the compounds in question, with the exception of the technique used by Monné and Slautterback (1951) which is founded on the successive use of two reactions for aldehydes in order to detect the carbonyls which appear as a result of periodic oxidation.

The method of Monné and Slautterback:

Dewaxed sections, treated with collodion where appropriate, and hydrated;
Oxidise using periodic acid as in the formulae given above;
Wash for 2 minutes in running water;
Rinse in distilled water;
Rinse in 70% alcohol;
Treat for 12-24 hours at laboratory temperatures with the solution:
    30% alcohol .... 100 ml
    2,4-dinitrophenylhydrazine .... saturated.
    aqueous 0.2 N solution of sodium acetate quant. suff. to neutralize the solution;
Wash in 17% alcohol repeatedly renewed;
Wash carefully in distilled water;
Treat with Schiff's reagent for 30 to 45 minutes;
Wash very vigorously in distilled water;
Give a long (10 minutes) wash in running water;
In appropriate instances, stain the nuclei with Groat's haematoxylin;
Dehydrate in absolute alcohol, clear and mount in a synthetic resin.

Certain structures containing carbohydrates which can be oxidised with periodic acid are stained in yellow, others in red.

Like the nuclear reaction of Feulgen and Rossenbeck, the periodic acid—Schiff reaction can be applied to pieces of tissue. Meyer (1960) considers that this procedure gives finer preparations and more precise evaluations than does the practice of the reaction on sections. For work with chick embryos of stages 11 to 17 of Hamburger and Hamilton, he advises the use of the following procedure.

Reagents:

- Gendre's fixative;
- Alcoholic solution of periodic acid, prepared by Hotchkiss' formula (1948); dissolve 0.4 g periodic acid in 35 ml absolute alcohol, add 5 ml of an 0.2 M aqueous solution of sodium acetate (27.2 g of the crystalline salt in 1000 ml of water) and 10 ml of distilled water; keep in the cold, and throw away at the slightest brown discoloration;
- Schiff reagent (any formula is suitable);
- Sulphur dioxide water for rinsing.

Working technique:

- Fix in Gendre's fixative at 4 °C;
- Wash for several days in 96% alcohol so as to eliminate all excess of picric acid;
- Oxidise the alcoholic solution of periodic acid for 15 to 20 minutes;
- Wash in distilled water for 10 minutes;
- Treat with Schiff's reagent for 30 minutes;
- Treat with sulphur dioxide water (three baths of 5 minutes);
- Wash in running water for 10 minutes;
- Dehydrate, clear in a benzenoid hydrocarbon, and embed in paraffin wax;
- Mount the sections after dewaxing, or dehydrate them for nuclear staining using the progressive iron lake of haematoxylin.

The presence of PAS-positive compounds is shown by the same stain as when the reaction is undertaken with sections.

The lead tetra-acetate-Schiff method follows procedures which differ mainly in the composition and the duration of action of the oxidising baths (Table 13). According to my personal experience, the best results can be obtained using the working technique advocated by Graumann (1953), the stages of which are as follows:

- Dewaxed sections, treated with collodion where appropriate, and hydrated;
- Wash in two baths, each of two minutes, of absolute alcohol;
- Wash in two baths, each of two minutes, of 8 N acetic acid;
- Oxidise for 15 minutes at laboratory temperatures with the following reagent, prepared immediately before use

    lead tetra-acetate .... 0.5 g
    8 N acetic acid (glacial acetic acid 50 ml, distilled water 50 ml) .... 100 ml

- Rinse rapidly in 8 N acetic acid;
- Wash for 15 minutes in running water;
- Rinse in distilled water;
- Treat for 20 minutes at laboratory temperatures with the Schiff reagent;
- Wash in sulphurous acid or in distilled water;
- Wash for 5 minutes in running water;
- In appropriate cases, stain the nuclei with Groat's haematoxylin;
- Dehydrate in absolute alcohol, clear, mount in Canada balsam or in a synthetic resin.

The positive result of this reaction is shown by a red or violet colour, comparable with the colours given by the PAS reaction.

The sodium bismuthate-Schiff technique follows the practice of Lhotka (1952).

> Dewaxed sections, treated with collodion if appropriate, and hydrated;
> Treat for 3 minutes at laboratory temperatures with the mixture
> > orthophosphoric acid .... 80 ml
> > distilled water .... 20 ml
> > sodium bismuthate .... 1 g
> > prepared immediately prior to use;
> Wash in running water for from 1 to 2 minutes;
> Treat for 15 seconds with normal hydrochloric acid to eliminate the precipitates of bismuth pentoxide;
> Rinse in distilled water;
> Treat for 10 minutes at the temperature of the laboratory with Schiff's reagent;
> Rinse in 3 baths of sulphurous acid or wash very vigorously in distilled water;
> Wash for from 5–10 minutes in running water;
> Stain the background where appropriate, dehydrate in absolute alcohol, clear in a benzenoid hydrocarbon, and mount in Canada balsam or in a commercial synthetic resin.

When this reaction is positive the structures containing compounds which can be oxidised by sodium bismuthate take on a red or violet colour.

Methods which use alkaline silver complexes are encumbered with all the practical defects of the argentaffin reaction, mentioned in Chapter 13; their advantage rests on the optical qualities of the preparations. The reduction of alkaline complexes to metallic silver results in more intense and more contrasted stains than are obtained with any other reaction of the aldehydes. To my knowledge, these methods have only been used for the histochemical detection of polysaccharides after chromic or periodic oxidation. We may recall, as does Lillie (1954), that a large number of structures which can be detected by the argentaffin reaction after periodic oxidation reduce the alkaline complexes of silver even when such an oxidation has not been put into effect. It stems from this that comparisons with control sections have not the same value for these techniques as they have for the methods set out earlier on.

Gomori's technique using silver-hexamethylenetetramine.

> Dewaxed sections, treated with collodion where appropriate, and hydrated;
> Oxidise for from 30 to 90 minutes (the time to be determined by trial and error) using a 5% aqueous solution of chromium trioxide, prepared immediately prior to use, or oxidise for from 5 to 10 minutes with a 0.5% aqueous solution of periodic acid;
> Wash for 5 minutes in running water (if the oxidation has been carried out with chromium trioxide verify that the yellow colour of the sections has been removed);
> Rinse in distilled water;

Treat in an oven at 37° with the following mixture, prepared immediately prior to use
stock solution of silver hexamethylenetetramine (p. 327) .... 25 ml
distilled water .... 25 ml
Holmes' buffer, pH 8.8 (a 1.23% aqueous solution of boric acid 30 ml, a 1.9% aqueous solution of borax 70 ml) .... 5 ml
Examine under the microscope every 15 minutes, and stop the action of the silver solution when the structures which are rich in carbohydrates show up in black, the background colour being a clear yellow;
Stop the reaction by rinsing in distilled water;
Tone for from 5 to 10 minutes with a 0.2% solution of gold chloride in distilled water;
Rinse in distilled water;
Treat for from 2 to 5 minutes with a 5% solution of sodium thiosulphate (hyposulphite);
Wash carefully (for about 5 minutes) in running water;
In appropriate cases, stain the background with Ramon y Cajal's trichrome, with safranine-picro-indigocarmine or with solid nuclear red-picro-indigocarmine;
Dehydrate in absolute alcohol, clear in a benzenoid hydrocarbon, mount in Canada balsam or in a synthetic resin.

The method of Arzac and Flores using silver-piperazine and silver carbonate.

Dewaxed sections, treated with collodion where appropriate, and hydrated;
Oxidise with a solution prepared immediately prior to use of 10% chromium trioxide for a period to be determined by trial and error (10 to 20 minutes), or oxidise for 5 to 10 minutes with a 0.5% aqueous solution of periodic acid;
Wash in running water for about 5 minutes (in cases where chromic oxidation has been used verify that all the yellow colour of the sections has been removed);
Rinse in distilled water;
Treat in an oven at 45° with a silver carbonate solution (p. 327), diluted to 1 in 10 with distilled water or with the silver-piperazine solution, diluted to 1 in 5 with distilled water and with the addition of 1 drop of a saturated solution of lithium carbonate for every 25 ml of solution; examine the condition of the sections every 15 minutes and stop the reaction when the reactive structures show up in black, the background remaining a clear yellow; the optimal duration of action of the silver complex is from 15 to 60 minutes according to the material;
Stop the reaction by rinsing in distilled water;
Tone with gold, fix in sodium hyposulphite and stain the background as in Gomori's technique;
Dehydrate in absolute alcohol, clear and mount in Canada balsam or in a commercial synthetic resin.

In both methods a positive result is indicated by an intense black colouration of the structures in which reducing groups, particularly carbonyl groups, have appeared following oxidation.

The other possible combinations of oxidative reactions of carbohydrates with procedures intended to discover carbonyl groups scarcely seem to be of practical interest. There is however an exception in the case of Scarselli's technique using p-phenylenediamine whose use is particularly tempting because of its sensitivity and its simplicity. The working technique is set out on page 369; the employment of this technique with a view to detecting carbohydrates obviously involves the periodic oxidation of the sections, carried out in the same way as for the PAS reaction; after washing, the oxidised sections are treated by the procedure described. This method does not seem to have been used by modern authors; according to my personal experiments it would be worthy of use, all the more so because treatment with gold chloride results in the stabilisation of the preparations, which can then be mounted after dehydration in alcohol and clearing.

THE METACHROMATIC REACTION

We know from the results set out in Chapter 13 that the metachromatic reaction discloses the presence in the structures which give rise to the phenomenon of electro negative groupings, capable of giving the reaction and distributed so that their density exceeds a certain threshold. The important role which this general method plays in the histochemical study of carbohydrates stems from the fact that some of the compounds in question, the acid polysaccharides, are in fact characterised from the chemical point of view by the presence of terminal electronegative groupings which are absent from other polysaccharides. Tests for metachromasia (metachromotropy) thus represent a means of distinguishing acid and neutral polysaccharides.

The first chemically identifiable chromotropes were in fact the sulphomucopolysaccharides (Lison, 1935, Jorpes, 1936) and in former times any metachromatic reaction was attributed to the presence of substances belonging to this group. Nowadays, we know that the sulphate grouping is not the only one capable of giving rise to this phenomenon and that in the particular case of carbohydrates carboxyl groups may also be responsible for it.

In any case, the tests for metachromasia represent one of the essential stages in the histochemical study of carbohydrates as they did in the past. Sulphomucopolysaccharides, sialomucins, the majority of mucopolysaccharides whose acid character is due to carboxyl groups are all metachromatic.

From the technical point of view, the application of the metachromatic reaction in the histochemical study of the carbohydrates calls for no special commentary. As I have remarked in Chapter 13, the attention of the histologist may be directed to the existence of metachromasia following the use of a large number of basic stains, but it is generally toluidine blue or azur A that are chosen during the systematic examination for chromotropic compounds. The method of use differs in no way from that which was described on p. 347 in relation to tests for tissular basophilia; it is nevertheless essential to examine the preparation before *and* after dehydration in absolute alcohol in order to be able to distinguish those metachromatic reactions which are resistant to alcohol from those which are eliminated by its action.

Studies in which the pH of the staining bath was varied indicated to Spicer (1962) that the metachromasia apparent at pH values lower than 1.5 was due to sulphomucopolysaccharides, whereas the clear metachromasia at pH 3 which was nevertheless absent at pH 1.5 indicated the presence of sialomucins, of non sulphated mucins with strongly dissociated carboxyl groups or of sulphomucopolysaccharides with most of their sulphate groups substituted. It is appropriate to remark that of all the metachromatropic reactions discernible in the animal body it is the metachromatic staining of the mast cells (tissular basophils, heparinocytes) which persists at the lowest pH values.

SULPHURIC OR PHOSPHORIC ESTERIFICATION

The sulphuric esterification of carbohydrates present in sections of animal tissue was used for the first time by Bignardi (1940), whose work seems to have escaped the attention of McManus and Mowry (1952) who considered themselves to have discovered this method. Phosphorylation was suggested by Landig and Hall (1956); it gives results equivalent to those using sulphuric esterification but does not seem to have been used on a large scale.

As Lison has very justly commented (1960, p. 171), these methods do not involve reactions specific to carbohydrates but are means for the detection of the alcohol group in general. Their principle consists of the esterification of the hydroxyl group of the alcohols by a strongly electronegative group (sulphate or phosphate), and then as a second stage the examination of the preparation for the appearance of a strong metachromatic basophilia. Naturally it stems from these considerations that the practical bearing of these methods is rather slight; they are nevertheless mentioned here because of their theoretical interest.

The earliest techniques for sulphuric esterification, which consisted of treating the sections, dewaxed and *dried*, with concentrated sulphuric acid for from 30 seconds to 1 minute, then washing them generously in running water and examining them by means of tests for metachromatic compounds, have been abandoned nowadays because of the corrosive nature of the treatment which has just been described. The following mixtures give better results:

- sulphuric acid-acetic anhydride in equal parts; the preparations, dewaxed and dried, remain for 3 minutes in the mixture and are then washed in water;
- sulphuric acid-ether in equal parts (Mowry) or 4 volumes of sulphuric acid to 1 volume of ether (Gomori); the sections remain in this bath for 2 to 6 minutes and are then washed in water;
- chlorosulphonic acid-pyridine (11 ml of chlorosulphonic acid and 100 ml of strictly anhydrous pyridine); the mixture is solid at ordinary temperatures, the sections should remain in it for 5 minutes at 70 °C; they are then washed in water;
- chlorosulphonic acid-acetic acid-chloroform (5 ml of chlorosulphonic acid, 10 of acetic acid, and 12 of chloroform); this mixture should be prepared immediately before use; the sections should remain in it for 5 minutes at laboratory temperatures and are then washed in water;
- sulphuric acid-acetic acid in equal parts (Lewis and Grillo, 1959); the sections, dewaxed and dried, remain in this mixture for 10 to 20 minutes; they are then gradually hydrated by passage through mixtures of sulphuric acid, acetic acid and water (6/3/1; 6/2/2; 5/1/4; 4/0/6), spending about 1 minute in each of the four mixtures; washing with water terminates the operation;

sulphuryl chloride acting in the gas phase; the dewaxed and dried sections are placed vertically in a Coplin vessel which has been well sealed, in the bottom of which about 1 ml of sulphuryl chloride has been placed; after 10 to 20 minutes they are taken out of the vessel by means of waxed forceps and washed in several baths of benzene, rinsed in absolute alcohol and then washed in water. Collodion treatment of the sections which have to undergo such a treatment is to be recommended. This latter technique of sulphuric esterification shows up glycogen in a very selective fashion.

The second stage of the technique is, in all cases, a test for compounds which have become basophilic—and metachromatic if the stain used gives rise to this phenomenon—following upon esterification. Most authors use the standard techniques with toluidine blue or azur A. Lewis and Grillo (1959) advise staining the sections with the following mixture:

M/10 solution of monopotassium phosphate	8 ml
N/10 hydrochloric acid	4 ml
1% solution of methylene blue	2 ml
Distilled water	26 ml

After 30 minutes in this staining bath, which keeps fairly well, the sections are rinsed in distilled water and treated for 1 minute with a mixture of equal parts of water and acetone, then dehydrated in acetone, cleared in a benzenoid hydrocarbon and mounted in Canada balsam or in a synthetic resin.

A positive outcome to the sulphuric esterification should be assessed by comparison with control sections which have not undergone the action of sulphuric acid but have been stained back to back with the esterified slides.

Evidently, the sulphuric esterification should abolish the PAS activity, increase the already existing metachromasia and bring to light the chromatropic properties of all the carbohydrates present in the sections. But the carbohydrates are not the only compounds to react; all the fats which have been maintained in place by the histological manipulations should also give the same reaction.

Phosphorylation is practised, according to Landing and Hall (1956), by treating the dewaxed and dried sections with pyridine containing phosphorus oxychloride to the extent of 1.5% for 3 hours at 60°C. The effects of this treatment are the same as those of sulphuric esterification.

The practical value of these procedures is not great but they may be of service, as Curran (1965) has noted, during the demonstration of certain glycoproteins or mucoproteins which are difficult to stain using other techniques.

FIXATION OF METALLIC IONS

Reactions which depend on the fixation of iron by carbohydrates endowed with electronegative groupings have been much in vogue since 1950, but it is appropriate to comment that the empirical use of these procedures dates back to the nineteenth century. According to Bensley (1934), Cl. Bernard was already using them then; methods for demonstrating the presence of mucins which correspond very closely to that of Hale have been used by List (1895) and P. Mayer (1896). An equivalent technique intended to distinguish neutral and acid mucopolysaccharides was put forward by Benazzi-Lentati (1941).

Since Hale's work (1946) the use of colloidal ferric hydrate has undergone a substantial number of modifications in detail, these differences principally concerning the preparation of the solution in which the ferric ions are carried; it is the composition of this solution which seems to be one of the essential features of this method. The publications of Gomori (1954), Lillie and Mowry (1949), Mowry (1963), Müller (1955, 1956), Rinehart and Abul-Haj (1951), Ritter and Oleson (1950), and Wolman (1956) contain many points of technical interest.

The principle of the method is simple; the ferric ions carried in the solution of colloidal ferric hydrate are fixed by the electronegative groupings of the acid mucopolysaccharides, that is to say the sulphate and carboxyl groupings; washing removes the excessive iron and the Prussian blue reaction enables one to detect that which has been solidly fixed to the tissues. Various background stains can be used and the combination with the PAS reaction enjoys a certain prestige among histochemists.

It is not hard to see that the results of using this method do not differ essentially from those which tests for basophilia give; the demonstration of acid mucopolysaccharides is very satisfactory, but other compounds endowed with electronegative groupings may fix the iron and react positively. False positives are a real risk and the staining of the nuclei under certain experimental conditions shows how difficult it is to define the limit between the histochemically significant detection of acid mucopolysaccharides on the one hand and the trivial observation of material with an affinity for iron on the other. The existence of other methods of detecting acid mucopolysaccharides removes much of the theoretical interest from procedures which rest on the fixation of ferric ions, but the morphological value of these methods cannot be contested and it is for this reason that it seems to me necessary to stress their utility here.

Preparation of colloidal solutions of iron hydrate.

This stage of the procedure is critical, the results obtained being to a large extent dependant on the quality of the reagent. Experiments using commercial solutions of ferric hydroxide represent a makeshift procedure which may be acceptable in work which is principally oriented towards morphological studies; in any histochemical study it is imperative to follow strictly the working technique for the preparation of solutions of colloidal ferric hydrate.

a) Technique of Rinehart and Abul-Haj. — Dissolve 300 g of ferric chloride in a litre of distilled water, add 400 ml of glycerine and then 220 ml of ammonia in small amounts with continual stirring; stir until dissolved. Dialyse in cellophane thimbles which are only half full against distilled water which should be renewed a dozen times in 72 hours. To this solution should be added at the moment of use a fifth of its volume of acetic acid.

b) Gomori's technique. — Prepare a mixture of equal parts of a 1% solution of medicinal iron saccharate and of 2% acetic acid. This mixture, which will keep for about a month, is used as it is.

c) Müller's technique. — Add 12 ml of a 32% solution of ferric chloride to 750 ml of distilled water kept at the boiling point. The solution keeps for several months; just before use a tenth of the volume of glacial acetic acid should be added.

We know from the work of Graumann and Clause (1958) that the selectivity with which acid mucosubstances can be demonstrated is greatly increased by increasing the acetic acid content. The authors who have just been mentioned suggest that, at the moment of use, 10 volumes of the solution of colloidal ferric hydroxide prepared according to Muller's formula, and 4 volumes of acetic acid, should be mixed. The mixture keeps for about one week, but there is, obviously, no great advantage in making up large quantities in advance.

d) Mowry's technique. — Add 4.4 ml of a 29% solution of ferric chloride to 250 ml of distilled water kept at the boiling point; allow it to boil until the liquid takes on a deep red colour. Dialyse for 24 hours against distilled water and filter. This stock solution can be used up to the moment where either a substantial precipitate or a distinct decolouration occurs. Prior to use 10 ml of the stock solution should be added to 18 ml of distilled water and 12 ml of glacial acetic acid.

We must stress the poor keeping qualities of solutions which have been diluted and treated with acetic acid; all these solutions, other than that of Gomori, should be diluted and have the acetic acid added immediately prior to use; any solution prepared on the previous day should be thrown away.

Method of use

Dewaxed sections, treated with collodion where necessary (a thin coating), and hydrated;
Treat with a dilute solution, to which acetic acid has been added, of colloidal iron for a period which varies according to the formula used

Rinehart and Abul-Haj	10 minutes
Gomori	30 minutes
Müller	10 minutes
Mowry	2 hours

Rinse in 10% acetic acid when using the formulae of Mowry or Gomori, wash in 5 baths of distilled water when using the formulae of Müller or Rinehart and Abul-Haj;

Treat for 10 minutes with the mixture consisting of equal parts of a freshly prepared 2% aqueous solution of potassium ferrocyanide and a 1 or 2% solution of hydrochloric acid;

Wash in several baths of distilled water;

In appropriate instances, stain the background by one of the techniques indicated in the section on the Prussian blue technique (p. 312);

Dehydrate in absolute alcohol, clear in a benzenoid hydrocarbon, mount in a synthetic resin (Prussian blue keeps poorly after mounting in Canada balsam).

Combination of the colloidal iron technique and the PAS reaction

(Ritter and Olsen, 1940)

Paraffin wax sections, taken from material fixed in formalin, in a formalin alcohol mixture or other customary fixatives, dewaxed, treated with collodion where appropriate, and hydrated;

Use the colloidal iron technique following the method of Rinehart and Abul-Haj;

After the wash which follows the Prussian blue reaction, use the periodic oxidative treatment and that using the Schiff reaction as in the method of McManus;

Stain the nuclei where appropriate in haemalum, or, better still, in Groat's haematoxylin;

Wash for from 2 to 5 minutes in running water;

Dehydrate in absolute alcohol, clear in a benzenoid hydrocarbon and mount in a synthetic resin.

Acid mucopolysaccharides show up in blue, neutral polysaccharides in a purplish-red. Obviously, other varieties of the colloidal iron technique can equally well be combined with the PAS reaction.

MARKER STAININGS

It seems to me appropriate to collect together in this section a certain number of procedures whose chemical mechanism cannot be unequivocally settled or whose range of specificity is very wide, but which are useful in histochemical studies on the carbohydrates. Certain classical "mucin" stains should unhesitatingly be rejected; the molybdic haematoxylin techniques of Held or of Clara, the mucicarmin and mucihaematin stains have been almost entirely eclipsed by other techniques and there is no reason to perpetuate their usage. The same comment holds good for glycogen staining, using the techniques of Vastarini-Cresi, Mayer, Fischer, etc... Staining with Best's carmine is still used for practical reasons. Although devoid of value when the polysaccharide is scarce, and distinctly less sensitive than the PAS reaction, this stain when applied to organs which are very rich in glycogen gives rise to clearer preparations than does PAS.

a) Staining with Best's Carmine

This is an empirical technique, whose chemical mechanism has not been properly elucidated, and which moreover has the awkward property of using a product as poorly defined from the chemical point of view as is carmine; I might add that the technique is one in which reverse staining is used which is always a source of inconvenience in histochemical practice. Its sole value is to allow us to obtain very clear preparations in cases where the abundance of glycogen results in opaque preparations being obtained when the PAS reaction is used. That is to say, that the technique using Best's carmine should be reserved for studies with a morphological orientation using tissues which are very rich in polysaccharides.

Reagents:

Stock solution of Best's carmine
- carmine .... 2 g
- potassium carbonate .... 1 g
- potassium chloride .... 5 g
- distilled water .... 60 ml

Boil the mixture in a sufficiently large receptacle (a great deal of froth is produced) for several minutes (until the colour is a very deep red and froth has ceased to be formed), allow it to cool and add 20 ml of ammonia;
Filter, keep in a refrigerator (the solution keeps for about 2 months);
Diluting liquid: equal parts of methyl alcohol and commercial ammonia;
Differenciator:
- methyl alcohol .... 4 volumes
- absolute ethyl alcohol .... 8 volumes
- distilled water .... 10 volumes

Masson's haemalum or Groat's haematoxylin.

Method of use:

Sections taken from material fixed in a fluid which preserves glycogen, dewaxed, treated with collodion and hydrated;
Nuclear staining with haemalum or Groat's haematoxylin;
Wash in running water;
Stain for about 10 minutes in the mixture
- stock solution of Best's carmine .... 1 volume
- diluting liquid .... 2 volumes

(prepare only the amount needed during the working session, diluted solutions of Best's carmine keep very poorly);
Without any further washing, differenciate directly by the differenciator to the point where all extraction of the dye ceases;
Dehydrate in absolute alcohol, clear in a benzenoid hydrocarbon, mount in Canada balsam or in a synthetic resin.

The nuclei are stained in blue or in black according to whether the sections have been treated with Masson's haemalum or with Groat's haematoxylin;

glycogen appears in a carmine red on a greyish or bluish background. Enzymatic control of the process is essential and one should not lose sight of the fact that too long a period in the staining bath may colour some of the mucopolysaccharides.

b) Staining with phthalocyanins of the alcian blue group

Since the introduction into histological practice of staining with alcian blue (Steedman, 1950), this method and its modifications has almost entirely supplanted the classical stains for mucins.

The stains we consider here (alcian blue, alcian green, alcian yellow, astra blue) belong to the class of copper phthalocyanins; their chemical composition is not disclosed by the manufacturers. Histological experience shows that these compounds, in certain respects, behave as basic dyes whilst devoid of the essential staining properties of these latter; in effect, they have no affinity for ribonucleins and only stain nuclei after certain pretreatments or in particular experimental conditions (material fixed for a long time or decalcified).

These properties explain the great selectivity of staining by the materials in question and justify their popularity; we should not hide from ourselves however the fact that the histochemical interpretation of the results so obtained is less easy than in the case of other procedures and that the users are always at the mercy of changes made in the manufacturing techniques. Mowry's memoir (1963) does indeed comment on the poor results obtained with samples of alcian blue supplied without any special warning and only a long correspondence with the supplier and with the chemical industry disclosed a hitherto undivulged modification of the manufacturing technique (see also p. 355, chapter 14).

Despite these defects, the copper phthalocyanins of the alcian blue group represent excellent stains for acid mucopolysaccharides. When applied without pretreatment they give results far superior to the older mucicarmine or mucihaematin stains; the results in question are substantially the same as those which Hale's method gives or which are given by procedures stemming from that method; they are also directly comparable with those of the metachromatic reaction. Nevertheless, as in the case of paraldehyde-fuchsin (see Chapter 14), various pretreatments can result in the appearance of a very strong affinity for the stains in question in structures which do not contain carbohydrates. Obviously we can only consider here those applications which are relevant to the histochemistry of the polysaccharides.

Using phthalocyanins of the alcian blue group, at a pH less than 3, without any pretreatment, results in an excellent demonstration of acid mucopolysaccharides, the "solidity" of the stain being sufficient to allow it to be combined with various background stains on the one hand or with the PAS reaction on the other.

Steedman's original working technique (staining for less than 1 minute with a 1% solution of alcian blue in distilled water) has been practically abandoned today. The various modifications now employed give equivalent results, as Lison (1960, p. 418) has noted. The technique advocated by Mowry (1956, 1963) has the advantage of simplicity and is the one I would recommend for adoption. The alcian blue solution should be made up to 0.1% for original samples and 0.5% for new samples (alcian blue 8GX) in 3% acetic acid; the pH of this solution is in the neighbourhood of 2.6. We need hardly add that the stain may, without any contra-indication, be dissolved in solutions of lower pH. The same concentrations give good results with the other phthalocyanins.

Staining with alcian blue following Mowry's technique:

> Dewaxed sections, treated with collodion where appropriate, and hydrated, taken from material fixed in a non osmic solution and not postchromated;
> Stain for from 10 minutes to 2 hours with a 0.1 to 0.5% solution of alcian blue in 3% acetic acid;
> Rinse in distilled water;
> Stain the background where appropriate with Groat's haematoxylin and van Gieson's picrofuchsin (p. 204);
> Dehydrate in absolute alcohol, clear in a benzenoid hydrocarbon, and mount in a synthetic resin.

In the absence of background staining with picrofuchsin, the acid mucopolysaccharides take on a more-or-less deep blue colour which sometimes tends towards green; the background stain in question always results in a trend towards a greenish colour. The stain is completely selective, gives rise to no opacity, and, in the very great majority of cases, the results obtained with it correspond to those obtained using the metachromatic reaction.

Combination of the alcian blue stain and the PAS reaction (Vialli, 1956; Mowry 1956):

> Dewaxed sections, treated with collodion, and hydrated;
> Stain as before with alcian blue;
> Rinse in distilled water;
> Oxidise using 0.5% periodic acid for 5 minutes;
> Wash for from 2 to 5 minutes in running water;
> Treat for 15 minutes with Schiff's reagent;
> Rinse in sulphurous acid or wash very vigorously in distilled water;
> Wash for from 5 to 10 minutes in running water;
> Stain the nuclei with Groat's haematoxylin;
> Wash for 2 minutes in running water;
> Dehydrate in absolute alcohol, clear in a benzenoid hydrocarbon, mount in Canada balsam or in a synthetic resin.

The acid polysaccharides which are rich in electronegative groupings and are PAS negative show up in blue, polysaccharides which are devoid of acid groupings show up in red, the co-existence of *vic*-glycol groupings and acidic groups being demonstrated by colours which range from purple to bluish purple.

The other phthalocyanins mentioned in this section give results which are identical with those which have just been set out for alcian blue, with minor modifications of colour. A combination of staining by alcian blue and alcian yellow, which is particularly of service in the study of acid mucopolysaccharides, is discussed in relation to the identification of these compounds.

c) Staining with alcian blue in saline solution

Scott and Dorling have been led to develop a technique for staining which applies the principal of a critical electrolyte concentration, already put to good use in the chemical separation of mucopolysaccharides, to their separation according to their acidity.

The principal of the technique consists in staining neighbouring sections with dilute solutions of alcian blue, buffered at pH 5.8, to which increasing amounts of magnesium chloride have been added. Under such conditions, the staining of slightly acid mucins is "extinguished" at concentrations of magnesium chloride less than 0.3 M, whereas that of very acid mucins only disappears at concentrations above 1.0 M.

Reagents:

1% freshly prepared aqueous solution of alcian blue 8GX;
5.0 M aqueous solution of magnesium chloride;
0.1 M sodium acetate buffer, pH 5.8;
To use, mix the solutions of alcian blue, magnesium chloride, buffer, and distilled water so as to obtain 50 ml baths whose alcian blue content corresponds to 0.05%, the molarity of the buffer being 0.025 M, and the molarity of magnesium chloride 0.05-1 M.

Working technique:

Dewaxed sections, treated with collodion where needed, taking great care to see that the coating of nitrocellulose is sufficiently thin, and hydrated;
Stain for one night, at laboratory temperatures, with the different solutions;
Rinse the sections individually in distilled water, set them aside for mounting or background staining in a bath of distilled water;
Dehydrate in absolute alcohol, clear in a benzenoid hydrocarbon and mount in a synthetic resin if the histochemical study of the structures, whose anatomy is already known, is the sole objective of the work; a background stain with the aluminium lake of nuclear fast red can be undertaken when the morphological study of the sections is also needed.

We know from Scott and Dorling's work (1965) that the mucin of the goblet cells of the rat ileum stain up to concentrations of magnesium chloride of 0.4 M, cartilage up to 0.6 M, mast cell up to 0.75 M, and the corneal stroma up to 1.0 M. As these authors have commented, their results are in agreement with biochemical findings.

d) Staining with paraldehyde-fuchsin

When applied to sections which have not undergone any particular pretreatment, this stain, whose affinity for certain electronegative groups has been described in Chapter 14, gives results which are substantially comparable with those which one obtains with alcian blue. The working technique described on p. 352 gives preparations in which the acid mucopolysaccharides take on an intense violet colour, the background of the preparation remaining substantially colourless. However, other constituents of the tissue which are devoid of acid mucopolysaccharides also stain with paraldehyde-fuchsin; elastic fibres constitute the clearest example of this. As a stain for acid mucopolysaccharides, paraldehyde-fuchsin has no advantage over the phthalocyanins of the alcian blue group.

CONTROL TESTS

The results of the techniques expounded in the preceding sections can be controlled by various methods, some of which depend on the blocking of carbonyl groups which appear in the polysaccharides following oxidation by various agents, others depend on the destruction, before the diagnostic reaction or stain, of the polysaccharide which is the object of study, and yet others depend on its chemical transformation. We might well add here that *the use of oxidative reactions in a histochemical study obliges the experimenter to compare sections, some of which have undergone the oxidising reaction whereas others have been kept for an equivalent time in the solvent, the subsequent treatment being rigorously identical for the two series of slides.*

a) Blocking reactions for the carbonyl groups

These reactions, which are described in Chapter 15, are of no great interest in histochemical tests for carbohydrates using oxidative reactions. In fact, the effective specificity of the Schiff reaction for aldehydes is sufficient for the blocking of these groups after the oxidation of wax embedded sections nearly always to give the negative result which the theory would predict. It is quite otherwise when the reactions take place in frozen sections, since the preservation *in situ* of some of the lipids and of their oxidative derivatives may represent a very real cause of error. Moreover, controls involving the blocking of aldehyde groups may be of service in this latter case even when the detection of the carbonyls is assured by the Schiff reaction.

The usefulness of such controls is evidently greater in cases where the carbonyls are detected by the argentaffin reaction, a method which is in no way specific for aldehyde groups and which rests quite simply on their reducing power. We know from the methodical study of Lillie (1954) that the comparison of results obtained after periodic oxidation with the Schiff reaction on the one hand and the argentaffin reaction on the other allows us to distinguish three categories of compounds which may be reacting.

Some of these, after periodic oxidation, give positive results with the Schiff reaction and with alkaline silver complexes, the two reactions are rendered negative by blockage of the carbonyl groups; results obtained with the two methods must then be due to the appearance of aldehyde groups following periodic oxidation.

Other compounds give the periodic acid-Schiff reaction, but cannot be detected by the argentaffin reaction when used after periodic oxidation.

Yet other compounds have an affinity for silver even without preliminary periodic oxidation and give the periodic acid-Schiff reaction, this last becoming negative when the aldehyde functions are blocked.

From the technical point of view, all the blocking methods considered in Chapter 14 can be used as controls between the periodic acid oxidation or that using other oxidising agents on the one hand, and the detection of carbonyl groups on the other.

b) Inhibition of oxidation by lead tetra-acetate

Staple (1955, 1957) has described the inhibition of oxidation by lead tetra-acetate by the addition to the oxidising bath of boric acid in sufficient quantities to result in a concentration of 0.01 M. Trials on a model and on sections of tissue containing chemically identifiable polysaccharides led this author to consider that boric acid formed complexes resistant to oxidation with the *cis*-glycol groups, this complex formation not taking place for *trans*-glycols; the latter thus remain detectable.

c) The decomposition of polysaccharides on sections

This decomposition which constitutes the point of the control reaction is obtained by means of enzymatic preparations. Among those which play a particularly important part are the amylase reaction, intended to serve as a control for the reactions and staining tests for glycogen, that using neuraminidase, which serves for the identification of sialomucins, and that of hyaluronidase, which allows us to recognise the occurrence of hyaluronic acid; other enzymatic reactions which have been put forward (chondroitinase, chondrosulphatase, pectinase, β-glucuronidase, extracts of *Flavobacterium heparinum*, ribonuclease, etc...) have given interesting results, but their use does not yet form part of current practice.

Tests with amylase. — Amylase treatments which are used for the identification of glycogen have long been practised in the form of the saliva test (see

Lillie, 1947, 1949 for a review of the older applications). The original working technique consisted in allowing filtered saliva to work in a damp chamber on the sections, and has happily been abandoned for less summary techniques. Most authors use commercial preparations of malt diastase which contain mixtures of α and β-amylase; the use of purified preparations of amylase, which are expensive, is not necessary in ordinary practice. We give here the simple and sure method of use of Lillie (1954).

Paraffin wax sections, dewaxed, but *not treated with collodion*, and hydrated;
Treat for 1 hour in an oven at 37 °C with a 1% solution of a commercial preparation of malt diastase in the following buffer

monopotassium phosphate monohydrate .... 0.8 g
anhydrous disodium phosphate .... 1.3 g
distilled water .... 1 litre
sodium chloride (optional) .... 8 g

(this buffer whose pH is 6 may be replaced by distilled water);
Wash in distilled water;
Dehydrate in absolute alcohol or in acetone;
Treat the sections with collodion;
Use whatever histochemical reactions or staining tests are required, comparing the results with those of control sections which have not undergone enzymatic digestion.

We may mention here that human saliva and most commercial preparations of malt diastase contain ribonuclease which is evidently of no importance when acting as a control for the demonstration of glycogen; one should nevertheless take it into account when considering the other stain affinities of preparations obtained in this way in order to avoid a source of error in experiments which are intended to examine at the same time glycogen and the ribonucleins.

Commercial preparations of malt diastase do not keep indefinitely, even when they are stored as a precaution at low temperatures and the required amount of solution is prepared immediately prior to use; it is wise therefore to check their efficacy by treating slides whose glycogen content is assured before using the preparation to study material which has not yet been examined.

Tests with sialidase (neuraminidase) of microbial origin are of increasing importance in the identification of sialomucins. The majority of authors use preparations obtained from cultures of *Vibrio cholerae* or of *Clostridium perfringens*. Preparations of this kind can be supplied by various institutes of bacteriology.

The enzymatic action lasts for from 6 to 24 hours, at 38 or 39°C; it should be carried out by covering the sections, which are placed in a damp chamber, with several drops of the enzymatic preparation. At the end of the chosen duration of action the excess liquid is removed with a pipette, the slides are carefully washed and then subjected to the reactions and staining tests appropriate for the demonstration of sialomucins (alcian blue-PAS, the metachromatic reaction, paraldehyde-fuchsin, the reaction with dimethyl-p-phenylenediamine, etc...). As in the case of the test using malt diastase, it is essential to compare the slides with those which have not undergone the action of the enzymatic preparation; to be rigorous, this comparison should be made with control slides treated with a solvent for the enzymatic preparation, so as to be able to distinguish between the destruction by the enzyme on the one hand and simple solution on the other.

The test with hyaluronidase was introduced into histological practice by Manozzi-Torini (1942). This enzymatic attack, which results in the depolymerisation of the hyaluronic acid, and then the cleavage of the glycoside linkages has been used by numerous authors in order to distinguish between hyaluronic acid and the other acid mucopolysaccharides. The results thus obtained are distinctly less unequivocal than those in which the other two enzymatic digestion tests which have just been mentioned are used, the essential reason for this state of affairs being the great variability of the effects which different commercial preparations of hyaluronidase can exert. In fact, biochemists have shown that hyaluronidase of microbial origin is in fact specific and that it only affects hyaluronic acid, whereas preparations of testicular origin also act on certain sulphomucopolysaccharides. As a result, from the practical point of view, the use of the hyaluronidase test in order to identify, histochemically, hyaluronic acid makes no sense unless the investigator has a tried and tested preparation of this enzyme; the origin and the characteristics of preparations of hyaluronidase used in a particular piece of work should always be most explicitly described.

The technique for using preparations of hyaluronidase closely follows that which has been described for amylase and neuraminidase. Most authors work in a damp chamber at 37°C using either commercial preparations or extracts prepared *ad hoc*, taken into solution in physiological saline or in buffers of a pH range between 4.8 and 7. The duration of action varies from one author to another from 30 minutes to 72 hours and the variability of the criteria of biochemical activity which serve to determine the strength of commercial preparations prevents any standardisation being attempted. For each new enzymatic preparation and for each new source of material trial and error methods are therefore essential.

d) *Chemical transformation of the polysaccharides*

The chemical transformation of polysaccharides, in sections, with a view to their identification, involves reversible acetylation and methylation which are important processes and used daily in this type of work; nevertheless benzoylation may also be used although this is a process rarely called into play in research on the polysaccharides.

According to Lillie (1954), **benzoylation** is practised in the following way.

> Dewaxed sections, passed through absolute alcohol, treated in a bath of pyridine for several seconds;
> Keep the sections for from 1 to 24 hours at 25 °C or from 30 minutes to 6 hours at 58 °C, in the mixture
>
> anhydrous pyridine .... 38 ml
> benzoyl chloride .... 2 ml
>
> Treat with two baths of absolute alcohol (20 to 30 seconds in each bath), pass through 96% alcohol, and hydrate the sections;
> Carry out the chosen histochemical reaction or diagnostic colour reaction, comparing the results with those given by sections which have been kept warm in anhydrous pyridine, without the addition of benzoyl chloride.

The time taken for the benzoylation of the hydroxyl groups, with a loss of their sensitivity to periodic oxidation, varies according to the material chosen. It is therefore useful in each particular case to investigate several slides which have been treated for periods intermediate between the extremes indicated above.

Reversible acetylation, which is much more widely used than is benzoylation, provides information on the carbohydrate, lipid or proteinaceous nature of compounds which react positively with PAS; we know from the data set out in the appropriate section of this chapter that substances belonging to the three groups which have just been noted above may, in principal, be responsible for a positive result of the reaction.

The method was put forward by Gersh (1949) during his work on the glycoprotein constituents of the Golgi apparatus, and has been put into practice and developed by means of the control reaction represented by the saponification of acetylated sections as used by MacManus and Cason (1950). These authors consider that only the *vic*-glycol groups undergo, in the experimental conditions defined by them (treatment of the sections with a mixture of acetic anhydride and pyridine, at laboratory temperatures for 45 minutes), acetylation of the two hydroxyl groups, saponification with a dilute soda or potash solution re-establishing the PAS activity.

This interpretation is universally admitted so far as the behaviour of the *vic*-glycol groups is concerned, but that of other groups, capable of oxidation by periodic acid, has given rise to debate. Most authors do not commit themselves on the behaviour of α-keto-groups, whose presence in compounds preserved on the sections embedded in paraffin rarely occurs; Lison (1953, 1950) considers that acetylation does not modify their reactivity. The same author comments that the activity of 1-hydroxy-2-alkylamine groups ought also to persist despite the acetylation. These two groups should thus be easily distinguished from the others since the *vic*-glycol groups are easy to acetylate as are the 1-hydroxy-2-amino groups. It is the distinction between the two groups, *vic*-glycol on the one hand and amino-alcohol on the other, which is the most controversial. According to MacManus and Cason (1950), acetylation abolishes the activity of the amino-alcohol groups, and saponification does not re-establish it; Pearse (1953) also takes this point of view, but Lison (1953) contests it. In fact, the chemical study of Kent and Whitehouse (1955) showed that the acetylation of the two amino-alcohol groups is in fact extremely easy, but that during saponification a clear distinction manifests itself between the acetic ester groups and amide groups formed during acetylation; the saponification of the first is easy but that of the second requires alkaline conditions and a temperature neither of which occurs under the working conditions of the histochemist. It follows from this that saponification only re-establishes one group oxidisable by periodic acid out of the two in the case of amino-alcohols so that there is a distinct weakening of the stain obtained by the PAS reaction. These ideas, which have been most opportunely brought to light by Hale (1957), should lead us to understand that the identification of groups other than the vic-glycols by means of reversible acetylation should not rest uniquely on the disappearance of the PAS activity after acetylation and on the reappearance of a colouration after saponification of the sections and the PAS reaction; the intensity of the colouration which reappears should also be taken into consideration. Since saponification of the amide groups is more difficult, the number of groups capable of periodic oxidation is reduced by half when sections containing amino-alcohol or alkylamino-alcohol groups are subjected to the two stages of the test advocated by MacManus and Cason. The very clear reduction of the staining reaction on acetylated sections which are then saponified represents the criterion for the presence in the structures under investigation of groups other than the vic-glycol. As a result, the comparison of sections treated with the PAS reaction and those which have undergone the two stages of reversible acetylation before being subjected to this technique give results analogous to those stemming from the comparison of the PAS reaction on the one hand and that of lead tetra-acetate on the other. In both cases the colour of those places where compounds rich in amino-alcohol groups occur is much more intense in sections treated simply with PAS than on the others. For this reason, reversible acetylation can be extremely useful.

We may add to the above that the test using reversible acetylation allows us to recognise the presence in sections of lipids oxidisable by periodic acid and which have survived the paraffin wax embedding. The bath of mixed acetic anhydride and pyridine in fact results in their extraction, and causes the complete disappearance of the reactivity to periodic acid-Schiff.

From the practical aspect, we may note that the working technique of MacManus and Cason (1950) has been abandoned by modern authors, all of whom recommend either durations of action which are longer or a higher working temperature. Lillie (1954) advises acetylation for 24 hours at laboratory temperatures or for 6 hours at 58°C. Graumann (1954) recommends a period of 24 hours, at laboratory temperatures, in the mixed acetic anhydride-pyridine. These authors consider that there is an "acetylation time" for the different compounds which can be detected by the PAS reaction. In fact, a methodical study of the part played by the time factor in the test using reversible acetylation showed that the duration of acetylation was very variable for one and the same carbohydrate according to the origin of the material and that substantial differences existed moreover between different carbohydrates (Gabe and Mme Martoja, 1956). The complexity of factors which might explain these differences (one might invoke the variability of the glycoproteide linkages according to the nature of the material) prevents us in any case from giving an acetylation time for any given carbohydrate. The same remark holds good for the saponification time which may vary, for one and the same carbohydrate, from 5 to 45 minutes.

The following working technique (Gabe and Mme Martoja, 1956), which we advocate for the practice of reversible acetylation, necessitates the use of five equivalent sections of the tissue under investigation.

Section A: Dewax, treat with collodion, hydrate, keep, for 3 hours, in distilled water at 37 °C;
Section B: Dewax, treat with collodion, rinse in pyridine and keep, for 3 hours, at 37°, in pure pyridine;
Section C: Dewax, treat with collodion, rinse in pyridine and keep, for 3 hours, in an oven at 37 °C, in the mixture used by MacManus and Cason.
 anhydrous pyridine .... 20 ml
 acetic anhydride .... 13 ml
 (this solution should be used only once);
Section D: The same treatment as for C, then rinse in distilled water, wash in running water for 1 minute, and treat for 45 minutes with a 0.1 N solution of potash or, according to the recommendations of Lillie (1954) with the mixture
 70% alcohol .... 8 volumes
 ammonia .... 2 volumes
Section E: Dewax, treat with collodion, and hydrate immediately prior to the use of the PAS reaction.

The five sections are subjected to the PAS reaction under rigorously identical conditions; the results are compared taking account of the intensity of the colours produced; they can be summarised according to the nature of the substance responsible for the activity in the form of a table (Table 16).

Table 16. — RESULT OF RESERVIBLE ACETYLATION OF THE COMPOUND RESPONSIBLE FOR THE PAS REACTION

	Slides				
	A	B	C	D	E
Carbohydrate rendered thoroughly insoluble during fixation	+	+	—	+	+
Carbohydrate rendered inadequately insoluble	—	— or +	—	— or +	+
Lipid	+	—	—	—	+
Protein	+	+	—	±	+

Reversible methylation, introduced into histochemical practice by Lillie's school (Fisher and Lillie, 1954; Spicer and Lillie, 1959) represents the most important among the methods to be discussed in this section. In fact, methylation acts as much on the orthochromatic or metachromatic basophilia as it does on the PAS reaction and the saponification of the methylated sections induces results which differ for sulphomucopolysaccharides and for mucopolysaccharides whose acidity is due to the carboxyl groups. The studies of Kantor and Schubert (1957) do in fact show that methylation results, in the case of sulphomucopolysaccharides, in the removal of the sulphate group which is replaced by a hydroxyl group so that it is impossible to re-establish the electronegative grouping by saponification; the carboxyl or phosphoryl radicals remain, on the other hand, attached to the molecule, so that it is possible to re-establish them by saponification.

The effects of methylation on the various tissue constituents have been defined in the major work of Fisher and Lillie (1954), and some of the conclusions of these authors have subsequently been confirmed.

The *PAS activity* is only abolished in certain cases and its weakening requires considerable durations of action (48 to 96 hours in methyl alcohol containing hydrochloric acid at 0.1 N molarity); on the other hand, the metachromasia disappears very quickly (in less than two hours at 58°C); *the cytoplasmic basophilia and that of the nucleoli* completely disappears in 4 hours at the most; *nuclear basophilia* may persist, though very much attenuated, when the duration of methylation is less than 24 hours; *the affinity of the nuclei for the progressive lakes of haematoxylin*, in particular for haemalum, persists unmodified even after 8 days of methylation in the warm or three weeks of methylation at laboratory temperatures; a methylation of 4 days in the warm does not modify the result of the nucleal reaction of Feulgen and Rossenbeck. These observations were made with tissue fixed in formalin; the time taken for the disappearance of cytoplasmic basophilia is slightly longer after fixation in Zenker's fluid, the others remaining unchanged.

We know from later work (MacManus and Mowry, 1960, Curran, 1964) that the affinity of acid mucopolysaccharides for alcian blue disappears a little less quickly than does their metachromasia; treatment for 3 hours, at 58°, might be needed.

In practical terms, reversible methylation is used in the following way.

Paraffin wax sections, dewaxed, treated with collodion and hydrated;
Treat in an oven at 58 °C for periods running from 2 to 12 hours (3 hours in general), with the mixture—
  concentrated hydrochloric acid .... 0.8 ml
  absolute methyl alcohol to make up to .... 100 ml
or (Kantor and Schubert, 1957; Lison, 1960) with methyl alcohol into which gaseous and dry hydrochloric acid has been bubbled);
Rinse rapidly in absolute alcohol;
Carry out a second treatment with collodion where appropriate (collodion is soluble in methyl alcohol);
Set by certain of the sections in distilled water;
Treat the remaining sections for 20 minutes with the solution
  potassium hydroxide in pellet form .... 1 g
  80% alcohol .... 100 ml
Wash in distilled water;
Carry out the appropriate colour reaction (alcian blue or tests for metachromasia, etc.) on the methylated sections and on those which have undergone boh methylation and saponification.

As Curran (1964) has remarked, the interpretation of the results of methylation should take account of the fact that this reaction may block the carboxyl groups of proteins, and hence change their electropolar nature; these macromolecules, when they have become electropositive, may enter into competition with the cations of the stain for the electronegative groupings of the mucopolysaccharides and thus inhibit the metachromasia.

Recent results, published since the French Edition of this book was published, require us to revise the interpretation given by Lillie's school. It so happens that replacement of methyl alcohol by inert solvents, such as cyclohexane or benzene, is compatible with the "methylation" of acid mucosubstances of the oviduct of *Triton* (Vilter, 1968); Vilter supposes, as a result, that the disappearance of the basophilia of the mucins in the experimental circumstances of Fisher and Lillie's methylation technique is due to their lactonisation rather than to their esterification. A wider study of material led Sorvari and Stoward (1970) to confirm this way of regarding the situation. The basophilia of a whole series of mucins is abolished after treatment with solutions of hydrochloric acid in methanol, ethanol, butanol, benzene or cyclohexane. In the great majority of cases, the results are equivalent to those obtained with Fisher and Lillies original technique; this fact makes it quite improbable that basophilia can be abolished by simple esterification of anionic groups.

After saponification, Sorvari and Stoward restored the basophilia due to the carboxyl groups, but that due to the presence of sulphate-esters remained suppressed. In a later investigation the same authors (Sorvari and Stoward, 1970) obtained supplementary evidence for the formation of lactones during the methylation procedure. They did in fact show that "methylated" mucosubstances did not regain their basophilia after saponification whenever this latter process was preceded by treatment at 4°C with a concentrated solution of sodium or potassium borohydride, substances which, *in vitro*, reduce lactones but not esters. The same results can be obtained by treating the sections, after "methylation" and before saponification, with hydroxylamine *in a neutral medium*; it is known that hydroxylamine, in neutral solutions, condenses with lactones but not with esters, to form hydroxamic acids. In both instances, the suppression of the liberation of anionic groups by saponification, a fact which explains the loss of affinity for azur A, is an argument of great value favouring the presence of lactones and not of esters in the structures rich in mucosubstances which have been subjected to methylation. Moreover, treatment of the methylated sections with very dilute soda (pH 9.5) affords a partial restoration of the affinity for azur A. We know that most of the glucuronic lactone rings can be opened quite easily at pH 9.5, whereas most esters, with the exception of the methyl esters of sialic acids of various kinds, only undergo alkaline hydrolysis at pH values above 10.

All these facts show that the simple explanations put forward originally to interpret the results of "reversible methylation", probably stand in need of revision. It seems wiser to dispense with the routine employment of this technique until further work has been done, despite the confirmation arising from the work of Sorvari and Stoward, that the basophilia due to carboxyl groups is the only one re-established after saponification of the "methylated" sections, in the material studied by these authors.

C. — HISTOCHEMICAL IDENTIFICATION OF DIFFERENT KINDS OF POLYSACCHARIDES

As has been remarked by Rosan and Saunders (1965), and Spicer and his collaborators (1965), the nomenclature of the carbohydrates contained in animal tissues has undergone a development which is different in the language of biochemists as compared with that of the histochemists, the disparity being particularly great in the usage of the terms mucopolysaccharide, mucosubstance and mucin. Individual chemical compounds can only be identified by the histochemist in a very small number of instances; most frequently the objective of the histochemical part of the work is to allocate the compounds studied to one or other of the groups of histochemically detectable carbohydrates. It would be all too easy to sit back and augment the number of difficulties which Spicer and his collaborators noted, by extending the framework of reference outside that of the tissues of mammals to which the American authors deliberately limited their article. Even a summary study of the "mucins" of the molluscs would bring to light compounds which cannot be classified in the categories proposed by Spicer (1960, 1963), or by Spicer and his collaborators (1965). Only close cooperation of biochemical and histochemical studies can remove this inconvenience.

It is nevertheless true that the attempt at a classification made by Spicer and his collaborators (1965) deserves to be taken widely into consideration and that the adoption of the nomenclature proposed by these authors would greatly increase the uniformity of the descriptions. It seems to me, then, indispensable to take account of it here.

GLYCOGEN

The demonstration by histochemical methods of this polyholoside in the sense of the chemists has been practised for more than a century but this does not mean that all the problems inherent in this demonstration can be considered as having been resolved.

The fixation of glycogen has given rise to an impressive number of publications, some of which are only of historical interest. Even the sharp debate concerning the diffuse or granular distribution of this polysaccharide in the cell has lost all its relevance since the electron microscope has solidly established the existence of glycogen in the cell, in the form of primary granulations, the dimensions of which are much below the possibilities of resolution under the light microscope (130 Å in diameter on an average); even secondary granulations (600 to 1,500 Å in diameter), which result from the agglomeration of the primary ones, are distinctly below the resolving power of the light microscope and only granulations of the third order, resulting from the aggregation of those mentioned above, are capable of being resolved. Nevertheless it is established that the best of the fixatives preserve the glycogen in the immense majority of cases in diffuse form within the cytoplasm, at least under the working conditions of light microscopy. As a result studies of the ultimate localisation of glycogen in certain organelles or in certain parts of the cell belong to ultrastructural cytology and not to histochemistry under the light microscope; this latter should content itself with determining the presence or absence of glycogen in a cell and even the estimation of the quantity to be found there can only be done to a very rough approximation.

The preservation of glycogen *in situ* results not from its precipitation but from the preservation of the protein web which holds it in place or to which it is chemically linked. Older fixative formulations using alcohol should be summarily rejected. Clarke's fluid and that of Carnoy, which have been mentioned in relation to general techniques, give satisfactory results for ordinary work; the same is true of Bouin's fluid, and that of Regaud; very satisfactory results can be obtained so far as glycogen is concerned using solutions of osmium tetroxide, but the preservation of the other tissue constituents is mediocre. It is admitted that, since the coming of the PAS reaction, most of the failures which have been noticed using topographical fixatives relate, not to the loss of glycogen, but to a badly stained preparation using Best's carmine. It has also been shown that the ease or difficulty with which glycogen is fixed varies greatly from one object to another. In the easy cases, all the customary liquid fixatives prepare glycogen in the cells where its abundance exceeds a certain threshold level for detection by the PAS technique. It is in the more difficult cases that recourse to fixatives devoid of corrosive sublimate and very rich in picric acid may be of special service. In this respect Gendre (1935) advises the use of a mixture of 80 volumes of 96% alcohol saturated with picric acid, 15 volumes of formalin and 5 volumes of acetic anhydride. This mixture is replaced at the end of several hours (4 to 24) according to the size of the pieces of fixed tissue, by 96% alcohol. Rossman's liquid (1940) contains 90 volumes of absolute alcohol saturated with picric acid to each 10 volumes of commercial formalin. It is used for from 12 to 24 hours, the pieces then being placed in 96% alcohol. It is appropriate to remember, for the record, that Pasteels and Leonard (1935) were led to use fixation in dioxane saturated with picric acid (30% of picric acid) in the particularly difficult case constituted by the preservation of glycogen in the gastrula of Amphibia.

The fixatives whose composition has just been described ensure a better preservation of glycogen than occurs when so-called topographical fixatives are used, but they preserve the tissue and cell structures in general very badly; moreover, they give rise to the classic phenomenon of polarization movement to a greater extent than occurs with aqueous fixatives, glycogen accumulating in each cell, at the pole which is furthest from the surface through which the fixative is penetrating.

When the preservation *in situ* of the glycogen is particularly difficult the investigator may need to have recourse to procedures which are certainly the best but not the most simple, namely freeze-drying and freeze-substitution. It is through the use of these two methods that we obtain the most faithful localisation on the scale of the light microscope. We should not lose sight of the fact that displacements of the glycogen under the effects of the fixative may go beyond the simple polarization (image de fuite), (Alkoholflucht of the German authors) and end up by causing the appearance of precipitates of the substance in the lumen of blood vessels, in the excretory ducts of glands, in the intercellular lacunae etc...

The rapidity with which glycogen is degraded during postmortem autolysis explains the need for prompt fixation; this need is as imperious for histochemical work as for quantitative studies of this substance using chemical methods.

The subsequent treatment of the pieces does not in principal require any particular precaution; it is at the moment of fixation that losses and movements are most to be feared. In the great majority of cases, the test for glycogen is made on paraffin wax sections, but it can take place on celloidin sections; it was even suggested before the PAS reaction came into use that the passage of the pieces of material in celloidin solutions (prepared with alcohol-ether or with methyl benzoate) favoured the preservation of this polyholoside; in fact, it may well stem simply from a better preparation of the blocks of tissue for staining with Best's carmine, but paraffin embedding passing through solutions of celloidin in methyl benzoate is, in any case, advantageous from the technical point of view and I would advise it most strongly.

The spreading of the sections may, in principle, be conducted in the usual fashion; it is only in exceptional cases that comparison with sections spread on alcohol shows a loss at the moment when this manoeuvre is carried out. Collodion treatment during the staining or the histochemical test is definitely required; where there is to be treatment with amylase, that with collodion should follow the action of this enzyme.

The histochemical demonstration in the strict sense of the term principally calls into play the PAS reaction; that with lead tetra-acetate or with sodium bismuthate whose range of action is narrower are only useful when the tissues examined are found to be very rich in PAS-positive compounds other than glycogen. When this latter substance is very abundant, the morphological study of the preparations may benefit from staining with Best's carmine. The classical stain using iodine is only useful in cases where the interpretation is contested; among the numerous formulae put forward the best is that of Mancini (1944), the working technique for which is as follows.

> Paraffin wax sections, coming from material fixed in a liquid which ensures the preservation of glycogen
> Dewax the sections;
> Cover them when they come out of the benzenoid hydrocarbon with a drop of vaseline oil saturated with doubly sublimed crystalline iodine; allowing it to act for from 3 to 24 hours;
> Take off the cover slip from the preparation, mop up the excess of vaseline oil around the sections, and allow the following mixture, which should be prepared immediately prior to use, to act for several minutes (2 to 5)
>   xylene .... 9 volumes
>   a 2% solution of mercuric iodide in
>   absolute alcohol .... 1 volume
> (the solution of mercuric iodide requires the addition of a trace of potassium iodide);
> Wipe the slide around the sections, replace a drop of vaseline saturated with iodine, replace the cover slip, wipe the edges and ring the cover slip.

Under these conditions, glycogen takes on the well known mahogany brown colour.

The strong PAS reactivity which disappears after the action of amylase and the positive result using the iodine technique suffice for the characterisation of glycogen. It is moreover appropriate to recollect that the PAS reactivity will obviously disappear when blocking of the aldehyde groups takes place between the oxidation and the action of Schiff's reagent; this blockage is difficult to obtain by the use of dimethylcyclohexanedione (dimedone) and Bulmer (1959) has put this peculiarity to good use; its chemical mechanism is still unknown but there is a highly selective demonstration of glycogen by the PAS reaction, even in cases where the sections are very rich in other PAS positive substances. The sections, after oxidation by periodic acid, are treated, for three hours at 60°C, with a 5% solution of dimedone in absolute alcohol, rinsed in absolute alcohol, rehydrated and submitted to the action of Schiff's reagent. Experience shows that glycogen is the only PAS positive substance to keep its activity under these experimental conditions.

We need hardly add that the PAS activity of glycogen resists the attack of other enzymes mentioned in the preceding sections; it disappears after acetylation but *completely* reappears after saponification. Glycogen, which is devoid of basophilia and is not chromotropic, acquires these properties after sulphuric esterification, under experimental conditions compatible with its preservation *in situ* (sulphuryl chloride, Lewis and Grillo, 1959). A result of the same kind can be obtained in certain cases by oxidation with chromium trioxide, but the practical interest of this latter method is negligible. It should be unnecessary to state that glycogen, in the absence of pretreatments capable of bringing into play electronegative groupings, is devoid of any of the histochemical characteristics of acid mucopolysaccharides.

The possibility of a quantitative determination of glycogen on sections can obviously scarcely be considered so long as the demonstration of this compound rests on colour tests whose chemical mechanism is unknown. Since the coming of the PAS reaction, various workers have tried to estimate glycogen histophotometrically; the results are rather discordant. According to some authors (Deane and collaborators, 1946), there is a good agreement between the histophotometric measures and chemical estimations in tissues whose glycogen content does not exceed 5%, but detailed precautions need to be taken during fixation; other authors (Eger, 1942; Gibb and Stowell, 1949) have far more reservations so far as the possibility of histophotometric determination of glycogen is concerned, and it seems reasonable that in the present state of our knowledge preference should be given to chemical methods of determination in all cases where the work is intended to go beyond the stage of an approximate estimation of the glycogen content of a tissue.

GALACTOGEN

This polyholoside whose hydrolysis gives rise to galactose, whereas that of glycogen gives rise to glucose, is not widely distributed in metazoan tissues. In addition to the albumen gland of the pulmonate gastropods, which is the essential site, modern studies have established its presence in certain vertebrate tissues.

Since the main work of Bauer (1933) showed the possibility of demonstrating galactogen by chromic oxidation, followed by the action of Schiff's reagent, the histochemical detection of this polysaccharide has been studied by various authors. The techniques have been set out by Grainger and Shillitoe (1952), whose results are summarised in Table 17.

According to my personal experience, which bears uniquely on the albumen gland of the pulmonate gastropods, the fixation of galactogen is much easier to secure than that of glycogen, none of the usual fixatives giving rise to true polarization images. Its preservation during embedding in paraffin is equally easy, but tissues which are very rich in galactogen have a strong tendency to harden. During reversible acetylation, galactogen behaves as does glycogen (Gabe and Mme Martoja, 1956). Its sulphuric esterification does not seem to have been studied.

Table 17. — FEATURES DIFFERENTIATING GLYCOGEN AND GALACTOGEN
(after GRAINGER and SHILLITOE)

Method	Glycogen	Galactogen
PAS	+	+
Best's carmine	+	+
Iodine	+	—
Metachromasia	0	+ (does not withstand dehydration)
Haemalum	0	0
Eosin	0	+
Mucicarmine	0	±
Silver-hexamethylenetetramine (Gomori)	+	±
Ruthenium red	dissolved	coloured
"Pectinase"	dissolved	dissolved
Saliva	dissolved	preserved
Malt diastase	dissolved	preserved

In practice, the positive result of the PAS method and of staining by Best's carmine, the absence of staining with iodine and its resistance to the action of malt diastase added to the negative result of reactions for mucopolysaccharides, serves to identify galactogen in paraffin wax sections. It is rare that an investigator would have to go so far as to bring into play staining with ruthenium red; this last method is applied in a way which is set out in works on botanical technique (see also p. 437).

CELLULOSE

Cellulose, which is very sparsely distributed in animal tissues, exists in fact only in the tunicates (tunicin). Its histochemical characteristics are extensively described in treatises on plant histochemistry. Its preservation in wax sections is ensured by any of the usual methods of fixation. The PAS activity is intense and persists after treatment with malt diastase; its behaviour during reversible acetylation is identical with that of glycogen. Treatment by Lugol's fluid, followed by the action of a mixture of two parts of sulphuric acid to one part of water (by weight), results in the appearance of an intense, but fugitive, blue colour, so that it is necessary to examine the preparations immediately, covering the reagent with a cover slip. In the same way, the violet colour obtained by mounting the hydrated sections in a mixture of 25 parts of zinc chloride (by weight), 8 parts of potassium iodide and 8.5 parts of distilled water is fugitive. We may moreover note that the fibres of cellulose are birefringent.

STARCH

This polyholoside also plays a rather minor role in animal histochemistry. The morphological characteristics of grains of starch and their behaviour under polarised light are too well known to need mention here. Fixation poses no special problems. Among the histochemical techniques allowing us to identify starch, the principal ones are the PAS technique, with a control using diastase, which results in the very rapid disappearance of the activity and the appearance of the well known blue colour after the action of solutions containing iodine alkaline iodides. Finally, we may mention the use of Gram-Weigert's method for staining starch black.

DEXTRAN

This is a water soluble polysaccharide made up of glucose units and used medicinally as a substitute for plasma in conditions of shock. Its histochemical study only arises during experimental investigations; it rests on the PAS activity exclusively in alcoholic media; the control reaction is carried out by extraction with water (a 5 minute passage of the control slides in distilled water). It was with tests for dextran in mind that Mowry and his collaborators (1952, 1953) developed the technique of periodic oxidation in alcoholic media, mentioned in the corresponding paragraph of this chapter. It is appropriate to comment that dextran-sulphate, an anticoagulant substance, is strongly metachromatic (Mowry, 1954), the search for metachromatic reaction obviously needing to take place in an alcoholic medium.

NEUTRAL MUCOSUBSTANCES

This term, put forward by Spicer and his collaborators (1965), designates the ensemble of neutral mucopolysaccharides, mucoproteins and glycoproteins according to the chemical classification: these are compounds whose identification and distinction into sub-groups raises the most difficult of all the problems which occur in the course of the histochemical detection of carbohydrates. In the present state of our knowledge there seem to be no means by which a clear cut division into the three categories of compounds can be made (the mucoids of older workers).

Under the working conditions of the histochemist, the need to identify neutral mucosubstances arises whenever PAS positive compounds are present which lose this activity after acetylation, but recover it after saponification of the acetylated sections, and at the same time resist the test with malt diastase and react negatively to tests for electronegative groupings. That is to say that neutral mucosubstances do not stain with alcian blue, do not take up paraldehyde-fuchsin applied without pretreatment, and show themselves to be incapable of fixing ferric ions in the experimental conditions defined in the preceding section. Sulphuric esterification and phosphorylation confer a strong metachromatic basophilia on neutral mucosubstances.

A condensation reaction of the aldehyde groups induced by periodic oxidation with dimethyl-p-phenylenediamine chlorhydrate leads to the formation of azomethines, in the case of neutral mucosubstances, so that structures rich in these compounds acquire a characteristic colouration, and, in certain cases, a clear fluorescence in ultra-violet light: this reaction which differs from that of Scarselli (1956), which was mentioned in relation to the detection of carbonyl groups, because it takes place in the absence of hydrogen peroxide, eventually stains the acid mucopolysaccharides with a colour which is different from that of the one first mentioned when the duration of action is prolonged (Spicer and Jarrels, 1961).

The working technique is slightly different according to whether we need to carry out relatively rapid staining or whether this should be prolonged. Staining of short duration confers on structures which contain neutral mucosubstances and which take up a red colour when the sections are treated with the technique using PAS and alcian blue, a brownish-orange colour as well as a yellow or orange fluorescence. When the reagent is allowed to act for more than 24 hours, most of the structures which contain acid mucopolysaccharides take on a greyish purple colour, and at the same time the brown colour of those structures which contain neutral mucosubstances becomes darker.

Short duration treatment (6 to 8 hours):

Dewaxed sections, treated where appropriate with collodion (a thin layer), and hydrated;
Oxidise for 10 minutes with a 1% aqueous solution of periodic acid;
Wash for 10 minutes in running water;
Treat for several hours with the reagent
  N,N-dimethyl-p-phenylenediamine chlorhydrate .... 0.1 g
  a citric buffer of pH 6.1 containing distilled water 76 ml; 0.1 M citric acid 9.6 ml; 0.2 M disodium phosphate 14.4 ml................. 100 ml
The reaction takes place at laboratory temperatures; there may be some advantage in allowing the sections to dry, placing the slides vertically whilst so doing, two or three times during the reaction;
Wash for 5 minutes in running water;
Dehydrate in absolute alcohol, clear in a benzenoid hydrocarbon, and mount in a synthetic resin.

Prolonged treatment (24 to 48 hours):

Proceed as above to the end of the treatment with the *p*-phenylenediamine based reagent;
Treat the sections for 10 seconds at the maximum with the mixture
70% alcohol .... 99.1 ml
concentrated hydrochloric acid .... 0.9 ml
Wash immediately for 2 minutes in running water;
Dehydrate in absolute alcohol, clear and mount in a synthetic resin.

According to Münch and Ernst (1964), the value of this technique as a means of distinguishing between neutral and acid mucosubstances is no greater than that of the combined PAS-alcian blue treatment, but the stains obtained after the prolonged action of the reagent allow us to make very fine distinctions between the various acid mucosubstances.

In addition to sulphuric esterification, which confers a strong metachromatic basophilia on the neutral mucosubstances, carboxylation, which was a method put forward by Shakleford (1962, 1963), allows us to introduce carboxyl groups and hence an affinity for toluidine blue, the resultant stain being, according to the circumstances, orthochromatic or metachromatic.

Carboxylation with *p*-hydrazinobenzoic acid is obtained by treating the sections, oxidised for 5 minutes with periodic acid and then washed, in a saturated solution of *p*-hydrazinobenzoic acid in anhydrous pyridine; the duration of the reaction is one hour at 58°C. The sections are then washed in alcohol, hydrated and subjected to the chosen reactions or diagnostic stains.

The same result can be obtained without preliminary periodic oxidation by treating the dewaxed sections for 1 hour in a saturated solution of succinic anhydride in pure pyridine at 58°C; the remainder of the operation proceeds as described above.

A third carboxylation technique described by Shakleford (1963) consists of treating the sections, after they have been subjected to periodic oxidation, with a saturated solution of phthalic anhydride in pure pyridine, at 58°C, for from 15 to 20 minutes.

A sulphonation technique which is also due to Shakleford (1963) brings into play the treatment of the sections after oxidation with periodic acid by a saturated solution of *p*-hydrazinobenzene-sulphonic acid in 5% acetic acid at laboratory temperatures for 1 hour. It is advisable to prepare the solution several hours in advance and to filter it before use.

In all three cases, Shakleford advises the use of dilute solutions (0.01%) of toluidine blue as the stain.

These procedures generally reinforce the histochemical characteristics and staining affinities of acid mucosubstances.

Chitin deserves special mention among the group of neutral mucosubstances; its importance as a constituent of the integument of arthropods, numerically the most important division of the animal kingdom, is well known, and its histochemical characteristics have given rise to some debate.

From the chemical point of view, chitin is a neutral mucopolysaccharide whose hydrolysis gives rise solely to acetylglucosamine. It is generally agreed that it consists of chitobiose entities, that is to say of N-acetylglucosamine radicals linked among themselves by 1,4-β-glycosidic links.

Such a chemical constitution would suggest a positive reaction to PAS; certainly it does not contain *vic*-glycol or amino-alcohol groups, but we know, since the work of Jackson (1944), that 1-hydroxy-2-acylamine groups can be oxidised by periodic acid and these theoretical predictions are in effect confirmed by the chemical studies of Jeanloz (1950). There are divergent opinions among histochemists. Some of them (Pearse, 1953, 1960), who depend entirely on the data of Brunet (1953), maintain that chitin is PAS negative. Others (Lillie, 1947, 1954; Mancini, 1950) note that the reaction can be positive in certain structures which are rich in chitin whereas others are negative. Hale (1957), who bases his arguments, with all the firmness one could wish, on chemical considerations in favour of the PAS activity of chitin, mentions that the method in question is universally adopted by mycologists to demonstrate chitin in fungi and, in accordance with the data of Richards (1952), considers that all the, negative results obtained by histochemists can be explained by sclerotisation that process of hardening which, by virtue of chemical transformations, causes the chitin to lose its activity.

Among the older methods of demonstrating the presence of chitin, most used rather drastic procedures incompatible with the preservation of the tissues as a whole; they need no mention here. The technique of Schulze (1922) may be of service. It can be carried out on sections of tissue which have undergone softening of the chitin with diaphanol, as described in the second part of this work. Sections taken from such pieces are covered with several drops of a mixture of two solutions, one of which contains 6.1 g of iodine, 10 g of potassium iodide and 14 ml of distilled water, and the second contains 60 g of zinc chloride and 14 ml of distilled water, the mixture of the two solutions having been filtered through glass wool before use. A violet colour appears either whilst in the mixture or after washing with water. The same technique gives a violet colour with cellulose and with its animal equivalent tunicin, but any confusion can be avoided by treating the sections successively with Lugol's fluid and dilute sulphuric acid. Under these conditions chitin takes on a brown stain, cellulose a blue one. The stains obtained with iodated zinc chloride, and those which the Lugol-sulphuric acid mixture give, fade rapidly; the slides should thus be studied immediately after mounting in water.

ACID MUCOSUBSTANCES

This group corresponds to that of the "acid mucopolysaccharides" of the classical nomenclature, the change of terminology having been proposed by Spicer and his collaborators (1965), as a result of comments by Rosan and Saunders (1965); the term "acid mucopolysaccharides" can rigorously be applied only in cases where the presence of polymers containing amino sugars has been disclosed by chemical analysis, that is to say principally in that of the connective tissue of the vertebrates. These authors also propose to maintain that usage in which the mucosubstances present in the epithelial cells are designated by the word "mucins" that of mucopolysaccharide being kept for compounds present in the connective tissue.

The identification of acid mucosubstances evidently rests on the demonstration of electronegative groups. Such compounds give the metachromatic reaction, stain with alcian blue and the other phthalocyanines of this group, and are capable of fixing ferric ions, losing all these properties after "methylation". Their behaviour with respect to the PAS technique is variable, some being PAS positive, others PAS negative; where it exists, the PAS activity disappears after acetylation.

The classification of the acid mucosubstances into categories poses very serious problems, all the more so because only in a very small number of cases does the histochemist dispose of sufficiently detailed biochemical information about the compounds whose presence he can detect in the sections. All modern authors maintain the classical distinction between mucopolysaccharides or sulphated mucins on the one hand and non-sulphated ones on the other.

A classification of the *sulphated mucosubstances* which is exclusively based on data acquired during a study of mammals has been proposed by Spicer (1963); it leads us to distinguish three categories.

The very acid sulphated mucosubstances stain with methylene blue or with azur A, applied according to the method described in relation to the measurement of the zone of isoelectric point, up to pH values in the neighbourhood of 0.5; they give a strong gamma metachromasia with toluidine blue; the affinity for alcian blue may be very feeble or negligible at pH 3. It is most frequently clearer at very low pH values; the affinity for paraldehyde fuchsin is very strong, the activity towards PAS being feeble or non existent.

A technique for double periodic oxidation, due to Scott and Dorling (1969) allows one selectively to demonstrate chondroitin-sulphates and other glycosamino-glycuronanes which are PAS negative under normal conditions.

These polysaccharides, which contain uronic acids linked in the 1 : 4 positions, are weakly oxidised by periodic acid, the slowness of the reaction being put to good use to enable us to distinguish them from neutral polysaccharides. The first periodic oxidation causes aldehyde groups to appear in neutral polysaccharides, the aldehydes then being reduced to alcohol groups by blocking with sodium borohydride. The second, and much the longer, periodic oxidation results in the formation of aldehyde groups from the glycosamino-glycuronanes, and these groups are then demonstrable by the use of Schiff's reagent.

Reagents:

    2% aqueous solution of sodium metaperiodate ($NaIO_4$), which should be kept in the cool and in darkness;
    1% aqueous solution of sodium borohydride ($NaBH_4$) which should be used in the 30 minutes following its preparation;
    Schiff's reagent;
    Where necessary, sulphur dioxide water for rinsing;

Working technique:

    Dewaxed sections, treated, where appropriate, with collodion, and hydrated;
    Oxidise for 1 hour at 30°C using the solution of sodium metaperiodate (primary oxidation);
    Rinse in distilled water; control sections, submitted to the PAS reaction at this stage of the reaction shows how strongly reactive are the PAS—positive structures;
    Treat for 3 minutes, at laboratory temperatures, with the sodium borohydride solution; control sections, carried through this stage of the reaction, show the disappearence of all PAS activity;
    Rinse in distilled water;
    Oxidise for 24 hours at 30 °C using the sodium periodate solution (secondary oxidation);
    Rinse in distilled water;
    Treat with Schiff's reagent for 30 minutes at laboratory temperatures;
    Rinse in the sulphur dioxide water (for frozen sections or freeze-dried sections) or generously in distilled water (for paraffin wax sections);
    Where appropriate, stain the background and mount as after the PAS reaction;

Sites of glycosamino-glycuronanes are stained reddish-violet.

Certain very acid mucosubstances acquire, as a result of methylation, a distinct PAS activity, which indicates that the sulphate radicals are situated in substances of this category on the *vic*-glycol groups; the other histochemical characteristics correspond to those of the first category.

The less acid sulphated mucosubstances lose all their affinity for methylene blue or azur A at pH values between 1 and 3; they take up alcian blue very strongly when it is dissolved in a solution of pH 3, and with toluidine blue give a metachromasia of type β. The affinity for paraldehyde-fuchsin is strong as is the PAS activity.

Non-sulphated mucosubstances owe their diagnostic histochemical characteristics to the presence of electronegative groupings with carboxyl functions (hexuronic and sialic acids). Staining with toluidine blue or with azur A confers on them an orthochromatic colour in certain cases; in others, one obtains a metachromasia of type β, veering more or less distinctly towards violet. This staining affinity, as well as that for methylene blue, does not show up when the pH of the staining solution is less than 3.4 or 3 (the extinction of methylene blue of Dempsey and his collaborators, 1949). Methylation causes this orthochromatic or metachromatic basophilia to disappear, saponification of the methylated sections re-establishing it. The affinity for alcian blue is generally very strong, that for paraldehyde-fuchsin being less so. All these compounds give the PAS reaction strongly. The test using hyaluronidase and that using neuraminidase will evidently permit us to identify hyaluronic acid and the sialomucins.

Ravetto (1964) has developed a technique for distinguishing between very acid and slightly acid mucosubstances, a technique which rests on staining with two phthalocyanines, used at different pH values. The working technique advocated by this author involves the use of alcian blue and alcian yellow.

> Dewaxed sections, treated with collodion and hydrated;
> Stain for 30 minutes, at laboratory temperatures, with the solution:
> alcian blue 8GX .... 0.5 g
> a sodium citrate hydrochloric acid
> buffer of pH 0.5 .... 100 ml
> Rinse for 10 seconds in the buffer of pH 0.5;
> Wash for two minutes in distilled water, several times renewed;
> Stain for 30 seconds in the solution
> alcian yellow GX .... 0.5 g
> the citrate hydrochloric acid
> buffer of pH 2.5 .... 100 ml
> Rinse rapidly in the buffer of pH 2.5;
> Wash in distilled water;
> Stain the nuclei where appropriate by the aluminium lake of nuclear fast red (p. 203);
> Wash in running water for 1 to 3 minutes;
> Dehydrate in absolute alcohol, clear in a benzenoid hydrocarbon, mount in Canada balsam or in a synthetic resin.

The very acid mucosubstances (sulphomucopolysaccharides in Ravetto's interpretation) are stained blue, the less acid mucosubstances (substances with carboxyl groups according to Ravetto) in yellow; intermediate colours indicate the presence of the two types of compound.

This method may be called into play to replace an older technique due to Wolman (1956) which depends on the successive treatment of the sections using the method by which ferric ions are fixed and then using a solution of colloidal gold, which is unstable and rather difficult to prepare.

According to a publication by Sorvari and Sorvari (1969) it is the concentration of the solutions of the two phthalocyanins and the duration of the staining that are the factors capable of modifying the stain obtained with any given mucin. The differences in question can be explained, on the one, hand, by the displacement of the first stain by the second when the latter is acting, and on the other hand by the incomplete saturation of the sulphate groups at the stage of staining with alcian blue, so that it is possible for alcian yellow to be taken up, and, lastly, by an inhibiting effect of the molecules of alcian blue, when combined with sulphate groups, on the combination of molecules of alcian yellow with the carboxyl groups. In fact, an examination of the table published by Sorvari and Sorvari shows that the differences of stain obtained by varying the dyestuff concentrations from 0.1%, to 1% are only slight for some materials but fairly marked for others. Differences of some importance only appear in this table when we compare the results obtained with 0.1% solutions on the one hand, and those from 5% solutions on the other. The same comment holds good for the duration of staining; only quite substantial differences result in a clear change of the stain obtained with the majority of materials.

A technique which uses the same stains as that of Ravetto, but which depends on the principal of a critical concentration of electrolytes, has been put forward by Staple (1967) to differentiate the biological polyanions discussed here. This technique involves, as a first stage, staining for 16 to 24 hours using an alcian blue solution (0.05%) buffered to 5.8 and having magnesium chloride (0.05–1.5 M) added to it, as used by Scott and Dorling (p. 414). Following this stain, the sections are rinsed in the buffer to which the required amount of magnesium chloride has been added so as not to allow any change in the molarity, and then stained for 30 minutes to one hour with a 0.05% solution of alcian yellow, buffered as for the alcian blue stain, with magnesium chloride (0.05 M) added to it. Under these conditions, the sites of polyanions which no longer take up alcian blue at any given concentration of magnesium chloride stain with alcian yellow. The advantage of this method over that of Scott and Dorling depends on the fact that the difference between the polyanions is disclosed, not by the negative fact of the disappearance of the stain, but by distinct stains.

Yamada (1970) suggests that a solutions of ruthenium red should replace alcian yellow in the double staining of mucosubstances; ruthenium red is a substance whose affinity for certain mucosubstances has been known since the end of the 19th century, but which is mainly employed in plant histology. The technique of this author, which closely resembles that of Ravetto, is carried out in the following way.

Reagents:

Hydrochloric acid/acetic acid, pH 1 (add concentrated hydrochloric acid to 3% acetic acid until a pH of 1 is achieved, this requires about 1 ml.);
0.5% solution of alcian blue in hydrochloric acid/acetic acid, pH 1;
3% acetic acid;
0.5% solution of ruthenium red in 3% acetic acid;

Working technique:

> Dewaxed sections, coated where necessary with a thin film of collodion, hydrated and rinsed in the mixed hydrochloric acid:acetic acid, pH 1;
> Stain for 30 minutes with the alcian blue solution;
> Rinse in hydrochloric acid/acetic acid, then twice in acetic acid;
> Stain for 5 to 20 minutes, the optimum to be ascertained by trial and error, with the acetic acid solution of ruthenium red;
> Rinse in 3% acetic acid, then in distilled water, dehydrate in absolute alcohol, clear in a benzenoid hydrocarbon and mount in a synthetic resin.

The stains vary from blue to red according to the predominance of very acid mucosubstances, as against those which are slightly acid, in the stained structures.

It is appropriate to mention that these polychrome techniques, such as that of Ravetto, that of Staple, or of Yamada, whose working technique has just been described, give results whose interpretation is not always easy. Although one can immediately make a distinction between the extreme stains, intermediate ones may be hard to classify and to compare one with another.

Despite its negative character, the disappearance of the affinity for a dyestuff, such as is obtained by causing solutions of alcian blue to act in buffers of different pH values, or by using the method of critical electrolyte concentrations (Scott and Dorling, 1965) can give results which are more nearly unequivocal.

To sum up, the procedures for distinguishing between sulphated and non sulphated acid mucosubstances, which have just been reviewed, depend on the same principle as the technique of the extinction of methylene blue or tests for the metachromatic reaction as a function of the pH of the staining bath; they turn to account the difference between the pK (the pH for which 50% of the radicals are ionised, 50% not being ionised) of the carboxyl groups on the one hand and of the sulphate groups on the other. That of the first is above 3, so that staining reactions diagnostic of the presence of anionic groups give negative results when the pH of the staining solution is distinctly less than that number. Nevertheless, we should not disguise from ourselves the fact that the dissociation of the sulphate groups can be influenced by the molecular configuration, and the neighbourhood of other radicals, etc..., so that the data of Spicer (1963) shows up zones of "overlap" of the results thus obtained, the sulphated mucosubstances being capable of behaving like some non sulphated mucosubstances. Data obtained by means of reversible methylation (the disappearance of the activity and its reappearance after saponification in the case of non sulphated acid mucosubstances, its permanent disappearance in the case of sulphated acid mucosubstances) seems to be much more significant in this respect but recent observations invite the greatest prudence as to the interpretation.

Under the working conditions of the histochemist the most reliable among the criteria for the identification of sulphated acid mucosubstances seems to be the incorporation of radioactive sulphur, followed by an autoradiographic study. Nevertheless, we must face the fact that even the employment of every one of these methods may leave the histochemist confronted with contradictions which only a chemical analysis can resolve; in fact we know of the existence, in the connective tissue of insects, of mucosubstances which behave as if they were sulphated, from the point of view of the incorporation of radioactive sulphur whereas reversible methylation tends to lead us to suppose that their acid character is due to carboxyl groups (Martoja, 1966); in all probability, it is the date obtained from autoradiographs which correspond to reality.

Another practical difficulty encountered even more frequently by the histochemist is the coexistence of several mucosubstances in any given structure. Certain results which appear to be discordant arising during a histochemical study of the cartilage of the Mammalia constitute a classical example. This possibility should always lead us to use as many histochemical reactions, staining reactions and various controls, as possible, before attempting to arrive at conclusions.

D. — THE PRACTICE OF HISTOCHEMICAL TESTS FOR POLYSACCHARIDES

The opportunity for the histochemical detection of polysaccharides may arise under a variety of conditions and all the considerations which we have developed in relation to the orientation of histochemical research in general are applicable to this particular case. No special mention needs to be made of the techniques to be used, since we have to appreciate the variations under defined circumstances of polysaccharides whose presence in the tissue under investigation is already known; in the same way, studies devoted to the methodology of the detection of a given polysaccharide do not need to be commented upon in this section. Another possibility which has to be considered is that of a systematic inventory of polysaccharides in tissues or in organs which have not yet been explored from this point of view, and we will suppose in general that the nature and the abundance of the material does not limit the number of fixations which can be made.

Among **the fixation techniques,** two are obligatory, namely that using an aqueous fluid, if possible without corrosive sublimate, and that using an alcoholic liquid (Bouin and Carnoy for example); in fact, experience shows that certain mucosubstances are better preserved by aqueous fixatives, others by alcoholic ones. When there is an overriding need for the perfect preservation of the tissue from the morphological point of view, the addition of a fixative based on potassium bichromate (Regaud, Orth, Kopsch) can be extremely useful.

Certain of the mucosubstances are in fact only fixed correctly from the cytological point of view by such liquids. We need hardly add that this bichromate fixation should be of short duration and followed by the traditional wash in running water. The practice of the histochemical reactions of the carbohydrates on post-chromed material is a makeshift to be avoided as far as is possible, since the oxidation which takes place during the time when the material is in the potassium bichromate bath can entirely modify the histochemical nature of the carbohydrates which it contains. The use of Gendre's or of Rossman's fluids, or better, of processes involving freeze drying or freeze substitution are useful in cases where the detection of glycogen must be irreproachable.

The embedding and the cutting of the sections calls for no particular comment; their spreading can be carried out in the great majority of cases according to traditional procedures; nevertheless, it is useful to practice the spreading on alcohol or else dry in order to be able to eliminate by the use of control sections the hypothesis of a loss of polysaccharides during spreading on gelatin-water or on albumin.

The choice of diagnostic reaction and stains is greatly aided by the use of the PAS reaction as a first step whether or not it is combined with alcian blue staining or with that of the metachromatic reaction to toluidine blue or to azur A. A clearly positive result of the metachromatic reaction will direct the subsequent investigation towards the acid mucosubstances and the presumption in favour of sulphated mucosubstances becomes very strong when the sites of the metachromatic reaction are also PAS negative or even stained by alcian blue. The absence of any metachromatic reaction even in sections examined after mounting in water should lead one to consider as a first approximation that the PAS reaction is due to the presence of neutral mucosubstances or of polyholosides whose type is glycogen. Procedures as simple as the test with malt diastase and iodine staining will suffice to confirm or invalidate this last hypothesis.

In cases where the positive result of the metachromatic reaction and the affinity for alcian blue sustain a presumption in favour of the presence of acid mucosubstances it is useful to verify the presumption by the fixation of ferric ions. Tests for metachromasia at different pH values, one of which is near to 3 and the other slightly less than 1.5, the test of "the extinction of methylene blue", provide information relevant to the pK of the electronegative groups responsible for the acid character and orients the studies either towards the identification of sulphated mucosubstances or towards that of mucosubstances which bear carboxyl groups. The results of the stain with alcian blue—alcian yellow following Ravetto's technique also helps us to distinguish between these two possibilities. Tests using enzymatic digestion (hyaluronidase, neuraminidase) allow us to identify hyaluronic and sialic acids.

It is when the techniques envisaged above lead us to suspect the existence of neutral mucosubstances in the structures under investigation that the remainder of the work becomes more difficult. We need hardly add that discrimination between glycoproteins and mucoproteins, which rests entirely on the results of a quantitative analysis, are outside the range open to a histochemist, and even the distinction between these two kinds of substance on the one hand and the "neutral mucopolysaccharides" of the chemical classification on the other hand can be of the greatest difficulty. The demonstration by other procedures of an accumulation of proteins in the structures where the PAS compounds which have to be classified are situated is perhaps an indication of the presence of glycoproteins in the broad sense of the term rather than of neutral mucopolysaccharides; in any case, it does not represent any proof of this idea since proteins and neutral mucopolysaccharides can perfectly well coexist. Sulphuric esterification and phosphorylation confer the same metachromatic basophilia on all these compounds; this remark also holds good for chromic oxidation when prolonged beyond the aldehyde stage.

It is appropriate to add to this that the interpretation of the results furnished by the PAS reaction can be aided by the practice of reversible acetylation, and that the taking into consideration of the colour obtained on one and the same structure by oxidation with periodic acid, with lead tetra-acetate and with sodium bismuthate often permits us to relate the appearance of carbonyl groups detectable by the Schiff reaction to the presence of *vic*-glycol groups or to amino-alcohol, alkylamino-alcohol or hydroxy-carboxyl groups.

The table of Spicer and his collaborators (1965) which is given as an appendix to the part of this work dealing with histochemical techniques includes proposals for the classification of the mucosubstances whose adoption would have the advantage of unifying the terminology employed in descriptions.

CHAPTER 18

HISTOCHEMICAL DETECTION OF FATS AND RELATED COMPOUNDS

The demonstration of certain fats by the reduction of osmium tetroxide is one of the oldest histochemical techniques (Schultze, 1865) and tests for lipid compounds on frozen sections have for a long time been part of the pathologists' and anatomists' routines. It is however true that the histochemical study of fats is distinctly less advanced than that of other organic compounds. As Lison (1960, p. 449) has very rightly stressed, the great majority of histochemical investigations have dealt with the least interesting among the fatty constituents of the animal cell, that is to say "adipose tissue" and the waste from lipid metabolism. Various attempts at the histochemical analysis of lipids linked to other cellular constituents (masked lipids, the histogenic lipids of Ciaccio, and the heterophasic lipids of Lison) are of considerable theoretical interest; in addition to the classical studies of Fauré-Fremiet (1901), Mayer and Schaeffer (1913), Ciaccio (1919 to 1936), we should also mention the more recent ones of the school of J. R. Baker (1941 to 1960). From the practical point of view, these investigations are no more than a promising start; they suggest a plan of campaign which might prove to be most fruitful but which has not yet provided any substantial addition to our knowledge and the procedures developed by the research workers in question are not yet of a status justifying their inclusion in the day to day practice of histochemistry.

One of the reasons for the retarded state of the histochemistry of fats as compared with that of other organic compounds is certainly the chemical heterogeneity of this type of substance, a heterogeneity which is abundantly reflected in the contradictions of the chemical nomenclature. Moreover, the most valuable of the chemical techniques useful in the study of fats cannot be adapted to the working conditions of the histochemist and practical difficulties which it would be dangerous to overestimate arise even when one tries to adopt procedures which at first sight seem completely suitable for investigations using sectioned material, that is to say the extraction by different solvent. To an extent which is even greater than for the polysaccharides, the coexistence of different kinds of fats in any given structure notably complicates the interpretation of the results from diagnostic stains and histochemical reactions. The properties of the constituents of mixtures of fats moreover are somewhat modified as compared with those of pure materials. We may add to this that fairly firm linkage with non lipid substances greatly modifies the characters of tissue fats, to the point of rendering them inaccessible to histochemical detection in a great number of cases.

All these observations will indicate the difficulties confronting the histochemical study of the fatty constituents of the animal cell.

The contradictions and disagreements of the chemical nomenclature relating to fats makes it necessary for us to review, at the earliest possible stage, the terminology generally used by histochemists and followed here. Then we review the techniques which permit of histochemical detection of the fats and then the distinctive characteristics of fatty compounds which are met with in animal histochemistry. Together with the study of the fats it seems logical to include that of the fat soluble vitamins (axerophthol, calciferol) and that of the oxidised derivatives of fats which form one of the most important of the groups of endogenous pigments, namely the chromolipoids in the broad sense of the term.

CLASSIFICATION OF FATS

All authors agree that the variability of the chemical nomenclature relating to fats exceeds that of all other areas in biochemistry. One and the same term is used with quite different meanings, often changing its meaning with the author and with the time in which it is used, so that the best practice often consists in renouncing its use altogether. The impossibility of a chemical definition of fats based on the structure and valid for all substances of the specified class affords an additional difficulty in the classification; this leads one to see why the authors and monographs are inconsistent.

It may be useful to mention that even the definition of the fats depends from the outset on a collection of characters relating to solubility; nowadays we know that these characters are no longer valid, some authentic fats being soluble in water, others, which are no less authentic, are insoluble in the classical "fat solvents". The chemical heterogeneity of the group is granted even by the classical authors; and it stems from this that "no one is capable any more of saying just what constitutes a fat" (Lison, 1960, p. 451). All classifications therefore contain an arbitrary element which we have to accept.

Certain terms, which were once much in use, are practically abandoned, such as that of "lipin" for lipids which are insoluble in acetone. Numerous authors still use the term "lipoid" and Debuch (1965) stresses the advantages which stem from designating by different words the adipose lipoids (*Fette* of the German nomenclature, *fats* of the anglo-saxon authors) and those which form an integral part of the protoplasm (*Lipoide* of german authors). In fact, the term "lipoid" has been used with meanings which are too widely disparate and its usage may be the source of misunderstandings to such an extent that it is better not to use it.

It is the classification put forward by Lison (1960) which is adopted here. This consists of dividing the fats as a class into seven groups of cmpounds.

The **glycerides** are triesters of glycerol with the fatty acids. Widespread within animal tissue, where they represent, in particular, reserves of energy, they differ from one another in the constitution of the fatty acids which esterify the hydroxyl groups of the glycerol. The saturated nature of these acids results in a higher melting point of the ester, which is thus solid at ordinary temperatures (*fat*); when rich in non saturated fatty acids there is a lower melting point such that the lipid is liquid at ordinary temperatures (*oils*); free *fatty acids* and their salts (*soaps*) are classed with the glycerides.

Waxes are esters of fatty acids with aliphatic alcohols having more than ten carbon atoms; they have only restricted importance in animal histochemistry although very abundant in certain secretory products (beeswax, the secretion of the preen gland of birds) or extracts from organs (the liver oil of fish), but their importance is much greater in plants.

Phospholipids are characterised by the presence of a phosphoric acid radical in the molecule which esterifies one of the hydroxyl groups of the glycerol; this phosphoric acid radical is moreover linked to an amino-alcohol or to an amino-acid. According to the nature of the latter and the number of hydroxyl groups of the glycerine which are esterified with fatty acids we can distinguish within the phospholipids, the lecithins (the two hydroxyl groups of glycerophosphoric acid being esterified by fatty acids, the phosphoric radical being linked with choline), the cephalins (the two hydroxyl groups of the glycerophosphoric acid being esterified with fatty acids, the phosphoric radical being linked to colamine in the colamine cephalins and to serine in the serine cephalins) and the plasmalogens (acetal phosphatides in the older nomenclature) (their chemical structure is different from those of lecithins and cephalins because in the one case the hydroxyl groups of the glycerophosphoric acid are esterified with an aldehyde radical, and in the other case with a fatty acid).

Sphingolipids contain an amino-dialcohol having 18 carbon atoms; this is sphingosine with one of the hydroxyl groups esterified with a fatty acid, the other, in the sphingomyelins, bears a phosphoric acid radical linked to choline, whereas in the cerebrosides it is linked to a hexose, and in the gangliosides to neuraminic acid and to hexoses, whether or not associated with hexosamines.

The **steroids**, which are characterised from the chemical point of view by a cyclopentaphenanthrene nucleus, are represented in the animal body by cholesterol and its esters as well as by the steroid hormones.

The carotenoids are hydrocarbons which are naturally coloured and which from the chemical point of view are characterised by cyclic or acyclic arrangements of isoprene radicals, so that conjugated double bonds exist in the molecule. These compounds belong to what used to be called the lipochromes. Vitamin A is included in the carotenoids.

The **chromolipoids**, whose chemistry is poorly known, are pigments derived by oxidation from the lipids. Solely identifiable in terms of their histochemical characteristics, these compounds still lack a rational classification. The ceroid pigment, the lipofuscins and hemofuscin are the principal representatives.

As Lison (1960, p. 455) has very rightly remarked, the chemical classification does not exhaust the problems which the classification of fats poses, from the histochemical standpoint. It is moreover essential to distinguish lipids which can be detected as such on tissue sections (free lipids or the metabolic lipids of Ciaccio) from those which, because of their association with non lipoid compounds, have substantially or entirely lost the characteristics which would permit of their histochemical detection. Such are the histogenic lipids of Ciaccio and the heterophasic lipids of Lison, the histochemical study of which seems at first sight to be the most promising since the group of homophasic lipids only includes fat reserves and waste products in addition to substances implicated in the metabolism of the steroid hormones. However it is precisely in the study of heterophasic lipids that there arises the greatest number of technical problems not yet resolved in a satisfying fashion.

PREPARATION OF THE TISSUES FOR A HISTOCHEMICAL STUDY OF LIPIDS

The difference between the homophasic and heterophasic lipids, in the sense of Lison, shows up during vital examination of tissues and cells. In fact, the homophasic lipids, which are hydrophobe and free within the cytoplasm, appear on vital examination as birefringent inclusions, whose appearance, without being truly characteristic, is somewhat evocative; the heterophasic lipids are not visible under such conditions.

Similarly, the conditions of fixation are very different in the two cases and will have to be considered separately.

Homophasic lipids by virtue of their hydrophobic nature are stable; their preservation in the tissue does not require any chemical transformation, so that the only precautions which need to be observed stem from their solubility in a certain number of the organic compounds used during the preparation of the tissues for histological examination. That is to say that the problem of the fixation of homophasic lipids as a first approximation reduces to the good preservation of the tissue and cell structures, a preservation which is obtained by using fixatives devoid of fat solvents (alcohol, chloroform, acetone, etc. . .). No other precaution is necessary in cases where the objective of the study is simply the morphological investigation of the free fats, but the possibility of chemical modification of the fats under the influence of the fixative must be remembered in truly histochemical investigations destined to result in the identification of the fats. One need scarcely worry about the passage of homophasic lipids into solution when fixation has been carried out with the 10% formalin generally used; this is far from true in the case of heterophasic lipids. The solubility of the lipids can be modified by fixation; this modification is particularly apt to arise in the case of phospholipids and its chemical mechanism is not entirely understood; from the practical point of view it results in a lessening of the solubility in the organic compounds customarily used for the extraction of fats, a diminution which may go so far as to preserve the lipids in paraffin wax sections. Moreover, the amount of lipids which can be distinguished within the inclusions by certain techniques (Fischler's haematoxylin, Ciaccio's technique and the Nile blue method of Lorrain Smith) increases after fixation in formalin, even where this is only slightly prolonged, this phenomenon probably being due to oxidation of the ethylenic linkages, resulting in the appearance of electronegative groups. The same phenomenon of oxidation results in the appearance of aldehyde groups whose presence lay at the origin of the interpretative errors mentioned in a subsequent section. The oxidation of fats by liquids based on potassium dichromate or chromium trioxide, the liberation of the aldehyde groups from the plasmalogens under the action of corrosive sublimate are mentioned for the record. We may add that the process of crystallisation during fixation can modify the results of staining by lysochromes and can cause the appearance of a birefringence under polarised light which was not present in the original condition.

From the practical point of view therefore, most of the aqueous fixatives lend themselves to the preservation of lipid inclusions *in situ*, when the morphological study of these inclusions is the sole objective of the work; a short-duration fixation in 10% formalin, neutralised as in the procedures given in the first part of this work, is the only method recommended in histochemical studies and the results thus obtained should always be controlled by examination of sections taken from fresh tissues; this last operation is much facilitated by the use of a cryostat or by arrangements for freezing the microtome blade.

We need hardly add that embedding in paraffin wax or in celloidin cannot be considered during a histochemical or even a morphological study of the fats; inclusion in gelatine is possible as is that in the water-miscible synthetic materials for embedding. The advantages and disadvantages of these latter embedding media were discussed in the corresponding chapter of the first part of the book.

In addition to sectioning in the cold, as mentioned above, we can use the freezing microtome which represents the principal way of making sections for a morphological or histochemical study of the fats. These sections may be manipulated without glue or else glued to the slides by one of the procedures described in relation to the manipulation of frozen sections. I might mention the usefulness of short-duration fixation (1 to 2 minutes) in 10% formalin, chilled to about 3° C, before any treatment of the cold-cut sections, excepting, obviously, those cases where we need to examine the possible action of this fixative on the tissular lipids.

The preservation *in situ* of the heterophasic lipids, in the sense of Lison, poses quite other problems. It happens that the compounds in question generally form part of structures which are difficult to preserve from the morphological point of view (the chondriome, the Golgi bodies, the membraneous systems, etc...); their unsaturated fatty acid content, which is often high, renders them particularly liable to oxidation and the presence of hydrophilic groups in their molecules permits them to form what are often very unstable links with other compounds. Unlike the homophasic lipids, they can pass into solution during fixation in aqueous fluids, so that there is a possibility of loss and consequent misinterpretation in the course of histochemical studies.

Among the fixative fluids intended particularly to avoid this loss during fixation we may mention in the first place the formaldehyde-calcium of Baker (1944) which was briefly mentioned in relation to the use of formalin as a topographic fixative. Turning to good use the well known idea that the presence of calcium ions in the medium inhibits the formation of myelinic figures, Baker put forward the idea of fixing heterophasic lipids, and in particular the phospholipids, by a mixture of 10 ml of 10% calcium chloride solution, 10 ml of commercial formalin and 80 ml of distilled water, excess pulverised calcium carbonate being added to the mixture. In the scheme put forward by Lillie and Laskey (1951), calcium acetate may replace the chloride, its buffering capacity allowing one to dispense with the neutralisation of the fixative. These authors dissolve 2 g of calcium acetate in 100 ml of 10% formalin. The addition of calcium salts to the osmic fixatives used in electronic microscopy has also been advocated (Chou and Meek, 1959) the better to conserve the lipids.

Another way of rendering the heterophasic lipids insoluble is represented by the action of potassium bichromate, acting either during the fixation or after it. This compound, which was used empirically by the older workers, renders the lipids insoluble to the point of permitting their preservation in certain cases in paraffin wax sections; there is still a possibility of staining them with lysochromes and there is, moreover, a fixation of chromium on the lipid molecules so that there is still a possibility for forming coloured lakes with solutions of haematein. The mechanism by which potassium bichromate renders "complexes" (other than the glycerides) insoluble is little known; apart from the oxidation of the double bonds of the unsaturated fatty acids, polymerisation may also play a part. In practice, this insolubilisation relates only to phospholipids and sphingolipids.

Some authors allow potassium bichromate to act during the fixation; Ciaccio (1926) advocates fixation for 2 hours in a mixture of 85 ml of a 5% aqueous solution of potassium bichromate, 15 ml of commercial formalin and 5 ml o acetic acid. Other workers only use this salt on fixed pieces of tissue, postchromatisation taking place, in Baker's technique, after about 6 hours fixation in formalin-calcium, and in the technique of Elftman (1954) after fixation for from 5 to 7 hours at 5° C in a 1% solution of osmium tetroxide in a sodium veronal buffer of pH 7.2.

Postchromatisation takes place at laboratory temperatures (5 to 8 days in a 3% aqueous solution of potassium bichromate) in Ciaccio's technique; Baker suggests treating the material for 18 hours at laboratory temperatures, and then for 24 hours at 60° with a 5% aqueous solution of potassium bichromate in which has been dissolved 1% of calcium chloride; Elftman advocates postchromatisation for 18 hours at 56° C in a 2.5% solution of potassium bichromate the pH of which is adjusted to 3.5 by means of a sodium acetate buffer or else in a 5% solution of mercuric chloride in which has been dissolved, immediately prior to use, 2.5% of potassium bichromate. We need hardly add that postchromatisation should be followed in all cases by careful washing in frequently renewed tap water or distilled water.

The "unmasking" of the "histolipoids" which take part in lipoprotein bonding was attempted by Ciaccio (1926 to 1936), either by means of fixatives with a heavy metal base or in treating the material, after fixation, with phenol, with alkalis or acids, with trypsin or with pepsin. These attempts were not successful and we have no means within the framework of current histochemical practice of obtaining an artificial lipophanerose.

The later handling of pieces of tissue fixed with a view to demonstrating heterophasic lipids may, according to the circumstances, include either the preparation of frozen sections or embedding in paraffin wax. We may recollect in this context that certain classical methods of neurohistology intended to show up myelin sheaths involve the preparation of celloidin or paraffin wax sections, the phospholipids whose demonstration is being sought having been rendered insoluble by postchromatisation.

A recent attempt at unmasking heterophasic lipids in mammalian and insect tissues is due to Wigglesworth (1971). This author uses tissue fixed in glutaraldehyde (a 2.5 or 5% solution in a cacodylate buffer, pH 7.4, with the addition of 2% sucrose) for two to three hours, or else with osmium tetroxide used in the way described for agar—paraffin wax double embedding (p. 95). Should this double embedding be practised, Steedman's ester-wax (his 1947 formula, p. 94) is to be preferred above any other medium of the paraffin wax type for embedding.

The sections, which should be 1 μ thick on an average, should be cut with a glass knife or a steel blade, and, prior to adhesion to the slide, should be treated with a very dilute solution of sodium hypochlorite obtained by diluting a commercial solution containing 10% of chlorine in the proportion of 1 : 100 with distilled water immediately before use. The pH of this diluted solution is of the order of 11.5. The duration of action varies from 15 seconds to 10 minutes, and it is obviously of interest to follow the progress of the 'unmasking' with time.

The sections are then caused to adhere to slides. After dewaxing, they can be stained as they are taken out of a bath of 70% alcohol, but it is often helpful to hydrate them and soak them in a dilute solution of sodium hypochlorite for about one minute, so as to allow this reagent to act on both face of the section.

The staining itself is done with Sudan Black B in 0.15% solution in 50% ethanol (at the moment of use, mix 0.2 ml stock solution of 2% Sudan black B in acetone with 3 ml of 50% ethanol.) After 10 minutes of staining with this solution, the sections are destained in 70% alcohol for about 30 seconds, rinsed in water and mounted in a medium miscible with water. Experience proves that this technique gives intensive staining at sites of heterophasic lipids; no stain is obtained unless the lipids are unmasked by sodium hypochlorite.

We might add that treatment with sodium hypochlorite renders heterophasic lipids accessible to extraction with a methanol—chloroform mixture.

THE HISTOCHEMICAL DETECTION OF LIPIDS BY MEANS OF LYSOCHROMES

Histological demonstration by means of lysochromes is the simplest and most effective method for the detection of lipids, but it gives little information about the chemical constitution of these compounds. Since its introduction by Daddi (1896) there have been numerous developments of this method; lists of the principal lysochromes are to be found in manuals of histochemical technique which have already been quoted frequently.

As I mentioned in the chapter which dealt in a general way with histological stains, lysochromes are not stains in the strict sense of the term. They have no auxochrome groups and are not ionised, but they confer on structures which contain a sufficient quantity of lipids a colour which is solely due to their solution in the lipids which become stained. Since it is due to a simple physical phenomenon and regulated by the partition coefficient between the stained lipid on the one hand and the solvent for the lysochrome on the other hand, this "stain" is obviously not produced if the lipid, whatever its constitution, is in a solid state.

Substances belonging to the anthraquinone group (Sudan blue, Sudan violet, BZL blue, Sudan green, oil blue N, carycinel red, cochineal), or azo-dyestuffs (Sudan II, III, IV or scarlet R, Sudan brown, Sudan red, permanent red R, oil brown D, oil red 0, oil red 4B, Sudan black B), or to the triphenylmethanes (alcohol blue) have been used by different authors; the list given above is in no way restrictive. Some hydrocarbons (3,4-benzopyrene, or anthracene) confer on the lipids a fluorescence which can be used for their histochemical detection.

Generally speaking, the colour of the lysochrome which is used is one element in determining it's choice for histochemical purposes, the intensity and the depth of colour obtained evidently influence the optical qualities of the preparations; the colour in the strict sense of the term, that is to say conferring the greatest light absorption, is to be taken into account, in particular, when it is desired to combine the demonstration of lipids with other stains or histochemical reactions; it is also necessary to take it into consideration when the preparations contain naturally coloured structures (pigments, etc...). Moreover, an essential quality of a good lysochrome is very high solubility in lipids; its affinity for the other constituents of the tissue or cells should be negligible, the solubility in the medium used for the stains sufficing to transfer an appreciable amount of "stain" into contact with the lipids, but this solubility should be much less than that in the lipids in order to obtain a high partition coefficient; it is this latter which determines the rapidity and intensity of the stain.

The choice of solvents gives rise to a serious problem; it happens that all the convenient media for lysochromes are at the same time lipid solvents, so that there is a danger of loss at the time of "staining". Ethyl alcohol in concentrations ranging from 40% to 70%, 70% methyl alcohol, 70% acetone, 50% isopropanol, isobutanol, ethyleneglycol, propyleneglycol, or diacetin (glycerol diacetate) have been suggested. In fact solutions in 70% ethyl alcohol can be used for ordinary work with no grave risk of losses due to dissolution of the lipids, especially if their action is not prolonged. In addition, the technique using supersaturated isopropanol solutions, due to Lillie and Ashburn (1943), is particularly advantageous.

As for the choice of lysochromes to use, the classical stains Sudan III and Sudan IV are nowadays certainly out of date; much their superiors are oil red O, oil red 4B, BZL blue and Sudan black.

This latter stain deserves special mention. It was introduced into histochemical practice by Lison and Dagnielie (1935) and gives a deeper and more intense stain than any other lysochrome and many authors consider it as clearly superior to the other substances of this group. A knowledge of its chemical formula, divulged in 1945, together with an appreciable amount of experimentation does nevertheless suggest that the results obtained by its use should be regarded with considerable circumspection. In fact, the structural formula of Sudan black B is characterised by the presence of two secondary amine groups, radicals which are known for their great reactivity, and on the face of it this information alone scarcely favours an "indifferent" character for this compound. Moreover, a chromatographic study shows that one can separate from commercial samples of Sudan black B no fewer than ten different fractions, some of which are endowed with a diffuse affinity for all the constituents of the tissue (see Schott and Schoner, 1964); in addition, experience shows that samples of this dye, used in the usual fashion for lipid staining, can show up mucopolysaccharides and proteins (Lillie and Burtner, 1953; Casselman, 1954; Fredricsson and his collaborators, 1958; Kutt and collaborators, 1959; Schott, 1962, 1964; Schott and Schoner, 1964). We know from the studies just cited that this occurrence takes place particularly with solutions which have been prepared for several weeks; Fredricsson and his collaborators have shown that acidification of the dye bath considerably increases the extent to which it is taken up by structures rich in proteins.

It is important to note within this framework of ideas that the dogma of the "chemical indifference" of dyestuffs of the Sudan family (this usage is intended to designate the lysochromes even if the term "Sudan" does not appear in the name of the compounds) has had doubt cast upon it by the discovery of "stable Sudanophilic substances" which are not extracted by alcohol. This phenomenon, discovered by Lillie and Burtner (1953), leads us to admit that there are firm bonds between the lysochrome, which in such cases would play the part of a true stain, and the stained structures. Moreover, Lillie (1965) advises considerable caution in cases where certain of the lysochromes give much more intense stains than do others and when after treatment with alcohol and a benzenoid hydrocarbon the relevant structures do not lose their stain.

A technique for the acetylation of Sudan black B, intended to reduce the intensity of the background colouration, has been developed by Lillie and Burtner (1953); the advantages of this procedure do not seem sufficient for it to be adopted for routine use.

TECHNIQUE OF STAINING BY LYSOCHROMES IN ETHANOL SOLUTION

The practical application of the observations which have just been set out needs to take into account the following facts.

The intensity of the stain obtained obviously increases with the lysochrome content of the solvent; it is therefore advantageous to work with solutions close to saturation, hence the necessity for avoiding any evaporation during the staining of the sections; such an event results in precipitates which are a great nuisance during the examination of the preparations. The solutions should be prepared some time before they are used; saturated solutions of the majority of the lysochromes contain less than 0.3%. We need hardly add that the staining solution should be filtered before it is used and that one should take care to avoid using solutions of Sudan black B which are too old; those of the other lysochromes keep much better.

Most lysochrome staining requires no "differentiation", in conformity with the theoretical mode of action of such compounds; Sudan black B is an exception to this and its use always results in a diffuse colouration of the tissues, and hence the necessity of extracting the excessive lysochrome by passage of the sections through 70% alcohol.

Only lipids whose melting point is not too different from the temperature at which the process is being carried out can dissolve lysochromes and take up a colour; it is therefore useful in doubtful cases to carry out the staining of the sections after they have been kept for about twelve minutes in tepid water (about 45°).

The ethanol content of the solvent should be reduced as far as is compatible with the solution of a sufficient amount of the lysochrome; this precaution heightens the partition coefficient between the solvent and the lipid which is to be stained. In practice, I would advise the use of 55 or 60% alcohol.

Staining by lysochromes other than Sudan black B:

} Frozen sections, free or stuck to the slides; where appropriate, paraffin wax sections, dewaxed and brought into water;

Treat for from 5 to 30 minutes with a freshly filtered saturated solution of the chosen lysochrome in 60% alcohol; the staining should take place in a closed receptacle (excavated blocks or Borrel tubes for paraffin wax sections, Petri dishes with snugly fitting covers for the frozen sections);

Transfer the sections rapidly into tap water; frozen sections which have not been treated with adhesive should be placed at the bottom of the receptacle; they will rise to the surface and unfold because of the change in surface tension;

Stain the background where appropriate (haemalum diluted to 30% with distilled water for red lysochromes, the aluminium lake of nuclear fast red diluted to one part in five with distilled water for blue lysochromes);

Wash in tap water;

Mount in a medium miscible with water.

The colour of the lipid preparations which one obtains in this way obviously varies according to the lysochrome chosen. As I have already remarked, Sudan III and scarlet R (Sudan IV) have only an historical interest at the present time. Sudan brown, Sudan red, oil red O and oil red 4B give much better results but according to my own personal experience the best lysochrome to use in aqueous alcoholic solution is BZL blue. Although it went off the market in 1954, this substance is again commercially available through certain suppliers of products for microscopy; used as just indicated it affords preparations which are hardly inferior so far as the depth and intensity of the staining is concerned but more easily obtained than the preparations using Sudan black B; rinsing with alcohol after treatment with the lysochrome is useless and the solutions keep for several years. This then is the stain that I would advise for use in all cases where the deep blue colour of the lipid preparations is not a nuisance.

Staining with Sudan black B:

Frozen sections, free or adhering to slides; where appropriate, paraffin wax section dewaxed and brought into water;

Treat for from 20 to 30 seconds with 50 or 60% alcohol;

Stain with the same precautions as for the other lysochromes with a saturated solution of Sudan black B in approximately 60% alcohol (this will not keep for more than a few weeks); the duration of staining may run from 5 to 30 minutes;

Transfer the sections into 50 or 60% alcohol, to extract the excess dye; it is generally advisable to keep the preparations in this fluid for about 30 seconds; it is not critical but the necessity for it is an inconvenience as compared with the other lysochromes;

Transfer the sections into tap water;

Where appropriate, stain the background with the aluminium lake of nuclear fast red diluted to one part in five with distilled water;

Wash in tap water and mount in a medium miscible with water.

STAINING TECHNIQUE USING LYSOCHROMES IN SUPER-SATURATED ISOPROPYL ALCOHOL SOLUTION

There are numerous advantages in the staining technique using super-saturated isopropyl alcohol solutions developed by Lillie and Ashburn (1943). The lysochrome concentration in the staining solution is high so that the duration of staining is short; all danger of extracting the lipids is obviated because the solutions used are diluted with water. The stock solutions can be prepared in advance and keep very well. A minor practical inconvenience results from the need to dilute the solution followed by its filtration, slightly before its use, the diluted solutions only keeping their staining power for from 2 to 3 hours.

Preparation of the stock solutions. — Dissolve the chosen lysochrome (all compounds of the Sudan family, including Sudan black B) to saturation point in 99% isopropyl alcohol (commercially pure isopropyl alcohol). According to the compound used saturation is attained with 250–500 mg for 100 ml of solution. Keep the solutions in well stoppered flasks; they keep for many months, even for years, without undergoing alteration.

Method of use:

> Frozen sections, free or adhering to slides; where appropriate, paraffin wax sections, dewaxed and brought into water;
> Treat for about 10 minutes with the solution
> stock-solution of the lysochrome .... 6 volumes
> distilled water .... 4 volumes
> stir for 20 to 30 seconds, allow to stand for about 12 minutes and filter;
> Transfer the sections which have been treated with a dilute solution of lysochrome into tap water;
> Where appropriate, stain the nuclei with a dilute solution of haemalum or with that of nuclear fast red;
> Wash in tap water;
> Mount in a medium miscible with water.

We may note that this method, as well as that using alcoholic solutions of the lysochromes, preserves the birefringence of anisotropic lipids, always providing, obviously, that the staining has been done with a compound other than Sudan black B and that the mounting medium does not contain substances likely to destroy the birefringence (for example, phenol).

All modern authors agree in attributing to the stains obtained after the use of lysochromes sufficient specificity for the needs of practical histochemistry; the interpretative difficulties which may arise during an analysis of the results of the technique using Sudan black B have been mentioned above. The sensitivity of the procedures is also quite satisfactory.

DEMONSTRATION OF LIPIDS USING FLUORESCENT LYSOCHROMES

Techniques for demonstrating lipids by treatment with fluorochromes, including phosphine 3R (Popper, 1944), 3,4-benzopyrene (Graffi and Maas, 1938; Berg, 1951) or anthracene (Ludwig, 1953), may be considered as complementary methods. They have no practical advantages over techniques using other lysochromes when the amount of lipids in the preparations exceeds a certain threshold but may be extremely valuable when there is a need to reveal the presence of very small quantities of these compounds. In practice, the sections are treated with an aqueous medium which suppresses all risk of loss by extraction due to the solvent and the sensitivity exceeds that of all other lysochrome stains. Countervailing this, an examination in ultraviolet light is necessary and the preparations do not keep.

Staining of lipids with phosphine 3R (Popper):

> Frozen sections, coming from material fixed in 10% formalin or fixed with the formaldehyde-calcium of Baker;
> Treat for about 3 minutes with a 0.1% aqueous solution of phosphine 3R;
> Rinse rapidly in distilled water;
> Mount in glycerine;
> Examine and photograph in ultraviolet light.

The presence of soaps, cholesterol, and lipids other than fatty acids is shown by a white fluorescence; the esters of cholesterol give this reaction.

Demonstration of lipids using 3,4 benzopyrene (Berg). — The benzopyrene solution is prepared in the following way: Add to 100 ml of a saturated and filtered solution of caffeine (approximately 1.5%) 0.002 g of 3.4 benzopyrene and allow it to stand for 48 hours at 37°C, filter and dilute with 100 ml of distilled water; allow it to stand for 2 hours and filter. This solution keeps for several months in a brown well stoppered flask in the cold.

The working technique is of the simplest:

> Frozen sections, taken from material fixed with dilute formalin or with formalin-calcium;
> Treat for 20 minutes with the benzopyrene solution;
> Wash rapidly in distilled water;
> Mount in water, examine and photograph in ultraviolet light.

All the lipid preparations, including the finest droplets, acquire a blue or whitish-blue fluorescence which is intense but fleeting.

As Lillie (1965, p. 460) has very rightly remarked, the lysochrome character of these fluorochromes is not evident and the control test using solvent decoloration followed by a fresh staining is quite as useful as in the case of stains of the Sudan family.

THE USE OF EXTRACTION TECHNIQUES IN THE HISTOCHEMICAL STUDY OF LIPIDS

Solubility, as a character, does not play the essential role which it has in analytical chemistry in the histochemical study of lipids. In fact, the classical definition of "lipids" of the chemists rests on solubility in a certain number of organic compounds combined with insolubility in water. Such characteristics are not to be found in the working conditions of the histochemist.

The histochemist often meets compounds which are authentically lipid on paraffin wax sections obtained after treatment of the pieces of tissue with dehydrating alcohols, a benzenoid hydrocarbon and the warm paraffin wax. Lison (1960) even notes the possibility of preserving certain lipids on celloidin sections, that is to say after weeks in mixtures of absolute alcohol and ether. The conditions under which the histochemist extracts are very different from those of the chemist and fixation can modify the solubility of the lipids altogether, either by acting on the compounds themselves or by imprisoning them in a protective web of denatured protein. Certain substances that the histochemist considers as lipid are in fact characterised by their insolubility in all the classical fat solvents; this is the case with the chromolipoids.

The reciprocal is also true; the histochemist often meets with compounds which are completely and easily soluble in alcohol, the benzenoid hydrocarbons and in chloroform but which are nevertheless not lipids.

Solubility then only plays a very minor role in the histochemical identification of the lipids.

The same remark holds good for the distinction between the categories of lipids arising from an examination of their differential solubility. This essential stage in any division of the lipids for a biochemical study is in fact only practised intermittently by histochemists; the results thus obtained are often disconcerting and their interpretation has given rise to much debate.

Among the tests involving differential solubility which are used to separate lipids in analytical chemistry, the insolubility of phospholipids and sphingolipids in acetone is the one from which most histochemists have sought to profit. As well as an older technique developed by Ciaccio (1931), the more modern method of use due to Keilig (1944) is succinctly described to provide a complete documentation.

CIACCIO'S TECHNIQUE
FOR SELECTIVELY RENDERING INSOLUBLE
THE PHOSPHO- AND SPHINGOLIPIDS

Fix for 24 hours in saline formalin or in a mixture of 25 ml of commercial formalin, 25 ml of water, 50 ml of acetone and 0.9 g of sodium chloride;

Treat the pieces of tissue for 1 hour in each of the following mixtures: acetone 70 volumes, a 10% aqueous solution of cadmium nitrate 10 volumes, distilled water 20 volumes;
acetone 80 volumes, a 10% solution of cadmium nitrate 10 volumes, water 10 volumes;
acetone 90 volumes, 10% solution of cadmium nitrate 10 volumes;

Treat the blocks of tissue for 24 hours with a mixture of 98 volumes of acetone and 2 volumes of a saturated solution of cadmium nitrate in absolute alcohol, this solution should be renewed 2 or 3 times;

Treat the blocks with mixtures of water and acetone in steadily decreasing concentration (acetone content 90, 80, 70, 60 and 50%), with cadmium nitrate added to give a final concentration of 1%;

Treat the tissue blocks for several hours with a mixture of equal parts of acetone and of a 5% aqueous solution of potassium dichromate;

Continue the treatment for 2 to 3 days at 37 °C with a 5% aqueous solution of potassium dichromate;

Wash for from 12 to 24 hours in running water;

Cut frozen sections or embed in paraffin and cut into sections;

Show up the pattern of lipids by means of a lysochrome (Sudan III, as recommended by Ciaccio, should obviously be replaced by Sudan black B, BZL blue or oil red);

Where appropriate, stain the background and mount in a medium which is miscible with water.

According to Ciaccio (1931), only the phospho- and sphingolipids will be preserved; rendering them insoluble by postchromatisation even permits one to preserve them on paraffin sections, all the other lipids having been extracted by the acetone treatments.

As Lison (1953, 1960) has commented, those few investigators who have tried to put this method of Ciaccio into operation have obtained results which are negative or difficult to interpret, so that it has been practically abandoned by modern authors.

KEILIG'S TECHNIQUE
FOR THE DIFFERENTIAL EXTRACTION OF LIPIDS

This technique which is closer to the working conditions of the chemist than is that of Ciaccio avoids some of the snags of the method recommended by the Italian author; in practice, the solvents are allowed to act on thin slices of unfixed tissue and their *modus operandi* is close to that of analytical chemical practice; moreover, the evaluation of the results takes place on frozen sections stained with Sudan black B, thus avoiding those errors which are associated with paraffin wax embedding.

Treat the thin slices (maximum thickness 3 mm) of fresh tissue with the following solvents:

cold acetone (for the extraction of glycerides and steroids);

boiling acetone (for the extraction of cerebrosides and the lipids which have been mentioned above);

boiling sulphuric ether (for the extraction of lecithins and cephalins);

a mixture of equal parts of methanol and chloroform maintained at boiling point (for the extraction of the totality of the lipids);

The hot extractions should take place in equipment with a reflux condenser (Soxhlet or Kumagawa apparatus) with all the precautions rendered necessary when handling highly inflammable solvents. The solvent should be renewed after 3, 6 and 12 hours of use;

Bring the tissue blocks into water, taking them through mixtures of water and alcohol having decreasing alcoholic contents;
Section on a freezing microtome;
Stain the lipids with Sudan black B;
Mount in a medium miscible with water.

All authors agree that the results are not generally as clear cut as are those obtained by chemical analysis. Indeed, the histochemical application of techniques involving differential extraction suffers from two serious defects, namely the modification of the solubility of the lipids when these compounds exist in mixtures in any given structure and the dispersion of the phospholipids during extraction by liquids which do not dissolve them; this second phenomenon results in displacements of such substances such as seriously diminish the morphological value of the results obtained.

A technique involving pyridine extraction, due to Baker (1944), and more particularly intended to serve as a control for the results given by the acid haematein method, has been described within the context of this last procedure.

HISTOCHEMICAL REACTIONS AND STAINS PERMITTING THE IDENTIFICATION OF CERTAIN LIPIDS

We know from the results set out in the preceding paragraphs that the demonstration of free lipids (homophasic lipids in the sense of Lison) by "staining" with lysochromes presents no major difficulty and that the sources of error in this method are minimal. The situation however is quite different when the objective of the work is the chemical identification of a group of lipids. Numerous interpretative difficulties arise when we have to determine the chemical constitution of lipidic inclusions, even though these may be easy to identify as such; the possibility of the coexistence, in one and the same structure, of various lipids whose physical and chemical properties can be modified because of their association together further complicates the task; in consequence, from the practical point of view, the results of the procedures described in this section should be interpreted with discretion and circumspection.

Following the example of Lison (1960), the different methods are grouped together according to the physical or chemical attribute upon which they rest.

OPTICAL ANISOTROPY

Examination under polarised light has for a long time been an integral part of the histochemical study of the lipids, but the errors of interpretation to which it can give rise are numerous. The excellent review of this question to be found in the three editions of Lison's work (1936, 1953, 1960) is accepted by all current workers and I feel that it is indispensable to summarise the principal ideas.

In the solid condition *all lipids* show a birefringence of the crystalline type *without a black cross* and with four extinction positions, a knowledge of which affords no indication about the chemical nature of the bodies thus detected. In the liquid state, glycerides and fatty acids are never birefringent; the cholesterids, phospholipids and sphingolipids when in a liquid state and within certain temperature limits (between the melting point and the so-called clearing point) appear in the form of birefringent spherocrystals giving rise to the phenomenon of the black cross.

So far as the lipids are concerned, then, it follows that the results of examination under polarised light can be modified as compared with the initial, fresh, condition by two factors, namely the crystallisation of the lipids which is accentuated by fixation in formalin and the change of temperature by comparison with that of the living animal. These factors should obviously be taken into consideration during the interpretation of the observed phenomena.

The investigator should moreover take account of the fact that staining by lysochromes does not modify the crystalline birefringence whereas it considerably attenuates that of the spherocrystals, these latter being transformed into solid crystals by most of the commonly used mounting media; this last phenomenon does not occur with glycerine. The abolition of all birefringence by mounting media containing phenol has already been remarked upon. One last fact which it is important to mention is the possibility that lipid inclusions may pass reversibly from the liquid state to the crystalline state by chilling or heating the preparation.

Such facts should influence the working technique when studying the optical anisotropy of lipids. An unstained preparation, cut from a fresh tissue block in all cases where such a practice is possible, and mounted in glycerine, is examined under the polarising microscope. There are then three possibilities.

a) The lipids, whose presence has been verified by staining a control section with a lysochrome, are isotropic and do not show up between crossed nicols or polaroids; such an observation of itself permits of no conclusion since the glycerides and fatty acids are never birefringent in the liquid condition, the cholesterids, phospholipids and sphingolipids may be isotropic either because the temperature is higher than their clearing point or because other physical factors inhibit the formation of spherocrystals. The slide should be chilled progressively and any changes which take place should be followed under the microscope. If the lowering of the temperature results in the appearance of a crystalline birefringence with four extinction positions and without a black cross no conclusion can be drawn, such a sequence being found with all lipids; but if the spherocrystals which give rise to the phenomenon of the black cross appear in the course of a suitable chilling the presence of cholesterids, phospholipids or sphingolipids is highly probable.

b) The lipids show up in polarised light but have a crystalline type of birefringence with four extinction positions during rotation of the stage through 360°. This observation by itself, as I have just mentioned, does not permit of any conclusion since all lipids may exist in this form. The slide is then progressively warmed. Under such conditions, the glycerides and the fatty acids pass directly from the crystalline birefringence to the liquid state when they are isotropic, whereas the cholesterids and phospho- and sphingolipids become spherocrystals (liquid crystals in the sense of Lehmann) with polarisation crosses.

c) The lipids show up in polarised light and show the black cross. We are then dealing with cholesterids, phospho- or sphingolipids existing as spherocrystals; the presence of glycerides and of fatty acids can be excluded. This birefringence with a black cross should disappear as the slide is warmed, the spherocrystals passing into the liquid state; chilling should further transform it into a birefringence of the crystalline type.

We may remark, as does Lison (1960), that the birefringence of heterophasic lipids shows up the molecular orientation of the systems to which it relates and has no bearing on their chemical nature.

DEMONSTRATION OF THE ACID NATURE OF LIPIDS

The demonstration of the "acid" nature of any given lipid inclusion has a definite histochemical interest since such information leads one to suspect the presence of free fatty acids, in particular of oleic acid, or of phospho- or sphingolipids or of chromolipids in the stained structures. This conclusion is undoubtedly valid only as a first approximation and exceptions to it have been mentioned in relation to one of the methods which permit us to reveal the presence of acid lipids; it is nevertheless true that tests for acidic groups constitute an essential stage of the histochemical study of the lipids.

The principal method for the histochemical detection of acid lipids is the classical technique of Lorrain Smith using Nile blue. In addition to that, I should like briefly to mention Feyrter's technique for staining "by mounting" (Einschlussfärbung) the interpretation of which is more delicate, and the older procedure of Fischler for demonstrating fatty acids; only the principle of this technique will be mentioned in a succinct fashion. It seems to me legitimate to mention in this section staining by phthalocyanines of the luxol solid blue type, which is a procedure whose histochemical value seems to be highly debateable, but whose morphological interest is undoubted.

The Nile blue method

The Nile blue method, used for the first time by Lorrain Smith, depends on the fact that a solution of Nile blue sulphate stains certain lipids blue and others pink; the first are the "acid lipids", the others are "neutral lipids".

The older explanations of this staining, which postulated the dissociation of the stain, with solution of the free base acting as if it were a lysochrome in the case of neutral fats, whereas it was supposed to give soaps which were stained blue in the case of acid fats, are no longer considered plausible. In fact, all commercial samples of Nile blue contain Nile red as impurity (Lison, 1935; Cain, 1947, 1950), a feeble base whose salts are completely hydrolysed by water so that the free base exists in aqueous solutions. This base is a lysochrome and on this account confers a pink tinge on all lipids. This tinge is however masked in the case of acid lipids by the blue colour due to Nile blue, a stain which is not taken up by neutral lipids.

It seems to me imperative to mention that the pink colour obtained under the working conditions of Lorrain Smith's method has the same significance as has the result of all "staining" by lysochromes and permits us to say that lipids are present in the structures shown up in this fashion. The blue colour, on the other hand, only indicates the presence of electronegative groups; in fact, Nile blue is a basic stain and shows up all acid groups whether lipidic or not. It is thus very important to verify, by means of some other method, that the structures which are stained blue by Lorrain Smith's method do indeed correspond to lipids. Moreover, we know from Cain's studies (1947), that Nile blue sulphate has this peculiarity in common with the lysochromes, that it will not stain any kind of lipid whatsoever when in the solid condition.

Among the numerous variations on the method of Lorrain Smith, that of Cain (1947) harmonizes most closely with the needs of histochemical research and it is the working technique of this author which I should like to see adopted.

Working technique:

Frozen sections, taken from material fixed in Baker's formol-calcium, with or without postchromatisation;

Treat a section with Sudan black B for a general demonstration of the free lipids;

Submit a section which is a near neighbour of the preceding one to extraction with pyridine (for example, for 1 hour at 60 °C) in order to dissolve the lipids as a whole take it into water and treat it with Sudan black B to verify the lipidic nature of the structures which were stained in the first section;

Treat a third section for 5 minutes, at 60 °C, with a 1% aqueous solution of Nile blue;

Wash rapidly in distilled water warmed to 60°;

Allow to stand for 30 seconds in 1% acetic acid at 60°;

Wash in water and mount in a medium miscible with water;

Treat a fourth section with a 1% solution of Nile blue for 5 minutes, then with a 0.02% solution of the same stain for 5 minutes, at 60°, thus ensuring the optimal conditions for the dissociation of Nile red;

Wash, differentiate in acetic acid, wash in water and mount as for the third section.

The comparison of sections stained with Sudan black B, with and without extraction by pyridine, allows one to identify the lipids; the comparison of the section stained with a concentrated solution of Nile blue on the one hand, and with the concentrated solution followed by the dilute solution on the other hand, enables one to sort out those rather rare cases where the neutral lipids are not stained by Nile red except in very dilute solutions. In any event, the acid lipids show up blue, the neutral lipids pink.

According to Menschik (1953), extraction by hot acetone, used after the Nile blue staining, allows one selectively to demonstrate the phospholipids in blue. The technique of this author includes staining for 90 minutes, at 60°C, with a saturated solution of Nile blue in a mixture of 500 ml of distilled water and 50 ml of 0.5% sulphuric acid, this mixture having been kept at boiling point for 2 hours before use. The sections are then rinsed in distilled water and placed in acetone brought up to 50°C but withdrawn from the source of heat immediately the sections are immersed in it; the sections remain in the acetone for 30 minutes and are then differentiated in 5% acetic acid for 30 minutes, washed and treated with 0.5% hydrochloric acid for 3 minutes, washed and mounted. Only the phospholipids will retain their blue colour under these conditions.

It is appropriate to mention, in relation to the interpretation of the Nile blue technique, that Cain's conclusions (1950) are not accepted without reservation by Lison (1960); this latter author notes in particular that lecithin does not stain blue by this method and that the "acid" nature of colamine-cephalin is uncertain; in the same way, the affinity of sphingomyelin for Nile blue seems dubious to Lison.

Tests for metachromasia

This test enables us selectively to demonstrate the presence of lipids, in particular in nervous tissue. In this way staining has succeeded with myelin, the characteristic granulations of the Schwann cells (Reich granulations), certain details of the structure of tactile corpuscles, and lastly pathological deposits of lipids. According to Lison (1960) the metachromasia of myelin is characterised by the slowness of its appearance, the optimum pH of the staining bath lying between 2 and 3, the progressive fading of sections mounted in water, and the instantaneous decolorisation with alcohol which nevertheless permits the preparation to be restained.

Naturally, tests for the metachromasia of the lipids are always made on frozen sections; the classical procedures described in relation to the metachromatic reaction on paraffin wax sections are quite suitable provided that the mounting always takes place in a medium miscible with water.

Staining by montage (Einschlussfärbung; Einschluss-mounting, not to be confused with Einbettung-embedding) as practised by Feyrter (1936) gives more striking preparations than does the metachromatic reaction using toluidine blue. It consists of sticking frozen sections on albuminized slides and covering them with several drops of a solution of thionine or of 1% cresyl violet in 0.5% tartaric acid, and then mounting them under a coverslip the edges of which are then sealed. The metachromasia may appear rapidly or in from 24 to 48 hours. The preparations keep for several weeks.

As for the interpretation of the results so obtained it seems imperative to me to recall that all compounds which bear sufficiently strong electronegative groups, whether of a lipid nature or not, may prove to be chromotropic under the conditions described above; we have therefore to verify by other methods, in particular by staining with lysochromes or by extraction with pyridine, that the metachromatic compounds we are studying are indeed of a lipidic nature. Once this fact has been established, it is appropriate to remark that glycerides, cholesterides and, in a general way, all "neutral" lipids never give the metachromatic reaction. In the case of the lipids of the nervous system this last reaction is due to compounds bearing sulphate and phosphate radicals, that is to say the sulphuric esters of cerebrosides and the phosphatids. The metachromasia of the first is the more intense.

In dealing with the metachromasia of lipids we may recall a technique for the simultaneous demonstration of free lipids and of non-lipid chromotropes (Arvy, 1958). The method follows that of Lillie for staining with oil red in a solution of isopropyl alcohol except that the isopropyl alcohol stock-solution of oil red O or oil red 4B is diluted for use, not with distilled water but, with a 0.5% solution of toluidine blue in distilled water. In this way we can demonstrate the free lipids on frozen sections, thanks to the lysochrome and the metachromatic stain of the non-lipid chromotropes; any metachromatic staining of the lipids is, obviously, masked by the red of the lysochrome.

Staining with copper haematoxylin

Staining with copper haematoxylin as used by Fischler (1904) was considered by its author as specific for fatty acids, which is manifestly inaccurate. The method involves the use of an aqueous solution of copper acetate as a mordant for the sections followed by staining with Weigert's solution of haematoxylin and lithium hydroxide followed by differentiation with borax-ferricyanide. Under these conditions, a blue colour would indicate the presence of fatty acids.

In fact, the fixation of copper ions, whatever the mechanism may be, results in the appearance of an affinity for haematoxylin; numerous structures which do not contain lipids give positive results; lipids not containing fatty acids may give positive results during tests on model structures, whereas negative results have arisen from experiments under the same conditions with mixtures which do in fact contain fatty acids. Although it has been somewhat complacently cited in certain recent texts, Fischler's haematoxylin should therefore be considered as being of no histochemical value.

Staining with phthalocyanins

Staining with phthalocyanins of the Luxol fast blue type (methasol fast blue) has been suggested by Klüver and Barrera (1953, 1954) for the morphological demonstration of myelin sheaths in paraffin sections. At one time considered by Pearse (1955) as being specific for phospholipids, the method in question in fact represents a morphological technique which it is impossible to interpret in chemical terms. Despite trials on model sections, which have included a relatively large number of substances (Pearse and Almeida, 1958), the mechanism of the staining reaction has not yet been elucidated. We do however know that numerous structures which are devoid of lipids can be stained under the technical conditions of this procedure and that all lipids with the exception of sphingomyelin may give rise to the stain in question. I have been led to mention this technique by the demonstration of structures rich in electronegative groupings using the luxol fast blue technique, whose morphological value is undoubted in relation to the detection of acid lipids.

Working technique:

Paraffin wax sections, taken from material fixed in formalin, in Bouin's fluid or in other aqueous fixatives, dewaxed, treated with collodion and brought into alcohol;
Treat for from 6 to 18 hours, at 60 °C, with a 0.1% solution of luxol fast blue or of methasol (and not methanol) fast blue 2G in 95% alcohol;
Rinse in 70% alcohol and bring into water;
Differentiate with concomitant microscopic inspection, using a 0.05% aqueous solution of lithium carbonate; the time taken varies greatly from one case to another;
Wash in tap water;
Stain the background with the aluminium lake of nuclear fast red, with Mayer's carmalum or with a 1% aqueous solution of neutral red, this latter background stain causes the blue colour to turn black or purple;
Dehydrate in absolute alcohol, clear in a benzenoid hydrocarbon and mount in a synthetic resin or in Canada balsam.

The firmness with which luxol fast blue stains is so great that other histochemical reactions or stains can be practised afterwards; it is particularly advantageous to associate this method with the PAS reaction.

In any case, the positive result as indicated by a more-or-less intense bluish tint does not constitute a proof of the existence of lipids in the stained structures. The chemical composition of the stain remains a secret and all the comments which were made in relation to alcian blue hold good in the case of luxol fast blue. From the practical point of view, we may stress the optical qualities of the preparations and the desirability of working with fresh solutions which have not been used more than twice.

DEMONSTRATION OF THE UNSATURATED NATURE OF LIPIDS

The presence of double bonds, often conjugated, in a large number of lipids is the basis of several methods allowing them to be demonstrated on sections, in particular reduction by osmium tetroxide, the addition of the halogens and reactions involving oxidation by peracids (performic, peracetic), followed by treatment with Schiff's reagent. To these methods may be added those based on the formation of peroxides during the oxidation of unsaturated lipids.

Reduction of osmium tetroxide

As I have noted, the reduction of osmium tetroxide is the oldest of the methods for demonstrating the presence of lipids, but it is far from being the case that its chemical mechanism has been fully elucidated. Regarded as a morphological technique the osmic blackening of lipids still plays a far from negligeable role at the present time, since this demonstration can be combined with techniques of fixation which are among the most reliable in cytological practice and which prepare the tissue admirably for the staining of the principal elements of the animal cell. Certain neurohistological techniques are also based on the osmic impregnation of lipids, but we should not forget that blackening under the action of solutions of osmium tetroxide is neither a general property of the lipids nor the exclusive prerogative of this group of compounds; in consequence this blackening does not prove the lipid nature of the structures which are shown up and its absence does not allow us to declare that lipids themselves are absent. From a practical point of view, the use of osmium tetroxide not only entrains the blackening of certain lipids but at the same time it renders the lipids sufficiently insoluble to permit of their being embedded in paraffin wax, and thus enabling us to obtain fine serial sections in which the lipids are well preserved and this desirable feature should also beset to the credit of the method.

From the histological point of view, osmic blackening can be used to distinguish some lipids from others provided that it is employed within the conditions which have been well defined by Cain (1950).

Indeed, a methodical investigation leads us to distinguish two distinct phenomena in the osmic blackening of the lipids; one of these phenomena is the primary blackening which takes place under the action of osmium tetroxide alone and without the intervention of any other reagents, whereas the secondary blackening occurs only when the osmium-treated pieces come into contact with ethyl alcohol as part of the dehydrating process.

Most authors consider that primary blackening indicates the presence of double bonds in the lipids which are shown up in this way; in other words, that it is diagnostic of radicals belonging to the olefinic series. It is within this category that Cain (1950) would set tests for osmic blackening under the influence of osmium tetroxide, acting on sections which have been fixed for a short time by Baker's formaldehyde-calcium, and which have been washed clear of any excess of formalin. Lison (1960) expresses some reservations in this respect and notes the absence of any close parallel between the intensity of the osmic blackening and the iodine index, which is a chemical expression of the degree of unsaturation of the lipids; the paucity of information concerning the complex formed between the lipids and osmium dioxide which results from the reduction of the tetroxide is also irritating in this context, but the validity of the primary blackening as a method of showing up double bonds in compounds whose lipidic nature has been otherwise verified can be accepted in the present state of our knowledge.

The mechanism of secondary blackening is still unknown; we may agree with Lison (1960) that the reaction involved is a reduction of the osmium tetroxide dissolved in the lipids by the alcohol and thus the secondary blackening in no way demonstrates the presence of double bonds. This phenomenon is thus incapable of interpretation in chemical terms and the same remark holds good for the different colours which lipidic inclusions show in paraffin wax sections coming from material which has been treated with osmium tetroxide; the classical assertion according to which the glycerides are stained black, the phospholipids and cholesterids brownish black or yellow does not conform to any recognizable reality.

It is appropriate to add that the behaviour of several lipids in the presence of osmium tetroxide can be entirely modified by the occurrence in the medium of oxidising agents such as chromium trioxide or the alkaline bichromates. Thus a normal myelin blackens under the action of solutions of osmium tetroxide whereas it does not become blackened by the action of chromic-osmic mixtures. This is the principle of Marchi's method which we deal with in relation to neurohistological techniques.

Addition reactions of the halogens

These reactions rest on the same chemical foundations as does the iodine index; in fact, two atoms of iodine are fixed by each double bond with the formation of dihalogenated addition derivatives. These derivatives, which are unstable, freely liberate the halogen whose occurrence can be detected in the form of the silver halide which may be reduced to the metallic state by a photographic developer. This is the principle of the method advocated by Barrolier and Suchowsky (1958) whose *modus operandi* is given below.

> Frozen sections taken either from fresh material or from that fixed for a short time in formalin;
> Treat for 5 minutes with a saturated aqueous solution of iodine chloride or with the mixture
>> potassium iodide .... 2.5 g
>> doubly sublimed iodine .... 1.25 g
>> distilled water .... 1 litre
>
> Wash for 30 minutes in distilled water, the washing liquid being frequently renewed;
> Treat for 20 minute with an N:5 solution (about 3.5%) of silver nitrate;
> Wash in distilled water;
> Treat for 10 minutes with N/10 nitric acid (about 0.6%);
> Wash in distilled water;
> Treat for from 10 to 20 minutes with a standard photographic developer based on metol-hydroquinone;
> Fix for from 10 to 15 minutes in the standard acid photographic fixative;
> Wash in tap water and mount in a medium miscible with water.

The structures containing unsaturated lipids show up in black.

A technique which depends on the same principle, but uses the fixation of bromine on the double bonds, has been described by Norton and his collaborators (1962). It comprises the following stages.

> Frozen sections taken from material fixed in Baker's formaldehyde-calcium and washed carefully in distilled water;
> Treat for 1 minute with the solution
>> bromine .... 1 ml
>> a 2% aqueous solution of
>> potassium bromide .... 388 ml
>
> Treat for 1 minute with a 1% aqueous solution of sodium bisulphite;
> Wash in 7 baths of distilled water;
> Treat for from 18 to 24 hours with the solution
>> silver nitrate .... 1 g
>> N/1 nitric acid (approx. 6.4%) .... 100 ml
>
> Wash in 7 baths of distilled water;
> Treat for 10 minutes with the photographic developer
>> Kodak dektol (concentrated solution) .... 1 volume
>> distilled water .... 1 volume
>
> Subject to prolonged washing in tap water, stain the background where appropriate and mount in a medium miscible with water.

The colour of structures containing unsaturated lipids varies from black to brown. From my own experience, this method is superior to that of Barrolier and Suchowsky as well as to another method which uses bromine, but in the gas phase (Mukherji and his collaborators, 1960). The bromine solution prepared according to the directions of Norton and his collaborators keeps for several weeks.

The results of these addition reactions of the halogens can be verified by extraction of the lipids, prior to the cutting of the sections, by the treatment of control sections with the procedures indicated but omitting the addition of halogen as well as by performic or periodic oxidation prior to the treatment with the halogen; all these test treatments should cause the activity to disappear.

Oxidative reactions using peracids

These reactions depend on the fact that performic or peracetic acids, potassium permanganate and chromic acid attack the double bonds with the formation of epoxides, peroxides, glycols and aldehydes. These latter compounds can be detected by one of the reactions mentioned in the chapter devoted to the detection of carbonyl groups; generally speaking, one has recourse to Schiff's reagent. This procedure which was described by Pearse (1951) and by Lillie (1952) is applicable to frozen sections and to those in paraffin wax, the choice between them being obviously dictated by the solubility relationships of the lipids which we have to detect. It is Lillie's variant which is the most used.

Performic acid is not sold as an industrial chemical, a fact which is easily explained by its instability; it should be prepared on the same day as it is to be used, according to the formula of Greenspan (1946).

> To 8 ml of the 90% commercial formic acid add 31 ml of 30% hydrogen peroxide (110 volumes), *taken from a bottle which has been opened for less than one week*, as well as 0.22 ml of concentrated sulphuric acid; allow to stand for 2 hours at a temperature which should not exceed 25°C and use on the same day.

Peracetic acid, which is more stable, is sold as an industrial chemical, but the ease of its preparation by means of Greenspan's formula (1946) is such that the experimenter may well prefer to make it for himself.

> Add 259 ml of 30% hydrogen peroxide and 2.2 ml of concentrated sulphuric acid to 95.6 ml of crystallizable glacial acetic acid. Allow to stand for from 1 to 3 days and then add 40 mg of disodium phosphate to stabilize it. The reagent keeps in a refrigerator for several months, 100 ml sufficing for the treatment of about 80 slides.

Working technique:

> Frozen or paraffin wax sections, the latter being optionally treated with collodion and hydrated;
> Treat for 1 to 2 hours with performic or peracetic acid;
> Wash for 10 minutes in water which is either running or frequently renewed;
> Treat with Schiff's reagent for from 10 to 15 minutes;

Wash in sulphur dioxide water (indispensable for frozen sections) or very energetically in distilled water (this most often suffices for paraffin wax sections);
Wash for 10 minutes in tap water which is either running or frequently renewed;
Stain the nuclei where appropriate with Groat's haematoxylin or with Hansen's ferric trioxyhaematein, if the lipids studied are very soluble in alcohol;
Wash for from 3 to 5 minutes in water which is either running or frequently renewed;
Mount in a medium which is miscible with water or dehydrate in absolute alcohol, clear in a benzenoid hydrocarbon and mount in a synthetic resin or in Canada balsam.

The reaction is positive when a reddish purple colour appears.

It is relevant to remark that treatment with performic or peracetic acid entrains the hydrolysis of the deoxyribonucleic acid which engenders a reddish stain in the nuclei, this being clear when the nuclei have not been stained with haematoxylin. This nucleal reaction is obviously independent of the presence of unsaturated lipids. In the same way, the interpretation of the results should take into account the fact that performic or peracetic oxidation can induce carbonyl groups to appear in molecules which are not lipidic; the presence of lipids in structures stained by these methods should thus be verified by means of other techniques, in particular, by extraction or by the use of lysochromes.

A control reaction, which allows us to verify the results obtained using the oxidative reactions which have just been described, is represented by bromination. This operation, which was put forward by Lillie (1953), involves the addition of halogens to carbon atoms bearing the double bond. In conformity with the advice of Lillie (1965 p. 185), the working technique of that author, which uses bromine water, should be replaced by that of Norton and his collaborators; this amounts to using the silver salts described above in the early stages of the technique for demonstrating double bonds, (up to the stage of washing with distilled water which follows treatment by the bromine-potassium bromide solution).

Demonstration of the peroxides formed during the oxidation of unsaturated lipids

The older finding that there is a positive reaction of certain lipids during tests for oxidases by the nadi mixture (α-naphthol and dimethylparaphenylenediamine) has been related by Lison (1936) to a direct non catalytic oxidation of the reagent by the peroxides formed from unsaturated lipids in contact with atmospheric oxygen. This formation of peroxides thus takes place in the same circumstances as those in which the compounds responsible for the pseudoplasmal reaction arise, as will be noted in one of the following sections.

Lison's technique for demonstrating positive lipids corresponds, detail by detail, with the M-nadi reaction of the classical authors; a slightly different technique, due to Dam and Granados (1945), uses 2,6-dichlorphenol-indophenol in the presence of haemin, which plays the part of a catalyst.

These techniques are principally of theoretical interest and have not entered into current histochemical practice.

DEMONSTRATION OF THE COMPLEXES FORMED BY LIPIDS WITH CHROMIUM COMPOUNDS

In addition to rendering certain lipids insoluble, probably through their polymerisation, potassium bichromate gives rise to the formation of complexes in which a chromium oxide is apparently bound to the diketones which result from the oxidation of the lipid. These compounds form particularly easily in the case of phospho- and sphingolipids whose conjugated double bonds lend themselves particularly well to this type of chemical reaction. By suitably regulating the action of the potassium bichromate, the reaction which has just been mentioned thus offers the possibility of the selective detection of the lipids in question through the formation of a chromic lake of haematin.

Such is the principle of Smith's method (1909), and that of Dietrich (1910), which are widely used in the classical studies on the histochemistry of the lipids; this method is derived from Weigert's technique for staining myelin. The working technique consists of treating frozen sections with an aqueous solution of potassium bichromate, then staining them with the acetic haematoxylin of Kultschitzky, and lastly differentiating by means of Weigert's borax-ferricyanide. This working technique was developed in particular by Baker (1944) and the postchromatisation was carried out on blocks of tissue, the preparation of the haematoxylin solution being set out in strict detail. The English author's technique using acid haematein has almost completely displaced the classical procedure, at least so far as its histochemical use is concerned. It is this technique which we set out at this point.

The acid haematein method

Fix in formol-calcium for from 6 to 18 hours, according to the size of the blocks of material;
Treat, without washing, with the solution
  potassium bichromate .... 5 g
  anhydrous calcium chloride .... 1 g
  distilled water .... 100 ml
for 18 hours at laboratory temperatures;
Transfer the pieces of tissue into a second bath of calcium-bichromate and keep them for 24 hours, at 60°C;
Wash in running water until the excess potassium bichromate has been eliminated (6 to 18 hours);

Where appropriate, embed in gelatin using Baker's technique (p. 92);
Cut the block into fine sections (10 μ or less) on a freezing microtome;
Treat the sections for 1 hour, at 60°, with the bichromate-calcium solution;
Wash in frequently renewed distilled water until the excess bichromate has been eliminated (about 5 minutes);
Treat for 5 hours, at 37°C, with the solution—

    crystalline haematoxylin .... 0.05 g
    distilled water .... 48 ml
    a 10% aqueous solution of
    sodium iodate .... 1 ml

(the weighings should be carried out on a precision balance, and the liquid measured using a pipette), bring to boiling point and allow to cool, add 1 ml of crystallizable acetic acid and use the solution on the day of its preparation;
Rinse in distilled water;
Treat for 18 hours, at 37°C, with the borax-ferricyanide differentiating solution

    potassium ferricyanide .... 0.25 g
    sodium tetraborate decahydrate .... 0.25 g
    distilled water .... 100 ml

(keep in a cool dark place);
Wash with care in distilled water (4 to 5 baths of a total duration of 10 minutes);
Mount in a medium miscible with water.

Structures containing phospho- and sphingolipids stain deep blue or black, but this colour is by no means confined to such compounds. All sites of heavy metals take on the same tint as do the mucins, the nucleoproteins and other protein-like compounds. It is thus indispensable to carry out a control reaction using the extraction technique which was developed by Baker (1944) along the following lines.

The pyridine extraction test

Fix control blocks of tissue as comparable as possible to those which have been treated in order to demonstrate phospho- and sphingolipids, using "weak Bouin's solution"

    saturated aqueous solution of picric acid .... 50 ml
    commercial formalin .... 10 ml
    acetic acid .... 5 ml
    distilled water .... 35 ml

for 20 hours;
Treat for some hours with 95% or 70% alcohol, renewed several times so as to eliminate the excess picric acid;
Treat for 30 minutes, at laboratory temperatures, with pure pyridine;
Treat for 24 hours, at 60°C, in a new bath of pure pyridine;
Wash for 2 hours in running water;
Proceed as for the acid haematein technique, starting from the treatment with the bichromate-calcium solution.

Extraction with pyridine results in the disappearance of the colour due to the presence of the lipids for which one is testing, the other structures being stained as in tissue which has not undergone this treatment; the stain taken up by the nucleus may even be reinforced.

Certain authors (Cain, 1950; Lison, 1960) consider the acid haematein technique as being truly specific for phospho- and sphingolipids while they insist on the necessity for taking into account only obvious stains and of not increasing the duration of postchromatisation, which is an essential stage of the method, nor of shortening the duration of the differentiation. Other authors have more reservations; for example Pearse (1960) says that the cerebrosides probably give positive results, that losses are practically inevitable at the time of fixation using formol-calcium and that further work is necessary before we can come down firmly in favour of the specificity of Baker's method for "lipins".

From the theoretical point of view, the indirect and inverted nature of the method is, evidently, intellectually unsatisfactory; there is nothing to guarantee *a priori* that the lipid constituents alone will retain chromium oxides after postchromatisation and comparisons made with sections taken from tissue extracted with pyridine in effect show that this is the case. Despite the very precise recommendations made by Baker, the process of differentiation introduces a subjective factor into our appreciation of the results, all the more so because the optimum duration of this stage of the method necessarily varies with the thickness of the sections.

Leaving aside its complexity, Baker's method has practical defects which in some cases may be considerable. It is true that postchromatisation on blocks of tissue represents a substantial advance on the classical method of Smith-Dietrich from the point of view of preserving the heterophasic lipids in position, but it renders necessary the practice of carrying out the extraction on a second block. Because of this, rigorously comparable sections may be difficult to obtain, especially in cases where the small size of the organs being studied makes it necessary to take the postchromatised block of tissue directly from one animal and the control block extracted with pyridine from a second animal. To all this we must add the nuisance from what, strictly speaking, is a morphological point of view, of having to compare sections taken from blocks fixed in different fluids, one of which is alkaline and the other acid.

We can therefore see why Baker's technique has not had quite the success which one might have expected it to enjoy during the years which followed its publication.

Most modern authors prefer to use, instead of Baker's method, "controlled postchromatisation", a procedure due to Elftman (1954), which is simpler and gives results which are equivalent to those of the preceding method.

Place rather thin slices of fresh tissue in the mixture
potassium bichromate .... 5 g
an M/5 solution of sodium acetate
(2.7% by weight) .... 7 ml
an M/5 solution of acetic acid
(1.2% by volume) .... 93 ml
and store them in an oven at 56°C leaving them there for 18 hours;
Wash for 6 hours in running water;
Dehydrate and embed in paraffin without special precautions;
Section the paraffin wax block, dewax it and hydrate it;
Stain for 2 hours, at 56°C, with the solution
M/5 acetic acid .... 98.5 ml
M/5 sodium acetate solution .... 1.5 ml
haematoxylin .... 0.1 g
potassium ferricyanide .... 0.005 g

the solution having been previously warmed to 56°C;
Wash in distilled water;
Dehydrate in absolute alcohol, clear in a benzenoid hydrocarbon and mount in a synthetic resin, or, if necessary, in Canada balsam;
Stain a section close to the preceding one in Sudan black B, and mount in a medium miscible with water.

Those lipids which have taken up chromium are stained in both sections. The lipids which have not taken up chromium show up only on the slides stained with Sudan black B, the non lipid structures which have taken up chromium being demonstrated solely on the slides stained with haematoxylin. The addition of potassium ferricyanide to the haematoxylin solution limits the extent of the stain; it is this addition which enables us to dispense with any differentiation.

The same technique is obviously applicable to frozen sections; when the investigator chooses this latter approach the blocks of tissue should be cut after the stage of washing in running water, the sections being stained on the one hand with acid haematoxylin and on the other with Sudan black B.

We should not lose sight of the fact that these techniques make use of a stain, haematoxylin, and that in consequence the results depend on the quality of the commercial sample.

DEMONSTRATION OF LIPIDS BEARING CARBONYL GROUPS

In all text-books of histochemical techniques the lipids bearing carbonyl groups occupy a place which in no way corresponds to their real importance, but which is accounted for by the substantial number of contradictions and misunderstandings with which the original publications dealing with this question were sprinkled. The importance of the problems raised by the demonstration of the aldehyde and ketone groups carried by the lipids, an importance which is particularly acute in the teaching of the subject, explains the interest that many authors attach to their study. Evidently there can be no question of retracing here the successive stages of a debate which at the present time is quite defunct; the texts of Lison (1960), Pearse (1960) and Clara (in Graumann and Neumann, 1965) affords an excellent entry into the literature on the subject of lipids which bear carbonyl groups.

Three categories of lipid compounds contain carbonyl groups and should, in principle, be accessible to histochemical detection through the demonstration of these functional groups; these categories are the plasmalogens (acetalphosphatides), the compounds formed from the oxidation of unsaturated lipids and the ketosteroids.

From the chemical point of view, the plasmalogens differ from the phospholipids in that their hydrolysis liberates aldehydes (palmitaldehyde, stearaldehyde, etc...) instead of fatty acids; their linkages with glycerophosphoric acid are of the semi-acid aldehyde type in the plasmalogens, and of the acid aldehyde type in the acetal phosphatides, the *in vivo* existence of this second group of compounds remaining uncertain.

These compounds which were discovered in 1924 by Feulgen's school are detectable in sections by the plasmal reaction (Feulgen and Voit, 1924). This method depends on the fact that mercuric chloride *very rapidly* sets off a hydrolysis of the plasmalogens liberating fatty aldehydes which can be detected using Schiff's reagent. Feulgen's school obtained its initial preparations using fresh tissue after a short treatment with corrosive sublimate and then with Schiff's reagent. The work to which I have just alluded was followed by a considerable number of publications and the general impression which one gets from reading them is that of an extraordinary degree of confusion. For the last fifteen years or so, under the influence of various authors, amongst which we should principally cite Cain (1949, 1950) and Hayes (1947, 1949), a return to the initial definition of the plasmal reaction has been universally agreed. Each of the three elements of the definition, as given above, has its own importance. Tests for plasmalogens should be carried out on sections or on spread preparations of fresh tissue, otherwise there is a grave risk of confusion arising from the appearance of carbonyl groups following the oxidation of unsaturated lipids; it is convenient to place all positive results obtained on fixed tissue in Lison's category of "pseudoplasmal" reactions. The action of corrosive sublimate should be of short duration; we now know that prolonged treatment with this reagent diminishes or abolishes the plasmal reaction and causes carbonyl groups to appear in structures which do not contain plasmalogens. Schiff's reagent should also act only for a short period since its acidity may result not only in a hydrolysis of the plasmalogens but also that of other compounds. We need hardly add that hydrolysis under the action of corrosive sublimate is the true criterion of the presence of plasmalogens, so that it is essential to compare sections treated by the plasmal reaction with control sections immersed directly in Schiff's reagent.

Among the modern variants of the plasmal reaction, two require mention here; one is the method of Hayes (1949) involving sections and the other that of Cain (1950) which is applicable to small blocks of tissue.

Plasmal reaction (Hayes technique)

Frozen sections of fresh tissue (use a cryostat or an apparatus for freezing the razor blade, where necessary), squash or smear preparations;

Wash with several (3 to 4) baths of a 0.9% solution of sodium chloride (in the case of mammalian tissue, for the tissue of other animals use an isotonic solution of the same salt);

Immerse some of the sections or smears in a 1% aqueous solution of mercuric chloride for from 2 to 10 minutes, the control sections or smears being placed for the same period in an isotonic solution of sodium chloride;

Treat the sections or smears after hydrolysis and the controls in a rigorously comparable fashion, but in different receptacles, with Schiff's reagent for from 5 to 15 minutes; this last period represents a maximum which should never be exceeded; only use Schiff's reagent which has not previously been used;

Rinse carefully in 3 baths of sulphur dioxide water;
Wash with care in running or frequently renewed water (for about 10 minutes);
Mount in a medium miscible with water; dehydration in alcohol followed by clearing and mounting in a synthetic resin is sometimes possible.

Nuclear staining using 0.5% methyl green in 0.5% acetic acid or using haemalum can be employed in certain cases; it should be practised after the bath in running water which terminates the reaction.

Plasmal reaction (Cain's technique)

Place very small and freshly dissected blocks of tissue in the mixture
  Schiff's reagent .... 1 volume
  an aqueous saturated solution of
    mercuric chloride .... 2 volumes
  sulphur dioxide water (a 10% solution
    of potassium metabisulphite 5 ml,
    N hydrochloric acid 5 ml, distilled
    water 90 ml) .... 1 volume
and keep them there for 15 minutes; treat the control blocks with the mixture of Schiff's reagent and sulphur dioxide water without corrosive sublimate;
Wash the blocks of tissue which have undergone hydrolysis and the controls with great care in 3 or 4 baths of sulphur dioxide water for a total duration of 10 minutes;
Fix for two hours with 10% formalin;
Cut frozen sections and, where appropriate, stain the background as in Hayes technique, mount in a medium miscible with water or dehydrate, clear and mount in a synthetic resin.

Naturally, it is very valuable to compare such sections with those treated for a general demonstration of lipids using a lysochrome; the presence of acetal-phosphatides is shown by the violet red colour characteristic of the restoration of the colour of Schiff's reagent.

Compounds derived from the oxidation of unsaturated lipids often bear aldehyde groups, stemming from the decomposition of the peroxides formed in a preliminary oxidative process. This sequence of reactions of lipids in fixed tissue or subjected to other treatments is particularly likely to occur in the case of phospholipids whose molecules contain fatty acids bearing numerous and conjugated double bonds. Oxidation in air, fixation in formalin or other fixatives, or treatment by ultra-violet light gives rise to the formation of these lipid derivatives bearing carbonyl groups, so that the positive result of the "pseudoplasmal" reactions are entirely devoid of significance, even though they may represent a serious source of error when the plasmal reaction is carried out without taking into account the essential points set out above.

It is this formation of compounds from unsaturated lipids, such as we have just mentioned, which lies at the origin of a passionate debate bearing on the possibility of the histochemical detection of ketosteroids. It happens that compounds of this group, whose carbonyl radical is to be found on positions 3,17 or 20, react with certain reagents for carbonyl groups, a fact which should *a priori* lead us to believe in the possibility of the histochemical detection of most of the steroid hormones of mammals. The use of reactions involving phenylhydrazines and 2-hydroxy-3-naphthoic hydrazine has indeed led a certain number of investigators to claim that the positive results obtained after fixation in the principal steroid-secreting endocrine glands of mammals do in fact demonstrate the presence of ketosteroids. Dempsey and his collaborators (1946-1949) do indeed attach the greatest importance, from this point of view, to the positive results of a group of tests (the battery of ketosteroid reactions) which include the uptake of Sudan dyes, solubility in acetone, optical anisotropy, primary fluorescence, the positive result of Liebermann's reaction, the positive colour reaction using Schiff's reagent and finally the positive result of the reaction with dinitrophenylhydrazine.

The essential source of error in this work rests in the fact that they in no way take account of the possibility that during fixation aldehydes will appear whose occurrence would explain the positive results of tests designed to detect carbonyl groups in just as convincing a manner as was found with the ketosteroids; we ought to remember in particular that these latter compounds do not give a positive reaction with Schiff's reagent, whereas a recolouration of this reagent corresponds rigorously to all the positive results obtained with substituted hydrazines.

The debate which we have just mentioned is now closed; we know from the detailed work of Albert and Leblond (1946, 1947, 1949), Claesson and Hillarp (1947) and of Karnovsky and Deane (1955) that certain elements of the "battery of reactions" intended to reveal ketosteroids can be found in sections taken from fresh material, whereas others appear only after fixation in formalin, which suffices to prove that the groups of reactions in question reveal different compounds. On the other hand, the chemical and histochemical study demonstrates the primary nature of all the carbonyl groups shown up by reactions which are said to reveal ketosteroids in the endocrine glands of mammals, a fact which definitively settles the question. All modern authors agree that the ketosteroids formed in the endocrine glands of vertebrates cannot be detected through the demonstration of their carbonyl groups; as Lison has noted (1960, p. 518), the concentrations of these hormones in the tissues which secrete them are such that it would be imprudent to count on their histochemical detection by any procedure whatever.

For the record, we may remark upon one consequence of the formation of aldehyde groups by the oxidation of unsaturated lipids, namely the possibility of staining the sites of these compounds with paraldehyde-fuchsin. We know, in fact, from the work of Holczinger (1957) that paraldehyde-fuchsin, applied after permanganate oxidation in an acid medium, intensely stains the regions of the adrenal cortex which are rich in lipids when the sections oxidised in potassium permanganate are decolorised using a solution of sodium bisulphite, whereas the result of the same staining reaction is entirely negative if the sections are bleached in oxalic acid. According to Holczinger, the explanation for this phenomenon, whose practical importance is but slight, lies in the formation of addition compounds of the aldehydes in the tissue with the sodim bisulphite, these compounds which carry the $-SO_3Na$ groups having an affinity for paraldehyde-fuchsin.

DEMONSTRATION OF THE CARBOHYDRATE CONSTITUENTS OF CERTAIN LIPIDS

Certain lipids, whose accumulation in the nervous tissue is characteristic of inherited diseases and which belong to the sphingolipid group (gangliosides, cerebrosides) contain sugars whose histochemical detection was attempted by Diezel (1954); in the course of his histopathological studies, this author used a variant of the method for detecting pentoses put forward by Roe and Rice (1948). The three techniques, of which I have no personal experience, are described below, following to the letter the data given by Diezel (1954).

The Molisch reaction:

Fix in formalin, or use frozen or paraffin wax sections according to the solubility of the lipids studied; the frozen sections are stuck to slides and dried, the paraffin wax sections dewaxed and dried;
Cover the sections with several drops of the mixture
    a 5% alcoholic solution of α-naphthol .... 0.5 ml
    2 N sulphuric acid .... 10 ml
    teepol .... 1 drop
do not add the coverslip but keep in an oven at 90°C for about 12 minutes;
Cover with a coverslip and examine immediately under the microscope.

The positive result of this reaction is a violet red colour which changes to grey in about 1 hour. As Pearse (1960) has noted, the effects of this treatment on the tissue are not as disastrous as one might have thought.

Brückner's reaction:

Fix in formalin, or cut frozen or paraffin wax sections, preparing the sections as for the Molisch reaction;
Cover the dried sections with several drops of the mixture
    a 2% aqueous solution of orcinol
    (3,5-dihydroxytoluene) .... 1 ml
    2 N sulphuric acid .... 10 ml
do not add a coverslip but place in an oven at 90°C for from 5 to 10 minutes;
Add the coverslip and examine immediately.

A red or bluish red colour which fades rather rapidly constitutes a positive result for this reaction.

Roe and Rice's reaction:

Fix in formalin, and prepare paraffin wax or frozen sections as for the Brückner reaction;
Immerse the slides for from 5 to 10 minutes, at 70–80°C, in a mixture prepared in the following way;

Saturate 100 ml of acetic acid with approximately 4 g of thio-urea; allow the excess solid to settle and remove it by decanting; add 2 g of bromo-aniline; keep out of light; the solution keeps for about a week;
Cover with a coverslip and examine under the microscope.

A rather fugitive red colour constitutes a positive result for this reaction.

DEMONSTRATION OF THE STEROL RADICAL

The biological importance of steroids is too well known to need mention here, but the possibilities for their histochemical detection are rather limited. Apart from the general characteristics already mentioned (staining by lysochromes at temperatures above the point of fusion, optical anisotropy of the same type as spherocrystals between the melting point and the clearing point) histochemical reactions of proven value exist only for the sterides (cholesterol and its esters, derivatives of vitamin D, etc...). A technique for demonstrating the steroid hormones, based on the oxidation, in the keto-aldehydes, of the α-keto group of the lateral chain characteristic of corticosteroids, has been described by Khanolkar and his co-workers (1958). This technique involves the preparation of frozen sections taken from fresh material, blocking the free aldehydes with aniline, oxidation using ferric chloride followed by washing in distilled water, and then the demonstration of the primary carbonyl groups using Schiff's reagent. Only those sites where corticosteroids are to be found will appear in a magenta red, the sex hormones and the cholesterol do not react. I have no personal experience of the method in question, whose theoretical specificity is considered by Pearse (1960) as being great.

The techniques for showing up cholesterol and its esters stem from two methods widely used in analytical chemistry, namely Liebermann's reaction using acetic anhydride-sulphuric acid and the Windaus reaction using digitonine.

The Liebermann—Burchard reaction is, in principle, applicable to work using sections and the first two editions of Lison's work (1936, 1953) give prominence to a technique which consists of covering the frozen sections, mounted on slides, with a mixture of equal parts of acetic anhydride and sulphuric acid and then placing a coverslip on the preparation which is observed immediately under the microscope. The greenish tint characteristic of a positive result does indeed appear but the solubility of cholesterol in the reagent explains the rapidity with which the colour diffuses, a rapidity such that even the taking of a photographic record of the preparation is frequently impossible. It is thus a microchemical reaction which does not meet the morphological needs of a histochemical technique; it demonstrates the presence in the section of cholesterol or of its esters without permitting us to study its localisation on the scale either of the organelle or of the cell.

The method of Schultz (1924) depends on the chemical data obtained by Lipschütz (1916); it consists of the transformation of cholesterol into oxycholesterol, either by exposing the section to bright light for from 3 to 4 days, or by treating it for from 2 to 3 days with a solution of iron alum; under such conditions the addition of a mixture of equal parts of acetic acid and concentrated sulphuric acid results in a green colour which is less fugitive than that given by the Liebermann—Burchard reaction. According to Reiner (1953), this reaction is only given by 7-hydroxycholesterol and by those steroids which are capable of being converted by oxidation into this substance, namely cholesterol and its esters, ergosterol and 7-dehydrocholesterol, but this greater specificity goes together with a lower sensitivity than that of the Liebermann—Burchard method.

In my opinion the best of the variations on Schultz's method is that due to Everett in which the tedious oxidation of iron alum is replaced by treatment of the sections using a concentrated solution of ferric chloride which allows us to reduce the duration of oxidation to several minutes.

Schultz's reaction (Everett's variation, 1945):

Frozen sections coming from fresh material or from material treated with formalin for a short period, the sections adhering to slides;
Treat for about 12 minutes with a 20% aqueous solution of ferric chloride;
Wash for 1 minute in water which is either running or frequently renewed;
Wipe the slide around the section and blot with absorbent paper;
Cover with several drops of a mixture of equal parts of acetic acid and concentrated sulphuric acid (the mixture keeps for several weeks);
Place a coverslip in position and examine immediately under the microscope.

The blue colour of structures containing cholesterol or esters of this compound changes progressively towards green; it is this change which is characteristic; the preparations will not keep for more than a few hours.

Other variations of Schultz's method do not, in my opinion, have any advantage over that which has just been described.

Adams' technique (Adams, 1951) which gives more intense stains than does Schultz's method gives positive results only with 3-hydroxy-Δ^5 (or $\Delta^{5,7}$) steroids and their esters; its specificity is illustrated by tests using models and by controls using extraction techniques but the chemical mechanism is still unknown.

Adams' reaction (1961):

Frozen sections coming from material fixed in calcium-formaldehyde, mounted on slides and dried;
Cover with several drops of a 0.1% solution of 1,2-napthoquinone-4-sulphonic acid in the mixture

> absolute alcohol .... 2 volumes
> 60% perchloric acid (handle with
>   great care) .... 1 volume
> commercial formalin .... 0.1 volumes
> distilled water .... 0.9 volumes
>
> Place the slide on a hot-plate or on the top of a metallic embedding oven for from 5 to 10 minutes; the colour which is red at the beginning changes towards deep blue;
>
> Discard the excess reagent, cover with several drops of perchloric acid, place a coverslip in position and examine under the microscope. These preparations cannot be mounted either in water or in the usual media miscible with water.

The intense blue colour of the sites of the sterols will last for several hours and change steadily towards a blackish grey.

The digitonin reaction, which is an adaptation of Windaus' technique, is extremely sensitive but shows up only the α-hydroxysterols and not their esters; among the variations of this method the most practically useful one is that of Lison (1936).

The digitonin reaction (Lison's variation):

> Frozen sections taken from material fixed in formalin or in calcium-formaldehyde, mounted on slides or free;
> Treat for several hours with a 0.5% digitonin solution in 50% alcohol;
> Rinse carefully in 50% alcohol;
> Wash in distilled water;
> Stain the background, where appropriate, or show up the fats using a lysochrome;
> Wash in water and mount in a medium miscible with water.

When this technique has a positive result crystals are formed in very characteristic needles or rosettes; the demonstration of these crystals is greatly facilitated by examination under polarised light. Staining the background using a lysochrome, as first advocated by Leulier and Revel (1930), is of considerable practical advantage; in fact, the birefringence of the cholesterol esters which do not form a complex with digitonin is greatly weakened or suppressed and these compounds take up the lysochrome, whereas the cholesterol-digitonin complex does not take up the stain and keeps its birefringence.

HISTOCHEMICAL CHARACTERISTICS OF THE PRINCIPAL CATEGORIES OF LIPIDS

The observations set out in the paragraph above, in particular the frequency with which mixtures of various lipids exist in one and the same structure, account for the difficulties with which the histochemical identification of these compounds is confronted. However, it seems to me to be useful to summarize the distinctive characteristics of the principal categories of lipids.

1° Glycerides

The glycerides are easily extracted by most organic solvents acting in the cold, in particular by ethanol and methanol, ether, chloroform and acetone. On sections of tissue the glycerides show up as isotropic droplets if the temperature is above their fusion point, or in the form of crystals if the temperature is less than their fusion point or if crystallization has taken place following fixation; in the solid condition, they are endowed with an optical anisotropy of the crystalline type with four extinction positions and with no polarisation cross. They are easily stained with all lysochromes provided that one works at a temperature above the fusion point. Potassium bichromate does not render the glycerides insoluble so that tests for them using the Smith–Dietrich method and its variations are negative. The deposits of glycerides in the animal body, such deposits being acid or neutral according to the presence or absence of free fatty acids, stain blue or pink by Lorrain–Smith's technique; this latter colour is virtually characteristic of "neutral fats" (triglycerides). Glycerides which are rich in oleic acid give rise to an intense primary blackening under the influence of osmium tetroxide; glycerides which are rich in palmitic or stearic acids undergo secondary blackening during the treatment of pieces of tissue with ethyl alcohol; the osmic blackening goes hand in hand with an insolubilisation which is generally sufficient to allow the material to be embedded in paraffin wax.

2° The phosphatide esters

The phosphatide esters are insoluble in cold acetone if they are pure; when mixed with other lipids, they may be carried off whilst such substances are passing into solution. They are endowed with a birefringence of the crystalline type when in the solid condition, and they show up as spherocrystals and exhibit the black cross at temperatures between the point of fusion and that of clearing, above which they become isotropic. They can be stained above the point of fusion by all lysochromes and are rendered insoluble by potassium bichromate and in this way they may be detected using Smith–Dietrich's technique and its variations. Even when rendered insoluble by potassium bichromate, their ability to dissolve lysochromes is not changed, and so such substances can demonstrate phosphatide esters on paraffin wax sections. They give rise to the phenomenon of secondary osmic blackening provided that the pieces of tissue do not contain potassium bichromate. The cupric phthalocyanins of the luxol fast blue group stain the phosphatide esters on paraffin wax sections. They are the "acid" lipids which are stained blue using Lorrain–Smith's technique and are chromotropic.

3° *Plasmalogens*

The plasmalogens are endowed with all the characteristics of the phosphatide esters which have just been mentioned, but are distinguished from all other lipids by the fact that they alone give the plasmal reaction; the various stages and conditions of this reaction, which have been set out in a preceding section, must be rigorously respected for the results to have any diagnostic value.

4° *Sphingolipids*

The sphingolipids, which only exist to a substantial extent in nervous tissue, are insoluble in cold acetone when they are pure; sulphuric ether extracts them at its boiling point. When they are liquid they can be stained with lysochromes and their birefringence has the same characteristics as has that of the phosphatide esters; the same remark is true, so far as their behaviour towards osmium tetroxide is concerned, and in respect of the action of potassium bichromate in rendering them insoluble. Like the phosphatide esters, the sphingolipids are "acid" and chromotropic. The presence of monosaccharides in the molecule explains the PAS activity which is clear after periodic oxidation of short duration for some of these compounds, whereas prolonged oxidation is necessary for others (Wolman, 1952, 1956, 1965). The reactions for carbohydrates mentioned in an earlier section (the reactions of Molisch, of Bruckner, and of Roe and Rice) give positive results.

5° *Steroids*

Steroids are easily extracted even by cold acetone; their examination under polarised light discloses characteristics identical with those of the phosphatide esters (crystalline birefringence in the solid state, spherocrystalline with a polarisation cross between the fusion point and the clearing point, optical isotrophy above this latter temperature). The steroids, which are shown up by all lysochromes when in the liquid condition, blacken in contact with osmium tetroxide; this blackening, unlike that of the phosphatide esters, is particularly marked when the medium contains potassium bichromate. Steroids which are "neutral" lipids are not rendered insoluble by potassium bichromate; Nile blue sulphate stains them pink and they are not chromotropic. They give the reactions of the sterol nucleus described in the preceding paragraph; other less widespread techniques have been suggested for their identification in sections (the method of Okamoto and his co-workers, 1944, using a mixed solution of iodides and iodates and sulphuric acid, and the method of Grundland and his co-workers, 1949, using bismuth trichloride).

Attempts to detect *vitamin D* (calciferol) and ergosterol (Seeger, 1939, 1940, 1942) have not given conclusive results.

6° Carotenoids

The carotenoids are isoprene derivatives which are grouped with the lipids because of their solubility characteristics. They are relatively soluble in cold alcohol and are very soluble in most other organic solvents. Their well known natural colour readily disappears under the action of even the less energetic oxidising agents. Their identification in sections depends on the one hand on the appearance of a violet blue or green colour with strong acids and on the other upon the violet colour which treatment by means of Lugol's solution confers on them. The classic reaction of Carr and Price, using antimony trichloride in chloroform solution, cannot be applied under the conditions of histochemical work since the carotenoids are very soluble in this latter medium. One property of the carotenoids, which has been put to the most fruitful use from the histochemical standpoint, is the primary green fluorescence of these compounds, which is relatively stable.

Vitamin A, which is a derivative of β-carotene, has the characteristics which have just been specified but it differs from other carotenoids by the very fugitive nature of its fluorescence; this peculiarity has been put to good use in Popper's (1944) histochemical studies.

Rhodopsin (retinin purple) is a chromoprotein whose prosthetic group is a carotenoid chemically related to vitamin A. Detection of the sites of this compound on paraffin wax sections is possible because it forms an insoluble precipitate with platinum trichloride in the compounds used in current histological technique (Stern, 1905); but the optical quality of the preparations so obtained leaves much to be desired so that various attempts have been made to stain them; the most recent and the best of these methods is due to Karli (1956) whose working technique follows below.

Demonstration of rhodopsin using Karli's technique:

The eye should be kept in darkness for 24 hours, and should be dissected in a feeble red light, and it should then be fixed using the mixture

commercial formalin (neutralized) .... 1 volume
a 2.5% solution of platinum
trichloride .... 4 volumes

the fixation, of 24 hours duration, should take place out of daylight;
Embed in paraffin wax with no particular precautions, section and cause the sections to adhere to the slide using the customary techniques;

Dewax the sections and hydrate them;
Stain the nuclei using haemalum, taking care to avoid over-staining;
Wash in running water (from 2 to 5 minutes);
Rinse in 60% alcohol;
Stain for 5 minutes in the solution
    60% alcohol .... 100 ml
    light blue (Lyon blue, spirit blue) .... 0.5 g
Rinse rapidly in tap water;
Differentiate using the mixture
    60% alcohol .... 2 volumes
    dioxane .... 1 volume
    agitating the slides, inspecting them under the microscope so as to lay bare the whole background of the preparation, only the external parts of the rods should remain strongly stained blue;
Dehydrate using 2 baths each of 1 to 2 minutes of pure dioxane;
Mount directly in Canada balsam.

Karli (1956) briefly mentions the possibility of replacing the very expensive material, platinum trichloride, with a 5% solution of potassium alum.

The demonstration of the external part of the retinal rods using this method is excellent, and the histophysiological data, as well as tests employing extraction techniques, indicate the reality of the relationship between this result and the presence of retinal purple, but the chemical mechanism of this colouration has not yet been elucidated although Vilter (1957) has attempted an analysis.

7° *Chromolipoids*

The chromolipoids do not constitute a category of compounds defined by common chemical characteristics. Most histologists, in conformity with the classical studies of Hueck (1912) and of Ciaccio (1915), subsume under this heading substances endowed with natural colours and derived from the oxidation of lipids. Difficulties associated with their extraction explain the virtually total lack of chemical data concerning the chromolipoids, compounds which are known under very various names (haemofuscin, lipofuscins, ceroids, wear and tear pigments, waste pigments, *Abnützungs-pigmente*, *pigmento di usura*, *pigments d'usure* and lipopigments). It would be most helpful if the term "lipochrome" were to be abandoned as it generates confusion, some authors also using it to indicate the carotenoids.

Despite the rarity and imprecision of the chemical data, the chromolipoids are of far from negligible histochemical interest since they are one of the main groups of endogeneous pigments and since a misunderstanding of their special characteristics can lead to serious interpretative errors.

One of their main characteristics is insolubility in lipid solvents; from the practical point of view this means that the compounds in question are generally available for study on paraffin wax sections and that they usually withstand methods of extraction which suffice to deprive the sections of all other lipid compounds.

The natural colour of the chromolipoids runs from a clear yellow to deep brown, practically black; these compounds are endowed with a yellow or brownish primary fluorescence. They are insoluble in water, in acids and alkalis, and generally withstand extraction by alcohol, benzene, or even ether, chloroform, or pyridine, they become stained using lysochromes and take up the basic dyes, this basophilia often being acid resistant which according to Berg (1951) suggests the presence of carboxyl groups. For the demonstration of this acid resistance most modern authors use the classic stain of Ziehl-Neelsen.

Ziehl-Neelsen's stain:

Paraffin wax sections, dewaxed, and where appropriate treated with collodion and hydrated;
Stain for 3 hours, at 60°C, in a closed vessel, using Ziehl's phenolic fuchsin (p. 202);
Wash for 1 to 2 minutes in running water;
Differentiate until all excessive fuchsin has been removed, where necessary making observations from time to time under the microscope, using the mixture
absolute alcohol .... 99 ml
concentrated hydrochloric acid .... 1 ml
in the case of vertebrate tissues, the differentiation should be taken to the point where the erythrocytes are a pale pink colour;
Wash for 1 to 2 minutes in running water;
Stain the nuclei with haemalum or with a 0.2% aqueous solution of toluidine blue;
Wash in tap water;
Dehydrate in absolute alcohol, clear in a benzenoid hydrocarbon and mount in a synthetic resin or in Canada balsam.

The structures which withstand acid treatment, particularly those which contain chromolipoids, are stained an intense red.

Amongst the other histochemical characteristics of the chromolipoids, one of the most important is the resistance of the natural colour to most oxidising agents; here is an important means of distinction from the melanins, pigments whose chemical nature is quite different but whose colour can be very close to that of the chromolipoids. Potassium permanganate, performic or peracetic acids, or hydrogen peroxide are the most frequently used of these "bleaching" agents. Hueck's (1912) technique depends on decolorisation using hydrogen peroxide, a technique which is very useful for the distinction between chromolipoids and melanins.

Hueck's technique for distinguishing between chromolipoids and melanins:

Paraffin wax sections, dewaxed, treated with collodion, and hydrated;
Stain for 30 minutes with a saturated aqueous solution of Nile blue sulphate;
Rinse in distilled water;

Treat for from 12 to 24 hours using a 3–10% (10 to 30 volumes) solution of hydrogen peroxide;
Wash in tap water;
Mount in a medium miscible with water.

The chromolipoids, which are "acid" lipids, are stained blue, the melanins are decolourised by treatment with hydrogen peroxide.

The reducing power of the chromolipoids is more or less intense according to the circumstances; in this context, they give positive results with the ferric ferricyanide reaction and, rather less clearly, with the argentaffin reaction. These methods should be put into practice according to the instructions given in Chapter 13. The fixation of halogens (bromine or iodine), when used according to the instructions given in relation to the study of unsaturated lipids, abolishes the reducing characteristic of the chromolipoids.

We know from a number of studies that the chromolipoids are PAS positive (see Clara, 1965, for a summary of the principal investigations); this reactivity is not due to the carbohydrate constituents but to the presence of unsaturated fatty acids. The same chemical feature explains the positive results of methods which employ performic or peracetic acid followed by the application of Schiff's reagent; the employment of these reactions has been described in relation to the demonstration of unsaturated lipids.

The chromolipoids themselves do not give the reactions of ionic iron, but ferruginous pigments may coexist with them thus rendering the interpretation of the results obtained in such instances very difficult.

The places where chromolipoids are to be found are often the seat of various enzymatic activities (carboxylic esterases, acid phosphatases, proteases).

Among the characteristics which enable us to distinguish chromolipoids from carotenoids the most important are the lower solubility of the first mentioned compounds, the absence of staining with iodine, and the blue stain with concentrated sulphuric acid.

We must, at this point, firmly insist on the schematic nature of the description of the histochemical characteristics of chromolipoids which has just been given. In fact, differences which are as important as they are difficult to interpret in the present state of our knowledge exist from one compound to the other. In conformity with the very tempting hypothesis of Pearse (1953, 1960) such differences would be associated with the various stages of a continuous evolution running from the scarcely oxidised chromolipoids up to those in which the degree of oxidation is very great. The colour of the substances, their resistance to extraction using lipid solvents, and their basophilia increase with the degree of oxidation. On the other hand, the sudanophilia becomes weaker while the reducing capacity increases; a clear activity under the technical conditions of the performic acid-Schiff technique exists only after a certain degree of oxidation has been attained and disappears in highly oxidised chromolipoids; the same is true for the primary fluorescence.

The principal types of chromolipoids, whose identification is particularly due to the histopathologists, are ceroid pigment, lipofuscins and haemofuscin.

Ceroid pigment, described for the first time by Lillie and his coworkers (1941), was noticed during dietary cirrhosis of the rat, and during experimental avitaminosis E, and in certain anaemic conditions.

This pigment is insoluble in most organic solvents and very resistant to acids and alkalis (to the latter compounds when cold) and is characterised by a greenish yellow fluorescence which slowly turns white and is suppressed by chromic oxidation or permanganate oxidation of the sections. All the usual lysochromes stain it on sections, whether frozen or in paraffin wax; Lorrain-Smith's technique confers on it sometimes a blue colour and sometimes a purple colour. It blackens under the influence of osmium tetroxide solutions and gives the argentaffin reaction weakly; the reaction to ferric ferricyanide is sometimes negative, sometimes positive. Tests for metallic iron in the globules of ceroid pigment most frequently give negative results but the opposite eventuality is possible.

Periodic, performic and peracetic oxidation result in the appearance of aldehyde groups which can be detected using Schiff's reagent; acetylation suppresses the PAS activity but not that of the Schiff-peracetic acid technique. The basophilia of the ceroid pigment disappears after benzoylation. The resistance to acids is very marked; staining using Ziehl's fuchsin persists even after two days of extraction in alcohol acidified with hydrochloric acid.

The lipofuscins, like the ceroid pigment, are endowed with a great resistance to extraction by organic solvents. They stain with lysochromes applied to paraffin wax sections, but the colour is often less intense than that of the ceroid pigment; the basophilia is often intense and acid resistant and the reducing capacity strong under the technical circumstances of the ferric ferricyanide reaction, but less so under the conditions of the argentaffin reaction. Osmic blackening and the activity of these compounds towards performic or peracetic acid-Schiff indicates that double bonds are present. Staining with Nile blue confers a blue colour on them. Methylation (6 hours at 60°C in a 0.1 molar hydrochloric acid solution in methanol) suppresses the basophilia whilst preserving the capacity for lysochrome staining and causes the tint produced by Lorrain-Smith's technique to turn pink.

Clear differences of dye affinities and of histochemical characteristics show us that the lipofuscins described in various organs represent not a single compound but a class of compounds; such differences are probably to be interpreted in the spirit of Pearse's hypothesis mentioned above.

Haemofuscin, a chromolipoid which exists mainly in the liver and spleen of patients suffering from haemochromatasia, has been distinguished from haemosiderin by v. Recklinghausen (1889). It is a pigment which can be stained by lysochromes on frozen sections but not on paraffin wax sections, and it has no resistance to acids. A technique for demonstrating this pigment, due to Mallory, comprises fixation in Zenker's fluid followed by embedding in paraffin wax; the sections are dewaxed and taken into water where they undergo nuclear staining using a progressive lake of haematoxylin and then staining for from 5 to 20 minutes in a 0.5% solution of basic fuchsin in a mixture of equal parts of distilled water and of 95% alcohol. The excess stain is extracted by differentiation in 95% alcohol (*not acidified*), the sections being thereafter dehydrated, cleared and mounted in Canada balsam or in a synthetic resin. Haemofuscin then appears intensely red, whereas the melanins and haemosiderin keep their natural colour.

DICHOTOMOUS KEYS FOR THE ANALYSIS OF LIPIDS

Lison's works (1936, 1953, 1960) include a dichotomous table for the analysis of lipids on sections; a more complete dichotomous key was published in Cain's review (1950); the two are reproduced here.

These dichotomous tables which cover most of the situations which the histochemist may encounter during studies of animal tissue may be of great service so long as the prescribed operations are carried out in the order indicated.

Dichotomous key for the histochemical identification of lipids
(CAIN, 1950)

Stage	After		See
1	—	Frozen sections of fresh tissue or fixed for less than 6 hours in formol-calcium; presence of crystals, droplets or bi-refringent granules	3
2	1	Idem. Absence of bi-refringent structures	7
3	1	Stain with Sudan Black B; substances stained (liquid lipids, fats)	11
4	3	Idem. Substances unstained (solid lipids or non-lipid bodies)	5
5	4	Extraction by various lipid solvents; objects dissolved (solid lipids)	9
6	5	Idem. Objects not dissolved NON LIPID STRUCTURES.	
7	2	Stained with Sudan Black B; diffuse staining	33
8	7	Idem. No staining ABSENCE OF DETECTABLE LIPIDS AFTER FIXATION WITH FORMOL-CALCIUM.	
9	5	Natural colouration of inclusions (solid carotenoids)	13
10	9	Absence of natural colour	19
11	3	Lipids with a natural colour	13

Stage	After		See
12	11	Lipids lacking a natural colour	15
13	11	Stained blue or blue-grey, fleetingly, with concentrated H_2SO_4; stained grey or blackish with Lugol's solution; stained blue fleetingly, with a chloroform solution of antimony trichloride; easy removal of natural colour by oxidation. CAROTENOIDS.	
14	13	Idem. Negative tests; stained red or not coloured with concentrated H_2SO_4; stained blue with Nile Blue. CHROMOLIPOIDS.	
15	12	Stained red with 1% Nile Blue. PRESENCE OF NEUTRAL LIPIDS	19
16	15	Stained blue with 1% Nile Blue. Acid lipids with or without neutral lipids	17
17	16	Stained weakly with Nile Blue (Probable presence of lipids)	19
18	17	Intense staining with Nile Blue. (Probable presence of fatty acids)	19
19	10 17 18	Positive Schultze reaction to acetic acid- sulphuric acid mixture, without previous oxidation; presence of PRODUCTS OF OXIDATION OF STEROIDS	31
20	19	Negative Schultze reaction to acetic acid -sulphuric acid mixture	21
21	20	Positive Schultze reaction to acetic acid and anhydride; presence of CHOLESTERYL GROUPINGS	23
22	21	Negative Schultze reaction	27
23	21	Positive reaction to digitonin; presence of BETAHYDROXYL STEROLS NOTABLY CHOLESTEROL.	
24	23	Negative reaction to digitonin; PROBABLE PRESENCE OF ESTERS OF STEROLS	25
25	23 24	Stained fairly stable blue with trichloracetic acid 24 (ERGOSTEROL)	31
26	25	Not stained or stained other than blue with trichloracetic acid	31
27	22	Presence of spherocrystals (probable existence of PHOSPHO- OR SPHINGO-LIPIDS)	29
28	27	Absence of spherocrystals	31
29	27	Positive reaction to acid haematin; presence of PHOSPHOLIPIDS.	
30	29	Negative reaction to acid haematin; presence of STEROLS *not detectable by the Schultze reaction* or of GALACTOLIPIDS.	
31	28	Positive reaction to acid haematein; presence of PHOSPHOLIPIDS.	
32	31	Negative reaction to acid haematein; presence of TRIGLYCERIDES WITH OR WITHOUT OTHER LIPIDS.	
33	7	Lipoids with a natural colour; consider firstly CAROTENOIDS and other chromolipoids	13
34	33	Absence of natural colour	19

Table of histochemical analysis of lipids
(LISON, 1953)

I. — Stain a frozen section, either fresh or fixed for a short time in formol calcium, with Sudan Black B.
   (*a*) Object stained blue black
      (lipid in liquid state) 11
   (*b*) Object not stained; restain at 50–60°C
     — object stained (solid lipid) 11
     — object not stained
        NO LIPID DETECTABLE WITHOUT UNMASKING

II. — Examine microscopically an unstained section, mounted in laevulose syrup.
   (+) The lipids detected by (I) have a natural colour (yellow, orange or brown).
      — Stained blackish green or brown with Lugol's iodine; decolourised slowly with chromic acid.
          CAROTENOIDS

      — These reactions are negative; stained red in certain cases by the action of sulphuric acid.
          CHROMOLIPOIDS

(+) The lipids detected in (I) without a natural colour
*— Positive Liebermann reaction
— positive digitonine reaction.
FREE CHOLESTEROL

— negative digitonine reaction.
CHOLESTERIDES

*— Negative Liebermann reaction
— An unstained section, mounted in levulose syrup, examined by polarised light, shows that the objects illuminated give a polarisation cross.
PHOSPHO- OR SPHINGOLIPIDS

— Objects not illuminated in these conditions or without giving a polarisation cross. Positive Smith-Dietrich x-reaction.

PHOSPHO- OR SPHINGOLIPIDS

Negative Smith-Dietrich x-reaction.
— Stained pink with Nile Blue.
SATURATED GLYCERIDES

— Stained blue or not stained with Nile Blue.
NON-SATURATED GLYCERIDES, PHOSPHO-OR SPHINGOLIPIDS, FATTY ACIDS —

CHAPTER 19

THE HISTOCHEMICAL DETECTION OF AMINO-ACIDS AND PROTEINS

The histochemical study of proteins is of particular consequence because it deals with substances which are virtually ubiquitous in the animal cell.

In the course of a histochemical study of carbohydrates, or that of fats, many examples arise of organelles or of products of cellular activity which are entirely devoid of some compound or other belonging to one of these two groups. This is in no way the case with proteins. Good methods for the histochemical demonstration of these compounds afford preparations in which "everything is stained"; only the different shades and intensities of the stain obtained allow us to differentiate the various cell organelles; only a few secretory products or stored materials are entirely devoid of histochemically detectable proteins. In consequence the preparations given by a histochemical study of proteins are not all that informative and the problem consists, not in testing for the presence of these compounds, but of their special accumulation in certain structures.

The rather deceptive nature of the histochemical study of proteins in general was well brought to light by Lison (1960, p. 306) who considered it as one of the factors which served to explain the small number of publications devoted to this aspect of histochemistry. As for the second factor invoked by Lison, that is, "fashion", the tendency to concentrate all efforts on the demonstration of enzymatic activity has grown, since 1960, to wholly unforeseeable proportions. As a result the amount of progress we have to report in terms of the histochemistry of proteins during the last dozen years or so is not very great.

Histochemical techniques applicable to the study of proteins in general aim either at demonstrating the peptide link, or at characterising the lateral or terminal active groups of amino-acids, or, lastly, at showing up the special electropolar nature of these compounds. The selective demonstration of certain amino-acids or the demonstration of characteristic electropolar features may result in the identification of certain types of proteins; results of the same general nature can be obtained by enzymatic digestion using sufficiently purified preparations, by extracting with chemical substances, or, in a still more elegant way, using the immuno-histochemical techniques already mentioned in the chapter devoted to histophysical methods.

THE FIXATION OF PROTEINS

The problems of a general nature which are posed by the histochemical fixation of proteins are confounded in practice with those of histological fixation in general; it is indeed true that the latter is secured fundamentally through the denaturation of tissue proteins. Moreover, the problems in question have already been discussed in the first part of this work as part of a general conspectus of histological fixation. Only what is, strictly speaking, the histochemical aspects of protein fixation will be mentioned here.

If the general mechanism of protein fixation is well known (see, in particular, Wolman's 1955 review), the action of various fixatives on the lateral or terminal active groups of polypeptide chains is much less so and the practical bearing of such knowledge is evident. It is indeed true that fixation obtained through the chemical blocking of these radicals is patently unsuitable for histochemical use because it abolishes the activity of the groups in question. The ideal fixative would immobilise protein molecules without their undergoing any morphological modification whatever and, at the same time, preserve unchanged the reactions of the active groups. Such an ideal seems unrealistic. Displacements of the protein chains, blocking of active groups, the liberating of other active groups are all in fact inevitable during fixation by chemicals and it may be useful to mention that freeze drying does not constitute fixation.

As Wolman (1955) has quite rightly emphasized, the "neutral" fixatives of classical authors denature the proteins in the same way as do any other fixatives; their use is all the more strongly contra-indicated because they are poor fixatives from the morphological point of view.

In the present state of our knowledge, it is not possible to set out genuine recommendations for the fixation of proteins for histochemical purposes. Most modern authors use fixatives which have proved their worth either by their good preservation of tissue structures in general or as cytological fixatives. Formalin, and mixtures in which it plays a part, topographical fixatives based on corrosive sublimate and cytological fixatives based on potassium bichromate, are used in the majority of histochemical investigations devoted to the proteins and the general impression which one gets from reading these publications is that of a choice which is all too often decided on an empirical basis or by slavish adherence to routine.

Recent work has shown that fixatives with a glutaraldehyde base are particularly advantageous when proteins are being studied by histochemical means.

It is apparent that one cannot count on free amino-acids or low molecular weight polypeptides being preserved in their original situations during the fixation of tissues for histochemical purposes. The losses in what are, properly speaking, proteins are quite slight; they have been evaluated by Kaufmann (1949) and by Hartleib and his colleagues (1956) as not exceeding 1%.

Other stages in the preliminary handling of the sections prior to treatment do not involve any particular requirements arising out of the histochemical demonstration of proteins. Many reactions can be carried out on frozen sections; embedding in paraffin wax is more suitable in cases where vigorous fixation or treatment at high temperatures must be used. Embedding in celloidin, followed by treatment of the sections without freeing them first from the embedding material does not seem to have been employed.

It is apposite to mention the advantages of working on rather thick sections when practising certain reactions whose sensitivity is rather limited .

THE HISTOCHEMICAL REACTIONS OF PROTEINS AS SUCH

Most of the techniques used by biochemists to characterise proteins are obviously inapplicable in histochemistry; they involve drastic procedures which are incompatible with the maintenance of the integrity of the tissue to such an extent that the morphological conditions under which histochemical work may be undertaken are not respected.

However, two methods may be singled out from those whose chemical validity seems to be well established, namely the biuret reaction and that of the carboxyl-α-acylamine groups, the first being specific for peptide links, whereas the second reveals the terminal groups of polypeptide chains.

The biuret reaction, which is well known to chemists, is difficult to apply in histochemical work because of its low sensitivity and the strong alkalinity of the reagent. Most modern authors advise the use of Sols' technique (1947) and they stress the need to work with thick sections.

The reagent is prepared by adding 2 ml of glycerine to 8 ml of a 5% solution of crystalline cupric sulphate pentahydrate and then adding 400 ml of 20% sodium hydroxide; the mixture is made up to one litre with distilled water.

Working technique.

Thick paraffin wax sections, dewaxed and hydrated;
Treat for 10 minutes at laboratory temperatures with Sols' reagent either pure or diluted with equal parts of distilled water;
Rinse in distilled water;
Dehydrate in absolute alcohol, clear in a benzenoid hydrocarbon, mount in a synthetic resin or in Canada balsam.

A bluish-violet colour indicates a positive result of the reaction; although highly significant from a chemical standpoint, this method is not very sensitive and modern authors only rarely use it.

The demonstration of terminal carboxyl groups in amino-acids, which was introduced into histochemical work by Barrnett and Seligman (1958), was developed by more recent authors (Karnowsky and coworkers, 1959, 1960, 1961; Geyer, 1962, 1964). These methods play no very substantial part in modern histochemical practice relating to the proteins, a fact which is in part due to the difficulty of getting the reagents needed to carry some of them out.

Barrnett and Seligman's technique for demonstrating terminal carboxyl groups in amino-acids depends on the transformation of acylamino-carboxy-acids into acylamino-methylketones under the influence of acetic anhydride in the presence of pyridine. The secondary carbonyl group which thus appears could not be demonstrated by the Schiff reagent and experience shows that this is indeed the case; detection by means of 2-hydroxy-3 naphthoic acid hydrazide, using the azo-reaction to show up the naphthol groups, nevertheless gives intense colours and, as Lison (1960, p. 203) has commented, such an intensity is rather surprising for a method believed to reveal only the terminal carboxyl groups of protein chains. We might add that esterification of the carboxyl groups by methylation using Lillie's method (p. 421) destroys the activity, a fact which obviously does not prove that terminal carboxyl groups alone react under the experimental conditions laid down by Barrnett and Seligman. In any event, the method consists of treating the sections by a mixture of acetic anhydride and pyridine and then demonstrating the carbonyl groups which appear by using 2-hydroxy-3-naphthoic acid hydrazide, the working technique being slightly different from that used by Ashbel and Seligman (1949).

Working technique.

Paraffin wax sections, taken from material the fixative for which will for preference have had a corrosive sublimate base, dewaxed and hydrated;
Treat for one hour, at 60°C, with a mixture of equal parts of acetic anhydride and anhydrous pyridine;
Wash in absolute alcohol and then in 50% alcohol;
Treat for 2 hours with the following solution which should have been prepared in the warm

    2-hydroxy-3 naphthoic acid hydrazide .... 50 mg
    acetic anhydride .... 2.5 ml
    50% alcohol .... 47.5 ml

Wash carefully in 50% alcohol (3 baths each of 10 minutes);
Treat for 30 minutes with 0.5 N hydrochloric acid (about 4%);
Rinse in tap water eliminating all excess of hydrochloric acid by several baths of 1% sodium bicarbonate in distilled water;
Wash in distilled water;
Place the preparations in 50 ml of a mixture of equal parts of absolute alcohol and 0.05 M phosphate buffer, pH 7.6; add, with continuous stirring, 5 mg of diazotizised *o*-dianisidine, allowing it to act for about 5 minutes;
Wash in distilled water renewed several times;
Mount in a medium miscible with water or dehydrate rapidly, clear and mount in a synthetic resin.

The presence of terminal carboxyl groups is shown by stains which vary from red to blue according to the abundance of the groups; this polychromy, which may be a nuisance when various regions of the preparation need to be compared, can be avoided by using a monocoupled diazonium salt.

The contrast between the intensity of the stain on the one hand and the number of carboxyl groups terminal to protein chains on the other, has already been mentioned in relation to Barrnett and Seligman's reaction but it also occurs in methods put forward by Geyer (1962, 1964), namely the epoxyether, the hydroxamate, and the carbodiimide reactions. Moreover, this latter author agrees that the techniques in question not only reveal terminal carbonyl groups but also at least some of the lateral carboxyl groups of the protein chains.

Only the principle of these three methods is mentioned here for the sake of completeness; it so happens that two of them require substances which are not commercially available so that the histochemist finds himself obliged to ask a sufficiently conscientious and competent chemist to synthesise them. The third method involves the use of compounds whose handling requires too many precautions for one to be able to advise its use in daily histochemical practice.

The epoxyether reaction, according to Geyer (1962), can be undertaken by treating paraffin wax sections, which have been dewaxed and dried, with a 2 or 5% solution of 1-(p-biphenyl)-1-methoxyethylene oxide in xylene. The reaction takes place at boiling point in an apparatus provided with a refrigerated reflux condenser and takes 30 hours. It results in the formation of ketoesters from the carbonyl groups with the liberation of methanol. The ketoesters so formed can be detected by 2-hydroxy-3-naphthoic hydrazide, as in Barrnett and Seligman's method.

The hydroxamate technique begins with the methylation of the sections carried out either by Fisher and Lillie's method, described in relation to the histochemical detection of polysaccharides, or by treating the sections with a mixture of 100 volumes of methanol and 4 volumes of thionyl chloride (for 2 hours at 56°C). After this esterification of the carboxyl groups the preparations are treated either with an alkaline solution of hydroxylamine chlorhydrate in an aqueous medium or with a mixture of an alcoholic solution of hydroxylamine chlorhydrate and sodium ethylate in an alcoholic medium. After washing in dilute perchloric acid, and then in alcohol, the sections are ultimately treated with a solution of ferric perchlorate in water and alcohol, so that a brownish red stain appears, due to the formation of a complex salt of iron by chelation with hydroxamic acid.

The carbodiimide reaction is derived from the technique of Sheehan and Hess (1955) for the synthesis of peptides. It involves treating the sections with a mixture of 1-cyclohexyl-3-(2-morpholinyl-(4)-ethyl)-carbodiimide-p-toluolmethylsulphonate and 2-hydroxy-3-naphthoic acid hydrazide, the solvent being a mixture of tetrahydrofuran, ethyl alcohol and water. After washing, the naphthol group attached to the carboxyl radicals is revealed by coupling with the diazo salt of *o*-dianisidine.

These three reactions give preparations whose optical appearance is satisfactory, adding to the attraction of having a well established chemical mechanism; it is nevertheless true that their practical conduct involves very serious difficulties. The reagents needed for the epoxyether and carbodiimide methods do not occur in commerce and must be synthesized as required; the preparation of sodium ethylate and in particular that of ferric perchlorate required by the hydroxamate reaction, involves risks such that it seems to me to be unwise to recommend the conduct of this technique to experimenters who do not have great experience of chemical work or who do not have a well equipped chemical laboratory available.

From the theoretical point of view, we might mention that the methods just discussed in this section do not detect the carboxyl groups of hexuronic acids.

In addition to these methods and to those which demonstrate the amine groups of α-amino-acids and on this account may also be considered as being general reactions of proteins (see the following section), we ought also to give brief mention, for the sake of completeness, to techniques whose chemical value is both debateable and debated, but which play a certain role in morphological research. These are the "precipitation reactions" using the nomenclature of Gomori (1952).

These techniques depend on the fact that proteins, even when fixed, are capable of remaining attached to certain substances which, *in vitro*, precipitate them vigorously, a further stage of the process being required for the demonstration of these substances. The principal methods in this group are those of Hartig-Zacharias, which depend on the fixation of potassium ferrocyanide by proteins, and that of Salazar, which puts to good use the affinity of proteins for tannins.

The opinions of modern workers are notably divergent as to the value of the procedures in question. Some of them (Gomori, 1952) emphasize the fact that we are not dealing with purely general methods for the demonstration of proteins but they consider that such methods may be helpful in certain cases. Others (Lison, 1960) deny any chemical value to the methods and regard them as simple morphological techniques depending upon special electropolar peculiarities of the proteins. Yet others (Pearse, 1960; Lillie, 1965) pass them by in silence, which amounts to excluding them from histochemical practice.

Many authors share the view expressed by Harms (1958) that tannophilia in the sense of Salazar indicates the presence of polysaccharides rather than of proteins.

There can be no doubt that their inability to explain coherently the procedures in question, on a chemical basis, effectively prevents us from using them as histochemical reactions; we have mentioned the two methods sketched above to remind readers of their existence and because of their morphological usefulness.

The Hartig-Zacharias method:

Paraffin wax sections, dewaxed, treated where appropriate with collodion and hydrated;
Treat for 10 minutes with a 1-5% solution (the concentration is not critical) of potassium ferrocyanide in 1% hydrochloric acid (prepare immediately prior to use);
Wash in distilled water renewed several times, examine under the microscope;
Treat for about 2 minutes with a 0.5-1% solution of ferric chloride in distilled water;
Wash in distilled water several times renewed;
Where appropriate, stain the nuclei using the aluminium lake of nuclear fast red;
Dehydrate in absolute alcohol, clear in a benzenoid hydrocarbon, mount in a synthetic resin or, where necessary, in Canada balsam.

The microscopic examination after the action of the potassium ferrocyanide solution allows us to locate free iron; in addition to that, structures which have retained ferrocyanide become blue under the action of ferric chloride.

Salazar's method:

- Paraffin wax sections, dewaxed, collodion-coated and hydrated;
- Treat for 15 to 20 minutes with a 5–10% tannin solution in 10% acetic acid;
- Wash carefully in distilled water;
- Treat for about 1 minute with a 0.5% or 1% solution of ferric chloride or of iron alum;
- Wash carefully in running water;
- Where appropriate, stain the background using a red nuclear stain;
- Dehydrate in absolute alcohol, clear in a benzenoid hydrocarbon and mount in Canada balsam or in a synthetic resin.

An affinity for tannins is disclosed by an intense black stain.

THE HISTOCHEMICAL DETECTION OF THE α-AMINO-ACID GROUP

As Lison (1960, p. 189) has commented, a certain number of histochemical reactions used for the detection of amino-acids do in fact demonstrate the occurrence of primary amine groups, the carboxyl radical of the amino-acids playing no part in the reactions in question. The practical consequences of this confusion are not serious so long as the work is carried out on paraffin wax sections, the principal source of theoretically possible error being the demonstration of the occurrence of the amine groups of colamine or of serine, which are constituents of certain lipids. It is, then, to the presence of proteins that we automatically attribute the positive results of general reactions for amino-acids, reactions which are in fact due to primary amine radicals.

Such reactions may be divided into three groups, namely condensation reactions with aldehydes giving rise to the formation of azomethines (Schiff bases), the condensation reaction with dinitrofluorobenzene and reactions depending on oxidative deamination.

REACTIONS DEPENDING ON THE FORMATION OF AZOMETHINES

The three reactions discussed here depend on the same principle, namely the condensation of amine groups with a primary carbonyl group carried by a molecule the remainder of which lends itself to histochemical detection.

The terephthalic aldehyde reaction (Danielli, 1953) involves condensation with a substance bearing two aldehyde groups, one of which reacts with the amine whilst the other is detected at a later stage by one of the classical reactions for aldehyde groups, for example the Schiff reaction.

The p-aminobenzaldehyde reaction (Danielli, 1953) uses a compound bearing a carbonyl group which gives rise to a condensation with the amine groups of amino-acids, and which itself carries a primary amine group; the latter is transformed, in the second stage of the reaction, into a diazonium salt under the influence of cold nitrous acid, coupling with a phenol or a naphthol leading to the formation of a coloured azo-dyestuff.

These two reactions, of undoubted theoretical interest, do not seem to have been adopted by modern histochemists, the reason for which is doubtless the impossibility of obtaining commercially the substances necessary to carry them out.

The third method of the group, namely ***the 3-hydroxy-2-naphthaldehyde reaction*** (Weiss, Tsou and Seligman, 1954) uses a compound which is available commercially but which is very costly. Its mechanism is the same as that of the two preceding methods, the naphthol group of the 3-hydroxy-2-naphthaldehyde being detected by coupling with a diazonium salt. The working technique involves the following stages.

Paraffin wax sections, dewaxed and hydrated;
Treat for one hour at laboratory temperatures with the following solution
    3-hydroxy-2-naphthaldehyde .... 20 mg
    acetone .... 20 ml
    veronal-hydrochloric acid buffer, pH 8.5 .... 30 ml
Wash in 3 baths of distilled water, of a total duration of 15 minutes;
Treat for 2 to 5 minutes with the solution
    diazotised *o*-dianisidine .... 25 mg
    veronal-hydrochloric acid buffer, pH 7.4 .... 50 ml
    (to be prepared at the moment of use);
Wash for 5 minutes in running water;
Dehydrate rapidly in absolute alcohol, clear in a benzenoid hydrocarbon and mount in a synthetic resin.

A red or blue colour, according to the abundance of the reactive groups, indicates that the result of the method is positive; with a monocoupled diazonium salt the preparations are monochrome and a quantitative appreciation is easier.

CONDENSATION REACTION WITH DINITROFLUOROBENZENE

2,4-dinitrofluorobenzene which was introduced as a reagent for primary amines in the course of investigations into the chemical constitution of insulin (Sanger, 1945–1949) has been applied to the histochemistry of proteins by Danielli (1953). This compound gives rise to the formation of condensation products with the amine groups of amino-acids, the phenol groups of tyrosine, imidazol groups and thiols. The natural colour of the condensation products with amines is yellow, other products of the reaction being colourless. Even the yellow colour is too pale for identification purposes on tissue sections; however, one of the nitro groups may be reduced to an amine group, following the suggestion of Danielli, Bell and Loveless (1953), and then diazotised and coupled with a naphthol so that a coloured azo dyestuff is formed.

The selective demonstration of amine groups requires that thiol groups present in the section should have been subjected to a preliminary blocking with one of the agents discussed in relation to the histochemical detection of these compounds; the detection of phenol groups of tyrosine and of imidazol is assured at the same time as is that of the primary amine groups.

The critical stage of the reaction is the reduction of the nitro groups to amines; the intensity of the final stain depends on the quality of this stage of the reaction. Chromous chloride, stannous chloride and sodium hydrosulphite have been suggested (Danielli, 1953; Pearse, 1953, 1960; Burstone, 1958) but all these agents are less effective than is titanium trichloride (Tranzer and Pearse, 1964); it is the variation due to these latter authors which we recommend here.

Reaction using 2,4-dinitrofluorobenzene (Tranzer and Pearse's technique):

Paraffin wax sections taken from material *not treated with osmium* or frozen sections, the latter having been dried in air; the paraffin wax sections are dewaxed and brought into absolute alcohol;
Treat for 16 to 20 hours, at laboratory temperatures, with the solution
  2,4-dinitrofluorobenzene .... 1 g
  absolute ethanol .... 100 ml
  N sodium hydroxide .... 0.2 ml
Wash in 4 baths of 96 or 90% alcohol (3 minutes for each bath);
Rinse in distilled water;
Treat for 15 to 30 minutes, at 37°, with the solution
  15% commercial solution of titanium trichloride .... 2 ml
  sodium citrate buffer (0.5 M, pH 4.5) .... 8 ml
Rinse in the buffer;
Wash in distilled water;
Diazotise for 5 minutes at 4°C with the mixture
  a 5% solution of sodium nitrite .... 8 ml
  N sulphuric acid .... 1 ml
Wash in distilled water chilled to 4°C;
Treat for 5 minutes, at 4°C, with a saturated solution of H-acid (1-amino-8-naphthol-3, 6-disulphonic acid) in a sodium acetate-sodium veronal buffer of pH 9 to 9.4;
Wash for 3 to 5 minutes in running water;
Dehydrate in absolute alcohol, clear in a benzenoid hydrocarbon, mount in a synthetic resin or in Canada balsam.

A positive result of the reaction is disclosed by a colour which varies between reddish and purple; the optical qualities of the preparations are excellent. From the point of view of their chemical specificity it is appropriate to recall that preliminary blocking of the sulphydryl groups allows us to avoid any reaction of such functions and that the application of the method to sections which have undergone such a blockage as well as blockage of the amine groups by nitrous acid will restrict positive results to the phenol groups of tyrosine and to imidazol groups.

REACTIONS DEPENDING ON OXIDATIVE DEAMINATION

The methods in this group are derived from colour reactions long used in analytical chemistry; the earliest of these techniques, the ninhydrin reaction, dates back, in effect, to Berg (1922) and represents the application of a technique due to Ruhemann (1911) by which amino-acids, polypeptides and proteins were detected through the violet or blue colour which these compounds give with the reagent in question.

The principle of all the methods to be discussed here is the elimination of the amine-group, under the influence of the reagent, with the release of ammonia and oxidation of the CH_2 group which bears the amine radical into a carbonyl. In some of these reactions the aldehyde group may be detected by one of the procedures dealt with in Chapter 14; in others, the appearance of a colour is due to the condensation of products of oxidative deamination with the reagent itself. The ninhydrin-Schiff, alloxan-Schiff and chloramine T-Schiff reactions all belong to the first set of possibilities, whereas the ninhydrin, alloxan and o-diacetylbenzene reactions belong to the second.

Techniques which do not involve the detection of primary carbonyls are only mentioned here in a very summary way. It so happens that the ninhydrin method (Berg, 1922) and that using alloxan (Romieu, 1925) are not very sensitive and the stains which they confer on the sections are too pale to allow of detailed study. The method using o-diacetylbenzene (Voss, 1940; Wartenberg, 1956), which is excellent, gives spectacular preparations but requires the use of a reagent which is not commercially available. For the sake of completeness we give its working technique.

> Paraffin wax sections taken from material fixed in a liquid which does not contain corrosive sublimate, dewaxed and brought into water;
> Render the sections alkaline by treating them for 5 to 10 minutes with the Michaelis sodium acetate-sodium veronal buffer of pH 8 to 8.2;
> Treat the alkaline sections for 30 to 60 minutes, at laboratory temperatures, with the mixture of equal parts of 2% o-diacetylbenzene in 70% alcohol and the Michaelis buffer, pH 8 to 8.2;
> Rinse rapidly in Michaelis buffer, pH 7;
> Wash carefully in distilled water several times renewed;
> Dehydrate in absolute alcohol, clear in a benzenoid hydrocarbon, mount in a synthetic resin or in Canada balsam.

The positive result of the reaction is shown by a colour which varies from red to purple or to violet.

Tests involving extraction and blocking reactions as practised by Wartenberg (1956) show that this reaction is specific, although its chemical mechanism has, as yet, not been elucidated.

Barka and Anderson (1963) also emphasize the advantages of the method of which, unfortunately, I have no personal experience. It seems to me probable that the only real reason to explain the fact that the o-diacetylbenzene method is not cited as of right in current histochemical practice is the impossibility of obtaining commercially the reagent necessary to carry it out:

$$\underset{(a)}{R-\underset{\underset{NH_2}{|}}{\overset{\overset{H}{|}}{C}}-C\overset{O}{\underset{OH}{\diagdown}}} + \underset{(b)}{\text{ninhydrin}} \rightarrow$$

$$\underset{(c)}{R-\underset{\underset{NH}{|}}{C}-C\overset{O}{\underset{OH}{\diagdown}}} + \underset{(d)}{\text{hydrindantin}} + H_2O$$

$$\underset{(c)}{R-\underset{\underset{NH}{\|}}{C}-C\overset{O}{\underset{OH}{\diagdown}}} + H_2O \rightarrow \underset{(e)}{R-C\overset{O}{\underset{H}{\diagdown}}} + CO_2 + NH_3$$

(a) = protein with terminal α-amino-acid; (b) = ninhydrin; (c) = imino-acid formed by the oxidation of the amino-acid; (d) = hydrindantin formed by the reduction of ninhydrin: it is the reaction of this substance with ninhydrin, in alkaline media, which results in the formation of the blue substance formed in Berg's reaction; (e) = aldehyde resulting from the decomposition of the imino-acid.

The practical value of methods involving the histochemical detection of aldehyde groups formed during oxidative deamination is much greater. These techniques use as deaminating agents substances which are easy to obtain and not costly; the detection of primary carbonyl groups is obviously a practice familiar to any histochemist. Moreover, the sensitivity of the methods is great and their specificity seems to be satisfactory even though their mechanism still gives rise to discussions.

The oxidative deamination agents which we need to consider here are ninhydrin, alloxan (mesoxalylurea) and chloramine T (sodium p-toluenesulphone chloramide). Sodium hypochlorite and calcium hypochlorite have also been suggested as deaminating agents, but we know from the work of Burstone (1955, 1958) that their effectiveness is less than that of chloramine T, especially so far as calcium hypochlorite is concerned. Financial considerations are also relevant in the choice of reagent; as Lison (1960) has commented, ninhydrin is the most costly of the three compounds; it also has the disadvantage of keeping badly even in the dry state, whereas alloxan keeps well so long as it is kept cold and sheltered from the light. Chloramine T is the least costly of the three reagents.

As for the detection of aldehyde groups formed during oxidative deamination the various reagents for aldehydes used by Chou and his colleagues (1955), Burstone (1955, 1958) and Surrey (1957) give equivalent results, but none of them have practical advantages over the Schiff reagent whose adoption is therefore strongly recommended.

The ninhydrin or alloxan-Schiff reaction (Yasuma and Ishikawa, 1953):

Paraffin wax sections, dewaxed, collodion-coated where appropriate and hydrated;
Treat for 16 to 20 hours, at 37°C, with the solution

ninhydrin	0.5 g
absolute ethanol	100 ml

or

alloxan	1 g
absolute ethanol	100 ml

The solutions should be prepared as required and used only once; the alloxan used should be white; the slightest pink tint to the powder is evidence of decomposition as a result of poor storage (heat, light) so that the sample should not be used;
Wash in running water for 2 to 3 minutes;
Treat with the Schiff reagent for 30 to 60 minutes;
Rinse in sulphur dioxide water or, very vigorously, in distilled water;
Wash for 10 minutes in running water;
Stain the nuclei with Groat's haematoxylin;
Wash for 3 to 5 minutes in running water;
Dehydrate in absolute alcohol, clear in a benzenoid hydrocarbon and mount in a synthetic resin or in Canada balsam.

A positive result of the reaction is shown by a stain which varies, according to the abundance of the primary amine groups present in the structures and deaminated by the ninhydrin or by the alloxan, from pink to magenta red. In the absence of nuclear staining with Groat's haematoxylin the nuclei often exhibit a red stain due to the nucleal reaction which is produced because of the acidity of the Schiff reagent; this is of frequent occurrence when the action of the latter reagent is prolonged for one hour.

The chemical interpretation of the alloxan or the ninhydrin-Schiff methods has, as I remarked above, given rise to debate. The explanation given by the authors of the method, which would involve the action of the reagents on free amino-acids, is inapplicable, as Lillie (1965, p. 247) has commented, to amino-acids which form part of peptide linkages. Moreover, Puchtler and Sweat (1962) stress the solubility of the aldehydes formed from amino-acids taking part in rather loose chemical linkages and they consider this a further reason to doubt the chemical value of Yasuma and Ishikawa's reaction. Whilst admitting that these criticisms are well founded, Kasten (1962) considered that the method had proved its worth; Glenner (1963) lays stress on the confirmation which is derived from the abolition of the activity by deamination with nitrous acid, but he remarks that the action of ninhydrin and of alloxan is, in all probability, a simple oxidative deamination and that in consequence the technique detects any primary amine group, a fact which should prevent us from considering it as being specific for α-amino-acids.

In practical work, the ease with which the reaction is carried out, the optical qualities of the preparations and the small number of sources of error, since proteins are the principal substances which bear amine groups that one is likely to find in animal tissues, lead us to consider that Yasuma and Ishikawa's technique deserves to be maintained among the general reactions of amino-acids. Naturally, its rigorous execution necessarily involves the comparison of the section treated as described above with two control sections, one of which has been subjected only to the action of the Schiff reagent and thus shows up any free primary carbonyl groups which may be present, whereas the other is subjected to the ninhydrin or the alloxan-Schiff reactions, the amine groups having previously been acetylated or destroyed by nitrous acid. Only when the results are negative on sections which have not been deaminated and acetylated, and positive following deamination alone, can one attribute them to the presence of primary amine groups.

The chloramine-T-Schiff reaction (Chou, 1953; Burstone, 1955):

Paraffin wax sections, dewaxed, collodion-coated and hydrated;
Treat for 6 hours, at 37°C, with a 1% aqueous solution of chloramine T or with a 10% solution of a commercial preparation of sodium hypochlorite;
Rinse rapidly in distilled water;
Treat for 3 minutes with a 5% aqueous solution of sodium thiosulphate;
Rinse in distilled water;
Treat with Schiff's reagent for about 30 minutes;
Rinse in sulphur dioxide water or wash vigorously in distilled water;
Wash for 10 minutes in running water;
Stain the nuclei with Groat's haematoxylin;
Wash for 3 minutes in running water;
Dehydrate in absolute alcohol, clear in a benzenoid hydrocarbon and mount in a synthetic resin or in Canada balsam.

The results are in every respect comparable with those given by the method of Yasuma and Ishikawa; the points made above in relation to the chemical specificity of this method are also valid for the chloramine T-Schiff reaction.

Experience proves that there is no chemical reason for preferring one of these two reactions to the other; the method using alloxan-Schiff is less damaging to the sections but more expensive than that using chloramine T-Schiff.

BLOCKING REACTIONS FOR PRIMARY AMINE GROUPS

These methods are control reactions for the techniques discussed earlier; their use suppresses the activity of the primary amine groups and should thus result in negative findings when used in conjunction with the methods described in the preceding section. It is also true that preliminary blocking of primary amine groups is indispensable when it is desired to use the 2,4-dinitrofluorobenzene reaction for the selective demonstration of the phenol groups of tyrosine, and imidazol groups.

Among the various methods which organic chemistry offers, histochemists principally use deamination with nitrous acid and acetylation.

Deamination with nitrous acid is generally carried out using van Slyke's method, adapted to histochemical technique by Lillie. It consists of treating the sections, when dewaxed and brought into water, for 1 to 12 hours, at laboratory temperatures, with the following solution, prepared just prior to use:

sodium nitrite	6 g
distilled water	35 ml
crystallisable acetic acid	5 ml

The sections are then washed in distilled water and subjected to different histochemical reactions or stains.

An interesting point is that this deamination technique, in addition to suppressing completely the activity of primary amine groups, also modifies certain stain affinities of the tissue and thus illustrates the mechanism of the staining reactions in question. In this way the affinity for azo-carmine and aniline blue in Heidenhain's azan stain disappears entirely, as does the eosinophilia of erythrocytes.

The acetylation of amine groups, obtained by treatment with acetic anhydride in the presence of pyridine, results in the transformation of these groups into N-acetylamines and abolishes their activity under the experimental conditions of the methods described in the preceding section. From the chemical standpoint, this acetylation should be effected under rigorously defined conditions if we desire it to operate selectively on the amine groups. We have indeed discussed the acetylation of glycol groups, using an acetic anhydride-pyridine mixture, in relation to the histochemical detection of carbohydrates (p. 419), and other basic organic groups can be acetylated by the mixture in question acting at a high temperature. Only acetylation in the cold and at pH values which do not exceed 8 is selective for primary amine groups; the acetylation of amine groups should therefore be conducted at temperatures around 0°. Most authors, in fact, seem to consider that the concomitant acetylation of other groups, in particular of glycols, is not a nuisance when the method is used as a control in the assessment of oxidative deamination or of any condensation in which amine radicals do not play a part, to such an extent that acetylation at laboratory temperatures or even at 37° by mixtures comparable to that of McManus and Cason is generally recommended.

The experimental conditions for the saponification of N-acetylated derivatives were discussed in relation to reversible acetylation as a control reaction for the PAS method (p. 419).

The acetylation of amine groups by mixtures of acetic anhydride, acetic acid and sulphuric acid is advocated by Lillie (1964, 1965). This author recommends the following working technique.

> Paraffin wax sections, dewaxed and brought into water;
> Rinse rapidly in crystallisable acetic acid;
> Treat for 3 to 5 minutes, at laboratory temperatures, with the mixture
> acetic anhydride .... 10 ml
> crystallisable acetic acid .... 30 ml
> concentrated sulphuric acid .... 0.1 ml
> (mix well by pouring several times from one receptacle to another);
> Wash for 10 minutes in running water;
> Treat the sections, together with those which have not undergone this operation, with appropriate histochemical reactions or marker stains for the presence of basic proteins

REACTIONS FOR THE SELECTIVE DETECTION OF CERTAIN AMINO-ACIDS

In addition to general reactions, allowing us to detect the presence of amino-acids and proteins through the demonstration of carboxyl and primary amine groups, the histochemist has at his disposal techniques which permit of the detection of certain amino-acids. In this context we might mention some techniques which are particularly important from the practical point of view because they allow us to demonstrate compounds whose biological importance is substantial, namely the reactions of the guanidyl group, characteristic of arginine, and the reactions of the imidazol group, enabling us to detect histidine, and of phenol and indol groups, allowing us to discover the sites of tyrosine and tryptophane, and lastly reactions of the thiol and disulphide groups which localise protein-bound sulphydryls histochemically.

DEMONSTRATION OF THE GUANIDYL RADICAL AND OF ARGININE

Guanidine $NH=C(NH_2)_2$ is represented in most proteins by an amino-acid, arginine; the richest in it are protamines and histones. The strongly basic nature of proteins rich in arginine stems from the fact that this amino-acid is provided with two primary amine radicals. The importance of protamines and histones as constituents of nuclear proteins explains the histochemical interest attaching to the detection of arginine; all the reactions are derived from the chemical technique of Sakaguchi and, apart from arginine, the only compounds that give it are galegine, agmatine and glycocyamine, compounds which are rarely met with. In practice, a positive result for the Sakaguchi reaction allows us to affirm that arginine is present.

This reaction depends on the appearance of a red or pink colour following treatment with α-naphthol and sodium hypochlorite or hypobromite in an alkaline medium; the chemical composition of the coloured compound has not been entirely elucidated but it is known (Baker, 1947) that the reaction is only positive when one of the hydrogen atoms of the primary amine group of the guanidine is substituted by a carbon chain, one of the hydrogen atoms of the other primary amine group being capable of substitution by a methyl group, as is the hydrogen of the secondary amine group.

The practical application of Sakaguchi's reaction comes up against severe difficulties which are partly associated with the harmful effect of the reagent, which is rich in sodium hypochlorite and alkaline, on the sections and also by the discolouration of the preparations due to an excess of hypochlorite, and lastly by the instability of the colour reaction once it has been obtained, permanent preparations being unobtainable. Mere consideration of the number of variants put forward shows how unsatisfactory the method is.

Among these variants, techniques which use α-naphthol (Baker, 1947; Thomas and Liebman, 1951) tend more and more to be replaced by techniques using 8-hydroxyquinolein (oxime) (Carver, Brown and Thomas, 1953), or those using 2,4-dichlor α-naphthol (McLeish and his colleagues, 1957; Deitch, 1961).

The Sakaguchi reaction (Carver, Brown and Thomas' variation):

Paraffin wax sections, taken from material fixed in a liquid not containing corrosive sublimate, dewaxed and collodion-coated and brought into 70% alcohol;
Treat for 15 minutes, at laboratory temperatures, using a mixture consisting of a 1% solution of 8-hydroxyquinolein (oxime) in
    absolute alcohol .... 1 volume
    distilled water .... 2 volumes;
Transfer the sections rapidly into the mixture
a commercial solution of sodium hypochlorite whose chlorine
    titre is 1.6 N .... 9.4 ml
    0.1 N caustic potash .... 15 ml
    distilled water to make up to 100 ml and leave them there for 60 seconds (this time should not be exceeded);
Transfer the sections rapidly into the solution
    urea .... 15 g
    0.1 N caustic potash .... 15 ml
    butanol .... 70 ml
    distilled water to make up to .... 100 ml
and leave them there for 10 seconds;
Transfer into a new bath of alkaline urea solution and leave the sections there for 2 minutes;
Treat with 2 baths of tertiary butanol (10 seconds and 4 minutes respectively);
Treat for 3 minutes with pure aniline;
Clear rapidly in a benzenoid hydrocarbon (10 seconds);
Mount in the mixture
    "Permount" (synthetic commercial resin) .... 4 volumes
    1% aniline solution in xylene .... 1 volume
    (other synthetic resins may be used instead of Permount).

A more-or-less intense orange colour indicates that the reaction is positive; the preparations pale rather rapidly.

The Sakaguchi reaction (the variation due to McLeish and co-workers):

Paraffin wax sections (fixation in Lewitzky's fluid, recommended by these authors, is not imperative), dewaxed and brought into water;
Treat for 6 minutes at laboratory temperatures or at 25° when the experimental conditions have to be rigorously standardized, using the following mixture, to be prepared immediately prior to use

a 1% alcoholic solution of 2,4-dichlor-α-naphthol .... 1 ml
1.2% sodium hypochlorite .... 2 ml
1% soda .... 47 ml

Rinse rapidly in a 5% urea solution in distilled water;
Treat for 5 minutes with 1% soda;
Mount in the mixture

glycerine .... 9 volumes
10% soda .... 1 volume

According to the investigations of McLeish and his colleagues, fading of the preparations takes place only to the extent of 3% in the first 8 hours so that histophotometric techniques may be applied; we may also add that the duration of fixation is to a large extent responsible for preserving the activity.

The Sakaguchi reaction (variation due to Deitch):

Paraffin wax sections, dewaxed, collodion-coated and hydrated;
Wash in 2 baths of distilled water;
Treat for 10 minutes, at laboratory temperatures, with the mixture

freshly prepared 4% solution of barium hydroxide .... 25 ml
1% solution of sodium hypochlorite, freshly prepared by diluting the 5% commercial solution with 4 parts of water .. 5 ml
1.5% solution of 2,4-dichlor-α-naphthol in tertiary butyl alcohol .... 5 ml

Pass the sections through 3 baths of the mixture

tertiary butyl alcohol .... 95 volumes
tributylamine .... 5 volumes

Clear in the mixture

xylene .... 95 volumes
tributylamine .... 5 volumes

Mount in the mixture

saturated solution of cellulose caprate in xylene ...... 9 volumes
tributylamine .... 1 volume

The red colour, indicating that the reaction is positive, will keep for 1 to 2 months.

DEMONSTRATION OF THE IMIDAZOL GROUP

Modern histochemical techniques offer no reaction capable of detecting imidazol groups to the exclusion of other radicals; imidazol is primarily present in histidine. The techniques proposed depend upon iodine pretreatments intended to block the phenolic radicals of tyrosine, this stage being followed by the use of the azo-reaction. Coupling with diazonium salts is in fact capable of disclosing the presence of imidazol groupings as well as of phenols.

In practice, the method due to Landing and Hall (1956), which was considered by those authors as specific for histidine, consists of a first stage in which the phenol groups of tyrosine are blocked, the sections so treated being subjected to Danielli's coupled tetrazonium reaction, described in relation to the detection of tyrosine. Comparison with sections which have not undergone iodine blocking does indeed show that the latter process abolishes the reactivity of certain structures or considerably attenuates it, but serious reserves have been formulated as to the true significance of the blocking in question. Lillie (1957) commented that iodine is introduced into the histidine molecule as well as into that of tyrosine; Lison (1960) considers that the "blockage" with iodine does not suppress the azoreaction of tyrosine; compounds formed during the blocking reaction are not sufficiently stable totally to prevent the azoreaction.

To these remarks we should add reservations concerning the significance of the method using double coupling, used for what is, properly speaking, detection. In addition to the source of error represented by unspecific adsorption, especially by proteins, of the azo-dyestuff formed during coupling the selectivity itself of the coupled tetrazonium reaction as a method for demonstrating aromatic amino-acids (tyrosine, tryptophane, histidine) is rendered rather dubious by recent research. It is, then, solely for the sake of completeness that we mention the working technique of Landing and Hall.

Landing and Hall's demonstration of histidine:

Dewaxed sections, treated where appropriate with collodion and hydrated;
Treat for 24 hours, at laboratory temperatures, with the solution
iodine .... 1 g
potassium iodide .... 2 g
distilled water .... 300 ml
3% ammonia .... 2 ml
Wash in running water, and then in distilled water, and lastly in 96% alcohol until the yellow colour has completely disappeared (avoid at all costs destaining with sodium thiosulphite which will totally break up the blocking of the phenolic groups);
Wash in distilled water and then in Michaelis' buffer, using sodium acetate-sodium veronal, of pH 9.2;
Carry out Danielli's coupled tetrazonium reaction (p. 509) comparing the result with that given by sections which have not been blocked with iodine.

DEMONSTRATION OF TYROSINE

The very wide distribution of tyrosine in proteins, its biological importance and its presence in clearly defined amounts in histones explains the interest attaching to the demonstration of this amino-acid on sections of tissue. Some of the methods discussed in the preceding paragraphs permit of this detection; in particular we have the 2,4-dinitrofluorobenzene reaction which is positive with amine groups and with the phenolic groups of tyrosine. Other methods to be discussed here include Millon's reaction, the coupled tetrazonium reaction of Danielli (1947) and the reaction of Morel and Sisley adapted to histochemical purposes by Lillie (1957) and Glenner and Lillie (1959).

Millon's reaction

This reaction, which chemists have known since the middle of the 19th century, detects the presence of hydroxyphenyl groups; positive results can be given by any compound not substituted in the *meta* position but in practice tyrosine is the only substance to react positively. The preparation of the reagent for histochemical purposes has been set out by Bensley and Gersh (1933); it is from the formula due to these authors that all the variations employed by modern histochemists are derived. The working technique of Baker (1956) is to be recommended for its simplicity; that of Pollister and Ris (1946) has the advantage of allowing us to estimate the histone content of the tissues.

Millon's reaction (Baker's technique):

Paraffin wax or celloidin sections adhering to slides and brought into water;
Place the slides in a pyrex beaker containing the following reagent

10% sulphuric acid .... 100 ml
mercuric sulphate .... 10 g

dissolve in the warm, allow to cool, make up to 200 ml and add 0.50 ml of an 0.25% aqueous solution of sodium nitrite;
Warm gently to simmering point;
Allow to cool to laboratory temperature;
Wash in 3 baths of distilled water (2 minutes for each washing);
Mount in a medium miscible with water or dehydrate with absolute alcohol, clear in a benzenoid hydrocarbon and mount in a synthetic resin.

A positive result of the reaction is shown by a colour which varies from red to reddish-yellow.

Millon's reaction (Pollister and Ris' technique).
— This method depends on the comparison of two slides carrying sections which are as comparable as possible, one of the slides being treated to demonstrate total tyrosine by Millon's

reagent with a trichloracetic acid base, whereas the other undergoes the same reaction in a reagent with a sulphuric acid base so that histones are extracted; the histones are evaluated by difference.

a) **Total tyrosine.** — Dewaxed sections, collodion-coated where appropriate and hydrated;
Blot with tissue paper;
Treat for 5 minutes, at 30°, with the following reagent, prepared immediately prior to use

3.6 N solution of trichloracetic acid	10 ml
distilled water	10 ml
mercuric acetate	1 g

Add 1 ml of a 1% sodium nitrite solution to 20 ml of the reagent and leave in an oven at 30°C for 25 minutes;
Remove the slides from the reagent, blot them with tissue paper;
Wash in 3 baths of 70% alcohol (total duration 15 minutes);
Dehydrate in absolute alcohol, clear in a benzenoid hydrocarbon and mount in a synthetic resin.

b) **Tyrosine in proteins other than histones,** — Dewaxed sections, treated with collodion and hydrated;
Blot with tissue paper;
Treat for 5 minutes, in an oven at 30°, with the reagent

10% sulphuric acid	100 ml
mercuric sulphate	10 g

diluted immediately prior to use with equal parts of distilled water;
Add 1 ml of a 1% solution of sodium nitrite to each 20 ml of reagent and leave to stand in an oven at 30° for 25 minutes;
Wash for 10 minutes in running water;
Dehydrate with absolute alcohol, clear in a benzenoid hydrocarbon and mount in a synthetic resin.

The technique of Pollister and Ris may be followed by a histophotometric study of the preparations, thus requiring detailed precautions as to the choice of sections which should be as comparable as possible. The measurement of the "blank" is made on a third slide, treated with one of the two reagents for 10 minutes, but omitting the addition of sodium nitrite. One can also treat the two slides which are to undergo the reaction with a first stage intended to measure the blank and then demount them and undertake any required reactions.

Danielli's coupled tetrazonium reaction

Danielli's coupled tetrazonium reaction (1947) does in fact depend on the principle of double coupling with diazonium salts, mentioned by Lison (1931). Originally it was considered that this method allowed a selective demonstration of tyrosine, tryptophane and histidine, as well as of purines and pyrimidines of the nucleic acid. The principle of the method is very simple. The azoreaction is undertaken using a double coupling salt, bearing two diazonium groups, one of which reacts with the phenol group present in tissue structures whereas the second is ultimately coupled with a naphthol so as to increase the depth and intensity of the azo dyestuff so formed. We know from Burstone's (1955) and Landing and Hall's (1956) investigations that the diazo-salt of benzidine used by the earliest workers can be replaced to advantage with diazotised o-dianisidine which is available in a stable form from the chemical industry. As for the naphthol to use for the second coupling, most modern authors have abandoned β-naphthol, which was first suggested, for H acid (1-amino-8-naphthol-3-6-disulphonic acid). It so happens that the azo dyestuffs formed with the first of these compounds (β-naphtholazobenzidine or β-naphtholazo-dianisidine) are very soluble in alcohol and in benzenoid hydrocarbons, whereas the azo dyestuffs obtained with H acid are much less so, so that it is possible to dehydrate with alcohol and to mount in an embedding mixture miscible with benzenoid hydrocarbons; in consequence the optical qualities of the preparations are much better. The reaction should then be practised in the following way.

> Paraffin wax sections, dewaxed, collodion-coated where appropriate and hydrated;
> Treat for 15 minutes, at a temperature around 4°C, with Michaelis' buffer solution using
> > acetate-veronal, pH 9.2, chilled to 4° .... 50 ml
> > the diazo-salt of o-dianisidine (fast blue salt B) .... 0.05 g
> > prepared immediately prior to use;
>
> Rinse in two or three baths of buffer at the temperature at which the coupling reaction took place;
> Treat for 15 minutes, at the same temperature, with the solution
> > H acid .... 0.1 g
> > Michaelis' buffer, pH 9.2 .... 50 ml
> Wash in running water for about 5 minutes;
> Dehydrate in absolute alcohol or in acetone, clear in a benzenoid hydrocarbon and mount in a synthetic resin or in Canada balsam.

The amount of H acid recommended here is ten times less than that suggested by Landing and Hall (1956). Experience shows that it is adequate to ensure coupling and that by this means adjustment of the pH may be avoided.

A colour which varies between yellow and purple shows that the reaction is positive; with β-naphthol the colours tend towards red and mounting should be carried out, when the slides are taken from the wash in running water, in a medium miscible with water.

$$R-\bigcirc-OH + HON-\bigcirc-\bigcirc-N_2OH \rightarrow$$
$$(a) \qquad\qquad (b)$$

$$R-\bigcirc-OH \atop {}^{\diagdown}N=N^{\diagup}\bigcirc-\bigcirc N_2OH + \bigcirc\!\bigcirc-OH \rightarrow$$
$$(c) \qquad\qquad\qquad (d)$$

REACTIONS FOR THE SELECTIVE DETECTION OF AMINO-ACIDS 511

(e)

(a) = protein with a terminal phenolic group; (b) = diazosalt of benzidine; (c) = azo-dyestuff formed after the first coupling reaction; (d) = bis-azo-dyestuff formed following the second coupling reaction.

The optical qualities of the preparations are excellent and this is indeed one of the great advantages of the method but the histochemical interpretation of the results should be revised in the light of modern knowledge.

In fact, Danielli himself suggested control reactions intended to increase the chemical specificity of the procedure. Treatment with dinitrofluorobenzene, undertaken in conditions which were described in relation to the use of that substance for the detection of amino-acids, suppresses the activity of the tyrosine under the conditions of the coupled tetrazonium reaction; only tryptophane and histidine remain detectable by this method. Performic oxidation suppresses the activity of tryptophane selectively; benzoylation (treatment of the sections in a rigorously anhydrous medium, for 10 to 16 hours, with a 10% solution of benzoyl chloride in pyridine) permits only the histidine to remain active.

However, *in vitro* trials, notably those of Zahn and his colleagues (1953) and of Howard and Wild (1957), show that proline, cystein, lysine and arginine can react under the experimental conditions of the method, such as were defined by Danielli, so that prudence would suggest that we should no longer use the coupled tetrazonium reaction as a means for the identification of aromatic amino-acids. It seems to be wise to follow Pearse (1960, p. 91–92) in considering it as a general reaction of proteins. It is in this context that the optical qualities of the preparations are particularly advantageous.

We might, moreover, recall the use made by Landing and Hall (1956) of the coupled tetrazonium reaction for the demonstration of histidine; the reservations formulated by modern authors have been mentioned in the corresponding section of this chapter.

Morel and Sisley's reaction

This reaction, which was adapted for histochemical use by Lillie (1957) and Glenner and Lillie (1959), depends on the diazotisation of tyrosine with nitrous acid at low temperatures and in darkness, the diazonium salt so formed being detected by coupling with an amino-naphtholsulphonic acid (S acid or H acid). The technique involves the following stages.

Paraffin wax sections taken from material fixed under conditions compatible with the preservation of tyrosine (formalin, Bouin, Carnoy, etc...), dewaxed, treated with collodion where appropriate and hydrated;
Treat for 16 hours, at about 3°C and *in darkness*, with the solution
    distilled water .... 28 ml
    sodium nitrite .... 2 g
    crystallisable acetic acid .... 1.7 ml
(*add the acetic acid last*);
Pass the sections through 4 baths of distilled water chilled to 3° (5 seconds for each bath);
Treat the washed sections for 1 hour, at 3°C and in darkness, with the solution
    70% alcohol .... 50 ml
    S acid .... 0.5 g
    caustic potash .... 0.5 g
    urea .... 1 g
(the urea of the reagent can be replaced by 500 mg of ammonium sulphamate);
Wash in 3 baths of 0.1 N hydrochloric acid (5 minutes per bath);
Wash for 10 minutes in running water;
Where appropriate, practise nuclear staining with haemalum or Groat's haematoxylin;
Wash for 2 to 5 minutes in running water;
Dehydrate in absolute alcohol, clear in a benzenoid hydrocarbon and mount in a synthetic resin or, where necessary, in Canada balsam.

A positive result of this method, which all modern authors agree in considering as being the best histochemical reaction for tyrosine, is shown by a stain which varies, according to the abundance of this amino-acid in the stained structures, from intense red to pink.

$$R-\bigcirc-OH + HNO_2 \rightarrow R-\bigcirc-OH \rightarrow$$
$$\hspace{4cm} \diagdown N=O + H_2O$$
       (a)   (b)

$$R-\bigcirc=O + 3 HNO_2 \rightarrow$$
$$\hspace{2cm} \diagdown NOH$$
       (c)

$$R-\bigcirc-OH + HNO_3 + H_2O$$
$$\hspace{2cm} \diagdown H=N-NO_3$$
       (d)

(*a*) = protein with a terminal tyrosine group; (*b*) = product of the nitroso-reaction; (*c*) = quinone-oxime tautomeric form of the foregoing; (*d*) = diazonium nitrate formed from (*c*) in the presence of nitrous acid; this compound is coupled with S acid to obtain the azo-dyestuff indicative of the presence of tyrosine.

We know from the systematic trials of Geyer (1962) that pretreatment of the sections with a 10% iodine solution in ethyl alcohol (1 to 6 hours) allows us to reduce to 1 hour the time needed for diazotisation of the sections in the mixture of sodium nitrite-acetic acid. The same author showed that the Morel-Sisley reaction was completely suppressed, as was that of Millon, following pretreatment of the sections by a solution of 0.1 ml of tetranitromethane in a mixture of 10 ml of pyridine and 20 ml of 0.1 N hydrochloric acid; after spending 6 hours at laboratory temperatures in this blocking bath, the sections are rinsed in 2 baths of absolute alcohol or acetone (5 minutes for each bath) and then washed for 10 minutes in running water, prior to undergoing the reactions.

DEMONSTRATION OF INDOLE GROUPS AND IN PARTICULAR OF TRYPTOPHANE

The histochemical demonstration of tryptophane is of interest because of the presence of this amino-acid in secretory products such as pepsinogen, chymotrypsinogen and trypsinogen, glucagon, thyroglobulin and gonadotropins, as well as in a large number of other constituents of tissue or products of cellular activity. The techniques which permit of this detection have undergone considerable development since the introduction of the dimethylamino-benzaldehyde method of Ehrlich into histochemical technique (Lison, 1933), and we currently dispose of methods which are satisfactory from the point of view of their chemical specificity and that of the optical qualities of the preparations.

Certain of the techniques put forward by the classical authors have only historical interest at the present time. Such is the case with Romieu's reaction using phosphoric acid and with the Voisenet-Fürth reaction using formalin-hydrochloric acid-sodium nitrite. The reaction involving nitrous acid-naphthylethylenediamine (Bruemmer, Carver and Thomas, 1957) is satisfactory from the chemical standpoint but the stains produced are unfavourable for a detailed study of the sections. The xanthydrol reaction (Lillie, 1957) was considered by its author as being of minor interest, so far as histochemical practice is concerned, because the stains produced are very pale when the fixatives used in his major work were employed. In reality, it gives very good results when the fixation is undertaken with mixtures having a glutaraldehyde base and should therefore be retained within modern histochemical practice, as should the rosindol reaction (Adams, 1957; Glenner, 1957) as well as that of Glenner and Lillie (1957) using p-dimethylamino-benzaldehyde with coupling to S acid.

We know from the investigations of Glenner and Lillie (1957) that the way in which fixation is done plays an essential role in the success of reactions intended to detect indole compounds. Pieces of tissue fixed in formalin can only be used if the fixation has been of short duration (about 10 hours); fixatives with a corrosive sublimate base entrain a considerable weakening of the activity, but this diminution, which is due to the formation of complexes which block the 2(α) carbon of the pyrrole group, disappears after treatment of the sections, for 5 to 10 minutes, at 37°C, with a 5% solution of sodium thiosulphate, a saturated solution of lithium carbonate in 70% alcohol or with a solution of dimercaptopropanol (BAL). Fixatives with a picric acid base will entrain the same loss of activity which is nevertheless capable of being reestablished by treatment for 10 minutes, at laboratory temperatures, with the alcoholic solution of lithium carbonate mentioned above. Fixatives with a potassium bichromate base entrain a severe loss, if not the disappearance of the activity, the phenomenon being irreversible. I would add to this, from my own experience, that fixatives containing trichloracetic acid are not particularly favourable to tests for indole groups. A better preservation of indole groups is assured by fixatives having a glutaraldehyde base.

1° The method using dimethylaminobenzaldehyde-diazo salt of S acid (Glenner and Lillie, 1957) depends on the same principle as Lison's (1933) main procedure, one molecule of the reagent giving rise to condensation with pyrrolenin (a tautomeric form of pyrrole). However, the violet colour so obtained is intensified by coupling the diaminobenzene radical of the reagent with the diazo-salt of S acid. According to Lison (1960, p. 254), this reinforcement is in fact not due to the formation of a coloured azo-dyestuff but simply to the oxidising action of the nitrous acid which is still present in the solution of the diazo salt of S acid, prepared according to the practices of the American authors. This remark in no way changes the practical value of the method, which is great; I would cordially advocate its use. The working technique involves the following stages.

Paraffin wax sections, taken from material fixed under the conditions defined above, and having undergone, where appropriate, one of the "reactivations" described;
Dehydrate with acetone, dry (the sections withstand the action of the reagent much better in a rigorously anhydrous medium);
Treat for 5 minutes, at about 25°, with the mixture, prepared immediately prior to use, of
  concentrated hydrochloric acid .... 10 ml
  crystallisable acetic acid .... 30 ml
  p-dimethylaminobenzaldehyde .... 1 g
Wash in 3 baths of crystallisable acetic acid (30, 60 and 60 seconds);
Treat for 5 minutes at a temperature between 15 and 20°C with the mixture, prepared immediately prior to use, of
  crystallisable acetic acid .... 40 ml
  the diazo salt of S acid or of safranin, freshly prepared
  (p. 377) .... 1 ml
Wash in 2 baths of crystallisable acetic acid (1 to 2 minutes each);
Where appropriate, stain the background with a 0.05% solution of basic fuchsin in crystallisable acetic acid and wash for 2 minutes in 2 baths of crystallisable acetic acid;
Clear in a mixture of equal parts of xylene and crystallisable acetic acid, eliminate the latter in 3 to 4 baths of pure xylene and mount in a synthetic resin (avoid mounting in Canada balsam).

A positive result of the reaction produces an intense blue colour; when the sections have been well dried prior to their immersion in the reagent, the preservation of the structures is good. The stains keep for a variable time and it is prudent to examine them and to photograph them without delay.

(a) = tryptophane; (b) = p-dimethylaminobenzaldehyde; (c) = condensation product; (d) = diazo-salt of S acid; (e) = azo-dyestuff formed as a result of coupling.

2° The rosindole reaction of Glenner (1957) also begins with the condensation of an indole nucleus with p-dimethylaminobenzaldehyde, but the intensity of the stain is increased by treatment with a mixture of hydrochloric acid and acetic acid in which sodium nitrite has been dissolved at the moment of use. The reaction is carried out in the following way.

> Paraffin wax sections, treated as for Glenner and Lillie's reaction and dried;
> Treat with the hydrochloric acid-acetic acid -p-dimethylaminobenzaldehyde mixture as in the preceding method; the initial formula of Glenner (1957, p. 298) envisaged a treatment of 3 minutes in a solution the solvent of which was a mixture of 5 ml of 60% perchloric acid, 1 ml of concentrated hydrochloric acid and 34 ml of crystallisable acetic acid, but Lillie (1965) considered the presence of the perchloric acid as being valueless;
> Transfer the sections directly into a Coplin jar, the bottom of which has been filled with 500 mg of sodium nitrite and into which, at the time of inserting the sections, a mixture of 5 ml of concentrated hydrochloric acid and 35 ml of crystallisable acetic acid has been poured; allow this mixture to act for 1 minute (*do not exceed this time*);
> Wash in 2 baths of crystallisable acetic acid (2 minutes altogether);
> Where appropriate, stain the background, clear and mount as in Glenner and Lillie's method.

A positive result for the method is also shown by the appearance of an intense blue colour; the comparison of the two procedures shows that the results are rigorously identical.

It is appropriate to comment that Adam's technique (1957) differs from that of Glenner only in the nature of the solvent used for the condensation with *p*-dimethylaminobenzaldehyde and for the oxidation by nitrous acid; this solvent is in both cases concentrated hydrochloric acid. The stains so obtained are perhaps a little more intense than with Glenner's method but the tissue structures generally withstand the action of concentrated hydrochloric acid less well than they do that of the acetic acid-hydrochloric acid mixture.

From the practical point of view, we may remark that solutions of *p*-dimethylaminobenzaldehyde in hydrochloric acid or in the hydrochloric acid-acetic acid mixture keep for about a month provided that they are kept in vessels with a ground glass neck and vaselined stoppers. The perchloric acid-hydrochloric acid-acetic acid mixture is less useful as a solvent for *p*-dimethylaminobenzaldehyde because the reagent keeps less well; the solutions of sodium nitrite should evidently be prepared as required at the time of use.

We know from trials, on models and on tissues, carried out by Glenner and Lillie (1957) that the techniques using *p*-dimethylaminobenzaldehyde are, from the standpoint of their chemical specificity, entirely satisfactory, thus confirming the opinions of Lison (1933, 1936, 1953, 1960); various possible sources of error of a chemical nature, in particular the possibility of condensation with other aromatic phenols or amines, are unlikely to arise under the conditions of histochemical practice.

As I commented above, the technique using xanthydrol, developed by Lillie (1957), is considered by all modern authors as being highly satisfactory from a chemical standpoint. The disadvantage of having a pale violet or blue colour when the result of the reaction is positive occurs only after certain fixations, such as with formalin and Bouin's fluid. After fixation with mixtures having a glutaraldehyde base the preparations are as good as those obtained using the techniques involving *p*-dimethylaminobenzaldehyde; they keep relatively well (for several months). We might add to this the advantage of having a very simple procedure.

Reagents.

A solution of xanthydrol (1 g in 36 ml of glacial acetic acid) to which, *at the moment of use*, 4 ml of concentrated hydrochloric acid are added for every 36 ml of solution (use only once);
A 0.05% solution of basic fuchsin (or new fuchsin) in glacial acetic acid.

Working technique.

Paraffin wax sections, taken from material fixed with a mixture having a glutaraldehyde base (the GPA of Solcia et al. (1968) serves very well), dewaxed and, on removal from the benzenoid hydrocarbon, passed through a bath of acetic acid;

Treat for 5 minutes in a mixture consisting of the solution of xanthydrol in hydrochloric acid;
Rinse in acetic acid;
Stain where appropriate with the acetic acid solution of basic fuchsin (new fuchsin);
Rinse in acetic acid;
Treat with a mixture of equal parts of xylene (or other benzenoid hydrocarbon) and acetic acid, and then in 4 baths of the benzenoid hydrocarbon.
Mount in a commercial synthetic resin, examine and photograph without delay.

A blue or violet colour indicative of the presence of indole groups generally keeps for 2 to 3 months and often for a longer period.

DEMONSTRATION OF THIOL AND DISULPHIDE GROUPS

The thiol and disulphide radicals are essentially represented in the animal organism by two amino-acids, cysteine and cystine; we ought to mention, since the contrary assertion occurs in the third edition of Lison's book (1960, p. 204), that the third sulphur-containing amino-acid, namely methionine, does not carry a thiol group and that it is not accessible to histochemical detection.

The importance of protein-bound sulphydryls as constituents of various structural materials of secretory products, of hormones and of enzymes is too well known to need recalling here and accounts for the interest attaching to the detection of these compounds in sections of animal tissue. In fact, the thiol groups are reliably detectable by a substantial number of histochemical reactions, some of which are very satisfactory from the point of view of their specificity and sensitivity; the disulphide groups which cannot be detected as such are easy to convert into thiols by a whole range of treatments which depend on reduction. The protein-bound sulphydryls thus represent one of the most satisfying chapters in the histochemistry of proteins in general.

All tests for protein-bound sulphydryls result in the demonstration of thiol groups; we should then give priority to a discussion of the techniques permitting of this detection before reviewing the conditions for fixation when these compounds are to be detected, as well as the ways of applying these reactions when the object of the work is the demonstration of disulphide groups. Control reactions which involve the blocking of active groups play a particularly important part in the histochemical study of protein-bound sulphydryls.

1° *Reactions for the histochemical detection of the thiol group*

The numerous methods proposed for the detection of thiol groups are divided by Pearse into eight groups, although the basis for this division is not clear from a reading of his text (1960, p. 99); more rationally, the classification of Lison (1960) distinguishes techniques based on the reducing capacity, on the formation of mercaptides, on the esterification of the thiol radical, and lastly on the oxidation of this radical.

Among the **reactions based on the reducing capacity** of compounds with a thiol group, the classic sodium nitroprusside is now only of historic interest. Its chemical specificity is satisfactory but its sensitivity is so low that the pioneers of histochemical investigations into the protein-bound sulphydryls used it on frozen sections which were 100 μ thick. Other reactions of protein-bound sulphydryls which are in current use also depend on the reducing capacity of thiols. These are the *ferric ferricyanide method* and that using *tetrazolium salts* in an alkaline medium.

The two reactions have been discussed with all necessary detail in Chapter 13 and their application to tests for protein-bound sulphydryls calls for no special comment. Among variations of the ferric ferricyanide method I would recommend in particular that of Adams (1956); it is Gomori's (1956) technique which gives the best results among techniques involving tetrazolium salts in alkaline media.

Naturally, these two reactions demonstrate the presence of reducing compounds in the structures which are stained and so they are not specific for proteins with a thiol group. The precursors of melanin, the secretory granules of the Kultschitzky cells of the intestine, those of the medullo-adrenal cells in cases where they have been preserved during fixation, and elastic tissue represent the main sources of error in mammalian tissue, but I need hardly add that this list is not complete. It is therefore necessary to verify in all cases, by the use of blocking reactions, that the reducing power observed as a result of applying one or other of these reactions does indeed indicate the presence of thiol groups.

A methodical comparison of the results given by the different histochemical reactions of protein bound sulphydryls, in any given mammalian tissue, led Gomori (1956) to note that the contrast afforded by the two techniques under discussion here is generally greater than that obtained with other methods, in particular with the DDD technique; moreover, this author emphasizes the fact that the reagents used in the ferric ferricyanide method penetrate very poorly into dense keratin, so that negative results can be obtained, whereas other techniques demonstrate the presence of a substantial amount of protein-bound sulphydryls.

In practice, the ferric ferricyanide method, which is simple and cheap, is to be recommended for ordinary work provided that we take into account its lack of chemical specificity; the technique using tetrazolium salts in an alkaline medium gives preparations of excellent optical quality and often gives better contrast than any other methods, but it has two disadvantages, namely the high cost of the reagent and the need to keep the sections in the alkaline medium for a rather lengthy period at 60°C.

Of the three **methods which are based on the formation of mercaptides** (thiolates) and used in the histochemical detection of thiols on the scale of light microscopy, that of Mauri, Vaccari and Kadavere (1954) using p-acetoxymercurianiline need not be discussed here because of its lack of specificity; Gomori (1956) has shown that the reagent recommended by the Italian authors has all the properties of an acid stain as well as having the capacity to form mercaptides. The two other reactions, those of Bennett (1948) using 1,4-chloromercuriphenylazo-2-napthol and that of Lillie and Glenner (in Lillie, 1965) using p-N,N-dimethylaminophenylmercuric acetate do have considerable chemical specificity.

Bennet's (1948) method consists of treating the sections taken from fresh or fixed tissue, or even small blocks of tissue, with a butyl or propyl alcohol solution of 1,4-chloromercuriphenylazo-2-naphthol (mercury orange, red sulphydryl reagent). The formation of mercaptide results in a yellow or orange colour in structures which are rich in thiol groups. The sections are then washed in propanol, cleared in a benzenoid hydrocarbon and mounted in a synthetic resin.

In addition to its simplicity, Bennett's method is attractive for its great chemical specificity; the only source of error resides in the possibility of staining the lipids because the phenylazonaphthol group confers on the reagent the properties of a lysochrome. Naturally, tests involving the extraction of lipids would allow us to settle any possible doubts without difficulty.

Nevertheless, practical disadvantages counterbalance the advantages. The colour of structures containing thiol groups varies from pale orange to a bright orange red and the preparations are not particularly advantageous from an optical point of view. Moreover, the synthesis of the reagent takes a long time and has a low yield; certainly it is possible to purchase it commercially but the difficulties of synthesizing it account for its relatively high cost.

These practical disadvantages doubtless explain why Bennett's method is not widely used and for these reasons I would not advise it for general use.

Lillie and Glenner's technique (Lillie, 1965) also depends on the formation of a mercaptide, but the synthesis of the reagent, which is not yet available on the market, is of the simplest; the mercaptide formed is, moreover, transformed in the second stage of the reaction into a coloured azo dyestuff, so that the optical qualities of the preparation so obtained are good.

The synthesis of p-N,N-dimethylaminophenylmercuric acetate is carried out in the following way.

Dissolve 32 g of mercuric acetate in 100 ml of distilled water; chill to 3°C and add small amounts at a time of a mixture of 12.5 ml of dimethylaniline and 100 ml of absolute alcohol, also chilled to 3°C. A yellow precipitate appears when the alcoholic solution is first added but redissolves when the receptacle is stirred; when about half the alcoholic solution of dimethylaniline has been added a dense white precipitate appears and ultimately occupies virtually the whole volume, except for a thin layer of yellow supernatant liquor in the receptacle, which should then be stoppered with a rubber bung, vigorously shaken so as to transform the curdy precipitate into a suspension and allowed to stand at the temperature of melting ice (4–3°C) for 12 hours. At the end of this time the precipitate is collected by filtration through paper, and washed in distilled water until the wash liquid ceases to react with ammonium sulphide (the presence of mercury is shown by a precipitate formed when several drops of a commercial solution of ammonium sulphide are added to the wash liquid). The washed precipitate is dried in a vacuum desiccator, at laboratory temperatures, for three to six days. The theoretical yield of the synthesis is 37.32 g; in reality, about 30 g of the reagent are obtained.

The working technique of Lillie and Glenner's reaction for thiol groups involves the following stages.

> Paraffin wax sections, for preference taken from pieces of tissue fixed in Carnoy's fluid, dewaxed, treated with absolute alcohol and immersed in isopropanol;
> Keep for 18 to 24 hours, at a temperature between 20 and 25°C, in a 0.7% solution of the reagent in isopropanol (this concentration corresponds roughly to that of a saturated solution);
> Wash in 3 baths of isopropanol;
> Wash in crystallisable acetic acid;
> Treat for 5 minutes, at laboratory temperatures, with the mixture
>   crystallisable acetic acid .... 38 ml
>   the diazo-salt of safranin, freshly prepared (p. 377) .... 2 ml
> Wash in 3 baths of crystallisable acetic acid or in 0.5 N hydrochloric acid (5 minutes in each bath);
> Dehydrate in absolute alcohol, clear in a benzenoid hydrocarbon and mount in a synthetic resin or in Canada balsam if the slides have been washed in acetic acid; introduce a 10 minute bath in running water between washing in hydrochloric acid and the dehydration in alcohol.

A positive result of the reaction is indicated by a deep red stain; background staining using a progressive lake of haematoxylin can be carried out after the wash in running water when the sections have been washed in hydrochloric acid after the coupling reaction; this last wash nevertheless carries some risk of detaching the sections, a risk which is greater than that run with acetic acid.

Investigations involving blocking reactions show that the method is of great chemical specificity; Lillie (1965, p. 275) further observed that treatment with a dilute solution of 2,3-dimercaptopropanol (24 hours at laboratory temperatures) completely destained preparations which were ready for mounting.

The group of **techniques which depend on esterification of the thiol radical** include two methods due to Barrnett and Seligman (1952, 1954) the stages of which are fairly similar, involving the reaction with 2,2'-dihydroxy-6,'dinaphthyl disulphide and that with 4-hydroxynaphthyl-N-maleilimide; a variation using naphtholiodoacetamide has been suggested by Barrnett, Tsou and Seligman

REACTIONS FOR THE SELECTIVE DETECTION OF AMINO-ACIDS 521

(1955). Only the first of the techniques in question has found an unquestioned place in modern histochemical practice; it represents one of the most widely used among methods for the detection of the thiol group.

(a) = protein with thiol group; (b) = DDD; (c) = thio-ether with a naphthol group; (d) = 6-thio-2-naphthol, a by-product of the reaction; (e) = diazo-salt of o-dianisidine; (f) = bis-azo-dyestuff formed by coupling the two diazonium groups with two molecules of thio-ether.

The principle of these three techniques consists in forming a thioester which carries a naphthol group whose existence can be detected by means of the azoreaction. The excess of reagent and the bi-products of the reaction are removed by washing in alcohol and ether. The working technique thus includes the following stages.

Paraffin wax sections, dewaxed, *collodion coated* and hydrated;
Treat for 1 hour at 50 to 60°C with the solution
    2,2'-dihydroxy-6,6'-dinaphthyl disulphide (DDD) ....25 mg
    absolute alcohol .... 15 ml
    Michaelis' buffer using sodium veronal-hydrochloric acid,
        pH 8.5 .... 35 ml
Allow to cool for 10 minutes at laboratory temperatures;
Rinse in distilled water;

Wash for 10 minutes in very dilute acetic acid (0.01%);
Dehydrate by passing through 70%, 96% and absolute alcohol;
Treat for about 1 minute with a mixture of equal parts of absolute alcohol and sulphuric ether;
Treat for 5 minutes with a bath of sulphuric ether;
Rehydrate the sections by passing through baths with a decreasing alcohol content; wash in distilled water;
Carry out the coupling reaction for 2 minutes in the freshly prepared solution

diazo salt of o-anisidine .... 50 mg
0.1 M Sörensen's buffer, pH 7.4 .... 50 ml

(chill the buffer to about 4°C before dissolving the diazonium salt);
Wash for 2 minutes in running water;
Mount in a medium miscible with water.

When the coupling is carried out according to the directions given above a positive result of the reaction is shown by a stain which varies from red (few thiol groups, coupling with a single diazonium group) to blue (numerous thiol groups, coupling with two diazonium groups). This polychromy of the preparations, which was considered to be an advantage by the authors of the method, is considered by most modern authors (see in particular Gomori 1956; Bahr, 1959) as a nuisance which hinders the semi-quantitative appreciation of the results. It is in fact advantageous to use a monocoupling diazonium salt; I would in particular recommend fast red B salt (the diazo-salt of 5-nitro-anisidine) and fast black K salt (the diazosalt of 4-amino-2,5-dimethoxy-4'-nitro-azobenzene) which give, respectively, red and black stains.

Mounting in Canada balsam or, better, in a synthetic resin is possible when the coupling has been undertaken with the diazo-salt of o-dianisidine, provided that the sections are dehydrated with acetone and not with ethyl alcohol; if other diazonium salts are used the mounting must be carried out in a medium miscible with water.

Nuclear staining with haemalum, Hansen's ferric trioxyhaematin (avoid Groat's haematoxylin because of its alcohol content) or the aluminium lake of nuclear fast red can be carried out after the washing which follows the coupling reaction.

The chemical specificity of the method is excellent and its sensitivity is quite satisfactory; it is, perhaps, this great sensitivity which explains why preparations obtained using DDD are less contrasty than those obtained using certain other techniques. At all events, the optical qualities of the preparations are excellent.

These advantages which justify the universal adoption of the DDD reaction for the demonstration of thiol groups should not cause us to lose sight of its two practical disadvantages. The first of these is the high cost of the reagent; the synthesis of DDD is complicated and of low yield, factors which will obviously influence its cost. We should add to this that each bath of the reagent can be used only once, the amount indicated in the formula being considered sufficient for the treatment of 9 slides. From my own experience the DDD content of the reagent can be reduced to 20 mg per 50 ml, but not below this amount. As to the second disadvantage, there is a grave risk that the sections may come loose from the slides during treatment with hot alkaline solutions of DDD and during the changes in surface tension inherent in the aqueous or alcoholic washes which follow this stage. This risk is particularly great for sections which are rich in bony or cartilaginous tissue, in cuticular structures or in muscle fibres. Moreover, careful treatment of the sections with collodion should be considered obligatory.

The methods in the last group, which depend on the *selective oxidation of disulphide linkages in cystine*, are considered by their authors as being reactions of this latter amino-acid. Their practical interest as means for the detection of protein-bound sulphydryls is not very great but the theoretical bearing of the discussions to which they have given rise is sufficient for them to be mentioned briefly here and they lie behind staining procedures of undoubted practical interest.

The origins of the methods in question stem from the work of Toennies and Homiller (1942) which showed that only the following amino-acids could be oxidised by performic acid; tryptophane, methionine and cystine, the oxidation of the latter giving rise to the formation of cysteic acid (alanine-β-sulphonic acid). The anionic groups, which are thus caused to appear in structures rich in cystine, should lead to an ortho- or metachromatic basophilia and to a capacity for fixing metal ions and an affinity for stains such as the cupric phthalocyanins of the alcian blue group and for paraldehyde-fuchsin. Experience shows that this is indeed the case. Moreover, tests for aldehyde groups using 2-hydroxy-3-naphthoic acid hydrazide or using Schiff's reagent give positive results (Pearse, 1951; Lillie, 1951). The basophilia, the affinity for phthalocyanins and that for paraldehyde-fuchsin are interpreted by most modern authors as demonstrating the formation of anionic groups following performic or peracetic oxidation, and the chemical mechanism discovered by Toennies and Homiller fully explains the origin of these strongly acid radicals. Nevertheless, we ought to say that results, which are in all respects comparable to those given by oxidation with the two peracids, can be obtained using an oxidising agent as vigorous and unselective as potassium permanganate in the presence of sulphuric acid. It is nevertheless true that a strong basophilia, a quite definite affinity for alcian blue and for stains of the same group and for paraldehyde-fuchsin or paraldehyde-thionin appearing after performic or peracetic oxidation may be indicative of the presence of a certain amount of proteins rich in cystine in the stained structures. This observation lies at the origin of a technique due to Adams and Sloper (1955, 1956) which was more particularly intended to demonstrate the hypothalamic neurosecretory product but which nevertheless gives positive results in any structure which is sufficiently rich in proteins containing cystine. The working technique of these authors involves the following stages.

> Paraffin wax sections, dewaxed, treated with collodion where appropriate, and hydrated;
> Oxidise for 5 minutes in freshly prepared performic acid (p. 467);
> Wash for 5 minutes in distilled water;
> Treat for 1 hour at laboratory temperatures with the solution
>
> | | |
> |---|---|
> | alcian blue 8GS | 1 g |
> | distilled water | 94.6 ml |
> | concentrated sulphuric acid | 5.4 ml |
>
> (the pH of the solvent which corresponds to 2 N sulphuric acid is 0.2);
> Wash for 5 minutes in running water;
> Dehydrate in absolute alcohol, clear in a benzenoid hydrocarbon and mount in a synthetic resin or in Canada balsam.

Structures which are rich in proteins containing disulphide groups, in particular the hypothalamic neurosecretory product and the cortex of hair, are intensely stained blue; the nuclei either stain weakly or not at all.

As Lillie (1965, p. 220) has commented, peracetic oxidation may, without any ill-effects, be substituted for performic oxidation. This avoids the use of a very unstable reagent which has to be prepared the same day as it is used and cannot be purchased commercially. We may also mention that other basic stains (thionin, azur A, toluidine blue etc...) can replace alcian blue. The content of this latter compound in the staining bath may be reduced, without ill-effects, to 0.1%; certain commercial samples of alcian blue are, moreover, not soluble to the extent indicated by Adams and Sloper.

When this technique is applied routinely to the material for which it was intended, that is to say the hypothalamo-hypophysial neurosecretory duct and the adenohypophysis of mammals, it gives results which can also be obtained using other oxidising agents which are much less selective such as potassium permanganate in a sulphuric acid medium. Many authors have deduced from this that the method of Adams and Sloper could, without untoward results, employ permanganate oxidation in an acid medium instead of the peracids, as was indeed suggested, right at the beginning, by Gomori (1941) for the selective staining of the B cells of the endocrine pancreas. This erroneous opinion was upheld in the French version of the present book. Data available since the publication of that work require a change of mind.

In fact, the comparison of the results obtained with secretory products rich in cystine (the hypothalamic neurosecretory product, the secretory product of the B cells of the endocrine pancreas) after oxidation by peracids on the one hand or after permanganate oxidation in a sulphuric acid medium on the other hand show a clear distinction between the two types of oxidation (Gabe, 1968, 1969).

In both cases, the two secretory products acquire an intense affinity for alcian blue, paraldehyde fuchsin, and other basic stains, this phenomenon being the basis for the selective staining techniques set out in the last part of the present work. But this basophilia goes hand in hand with the appearance of chromatropic properties when the oxidation has been carried out with peracetic or performic acids. A metachromasia of the gamma type which withstands dehydration by alcohol can be obtained by staining with basic blues of the thiazine family. On the contrary, permanganate oxidation in a sulphuric acid medium results in an orthochromatic basophilia, as has been known for a long time, when the pH of the thiazine solution is above 4.2, and to a feeble and unstable metachromasia, verging on orthochromasia during dehydration, when the pH of the solution is below 4.2 (Fujita and Takaya, 1968). Moreover, the extinction pH of this basophilia differs in the case of the B cells of the endocrine pancreas according to the procedure used for oxidation. The metachromatic basophilia and the affinity for alcian blue shown at a pH of 1 when the sections have been oxidised using potassium permanganate in a sulphuric acid medium are only clear at pH values above 2.6 when the oxidation is carried out using peracids. In the case of the hypothalamic neurosecretory product, which is much richer in protein-bound sulphydryls, such a difference, dependent on the type of oxidation, is not observed, the basophilia and the affinity for alcian blue being strong at pH 1 even when the oxidation has been carried out using peracids; this fact is consistent with Adams and Sloper's original observation (1955). In the same way, the intensity of the background stain is always greater after permanganate oxidation than after oxidation using performic or peracetic acid.

We may therefore legitimately conclude that the two kinds of oxidation result in the formation of different anionic groups.

Even though the technique of Adams and Sloper results in the demonstration of structures rich in cystine or cysteine with magnificent selectivity, its chemical specificity cannot be considered great. The staining of those anionic groups which preexist in the sections is possible even at the very low pH values recommended for staining with alcian blue so that it is necessary to compare the sections with unoxidised controls; moreover, although the selectivity of performic or peracetic oxidation for cysteine, methionine and tryptophane is very great, compounds other than these amino-acids may be oxidised in the sections.

The value of performic or peracetic oxidation for the demonstration of secretory products rich in sulphur-containing amino-acids is substantial; the basophilia and chromatropism which appear under these conditions allow us to obtain strikingly selective stains. Although it seems plausible to suggest that such results do indeed indicate the presence of cystine or of cysteine the converse is not automatically true and compounds rich in anionic groups other than cysteic acid may give rise to the same orthochromatic or metachromatic basophilia. It seems prudent therefore to include the method of Adams and

Sloper in that group of marker stains the results of which require confirmation by methods with a greater chemical specificity.

As for the positive result given by the performic (or peracetic) acid-Schiff reagent methods, in the cortex of hair, its practical bearing is none too wide and its chemical interpretation is still the subject of debate. According to Pearse (1960) its reactivity could be due either to carbonyls or to cysteic acid or to the sulphinic acid corresponding to it; but according to the results of Lillie's school (see Lillie, 1965, p. 184) it relates to the demonstration of carbonyls formed by the oxidation of compounds with a double bond which bear no relation to proteins with a disulphide group.

2° Preparation of tissue for detection of protein-bound sulphydryls

The procedures preparatory to the histochemical reactions discussed in the preceding section should take account not only of the general needs of histological fixation but also of certain biochemical peculiarities of protein-bound sulphydryls. It is in fact known that not all the protein-bound sulphydryls of the cell are directly accessible to reagents for these compounds and that the demonstration of some of them requires a true "unmasking". We may follow Barron Guzman (1951) in distinguishing free thiol radicals directly detectable by all the usual reagents, "inert" radicals directly detectable only by some of these reagents and, lastly, masked radicals which cannot be demonstrated by any reagent without appropriate pretreatment. These biochemical ideas have been confirmed by histochemists; we know that certain thiol groups cannot be detected in fresh tissue whereas their detection after fixation poses no special technical problems (see in particular Barrnett and Roth, 1958).

Another essential point is the lability of the thiol group; in fact, the transformation of thiols into disulphides takes place with great ease under the influence of very mild oxidising agents and even by exposure to air; that is to say, it may happen during the preparation of sections, during their spreading, their washing, etc. Whilst on this subject we might note that the amount of alkaline hypochlorite present in some tap water is sufficient to induce this transformation (Gomori, 1956). In consequence the fixation of pieces of tissue should not be carried out in the same way in cases where the investigator needs to preserve the distinction between thiol and disulphide groups present in the tissue as when the object of the work is to test for total protein-bound sulphydryls.

The best preservation of proteins with a thiol group directly accessible to histochemical detection is obtained by fixation with trichloracetic acid. The stabilising action of this acid has been put to good use by classical authors whose fixative was a 5% aqueous solution of trichloracetic acid. Modern authors generally prefer to use 80% alcohol to which 1 gram of trichloracetic acid has been added for every 100 ml. The preservation of the thiol disulphide ratio in the tissue is satisfactory but the quality of fixation leaves much to be desired from the morphological standpoint and we have to come to terms with substantial losses of protein-bound sulphydryls because of the destruction of many structures, in particular of the secretory products. However this may be, the procedures preparatory to the manufacture of sections (dehydration, clearing, embedding in paraffin wax) and sectioning on a microtome, together with spreading, require no particular precautions.

Fixation in formalin, whether or not it is neutralised, and whether or not it is saline, has been recommended by a certain number of authors. In theory, treatment with this reagent results in blocking the thiol groups in the form of thiazolidine-4-carboxylic acid, but this is an easily reversible reaction and washing with aqueous fluids is generally sufficient to reactivate the thiol groups present in the sections. Losses are nevertheless substantial and I subscribe entirely to the opinion of Lillie (1965, p. 208) who does not recommend this fixative in cases where tests for protein-bound sulphydryls represent a major part of the work.

Clarke's and Carnoy's fluids, already discussed as topographical fixatives, are quite suitable in cases where the distinction between protein-bound sulphydryls and proteins with disulphide links plays an important part in the work. The results may be greatly improved by cold fixation and by shortening the time spent by the pieces of tissue in hot paraffin as far as possible (vacuum)

Fixatives with a mercuric chloride base were, formerly, automatically rejected because of the danger of mercaptide formation, since such a blocking would cause the thiol groups to be inaccessible to any histochemical reactions. In fact, experience shows that the mercaptides formed during the fixation of the tissue are easily decomposed by reducing agents so that the -SH groups are liberated; but this reduction also transforms the disulphide groups into sulphydryls, so that it becomes impossible to distinguish the two kinds of sulphur-containing radical. These fixatives, therefore, can only be used when the object of the work is the detection of the total protein-bound sulphydryls.

Fixation in Bouin's fluid is compatible with tests for protein-bound sulphydryls; experience shows that losses are much greater using Duboscq-Brazil's fluid whose use I would not recommend.

Short-term fixation using cytological fixatives without osmium tetroxide permits us easily to detect protein-bound sulphydryls, but post-chromatisation should be avoided at all costs; it makes the reduction of -S-S- groups into -SH groups impossible.

3° *Reduction of disulphide linkages to thiol groups*

This procedure, the importance of which stems from the considerations outlined in the preceding section, has the result of rendering accessible to histochemical detection the whole of the cysteine *and* cystine which are preserved in the sections; it immediately effaces any distinction between the two amino-acids and should thus be avoided in all cases where this distinction is one of the objectives of the work. In addition, this reduction renders accessible to histochemical detection thiol groups which are blocked in the form of mercaptides with a mercury salt base.

Numerous reducing agents have been proposed; only the most effective are mentioned here.

Alkaline sulphides (ammonium or sodium sulphide, in 5% aqueous solution) are generally used at laboratory temperatures or at 37°C; the duration of the treatment is from 2 to 3 hours at laboratory temperatures, 1 hour at 37°. The high pH of the reducing solution (about 9.5) necessitates an extremely careful treatment of the sections with collodion. Naturally, every precaution should be taken to ensure that the room is well aired (do not forget that hydrogen sulphide is highly toxic) and that the last traces of the reducing fluid must be eliminated from the sections before the histochemical reactions are undertaken, especially those which depend precisely on the demonstration of reducing capacity. This washing should be conducted with distilled water or a 1% solution of acetic acid in tap water; it is in distilled water to which 1% of acetic acid has been added that the sections should be allowed to stand if necessary so as to forestall any new oxidation of the thiol groups to disulphides.

Alkaline cyanides, which have been much commended by certain authors, are considerably less active than other reducing agents and I would not recommend their use; those who are keen on this technique use 10% solutions of sodium or potassium cyanide.

Sodium hydrosulphite, which is a highly vigorous reducing agent but very harmful to the sections, should not be used.

Thioglycollic acid, which has been recommended by the majority of authors, is used as a 0.2 to 0.5 M aqueous solution, the pH being adjusted to 8, at the moment of use, with 0.1 N soda; the reaction takes place at 37° and generally requires three to four hours; it should be followed by careful washing in water to which acetic acid has been added and then in distilled water. We may mention that Lillie (1965) preferred to use a 10% solution of sodium thioglycolate, adjusted with soda to a pH of 9.5; treatment for 10 minutes at laboratory temperatures was sufficient to ensure reduction.

Thioglycerol (thiovanol), which is very effective and easy to use, has the single disadvantage of being rather costly. This reduction, which was introduced by Gomori (1956), takes place in an oven at 37° for about 12 hours, the reagent containing 2 to 3 ml of thioglycerol, 40 ml of distilled water and 10 ml of a borax-boric acid buffer of pH 8.5 to 9.1. On removal from the reducing bath the sections are washed in water treated with acetic acid and, where appropriate, allowed to stand in that fluid.

Thiolacetic acid and **dimercaptopropanol** (BAL) which are very effective reducing agents are hardly used at all; the cost of the second of these substances is relatively high and neither presents advantages over other reducing agents.

In practice, reduction with alkaline sulphides or with thioglycerol are quite satisfactory provided that all traces of the reducing compound are eliminated with great care prior to the practice of the reactions themselves and provided that the sections, once reduced, are not allowed to stand for an excessive length of time. For financial reasons, I would recommend that reduction with thioglycerol should be reserved for difficult cases.

4° *Blocking reactions for thiol groups*

A negative result after blocking of the thiol groups represents an indispensable control reaction for any test for protein-bound sulphydryls, this remark being particularly essential in cases where the histochemical detection is being done with reactions which simply disclose reducing capacity (ferric ferricyanide, tetrazolium salts in an alkaline medium). The simplest blocking agents are iodine and corrosive sublimate but in both cases the reactions are readily reversible, especially if the reagent used for the detection of protein-bound sulphydryls contains an alkaline cyanide (methods involving tetrazolium salts). Blocking with ethylmaleilimide, with sodium monoiodo-acetate or with chloropicrin are much more effective and should be preferred to the preceding reducing agents in any doubtful case.

Blockage with iodine takes place at temperatures around 25 °C, in practice at laboratory temperatures. The sections are kept in an iodine-iodide solution containing 0.038% iodine and 0.033% potassium iodide, the pH being adjusted to 3.2 with 0.01 N hydrochloric acid; the duration of action is about 4 hours.

Blocking with mercuric bichloride involves keeping the sections in a saturated aqueous solution of this salt (about 7%), at laboratory temperatures for a time varying from one to five hours; even longer periods may be needed in some instances.

Blocking with ethylmaleilimide involves keeping the sections for four hours at 37°C in a 1.25% (0.1 M) solution of this compound in a Sörensen phosphate buffer of pH 7.4.

Blockage with sodium iodo-acetate may be carried out by treating the sections for about twenty hours, at 37°C, with a 0.1 M solution (about 2%) of iodo-acetic acid, adjusted to pH 8 with N/1 soda.

Blockage with chloropicrin is carried out at laboratory temperatures in a 0.5% solution of this compound in 30% alcohol; the period of action varies around four hours.

5° *The practice of histochemical tests for protein-bound sulphydryls*

The possibility of demonstrating protein-bound sulphydryls may suggest itself, *a posteriori*, during the examination of sections made with a view to other histochemical reactions or stains; valid results can be obtained in such cases with sections taken from the same tissue block provided that it is not material which has been osmicated or post-chromatised. In other cases, such tests represent the essential objective of the work and this requirement is known prior to the fixation of the pieces of tissue. The working technique thus varies according to whether the distinction between cysteine and cystine does or does not represent an essential objective of the work. In cases where this distinction forms an essential part of the work, we cannot avoid having recourse to alcohol-trichloracetic acid as a fixative, but it seems wise to me to control the results with a fixative such as Bouin's fluid which ensures better preservation of the tissue, without in any particular way stimulating the oxidation of cysteine into cystine. Recourse to Carnoy's fluid is also indicated, this latter fixative being clearly superior to Bouin's fluid so far as the "chemical" preservation of protein-bound sulphydryls is concerned, but distinctly inferior to it for the morphological preservation of certain secretory products (granulations of the pancreatic islet cells, neurosecretory products, pancreatic zymogene etc...).

In many cases the necessity of conserving certain structures, notably of secretory products or of cell organelles, compels us to forget about the distinction between cysteine and cystine, only total protein-bound sulphydryls being capable of identification after reduction of the sections by one of the techniques described in the preceding section.

As to the choice of reactions, I would recommend the ferric ferricyanide technique as a first approximation, its results being controlled by the method of Lillie and Glenner using p-N,N-dimethylaminophenylmercuric acetate and the technique of Barrnett and Seligman using DDD.

In all cases where the reduction of the sections is not imposed by the choice of fixative it is advisable to carry out the histochemical detection, properly speaking, simultaneously on slides some of which have undergone the reduction of disulphide links to thiol groups, whereas the others have simply been dewaxed and brought into water at the required moment. It is the comparison between these two sets of slides which allows us to evaluate by difference the part played by proteins bearing disulphide groups in the result of attempts to detect total protein-bound sulphydryls. In any case, the results should be controlled by blocking reactions with one of the techniques mentioned in the preceding section. Naturally, this blockage should take place prior to what, properly speaking, is the histochemical reaction but after the reduction in cases where it is intended to examine the validity of the histochemical technique.

We can thus set out the operations in the following scheme.

a) **Detection of protein-bound sulphydryls** (thiol groups only): using material fixed in Carnoy's or Bouin's fluid or in trichloracetic acid-alcohol compare the results obtained on the one hand with sections which have directly undergone the reaction and on the other hand on sections which have undergone the reaction after blocking; positive results without blocking and negative results on sections which have undergone this treatment can be attributed with safety to the presence of thiol groups.

b) **Detection of total protein-bound sulphydryls** (thiols and disulphides): after suitable fixation compare the results obtained, on the one hand with sections which have undergone reduction by one of the agents mentioned above, and on the other on sections which have undergone reduction and then blocking of the thiol groups. Positive results without blocking, and negative results after it, may be attributed to the presence of protein-bound sulphydryls or of disulphide groups, no distinction being possible between these two categories.

c) **Distinction between protein-bound sulphydryls and disulphide links:** after fixation in a fluid which allows us to detect thiols without reduction compare the results obtained on the one hand by the use of histochemical reactions directly practised, their validity being controlled by blocking reactions, and on the other through reduction followed by the same histochemical reactions, the validity of the result being tested by a blocking reaction inserted between reduction and what properly speaking is the histochemical reaction. Positive results before and after reduction disclose the presence of thiol groups, those which do not appear until after this reduction disclose the presence of disulphide groups.

DEMONSTRATION OF ELECTROPOLAR FEATURES OF PROTEINS

The histochemical techniques which allow us to explore the electropolar features of tissue constituents (the histochemical study of acidophilia, of basophilia, and estimation of the zone of the isoelectric point) were described in Chapter 13 of this work. Their use is not restricted to proteins; but since these compounds are the principal amphoteric constituents of the animal cell such procedures are particularly valuable for them, although the histochemical study of polysaccharides also benefits greatly from their application.

TESTS FOR ACIDOPHILIA AS A METHOD FOR THE IDENTIFICATION OF PROTEINS

Primary amine groups are the most numerous of the electropositive (basic) radicals of the animal cell; two other radicals with the same charge, namely imidazol and guanidyl groups, serve equally with them to account for the acidophilia of tissue proteins and it is easy to understand why histologists have tried to detect and even to undertake a semi-quantitative estimation of proteins, especially histones, through the demonstration of their acidophilia under well defined experimental conditions, that is to say by staining solutions whose pH is distinctly lower than the pH of the carboxyl radicals so as to ensure the ionisation of all electropositive groups.

Such facts justify the practice of classical histologists who agreed that highly acidophilic structures were rich in proteins; they find their expression in techniques for the estimation of total acidophilia in the sense of Lison (1960) the principles of which, and in particular Deitch's (1955) method, were dealt with in Chapter 13.

Tests for acidophilia under very special conditions of pH, different from those which have just been mentioned, were put forward by Alfert and Geschwind (1953) for the selective demonstration of histones. Because basic radicals predominate in the lateral groups of these proteins their isoelectric point is distinctly higher than that of other proteins, whence the theoretical possibility of demonstrating them using an acid stain acting at a pH which is sufficiently high to suppress the acidophilia of other proteins through the ionisation of all the carboxyl groups, whereas the amine groups on the other hand pass into the unionised condition. The desire to avoid any competition between the basic groups of the proteins to be demonstrated, and the nucleic acids, led the authors of the method to carry out a trichloracetic acid extraction prior to staining. Fast green FCF is used as the anionic stain. The technique thus includes the following stages.

Paraffin wax sections taken from material fixed for 3 to 6 hours in neutral 10% formalin, washed in running water, and then embedded in the usual way; dewaxed, treated with collodion and brought into water;

Extract the nucleic acids by keeping the sections for 15 minutes, over a steam bath, in a 5% aqueous solutions of trichloracetic acid;

Wash with 3 baths of 70% alcohol, each of 10 minutes duration, and then in distilled water;

Stain for 30 minutes with the solution
 distilled water .... 100 ml
 fast green FCF .... 0.1 g
0.1 N soda as required to make a solution of pH 8.1 (a very small quantity suffices);

Wash for 5 minutes in distilled water;

Dehydrate in 96% alcohol and then absolute alcohol, clear in a benzenoid hydrocarbon and mount in a synthetic resin.

Structures containing basic proteins (in particular histones and protamines) are stained green; the method is capable of histophotometric applications.

A formula of Spicer and Lillie (1962) rests on the same principle, but these authors do not carry out the trichloracetic acid extraction of the nucleic acids, replacing the fast green FCF of the stain bath by Biebrich scarlet and dissolving this stain in soda-aminoacetic acid buffers of the required pH, using a 0.01% concentration. The staining lasts for 30 to 90 minutes, the sections being then dehydrated directly in alcohol, cleared and mounted in a synthetic resin.

The technique using bromphenol blue (Mazia, Brewer and Alfert, 1953) is derived from Durrum's stain (1950) put forward for the identification of protein spots in microelectrophoretic bands. The staining soluton contains 1 gram of mercuric chloride and 0.05 grams of bromphenol blue in a 100 ml of 2% acetic acid; it is allowed to act for 25 hours at laboratory temperatures prior to washing for 5 minutes with 0.5% acetic acid, the dehydration which precedes mounting in a synthetic resin being carried out in tertiary butanol.

Most modern authors agree in seeing only staining with an acid dye in this technique; there is no argument if favour of any specificity whatever of this procedure for proteins.

THE EVALUATION OF THE TISSUE ZONE OF THE ISOELECTRIC POINT IN THE HISTOCHEMICAL STUDY OF PROTEINS

The approximate estimation of the zone of the isoelectric point using variations of the acidophilia and basophilia of the structures as a function of the pH of the stain bath have been discussed and described from the technical standpoint in Chapter 13 of this work, so that we need not dwell on it longer. Only the bearing of this method on the histochemistry of proteins needs to be considered here.

Even making full allowance for all the criticisms formulated in respect of Pischinger's method, it still remains one of the most valuable for defining certain characteristics of the proteins contained in this or that structure. It is indeed true that the procedures carried out prior to the staining itself may displace the isoelectric point of tissue proteins and that this displacement does not necessarily occur in the same sense for all the proteins in a section; the chemical constitution of the stain, the ionic strength of the stain bath and other factors discussed in the corresponding section of Chapter 13 should not, indeed, be forgotten, and we should not expect to deduce an isoelectric point identical with that measured by electrocataphoresis from changes in the affinity for dyes as a function of pH. However, such reservations do not detract from the true significance of the method which is to furnish the histochemist with a precise and easily codifiable means of comparing the proteins contained in tissue or cell structures. Moreover, experience shows that displacements of the isoelectric point resulting from pretreatments are constant for any given protein; the conditions of the stain itself are easy to codify rigorously. A curve showing staining as a function of the pH, which presents notable features as compared with the "average", may then become a criterion for the identification of any given protein; any quite disparate behaviour of the structures contained in the same sections during staining at suitably chosen pH values may indicate an important difference in the chemical constitution or in the physico-chemical characteristics of the substances responsible for the dyestuff affinities under examination. Merely by visual inspection of the preparations the histologist can begin to discriminate between the cell and tissue constituents; an objective study of absorption curves, obtained under conditions compatible with quantitative work may become in the future one of the essential elements in the histochemical study of tissue proteins.

THE IDENTIFICATION OF CERTAIN PROTEINS BY ENZYMATIC DIGESTION

The selective attack on certain structures by enzymatic preparations represents a very old method, much to the taste of histologists at the end of the 19th century, and subsequently fallen into desuetude. Recent authors have tried to restore this procedure to favour, applying it to the histochemistry of proteins, in an attempt to profit by the commercial availability of highly purified or even crystalline enzymatic preparations. Trypsin, chymotrypsin and pepsin, collagenases and elastase are the principal enzymes recommended for the histochemical study or proteins.

However tempting the method may be from the theoretical standpoint, and despite the achievement of substantial successes in other domains of histochemistry through the use of enzymatic preparations as reagents (amylase, sialidase, ribonuclease, etc...), its value for the histochemistry of proteins is as yet slight.

The principal difficulty that arises during the use of proteolytic enzymes as histochemical reagents lies in the contamination of these preparations by other enzymes. We may follow Lison (1960) in remarking that the older histologists considered that digestion by trypsin was one of the essential characteristics of nucleins, this error being explained by the contamination of almost all commercial preparations of trypsin then on the market by ribonuclease. In fact, crystalline trypsin has no effect whatever on ribonucleins. But even crystalline preparations cannot be guaranteed from this point of view. It is, indeed, known that crystalline trypsin is usually contaminated with collagenase (Reech, 1954).

Moreover, the procedures undertaken prior to section cutting may substantially modify the properties of the proteins contained in various structures; their attack by enzymes may be rendered easier or hindered because of chemical or physico-chemical changes undergone during fixation or during the other manipulations to which the pieces of tissue have been subjected. Consequently, the results obtained by in vitro biochemical work, often on purified proteins, cannot be directly transposed into the domain of histochemistry.

It is thus essential when using enzymes for the histochemical identification of proteins to take account of the reservations some of which have been set out in timely fashion by Lillie (1965).

The difficulty of purifying enzymes prevents us from considering the destruction of any given structure by an enzymatic preparation as constituting a formal proof of the presence in that structure of the specific substrate of the enzyme used. Conversely, the absence of attack on a particular structure by an enzyme whose effectiveness has been demonstrated does indicate that the substrate of the enzyme in question is absent from that structure. Naturally the specificity of the enzymatic action should be verified by controls in which the solvent is used alone or the enzymatic preparation is subjected to the action of a specific inhibitor, controls which should be without effect on the structures studied. Moreover, any possible modification of the chemical and physico-chemical characteristics of structures containing the substrate for the enzyme should be examined by causing the enzyme to act on sections taken from pieces of tissue fixed in various fixatives and, where necessary, by having recourse to freeze drying as a technique for the preparation of the sections.

Trypsin (optimal pH 7 to 8), *chymotrypsin* (optimal pH around 8) and *pepsin* (optimal pH around 2) are endopeptidases capable of hydrolysing the peptide link not only at the extremity of polypeptide chains but within these chains. Trypsin acts primarily on peptide links which involve the carboxyl group of basic amino-acids, such as lysine and arginine, whereas pepsin attacks links involving the carboxyl groups of dicarboxylic acids (aspartic and glutamic acids); chymotrypsin primarily attacks liaisons which involve the carboxyl groups of aromatic amino-acids. The presence in most tissue proteins of all three types of amino-acid just mentioned removes much of the value from this distinction at least in so far as it relates to the histochemical identification of proteins.

Lillie (1965) gives the following technical details for the use of these enzymes.

Fix the tissues to be studied in absolute alcohol, Carnoy's fluid, or a formalin alcohol mixture, for a period not exceeding 18 hours; avoid prolonged fixation in aqueous media at all costs; never use material fixed in fluids with a potassium bichromate base;

Embed in paraffin wax (avoid the use of celloidin), cut into sections, spread and dewax as usual; the use, for enzymatic digestion, of sections which have not been dewaxed may be considered;

Treat control sections with the solvents alone, namely
0.01 M phosphate buffer of pH 7.6 containing 0.01% of sodium fluoride and 0.4% of sodium chloride for the trypsin;
0.1 N hydrochloric acid for the pepsin;
a 0.01 M phosphate buffer of pH 7.6 for the chymotrypsin and the papain;

Treat the sections subjected to digestion with the same solvents in which the enzymatic preparation has been dissolved at a concentration of 0.1%;

Undertake the stage of digestion at 37°C for a time varying between 30 minutes and 16 hours according to circumstances;

Submit control preparations and those treated with enzymes to techniques intended to demonstrate the structures under investigation.

Collagenase, an enzyme of microbial origin, selectively attacks collagen, reticulin and gelatin. It has yet to be isolated in the pure state. Its action is suppressed by fixation in formalin; material which is to be digested by it should, then, be fixed in alcohol. The activity of the preparations varies a great deal according to the strain of *Clostridium* the filtrates from cultures of which have been used for the extraction. The optimum pH is near neutrality for most preparations of microbial collagenase; inactivation by phosphate base buffers has been mentioned by certain authors and Lison (1960) suggests the use of borate buffers to regulate the pH. The duration of action cannot be laid down and trial and error methods are necessary when collagenases are used for histochemical purposes; the ease with which collagen fibres can be identified by a whole series of procedures markedly detracts from the value of collagenases as a means of detecting collagen histochemically.

Elastase, an enzyme which selectively attacks elastin and the keratohyalin granules of epidermal cells, can be extracted from commercial preparations of trypsin in which it is a contaminant (Balo and Banga, 1949, 1950). The optimum pH is of the order of 9, the action being fairly rapid (less than 1 hour at 37°); unlike preparations of collagenase, elastase is not inactivated by phosphate so that Sörensen buffers, sodium acetate buffers or sodium bicarbonate buffers dan be used.

Modern work shows (see Loven, 1963 for a bibliography) that elastase is in reality a complex of enzymes and that at least part of its action is not on the molecules of proelastin but on the mucopolysaccharide cement which links them to one another.

The histochemical applications of elastase attack seem to be of the slightest and it scarcely seems likely that this enzymatic digestion will have much of a future in vertebrate histochemistry, since the vertebrates are animals whose elastic tissue has well defined characteristics which are easy to demonstrate; the use of this procedure may be worth-while in the study of the connective fibres of various invertebrates, especially molluscs and arthropods.

THE IDENTIFICATION OF PROTEINS BY DIFFERENTIAL SOLUBILITY

The distinction of classes or proteins by means of solubility differences plays an essential role in the biochemical study of these compounds but this is in no way the case in their histochemical study. As was the case with digestion by enzymes, the extraction of proteins using appropriate solvents was fashionable with the older histologists and a reading of the works of P. G. Unna (see in particular the article by this author in the 2nd edition of the "Enzyklopädie der mikroskopischen Technik", 1926) illustrates the aberrations which may stem from an excessive enthusiasm for refining pretreatments of the tissues and the staining of sections. More recent attempts at extraction have been followed not by stains but by general reactions for proteins yet objections of principle need to be formulated with respect to any such methods.

Naturally extraction carried out on sections taken from fixed tissue is meaningless when it comes to the identification of proteins; the denaturation of these compounds and their immobilisation is the very objective of fixation by chemical substances; it seems justified to apply the method solely to sections which have not been denatured and which are taken from freeze dried tissue or to unfixed cryostat sections.

Even in this case however theoretical objections arise; in fact, the degree of solubility of any given protein in the solvent used varies according to the type of macromolecular association, and the solubility of the structured protein, *in vivo*, is not necessarily identical with that of the extracted and purified protein that the biochemist studies. From the chemical point of view the association of proteins with other compounds may completely modify its solubility characteristics, this particular trap being common to questions of the solubilisation of proteins and that of other classes of compounds met with in histochemical work. From the morphological point of view, many tests of solubility, which necessarily need to be practised on fresh tissue or on sections which have not been denatured and have been obtained after freeze drying, alter the structures to the point of depriving their histochemical examination of all validity.

The use of techniques for differential solubilisation is thus restricted to very special cases and even there valid results are not generally obtained except in association with histochemical, physiological and biochemial techniques; the work of Barrnett and his colleagues on the adenohypophysial hormones provides us with an example of this.

It does, then, seem to me to be legitimate to suggest that these techniques have not so far ensured themselves a place in modern histochemical practice.

CHAPTER 20

HISTOCHEMICAL DETECTION OF NUCLEOPROTEINS AND METALLOPROTEINS

The desire to avoid excessive fragmentation of the subject matter leads me to bring together, into a single chapter, methods the practical importance of which is considerable together with techniques which are only occasionally used; it so happens that the demonstration of nucleic acids represents one of the most important chapters for the histochemist, whereas the detection of chromoproteins containing metals has only a limited part to play. This association is, however, justified from the point of view of chemical classification, because in both cases we have to deal with heteroproteins in the sense of the older nomenclature (conjugated proteins of English speaking authors) which contain not only proteins but prosthetic groups.

HISTOCHEMICAL DETECTION OF NUCLEIC ACIDS

From the chemical standpoint, nucleoproteins represent an association of basic proteins (protamines, histones) with nucleic acids which are polynucleotides whose degree of polymerisation varies from one to the other. The fundamental unit of the nucleic acids is the mononucleotide which contains one molecule of phosphoric acid, one molecule of pentose, ribofuranose in the case of ribonucleic acid, deoxyribofuranose in the case of deoxyribonucleic acid, as well as a purine base (adenine, guanine) or a pyrimidine base (thymine, uracil, cytosine).

Numerous general reviews set out the degree of progress recently achieved in the chemistry and biochemistry of nucleic acids. The work of Chargaff and Davidson (1960) competently puts together what was known at that time. The number of more recent publications is such that any attempt to list them would be condemned in advance to be absurdly incomplete. Because of their topicality, the essential biochemical ideas concerning nucleic acids will, therefore, be supposed to be known.

Among the histochemical techniques used for the study of nucleoproteins, some aim at detecting the essential amino-acids of basic protein of the histone type (the tyrosine and arginine reactions) or at demonstrating some of their electropolar features. These methods were studied in Chapter 18.

Other techniques attempt more particularly to detect nucleic acids and to put to good use the characteristics of the three constituents of the mononucleotides, namely the purine or pyrimidine bases, ribose or deoxyribose, and phosphoric acid.

The detection of nucleic acids by absorption histospectrography in the ultraviolet depends on the presence of purine and pyrimidine bases: this technique has been the subject of a magnificent series of investigations by Caspersson and his school. Such detection permits of no discrimination between deoxyribonucleic and ribonucleic acids.

The presence of the phosphoric acid radical confers an electronegative character on the nucleic acids and thus explains their basophilia. Numerous methods have been put forward for the demonstration of this basophilia which in no case takes on the value of a chemical reaction because the nucleic acids are far from representing the only category of basophilic compounds that one is liable to meet in sections of animal tissue. This amounts to saying that the results so obtained must be subject to control by other methods. Basophilia, in itself, permits of no distinction between the two classes of nucleic acids, such a distinction can however be obtained through the selective extraction of ribonucleic acid. It is, moreover, appropriate to recall that staining with mixtures of basic dyes allows us to confer different colours on the sites of the two nucleic acids, the results of such stains having an undoubted diagnostic value but needing confirmation by tests involving extraction.

The presence of a carbohydrate (deoxyribose, ribose) in the molecule of the mononucleotide is put to good use for the detection of nucleic acids by certain colour reactions of monosaccharides which often give rise to different colours for the two types of nucleic acid. Moreover, the chemical constitution of deoxyribose shows us that it is possible to liberate carbonyl groups by careful acid hydrolysis so that it becomes possible to detect deoxyribonucleic acid using reagents for aldehydes; such are the nucleal reactions.

DEMONSTRATION OF NUCLEIC ACIDS THROUGH THEIR ULTRAVIOLET ABSORPTION

The study of nucleic acids represents the principal field of application of ultraviolet absorption microspectrography; the general principles of the method were described in the chapter devoted to histophysical techniques and there is no need to devote more space to the subject. Such methods, which are very sensitive, are of excellent chemical specificity because the nucleic acids are the only ones, of all the compounds endowed with a strong absorption in the region of 2,600 Å, to be preserved in paraffin wax sections. A controlled extraction (10 minutes in 5% cold trichloracetic acid) is sufficient to allow this detection to take place and gives every guarantee required by a quantitative study (Panijel, 1951).

The substantial interest attaching to the method resides in the possibility of making a quantitative study of the nucleic acids, particularly of ribonucleic acid which is only capable of qualitative investigation by other histochemical techniques. There are numerous sources of error; various procedures have been devised for taking these into account and for limiting their effects. Some of these sources of error were mentioned in relation to the outline of the general principles of ultraviolet absorption microspectrography. In any event, the equipment needed for this type of work is such that only specialised research establishments can follow it up seriously. I feel, therefore, that there is no point in giving details of techniques which are only handled in an up-to-date fashion by a small number of narrow specialists.

The absorption curves of deoxyribonucleic and ribonucleic acids show no noticeable differences; the distinction between the two types of nucleic acids must, therefore, be undertaken by tests involving extraction, notably using adequately purified enzymatic preparations, and by the practice of nucleal reactions.

DEMONSTRATION OF NUCLEIC ACIDS THROUGH THEIR BASOPHILIA

The selective staining of "nucleins" by basic dyes has been well known to histologists since the end of the nineteenth century and a large number of topographical or cytological techniques depend on this basophilia. Many progressive or regressive techniques intended to demonstrate selectively the nuclei and the different cytoplasmic sites of ribonucleic acid (the ergastoplasm, the Nissl body, etc...) depend on the use of basic dyes, thiazines of the thionine family, safranine, cresyl violet, safranine and the basic triphenylmethanes being the most widely used. We might mention that an affinity for a haematoxylin lake, whether progressive or regressive, cannot in any way be automatically considered as if it were a true basophilia.

Merely knowing the mechanism of the basophilia of nucleic acids should deter us from a useless discussion about the supposed "specificity" of this dyestuff affinity for the compounds in question. Obviously, other acid groups present in the sections can retain cationic dyestuffs through the same mechanism as do the nucleic acids and only an exclusive study of objects in which the nuclei and ergastoplasm respresent the sole sites of substances of an acidic nature can explain the enthusiasm with which renowned research workers have maintained that certain dyes, such as methyl green or gallocyanine, are "specific" for nucleic acids. However, when the disappearance of this basophilia after enzymatic or non-enzymatic extraction supplements the result of staining by itself, the total result is highly significant and allows us to affirm that nucleic acids are present in the basophilic structures.

From the technical standpoint, the methods mentioned in relation to the study of tissue basophilia in general (p. 339) give good results in the case of nucleic acids. It is obviously desirable to work at a rather low pH, distinctly below the isoelectric point of the common tissue proteins, when we need to demonstrate nucleic acids with a high degree of selectivity; using safranine and thiazines of the methylene blue group very good results are obtained by staining in a medium buffered to pH values between 3.75 and 4.2; Walpole buffers with sodium acetate-acetic acid or McIlvaine-Lillie buffers using disodium phosphate -citric acid are quite suitable. I might mention how useful it is to stabilise the stain with ammonium molybdate when thiazines are used (thionine, toluidine blue, azur, etc...).

Two basic dyes deserve special mention, namely methyl green and the chromic lake of gallocyanin; these have indeed a particularly high selectivity for nucleic acids. Moreover, staining with the chromic lake of gallocyanin has substantial practical advantages and has been suggested with a view to quantitative studies. Although less advantageous, staining with methyl green has also been used by some authors for histophotometric research.

Staining nucleic acids with the chromic lake of gallocyanin

Gallocyanin is a stain of the oxazine group whose introduction as a nuclear stain, in the form of the chromic lake, dates back to Becher (1921); the chromic lake of gallocyanin was recommended by Einarson (1932) for demonstrating the Nissl bodies of the nerve cell and it is generally recognised at the presen time as being one of the most useful of the selective stains for nucleic acids.

We must firmly declare, at the outset, that the chemical significance of an affinity for gallocyanin is in no way superior to that of any other way of detecting basophilia. The chromic lake of this oxazine is a dyestuff but not a histochemical reagent and the results obtained, in common with the detection of basophilia in general, fall into the group of marker stains. Even a quick examination of mammalian tissue shows that sulphomucins and mast cell granules stain with the chromic lake of gallocyanin with an intensity in no way inferior to that with which nucleic acids stain; the stain obtained in the two cases is slightly different with most commercial samples of gallocyanin.

Even though the chemical significance of staining with gallocyanin is in no way superior to that attributed to the stains obtained with other basic dyestuffs, the practical advantages of the method are substantial. Indeed the stain is quite easy to prepare and keeps well (2 to 3 months); staining is fully automatic and requires no supervision; the duration of staining is not critical, the results scarcely varying for durations between 24 hours and one week; once obtained, the stain withstands the action of acids, alkalis and all the organic solvents used for dehydration and mounting the preparations. Staining with gallocyanin therefore represents the ideal method in instances where numerous slides need to be stained serially, strictly equivalent and perfectly reproducible results being obtained without any intervention of the experimenter. We might add to this that work done by Sandritter's school (1953 to 1955) shows that there is indeed a stoichiometric relationship between the intensity of the stain and the amount of nucleic acid present in the models used for the experiments in question. Despite the reservations formulated by Lison (1960) who objected to the practice of transposing such results, obtained *in vitro*, to the practical conduct of histophotometry on sections, the working conditions following gallocyanin staining seem, *a priori*, more favourable than they are when any other stain is used, for in such cases the stoichiometric relationship which has just been mentioned certainly does not exist.

The chromic lake of gallocyanin is prepared by dissolving 0.15 g of the stain in 100 ml of a 5% aqueous solution of chrome alum; the mixture is brought to the boil and simmered for 2 to 3 minutes; there is a wide tolerance for this stage of the operation because lengthening the simmering to 20 minutes in no way changes the quality of the stain (Sandritter and Diefenbach, 1953). The solution is then chilled and filtered; I would recommend a 24 hour wait prior to filtration as experience shows that a rather fine precipitate can form, sometimes several hours after the boiling has been arrested; if filtration is carried out too early it will then have to be done again the next day. The volume of the filtrate is made up to 100 ml. This staining lake keeps for several months.

The staining itself is of the simplest and involves the following stages.

Paraffin wax sections, taken from material fixed in one of the ordinary fixatives (avoid pieces of tissue treated with osmium and those which have undergone prolonged postchromatisation), dewaxed, treated where appropriate with collodion, and hydrated; the method may be applied to celloidin sections provided that they are stuck to slides and that the embedding material is dissolved away;

Keep the sections for 24 to 48 hours (even if this period is substantially exceeded no untoward effects will ensue) in the chromic lake of gallocyanin whose preparation was described above;

Wash for 5 minutes in running water;

Dehydrate in absolute alcohol, clear in a benzenoid hydrocarbon and mount in Canada balsam or in a synthetic resin.

The preparations keep extremely well; structures containing basophilic compounds take on a bluish-black colour which is highly advantageous from the optical point of view. It is both possible and useful to use background stains consisting of acid yellow dyestuffs, Van Gieson's picrofuchsin or picric acid-thiazin red in cases where the work is done for morphological purposes; they are not generally employed when the preparations are made with a view to studying the nucleic acids.

A disadvantage common to staining with the chromic lake of gallocyanin and all other histological stains is the need to have at one's disposal a commercial sample of the dye of high quality.

The pH of the chromic lake of gallocyanin, prepared according to the instructions given above, is around 1.64. In consequence, only acid groups which are ionised under these conditions of pH are demonstrable by the staining technique just mentioned. According to Einarson (1951), the pH of the staining solution may be lowered to 0.83 by the addition of N/1 hydrochloric acid or raised to the region of 4 by the addition of N/1 soda. Evidently such manoeuvres are devoid of practical interest when the staining is conducted to demonstrate nucleic acids. I might mention that solutions of gallocyanin rendered alkaline with soda do not keep for more than 7 days.

The staining of nucleic acids using methyl green

The staining of nuclei with methyl green was recommended by Carnoy as early as 1879 and under certain experimental conditions it may be of remarkable selectivity; the use of this substance of the triphenylmethane group is advocated in a whole series of formulae. Those which serve purely morphological ends are discussed in that part of this work which deals with general cytological technique; only the applications of methyl green to the histochemical study of nucleic acids are mentioned here.

Although it is true that methyl green stains the nuclei with great selectivity and that this dyestuff affinity seems to be linked to the presence of a deoxyribonucleic acid whose degree of polymerisation exceeds a certain threshold many other structures take up this stain. The granulations of mast cells, certain mucins, the ground substance of cartilage are the best known examples, but it would be easy considerably to extend this list. Contrary to an idea which is not only inaccurate but very widespread, methyl green, *used alone*, intensely stains structures rich in ribonucleic acid. The selectivity of this stain for nucleic acids is certainly not greater than that of thiazines of the methylene blue group.

To these findings we have to add the practical disadvantages of methyl green. The great majority, not to say the entirety, of commercial samples of the stain are contaminated with methyl violet so that it is necessary to extract this impurity in all instances where pure stains are desired and, *a fortiori*, when the stain is used as a marker technique for the presence of nucleic acids. The purification in question puts to good use the great solubility of methyl violet in chloroform, which is a liquid which does not dissolve methyl green. Many authors recommend chloroform extraction of the aqueous solution of methyl green in a separating funnel, a procedure which has the disadvantage of leaving the experimenter in ignorance of the effective concentration of methyl green in the solution which he will use for critical purposes. It seems to me by far preferable to follow the recommendations of Pollister and Ris (1946) by carrying out the extraction on powdered methyl green. The required amount of the stain is shaken with two to three volumes of chloroform in a glass recipient; it is better to use several small amounts of the solvent rather than to increase the volume and reduce the number of samples added. When chloroform extraction gives only a colourless or very pale violet liquid, the powder, after separation by decantation, is rapidly dried in an oven and then dissolved in distilled water to a concentration of 1%. Experience does indeed show that aqueous solutions of methyl green keep very well whereas methyl green, when dry, is progressively transformed into methyl violet.

It is also appropriate to mention that methyl green is very sensitive to alkalis so that it is helpful to preserve the solutions in waxed flasks or in hard glass (pyrex, jena) receptacles. Stains made with this substance generally keep rather poorly, this state of affairs being scarcely improved by the substitution of the currently available synthetic resins for Canada balsam; this is probably due to destaining under the influence of the alkali liberated into the medium by the soft glass of the carrier slide.

The requirements of methyl green in terms of the fixation of the tissue are greater than are those of most of the basic dyes mentioned in this chapter. Staining always fails on material treated with osmium and gives poor results after postchromatisation; fixatives with a picric acid base do not allow us to obtain correct stains, a fact which is, in all probability, due to the depolymerisation of deoxyribonucleic acid under the influence of the fixative. Material fixed in formalin or in formalin-treated alcohol also gives mediocre results. The most suitable media are Clarke's and Carnoy's fluids and mixtures with a corrosive sublimate and acetic acid base.

Among staining techniques, only that due to Pollister and Leuchtenberger (1949) is mentioned here. The stain recommended by these authors differs from the classical Pappenheim-Unna mixture using methyl green-pyronine in the absence of this latter stain.

Paraffin wax sections taken from material fixed in Clarke's or Carnoy's fluids, dewaxed, treated with collodion where appropriate and hydrated;
Stain for 15 minutes with the mixture
    1% aqueous solution of methyl green .... 25 ml
    phenol .... 0.5 g
    glycerine .... 20 ml
    96% alcohol .... 25 ml
    distilled water .... 100 ml
(keeps well in a pyrex flask in the dark);
Rinse in iced distilled water;
Blot with tissue paper;
Dehydrate in two baths of tertiary butyl alcohol (total duration 12 hours);
Clear in a benzenoid hydrocarbon, mount in a synthetic resin or where necessary in Canada balsam.

When a quantitative study is not the object of the staining the dehydrating step preceding the mounting may be carried out with absolute alcohol.

This staining process results in a very selective demonstration of polymerised deoxyribonucleic acid provided that the precautions mentioned above have been taken following the fixing of the tissue. Its value as a diagnostic technique is no greater than that of any other method of detecting basophilia using other dyes and its use in histophotometric studies has given rise to quite vigorous criticism (Mayersbach, 1956; Lison, 1960).

In practice, the demonstration of nucleic acids by virtue of their basophilia is a marker stain; its value is undoubted but the results do not take on their full significance until controls by extraction have shown that the basophilia in question is indeed due to these acids and not to other anionic groups present in the structures. The practical interest attaching to staining with thiazines, used at a rather low pH value, is that of rapidly providing very clear preparations, in which structures rich in sulphomucopolysaccharides are simultaneously demonstrated because of their metachromasia. The advantage of the gallocyanin rests in the absolute security with which the method can be conducted in the absence of any differentiation and in the great resistance with which the stain withstands all the reagents used in histological technique. It is therefore this latter technique which is the method of choice in all cases where we need to demonstrate nucleic acids on a large number of slides the homogeneity of whose staining is required.

DEMONSTRATION OF NUCLEIC ACIDS BY STAINING WITH TWO BASIC DYES

The principal method of this group, and the only one which most histochemical works mention, was developed empirically. It was in 1899 that Pappenheim noticed the green colour of the nuclei and the red colour of the basophilic cytoplasm, notably of these of the plasmocytes, obtained by treating blood smears or sections of haematopoietic organs with a solution containing two basic dyestuffs in water-alcohol solution, these dyestuffs being, a triarylmethane, methyl green, and pyronine, a substance which belongs to the xanthene group. The initial formula of Pappenheim was developed by Unna (1910) through the introduction of a small quantity of phenol into the dye bath so that it is customary to describe staining with methyl green-pyronine under the name of the Pappenheim-Unna method. When used on a small scale, principally in the study of mammalian haematopoietic organs, this technique enjoyed a considerable vogue following the work of Brachet (1940, 1941) to whom we owe the substantial merit of having introduced control techniques involving ribonuclease preparations. Even though the green colour of nuclei stained with methyl green is not specific for deoxyribonucleic acid, and the affinity for pyronine is of no greater significance than is that of ribonuclein for any other basic dye, the detection of pyroninophilia, abolished by treatment with ribonuclease, allows us formally to affirm the existence of ribonucleic acids in the structures stained with pyronine.

The mechanism of this "differential basophilia" which is highly advantageous from the morphological point of view has remained unknown for several years; the question has as yet not been entirely clarified but experimental work enables us to attempt an interpretation. We do in fact know (Gerola and Vannini, 1948, 1949; Mayersbach, 1956) that when used alone each of the two dyes of the Pappenheim-Unna mixture is capable of staining the two kinds of nucleic acids but that these two dyes differ slightly in the way in which their staining capacity is modified when the pH of the solution changes. The affinity of structures rich in nucleic acids diminishes substantially when the pH of the methyl green solution is lowered below 4.3; with solutions of pyronine this decreasing affinity only takes place in the region of pH 2.8. In the same way, it is staining with pyronine which predominates at low pH values when a mixture of the two stains is used, whereas staining with methyl green predominates at high pH values. It seems, therefore, legitimate to consider that basophilic structures stain with pyronine when they do not fix methyl green and do not stain with pyronine when they do fix methyl green. The pH range between 4 and 5 comprises the "favourable" zone in which the distribution of the two stains between structures which are primarily rich in deoxyribonucleic acid or which contain ribonucleic acid results in the desired differentiation of colour. There is in this way an *a posteriori* justification for the introduction of a small amount of phenol into the dye bath.

The technique of staining with methyl green has undergone a substantial number of modifications, a fact which, of itself, illustrates the practical difficulties with which various experimenters have met in the course of carrying out the technique.

The first essential feature, which many authors have been wrong to neglect, is the fixation of the tissues. Staining with methyl green-pyronine never succeeds on material treated with osmium or postchromated; it is impossible to carry it out after fixation in liquids with a picric acid base; fixation in formalin gives rise to very mediocre preparations and formalin-alcohol is hardly better. The best solution is to fix the pieces of tissue for a rather short period (less than 24 hours) in Clarke's or Carnoy's fluids; a *short duration* fixation in Zenker's fluid or, better, in those of Helly, Maximow, or Regaud, is compatible with the use of the Pappenheim-Unna stain; fixing in alcohol is suitable as a preparatory stage for staining but the results are disastrous from the morphological standpoint and alcohol fixation cannot therefore be recommended. I might mention that these observations concerning fixation relate solely to stages preparatory to Pappenheim-Unna staining and have no bearing on the problem of maintaining the nucleic acids *in situ;* it is almost impossible to obtain the desired result after fixing in Bouin's fluid whereas staining with toluidine blue or gallocyanin succeeds well under these conditions.

The quality of the stains used, in particular that of pyronine, is a factor bearing on the success of the process, a factor which often lies outside the control of the experimenter. All publications dealing with the technical problems stress the need to use a pyronine sample capable of withstanding aqueous washing and, if possible, alcoholic dehydration. I might add that the best brands of this stain are no longer available on the European market; the only practical solution consists in trying out a sufficient number of samples from various sources and keeping those which are satisfactory. Evidently, methyl green should undergo the chloroform extraction intended to remove methyl violet from it.

The technique for staining itself does not have the importance which many authors have seen fit to accord it. When fixing has been properly chosen and carried out, when the dye bath has been prepared with materials of good quality, Unna's technique gives results which in all respects are the equivalent of those of more highly developed methods, notably those which involve working in a buffered medium. I should therefore say, at the risk of appearing retrograde and reactionary, that my preference is for the original formula. The techniques of Kurnick (1955) and Lison (1960) are nevertheless mentioned here so that I should not be accused of favouritism.

Staining with methyl green-pyronine (Unna's technique):

> Paraffin wax sections, taken from material fixed as noted above, dewaxed, treated with collodion where appropriate and hydrated;
> Stain for 5 minutes at laboratory temperatures with the solution
>
> | | |
> |---|---|
> | methyl green (extracted with chloroform) | 0.15 g |
> | pyronine G (Y) or B | 0.25 g |
> | 96% alcohol | 2.5 ml |
> | phenol | 0.5 g |
> | glycerine | 20 ml |
> | distilled water .... to make up to | 100 ml |
>
> (dissolve the solid ingredients in the water-alcohol-glycerine mixture, and keep *away from light* in a hard glass flask (pyrex, jena); it keeps for several months);
> Rinse very rapidly in distilled water (optional);
> Blot with tissue paper;
> Dehydrate rapidly in absolute alcohol, clear in a benzenoid hydrocarbon and mount in a synthetic resin or in Canada balsam.

Nuclear structures containing deoxyribonucleic acid stain a more or less obvious green according to the sample of methyl green used; the nucleoli and cytoplasmic structures containing ribonucleins stain an intense red; such colours do not represent histochemical reactions. In fact, mucins stain either with methyl green or with pyronine, the latter giving, according to the sample used, a more or less clearcut yellow metachromasia. Other structures containing acid groups may take up one or other of the dyes, only control extractions allowing us to be sure of the identification of nucleic acids.

Over-staining of the cytoplasm in a diffuse pink may occur with some of the older formulae put forward for purely morphological ends and may be avoided by reducing the staining time to five minutes; the authors of such methods did, indeed, have in mind an alcoholic (96%) differentiation which cannot be considered when the method is used for histochemical purposes. According to Lillie (1965), the small amount of 96% alcohol added to the stain is without effect whereas the phenol and glycerine are important.

Staining with methyl green-pyronine (Kurnick's technique). — This author's formula involves chloroform extraction of the methyl green and of the pyronine. 2% aqueous solutions of these stains are therefore extracted in separating funnels with chloroform until all the impurities have passed into the latter solvent.

Paraffin wax sections, treated with collodion where appropriate and hydrated;
Stain for 6 minutes with the mixture
- methyl green solution .... 7.5 ml
- pyronine solution .... 12.5 ml
- distilled water .... 30 ml

Blot with tissue paper;
Dehydrate in 2 baths of normal butyl alcohol, each lasting for 5 minutes;
Clear in xylene;
Treat for 5 minutes with white cedar wood oil;
Mount in a synthetic resin.

Staining with methyl green-pyronine (Lison's technique). — This variation of the method involves the preparation of a stock solution (1.5 g of methyl green, 2.5 g of pyronine, 200 ml of distilled water) which has been subjected to chloroform extraction. Staining takes place at the temperature of melting ice, thus increasing the intensity of the stains. Dehydration is carried out with tertiary butanol.

Paraffin wax sections, dewaxed, treated with collodion and hydrated;
Stain for 30 to 60 minutes, in the cold, with the mixture
- stock solution .... 20 ml
- M/10 phosphate buffer, pH 4 to 5.5 .... 20 ml
- distilled water .... 60 ml

Rinse for 2 to 3 seconds in running water;
Blot with tissue paper;
Dehydrate, with stirring, for 5 seconds in tertiary butyl alcohol;
Clear in xylene and mount in a synthetic resin.

The staining in the cold was inspired by the finding of Rosenbaum and Deane (1959) that staining with basic dyes has a negative temperature coefficient, that is to say is favoured by low temperatures. This precaution, the long duration of the staining and the extreme rapidity of the dehydration advised by Lison might lead us to think that this author had at his disposal, when he was developing his variation of the staining technique, a particularly poor quality sample of pyronine.

From the histochemical standpoint, the methyl green-pyronine method is not superior to other techniques capable of detecting basophilia; its great worth resides in the clear cut distinction between the two groups of nucleic acids. With this in mind the technique renders considerable service when nuclear structures are being studied and I rather tend to consider it as being quite irreplaceable in difficult cases. Its value is still further increased by the ease with which control reactions involving enzymes can be used, at least so far as ribonucleic acid is concerned.

Various authors have tried to replace one or other of the mixed stains in the Pappenheim-Unna formula by related compounds. In this way iodine green, ethyl green (a chloroform extraction is useful in both cases) or malachite green (the fast green of certain suppliers not to be confused with fast green FCF which is an acid stain) have been put forward to replace methyl green. The pyronine can be replaced by acridine red; this substitution, in my opinion, is of only minor interest because the same practical problems arise as in the case of pyronine when it comes to obtaining suitable samples.

NUCLEAL REACTIONS

It is customary to designate under the name of nucleal reactions those which depend on the presence of ribose or deoxyribose in the mononucleotides. These two carbohydrates may be detected by virtue of the different colours obtained through a condensation reaction with 9-methyl (or 9-phenyl)-2,3,7-trihydroxy-6-fluorone as used in the method of Turchini, Castel and Khau Van Kien (1943), the only nucleal reaction to give positive results with the two groups of nucleic acid. The other reactions only reveal the presence of deoxyribose and permit no more than the detection of deoxyribonucleic acid. In both cases the first stage of the reaction is a controlled acid hydrolysis which as a first step detaches the purine bases (adenine, guanine), and then in a second step the pyrimidine bases (thymine and cytosine of deoxyribonucleic acid, uracil and cytosine of ribonucleic acid) attached to carbon atom 1 of the sugars mentioned above.

The nucleal reaction of
Turchini, Castel and Khau van Kien

This reaction is not used very often, the reason for its restricted use being, doubtless, the need to synthesize the reagent. Such a process is no longer necessary as 9-methyl-2,3,7-trihydroxy-6-fluorone and the corresponding phenyl derivative is commercially available in the pure state.

As I noted above, the principal interest of the technique is that of ensuring the simultaneous demonstration of the two nucleic acids. However, the specificity of the reaction is less well established than is that of the other nucleal reactions so that histochemists tend to be somewhat reticent about it. We need also to consider that the duration of the acid hydrolysis recommended by Turchini and his colleagues to obtain the "nucleal" reaction on the one hand or for demonstrating ribonucleic acids (the "cytoplasmal" reaction) on the other hand are rather different so that the real point of the method, namely the simultaneous detection of the two types of nucleic acids, is not always attained. This hydrolysis is effected by N/1 hydrochloric acid in an alcoholic medium (concentrated hydrochloric acid, d - 1.19, 8.25 ml, 96% alcohol to make up to 100 ml), at laboratory temperatures; Table 18 sets out the durations recommended for any given fixative and according to the result desired.

Table 18. — DURATION (in minutes) OF THE HYDROLYSIS FOR THE REACTION OF TURCHINI, CASTEL AND KHAU VAN KIEN

Fixative	Nucleal reaction	Cytoplasmal reaction
Helly	22 to 25	16 to 18
Zenker	18 to 22	15 to 18
Navachine	20 to 25	16 to 20
Sanfelice	20 to 25	16 to 20
Carnoy	7 to 9	5 to 7
Formol	7 to 8	5 to 7
Bouin	7 to 8	5 to 7

The hydrolysis recommended by Blackler and Alexander (1952) is much more vigorous; these authors recommend hydrolysis in an aqueous medium, using normal hydrochloric acid, at 60°C, the time varying between 5 and 12 minutes. This way of proceeding gives better results, in my personal experience, than does hydrolysis at laboratory temperatures but the optimum time varies with the way in which the tissues have been fixed and needs to be adjusted by trial and error.

Similarly, the conduct of what is, properly speaking, the reaction itself is easier to standardise when Blackler and Alexander's technique is followed; it is therefore the one whose adoption I would recommend.

   Paraffin wax sections, dewaxed, treated with collodion and hydrated;
   Hydrolyse at 60°C with normal hydrochloric acid;
   Wash for several seconds (15 to 20) in 80% alcohol;
   Treat for 4 to 14 hours (10 hours on an average) with the solution
      9-phenyl (or 9-methyl)-2,3,7-trihydroxy-6-fluorone .... 0.5 g
      96% alcohol .... 99 ml
      concentrated sulphuric acid 1   ml
      (filter before use);
   Treat for 2 minutes with a 1% aqueous solution of sodium carbonate;
   Wash for 2 minutes in distilled water;
   Dehydrate with a mixture of equal parts of acetone and water and then with pure acetone;
   Clear in a benzenoid hydrocarbon and mount in a synthetic resin.

Under these conditions deoxyribonucleic acid gives a stain varying between blue and purple, ribonucleic acid staining reddish or orange. Evidently all those controls which depend on the selective extraction of one or the other of the nucleic acids may be applied.

We may mention that alcoholic dehydration, recommended in the original formula, results in some extraction of the stain; it is possible that the introduction of dehydration with acetone is the main factor capable of explaining the superiority of Blackler and Alexander's variation.

The nucleal reaction of Feulgen and Rossenbeck

This technique, which was invented in 1934, is one of the most valuable available to the histochemist. A large number of publications are devoted to it; in addition to works dealing with histochemical techniques, the reviews of Lessler (1953), and of Kasten (1960, 1961, 1962) are a great help in directing attention to the literature dealing with the chemical mechanism and the biological significance of the reaction of Feulgen and Rossenbeck; evidently, only those ideas which are essential and which are of some practical consequence can be discussed here.

The reaction of Feulgen and Rossenbeck (the mention of these two names is not merely just but helps to avoid confusion with the reaction of Feulgen and Voit (which is the plasmal reaction)) involves two essential stages, namely the hydrolysis whose effect is to liberate purine bases, and subsequently pyrimidine bases, and the detection, by means of a reagent for aldehydes, that of Schiff, of the carbonyl group so produced.

> The chemical interpretation of the technique has given rise to much debate, because the deoxyribose does not bear a carbonyl group; however, the use of any of the blocking reactions shows that it is indeed an aldehyde function which is detected in the second stage of Feulgen and Rossenbeck's method. Most modern authors consider, with Overend and Stacey (1949), that the liberation of carbon atom 1 of the deoxyribose renders possible an equilibrium reaction between the furanose form of this pentose and its aldehyde form, this latter being responsible for restoring the colour of the Schiff reagent.
>
> The history of the reaction of Feulgen and Rossenbeck is strewn with periodical attacks led either by chemists or by histologists, such attacks tending to cast doubt on the chemical specificity or the localising value. It would serve no useful purpose to deal with this subject at length because Feulgen and Rossenbeck's nucleal reaction has survived all such attempts and all modern authors agree in according to it great chemical specificity and a substantial localising value. This specificity is, obviously, only valid when both stages of the method are taken into account; it is the entire sequence of acid hydrolysis-appearance of the red colour under the influence of the Schiff reagent, which represents the nucleal reaction of Feulgen and Rossenbeck; contrasts with a control slide which has not been hydrolysed will avoid errors of commission represented by the presence of free aldehydes in the preparation.

From the practical point of view, the two stages of the reaction need to be considered separately, all the more so because numerous authors have suggested the replacement of the Schiff reagent by other substances capable of detecting the presence of carbonyl groups.

a) In the original technique **the hydrolysis** is carried out on sections of tissue fixed with liquids which contain neither aldehydes nor oxidising agents; it should be conducted at 60°C, in Normal hydrochloric acid (concentrated hydrochloric acid, $d=1.19$ 8.2 ml; water to make up to 100 ml). The optimal duration should be determined by trial and error.

Each of these points has undergone substantial changes; the use of fixatives containing formalin or oxidising agents is without harmful effect, the hydrolysis may be practised at other temperatures and with other acids, the duration of the hydrolysis, lastly, may be determined exactly by prior experiment especially after certain fixatives have been used.

The choice of **the fixative** for the nucleal reaction of Feulgen and Rossenbeck is dictated by a variety of considerations. It is obviously desirable to have an impeccable preservation of the structure since the study of the preparations will be dealing with fine morphological detail. Moreover, the duration of hydrolysis is strictly conditioned by the fixation, the margin of tolerance as compared with the optimum being slight after certain fixatives and much larger after others; it is obviously this second condition which is the most advantageous. Some fixatives, in particular Bouin's fluid and that of Duboscq-Brazil entrain a marked depolymerisation of the deoxyribonucleic acid and their use is not advisable for this reason. As in many other cases, the best histochemical results are obtained when fixatives recognised as being the best from the cytological point of view are used.

Most modern authors conduct their hydrolysis by means of normal hydrochloric acid, at 60°C, for periods which have been set out by Bauer (1932). Table 19, which is made up from the data of various authors and my own personal experience, summarises these recommendations.

Table 19. — DURATION OF THE HYDROLYSIS BY MEANS OF NORMAL HYDROCHLORIC ACID AT 60°C (LIQUID PREVIOUSLY BROUGHT TO THIS TEMPERATURE)

Fixative liquid	Duration (in minutes) of the hydrolysis		
	minimum	optimum	maximum
Apathy	4	5	8
Bouin-Allen (B15)	19	22	40
Bouin-Allen-sublimed	10	14	25
Carnoy	4	6	8
Champy	16	25	40
Clarke	4	6	8
Flemming	16	36	60
Formol	5	8	12
Heitz	16	25	40
Helly	4	8	16
Maximow	4	8	16
Petrunkevitch	2	3	6
Regaud	6	14	60
Sanfelice	3	6	60
Heidenhain's Susa	12	18	25
Telliesnitzky	8	12	20
Zenker	4	5	12

In this table the minimum time corresponds to the period for which the sections remain uncoloured when passed through the Schiff reagent, the optimum corresponding to that which generally gives the most intense stains, and the maximum to that beyond which a considerable weakening of the reaction sets in.

The particularly long period needed to obtain the maximum stain after fixing in Flemming's fluid deserves special mention; Lison (1960 p. 368) and Pearse (1960, p. 823) recommend a hydrolysis for 16 minutes when using this fixative but this is indeed a copying error and corresponds in fact to the minimal time suggested by Bauer.

Bouin's fluid does not appear in this table and its use is not recommended; in cases where the nuclear reaction of Feulgen and Rossenbeck has to be applied to material fixed in this fluid I would recommend a very short hydrolysis (2 minutes); the period of 12 minutes recommended by Lison (1960, p. 368) is undoubtedly a printer's error which escaped correction in the proofs; it will indeed ensure the complete extraction of the deoxyribunucleic acid which will already have been considerably depolymerised during fixation.

It is imperative not to forget that the choice of the hydrolysis time is in fact a compromise; in effect, the extraction of the purine bases with the liberation of potential aldehyde groups goes hand in hand with the depolymerisation of the nucleic acids and their extraction; histones are also extracted. Such extraction will be the determining factor when the hydrolysis is too prolonged, a possibility to be avoided at all costs when carrying out the reaction because it results in the weakening, and eventually the disappearance, of the stain in structures containing deoxyribonucleic acid.

From the practical point of view it is evidently best to use those fixatives for which the difference between the optimum hydrolysis time and the maximum time tolerated is the greatest and I would recommend the use of such fixatives whenever the need to use the nucleal reaction can be foreseen at the time the tissue is fixed; an examination of Table 19 clearly shows that such fluids are, moreover, excellent cytological fixatives and this fact is certainly more than a coincidence.

The replacement of hydrochloric acid by other acids has been suggested by a certain number of authors, Sharma (1951) uses trichloracetic acid, Di Stefano uses perchloric acid, Hashim (1953) uses phosphoric acid; the practical advantages of such substitutions are not at all evident. The method of Barka and Dallner (1956) deserves special mention from this point of view because the duration of the hydrolysis may vary between 15 and 60 minutes without any noticeable influence on the intensity of the final stain. These authors dehydrate the dewaxed sections with alcohol and then pass them through carbon tetrachloride and hydrolyse them at laboratory temperatures with a solution of 1 ml of bromine in 39 ml of carbon tetrachloride. The sections are washed at the end of the hydrolysis in carbon tetrachloride and passed into absolute alcohol, hydrated, treated with a 5% aqueous solution of sodium thiosulphate, and washed in running water and then subjected to the action of the Schiff reagent. The only practical disadvantage of the method is the need to handle a toxic and volatile substance whose use and storage in the laboratory requires precautions which it would perhaps be better not to impose on those not familiar with chemical manipulations.

Much more promising are the recent attempts to conduct the hydrolysis at laboratory temperatures. This way of working was already advised by Di Stefano (1952) for perchloric acid hydrolysis and by Hashim (1953) for phosphoric acid hydrolysis and has been applied to hydrochloric acid hydrolysis by Itikawa and Oguro (1954), Kasten (1960), Jordanov (1963), and Decosse and Aiello (1966). These latter authors used 5 N solutions of hydrochloric acid acting at laboratory temperatures, the concentration of acid corresponding substantially to that recommended by their precursors. A histophotometric study confirms the impression obtained from simple visual inspection of the preparations by the authors just cited, namely, that the preservation *in situ* of the deoxyribonucleic acid is much better after hydrolysis at laboratory temperatures, the factor of temperature playing the principal role in the extraction which takes place during hot hydrolysis. In the experiments of Decosse and Aiello, which were conducted on blood smears fixed with a mixture of 85 parts of methanol, 10 parts of formalin, and 5 parts of acetic acid, the maximum intensity of the nucleal reaction is obtained after hydrolysis in N/1 hydrochloric acid, in the warm, at the end of 12 minutes and there is a significant drop after the 24th minute. With hydrolysis at 26° in 5 N hydrochloric acid, the reaction reaches its peak after 40 minutes of hydrolysis and only begins to diminish after 120 minutes in the acid bath.

Obviously this greater tolerance is highly advantageous and it would be most interesting to conduct trials on various materials, with simultaneous variation of the fixatives used.

However this may be, the hydrolysis should be stopped by washing in cold water whenever it has been practised with a dilute acid; in the case of Barka and Dallner's technique it is washing in carbon tetrachloride which terminates the action of the bromine.

b) **The action of the Schiff reagent** calls for no particular comment; it takes place in the way set out in Chapter 14. Any of the formulae recommended for the preparation of the Schiff reagent will serve; my personal preference is for that of Graumann; the reagent of this author is less rich in hydrochloric acid than the others, so that there is less risk of hydrolysing the deoxyribonucleic acid of the control sections. Recommendations as to the duration of the reaction vary a great deal from one author to another; in practice it is never useful to exceed one hour when the reaction is carried out on sections. Washing in sulphur dioxide water is recommended by most histochemists; it may be replaced by very vigorous washing in distilled water when the nucleal reaction of Feulgen and Rossenbeck is carried out on thin sections, but should be regarded as a necessity when working with thick sections and, *a fortiori*, when using blocks of tissue.

Various background stains can be used after the nucleal reaction of Feulgen and Rossenbeck. Most authors recommend staining with a dilute solution (0.01% or less) of light green which is a rather summary procedure. Rapid passage (10 to 15 seconds) through picro-indigocarmine (p. 201) gives preparations in which the staining is comparable with that produced by Ramon y Cajal's trichrome, with the exception that the red stain is strictly limited to structures containing deoxyribonucleic acid. Yet more highly polychrome preparations can be obtained by treating the sections, following the practice of Huber (1946), with phosphotungstic acid and a mixture of aniline blue and orange G as used in Heidenhain's azan. The passage through phosphotungstic acid can be reduced to 10 minutes, that in Heidenhain's blue should not exceed 5 minutes because of the risk that the aniline blue will invade the nuclei.

When Feulgen and Rossenbeck's reaction is practised for histochemical purposes the sections can be mounted without background staining and this procedure is necessary on any occasion when a histophotometric study is the objective of the work.

As I have mentioned it is the entire hydrolysis-Schiff reaction which characterises the nucleal reaction of Feulgen and Rossenbeck. The results should therefore be compared with control slides which have undergone only the action of the Schiff reagent. The hydrolysis associated with the acidity of this reagent may constitute a source of error; it is therefore advisable not to prolong unnecessarily the period spent by the control slide in the bath of reagent.

It is appropriate to mention that the nucleal reaction of Feulgen and Rossenbeck can be carried out on pieces of tissue and gives excellent bulk staining. Voss (1926) advises the following periods of action for mice embryos at the 15th to 16th day of gestation:

Hydrochloric hydrolysis	75 minutes in normal hydrochloric acid at laboratory temperatures;
idem.	105 minutes in an oven at 55°C;
Washing with sulphur dioxide water	15 to 20 minutes at laboratory temperatures;
Schiff reagent	4 to 5 hours at laboratory temperatures;
Washing in sulphur dioxide water	16 to 18 hours at laboratory temperatures

Dehydration with alcohol, clearing and embedding in paraffin wax without special precautions; pieces of tissue of sufficiently small size may be mounted *in toto*.

The nucleal reaction on paraffin wax sections is conducted in the following way:

- Sections taken from material fixed as required by the needs of the method, dewaxed; *treated with collodion,* and hydrated;
- Hydrolysis with hydrochloric acid in an oven at 60° for a time which varies with the fixative used; the temperature requirements are very strict, a drop of one or two degrees resulting in a substantial increase in the duration of the hydrolysis;
- Wash in tap water;
- Apply the Schiff reagent (it is of no advantage to exceed one hour in general);
- Wash in sulphur dioxide water or, very vigorously, in distilled water;
- Wash in running water (5 minutes);
- Where appropriate, stain the background with light green, picro-indigocarmine or phosphotungstic acid-Heidenhain's blue;
- Dehydrate in absolute alcohol, clear in a benzenoid hydrocarbon and mount in a synthetic resin or in Canada balsam.

As I have remarked, the specificity of the method is considerable and we know from a whole series of investigations that losses during hydrolysis are insignificant provided that the periods recommended for this stage of the reaction are not exceeded. A stoichiometric relationship exists between the deoxyribonucleic acid content and the intensity of the stain so that the nucleal reaction of Feulgen and Rossenbeck represents the epitome of techniques for use in histophotometric studies.

All modern authors agree in recognising that Feulgen and Rossenbeck's reaction occupies pride of place in the development of our knowledge relating to the nucleic acids and that cytology, physiology, biochemistry, and genetics have greatly profited from the results acquired through its use. However, some consider that its practical importance is not very great. Pearse (1960, p. 194) considers that "for the histologist Feulgen's reaction is less useful in practice than theoretical considerations would suggest. Most usually we need to apply it solely to be able to say with certainty that any given basophilic inclusion does not contain deoxyribonucleic acid." This assertion is not at all surprising coming from a worker who is largely experienced with the techniques of pathological anatomy, the daily task of which is the examination of human tissue and of that of the few mammals currently used in physiological experiments, but it is very far from corresponding with reality. Even if the exploration of the main mammalian tissues no longer has surprises for us so far as the nuclear structures are concerned, it is quite otherwise in numerous invertebrate tissues where the analysis of the nuclear structures would be impossible without the nucleal reactions; comparative histology offers us a rather large number of examples of nuclei whose very identification as such cannot be made with certainty without employing nucleal reactions. It seems therefore legitimate to me to affirm that the nucleal reaction of Feulgen and Rossenbeck, together with related procedures, represents, now as in the past, a group of techniques which any histologist who seeks to work outside the narrow framework of mammalian tissue is called upon to use virtually day by day.

Other nucleal reactions

The methods requiring mention in this section differ from the nucleal reaction of Feulgen and Rossenbeck in the means adopted for showing up the aldehyde groups liberated during hydrochloric acid hydrolysis, that is to say that all the technical considerations relating to the first stage of the method remain valid.

Some of the replacements for Schiff's reagent by other means for detecting aldehydes are mainly of theoretical interest because their success confirms the chemical mechanism of the reaction, which was briefly set out in the preceding section; this is true of Pearse's technique (1951), which was itself derived from a technique used by Danielli (1947) involving 2,4-dinitrophenylhydrazine and also the use of alkaline silver complexes with which various authors have experimented (Bretschneider, 1949; Bradfield, 1954; Jurand and coworkers, 1959; Bryan, 1964). Danielli's technique consists in detecting the aldehyde groups with 2,4-dinitrophenylhydrazine after hydrochloric acid hydrolysis, whereas Pearse's consists of practising this detection with 2-hydroxy-3-naphthoic hydrazide after the same hydrolysis. The technical recommendations given in Chapter 14 suffice to carry out these reactions whose practical interest is slight. The same remark seems to me to hold good for methods involving the silver complexes which are neither more reliable nor more specific than that of Feulgen and Rossenbeck; from the theoretical standpoint, it is appropriate to mention that some authors have, until quite recently, contested the very possibility of detecting thymic acid (apurinic acid) through the reduction of alkaline silver complexes by its aldehyde group. Lison (1960, pp. 168 and 367) still maintains this point of view.

Other replacements, notably those which draw upon equivalents of the Schiff reagent have, on the contrary, a far from negligible practical bearing either because they give more intense stains than does the reaction of Feulgen and Rossenbeck, and so facilitate the study of certain details of the structure, or because the use of a stain other than a red one allows us to combine the nucleal reaction with other stains or histochemical reactions, whilst preserving its chemical significance.

It is this possibility which illustrates the usefulness of reagents equivalent to that of Schiff, already mentioned in the chapter dealing with the detection of carbonyl groups; we must not lose sight of the fact that the earliest of these equivalents was developed precisely with a view to the use envisaged here. Among the numerous possible combinations three have sufficient practical bearing to be described here, namely the nucleal reaction with thionine- (or azur A)-sulphur dioxide (DeLamater, 1948, 1951), the technique of Himes and Moriber (1956) and that of Benson (1966).

The nucleal reaction with thionine- (or azur A)-SO$_2$ of DeLamater. — In this technique the equivalent of the Schiff reaction is a 0.25% aqueous solution of thionine or azur A to which, prior to use, thionyl chloride has been added (One drop for 10 ml of the thionine solution, two drops for 10 ml of azur A); the reagents keep poorly and one should not prepare substantial amounts in advance. DeLamater's formula, developed for studies on unicellular organisms and microbes, does not employ a background stain; when it is applied to the study of metazoan tissue it is obviously useful to complement the demonstration of deoxyribonucleic acid with a cytoplasmic stain; from my own personal experience Van Gieson's picro-fuchsin gives very good results, the technique for applying it being comparable with those already described in relation to the selective staining of collagen fibres. Naturally, any other red cytoplasmic stain can be used provided that the staining is of short duration with sufficiently dilute solutions to avoid clogging the preparations. The working technique thus involves the following stages.

> Dewaxed sections, treated with collodion and hydrated
> Carry out hydrochloric acid hydrolysis following the recommendations given in relation to the nucleal reaction of Feulgen and Rossenbeck;
> Wash in distilled water;
> Treat for about one hour with a freshly prepared solution of thionine-thionyl chloride or azur A-thionyl chloride;
> Rinse in sulphur dioxide water or, very vigorously, in distilled water;
> Wash for 5 minutes in running water;
> Stain the background with Van Gieson's picrofuchsin or with any other cytoplasmic stain giving good contrasts with the nuclear stain;
> Dehydrate in absolute alcohol, clear in a benzenoid hydrocarbon and mount in a synthetic resin or in Canada balsam.

We may remark that the addition of thionyl chloride does not result in the decolorisation of the initial solution as in the case of the Schiff reagent; but this solution nevertheless acquires the properties required.

The results of the technique are comparable with those of the nucleal reaction of Feulgen and Rossenbeck with the exception that the staining of the structures containing deoxyribonucleic acid is more intensely blue, very deep and highly favourable to the study of fine details of the structure. In most cases strongly acid mucosubstances also take up a strongly metachromatic stain which cannot, however, represent a source of error.

Himes and Moriber's technique. — This excellent method, which should be most widely deployed, brings together a nucleal reaction and the PAS reaction, a combination already suggested by Van Duijn (1956) but the basic proteins are further stained with naphthol yellow S. The technique uses the following **reagents**:

a) azur A-SO_2: dissolve 1 g of azur A in a 100 ml of bleaching fluid (see below); this keeps for several weeks provided that prior to each use several drops of a 10% aqueous solution of potassium or sodium metabisulphite are added;

b) bleaching fluid: add 5 ml of a 5% aqueous solution of potassium or sodium metabisulphite and 5 ml of normal hydrochloric acid to 90 ml of distilled water (this reagent should be prepared afresh prior to use);

c) periodic acid: dissolve 0.8 g of periodic acid in 90 ml of water and add 10 ml of a 0.2 N aqueous solution of sodium acetate (this solution keeps rather poorly and should be prepared fresh prior to use);

d) Schiff's reagent: the authors of the technique recommend that this should be prepared according to Stowell's formula but any of the others will do;

e) naphthol yellow S solution: dissolve 1 g of the stain in a 100 ml of 1% acetic acid (this keeps indefinitely; it should be diluted at the time of use with 1% acetic acid in the proportions of 1/50; the dilute solution keeps distinctly less well than the stock solution).

The working technique involves the following stages:

Paraffin wax sections, treated with collodion where appropriate and hydrated;
Hydrolyse with normal hydrochloric acid at 60°C following the recommendations given in relation to the nucleal reaction of Feulgen and Rossenbeck;
Rinse carefully in distilled water;
Treat with azur A-SO_2 for 5 minutes at laboratory temperatures;
Rinse in distilled water;
Treat with 2 baths of the bleaching fluid (2 minutes for each bath);
Rinse in distilled water;
Oxidise for 2 minutes in periodic acid;
Rinse in running water;
Treat for 2 minutes with Schiff's reagent;
Rinse in distilled water
Treat for 2 minutes in each of 2 baths of bleaching fluid;
Wash in running water;
Stain for 2 minutes in the diluted naphthol yellow S solution;
Rinse in water;
Blot with tissue paper, dehydrate with 2 baths, each of 10 minutes, of tertiary butyl alcohol, clear in a benzenoid hydrocarbon, mount in a synthetic resin or in Canada balsam.

The nuclei are stained blue or green, the structures containing PAS-positive compounds in red, those containing basic proteins are yellow.

Benson's method. — This recent technique depends on the same principles as does that of Himes and Moriber but differs in the addition of an alcian blue stain so that it is capable of demonstrating mucopolysaccharides and acid mucins in a fashion comparable to that of Mowry's method using alcian blue-PAS; the nucleal reaction is conducted with azur A-SO_2 and the staining of structures rich in acid proteins with Deitch's naphthol yellow S is maintained.

The following **reagents:** are involved.

a) azur A-SO_2: dissolve 0.5 g of azur A in a 100 ml of a bleaching fluid containing 5 ml of normal hydrochloric acid, 5 ml of a 10% aqueous solution of sodium metabisulphite and 90 ml of water; the content of azur A is therefore half as much less than that of Himes and Moriber's technique;

b) alcian blue solution: dissolve 0.1 g of alcian blue 8GX in a 100 ml of 0.01 N hydrochloric acid and adjust the pH to 2 by the addition of a small amount of hydrochloric acid or of soda;

c) Schiff's reagent: it is recommended that this be prepared according to Stowell's formula but the others will serve;

d) periodic acid: a 0.5% aqueous solution of this compound;

e) naphthol yellow S: dissolve 0.01 g of the stain in a 100 ml of 1% acetic acid.

The **working technique** is also close to that of Himes and Moriber's method.

> Paraffin wax sections, treated where appropriate with collodion and hydrated;
> Hydrolyse in 5 N hydrochloric acid at laboratory temperatures; the optimum time, which is about 9 minutes under Benson's experimental conditions using pieces of tissue fixed in 10% formalin containing 0.5% of cetylpyridinium chloride, should be determined by trial and error and its adjustment represents the critical stage of the technique;
> Wash for one to two minutes in running water;
> Treat for 10 minutes in azur A-SO_2 solution;
> Wash in 2 baths, each of 10 minutes, of the bleaching fluid;
> Wash for one to two minutes in running water;
> Stain for 10 minutes with the alcian blue solution;
> Rinse in 0.01 N hydrochloric acid for one minute;
> Wash in running water for one to two minutes;
> Oxidise with periodic acid for 5 minutes;
> Wash in running water for one to two minutes;
> Treat with the Schiff reagent for 10 minutes;
> Wash in 2 baths, each of 2 minutes, of the bleaching fluid;
> Wash in running water for one to two minutes;
> Stain with a dilute solution of naphthol yellow S for one to two minutes;
> Wash in 1% acetic acid for 2 minutes;
> Blot with tissue paper, dehydrate with tertiary butanol, clear in a benzenoid hydrocarbon and mount in a synthetic resin or in Canada balsam.

Structures containing deoxyribonucleic acid are stained an intense blue, acid mucosubstances stain clear blue or green, and PAS-positive compounds stain red or violet whereas formations containing basic proteins stain yellow.

The weak point of the method is obviously the use of azur A and alcian blue in the same stain; because of this the hydrochloric acid hydrolysis must be adjusted with the greatest care or else we shall obtain too clear a blue stain or even a greenish one in structures containing deoxyribonucleic acid so that the demonstration of the nuclei will be poor; an insufficient hydrolysis will result in a purple nuclear stain which is also disadvantageous.

We may ask ourselves how far the return from the method may be improved by substituting alcian green for alcian blue; in the same way, essays carried out using a reagent equivalent to that of Schiff giving stains very different from those given by other reagents or stains might be well worth trying.

TECHNIQUES FOR THE EXTRACTION OF NUCLEIC ACIDS

We have mentioned several times in the preceding sections of this chapter that some of the techniques for demonstrating nucleic acids are of chemical significance only when they follow tests involving the selective extraction of the substances to be detected. This applies primarily to the detection of nucleic acids through their basophilia. An affinity for these latter compounds simply shows that there are electronegative groups in the stained structures and it is the disappearance of this dyestuff affinity after extraction which shows that it is indeed due to nucleic acids. We can therefore understand the essential part played by extraction techniques in the histochemical study of nucleic acids, especially when the presence of these compounds has not been disclosed by the nucleal reaction or by ultraviolet absorption microspectrography; but even these latter techniques benefit from being confirmed in really difficult cases through the action of specific enzymes or other agents capable of ensuring the selective extraction of nucleic acids.

Such extraction may be ensured with great selectivity using the enzymes ribonuclease and deoxyribonuclease; there are, moreover, techniques allowing the extraction by acids of the entirety of the nucleic acids; the selective extraction of ribonucleic acid by acids has also been suggested. We need to consider each of these techniques in turn.

Extraction with ribonuclease

Extraction with ribonuclease which selectively involves ribonucleic acid is the oldest of the histochemical applications of techniques for the extraction of nucleic acids. It was introduced by Brachet (1940) and raises the value of staining with methyl green-pyronine and that of other techniques for detecting basophilia to the level of histochemical reactions for ribonucleic acid.

In conformity with Greenstein's (1944) opinions, most modern authors consider ribonuclease as a depolymerase; its activity under the working conditions of the histochemist is therefore associated with the fragmentation of the macro-molecules of ribonucleic acid into entities of smaller size which can be dialysed and extracted from the sections with a solvent. Discussions have taken place as to the specificity of this action, discussions whose interest for the histochemist is slight since they concern the effect of highly purified preparations such as are rarely used in work with tissue sections. Even crystalline preparations are endowed with some proteolytic activity; it has, moreover, also been noted that very pure preparations of ribonuclease may, after hydrochloric acid hydrolysis, depolymerise and transfer into solution thymic (apurinic) acid, formed during the hydrolysis of deoxyribonucleic acid.

Nevertheless, such observations have no very great bearing on the histochemist's work; for him the commercial preparations of ribonuclease currently available are sufficiently selective for their correct application to afford him all the required guarantees. The older methods of preparation of active extracts starting from the pancreas have been almost entirely abandoned in favour of the purified samples available from industrial chemical firms; it is true that their cost is by no means negligible but the amounts used are so small that their careful employment will not bite too deeply into the laboratory budget.

From the technical standpoint, we may draw attention to a source of error common to extraction with ribonuclease and to that using other digestive enzymes, namely the simple dissolution of some substances by the solvent. In the particular case of ribonuclease we should not lose sight of the fact that fixing in Clarke's or Carnoy's fluids, which represent the best preparation for staining with methyl green-pyronine, will render the ribonucleins insoluble to an extent which is not sufficient for these compounds to withstand prolonged extraction in hot water. As a result the test should be of short duration when the material has been fixed with these fluids and should be supplemented by treatment of the slides with the solvent alone. Sections taken from material fixed in Bouin's fluid generally give rise to no dissolution of the ribonucleins so long as extraction with hot water does not last for more than two hours. In the case of slides taken from material fixed with a fluid having a potassium bichromate base even the ribonuclease treatment needs to be prolonged for several hours (Stowell and Zorzoli, 1947).

I am entirely in agreement with Lison (1960, pp. 390–391) in discarding some of the refinements recommended by certain authors as of no avail in the practice of digestion with ribonuclease for histochemical purposes. The use of distilled water as the solvent for the enzymatic preparation causes not the slightest harmful effect. The working technique should then be developed in the following way.

> Paraffin wax sections, dewaxed, *not treated with collodion* (even a very thin film of nitrocellulose will completely block the action of the enzyme), and hydrated;
> Treat in a high humidity, at 37°C, sections on slides which have undergone the action of the enzyme with a solution of purified commercial ribonuclease dissolved in distilled water to concentrations of 1/100,000 to 1/10,000; control sections should undergo, under the same experimental conditions, the action of distilled water alone; the duration of action should vary according to the fixative (less than one hour for material fixed in Carnoy's or Clarke's fluids, about 90 minutes for material fixed in Bouin's fluid, 3 hours for material fixed in Zenker's or Helly's fluids); avoid conducting the treatment at temperatures above 50°C which certain enzymatic preparations withstand very poorly;
> Rinse in distilled water;
> Undertake the staining chosen for demonstrating the basophilia simultaneously on slides treated with ribonuclease, with distilled water, and on slides which have been freshly dewaxed and hydrated.

Only that basophilia which exists on slides which have not been extracted, which is nevertheless entirely suppressed following ribonuclease treatment, discloses the presence of ribonucleic acid. The comparison of the slide treated with distilled water with that which has been subjected to the action of ribonuclease on the one hand or that which has been simply dewaxed and stained on the other hand allows us to discover whether any dissolution of the ribonucleins has taken place in the hot water.

> As I remarked above, the preparation of ribonuclease by the histochemist, beginning with the ox pancreas, is no longer of practical interest since satisfactory commercial preparations have been put on the market at a reasonable price. The technique for such extraction is nevertheless given for the sake of the record in case the obtaining of commercial ribonuclease gives rise to difficulties.
> Pass the freshly dissected ox pancreas through a mincer and suspend it in one or two volumes of 0.1 N acetic acid, allowing it to remain for about 12 hours; boil for 10 minutes and filter; neutralise the filtrate with soda, adjust the pH to 7.2 to 7.4; remove the precipitate which forms by filtering; dialyse for about 24 hours against distilled water; centrifuge and keep in a refrigerator without using toluene. This preparation keeps its activity for several weeks.

Extraction with deoxyribonuclease

This extraction by the depolymerase, acting selectively on deoxyribonucleic acid, has nothing like the same importance as has extraction by ribonuclease when regarded as a histochemical technique, this state of affairs being associated with several factors.

It so happens that the purification of deoxyribonuclease is much more difficult than is that of ribonuclease; as a result many commercial preparations are endowed with a proteolytic activity which renders them unsuitable for histochemical use; in any event the cost of deoxyribonuclease preparations considerably exceeds that of ribonuclease. The technique for purification, set out by McCarty (1946) and by Kunitz (1948), is too complicated to be used in laboratories which are not specialised in this topic.

Moreover, the effect on the sections is less regular than is that of ribonuclease. Apart from variations from one brand to another or from one sample to another numerous trials have shown that only material fixed with alcohol, with acetic acid or with mixtures of these two liquids are really suitable for the application of the extraction test. Many liquid fixatives—amongst these are the best cytological fixatives—render the tissue quite unsuitable for the extraction in question; it is generally agreed that such resistance to enzymatic action is associated with the links which deoxyribonucleic acids form with the proteins during fixation.

We may add that the need for control reactions using specific extractions is much less marked in the case of deoxyribonucleic acid than in that of ribonucleic acid because the nucleal reactions, in particular that of Feulgen and Rossenbeck, provide us with a truly specific demonstration of the first of these two acids.

Kurnick (1952) recommends the use of a solution of deoxyribonuclease containing 2 mg per 100 ml, the solvent being the tris-buffer of Gomori, of pH 7.6; the formula of Love and Rabotti (1963) recommends half that amount of the enzyme in the same buffer at pH 7.3, magnesium chloride being added as an activator. For material fixed in Carnoy's fluid the optimal duration of action is about 2 hours.

The general extraction of nucleic acids

Such extraction may be obtained by treating the sections, under well defined experimental conditions, with acids. The most fashionable acids for this purpose are trichloracetic and perchloric.

Trichloracetic extraction in the warm, as recommended by Schneider (1945), is an integral part of the technique due to Alfert and Geschwind for staining basic proteins with fast green FCF; it was mentioned in this context in Chapter 18. It is generally advisable to treat the dewaxed and hydrated sections or smears with a 5% solution of this acid in distilled water, using a water-bath at 90°C; the average duration of the reaction is 15 minutes, but it may be useful to adjust this, particularly in relation to the way in which the material has been fixed; it is not advisable to conduct this extraction after fixing in Flemming's fluid (Kaufman et al., 1954).

Perchloric extraction of the two nucleic acids is also carried out in the warm; following the investigations of Ogur and Rosen (1949) treatments for 20 minutes, at 70°C, with 10% perchloric acid are used.

These authors commented on the risk of a concomitant extraction of proteins but this danger does not seem to be great, the two procedures being fairly specific for nucleic acids. Their main application is however not the use as controls for the detection of nucleic acids but for removing these compounds during histochemical investigations on other substances in cases where the basophilia or electropolar nature of the nucleic acids may hinder the investigation.

Selective extraction of ribonucleic acid

This selective extraction of ribonucleic acid by mineral or organic acids, by buffer solutions and even by water has been put forward by several authors, particularly at the time when it was difficult to obtain sufficiently pure commercial samples of ribonuclease. All these procedures depend on the greater solubility of the ribonucleic acids. The methods in question are obviously less specific than is a direct attack by the ribonuclease; most of the substances suggested dissolve many of the compounds in the sections, such compounds bearing no relationship to the ribonucleins, and we can understand why they have been abandoned in favour of ribonuclease. It seems, however, useful to mention some of these procedures which may be of use as "emergency methods" in cases where the investigator has no ribonuclease at his disposal.

Normal hydrochloric acid used under the conditions for hydrolysis in the nuclear reaction extracts the whole of ribonucleic acids in 3 to 10 minutes at 60°C (Pouyet, 1949, Vendrely, 1949); the deoxyribonucleic acids are only extracted in a period ranging from 20 minutes to one hour.

10% perchloric acid, which ensures rapid extraction of all the nucleic acids when used in the warm, extracts ribonucleic acids in from 4 to 18 hours, at 4°C, the extraction of the deoxyribonucleic acids requiring a much longer period (Ogur and Rosen, 1949).

Nitric, hydrochloric and sulphuric acids, used at 4°C, in 2 M concentrations, ensure the same selective extraction.

Sörensen phosphate buffer, of pH 6.75, acting for 45 minutes at 58 °C, and the tris buffer of Gomori, of pH 7.5, acting at the same temperature for 2 hours, enable us to reach the same result (Seigel and Worley, 1951; Kurnick, 1952).

THE PREPARATION OF THE TISSUES
FOR DETECTION OF NUCLEIC ACIDS

Some of the requirements to be considered during the preparation of material intended for the histochemical study of nucleic acids are common for all histochemical investigations, these include the need to preserve the compounds we wish to investigate *in situ* and to respect the morphology of the tissues and cells. Moreover, some of the techniques reviewed in the preceding sections require fixation by special fixatives so that a knowledge of the methods required subsequently may be useful or even indispensable at the time the material is dissected.

We know from a coherent body of research that the preservation *in situ*, in the chemical sense of the term, of deoxyribonucleic acid at the time of fixation is satisfactorily secured by most of the usual fluids. Because of its polymerisation and the firm links which it forms with proteins this acid is easy to fix; once fixed it is kept in place and the procedures prior to section cutting hardly involve the risk of losses. But conservation in the morphological sense of the term is not equally good after all the fixative procedures and the quality of the preparation for nuclear reactions and other techniques must also be taken into consideration during fixation. It is essential to use Clarke's or Carnoy's fluids when the experimenter can foresee the need for methyl green-pyronine staining for the detailed analysis of complicated nuclear structures. These fluids ensure the best preparation for Pappenheim-Unna staining and the results of the nucleal reaction on sections prepared after this fixative are also acceptable. Bouin's fluid is suitable especially in cases where only tests for basophilia with controls involving extraction by ribonuclease form part of the project; it is indeed only a poor preparation for nuclear reactions and quite unsuitable for methyl green-pyronine staining. When nucleal reactions are the essential objective of the work, fluids such as those of Regaud, Sanfelice, and Flemming are entirely suitable; Champy's fluid also allows for very serviceable nucleal reactions but the size of the tissue pieces should be very small and one may encounter irregularities in the fixation.

The fixing of ribonucleic acids poses more complex problems, especially the cytoplasmic localisation of these compounds. Their degree of polymerisation, which is distinctly less than that of deoxyribonucleic acid, explains why they are lost by solution, expecially if the fixation is of long duration; some authors consider that these losses may also occur during the procedures preparatory to section cutting whereas others are quite confident in this respect. Decalcification practically always goes hand in hand with a more-or-less severe loss of ribonucleic acids; the technique for decalcification recommended by Hamberger and Hyden (1945), which consists of a short fixation in Carnoy's fluid, and then immersing the tissue blocks in a 0.05 M solution of lanthanum acetate in 20% acetic acid, is little used; it is, in any case, only suitable for very small blocks of tissue. As for the special requirements stemming from the techniques to be used, the employment of methyl green-pyronine necessitates the use of Carnoy's fluid, that of Clarke, or if need be those of Helly, Maximow or Regaud reducing as far as possible the period spent by the tissue blocks in these fluids. The other staining techniques reviewed in this chapter can be employed after any of the common fixatives. Whatever course is adopted, and whatever the fixative chosen, the ribonucleic acids are never rendered as insoluble as are the deoxyribonucleic acids and losses may take place even during treatment of the sections.

It may be helpful to note that fixing in formalin, whether dilute or saline, but without other fixatives incorporated, is not a very good preparation for the study of nucleoproteins.

Apart from the restrictions mentioned above, the techniques of handling preparatory to section cutting require no special consideration. Most of the techniques which allow us to study nucleoproteins involve paraffin wax sections but many of these methods are capable of accommodating celloidine sections from which the embedding material has been removed, or even frozen sections.

HISTOCHEMICAL DETECTION OF METALLOPROTEINS

In practical terms, the histochemical detection of metalloproteins reduces to the demonstration of haemoglobin. Despite the considerable interest attaching to their study, the other metalloproteins acting as respiratory pigments cannot be detected, in the present state of our knowledge, using histochemical techniques in which confidence can be placed. Only techniques for the detection of haemoglobin are therefore reviewed here, its metabolic products being discussed in the following chapter.

Tests for haemoglobin can be carried out either on fresh tissue or after fixation. It is the first of these two courses that offers the best guarantees of chemical validity, since histological fixatives do not always preserve this tetrapyrrolic pigment; however, the preparations so obtained are not permanent so that older techniques involving fresh tissue have been abandoned in favour of those which use fixatives.

Among the fixatives capable of preserving haemoglobin the best are Lison's formalin-lead acetate (1929) containing 90 ml of water, 10 ml of neutralised formalin and 2.5 g of lead acetate, as well as Slonimsky and Lapinsky's (1927) fixative involving formalin and potassium ferricyanide which contains 90 ml of water, 2 to 4 g of potassium ferricyanide and 10 ml of neutralised formalin. Neutralised formalin is also suitable; acid fixatives should not be used and the same is true of those which contain heavy metals.

The histochemical detection itself can be ensured either through histospectroscopy or by putting to good use the peroxidase properties of haemoglobin. We can add to these procedures those in which use is made of the particularly high isoelectric point of haemoglobin (Fautrez and Lambert, 1936).

HISTOSPECTROSCOPY

The histospectroscopic method involves either testing for the characteristic absorption spectrum of oxyhaemoglobin (about 5.400 and 5.800Å) using an ocular spectroscope, or the demonstration of the characteristic line at 4.150Å (Soret's line) using an ultraviolet spectrograph.

The use of an ocular spectroscope, as once practised, represents a first attempt which cannot be considered as truly histochemical since it does not permit us to localise material on the cellular scale. Ultraviolet spectrophotometry, on the other hand, has led to some important discoveries (Thorell, 1947; Carvalho, 1954; Barer et al., 1950); it even allows for the quantitative estimation of the amount of haemoglobin contained in an isolated cell. This technique obviously requires complex apparatus; it cannot be considered as a routine technique and is accessible only to specialised laboratories; it hardly seems worth while therefore for me to stress its use.

PSEUDO-PEROXIDASE PROPERTIES

Pseudo-peroxidase activity (the thermostable capacity for catalysing the transfer of hydrogen from a donor to a peroxide) is a feature of haemoglobin and of some of its derivatives (oxyhaemoglobin, carboxyhaemoglobin, methemoglobin, haematin, haemochromogen); it does not occur in haematoporphyrin, haematoidin or haematosiderin. Such properties, which it is easy to distinguish from the action of true peroxidases because they are thermostable (according to Lison (1960) they persist even after 20 minutes of heating at 180°C), can be put to good use for the detection of haemoglobin and its derivatives as set out above by any of the reagents for peroxidases. In practice we use certain of the benzidine reactions and in particular those procedures which involve zinc-leucobases. Fixing in formalin-lead acetate which transforms haemoglobin into haematin and fixing in formalin-potassium ferricyanide, which transforms it into methemoglobin are compatible with the conduct of these reactions as is fixing in neutralised formalin. Because of the sensitivity of haemoglobin to acids in the fixative, dilution of the formalin with a phosphate buffer is recommended. Lillie (1965) recommends mixing 100 ml of commercial formalin with 900 ml of distilled water and adding 4 g of anhydrous monosodium phosphate together with 6.5 g of anhydrous disodium phosphate.

When the nature of the material permits, the conduct of these reactions on frozen sections reduces the risks of failure or of loss; embedding in paraffin wax is, nevertheless, possible in most cases; so far as I know, the methods discussed here have never been used with celloidin sections.

Among the numerous variations of *the benzidine reaction*, I recommend in particular that of Slonimsky and Lapinsky whose working technique is as follows.

> Fix in formalin-potassium ferricyanide, freshly prepared;
> Cut frozen sections, the thickness of the sections may be substantial (more than 100 μ) when the method is conducted with a view to demonstrating blood vessels; tissue blocks one dimension of which is very small may be treated as a whole;
> Wash the sections in frequently renewed distilled water so as to remove the last traces of the fixative;
> Treat the sections with the following reagent, freshly prepared
> dissolve one g of benzidine in 25 ml of 96% alcohol, add, drop by drop, one ml of 30% hydrogen peroxide and then 9 ml of 70% alcohol and leave the sections there until the deep brown stain characteristic of the presence of haemoglobin appears;
> Wash rapidly in 96% alcohol, dehydrate in absolute alcohol, clear in a benzenoid hydrocarbon and mount in Canada balsam or in a synthetic resin.

The sections may also be mounted in a medium miscible with water; the alcoholic washing which follows the reaction should, in such cases, be replaced by washing in distilled water. Mounting after dehydration and clearing is the most advantageous when the reaction has been conducted using thick sections.

The method recommended by Lison (1930) differs slightly from that which has just been set out in the composition of the reagent, which is prepared by dissolving, at boiling point, 0.1 g of benzidine in 10 ml of water and then adding, after cooling to 60°C, 20 ml of commercial 12 volume hydrogen peroxide. The reaction takes place at 60°C and lasts for five minutes. We need hardly add that fixing with formalin-lead following Lison's technique may be used in the place of the fixative consisting of formalin-ferricyanide; in such cases, it is often useful to remove any precipitate of lead which the sections may contain prior to the reaction by washing them for several minutes in 5% nitric acid. Tissue blocks fixed for a short time in neutralised formalin, diluted as is usual, in saline formalin, or in formalin buffered with phosphates, is also suitable in most cases.

The techniques involving zinc-leucobases introduced by Lison (1931) are much superior to the benzidine reaction, not only so far as the optical qualities of the preparations are concerned but also from the standpoint of their stability. They depend on the possibility of transforming a certain number of dyestuffs into leuco-derivatives under the action of nascent hydrogen, these leuco-derivatives playing the part of hydrogen donors during the reaction so that the transfer of hydrogen to the peroxide results in the regeneration of the initial colour. The most used substances are acid fuchsin, various acid violets (Lison, 1931), patent blue (Fautrez, 1936) and cyanol (Dunn, 1946). It is the two latter of these dyestuffs, which are closely related chemically, which give the best results.

The preparation of the zinc-leucobases is carried out in the following way.

> Mix 1 g of patent blue or of cyanol in an Erlenmeyer flask, with 10 g of powdered zinc, 100 ml of distilled water and 2 ml of acetic acid; bring to the boil and maintain at boiling point until the solution becomes straw- or amber—coloured; it is often helpful to restrict the entry of air by covering the mouth of the flask with a small funnel; preserve in a well stoppered flask leaving in the zinc which has been used for the preparation and, after chilling, add a further 2 ml of crystallisable acetic acid. The zinc-leucobases of acid fuchsin keep for little longer than one week but can be rendered suitable for re-use if boiled again with the zinc powder; the leucobases of patent blue and of cyanol are much more stable usually keeping for more than one year.

The working technique of the reaction involves the following stages.

> Fix with one of the fluids recommended for the preservation of haemoglobin; cut frozen sections or embed in paraffin wax reducing as far as possible the time taken for dehydration, clearing and the period spent in hot paraffin wax; section cutting and spreading are carried out as usual; tissue blocks of sufficiently small size may be treated as a whole;
> Treat the frozen or paraffin wax sections taken from material fixed in formalin-lead, with 5% nitric acid to dissolve the precipitate of lead and wash with care in distilled water; omit this stage for material fixed in formalin-ferricyanide or in buffered formalin;
> Treat the sections for 5 to 10 minutes using the following mixture prepared immediately prior to use—
> the stock solution of the zinc leucobase,
>   freshly filtered .... 10 volumes
>   12 volume hydrogen peroxide (3%) .... 1 volume
> Wash in tap water;
> Stain the background with the aluminium lake of nuclear fast red or with any other red nuclear stain;
> Spread the frozen sections on slides, dehydrate in absolute alcohol, clear in a benzenoid hydrocarbon and mount in balsam or in a synthetic resin.

A positive result of the reaction is shown by an intense blue or green colour and keeps very well; the optical qualities of the preparations are by far superior to those involving sections treated with the benzidine technique.

The method of Fautrez and Lambert for staining haemoglobin is, it must be said, far from having the value of a histochemical reaction, but the selectivity of the colour obtained is much superior to that given by other staining procedures based on the eosinophilia of haemoglobin or on its siderophilia after staining with ferric haematoxylin. The technique of Fautrez and Lambert depends on the fact that the isoelectric point of haemoglobin is particularly high (6.8), whereas that of most other tissue proteins is around 4. Under such circumstances, the acidophilia of haemoglobin is shown even at the pH of the dye bath, when that of the other tissue proteins is either suppressed because of the total dissociation of the ionisable carboxyl groups, the amine groups passing into the unionised condition, or strongly depressed because of the great predominance of the carboxyl groups among the ionised reactive radicals. Experience shows that the difference between the isoelectric point of haemoglobin and that of other tissue proteins is maintained even during fixation by any of the usual fluids (Bouin, formalin, etc.) so that it is particularly easy to apply the staining technique of Fautrez and Lambert whose working technique is as follows.

Paraffin wax sections, treated with collodion where appropriate, and hydrated;
Stain for one to 24 hours in the mixture
- carmalum .... 1 volume
- a 1% aqueous solution of cyanol .... 1 volume
- McIlvaine's buffer, pH 6.4 .... 1 volume

Wash in McIlvaine's buffer, pH 6.4;
Differentiate in 70% alcohol until the sections are generally of a red colour (several seconds);
Dehydrate in absolute alcohol, clear in a benzenoid hydrocarbon and mount in Canada balsam or in a synthetic resin.

We may mention that Lison (1953, p. 462; 1960, pp. 771-772) suggests a procedure for preparing the carmalum which is in fact, that of Grenacher's alum carmine (Boil for 2 hours a mixture of 3 g of potassium alum and 2 g of carmine in 100 ml of water, filtering after chilling). Remember that P. Mayer's carmalum is prepared from an acid carmine base and that its potassium alum content is very high. In practice, both solutions are suitable and equivalent results are obtained with a dilute (0.01%) solution of safranine.

CHAPTER 21

HISTOCHEMICAL DETECTION OF SOME PRODUCTS OF PROTEIN METABOLISM

It seems to me sensible to bring together in this chapter the procedures intended to demonstrate compounds whose functional significance is very diverse but which have in common one essential biochemical characteristic, namely, close relationships with protein metabolism. Some of the substances in question are waste products such as urea and the purines; others represent neurohumoral agents in the sense of Welsh (1956, 1959) such as the catecholamines, histamine and 5-hydroxytryptamine (serotonine, enteramine); and still others are endogenous pigments (melanins, haematoidin, haemosiderin, bile pigments, and porphyrins.

COMPOUNDS ASSOCIATED WITH THE METABOLISM OF PHENYLALANINE AND TYROSINE

It is known that close chemical links exist between the two aromatic aminoacids which have just been mentioned and a whole series of compounds such as the catecholamines and other biogenic amines and melanins. These compounds are of substantial biological interest, so that techniques which allow us to demonstrate them selectively are of real value. In addition to techniques which have been known for a long time, and which are mentioned below, the fluoroscopic identification of biogenic amines has become of considerable importance during the last ten years without in any way becoming a routine method available to all laboratories. We begin by setting out its general principles.

FLUOROSCOPIC DETECTION OF BIOGENIC MONOAMINES

The histochemical detection of biogenic amines by treatment with formaldehyde followed by examination under a fluorescent microscope has, during the last twelve years or so, given rise to a substantial number of publications. The method, which has very great successes to its credit, is of considerable sensitivity and allows us to distinguish the different monoamines from one another. However, it requires apparatus which is not available in all histological laboratories and the technique needs to be carefully considered in the light of each new specimen subjected to it. Moreover, it may not be unhelpful to recall that the preparations are far from permanent.

The theoretical foundations of the technique and its practical application are set out in excellent recent reviews (see, in particular, Corrodi and Johnson, 1967; Falck and Owman, 1965; L'Hermite, 1969). Moreover, this account of the method, of which I have no personal experience, is deliberately restricted to the basic concepts.

It was in the course of histochemical investigations on the monoamines of the nervous system that Hillarp discovered the possibility of adapting to histochemical practice the condensation reactions with formaldehyde of the indolamines (Mannich's reaction) and the catecholamines (the Pictet-Spengler reaction). This general reaction of beta-arylethylamines with a compound bearing a primary carbonyl group results in the formation of derivatives of tetrahydroisoquinoline; the dehydration of this compound yields 3,4-dihydroisoquinolinic compounds which, after undergoing an equilibration reaction, give rise to the corresponding quininoid derivatives which are endowed with an intense fluorescence at 480 mμ. Experience shows that this reaction proceeds very easily under conditions which are compatible with maintaining the integrity of the tissues when formaldehyde is acting in a dry medium and in the presence of a film of dry protein, that is to say under the conditions obtaining when a section, a slice of tissue, dissociated material, or a smear are subjected to the action of formalin vapour. Falck's (1962) work has shown that the technique may be applied to freeze-dried tissue.

The chemical conditions for ring formation involving the Pictet-Spengler reaction are fulfilled by 3-hydroxylated beta-phenylethylamines such as dioxyphenylalanine, dopamine, noradrenaline, and adrenaline, as well as the m-tyramines of biological importance (m-tyrosine, m-tyramine etc...). Under the same experimental conditions tryptamine and a large number of its derivatives undergo the Mannich condensation to give tetrahydro-beta-carbonyls which may also be detected through their fluorescence. The two types of fluorophors have the same peak activation between 390 and 410 mμ. But the fluorescence spectrum of the dihydroisoquinolines formed by the condensation of catecholamines has a peak at 480 mμ whereas that of the dihydrocarbolines formed by the condensation of the tryptamine derivatives has a peak 30 to 40 mμ higher. Under such conditions the two types of fluorophor can be distinguished by the colour of their fluorescence which are, respectively, green and yellow, provided that a second filter with strong absorption below 490 mμ is used to eliminate the blue component.

The technique for the preparation of the tissues is regulated by the fundamental requirements of the procedure, namely that the reaction must take place in the dry. Modern authors (see in particular Falck and Owman, 1965) are inclined to explain the low sensitivity of certain classical reactions of the catecholamines, such as the chromaffin reaction, by the fact that they are taking place in a liquid medium.

Once the samples of tissue have been desiccated (squash preparations, smears, sections obtained from fresh tissue by the technique mentioned on p. 699, and freeze-dried tissue) they are sealed in a receptacle with paraformaldehyde and placed in an oven at 60 to 80°C. Generally speaking 5 g of paraformaldehyde is allowed for a receptacle of one litre volume. All authors emphasize the critical importance of the water content of the paraformaldehyde, a compound whose depolymerisation liberates the formaldehyde needed for condensation with the catecholamines or the indolalkylamines. The degree of hydration of the paraformaldehyde is generally regulated by keeping it under a vacuum followed by storage in containers containing mixtures of concentrated sulphuric acid and water. As Falck and Owman have commented the reaction is more intense when the paraformaldehyde is kept in a medium of relatively high humidity but it is under these conditions that the diffusion of the biogenic amines which are to be demonstrated is the greatest. The compromise between the requirements of a satisfactory condensation and as little diffusion as possible necessitate trial and error runs for each tissue and the optimum may not be the same for the different parts of the same tissue.

As Falck and Owman (1965) have commented this treatment with formaldehyde vapour not only gives the desired reaction but also fixes the tissues in a satisfactory manner and these authors suggest the possibilities of using it for other histochemical reactions or histological techniques when applied to lyophilised tissue.

The pieces of tissue are embedded as in the standard technique for freeze-drying; squash prep rations or smears may be mounted and examined as soon as the treatment with formaldehyde vapour is complete.

The sections are stuck on to slides dry. The mounting of any preparation may be carried out with Merck's Entellan; in the case of paraffin wax sections a small amount of xylene should be added to the medium (approximately 0.5 ml for 10 ml of the mountant) and it is warmed for several minutes on a hot plate at 50°C to dissolve the paraffin wax. When the objective of the work is a histochemical study of adrenaline, mounting should be carried out in paraffin oil and the warming on the hot plate should last longer to ensure the dissolution of the embedding medium.

The examination of the preparations may take place immediately after mounting. It can be done with the standard equipment for fluorescent microscopy using a mercury vapour lamp whose light is filtered through a heat filter and an excitation filter of the Schott BG 12 type. Falck and Owman recommend as a terminal filter the Schott OG 4 type. Evidently, immediate photography of the preparations is essential.

The distinction between the different monoamines is evident from an examination of the preparations.

The fluorophors formed by condensation of catecholamines or of dopamine with formaldehyde vapour give a green fluorescence, sometimes with a slight tendency to a yellowish tint whereas the fluorescence associated with the condensation of indolamines is intensely yellow. This distinction may, however, be difficult in the case of cells which are very rich in catecholamines.

The fluorophors formed by the condensation of catecholamines are much less sensitive to ultra-violet light than are those formed from the condensation of indolamines; the fluorescence associated with these latter compounds may have faded after one minute's examination but obviously the persistence of the fluorescence depends on the amount of the compound initially present.

It is appropriate to mention that diffusion caused by too high a water content of the paraformaldehyde used for condensation is much more marked in the case of catecholamines than it is for the indolamines.

Adrenaline may easily be distinguished from other catecholamines by the fact that its fluorophor dissolves in all mounting media except for paraffin oil.

In addition to the sense of security which stems from our thorough knowledge of the chemical mechanism of the reaction the main advantage of the technique for fluoroscopic detection of biogenic amines is its very great sensitivy; the recent results of Owman and Ljungdahl (1972), using sections cut without freezing, allow us indeed to hope for still further improvements in this sensitivity by comparison with those obtained by freeze-drying. The preparations are however not permanent, the study of any given tissue requiring developmental investigations which may turn out to be rather lengthy and we cannot consider this procedure as suitable for a routine method in non-specialised laboratories or as a technique which can be used occasionally by experimenters who do not possess the special training required.

HISTOCHEMICAL DETECTION OF CATECHOLAMINES

All techniques for the histochemical detection of catecholamines depend on the presence of the phenol group in these compounds; the theoretical specificity of the reactions in question is not great because the number of chemical compounds capable of reacting is substantial, but the effective specificity, taking account of the morphological data on the one hand and of the data obtained from analytical biochemistry on the other, is quite adequate for the needs of practical histochemistry. The very substantial majority of histochemical investigations of the catecholamines relate to adrenalin and noradrenalin. Falck, Hillarp and Torf (1959) detected dopamine by one of the techniques which disclose the presence of the two compounds just mentioned; new investigations in this field are much to be desired.

The histochemical detection of catecholamines is dominated by the need for adequate fixation of the tissue; in fact, noradrenalin and adrenalin are localised *in vivo* in cytoplasmic granules which are more or less well preserved by a large number of liquid fixatives, but the maintenance of catecholamines in place can only be ensured by a chemical change which involves the practice of histochemical reactions on fresh tissue. The presence of appropriate reagents in the fixative is indispensable. From the practical point of view, it follows that the need for the investigation of these compounds must be foreseen at the time that the tissue is dissected and that it regulates the choice of certain fixatives.

Adrenalin and noradrenalin are *o*-diphenols and should, in principle, be detectable by any reactions for the phenol group which were reviewed in Chapter 16, but the special requirements of fixation mentioned above explain the difficulties of applying the azoreaction in practice as this procedure is poorly adapted to work involving pieces of tissue. The same remark holds good for the indoreaction and for that of Gibbs; the argentaffin reaction has been applied by numerous workers to the detection of adrenalin in pieces of tissue, but the alkalinity of the reagent allows us to understand why the results obtained at the cellular level are mediocre. The pheochrome reaction is the method of choice in the particular case we are considering here.

Simultaneous demonstration of adrenalin and noradrenalin

The classical pheochrome reaction involving fixation in a fluid with a potassium bichromate base, and for preference not containing corrosive sublimate (the fixatives of Orth, Kopsch, Regaud, etc...), followed by postchromatisation, washing in water, and then embedding in paraffin wax, confers a yellow or brown stain on structures containing one or other of the two catecholamines. It is advisable to shorten, as far as possible, the time spent by the pieces of tissue in the hot paraffin and cutting on a freezing microtome is advisable in all cases in which the examination is to be conducted without background staining.

In fact, the optimal conditions for the pheochrome reaction are not realised when the classical procedures are used. The methodological studies of Hillarp and Hökfelt (1955) have shown that the stains obtained are much more intense when the pieces of tissue are treated in a preliminary stage with a mixture of aqueous solutions of potassium bichromate and chromate, at pH values around 5.6, and then fixed in formalin. It is the technique of the Swedish authors which I would cordially recommend in all cases where a slice of the tissue to be examined can be devoted exclusively to tests for catecholamines.

The technique of Hillarp and Hökfelt for the demonstration of noradrenalin and adrenalin:

> Treat pieces of fresh tissue, whose least dimension does not exceed 1 mm, for 48 hours, at laboratory temperatures, with the mixture 5% aqueous solution of potassium bichromate .... 10 volumes
> 5% aqueous solution of potassium chromate .... 1 volume
> (the pH of the mixture is 5.6);
> Fix in 10% formalin;
> Cut frozen sections or dehydrate, clear and embed in paraffin wax, reducing as far as possible the time spent by the pieces of tissue in the hot paraffin; cut the material embedded in paraffin wax without special precautions.

A positive result of the reaction is shown by a stain varying between brownish yellow and brown; it often happens that cells containing noradrenalin, which are lighter, can be distinguished on sections of the medullo-adrenal subjected to this reaction from adrenalin-containing cells which are darker.

Indeed it does often happen that the paleness of the sections is a nuisance during their examination especially when the pheochrome reaction has been applied in the classical way. Numerous background stains have been put forward and some histochemical reactions allow us substantially to improve the optical qualities of the preparations without losing any of the chemical significance of the results obtained.

A background stain involving toluidine blue confers a green stain on cells which contain substances which have reacted positively whilst still allowing us to demonstrate the nuclei; we may either stain with a solution containing 0.2% of toluidine blue in distilled water followed by a short differentiation in 1% acetic acid prior to the dehydration and mounting of the sections, or we may employ a solution of the same concentration in Walpole's buffer of pH 4.2 which is to be recommended for tests of the basophilia of the tissue, this latter technique allowing us to dispense with any differentiation prior to the dehydration and mounting of the sections.

Staining with iron haematoxylin or Altmann's fuchsin, described among the general cytological techniques, very often gives an excellent demonstration of sites of substances which have reacted positively to the classical pheochrome reaction.

The best way of improving the contrasts is to follow the chromaffin reaction either with tests for reducing groups using the ferric ferricyanide method or with the PAS reaction. The first of these two reactions can be carried out using one of the variations described in Chapter 14; I would recommend particularly that of Adams. Instead of the brownish yellow of the pheochrome reaction a dark blue-green stain is obtained at sites which have reacted positively. This procedure can be applied just as well to frozen sections as to paraffin wax ones. Using the PAS method, when carried out according to the recommendations of Chapter 17, stains varying from pink to greyish red can be obtained.

From the theoretical standpoint, it is appropriate to remark that the precipitate obtained by mixing *in vitro* a solution of potassium bichromate with one of adrenalin, catechol, or dioxyphenylalanine (dopa) strongly reduces mixtures of ferric chloride and potassium ferricyanide; the pheochrome reaction thus goes hand in hand with the preservation of the reducing power of catecholamines. As for the positive result of the PAS method applied after the pheochrome reaction, Lillie (1965) follows on from a suggestion of Hudson in considering that the oxidation involves carbon atoms which bear quinone groupings in the adrenochrome formed during the reaction; such carbon atoms would be oxidised to CO_2 and the adjacent carbon atoms would give rise to carbonyl groups. The reaction can only take place in the presence of a substantial excess of periodic acid but this condition is to be found in the course of histochemical practice.

It is appropriate to recall that other oxidising agents can be substituted for potassium bichromate during the pheochrome reaction; positive results are indeed obtained with potassium or sodium iodate (Gérard, Cordier and Lison, 1930). Mixtures of formalin and potassium iodide give preparations which are comparable, from the point of view of the localisation obtained, with those obtained using the classical pheochrome reaction and the theoretical bearing of this fact has been discussed in relation to the histochemical detection of phenols in general; from the practical point of view, the stains are paler than those of the pheochrome reaction using potassium bichromate so that the method is but little used.

Selective demonstration of noradrenalin

Two recent techniques allow us to demonstrate noradrenalin selectively and the distinction of cells in the medullo-adrenal of mammals or the adrenal tissue of other vertebrates, cells which contain one or other of the two catecholamines, can also be assured. These techniques are those of Hillarp and Hökfelt (1954, 1955) and that of Eränko (1954, 1955, 1960).

The method of Hillarp and Hökfelt depends on the fact that only cells containing noradrenalin are stained yellow or brown when treated with a solution of potassium iodate *used without other adjuvants*. The compound so formed, whose chemical constitution is in all probability close to that of the adrenochrome polymers which are formed during the classical pheochrome reaction, is soluble in substances used for paraffin wax embedding; it is therefore indispensable to section the tissue on a freezing microtome.

The reaction is rather slow and experience shows that it cannot be used for thin sections cut from fresh tissue (a freezing microtome or a cryostat). All modern authors use saturated solutions of potassium or sodium iodate in distilled water; the solubility of the two compounds is practically the same between 20 and 30°C (between 9 and 11%) and the results obtained are equivalent; moreover, Lillie (1965) considers that there is no reason to prefer potassium iodate to the sodium salt except when the reaction is carried out below

15°C, since potassium iodate is the more soluble of the two salts at lower temperatures. The working technique involves the following stages.

> Treat the pieces of tissue, of very small size, (one dimension less than 2 mm) for 24 hours, at laboratory temperatures, using a saturated aqueous solution of potassium or sodium iodate (about 10%);
> Transfer the tissue pieces for 24 hours in 10% formalin;
> Cut on a freezing microtome;
> Rinse the sections in tap water;
> Where appropriate, stain the nuclei with the aluminium lake of nuclear fast red or haemalum (dilute solutions used as for background staining after the demonstration of lipids by a lysochrome);
> Wash in tap water whenever background staining is to be practised;
> Mount in a medium miscible with water; rapid dehydration in absolute alcohol, followed by clearing and mounting in Canada balsam is possible.

A positive result of the reaction is shown by a fairly intense brown stain which recalls that obtained using the classical pheochrome reaction. We must emphasize that the brown staining is only diagnostic of the presence of noradrenalin when the iodate of the alkali metal chosen acts without any adjuvant; in the presence of formalin both catecholamines give the reaction.

The specificity of the reaction cannot be considered as complete; the authors of the technique themselves comment that dioxyphenylalanine, 5-hydroxytryptamine, and probably other substances are capable of giving it but these substances only exist in infinitesimal quantities in the medullo-adrenal cells. Adrenalin does not react or reacts so weakly that the technique of Hillarp and Hökfelt gives excellent contrasts between cells containing one or other of the two catecholamines. The slowness of the reaction does nevertheless give rise to the possibility of some weak diffusion; we must in this context recall that the solution of potassium iodate in which pieces of tissue rich in noradrenalin are immersed often becomes pink in 24 to 48 hours. Experience shows that the size of the pieces of tissue substantially modifies the quality of the reaction. Hillarp and Hökfelt consider that it is possible to treat the adrenal glands of the cat as a whole; it seems to me preferable to reduce the dimensions of the pieces of tissue still further, and to treat only pieces whose maximum dimension is less than 2 mm without further slicing.

We may note that Cattaneo (1958) has shown that the brown stain obtained using potassium or sodium iodate solutions is only specific for noradrenalin at highly alkaline pH values; according to this author the reaction takes place with noradrenalin alone at pH values close to 10 and with adrenalin alone at pH values less than 3. This view is contested by most modern authors and all attempts to reproduce the demonstration of adrenalin using acidified solutions of potassium iodate seem to have failed.

Eränkö's method depends on the fact that noradrenalin forms an insoluble compound with formalin, a compound which it is easy to detect on frozen sections because of its particularly intense greenish fluorescence. Adrenalin does not give this reaction and it is agreed that the substitution of one of the hydrogens of the amine group in this latter catecholamine by a methyl radical, slows down or inhibits the formation of the tetrahydro-isoquinolinic compound responsible for the fluorescence.

The formation of this latter compound is sufficiently rapid for the method to be used, unlike that of Hillarp and Hökfelt, on frozen sections of fresh tissue cut in a cryostat; it can also be applied to pieces of tissue and then amounts to fixing them in Baker's calcium-formaldehyde, cutting them on a freezing microtome and then examining the unstained sections in a fluorescence microscope.

Eränkö (1960) also notes two other ways of selectively demonstrating cells in which the fluorescent derivative of noradrenalin is formed, namely the azo-reaction and the argentaffin reaction. In cases where the experimenter does not possess a fluorescence microscope sections taken from formalin treated material can be subjected to the azo reaction or the argentaffin reaction after sectioning on a freezing microtome, using the working techniques given in Chapter 15. From my own experience coupling with diazo o-anisidine (fast blue B salt) or the diazo salt of 5-nitro-anisidine (fast red B salt) and the argentaffin reaction using Lillie and Burtner's variation is highly suitable.

The osmium-iodide technique of Champy and Coujard

This method (Champy, 1913) which was described as a technique for demonstrating certain nerves depends on fixation in a mixture of osmium tetroxide and potassium iodide and was considered by Coujard and Champy (1941), Champy and Coujard (1945), Hatem (1955), Champy and Hatem (1955) as a histochemical reaction for compounds bearing a phenol group, in particular the sympathomimetic catecholamines.

According to the authors of this technique, of which I have no personal experience, when the two substances are mixed a complex is formed in equilibrium with potassium iodide and osmium tetroxide, one of the essential chemical properties of this complex being a practically instantaneous reduction by ortho- and para-diphenols. From the practical point of view it follows that the superficial zones of pieces of tissue immersed in the mixture simply undergo fixation by osmium tetroxide, whereas the reduction of the complex which penetrates further results in the selective demonstration of the medullo-adrenal cells of mammals, of melanic pigments, of enterochromaffin cells, of the poison glands of amphibia, and of adrenergic nerves. In tissue which has been well fixed these structures appear intensely black, the background being stained pale yellow; too long a fixation results in non-specific reduction phenomena which remove all significance from the results so far as the presence of phenolic compounds is concerned.

The working technique involves the following stages.

Fix pieces of tissue of conveniently chosen size for 24 to 48 hours (the optimal duration to be determined by trial and error), at between 10 and 15°C, with the mixture—

a 2% aqueous solution of osmium
tetroxide .... 1 volume
a 3% aqueous solution of potassium iodide .... 3–4 volumes

Dehydrate rapidly, embed in paraffin wax;
Cut the tissue into serial sections, rejecting the superficial regions;
Dewax and mount in Canada balsam or in a synthetic resin;

The value of the procedure as a morphological technique is undoubted but its chemical significance has given rise to discussions and to criticisms. Among modern authors some do not mention it as a histochemical technique (Gomori, 1952; Lillie, 1965); others (Lison, 1953, 1960; Pearse, 1960) have reservations as to its specificity remarking that the ability to reduce the osmium-iodide complex is in no way the prerogative of o- and p-diphenolic compounds. A variation of the technique is described amongst those for studying the nervous system.

THE HISTOCHEMICAL DETECTION OF MELANINS

The melanins are pigments whose natural colour varies between yellow and black, with brown and violet as intermediate colours. From the chemical point of view, these compounds are closely linked to the metabolism of phenylalanine and of tyrosine; they are widely distributed in animals and can be met with in most tissues and cells. It is customary in vertebrate histology to distinguish melanophor cells in which these pigments are secreted and melanophage cells where they accumulate as a result of the processes of phagocytosis or of cytocrinia in the sense of P. Masson.

The natural colour of the melanins to some extent assists their identification. Moreover, some of their physical characteristics are highly diagnostic. They are in fact compounds insoluble in any of the organic solvents used during histological manipulation so that they are impeccably preserved on paraffin wax sections or in celloidin. This character is, moreover, common to the melanins and to sufficiently highly oxidised chromolipoids (see p. 485). In addition, the melanins withstand organic or mineral acids, even when concentrated; their passage into solution can be obtained through the action of concentrated alkalis but naturally this procedure is incompatible with the preservation of the integrity of the sections.

Among the chemical characteristics of melanins one of the most important is the ease with which oxidation destroys their colour. This procedure (depigmentation, decolouration) may be carried out either for what are properly speaking histochemical ends or to identify pigment granules or more especially to ensure a distinction between melanins and lipofuscins (Hueck's method, p. 484), or again to remove too abundant a pigment which may hinder the detailed cytological study of the preparations.

Methods for bleaching

Hydrogen peroxide is used as a decolourising agent for melanin in Hueck's technique, which has been examined in relation to the demonstration of chromolipoids. It acts rather slowly, but has the advantage of preserving the tissues in their integrity. It is the method of choice in cases where the melanic granules are not very abundant. Paraffin wax sections are dewaxed, treated with collodion and hydrated and then placed for 24 to 48 hours in 3 to 10% (10 to 30 volume) hydrogen peroxide. It is easy to follow the progress of the depigmentation by examining the sections under a microscope. Once the desired result is obtained, the sections are washed in tap water and then subjected to stains or other histochemical reactions as required.

Chlorine is a very effective bleaching agent. Among the numerous formulae put forward for its use, the best is that of P. Mayer. Crystals of potassium chlorate are placed at the bottom of the receptacle used for staining the sections (Borrel tubes, Coplin jars, etc...); the receptacle is filled with 50% alcohol and 1 to 2 ml of concentrated hydrochloric acid are added by means of a pipette reaching to the bottom of the receptacle so as to bring the acid into contact with the crystals of potassium chlorate. The sections are then placed in the receptacle and this is thoroughly closed. Depigmentation is generally complete in 24 hours.

Bromine, which is also very effective, is most often used in the formula due to Mawas. The sections spend 12 to 24 hours in a mixture of 100 ml of distilled water and 50 drops of bromine. They are then washed in water.

Chlorine dioxide is considered by many authors as being one of the best bleaching agents but has the practical disadvantage of needing to be prepared by the experimenter. This is done in the following way (Grynfeltt and Mestrézat).

Dissolve 50 g of barium chlorate by warming to about 50°C in 70 ml of distilled water, *allow to cool*; add, little by little and only when chilling is complete, a mixture of 8.5 ml of concentrated sulphuric acid and 40 ml of distilled water. A massive precipitate of barium sulphate is formed, chlorine dioxide passing into solution. The precipitate is removed by decantation and the supernatant liquor is preserved in a flask with a ground glass stopper which should be kept in the cold and darkness.

In use, 60 ml of distilled water are mixed with 8 ml of this solution of chlorine dioxide. The sections remain in it for 10 to 12 hours; they are then rinsed in 70% alcohol and again in water.

Chlorine dioxide, used in solution in nitric acid or in acetic acid (diaphanol) is a particularly vigorous depigmentation agent but its destructive action on the tissue structures reduces the number of cases where it is used to those in which the other methods appear to be ineffective. Sections are treated for 24 hours in well stopped receptacles and in darkness, with a commercial solution of diaphanol or with one of the mixtures with a chlorine dioxide base indicated in Chapter 10.

Chromium trioxide (chromic acid) acting in a 5% aqueous solution is an effective and inoffensive bleaching agent for tissue structures but its action may have inexplicable irregularities as Lillie (1965) remarked; this author introduced chromic acid to the ranks of depigmenting agents.

Potassium permanganate used in a 0.25% aqueous solution is also an excellent depigmenting agent. In most cases, bleaching is obtained in less than 4 hours. From my own experience this time may be reduced to several minutes by using the permanganate-sulphuric acid mixture recommended by Gomori (1941) as a preliminary treatment in certain staining procedures (p. 759) in place of the 0.25% aqueous solution. However this may be, the sections which have just been treated with potassium permanganate are rinsed in water and then destained in a 4% aqueous solution of oxalic acid or with a 3 to 5% aqueous solution of sodium metabisulphite; they are then washed for 2 to 5 minutes in running water. Obviously such an oxidation substantially modifies certain of the affinities for dyestuffs.

Performic and peracetic acids, whose introduction for depigmentation is also due to Lillie, are very effective. The need to prepare performic acid immediately prior to use obviously leads us to prefer the use of peracetic acid which may be prepared in advance and kept in reserve. The sections, dewaxed, treated with collodion and hydrated, are allowed to spend 1 to 24 hours in the acid according to the circumstances; it is rare that total depigmentation requires more than 8 hours (ocular melanins). The operation is terminated by washing in tap water.

It is unnecessary to add that the action of oxidising agents, such as all the bleaching agents, is not restricted to melanins. The affinities for dyes and the histochemical characteristics of certain cell and tissue constituents are profoundly modified following these treatments and it is essential to take account of these changes when interpreting the results.

Another chemical characteristic of the melanins, which is widely used in histochemistry for the identification of these compounds, is their reducing power. The ferric ferricyanide method and the argentaffin reaction, applied as in Chapter 14, give strongly positive results with these compounds and any variant of these two reactions can be used when we have to identify small and not too numerous granules. We must not lose sight of the fact that the reduction of ferric chloride, which is the chemical basis of the ferric ferricyanide method, is a property common to melanins and chromolipoids, so that this method is non-operational for the distinction between the two groups of pigments. The argentaffin reaction, involving alkaline silver complexes, is very rapidly and energetically given by melanins, whereas lipofuscins give negative or weakly positive results according to their degree of oxidation. In doubtful cases, tests for the reduction of silver nitrate in an acid medium may be very useful. The working technique which follows is that recommended by Lillie (1965).

> Dewaxed sections, treated where appropriate with collodion and brought into water;
> Treat for one hour or more, at 25°C and in darkness, with the solution
>
> silver nitrate .... 1.7 g
> Walpole's buffer (sodium acetate-acetic acid), pH 4 .... 100 ml
>
> Wash in distilled water;
> Wash rapidly in a 5% aqueous solution of sodium thiosulphate;
> Wash for 10 minutes in running water;
> Stain the background where appropriate (safranin, basic fuchsin, the aluminium lake of nuclear fast red, etc. ...);
> Dehydrate in absolute alcohol, clear in a benzenoid hydrocarbon and mount in Canada balsam or in a synthetic resin.

The blackening of cutaneous melanins is generally obtained in about 12 minutes but other sites of these pigments are not revealed before one hour. In any case, the positive result is shown by an intense black stain. Certain melanins (trichoxanthin, neuromelanin) react poorly under these experimental conditions and should be tested for, using variations of the argentaffin reaction involving alkaline silver complexes.

The capacity of melanins to fix ferrous ions has been put to good use by Lillie (1955) when developing a technique for their detection on paraffin wax sections, applicable to material *fixed in fluids containing neither potassium bichromate nor chromium trioxide*. This technique involves the following stages.

> Dewaxed sections, treated where appropriate with collodion and hydrated;
> Treat for one hour, at laboratory temperatures, with a 2.5% aqueous solution of crystalline ferrous sulphate;
> Wash in 4 baths of distilled water (5 minutes per bath);
> Treat for 30 minutes with the solution
>
> potassium ferricyanide .... 1 g
> distilled water .... 99 ml
> acetic acid .... 1 ml
>
> Rinse in 1% acetic acid;
> Where appropriate, stain the background with van Gieson's picrofuchsin (p. 204); avoid staining with haematoxylin lakes;
> Dehydrate in absolute alcohol, clear in a benzenoid hydrocarbon and mount in a synthetic resin or, if necessary, in Canada balsam.

A positive result of the reaction is shown by a deep green stain, the background being either a very pale green or stained with picro-fuchsin.

Among the negative characteristics of melanins it is appropriate to mention that these compounds give neither the reactions of tyrosine nor those of tryptophane; the azoreaction also gives negative results. Tests for iron remain negative as do those for nucleic acids; only a few melanins react weakly with PAS and all other oxidation reactions of carbohydrates give entirely negative results.

Staining with dilute solutions of azur A confers a green stain on melanins and this tinctorial affinity withstands prolonged methylation (24 hours at 60°C), whereas the basophilia of the lipofuscins disappears very rapidly when subjected to methylation.

COMPOUNDS RELATED TO THE METABOLISM OF TRYPTOPHANE

Among the derivatives of tryptophane which need to be considered here, the main one is 5-hydroxytryptamine (serotonine, enteramine) whose histochemical detection has given rise to a large number of recent publications. The physiological importance of the substances in question is too well known to need mention here; in the same way, the histological and physiological arguments which lead us to consider the enterochromaffin cells as the principal site of their secretion are also well known.

It is the histochemical interpretation of the characteristics of the granulations which are contained in the cytoplasm of the elements in question, which represents the substance of the debate concerning the histochemical detection of serotonine; the question is whether they are or are not diagnostic of the presence of 5-hydroxytryptamine. It is by feedback processes and by causing a diversity of methods to converge that protagonists of the view that histochemical reactions can indeed disclose the presence of serotonine seeked, in the past to sustain the approach that they adopt. In consequence, such considerations should, when considered rigorously, remain outside a text-book of strictly technical orientation. However, the debate is an important one and the demonstration of enterochromaffin cells (Kultschitzky cells, argentaffin cells, etc...) plays such a role in histophysiological studies on the intestine and in anatomical-pathological studies on carcinogenic tumours that it seems to me difficult not to follow, in this matter, the example given by all modern manuals of histochemistry.

The secretory granules of the Kultschitzky cells, whose morphological characteristics patently do not need to be described here, are revealed by a whole series of histochemical reactions. Their reducing power is attested by the strongly positive result of the ferric ferricyanide method considered by Lillie (1961, 1965) as being the most sensitive and the simplest of techniques for their demonstration; the argentaffin reaction and that using tetrazolium salts in an alkaline medium also give positive results and it is the degree of the argentaffin reaction which has generally been used since the time of Masson (1914) for demonstrating the cells in question. The pheochrome reaction, the azoreaction, Lison's indoreaction and that involving alkaline thioindoxyl (Pearse, 1956) which depends on coupling this substance with a quinone-imine, formed during the transformation undergone by the serotonine in the course of formalin fixation, are all positive and this collection of data is in accordance with the hypothesis according to which such reactions would indicate the presence of 5-hydroxytryptamine in the secretory granules of the enterochromaffin cells. The existence of a yellow fluorescence after fixation in formalin was observed for the first time by Hamperl (1934) and also fits in with this hypothesis.

To this collection of what are properly speaking histochemical results we need to add the physiological and pharmacodynamic data patiently accumulated by Vialli's school, notably by Erspamer; this very fine collection of investigations has persuaded research workers (see Vialli, 1963, for a bibliography) to strengthen to no small degree the hypothesis according to which the enterochromaffin cells are the site of secretion of serotonine.

The investigations of Lillie's school (see Lillie, 1961, 1965 for a bibliography) do, nevertheless, bring to light a serious interpretative difficulty. It so happens that *in vitro* tests show that 5-hydroxytryptamine reacts strongly under conditions in which indol groups can be demonstrated, as described in relation to the detection of tryptophane (p. 513), a formalin pretreatment in no way modifying this activity; moreover, the reactions in question (the rosindole reaction, the reaction with *p*-dimethylaminobenzaldehyde with coupling to the diazo salt of S acid) always give negative results with the specific granules of the enterochromaffin cells which are nevertheless easy to demonstrate on the same sections by means of the azoreaction. Glenner and Lillie (1957) noted a diffuse reaction of the cells in carcinogenic tumours, but emphasized the absence of any reactivity of the normal enterochromaffin cells of the intestine. Lillie (1965, p. 238) considers in consequence that the presence of a diphenolic compound of the catechol type in the granulations of the enterochromaffin cells is highly probable, the hypothesis of a *para* configuration cannot be discounted formally but the presence of the indol group may not be detectable by histochemical methods. The author mentioned, deduces from this that the positive result of the azoreactions of the enterochromaffin granules may disclose the presence of a compound other than 5-hydroxytryptamine.

The interpretative difficulty which has just been stressed has been resolved through the use of fixatives containing aldehydes other than formaldehyde. In fact, the investigations of Solcia and Sampietro (1967) have shown that the granules of the enterochromaffin cells after fixation in mixtures with a glutaraldehyde base give not only the azoreaction and the argentaffin reaction but the general reactions of indolic compounds, notably those of *p*-dimethylaminobenzaldehyde and of xanthydrol. This information completely confirms Vialli's (1966) conception of the negative character of tests for indol groups after fixation in formalin as being due to the "denaturation" of the 5-hydroxytryptamine.

Work by Geyer (1968) adds supplementary information concerning the changes of the serotonine molecule during fixation by various aldehydes. Fixation in formalin, in the gaseous or liquid condition, results in the appearance of the yellow fluorescence described in relation to the fluoroscopic demonstration of monoamines. Mannich's ring formation, the first stage in the formation of the carboline responsible for this fluorescence, results in the disappearance of all the histochemical reactions of the indol group which depend on the non-substitution of carbon atom 2 in the molecule. Naturally, the results of the azoreaction of the argentaffin reaction and of the ferric ferricyanide reaction, which are conditioned by the hydroxyl group of 5-hydroxytryptamine, remain positive despite substitution on carbon atom 2.

It is easy to understand why the Mannich reaction cannot take place in terms of the structural formula of the other aldehydes used by Geyer (acrolein, acetaldehyde, glutaraldehyde). Carbon atom 2 then remains free. The study of the preparations does indeed show that tests for indol groups *and* the normal histochemical reactions of polyphenols give strongly positive results but that fluorescence is totally absent.

COMPOUNDS RELATED TO THE METABOLISM OF HISTIDINE

Among the compounds directly related to the metabolism of histidine, only histamine seems to have been the subject of histochemical research, experiments intended to detect it dealing only with the mast cells (tissue basophiles, Mastzellen, labrocytes), the concomitant presence of heparin and of histamine in the granulations of the cells being inferred from a whole collection of physiological, pharmacodynamic and biochemical data.

An early technique, due to Schauer and Werle (1959) depended on the precipitation *in situ* of the histamine by prolonged immersion of the pieces of tissue in a solution of Reinecke's salt. Thus rendered insoluble, the histamine is demonstrated by coupling with a diazonium salt. The preservation of the tissue structures leaves a lot to be desired and the scheme indicated by the German authors seems not to have been followed, all the more so as this way of demonstrating histamine lacks chemical specificity.

Lagounoff and his colleagues (1961) recommend immediate freezing of the tissue in isopentane chilled in liquid nitrogen; these pieces of tissue are then dried at low temperatures, transfered to a desiccator furnished with paraformaldehyde and placed in an oven at 60°C so as to ensure fixation in formalin vapour. This result is obtained in 4 to 96 hours, according to the size of the fragments. The tissue fragments are then embedded in paraffin wax (for preference in a vacuum oven), cut into sections and stuck to slides in the usual way. Under these conditions, the azoreaction with the diazo salt of *p*-bromaniline, or certain stable commercial diazonium salts, the ferric ferricyanide reaction and the argentaffin reaction give strongly positive results; moreover, the appearance of an intense greenish-yellow fluorescence is also observable. The pheochrome reaction remains negative, as do all techniques for demonstrating tryptophane.

Results of the same kind, but distinctly weaker, are obtained by fixing the tissues in dilute formalin (10%). These authors agree that the facts just set out may be explained coherently by supposing that an addition compound is formed from the formalin and the histamine of the tissues, this addition compound being tetrahydropyridino-iminazol. Such a condensation reaction has been known to biochemists for a long time and the interpretation seems to be plausible but the concomitant presence in the mast cells of tyrosine or tyramine could represent a serious source of error.

A simpler method, described by Juhlin and Shelley (1966) requires the use of fresh tissue (free-hand sections, suspensions of cells spread upon slides, and brought into a virtually desiccated condition). The sections or smears are covered with a 1% solution of phthalaldehyde in xylene; after three minutes this solution is replaced by tetrahydrofurfurol and the preparations are examined under a fluorescence microscope. The presence of histamine is shown by a yellow fluorescence which keeps for about a quarter of an hour.

In fact, the major histochemical problem posed by the detection of histamine is its preservation *in situ*; we have to deal with a substance whose molecule is of small size, diffuseable and soluble in water, so that right from the start we may have reservations as to the validity of the results obtained. The clearest results have been obtained in mast cells where the histamine exists in large amounts. Juhlin and Shelley do, moreover, report positive results in blood vessels, blood corpuscles, and gastric mucosa.

The interest of these methods is great but their entry into current practice will have to await further investigations.

COMPOUNDS RELATED TO THE METABOLISM OF HAEMOGLOBIN

The catabolism of haemoglobin occurs *in vivo* in ways which are rather different from those which occur *in vitro*; in fact, the latter degradation results in the separation of the protein constituent, the globin, the prosthetic group (haem, haematin) losing its iron to give haematoporphyrin. *In vivo* haematin and haematoporphyrin virtually never appear in tissue.

It is classical to distinguish the normal products of the catabolism of haemoglobin into haemosiderins and bile pigments, according to whether they do or do not contain iron. To the study of such substances we may add that of the malarial pigment, which is pathological, and that of the formol pigment whose appearance represents a fixation artefact.

THE HAEMOSIDERINS

The haemosiderins (rubigen, ochre pigment, ferratin, ferrin, siderin) are pigments whose colour varies from yellow to rust, passing through ochre. When free they may be distinguished from protosiderins (Lillie, 1948) which have the same histochemical characteristics that exist in the cells in a diffuse form.

Their *solubility characteristics* are highly indicative. We are dealing in fact with substances which are insoluble in water, in alkalis and in most organic solvents, but freely soluble in the cold in acids, though often rendered hard to dissolve by fixation.

Their *major histochemical characteristic* is the presence of ferric iron in the ionic condition or easily unmaskable. The detection of this cation involves procedures described in Chapter 13. It is appropriate to recollect the ease with which the iron contained in the haemosiderin can be extracted; this being particularly valuable when it is desired to study the chemical substances with which it is associated. The extraction is generally complete after treatment of the sections for three hours, at laboratory temperatures, with a 5% aqueous solution of oxalic acid; the importance of this organic substrate was mentioned in Chapter 13.

Among the other histochemical characteristics of the haemosiderins, which are particularly valuable for distinguishing them from pigments of the same colour but of a different chemical nature, we may mention the absence of any depigmentation by oxidising agents, the absence of a reducing capacity and the absence of any staining with lysochromes. These features ensure the easy distinction of the haemosiderins on the one hand and the melanins and chromolipoids on the other; these latter compounds may however pose difficult problems when they contain iron.

Gedigk and his collaborators have shown (see in particular Gedigk and Strauss, 1953) that the iron in haemosiderin deposits is linked to a complex organic substrate which contains, in particular, carbohydrates and proteins;

the reactions of these compounds become strongly positive after extraction of the iron with oxalic acid.

As I mentioned in relation to the histochemical detection of iron, ferritin, which is the principle way in which iron used by the organism is deposited in mammals, escapes detection by the reactions of this cation; in fact, haemosiderin represents excess iron.

BILE PIGMENTS

Bile pigments may appear, in pathological conditions, within the tissues in the free form, crystallised or amorphous but always extra cellular, as the substance *haematoidin*, whose chemical constitution is identical with that of bilirubin. Moreover, bilirubin itself may exist within the cells.

Haematoidin shows up either in the form of granules or spheroids, or in the form of rhombic crystals or platelets, or of bundles of needles; the essential sites are those of old haemorrhages. Such masses are insoluble in water, alcohol, ether, or dilute acids, but soluble in alkalis, chloroform, and carbon tetrachloride. Tests for iron by any technique (ionic, masked, etc...) give negative results which is evidently in agreement with the chemical information on the constitution of bilirubin. Oxidising agents do not bleach haematoidin which, moreover, has no affinity for acid or basic dyes used in normal histochemical practice and which does not absorb lysochromes. Kutlick (1958) notes that haematoidin and bilirubin reduce alkaline silver complexes but that the silver deposits so formed may be dissolved by passing the preparations through a solution containing 5 g of potassium ferricyanide and 0.5 g of sodium hyposulphite in 100 ml of water, without the natural colour of the pigments reappearing because they have been transformed into maleinimides; any other argentaffin pigment will, under these conditions, regain its natural colour thus representing an important element for the differential diagnosis.

Techniques which assure the histochemical demonstration of **bile pigments** depend on the oxidation of bilirubin to biliverdin; Stein's (1935) technique was the earliest of these procedures. It may not be unhelpful to mention, for the record, that Gmelin's classical reaction does not satisfy the morphological requirements of histochemical research. Some of the techniques deriving from that of Stein may be applied to paraffin wax sections; others, notably that of Glenner (1957) necessitate the sectioning of fresh tissue. The techniques of Stein, Kutlick and Glenner are set out here.

Stein's method for the demonstration of bile pigments:

Paraffin wax sections, taken from material fixed in formalin or alcohol;
Treat for 12 to 18 hours with the mixture
  Lugol's fluid .... 2 volumes
  tincture of iodine BP .... 1 volume
Wash for 5 minutes in running water;
Treat for 30 seconds with a 0.5% aqueous solution of sodium thiosulphate;
Wash for 5 minutes in running water;
Stain the nuclei with a red stain (I would particularly advise the use of the aluminium lake of nuclear fast red which is much superior to the carmalum specified in the original formula);
Wash for 2 minutes in running water;
Dehydrate *in acetone* (avoid alcohol) clear in a benzenoid hydrocarbon and mount in Canada balsam or in a synthetic resin.

The positive result of this reaction is shown by a deep green stain.

Kutlik's method for demonstrating bile pigments:

Paraffin wax sections, taken from material fixed in formalin, alcohol or in Carnoy's fluid, dewaxed and brought into water;
Treat for 15 minutes with a 5% aqueous solution of iron alum or for 10 minutes with a 5% solution of ferric chloride in 2% acetic acid;
Rinse rapidly in distilled water;
Rinse in 80% alcohol;
Where appropriate, stain the background with a 1% solution of brilliant yellow in 96% alcohol;
Wipe with blotting paper, dehydrate in acetone (avoid the action of absolute alcohol), clear in a benzenoid hydrocarbon and mount in Canada balsam or in a synthetic resin.

The green colour of the bilirubin is no clearer than it is in Stein's technique but the duration of the oxidation is substantially reduced in relation to that method.

Glenner's method for demonstrating bile pigments:

Sections of fresh tissue (with a chilled blade or in a cryostat), adherent to slides and dried in air;
Treat the dry sections for 15 minutes with the mixture
  hydrochloric acid-monopotassium phosphate buffer,
  pH 2.2 .... 1 volume
  0.1 M (2.94%) potassium bichromate solution .... 1 volume
Wash for 5 minutes in running water;
Fix for 20 minutes in calcium formaldehyde;
Wash for 5 minutes in running water;
Stain the background where appropriate, dehydrate with acetone, clear and mount in a synthetic resin.

As with the preceding techniques, that of Glenner results in a deep green stain.

A variant of Glenner's method allows the simultaneous demonstration of bile pigments, of free iron, and of free lipids. The working technique involves the following stages.

Frozen sections from fresh tissue, treated as in the preceding techniques;
Immerse the dry sections for 5 minutes in a 2% aqueous solution of potassium ferrocyanide;
Replace this solution with a mixture of equal parts of a 2% aqueous solution of potassium ferrocyanide and 5% acetic acid;
Leave the sections in this mixture for 20 minutes;
Wash in running water for about 2 minutes;
As in the previous variations, treat the sections with the acid solution of potassium bichromate;
Wash in running water for about 2 minutes;
Stain the free lipids with a supersaturated solution in water-propyl alcohol of oil red O (p. 453);
Wash for 5 minutes in running water;
Mount in Apathy's syrup or in any other medium miscible with water.

The free lipids (including chromolipoids) take on a red colour, the haemosiderin is stained blue and the bile pigments in deep emerald green.

We may recollect, as does Lillie (1965, p. 397) that the bile pigments encountered by the histopathologist in human material are often present in the same state as biliverdin, the green colour undergoing no changes when oxidised by one of the procedures mentioned above.

PORPHYRINS

The porphyrins may be recognised on tissue sections through the intense red or orange fluorescence which they exhibit in ultraviolet light; it is these compounds which account for most instances of primary fluorescence of this colour but naturally their identification requires a study of the fluorescence spectrum. The principle of the method has been briefly described in the chapter devoted to histophysical techniques; the publications of De Lerma (1958, 1963) carry an exhaustive bibliography on this topic.

WASTE-PRODUCTS OF PROTEIN METABOLISM

Among these compounds, urea and the purines and, in particular, uric acid and its salts have been the subject of histochemical investigations.

THE HISTOCHEMICAL DETECTION OF UREA

The interest attaching to the demonstration of the main nitrogenous waste-product of mammals on sections is obvious, but we must recognise that none of the methods put forward is satisfactory and that the conditions for this particular demonstration are, *a priori*, as unfavourable as possible. It is, in fact, vain to try to immobilise *in situ* a molecule of as small a size and as diffuseable as that of urea. Leschke's method using mercuric nitrate and Oliver's method using xanthydrol are mentioned for the record but their use as procedures for localisation at the cellular level is anything but advisable.

Leschke's (1914) method consists of fixing the tissues in a mixture of equal parts of a saturated aqueous solution of mercuric nitrate and 2% nitric acid. The author of the technique relied on the precipitation *in situ* of urea in the form of a mercuric complex. The pieces of tissue were then hydrated, embedded in paraffin wax and cut into sections, these being treated so that the mercury can be detected with an aqueous solution of hydrogen sulphide (distilled water saturated with gaseous H_2S). It is unnecessary to stress the lack of chemical specificity and the absence of any localising value of this method.

The xanthydrol method is tempting because of its rigorous chemical specificity; derived from the classical analytical reaction of Fosse, it rests on the formation of crystals of dixanthylurea in an acid medium, the form and assemblage into partially interpenetrating crystalline clusters being highly characteristic of urea. However, the formation of these crystals is slow, the xanthydrol is a molecule of rather large size, only slightly diffusible, whereas the contrary is true for the urea, and the examination of the preparations obtained using this procedure often shows crystalline rosettes whose size substantially exceeds that of the cells in which the presence of urea is sought. We have to deal in fact with a rigorously specific microchemical reaction which does not, however, fulfil the morphological conditions required of a histochemical technique. We may moreover note that the reaction takes place in fresh tissue and that it rather poorly preserves the tissue structures. Most modern authors use Oliver's variation (1921). Pieces of tissue of small size are immersed for 6 to 12 hours in a solution of 6 g of xanthydrol in a mixture of 35 ml of absolute alcohol and 65 ml of crystalliseable acetic acid (use fresh xanthydrol and prepare the solution at the time of use, allowing it to become tepid in order to dissolve all the xanthydrol, and then filter after chilling); dehydration and embedding in paraffin wax as well as the spreading of the sections call for no particular precautions; background stains may be used. The best identification of the crystals of dixanthylurea is afforded by examination under polarised light. As Lillie (1965) remarked, freeze-substitution is possible when this method is used.

HISTOCHEMICAL DETECTION OF PURINES

The histochemical detection of free purines is only possible with deposits of these compounds formed *in vivo*, their precipitation at the time of fixation being illusory in the current state of our knowledge. It is, therefore, mainly guanine, uric acid and the urates which are amenable to histochemical investigation.

Classically the disadvantages of highly acid fixatives during the preliminary stages of tests for purines come to mind and this remark is certainly justified.

when fixation takes place in an aqueous medium; in alcoholic media the acidity of the fixative is much less noxious. In practice, the best results are obtained by using formalin alcohol or Carnoy's fluid. Embedding may be undertaken in paraffin wax without particular precautions; it is recommended not to prolong the treatment of the sections with hot water at the time of spreading the sections but it is rarely useful to go so far as to spread them out dry.

Among the techniques for demonstrating purines the classical technique of Saint-Hilaire based on the formation of cuprous salts of these compounds, the copper then being detected by the potassium ferrocyanide method, is associated with so many causes of error that it seems reasonable to abandon it.

Other histochemical features of the purines are used in order to demonstrate them on sections. These are their basophilia and their reducing power. Techniques for staining using progressive lakes of haematoxylin or various preparations with a carmine base depend on the basophilia of deposits of uric acid and urates; these techniques are obviously devoid of all histochemical significance. Tests for basophilia using the procedures indicated in the appropriate chapter of this work may furnish an argument in favour of the presence of purines but they can in no way constitute a proof.

The same remark holds good for the argentaffin reaction when given by structures which may contain purines, but the number of argentaffin compounds present in the tissues is much less than the number of basophilic compounds, so that the probability in favour of the presence of purines is distinctly greater when the positive results are obtained with this method, especially if, in addition, the morphological characteristics of the structures are taken into account. The need to carry out the reaction in conditions which preserve its histochemical significance should lead us to reject the procedure of De Galantha (1935) which finds favour with anatomo-pathologists, since it brings into play a reducing agent. It is the silver-hexamethylenetetramine technique of Gomori which gives the best results. The working technique may be conducted in the following way.

Paraffin wax sections, taken from material fixed in alcohol, formalin treated alcohol, or Carnoy's fluid, spread with the precautions mentioned above, dewaxed and washed in absolute alcohol;

Treat the sections taken from the absolute alcohol with the silver hexamethylenetetramine solution buffered to pH 8–9, and previously brought to 37°, for about 30 minutes;

Rinse in distilled water;

Rinse rapidly with a 5% solution of sodium thiosulphate;

Rinse in tap water;

Where appropriate, tone with gold chloride in a non-acetified 0.2% aqueous solution;

Rinse in distilled water;

Where appropriate, stain the nuclei with a red stain (safranine, basic fuchsin, the aluminium lake of nuclear fast red);

Dehydrate in absolute alcohol, clear in a benzenoid hydrocarbon and mount in Canada balsam or in a synthetic resin.

Under these experimental conditions, the deposits of urates take on an intense black stain and the presence of large quantities of calcium salts represents the only source of error giving rise to serious disquiet. The small quantities of silver phosphate or carbonate which might disclose the presence of these calcium salts are in fact soluble in the alkaline silver complex and only more substantial amounts run the risk of creating a nuisance. In fact, it is easy to make the distinction because the calciferous deposits are easily extracted from the sections by a short treatment with a dilute acid and they usually withstand treatment with alkalis, whereas urate deposits withstand treatment by dilute acids and are very rapidly dissolved by aqueous solutions of lithium carbonate.

The murexide reaction, which is positive with uric acid, xanthine and guanine, but negative with adenine and hypoxanthine, depends on the appearance of a violet stain when the section is covered with a drop of concentrated nitric acid, warmed to the point of evaporation, and then treated with ammonia vapour. Naturally this is a drastic procedure, unworthy of the dignity of a histochemical technique; not only that but its sensitivity is rather slight.

The distinction between guanine and uric acid depend on the solubility haracteristics. It so happens that guanine is very soluble in mineral acids, nsoluble in organic acids, very soluble in alkalis except for ammonia and insoluble in piperazine hydrate, whereas uric acid is insoluble in mineral acids, soluble in alkalis except for ammonia, and soluble in piperazine hydrate. In doubtful cases the solubility of guanine in aqueous solutions of iron alum (Millot, 1923) affords an additional criterion for discrimination.

CHAPTER 22

THE HISTOCHEMICAL DETECTION OF THE PRINCIPAL ENZYMES

Of all the branches of modern histochemical research histoenzymology is certainly the one which gives rise to the greatest number of publications; very often, whole issues of the major histochemical journals do not contain a single original paper dealing with results outside the scope of histoenzymology. An attempt to classify modern histochemists by their speciality would lead to the discovery that the substantial majority were histoenzymologists and this branch of histochemical technique is perhaps the only one for which specialised treatises have been published.

This orientation of histochemical research which was clearly indicated by Lison (1960) has become even more marked since the appearance of his book. The attraction which an ever growing number of research workers finds in the histochemical detection of enzymes results in such a flood of contradictory publications that only a specialist is in any position to discriminate with certainty between soundly based results, doubtful findings, and mistakes.

From an individual point of view, specialisation in histo-enzymology is to all appearances a logical and coherent attitude; what seems to me to be much less certain is that the wholesale commitment, some of whose consequences have just been mentioned, represents an attitude which is truly rational and justified by its results. It is perfectly understandable that the magnificent successes of biochemical enzymology have led histochemists to try to adapt enzymological techniques to their working conditions, but the desire to be "in the fashion" and to jump on the band wagon also plays a part in determining the selection of histo-enzymology by many research workers.

The concentration of all the efforts of a research worker or of a team on methodological programmes is rather unusual in other sections of histochemical research; it is on the contrarie quite normal in the case of histo-enzymology. The main objective is the development of techny ques for detection and those histo-enzymologists, who try themselves to put to good use th- techniques which they have invented or developed by applying them to biological problems, are certainly not in the majority.

This inflation of methodological publications represents only one of the peculiarities of histoenzymology when compared with other sectors of histochemical research. The methodology of the histo-enzymologist's work is clearly different from that obtaining in other histochemical investigations and this state of affairs clearly explains the present development of a tendency for histoenzymology to become a distinct subject.

It is indeed true—and this is an essential feature of which we should never lose sight—that *the histo-enzymologist is so far unable to detect enzymes themselves but only the products of their action on substrates contained in the reagents.* The detection of the proteins which constitute the enzymes as chemically defined substances has been secured in some cases through immuno-histochemistry; the number of unquestionable results obtained by this technique is not great because it is an essential preliminary step to obtain enzymatic preparations which are rigorously pure. The general use of this procedure seems to be reserved for a somewhat distant future. Instead of being able to localise enzymes as chemical substances the histo-enzymologist must therefore have recourse to much more indirect procedures than most of the reactions studied in the preceding chapters; his labours are therefore much increased, the sources of error become more numerous and the interpretation of the results shows this all too clearly.

One of the first consequences of what we have just discussed is the need to preserve the activity of the enzymes on sections subjected to histo-enzymological techniques; any denaturation which results in a loss of activity is intolerable for the histo-enzymologist who, because of this, is obliged to do without the best morphological fixatives, everything being deliberately sacrificed to the special chemical conditions of histochemical work. From the practical point of view the activity of the enzymes is often preserved at the expense of changes in the cell and tissue morphology which prevent their being studied at the cytological level. Very frequently the histo-enzymologist is unable to keep any material in reserve. The time schedule of his work is particularly demanding and the use of material taken from animals other than those commonly kept alive in laboratories may give rise to substantial practical difficulties.

The indirect nature of histo-enzymological reactions at the present time also confer special characteristics on histo-enzymological research. Very often any given enzyme is capable of acting on several substrates and the converse is also true, one single substrate can be affected by several enzymes. The danger of diffusion of the enzyme itself during the manipulations exists as in any other histochemical research; moreover, the danger of diffusion of reaction products by which the enzymatic activity is detected is at least as great. It is therefore, easy to understand the care taken by various authors to investigate reactions whose reaction products are as little soluble, as slightly diffusible and as substantial as possible.

As I remarked in the introduction, any attempt at a methodical account of modern histo-enzymological literature would far exceed the scope of this work and of my own capacities; it would moreover be wasted labour. It is in the field of histo-enzymology that the review literature is the easiest to come by of any sector of histochemistry. In addition to the long sections devoted to histoenzymology in modern textbooks of histochemical technique, specialised monographs (Arvy, 1957/58; Burstone, 1962; Deane et al., 1961; Greenberg, 1960; Mehler, 1957; Sumner and Sommers, 1953) greatly facilitate an entry into the topics;

the considerable part devoted to histo-enzymology in all histochemical journals has also been mentioned. Further, the account of histo-enzymological techniques attempted here is voluntarily restricted to those concepts which seem to me to be indispensable for the unspecialised histologist. It is, nevertheless, true that the general conditions for investigations of enzymatic activity should be set out succinctly before reviewing the main techniques for demonstrating enzymatic activity corresponding to the hydrolases, transferases and oxi-reductases in Hoffmann-Ostenhof's (1954) classification.

THE PREPARATION OF TISSUES INTENDED FOR HISTO-ENZYMOLOGICAL RESEARCH

One clear result of the facts mentioned above is that modern histo-enzymology is characterised by the deliberate sacrifice of the morphological requirements of histochemical research. The preservation of those enzymatic activities which are to be investigated predominates over any other consideration during the treatment of the tissue. In most cases this state of affairs precludes investigations at the level of the organelle or even of the cell; as Lison (1960, p. 532) has quite rightly commented, the attempt to localise enzymatic activity can in no case be more successful than the preservation of the tissue and cell structures.

The preservation of that enzymatic activity which requires to be demonstrated and the maintainance of its localisation are equally important for the histo-enzymologist. Experience shows that difficulties which may be met with vary greatly according to circumstances; some enzymes remain detectable after embedding in paraffin wax, carried out without special precautions; others are seriously modified even by freezing the tissue, undertaken with a view to section cutting; the extent to which diffusion takes place is also very variable according to the circumstances.

Certain enzymes can only be studied on fresh tissue; in such cases the only solution is to cut the sections after freezing, using a Schultz-Brauns microtome or a cryostat. It is easy to imagine the amplitude of the displacements to which substances may be subjected when frozen, unfixed sections are treated with different reagents, and this explains the range of precautionary measures with which the investigator must surround himself when studying this kind of preparation at the level of the cell.

In other cases, chemical fixatives can be used; it is always helpful to fix at low temperatures (0 to 4°C). Absolute alcohol, acetone, 10% formalin, whether saline or not, formalin-chloral hydrate, formalin-pyridine, and even mixtures of formalin and acetic acid have been suggested. The advantages of fixation by aldehydes other than formalin (glutaraldehyde, acrolein, etc...) have been mentioned in the general comments on fixatives (p. 52). Dehydration using acetone or even ethanol is compatible with the preservation of the activity of certain enzymes. Of all the stages prior to the preparation of paraffin wax sections, it is the time spent at high temperatures in this substance which is the most harmful. There is, therefore, general agreement on this subject at the present time; it is always better to work on frozen sections than on those in paraffin wax; when the latter course cannot be avoided everything possible should be done to shorten the time spent by the pieces of tissue in the oven (tissue blocks of very small size, vacuum embedding, etc...).

It is hardly necessary to add that the maintainance of the chemical properties which serve for the detection of enzymes is not the only essential feature which has to be taken into account during the preparation of the tissue; to prevent the enzyme from moving is as important as to preserve its activity. From this point of view, the classical distinction between lyo-enzymes and desmo-enzymes (Willstätter and Rohdewald, 1932) is as important as it ever was. It so happens that during fixation losses of lyo-enzymes may take place quite apart from any chemical action of the reagents used at this stage; losses may also take place when the tissue blocks are allowed to stand in a "physiological" fluid. Nachlas and his colleagues have shown that 60% of alkaline phosphatase activity, 48% of acid phosphatase activity, 65% of leucine-aminopeptidase activity and only 5% of B-glucuronidase activity in mammalian tissue corresponds to desmo-enzymes. Such proportions are obviously accentuated after fixation, the lyo-enzymes having been either lost or rendered insoluble. From the histochemical standpoint displacements of the lyo-enzymes at the time that the tissues are treated may result either in overestimation due to false localisation or to underestimation due to solution in the reagents. There is all the more cause to be worried about displacement of the enzymes when sections of fresh tissue are incubated in substrates without having undergone fixation even of short duration.

From the point of view of histo-enzymological technique freeze-drying is a step of great theoretical value but the practical limitations of the method, mentioned in the first part of this work, apply as much to the detection of enzymes as to other techniques. Denaturation of the sections should be undertaken before they are incubated in substrates, unless we wish to find ourselves in the same difficulties as when working with fresh tissue.

The solution adopted for the preparation of tissues for the demonstration of enzymes is, therefore, always a compromise between contradictory requirements, the working techniques recommended in various special cases being sketched in the following sections.

THE GENERAL COURSE OF HISTO-ENZYMOLOGICAL REACTIONS

All modern histo-enzymological reactions depend on the same fundamental principle which consists of the incubation of the preparation in a medium containing the substrate for the enzyme under investigation as well as substances intended to control the pH at the level required and, where necessary, activators. The choice of the subtrate is essential for success because one of the reaction products should be on the one hand *coloured or capable of giving rise to a colour reaction* and on the other hand *insoluble in water and in the lipids of tissues* so that it does not behave as a lysochrome, *with a substantial but not selective affinity for proteins, and lastly devoid of any strongly polar nature.* It is easy to see how difficult it is to secure all these conditions, especially when we have to add the need to use a substrate which is sufficiently soluble in water for the enzymatic reaction and of a sufficiently low molecular weight to penetrate rapidly and in sufficient concentration at the site of the activity of the enzyme.

In a substantial number of cases it is impossible to realise all the conditions which have just been specified and the histo-enzymologist must then face the prospect of working with substrates which give rise to enzymatic reactions whose products are soluble but whose precipitation *in situ* (capture) may be secured, as fast as the material is produced, by adding suitably chosen compounds to the incubating bath. In this way anions liberated by the enzymatic reaction may be immobilised at the place where they are formed, by adding to the incubating bath the salt of a metal which forms insoluble salts with these anions. When the reaction product is a phenol or a naphthol the addition to the incubating medium of a diazonium salt ensures not only that it is rendered insoluble but also that there is a colour reaction through the formation of an azo dyestuff. In the course of enzymatic reactions which liberate indoxyl derivatives these may be immobilised by oxidation and transformation into dyes of the indigo group.

In addition to the substrate for the enzymatic reaction (primary reaction), a buffer intended to stabilise the pH, and possibly an activator for the enzyme, the incubation should therefore contain in many cases an immobilising agent for the product of the primary reaction. Naturally the whole should have a certain stability in the chemical sense and none of the substances present should behave as an inhibitor of the enzyme under investigation; specific inhibitors may on the other hand be deliberately added to the medium in order to investigate the reaction.

Immobilisation by metal ions is the oldest technique for capturing the primary reaction product. It is still used in a certain number of instances giving results distinctly inferior to those obtained by capturing with diazonium salts which was introduced into histo-enzymological technique by Menten and his colleagues (1944). This second technique, however, is not without its disadvantages; the principal ones are the chemical instability of diazonium salts in solution, their inhibiting action towards certain enzymatic reactions and the fact that pH values needed for the coupling reaction do not always correspond to the optimal pH of the primary reaction. The practical disadvantages which we have just mentioned have led certain authors to develop techniques for post-coupling which use, for the primary reaction, substances which liberate insoluble phenols or naphthols which are precipitated *in situ*. Once this primary reaction is complete coupling with a suitably chosen diazonium salt may take place under optimal conditions of pH and temperature since we no longer have to worry about the needs of the enzymatic reaction. However, we should not fail to recognise that this theoretical advantage may be counter-balanced by the disadvantage stemming from the danger of unspecific adsorption of the primary reaction products; over-estimation is in such cases to be feared.

Techniques using indoxyl esters, which were introduced by Barrnett and Seligman (1951) and greatly developed by Holt and his colleagues (1952, 1955), depend on the fact that the indoxyl liberated during the primary reaction oxidised to indigo a substance which is at once coloured and insoluble. The main recent improvements to this technique consist of the introduction of radicals which increase the insolubility of the indoxyl molecule and the addition to the incubating medium of catalysts for the oxidation which will accelerate the transformation of indoxyl into indigo, and thus diminish the risk of diffusion.

Whatever the circumstances, histo-enzymological work takes place in technical conditions which are more difficult than those of other histochemical methods. Even the most "indirect" of the procedures discussed in the preceding chapters, even those which depend on a complicated sequence of reactions are basically founded on the chemical modification of the molecule we wish to detect. It is quite otherwise with histo-enzymological methods; none of the latter include a reaction which effectively changes the enzyme molecule we wish to detect. The products of the primary reaction and, *a fortiori*, those of the capturing reactions are by definition independent of the enzyme which gave rise to them and, because of this, may undergo much more substantial displacements than the products of other histochemical reactions. The need for accuracy in localisation is particularly difficult to secure and to investigate in histo-enzymological reactions. When the product of the enzymatic reaction (primary reaction) is insoluble, its formation is a reaction of order zero from the chemical kinetic standpoint and is therefore independent of the concentration of the substrate and uniquely dependent on the enzymatic activity; however, the precipitation of this reaction product only takes place when its concentration exceeds a certain threshold so that the possibilities for diffusion are all the greater when the enzymatic activity and the solubility of the reaction product are weaker. Errors of over, or under, estimation may also stem from displacement of the reaction product and from its affinity for structures where there is no enzymatic activity. Moreover, precipitation may take place in the form of granules or even crystals which are a great nuisance when studying organelles. When the primary reaction product has to be immobilised by means of a second reaction, which is itself of the first order in the chemical kinetic sense (rate proportional to the concentration of the reaction product), the accuracy of localisation is all the greater when the speed of the rate of the capturing reaction and the substantivity of the substance to be demonstrated are greater and the solubility is weaker (Holt, 1958).

These theoretical observations are very widely taken into account during the synthesis of substrates for histo-enzymological research. The introduction into the molecules of functional groups whose presence increases the substantivity and diminishes the solubility has indeed resulted in spectacular progress, a consequential disadvantage being the often great increase in the cost of the materials.

To terminate this section, it is appropriate to stress the difficulties which may arise when we have to decide how good a histo-enzymological preparation is. As Lison (1960) and Burstone (1963) have quite rightly commented, a tendency to consider that clear, "sharp" localisations are necessarily good is not above criticism. This way of looking at the results of histo-enzymological techniques, which is directly inspired by criteria which are perfectly valid when judging the results of a staining procedure, amounts to the proposition that the distribution of enzymes within a cell is never diffuse, an interpretation which is patently false on the scale of light microscopy. We should never forget that particularly clear cut images may result from under-estimation, activity weaker than that of the structures which have been shown up having been lost during the manipulation. Images which are just as clear may correspond to over-estimation and simply result from a very high substantivity for the stained structure of substances which have diffused during the primary reaction or during the capture reaction.

In fact, criteria for validity which are much more important than just the clarity of images stems from taking into consideration the mechanism of the reactions and from the study of the chemical properties of the substrata. In histo-enzymological practice the value of cross checking the results obtained using methods which are based on different chemical principles is particularly great. In any event, histo-enzymological preparations should always be compared with controls obtained in an incubation medium which is the same except for the fact that the enzymatic activity has been inhibited using as specific an inhibitor as possible.

Naturally the value of any histo-enzymological publication is greatly increased when its text includes all the details necessary for the reproduction of the results (the conditions under which the reaction has been carried out, the nature and origin of the substrate, a precise indication of the inhibitors used).

HISTOCHEMICAL DETECTION OF HYDROLASES

The hydrolase group in the Hoffmann-Ostenhof classification is characterised by its capacity to catalyse the transfer of an exchangeable group to water, the general scheme of the reaction being

$$R{-}R' + H_2O \rightleftharpoons R{-}OH + R'{-}H$$

Among the numerous enzymes of this group we may mention here the phosphatases, carboxylic esterases and glycosidases, and the peptidases and phosphamidases whose activity can be detected histochemically.

A. — PHOSPHATASES

Some of these enzymes, whose common property is the catalysis of the hydrolytic cleavage of phosphoric esters, are specific only in the way in which they form links and may act on substrates which are very different from one another in various chemical characteristics (unspecific phosphatases); other enzymes of the same group which are said to be specific act only on well defined substrates.

If we take into consideration the optimum pH we are led to distinguish acid and alkaline phosphatases which may be either specific or unspecific.

The most important of the alkaline phosphatases accessible to histochemical detection are the unspecific alkaline phosphomonoesterase (phosphatase A_1 or I of the classical biochemists), 5-nucleotidase, and adenosinetriphosphatase; techniques for the detection of pyro- and metaphosphatases which are still subject to debate are not mentioned here.

NON-SPECIFIC ALKALINE PHOSPHOMONOESTERASE

This was in fact the first enzyme whose activity was detected histochemically, the celebrated experiments of Robison and his colleagues (1923) on the "bone enzyme" representing a histochemical demonstration. The techniques of Gomori (1939) and Takamatsu (1939) depend on the same principle. Since these investigations the detection of the enzyme activity in question has given rise to an impressive number of publications. The methods put forward can be brought together schematically under five headings, which are, the deposition of acid calcium phosphate ($CaHPO_4$) at the site of enzyme activity, the deposition of naphthyls with simultaneous coupling, the deposition of naphthyls with postcoupling, the deposition of azo-dyestuffs, without coupling and the deposition of indigo. Techniques which depend on the three last headings are of only theoretical interest in the case of the enzyme activity discussed here; they are described in histochemical text-books (see in particular Lison, 1960; Pearse, 1960; Barka and Anderson, 1963) and in the specialist monographs cited at the beginning of this chapter. The techniques involving acid calcium phosphate and the naphthyls are on the other hand widely employed and should be described here.

Techniques using sodium glycerophosphate

This is the classical method of Gomori (1939) and Takamatsu (1939) from which numerous variations are derived. The principle is simple. The sections are incubated at about 37°C in a medium which, in addition to a sodium veronal buffer intended to keep the pH around 9.4, also contains sodium glycerophosphate, calcium nitrate and sulphate or magnesium chloride to act as activators of the enzyme. Under these conditions the phosphate ions, liberated during the primary reaction, react with the calcium ions introduced with the calcium nitrate present in the medium to give calcium phosphate which is insoluble in an alkaline medium. The reaction is completed by the histochemical demonstration of the calcium phosphate so formed and comparison of the results with control preparations in which either the incubation is carried out in a medium to which a specific inhibitor has been added or in which the enzymatic activity has been destroyed by heat prior to incubation.

A whole series of investigations shows that the chemical specificity of the method is satisfactory but that its value for localising the enzyme is marred by sources of error, the principal of which is the diffusion of the primary reaction product and even of that of the capture reaction. Nuclear sites for non-specific alkaline phosphatase have been described after the application of the sodium glycerophosphate technique and these results are considered by the great majority of modern specialists as being diffusion artefacts. Other sources of error, such as confusion between the deposition of calcium phosphate associated with the reaction and pre-existing deposits of calcium or other metals capable of reacting while calcium is being demonstrated are much easier to avoid.

Among the numerous ways of preparing the substrate I would recommend Barger's (1947) formula the principal practical advantage of which is to use two solutions which keep for months or even for years when a few drops of chloroform are added and when they are stored at low temperatures (about 4°C). The solution A consists of 2% sodium β-glycerophosphate, the solution B contains 5 grams of sodium veronal (sodium diethylmalonylurea), 5 grams of anhydrous calcium chloride or the nitrate of the same metal, and lastly 0.5 grams of magnesium sulphate for every 1000 ml of distilled water. At the time of use 25 to 30 ml of solution A are added to 50 ml of solution B. The mixture keeps less well than do the stock solutions.

Stoelzner's method using cobalt nitrate seems to me preferable to any others for the detection of calcium phosphate deposited as a result of the sequence primary reaction-capture reaction. It has the advantage of being more rapid and less costly than von Kossa's method which is recommended by some authors; the stains which it affords are clearer than those obtained by staining with sodium alizarin-sulphonate or with purpurin; the demonstration of calcareous deposits by examination in polarised light has no practical advantages. The substitution of lead nitrate for cobalt nitrate followed by the detection of this metal using the sodium rhodizonate technique or by staining with gallamine blue, the use of glycerophosphate labelled by means of a radioactive tracer followed by autoradiography are both of no interest for routine work.

The reaction may be applied to sections of fresh or fixed tissue, to smear preparations or even to small tissue blocks (spread membranes, etc...). Incubation takes place at 37° to 40°C. The following precaution should be taken during incubation and the detection of calcareous deposits in order to reduce diffusion artefacts as far as possible. *Collodion treatment* of sections adhering to slides is always useful; *the incubation time* should not be excessive (about 20 minutes at the most for frozen sections treated in staining baths, 30 minutes to 2 hours for sections adhering to slides); *careful washing* in tap water which should not be acid, or with a dilute solution of sodium veronal (2 ml of a 2% solution for every 100 ml of distilled water) helps to eliminate diffuse stains. We must emphasize the serious drawbacks attaching to prolonged incubation as was formerly practised, which generates gross artefacts through the diffusion of the calcium phosphate. During the Stoelzner reaction intended to reveal calcium phosphate it is patently necessary to wash carefully after treatment with the cobalt salt.

The *working technique* includes the following stages

> Paraffin wax sections, treated with collodion and hydrated, frozen sections, free or adhering to slides, smear preparations, etc...
> Treat for 20 minutes to 2 hours, at 37°, in Barger's incubation bath or one of the numerous other mixtures suggested;
> Wash carefully (about 5 minutes) in frequently renewed tap water;
> Treat for 3 to 5 minutes with a 2% solution of cobalt nitrate in distilled water (the acetate or the chloride of the same metal can equally well be used);
> Wash with great care in frequently renewed tap water;
> Treat for 1 to 2 minutes with a dilute solution of ammonium sulphide (about 1 ml of a commercial 20% solution in 50 ml of tap water);
> Wash carefully in tap water;
> Stain the background, where appropriate, using the aluminium lake of nuclear fast red;
> Wash in running water;
> Dehydrate in absolute alcohol, clear in a benzenoid hydrocarbon and mount in Canada balsam or in a synthetic resin.

The presence of calcium phosphate deposits diagnostic of enzymatic activity is shown by a black stain but naturally any sites of calcium carbonate or phosphate will be shown up irrespective of the reaction; in the same way any ferruginous inclusion and, more generally, any structures containing a metal with a black sulphide are detected by this technique. Moreover experience shows that the fixation of cobalt by structures rich in acid groups, in particular by mucosubstances, may result in a black stain unrelated to the presence of alkaline phosphomonoesterase activity.

Some of these sources of error can be eliminated by comparison with control slides which constitutes an obligatory stage in all histo-enzymological research. The incubation of the sections in a bath containing all the ingredients mentioned above with the exception of sodium glycerophosphate, such as the early authors practised, is not very satisfactory from a theoretical point of view because it leads us to compare sections which have undergone very different treatments. Nowadays it is preferable to add an inhibitor (potassium cyanide at 0.01 M concentration or, better, cysteine chlorhydrate at 0.004 M concentration) to the incubating bath in which the control sections are kept; a still more elegant technique due to Danielli (1948) consists of inactivating the enzyme by keeping the control sections in distilled water warmed to 90°C; it is sufficient to keep them there for 3 minutes and experience shows that the risk of loosening the sections is minimal, especially if they have been treated with collodion. The adoption of this latter working technique allows all the sections to undergo the same treatments and the demonstrative value of the results is substantially improved.

The distinction between pre-existing calcareous deposits and those which indicate the presence of enzymatic activity can be made by revealing the first using Stoelzner's reaction with cobalt nitrate prior to incubation (Wachstein,

1952); the sections are then washed, incubated, treated with cobalt nitrate, the cobalt phosphate so formed being revealed with dithioxamide (p. 317) giving a brownish yellow stain very different from that given by Stoelzner's reaction. the pre-existing calcareous inclusions can be eliminated (Gomori, 1952) by treating the sections prior to incubation for about twelve minutes with a citrate buffer of pH 4.5 to 5; prolonged washing in tap water (about 10 minutes) should precede incubation in the substrate.

The simultaneous demonstration of alkaline phosphatase activity and of free iron can be performed in the following way (Arvy and Gabe, 1949).

> Carry out the test for alkaline phosphatase activity using the Gomori-Takamatsu method but prolonging for 15 minutes the time spent by the sections in the dilute solution of ammonium sulphide;
> Rinse in tap water;
> Treat the sections with the potassium ferricyanide-hydrochloric acid mixture for the demonstration of free iron using the Turnbull blue reaction (p. 313);
> Rinse in distilled water;
> Stain the background as in tests for free iron, dehydrate in absolute alcohol, clear in a benzenoid hydrocarbon and mount in a synthetic resin.

Inclusions containing iron appear blue, the calcareous deposits, whether pre-existent or diagnostic of alkaline phosphomonoesterase activity, appear black; this technique may be applied after Koelle's technique for demonstrating cholinesterases (Arvy, 1964).

Naturally, any confusion between pre-existing metalliferous inclusions and the sites of alkaline phosphatase activity is excluded when the latter is revealed by methods involving naphthylphosphates, a comparison of these preparations with those given by the Gomori-Takamatsu method being a supplementary control method.

The detection of alkaline phosphomonoesterase activity using the sodium glycerophosphate-cobalt nitrate technique has advantages, the most important of which are the moderate price of the substances necessary for the reaction and the ease with which they can be obtained. However the incubation periods are longer than with methods using naphthylphosphates, the incubation has to be carried out in the warm and, above all, diffusion artefacts are much more to be feared than with procedures which result in the formation of coloured azo dyestuffs. It would perhaps be an excessive reaction to discount altogether the use of the glycerophosphate-cobalt nitrate reaction but the superiority of techniques involving naphthylphosphates is agreed by all modern histochemists.

Techniques involving naphthyl phosphates

These techniques, derived from the method of Menten, Junge and Green (1944), whose superiority over those involving sodium glycerophosphate has just been stressed, have been subjected to successive developments the principal stages of progress being the use of α-naphthylphosphates instead of the β-naphthylphosphates used at the beginning, the choice of diazonium salts particularly suitable for coupling and lastly the development of substrates whose base is 3-hydroxy-2-naphthoic acid anilide (the naphthol AS compounds of the American industrial nomenclature, the brenthol AS compounds of the English nomenclature).

One advantage of the techniques considered here over the sodium glycerophosphate technique springs immediately to mind; in effect, the capture reaction and the colour reaction intended to demonstrate the primary secretory product are one and the same. The naphthol liberated at the site of phosphatase activity is precipitated by coupling with the diazonium salt present in the incubating medium, this precipitate being coloured. We may add to this that the reaction takes place at laboratory temperatures and that it is much more rapid than that with glycerophosphate; no metalliferous inclusion can simulate phosphatase activity and the azo-reaction of the proteins, which is automatically obtained at the same time as is the detection of the phosphomonoesterase, gives rise to much clearer stains so that no confusion is possible. Factors in the success of the method are solubility in the substrate, the insolubility and the substantivity of the naphthol formed during the primary reaction, the rapidity of the coupling reaction and the substantivity of the azo dyestuff which is the final product of the reaction. Obviously it is very difficult to satisfy all these needs. The α-naphthylphosphates used currently have the advantage over their β-isomers of being less soluble when combined into an azo dyestuff so that there is less risk of diffusion. The prototype is Gomori's reaction (1951) using sodium α-naphthylphosphate whose use I would cordially recommend for routine work. The replacement of this substrate by phosphate of naphthol AS compounds results in an improvement of the substantivity and a distinct lessening of the solubility of the reaction product (Burstone, 1958, 1962) but the disadvantages counterbalance the advantages. In fact, the phosphates of naphthol AS compounds are very slightly soluble in water so that the substrates have to be prepared from stock solutions in N,N'-dimethylformamide, whereas sodium α-naphthylphosphate dissolves very readily in distilled water; the molecules of the phosphates of naphthol AS compounds are distinctly more voluminous than those of sodium naphthyl phosphate and carry numerous polar groups which slow down the build-up of the required concentration of substrate for the primary reaction at sites where there is phosphatase activity, as Pearse (1960) has quite correctly noted. Moreover, coupling with diazonium salts is very slow in the case of the naphthol AS compounds, the risk of diffusion which results being, therefore, counterbalanced by their slight solubility and their high substantivity. From the practical point of view, we should add to this that naphthol AS compounds are more costly and more difficult to obtain than sodium naphthylphosphates; as for the phosphates of these compounds only a few are commercially available at far from negligeable prices and in most cases the histochemist is obliged to prepare them himself.

The choice of the diazonium salts used for the coupling reaction deserves special mention; to some extent at least it conditions the speed of this stage of the reaction as well as the substantivity of the azo dyestuff formed; moreover, the optimum pH of the coupling reaction is not the same for all the diazonium salts and does not necessarily coincide with the optimum pH of the primary reaction. Moreover, all diazonium salts may behave as inhibitors of alkaline phosphatases when present at too high a concentration. We should not forget that only the azo dyestuffs obtained, in the case of the Gomori reaction, by coupling with the diazo salt of o-dianisidine are insoluble in ethyl alcohol and in benzenoid hydrocarbons so that it is possible to mount in Canada balsam or in equivalent synthetic resins. In all other cases mounting in a medium miscible with water is obligatory. We know from the systematic studies of Gomori (1952), Goessner (1958) and Pearse (1960) that in addition to fast blue B salt (the diazo salt of o-dianisidine),, fast blue BB salt, variamine blue B salt, fast blue RR salt, fast red RC salt, and fast red TR salt are most suitable for the coupling reaction in the technique which involves sodium α-naphthyl phosphate. As for techniques using the naphthol AS compounds, Burstone (1958–1962) particularly recommends fast blue RR salt and red violet LB salt, the mounting in both cases having to be carried out in a medium miscible with water.

In practice, the sodium α-naphthylphosphate method, due to Gomori (1951, 1952), is as valuable as ever; the "sharpness" of preparations obtained using the technique involving naphthol AS compounds after Burstone (1958, 1962) is slightly better but the "return" from these preparations does not exceed that provided by the preceding method to an extent sufficient to justify the erection of techniques using phosphates of the naphthol AS compounds into routine procedures.

The method using sodium α-naphthylphosphate is mentioned here with minor modifications as compared with the original working technique of Gomori; the principal of these are the reduction to 10 minutes of the duration of incubation, the suppression of differentiation in acid alcohol, intended to clear the background, and the introduction of iodine green as a nuclear stain. The working technique thus includes the following stages.

> Frozen sections, treated in staining baths or adhering to slides, smears, paraffin wax sections, dewaxed, treated with collodion and hydrated;
> Treat for 10 minutes, at laboratory temperatures, with the reagent prepared *immediately prior to use* in the following way;
> dissolve 10 mg of sodium α-naphthylphosphate in a few ml of distilled water, make up to 45 ml with chilled distilled water at the temperature of melting ice; add 5 ml of 4% borax solution (sodium tetraborate decahydrate) (this concentration corre-

ponds roughly to saturation at 20°C) and 2 to 3 drops of a 10% solution of magnesium chloride or sulphate;

dissolve 20 mg of the diazo salt of *o*-dianisidine in this mixture; the filtration recommended in the original formula is of no value in most instances;

Wash in tap water which is either running or repeatedly renewed;

Stain the nuclei using a 0.5% aqueous solution of iodine green for 3 to 4 minutes;

Rinse in distilled water;

Dehydrate in absolute alcohol (a violet impurity with which most commercial samples of iodine green are contaminated is extracted from the sections by this manoeuvre), clear in a benzenoid hydrocarbon and mount in Canada balsam or in a commericial synthetic resin.

The background stain using iodine green which gives preparations with a better contrast than those using carmine alum or haemalum, as recommended by Gomori, should be omitted if it is desired to mount in a medium miscible with water, thus avoiding dehydration, unless the violet impurity has been removed from the dye first by extraction with chloroform.

Under these experimental conditions the presence of alkaline phosphatase activity is shown by a deep purple or black stain, the nuclei being stained green, the yellow colour of the background corresponding to the azo reaction of proteins. Control sections should undergo the same treatment after having been kept for 2 or 3 minutes in distilled water brought to 90°C.

Burstone's technique using the phosphates of substituted naphthol AS derivatives, includes as a first step the preparation of the phosphate from commercial samples of naphthol AS; the most suitable are napthol AS-MX, AS-TR and AS-CL in the American nomenclature.

The substrate is prepared in the following manner:

Suspend 5 g of the selected naphthol AS in 50 ml of tetrahydrofuran *free from hydroquinone*; add about 300 ml of versene (sodium ethylene-diamine-tetraacetate), 50 to 100 mg of sodium laurylsulphate, two grams of sodium chloride and 5 ml of phosphorous oxychloride ($POCl_3$); add, with stirring, two to three ml of pure pyridine;

Pour the mixture, whilst still stirring, into a 1 litre beaker and allow it to evaporate under a jet of air until a clear syrup is formed; add three or four cubes of ice (prepared with distilled water) whilst still vigorously stirring the mixture;

After 5 minutes stirring, add about 500 ml of chilled distilled water and mix vigorously; in certain cases, a voluminous pulverulent precipitate is formed, in others a tarry or rubbery mass is formed which shows a distinct tendency to harden;

Fragment, where necessary, the tarry masses by crushing them in chilled distilled water, collect the fine precipitate by filtration with the aid of a water pump and wash several times with cold water; this crude preparation can be purified by dissolving in tetrahydrofuran and precipitation with petroleum ether, but experience shows that the impurities so eliminated do not interfere with its useful histochemical purposes;

For the detection of alkaline phosphomonoesterase activity prepare a solution of 50 mg of naphthol AS phosphate in 20 ml of N,N'-dimethylformamide, add 20 ml of water and adjust the pH to 8.0 with an M/1 solution of sodium carbonate. Then add 600 ml of distilled water and make up to 1,000 ml with a "tris" buffer of pH 8.3. The opalescent liquid so obtained keeps for several months, even at laboratory temperatures.

The ***working technique*** is similar to that of Gomori's method using sodium naphththylphosphate.

> Frozen sections adhering to slides or paraffin wax sections, dewaxed and hydrated;
> Treat for 5 to 30 minutes, at laboratory temperatures, with the solution of naphthol AS phosphate mentioned above, to which 1 mg per ml of the chosen diazonium salt (red-violet fast LB, fast blue RR, fast red RC or fast red TR) has been added;
> Rinse in tap water and mount in a medium miscible with water; Burstone particularly recommends a polyvinylpyrrolidone medium, prepared in the following way; dissolve 50 g of polyvinylpyrrolidone in 50 ml of distilled water, allow to stand for about 12 hours, and add 2 ml of glycerine and one crystal of thymol.

The sites of alkaline phosphomonoesterase activity are shown up with striking selectivity by an intense blue or red colour according to the diazonium salt chosen; the precision of the images exceeds that afforded by any other technique.

Preparation of tissues intended for the demonstration of non specific alkaline phosphomonoesterases

Of all the enzymes accessible to histochemical detection non-specific alkaline phosphatase is probably the easiest to preserve, this state of affairs explaining in part the substantial number of publications devoted to it.

Fixation of tissue pieces can be done in 10% formalin, whether saline or not, Baker's formaldehyde calcium, Danielli's formaldehyde pyridine (80 ml of 80% alcohol; 20 ml pyridine; 4 ml formalin), 96% or absolute alcohol, or acetone. The two last fixatives should only be used when it is desired to embed the tissue in paraffin wax; in other cases, mixtures with a formalin or other aldehyde base are much to be preferred. Whatever fluid is used the fixation should be of *short duration*; it is indispensable to carry it out *in the cold* (0 to 4°C). Freeze drying can obviously be used as can sectioning in a cryostat, the sections undergoing a short fixation (a few minutes) in 10% formalin chilled to the temperature of melting ice. The size of the tissue blocks fixed by the chemical fixatives should be adopted to the requirements of the duration of fixation; this latter should not under any circumstances exceed 24 hours in the cold and it is desireable to reduce this period.

Frozen sections, taken from material fixed in formalin, can be incubated in staining baths or stuck to slides; thorough washing in tap water intended to remove the fixative is plainly needed before incubation.

The dehydration of tissue fixed in alcohol is carried out in absolute alcohol; the material fixed in acetone is dehydrated in two to three baths of acetone. It is desireable to change the dehydrating agent three or four times to shorten the duration of this stage for which 12 hours represents the average duration and 24 hours a maximum which should not be exceeded. The quality of the sections is much improved by following the dehydration with a passage for 12 to 24 hours in a 1% solution of nitrocellulose dissolved either in acetone or in a mixture of equal parts of absolute alcohol and ether. On being removed from this bath or from the last dehydration bath the tissue blocks are cleared in two or three baths of benzene, the total duration of treatment not exceeding two hours.

Embedding in paraffin represents the manoeuvre which of all those preparatory to the section cutting causes the greatest losses of enzymatic activity. It is therefore most important to reduce its duration, as far as is at all possible, either by still further fragmentation of the tissue block or by working in a vacuum oven. Everything possible should be done to obtain as rapid a penetration as possible in the embedding material and the period spent in hot paraffin should in no case exceed two hours. The pouring of the block requires no special precautions. It is advantageous to keep the blocks in the cold if they are not needed for immediate sectioning but this precaution may not always be necessary.

Section cutting of material fixed in alcohol or acetone is often difficult; it is adviseable not to cut the sections too thinly and to spread them rapidly on a hot plate brought to as low a temperature as possible so as to reduce losses of enzymatic activity. Adhesion to slides can be done with gelatine water or with Mayer's albumin. Once stuck, the sections should be *dried cold* (about 4°C) and put to incubate as soon as possible, the losses of enzymatic activity on ribbons or sections adhering to slides set aside in free air being rather rapid.

Dewaxing and hydration of sections intended for incubation may be conducted in the usual way; it is recommended that the slides should be warmed on a suitably adjusted hot plate until fusion begins in the paraffin (*and not beyond*) prior to immersing them in the benzenoid hydrocarbon intended to dissolve the embedding material. Treatment with collodion is recommended.

Tests for alkaline phosphomonoesterase activity in calcified tissues are made possible by the development of **decalcifying liquids which do not entirely destroy enzymatic activity** but we should not disguise from ourselves the fact that the techniques suggested do result in considerable losses.

Lorch (1946) recommends treatment of pieces of tissue whose dimension should not exceed a few millimetres, after 24 hours fixation in alcohol or acetone, at 0° to 4°C with the following liquid

crystalline citric acid	14.7 g
0.2 N soda	700 ml
0.1 N hydrochloric acid	300 ml
1% zinc sulphate solution	2 ml
chloroform	0.1 ml

The decalcifying action may last for 3 to 10 days; it is checked by careful washing in frequently renewed distilled water before the reactivation bath described below is applied.

The fluid devised by Greep and his colleagues (1948) also gives good results. Blocks of tissue, fixed as before, are treated for 2 to 10 days with a mixture of equal parts of 2% formic acid and a 20% solution of sodium citrate.

Washing in running or frequently renewed water (for about 5 minutes) eliminates the decalcifying agent and the pieces of tissue are then placed in the reactivation bath.

Two other formulae are recommended by Lillie (1954, 1964), namely a citrate buffer of pH 4.5

N hydrochloric acid	540 ml
N solution of sodium citrate	460 ml

and a buffer of the same pH with a citric acid and ammonium citrate base

N solution of citric acid (about 7%)	50 ml
N solution of ammonium citrate (about 10% of the dehydrated salt)	950 ml
1% solution of zinc sulphate	2 ml
chloroform	0.1 ml

The time needed for decalcification is the same as with the preceding formulae; the washing intended to remove the decalcifying agent can be carried out in tap water or in distilled water.

A formula due to Freiman (1954) involves the decalcifying action of versene (ethylene-diamine tetraacetic acid). Pieces of tissue fixed in acetone or alcohol are treated for 24 hour at 4°C with the solution

versene	5 g
distilled water	100 ml
N soda	to adjust the PH to between 6.0 and 6.5

Where necessary, the decalcification may be prolonged, by changing the liquid, at laboratory temperatures; it can last up to 21 hours without the total destruction of alkaline phosphomonoesterase activity. Washing in water is followed by the reactivation bath.

The reactivation of alkaline phosphomonoesterases is secured by spending several hours in an alkaline fluid prior to dehydration. Among the different techniques put forward I recommend that of Lillie (1954) which consists of treating the tissue for 6 hours at 37°C in the mixture

distilled water	100 ml
sodium veronal	1 g
glycine	75 mg

On removal from the bath, the tissue is washed for 1 to 2 hours in running water before dehydration is begun.

For the record I might mention that none of the recommended treatments for softening cuticular structures is compatible with the preservation of phosphatase activity.

ADENOSINE-TRIPHOSPHATASES

These enzymes, whose multiplicity is agreed by most biochemists, catalyse the hydrolysis of adenosine-triphosphate into adenosine-diphosphate and orthophosphoric acid. The first attempts to detect histochemically adenosine-triphosphatase activity are due to Glick and Fisher (1945, 1946), Soulairac and Desclaux (1949) and Gomori (1950). The introduction of control reactions using specific activators or inhibitors (Padykula and Herman, 1955) represents a substantial measure of progress compared with the older methods. Sulphydrilated compounds such as 2,3-dimercapto-1-propanol (BAL) or cysteine strongly inhibit the non-specific alkaline phosphomonoesterase and activate adenosine-triphosphatase, whereas agents which block the sulphydryl groups inhibit the latter enzyme. The great majority of modern authors consider that such a control reaction is essential for the histochemical detection of the enzyme with which we are concerned; the need arises from the fact that non-specific alkaline phosphomonoesterase may catalyse the hydrolysis of adenosine-triphosphate.

It is generally agreed that the technique of Padykula and Herman and that of Wachstein and Meisel (1957) give equivalent results. The two depend on the same principle as Gomori's method using sodium glycerophosphate but the capture of the phosphate ions is made by calcium in the technique of Padykula and Herman, and by lead in that of Wachstein and Meisel.

The technique of Padykula and Herman

These authors worked with sections of fresh tissue cut on a freezing microtome and treated in dishes or adhering to slides but experience shows that a short fixation in neutralised and chilled (about 4°) 10% formalin, followed by sectioning on a freezing microtome, will do perfectly well. Only freeze-dried tissue can be embedded in paraffin wax.

Incubate for from 5 minutes to 3 hours, at 37°C, in the following substrate which should be prepared immediately prior to use a 0.1 M solution (2.062 g/100 ml) of
sodium veronal .... 20 ml
a 0.18 M solution (1.998 g/100 ml) of calcium chloride ... 10 ml
distilled water .... 30 ml
adenosine-triphosphate (the disodium salt) .... 152 mg
Stir until dissolved, adjust the pH immediately to 9.4 with 0.1 M soda, make up to 100 ml with distilled water. Filter if the liquid is cloudy;

Wash in 3 baths of a 1% calcium chloride solution;
Treat for 3 minutes with a 2% solution of cobalt chloride;
Wash carefully in distilled water;
Treat for 1 to 2 minutes with a dilute solution of ammonium sulphide;
Wash in frequently renewed water, stain the background (carmalum, the aluminium lake of nuclear fast red);
Dehydrate with absolute alcohol, clear in a benzenoid hydrocarbon and mount in a commercial synthetic resin or in Canada balsam;
The presence of adenosine-triphosphatase is shown by a black stain;
The pseificity of the localisation obtained should be checked by blocking the reaction; the following technique is recommended by Padykula and Herman (1955);
Incubate the control slides in a substrate prepared as above but containing, in addition, 0.0025 M p-chloromercuribenzoate for 15 minutes; continue the incubation in a substrate without the inhibitor, after rinsing in distilled water, should a longer period be needed to obtain a clear reaction (prolonged contact with the inhibitor induces an irreversible blocking of the adenosine-triphosphatase activity);
Wash the sections in the calcium chloride solution and use some of them to verify that the reaction has been inhibited by means of Stoelzner's reaction which should be negative;
Incubate the remaining sections which have undergone the action of the inhibitor in a substrate to which 4.9×10^{-3} M of 2.3-dimercapto-1-propanol have been added, for 30 to 40 minutes;
Wash in the solution of calcium chloride and, by means of Stoelzner's reaction, verify that the thiol group has been reactivated.

The technique of Wachstein and Meisel

The conditions for fixing are the same as for the preceding technique; these authors comment that the incubating time is longer after fixation in formalin followed by frozen sectioning than after the sectioning of fresh tissue; they also mention the fact that human tissue generally requires a longer period of incubation than does material taken from the small so-called laboratory mammals.

Incubate for from 5 to 180 minutes, at 37°C, in the following substrate, prepared *immediately prior to use*
solution of 125 mg/100 ml of adenosine-triphosphate .... 20 ml
a tris-maleate buffer, pH 7.2 .... 20 ml
a 2% solution of lead nitrate .... 3 ml
a 0.1 M solution of magnesium sulphate .... 5 ml
distilled water .... 2 ml
Mix the constituents in the order indicated, adjust the pH if necessary and filter if the mixture is cloudy;
Wash in distilled water;
Treat for 1 minute with the dilute solution of ammonium sulphide;
Wash for a long time in tap water;
Mount in a medium miscible with water.

A positive result of the reaction is shown by a stain varying between brown and black. As Lison (1960) has remarked, one of the practical disadvantages of the two methods is the need to use a substance as unstable and costly as adenosine-triphosphate.

5-NUCLEOTIDASE (ADENOSINE-5-PHOSPHATASE)

This enzyme which has been known to biochemists since the time of Reis (1934) hydrolyses purine- and pyrimidine-nucleotides into nucleosides. It was first demonstrated histochemically by Gomori (1949) whose technique is very close to that using sodium glycerophosphate for the detection of non-specific alkaline phosphomonoesterase activity. The method in question retains its value; we give it below therefore, at the same time as a variation due to Wachstein and Meisel (1954) whose capture reaction uses lead.

Gomori's technique

Frozen sections, taken from tissue which is either fresh or fixed in 10% formalin, chilled to 4°C, or paraffin wax sections, obtained after freeze-drying or after fixing in cold acetone and rapid embedding, may be used.

Incubate for 2 to 5 hours, at 37°C, in the following substrate
adenosine-5'-phosphate (muscle adenylic acid) .... 20 mg
0.1 or 0.2 M tris-hydrochloric acid buffer, pH 8.3 .... 20 ml
2% solution of calcium chloride .... 20 ml
10% solution of magnesium sulphate .... 3 drops
Wash with care (for a few minutes) in tap water;
Treat for 2 to 5 minutes with a 2% solution of cobalt nitrate, chloride or acetate;
Wash carefully in tap water;
Treat for 1 to 2 minutes with the dilute solution of ammonium sulphide;
Wash carefully in tap water, stain the background and mount as when investigating non-specific alkaline phosphatase activity.

A positive result of the reaction is shown by a black stain, due to the formation of cobalt sulphide. The experimental sections are compared with controls, incubated in a substrate in which the adenylic acid has been replaced by sodium glycerophosphate; only active sites which are positive on the first section and negative on that with glycerophosphate can safely be attributed to the exclusive presence of the 5-nucleotidase.

Wachstein and Meisel's technique

Directions for the preparation of the sections are as for Gomori's technique. When the work is carried out on sections of fresh tissue, these should be collected directly into the incubating medium, incubated and fixed in 10% formalin for 30 minutes immediately after incubation.

Incubate for 30 minutes to 2 hours in the mixture
  1.25% solution of adenosine-5-phosphate .... 10 ml
  0.2 M tris-hydrochloric acid buffer, pH 7.2 .... 5 ml
  0.2% lead nitrate solution .... 30 ml
  0.1 M magnesium sulphate solution .... 5 ml
Where appropriate, fix in 10% formalin for 30 minutes;
Wash carefully in distilled water;
Treat with the dilute solution of ammonium sulphide;
Wash carefully in tap water;
Mount in a medium miscible with water.

A positive result of the reaction is shown by a brown colour which corresponds to lead sulphide.

NON-SPECIFIC ACID PHOSPHOMONOESTERASE

The histochemical detection of this enzyme, which probably corresponds to phosphatase A_2 or II of the biochemists, gives results which are much less satisfactory than those which have just been reviewed in relation to alkaline phosphatases. The preservation of the enzymatic activity on sections is more difficult and the lower optimum pH lies at the origin of a series of practical disadvantages the rational solution to which is rather difficult to find.

The enzyme whose optimum pH is around 5 is inactivated by ethyl alcohol and by a whole series of mineral salts (potassium cyanide, zinc sulphate, 0.001 M cobalt sulphate, 0.01 M sodium fluoride) and by ammonium molybdate. It is more sensitive to heat than are the alkaline phosphatases and only poorly withstands embedding in paraffin wax and even spreading the sections on too warm a hot plate may lie at the origin of irregular results through the loss of enzymatic activity.

From the standpoint of the preparation of the tissues, fixing in chilled acetone at the temperature of melting ice, followed by dehydration in acetone and very rapid embedding in paraffin wax, is a makeshift solution to be used only when the examination of serial sections is absolutely indispensable or when the detection of this enzyme is peripheral to the major objectives of the work. Freeze-drying with embedding in paraffin wax gives much better results as does short duration fixing (less than 16 hours) using 10% neutralised and chilled formalin. Obviously sectioning of fresh tissue in a cryostat with rapid fixing of the sections using chilled 10% formalin also represents an excellent solution.

Sections in paraffin wax may be dewaxed using a benzenoid hydrocarbon but the latter should be flushed out with acetone and not with alcohol which inactivates acid phosphatases. Similarly the 0.1% solution of collodion used for treating the sections should be prepared with acetone and not with the alcohol-ether mixture.

As in the case of alkaline phosphatases it is necessary to distinguish techniques for detecting the enzyme which depend on the capture of the phosphate ion using a salt added to the incubating medium, and techniques which depend on the capture of naphthol liberated by the primary reaction, coupling being carried out simultaneously or at a later stage. Techniques for post-coupling have not given very encouraging results in the case of acid phosphatases so that only techniques using heavy metal salts and those using diazonium salts with simultaneous coupling are discussed here.

Gomori's technique using lead nitrate

This is the oldest (Gomori, 1941) of the techniques for detecting non-specific acid phosphatase activity. Its principle rests on that of the Gomori-Takamatsu reaction for alkaline phosphomonoesterases but the need to work at a pH near 5 involves modifications of the working technique since calcium phosphate is soluble under these conditions. The capture of phosphate ions is therefore afforded by lead phosphate through the introduction of lead nitrate into the incubating bath. Washing eliminates the excess of this latter salt and lead phosphate is developed in the form of a sulphide, which is brown, by treating the sections with a dilute solution of ammonium sulphide. The same procedure, with the addition to the substrate of 0.0042 to 0.042% (0.001 M to 0.01 M) of sodium fluoride gives control preparations. The irregularity of the results already mentioned led Gomori (1950, 1952) to modify certain stages of the method and it is the latest of the variations put forward by this author which is given here.

> Frozen sections, taken from fresh tissue or tissue fixed in chilled 10% formalin adhering to slides or as sections in paraffin wax, dewaxed with the precautions mentioned above.
> Treat in an oven at 37°C for 1 to 24 hours with the substrate prepared in the following manner:
> dissolve 0.6 g of lead nitrate in 500 ml of 0.05 M sodium acetate buffer, pH 5 (285 ml of a 0.41% sodium acetate solution and 215 ml of a 0.3% acetic acid solution); add 50 ml of a 3% solution of commercial sodium glycerophosphate. The liquid becomes cloudy, the amount of precipitate being determined by the relative abundance of the B isomer in a commercial sample. Place the solution in an oven at 37°C and keep it there for 24 hours, filter and add a small quantity of distilled water to forestall precipitation through evaporation. The mixture keeps for several months provided that it is kept cold; it should be thrown away if any fresh cloudiness appears;
> Rinse carefully in distilled water (the lead nitrate precipitates with tap water);
> Wash for 1 minute in 1% acetic acid;
> Wash for 1 minute in distilled water;
> Treat for 2 minutes with the dilute solution of ammonium sulphide;
> Wash in tap water and where appropriate stain the background (aluminium lake of nuclear fast red, iodine green, etc...);
> Dehydrate in absolute alcohol, clear and mount in a synthetic resin; the use of benzenoid hydrocarbons as clearing agents and solvents for the resin is not recommended by Gomori who considers that the stain due to precipitates of lead sulphide becomes paler in these fluids; automobile spirit or tetrachlorethylene do not have this disadvantage.

A positive result of the reaction already perceptible when the slide is removed from the incubating fluid because of the chalky colour of the deposits of lead phosphate finally gives a black stain in the completed preparation.

Among the disadvantages of this method the irregularity of the results already mentioned above is, according to certain authors, associated with differences in the treatment to which the sections are subjected at the moment of adhesion to slides; Goetsch and Reynolds consider that Meyer's albumin inactivates the enzyme and recommend that adhesion should be carried out using distilled water. Experience does indeed prove that these irregularities are much less serious when working with frozen sections, the incubating time being then reduced to 30 minutes for tissues which are very rich in acid phosphatase and 1 to 2 hours for others.

Fixation of the lead ions of the incubating medium on structures devoid of enzymatic activity gives rise to false positive reactions with depressing regularity. This "lead effect" is to some extent reduced through washing in acetic acid, introduced by Gomori in the last variation of his method; naturally comparison with control sections avoids this interpretative error.

Diffusion artefacts exist as they do when demonstrating alkaline phosphomonoesterases using the glycerophosphate method.

Many histo-enzymologists consider that Gomori's method using glycerophosphate-lead nitrate is of only historical interest at the present time; others still use it but all consider that techniques involving naphthol phosphates with simultaneous coupling using diazonium salts are incontestably superior.

Techniques using naphthol phosphates

The principle of these methods is the same as that of the technique due to Menten and his colleagues described in relation to the detection of alkaline phosphatases but the use of histochemical tests for acid phosphomonoesterases meets with numerous difficulties associated with the need to work at relatively low pH values so that the coupling which simultaneously ensures the capture of naphthols and their demonstration in the form of azo dyestuffs is considerably slowed down. It is also easy to understand why the first attempts due to Seligman and Manheimer (1945) which depended on the use of calcium α-naphthylphosphate were not very encouraging, diffusion artefacts being enormous. The technique of Grogg and Pearse (1952) using sodium α-naphthylphosphate is better without being entirely satisfactory; the working technique is indicated below. It is the technique of Burstone (1958, 1962) using the phosphates of naphthol AS compounds which surpasses all others by the precision with which it localises enzymes. All the techniques which have just been mentioned can be applied to frozen sections taken from fresh tissue (cryostat, microtome with a chilled blade) or fixed for a short time in 10% neutralised and chilled (about 4°) formalin; paraffin wax sections taken from freeze-dried material serve equally well. Fixation in acetone is a make-shift solution.

Grogg and Pearse's technique is applied to frozen sections, attached to slides without any adhesive whatever, the adhesion being secured by about one hour's drying at laboratory temperatures.

> Incubate the sections for a few minutes to one hour, at 37°C, in the following mixture: dissolve 20 mg of sodium α-naphthylphosphate in 20 ml of Michaelis' veronal-acetate buffer or that of Walpole, at 0.1 M, of pH 5; add 1.5 g of polyvinylpyrrolidone and stir until dissolved. Add about 20 mg of fast garnet GBC (the diazo salt of *o*-amino-azotoluene), stir well and filter; the mixture will not keep beyond one or two hours;
> Wash for one to two minutes in running water;
> Stain the nuclei with haemalum;
> Wash in tap water;
> Mount in a medium miscible with water (the azo dye formed is soluble in alcohol and in benzenoid hydrocarbons).

A positive result of the reaction is shown by a brownish red stain; the peculiar, even crystalline, appearance of the precipitate, which is almost inevitable once the incubation period has exceeded a few minutes, detracts from the precision of the images obtained.

Burstone's technique uses the phosphates of naphthol AS-BI, AS-TR, AS-CL, or AS-MX, prepared where necessary from the corresponding naphthols using the method suggested for the alkaline phosphomonoesterases (p. 608); it can be applied like Gomori's method using glycerophosphate-lead nitrate to frozen sections or to paraffin wax sections obtained after freeze-drying or a fixation of short duration in chilled acetone; the precautions indicated so far as dewaxing is concerned remain valid.

> Incubate the sections for from 30 minutes to 8 hours, at laboratory temperatures or at 37°C, in the following mixture;
> dissolve about 5 mg of the chosen naphthol AS phosphate in 0.25 ml of N,N'-dimethylformamide or dimethylsulphoxide; add 25 ml of distilled water and 25 ml of 0.2 M Walpole buffer, pH 5.2; dissolve 30 mg of fast red-violet LB salt in this mixture, stir and filter; add 2 drops of a solution of manganese chloride $MnCl_2$ which activates the enzyme; other diazonium salts, in particular fast red 3G salt and fast scarlet GG salt can equally well be used;
> Wash carefully in tap water;
> Stain the background where appropriate with a dye chosen because of the stain obtained after coupling;
> Mount in a medium miscible with water.

A positive result of the reaction is shown by stains which vary according to the diazonium salt used from brownish red to blue-black. The precision with which sites of enzymatic activity are demonstrated exceeds that of any other method.

PHOSPHAMIDASE

The existence of an enzyme capable of catalysing the hydrolysis of phosphocreatine and, more generally, that of N substituted phosphoric amides was discovered by Waldschmidt-Leutz and Köhler (1933) and by Ichihara (1933) using biochemical techniques. The first method of histochemical detection, founded on a principle identical with that of the sodium glycerophosphate-lead nitrate method for demonstrating non-specific acid phosphomonoesterase, is due to Gomori (1949), the substrate used being the ammonium salt of *p*-chloranilidophosphonic acid. The commercial availability of this compound represents a distinct simplification of the working technique for the user of this method; some details of the latter have been developed by Meyer and Weinmann (1955); this latter variation is also described here.

We may also comment that attempts to demonstrate phosphamidase with substrates containing the diamides of naphthol-AS-phosphoric acids seemed encouraging to Burstone (1958, 1962).

Gomori's technique

This method may be applied to paraffin wax sections taken from material fixed in acetone or freeze-dried; the sections are dewaxed and brought into water; their treatment with collodion is possible if an acetone solution of collodion is used.

> Incubate for 2 to 8 hours, at about 40°C, in the following medium:
> a 0.1 M solution of ammonium chloranilidophosphonate ... 2 ml
> a maleic acid buffer of pH 5.6 (dissolve 5.8 g of maleic acid in 500 ml of water adding 62 ml of normal soda and make up to 1 litre) .... 50 ml
> a 0.1 M solution of lead nitrate .... 1.5 ml
> a 10% solution of manganese chloride ... several drops (allow to stand for 30 minutes in an oven at 60°C, filter);
> It is essential to arrange the slides so that the side bearing the sections is underneath;
> Rinse in distilled water and wipe away the white precipitate deposited on the slide away from the sections;
> Where appropriate, wash the slide in a citric or acetic buffer (0.1 M, pH 4.5) until the diffuse precipitate which covers the sections is dissolved;
> Rinse in tap water;
> Treat with a dilute solution of ammonium sulphide for 1 to 2 minutes;
> Wash in running water for about a minute;
> Where appropriate stain the background and mount taking the same precautions as during the demonstration of acid phosphomonoesterases using the lead method.

A positive result of the reaction is shown by a black stain due to lead sulphide formed by the action of ammonium sulphide on the lead phosphate deposited during the reaction. The inspection of the preparations may be rendered very unsatisfactory by diffuse precipitates and their solution by a buffer of pH 4.5 carries an obvious risk of entraining losses of the reaction product. Most authors recommend that two sections of the mouse encephalon should be stuck to the same slide as the sections under investigation; the encephalon is an organ rich in phosphamidase and the enzyme may be inactivated on one of the sections (to be placed at one end of the slide) by immersing it, prior to dewaxing, in 10% nitric acid for 90 minutes. The washing in a citrate buffer should be stopped, during this procedure, as soon as the section treated with nitric acid is entirely clear.

It is appropriate to remark that ammonium chloranilidophosphonate is sold in sealed ampoules and that its aqueous solutions keep very poorly.

Meyer and Weinmann's technique

This technique, intended for use on sections prepared as for Gomori's method, differs in respect of the substrate; this is the sodium salt of p-chloranilidophosphonic acid, prepared from the acid, which is a rather stable and commercially available substance. 2.08 g of this acid are dissolved in 15 ml of normal soda; the solution is made up to 100 ml with distilled water;

> Incubate the sections, at 42°C, for three hours or longer in the medium prepared in the following way;
> > dissolve 534 mg of maleic acid in 5 ml of N soda, making up to 100 ml with distilled water; add 175 mg of sodium chloride and 94 mg of lead nitrate; warm gently until the precipitate formed re-dissolves, chill, filter; add 4.5 ml of the sodium salt of chloranilidophosphonic acid, warm to 44°C, and filter;
>
> Rinse in distilled water;
> Where appropriate, wash in the citric acid buffer of pH 4.5 (the precautions mentioned in relation to Gomori's technique remain valid); Meyer and Weinmann consider that this "differentiation" is only useful when the incubation is prolonged beyond three hours;
> Wash in distilled water;
> Treat with a dilute solution of ammonium sulphide;
> Wash in running water;
> Carry out a background stain and mount as for Gomori's technique.

A positive result is shown by a black stain disclosing the presence of lead sulphide.

GLUCOSE-6-PHOSPHATASE

This enzyme which is characterised from the biochemical standpoint by its catalysis of the cleavage of glucose-6-phosphate into glucose and orthophosphoric acid has an optimum pH around 6.5, is very thermosensitive and quite rapidly inactivated by acids. Its investigation requires the use of sections taken from fresh tissue, sectioned on a cryostat or on a microtome with a chilled blade.

Chiquoine's (1955) technique and that of Wachstein and Meisel, mentioned below, depend on the capture by lead of orthophosphate ions, liberated during the primary reaction whose substrate is potassium glucose -6-phosphate now commercially available so that histo-enzymologists are no longer compelled to prepare it from barium glucose-6-phosphate, which was once the sole means available.

Chiquoine's technique

Frozen sections from fresh tissue, treated in baths or adhering to slides;
Incubate for 5 to 15 minutes, at 32°C, in the following mixture:
    a 1% solution of potassium glucose-6-phosphate ...... 1 volume
    a 2% solution of lead nitrate .... 2 volumes
    normal potash .... to adjust the solution to pH 6.7
Wash in distilled water;
Treat with the dilute solution of ammonium sulphide;
Wash in running water;
Where appropriate fix in 10% formalin;
Wash in tap water;
Mount in a medium miscible with water or dehydrate and mount with the same precautions as are needed during the demonstration of acid phosphomonoesterases using the lead technique.

A positive result of the reaction is shown by a brown or black stain.

Wachstein and Meisel's technique

This technique differs from the preceding one only in the adoption of a tris-hydrochloric acid buffer to regulate the pH; the requirements concerning the preparation of the tissue are as for Chiquoine's method.

Incubate the sections for 5 to 15 minutes, at 32°C, in the following mixture:
    a 0.125% solution of potassium glucose-6-phosphate ...... 20 ml
    a tris-hydrochloric acid buffer, pH 6.7 .... 20 ml
    2% lead nitrate solution .... 3 ml
    distilled water .... 7 ml
Rinse in distilled water;
Treat with a dilute solution of ammonium sulphide;
Wash in tap water;
Fix in 10% formalin;
Mount in a medium miscible with water.

As in Chiquoine's technique, a positive result is indicated by a stain which varies between brown and black.

The inactivation of the enzyme on slides intended to serve as controls may be carried out using heat or by treatment with an acid; alkaline fluorides, arsenates and 1,5-sorbitane-6-phosphate are the best known of the chemicals which may be used as inhibitors.

B.-CARBOXYLIC ESTERASES

This group includes esterases which catalyse the hydrolysis of carboxylic esters, the general scheme of the reaction being

$$RCOOR' + H_2O \rightleftharpoons RCOOH + R'OH$$

All the authors of specialist monographs stress the great complexity of this group of enzymes; none of the classifications put forward for histochemically detectable carboxylic esterases can be regarded as being entirely satisfactory. It is customary to distinguish cholinesterases, which are eserine sensitive (inhibited by eserine at 10^{-5} M, or 2 mg per litre); aliesterases, which are eserine resistant and hydrolyse mainly the esters of aromatic fatty acids or short chain aliphatic fatty acids (fewer than 8 carbon atoms); lipases, which are eserine resistant and more particularly hydrolyse the esters of long chain aliphatic fatty acids. The aliesterases are inhibited by bile salts at a concentration of 0.5%, whereas the lipases are activated by these compounds at the same concentration.

Lison (1960 p. 564) quite rightly stresses the difficulties met with during the histochemical identification of the various carboxylic esterases; the range of action of each of these enzymes on diverse substrates is quite extensive so that the results of control reactions using specific activators and inhibitors counts for much more than does the choice of substrate when it comes to recognising the nature of a carboxylic esterase. The preference of cholinesterases for the esters of choline, that of aliesterases for aromatic fatty acid esters and that of lipases for long chain fatty acid esters is by no means absolute. If we take into account the variability of the properties of these enzymes in different organs the results become of such complexity that most recent authors content themselves with defining the histochemical activity detected by the name of the substrate and an indication of the control reactions used, speaking for instance of α-naphtholesterases which are eserine resistant, etc...

CHOLINESTERASES

The enzymes of this group are defined by their great sensitivity to eserine (physostigmine); concentrations of the order of 10^{-6} M of the compound in question inhibit them entirely, whereas other carboxylic esterases are only slightly affected by much stronger concentrations (10^{-3} M). Fixation in acetone, at 4°C, destroys cholinesterase activity in three to four hours, whereas the other carboxylic esterases withstand fixation in this liquid for up to 24 hours.

The classification of cholinesterases has given rise to much debate, an account of which would be out of place here. Most modern authors agree on the distinction between acetylcholinesterases ("true" or specific cholinesterases) and non-specific cholinesterases (pseudocholinesterases) (Augustinsson and Nachmansohn, 1949). The first group specifically hydrolyses acetylcholine and acetylthiocholine, the others act on any choline ester, including the two compounds just mentioned.

In fact the specificity of action on the substrate is not all that strict; the demonstration of these enzymes on sections may be secured by methods in which the substrate is represented by lauryl- or myristoylcholine (Gomori, 1948), acetyl- or butyrylthiocholine (Koelle and Friedenwald, 1949), indoxyl acetates (Holt and Withers, 1952), naphthyl acetates (Ravin et al., 1953, Chessick, 1953), and thiolacetic acid (Crevier and Bélanger, 1955, Wachstein et al., 1961). It is therefore easy to understand the importance attaching to the use of specific inhibitors when undertaking the histochemical detection of cholinesterases. Among these inhibitors the most important are tetra-isopropylpyrophosphoramide (iso-OMPA), which acts irreversibly at a concentration of 10^{-5} M on non-specific cholinesterases without affecting acetylcholinesterase, as well as the methylsulphate of ethopropazine (lysivane) whose inhibitory action, which is equally effective on non-specific cholinesterases, is reversible, the effective concentration being 3×10^{-5} M. Table 20 which follows Pearse (1960) gives a summary of the essential data available.

Table 20. — SUBSTRATES AND INHIBITORS IN HISTOCHEMICAL DETECTION OF CHOLINESTERASE ACTIVITY
(after Pearse, simplified)

Enzymes	Substrates	Inhibitors
Acetylcholinesterases (true or specific cholinesterases)	-naphthylacetates -acetylthiocholine o-aceto-indoxyls myristoylcholine (weakly hydrolysed) butyryl-thiocholine (very weakly hydrolysed)	diisopropylfluorophosphate (DFP), 10^{-5}M di-iodide of 1 : 5-*bi* (4-trimethyl ammoniumphenyl) pentane-3-one (62C47) 10^{-5}M di-iodide of 1 : 5-*bi* (4-allyl-dimethylammoniumphenyl) pentane-3-one (284C51) 10^{-5}M
Pseudocholinesterases (non-specific cholinesterases, butyrocholinesterases)	naphthylacetates acetylthiocholine butyrylthiocholine myristoylcholine o-aceto-indoxyls	diisopropylfluorophosphate (DFP) 10^{-6}M N-*p*-chlorophenyl-N-methyl-carbamate of M-hydroxyphenyltrimethylbromide of ammonium (Nu-1250) 10^{-5}M tetra*iso*propylpyrophosphoramide-(*iso*-OMPA) 10^{-6}M methosulphate of ethopropazine (lysivane) $3 \cdot 10^{-5}$M

Numerous other inhibitors have been put forward; the reader is referred to specialised monographs for their characteristics. Apart from eserine which is added in the form of a salicylate to the incubating medium the inhibitors are used as pre-incubation baths, dissolved at the required molarity in the buffer which serves for the incubation properly speaking; their action takes place at the same temperature as what is properly speaking the histochemical reaction.

Among the methods for detecting cholinesterases those using naphthol acetates and *o*-aceto-indoxyls may be carried out as for tests for non-specific esterases, the identification of the cholinesterases being secured by control reactions using inhibitors. The technique using myristoylcholine, due to Gomori (1948), has now only historical interest. It copies a technique for the detection of alkaline phosphomonoesterases, the substrate being the choline ester of myristic acid (that of lauric acid may equally well be used), the fatty acid liberated during the primary reaction being precipitated in the form of its cobalt salt which is then detected by the Stoelzner reaction. This method has been abandoned by the great majority of modern histochemists because of its low sensitivity. The most used among the techniques for demonstrating cholinesterase stem on the one hand from the method of Koelle and Friedenwald (1949) or on the other hand that of Crevier and Bélanger (1955). Among the variations of the first method, three are discussed here, namely that of Coers (1953) which was developed specially for the study of myoneural synapses, that of Gerebzoff (1953) which is useful in investigations on tissues whose activity is very variable, and lastly that of Arvy (1962).

The preparation of the tissue includes in all three cases a short fixation in 10% neutralised and chilled formalin; most authors advise that this should not exceed six hours. *Chilled acetone as a fixative should not be used*; to work on sections of fresh tissue as recommended by Koelle is an unnecessary complication but sections cut on a cryostat and fixed for a short time in diluted and chilled formalin are entirely suitable.

Coers' technique

Wash the frozen sections whose thicknes may be as great as 100 μ for 30 minutes, in distilled water;
Incubate for 10 to 60 minutes at 37°C in the following mixture
    a 3.75% solution of amino acetic acid .... 0.2 ml
    a 0.1 M solution of copper sulphate (2.5% of the crystalline salt) .... 0.2 ml
    0.1 M Walpole buffer, pH 5 .... 5 ml
    distilled water .... 3.8 ml
    a solution of acetylthiocholine copper salt .... 0.8 ml
(this latter solution to be added at the moment of use is prepared by mixing in a centrifuge tube 15 mg of acetylthiocholine iodine, 0.78 ml of distilled water and 0.26 ml of a 0.1 M solution of copper sulphate; the precipitate is removed by centrifugation and the clear supernatant liquid collected);
Wash in distilled water;
Treat for 5 minutes with the dilute solution of ammonium sulphide;
Wash in tap water;
Spread the sections onto slides, dehydrate in absolute alcohol, clear and mount in a synthetic resin or in Canada balsam.

A positive result of the reaction is shown by a black stain due to the presence of copper sulphide.

Gerebzoff's technique

Refix the frozen sections for 30 minutes in neutralised 10% formalin;
Wash in 2 baths, each of 20 minutes, of distilled water;
Incubate at 37°C, for a maximum of 2 hours, in the medium
- Walpole buffer of pH 5, 6.2 or 6.8 .... 2.9 ml
- distilled water .... 1.9 ml
- a 3.75% solution of amino-acetic acid .... 0.1 ml
- a 0.1 M solution of copper sulphate .... 0.1 ml
- a solution of cupric acetyl- or butyrylthiocholine .... 0.4 ml

(to prepare this solution, mix 15 mg of acetylthiocholine iodide or 18.5 mg of butyrylthiocholine iodide in a centrifuge tube with 0.78 ml of distilled water and 0.26 ml of 0.1 M copper sulphate; centrifuge for about 12 minutes at about 3,500 r.p.m. and remove the supernatant fluid with a pipette);

Wash in distilled water (for a maximum of 1 minute);
Treat for 5 minutes with a dilute solution of ammonium sulphide;
Wash in tap water;
Mount in a medium miscible with water or dehydrate, clear and mount in balsam.

As in Coers' variation, a positive result is shown by a black stain, due to the deposition of copper sulphide. The lowest pH (5) is recommended for tissue which is very rich in cholinesterase, the highest for tissues which are poor in it and the intermediate pH for tissues of average activity.

Arvy's technique

The frozen sections are washed and incubated in the following bath for, at the most, 6 hours, at 37°C
- Walpole's buffer, 0.1 M, pH 6.5 to 6.8 .... 50 ml
- a 3.75% solution of amino-acetic acid .... 2 ml
- a 0.1 M solution of copper acetate .... 2 ml
- a solution of the chosen cupric thiocholine .... 10.5 ml

(to prepare this solution, dissolve 150 mg of acetylthiocholine iodide or 185 mg of butyrylthiocholine iodide in 8 ml of distilled water, add 2.5 ml of 0.1 M copper acetate, centrifuge, and collect the supernatant liquor);

Wash in distilled water;
Treat with the dilute solution of ammonium sulphide;
Wash in tap water;
Mount in a medium miscible with water or dehydrate, clear and mount in Canada balsam or in a commercial synthetic resin.

The presence of cholinesterase is shown by a black precipitate of copper sulphide.

These three variations as well as numerous other procedures derived from the original technique of Koelle and Friedenwald depend on the same principle; the enzyme liberates thiocholine which gives a precipitate of copper thiocholine in the presence of copper ions in the incubating medium; this cupric thiocholine is revealed by transformation into copper sulphate.

It is appropriate to remark that this latter transformation was omitted in Holmstedt's (1957) variation; this latter author did indeed consider that the precipitate of cupric thiocholine was easy to discern under the light microscope.

The localising value of techniques using cupric thiocholine have been much discussed by Malmgren and Sylven (1955); according to these authors the precipitate which corresponds to the capture reaction is that of the sulphate of cupric thiocholine which is soluble in an alkaline medium and less soluble in an acid medium; *in vitro* tests showed the Swedish authors that this compound when treated with an ammonium sulphide solution redissolved before the appearance of the copper sulphide precipitate. In consequence Malmgren and Sylven consider that only the very small rod shaped crystals have any true localising value as their growth results in rather large crystalline needles, especially when the medium is saturated with cupric thiocholine. The conversion into sulphide thus diminishes the localising value of the technique and *there can be no question of wanting to convert it into a quantitative method*. In spite of these criticisms and those of Holt and Withers (1952), and of Ravin, Zacks and Seligman (1953), most modern authors consider that Koelle's method and its variations give valuable localisation on the scale of the light microscope.

The three variations mentioned above can obviously be combined with controls using inhibitors in the form of pretreatments for the control slides; *it is appropriate to remind readers of the toxicity of all anticholinesterases and of the precautions to be taken during their handling.*

Diisopropylfluorophosphonate, which is often used as a specific inhibitor for cholinesterases, is employed at 10^{-7} M, the inhibiting bath being prepared by diluting a 0.1 M stock solution in anhydrous propylene-glycol.

The technique using thiolacetic acid (thioacetic, or thiacetic) depends on the discovery by Wilson (1951) of the ability of acetylcholinesterase to catalyse the hydrolysis of thiolacetic acid with the formation of acetic acid and hydrogen sulphide. Crevier and Bélanger (1955) developed from this a very ingenious technique for the histochemical demonstration of enzymes, the capture of the hydrogen sulphide liberated during the primary reaction being secured by the addition of lead ions in the form of lead nitrate to the incubating medium, so that the capture reaction and the demonstration of its product go hand in hand. Despite the excellent results reported for the motor plates of mammalian striated muscle this method seems to have been neglected until it was taken up again by Wachstein et al (1961) to whom we owe not only technical developments but also a careful study of the effects produced by different inhibitors and a comparison with methods for demonstrating non-specific esterases.

The technique of Wachstein et al.

The incubating medium recommended by these authors should be prepared from two solutions:

SOLUTION A: Pour 0.15 ml of thiolacetic acid in 5 ml of water, adjust the pH to 5 with 0.1 N soda (about 5 ml) and make up to 100 ml with 0.2 M Walpole's buffer of pH 5.5. This solution keeps poorly and the formula recommends the preparation of so large an amount in order not to involve the pipetting of too small a quantity of thiolacetic acid.
SOLUTION B: Dissolve 0.5 g of lead nitrate in 100 ml of distilled water; this solution is stable.

For use, add, drop by drop, 1 ml of solution B to 20 ml of solution A, allow to stand for a few moments, centrifuge and use the supernatant liquid; it may be helpful to change the incubating bath every 20 minutes to avoid the formation of precipitates.

The technique may be applied to frozen sections, cut on a cryostat from fresh tissue, or to frozen sections cut after a short fixation in Baker's formaldehyde-calcium at low temperatures (4°C approximately).

The sections are incubated for 5 to 120 minutes, at laboratory temperatures (23 to 25°) and rinsed in distilled water; they may be mounted without background staining in a medium miscible with water or, after dehydration and clearing, in a commercial synthetic resin. Various stains may also be applied.

A positive result of the reaction is shown by a black stain.

We know from the detailed study of Wachstein *et al.* that thiolacetic acid is hydrolysed under the experimental conditions defined above not only by acetylcholinesterases but by non-specific esterases and by C-esterases (which withstand E 600); in the presence of sodium taurocholate this acid is also hydrolysed by a pancreatic lipase.

We are therefore concerned with a reaction with a very wide range of specificity whose localising value is undoubted but which only permits the identification of the enzymes responsable if adequate control reactions with inhibitors are used.

NON-SPECIFIC ESTERASES

These enzymes are characterised by their resistance to eserine (concentrations lower than 10^{-3} M of this compound in no way effect them). Their distinction from the lipases is not as clear cut as in the classical scheme mentioned at the beginning of this section and they are divided by recent authors into three groups according to their ability to catalyse the hydrolysis of butyrates, and their sensitivity to organo-phosphorous compounds, the most widely used of which is diethyl-*p*-nitro-phenylphosphate (E 600) and the inhibiting or, possibly, the activating effect of compounds such as p-chloromercuribenzoate and phenylmercuric chloride. By these means we can distinguish A-esterases, which are more active towards acetates than towards butyrates and withstand concentrations of E 600 less than 10^{-3} M (the arom-esterases of Aldridge, 1953); B-esterases, which are also active towards acetates and butyrates and are inhibited by concentrations of E 600 less than 10^{-5} (the aliesterases of Aldridge, 1953), and lastly the C-esterases (Bergmann *et al.*, 1957), sensitive to organo-phosphorous compounds but activated by the p-chloromercuribenzoate, an inhibitor of cholinesterases and of all other non-specific esterases. Table 21, simplified from Pearse (1960), summarises these findings.

Table 21. — Distinctive characters of groups of non-specific esterases
(after Pearse, 1960, simplified)

Enzymes	Substrates	Inhibition completed by	Activation
A-esterases arom-esterases, organo-phosphate resistant esterases	acetates of naphthyl, of naphthols AS, of indoxyl	E 600, 10^{-2}M $CuSO_4$, 10^{-3}M p-chloromercuri-benzoate, 10^{-4}M $AgNO_3$, 10^{-2}M	cysteine 10^{-3}M
B-esterases ali-esterases organo-phosphate sensitive esterases	acetates of naphthyl, of naphthols AS, of indoxyl	E 600, 10^{-5}M Mipafox, 10^{-3}M $AgNO_3$, 10^{-2}M	cysteine 10^{-3}M
C-esterases	acetates of naphthyl, of naphthols AS, of indoxyl	β-phenylpropionic acid, 10^{-2}M $AgNO_3$, 10^{-2}M	phenylmercuric chloride, 10^{-4}M p-chloromercuri-benzoate, 10^{-4}M

Some of the techniques already discussed in relation to the histochemical detection of cholinesterase activity also afford evidence for the existence of non-specific esterases; this is true of methods using thioacetic acid (p. 626); moreover, esterase activity can be detected by techniques involving naphthyl acetates, naphthol AS acetates and indoxyl acetates; the two first groups of methods depend on a capture reaction in which coloured azo-dyestuffs appear through simultaneous coupling with diazonium salts, those of the latter group depend on the oxidation of indoxyl with the formation of insoluble dyes of the indigo group.

The earliest of these techniques for the detection of non-specific esterases depending on simultaneous coupling with a diazonium salt is due to Nachlas and Seligman; it involves the use of β-naphthyl acetate as a substrate. Some serious disadvantages, such as the solubility of the reaction product and its weak substantivity have led to this substrate being abandoned in favour of α-naphthyl acetate (1-naphthol) (Gomori, 1950). Among the variations of this technique that due to Burstone (1956) is discussed here. Further developments of this technique are associated with the use of naphthol AS acetates (Gomori, 1952), of substituted naphthol AS acetates (Burstone, 1957; Goessner, 1958), the substantivity of the reaction product being still greater.

It is appropriate to mention, when speaking of these methods, that a practical problem arises during the coupling reaction intended to precipitate *in situ* the naphthols liberated by the primary reaction; it so happens that the optimum pH of the primary reaction is close to neutrality, a pH zone in which coupling is slow for most diazonium salts, so that there is a considerably increased risk of diffusion of the reaction product. This is the reason why most recent authors prefer to use fast garnet salt GBC and fast corinth salt LB which couple well at pH values as low as 6.5, in this way deliberately accepting the disadvantage which stems from the granular appearance of the coloured precipitate which indicates a positive result of the reaction.

Preparation of the tissues

It is possible to test for non-specific esterase activity after fixing in acetone, provided that this is carried out with the precautions recommended in relation to alkaline phosphatases, followed by embedding in paraffin wax; however some of these enzymes are sensitive to ethyl alcohol so that it is necessary to flush out the benzenoid hydrocarbon used for dewaxing by means of acetone and not alcohol; collodion treatment of the sections should be undertaken using a nitrocellulose solution in acetone and not in alcohol-ether. The preservation of enzymatic activity is much better after a short fixation in 10% formalin or in Baker's formaldehyde-calcium chilled to 4°C and followed by section cutting on a freezing microtome; it is often desirable to stick the sections to slides and to allow them to dry in air rather than to treat them in baths. Freeze-drying with embedding in paraffin wax is equally suitable as is the cutting of fresh tissue on a cryostat with a short fixing of the sections adhering to slides or on coverslips (10% formalin or formaldehyde-calcium).

Techniques involving naphthylacetates

Burstone's technique using α-naphthyl acetate (1-naphthol):

Incubate the sections, prepared as described above, in the following medium prepared immediately prior to use

a 1% α-naphthyl acetate solution in methyl alcohol .... 1 ml
chilled distilled water .... 50 ml
0.2 M Sörensen buffer, pH 8 .... 5 ml
the diazo salt of o-dianisidine .... 25 mg

(The solution of α-naphthyl acetate keeps for some time provided that it is kept cold; when it is added to distilled water the liquid becomes cloudy but clarifies again on agitation; the appearance of a violet colour after the addition of fast blue B salt shows that the substrate has changed with the liberation of α-naphthol and that the sample used should be discarded). There is every advantage in incubating at a temperature below 20°C and in not prolonging the time for which the medium is allowed to act beyond that needed to obtain the required colour, because the substantivity of the reaction product is not very great; the sections may be examined under a microscope during the reaction.
Wash for 3 to 5 minutes in running water;

Stain the background where appropriate; I recommend the technique using iodine green, discussed in relation to alkaline phosphatases, whenever dehydration with acetone is possible; use the aluminium lake of fast nuclear red in other cases;
Dehydrate in acetone, clear in a benzenoid hydrocarbon and mount in a synthetic resin or in Canada balsam; it is also possible to mount directly in a medium miscible with water and this procedure becomes necessary in all cases where the coupling has been carried out using a diazonium salt other than that of *o*-dianisidine (fast blue RR salt and fast red RC salt give very good results).

A positive result of the reaction is shown by a colour which varies between violet and black; the precision with which the enzymes can be localised is greater than the first set of techniques involving simultaneous coupling with β-naphthyl acetate, but less than the methods involving naphthol AS acetates. The principal advantage of this technique, which at the time of writing is still suitable for routine work, is the ease with which the substrate can be obtained and its modest price.

Gomori's technique using naphthol AS acetate:

Incubate the sections in the following way, at laboratory temperatures in the medium which should be prepared *immediately* prior to use,
mix 1 ml of a 1% naphthol AS acetate solution in a mixture of equal parts of acetone and of propylene glycol (this stock solution keeps for some time provided that it is kept in a refrigerator) and 10 to 15 ml of propylene glycol, stir and make up to 50 ml with distilled water added in small amounts at a time with continual stirring; add about 5 ml of 0.2 M Sörensen buffer, pH 6.5, and then 20 to 50 mg of fast garnet GBC salt; stir and filter. From personal experience, the preparation can be simplified by dissolving at the time of use 0.01 g of naphthol AS acetate in one to two ml of acetone and by progressively making up to 50 ml with distilled water before adding the buffer and the diazonium salt. The time for incubation may vary between 30 and 120 minutes, the sections may be examined under the microscope during the reaction;
Wash in tap water (one to two minutes);
Where appropriate, stain the nuclei with haemalum;
Wash in running water (one to two minutes);
Mount in a medium miscible with water.

A positive result of the reaction is shown by a red precipitate which is, to a greater or lesser extent, dark and granular; diffusion artefacts are slighter than when using the methods involving α-naphthyl acetates, so that it is then possible to prolong the incubation time; Gomori (1952) therefore recommends the use of this method when working with paraffin wax sections.

Burstone's technique using naphthol AS — D acetate. — As its author noted, this technique is particularly advantageous for working with frozen sections taken from material fixed in chilled formalin.

> Incubate the sections for 10 minutes to several hours in the following mixture prepared *immediately* prior to use.
> Place about 5 mg of naphthol AS-D acetate in a 50 ml conical flask, add 0.5 ml of acetone or of N,N'-dimethylformamide, and stir until it is dissolved; add 25 ml of distilled water and 25 ml of tris-hydrochloric acid buffer, pH 7.1, and then 20 to 40 mg of fast garnet GBC salt; stir until dissolved, filter using a fast filter.
> The medium is unstable at pH values above 7.1; working in an alkaline medium should therefore be avoided, especially for prolonged incubation; the incubation should take place at laboratory temperatures;
> Wash in tap water (one to two minutes);
> Where appropriate, stain the background;
> Mount in a medium miscible with water.

The incorporation of 10^{-5} M eserine salicylate into the incubating medium allows us to inhibit cholinesterase activity and to obtain only that of non-specific esterases. A positive result of the reaction is shown by a vivid red precipitate.

Burstone's technique using naphthol AS—LC acetate. — This technique is particularly intended for work using paraffin wax sections, taken from freeze-dried material, or that fixed in chilled acetone.

> Incubate the sections, at laboratory temperatures, in the following substrate prepared *immediately prior to use*—dissolve about 20 mg of naphthol AS–LC acetate in 2 to 4 ml of N,N'-dimethylformamide or dimethylsulphoxide, add 5 to 10 ml of monoethylethyleneglycol and then 10 ml of the tris-hydrochloric acid buffer of pH 7.1; make up to 50 ml with distilled water, add 20 to 30 mg of fast garnet GBC salt or fast corinth LB salt, stir and filter. The incubating time varies between 10 and 60 minutes;
> Wash in tap water (1 to 2 minutes);
> Where appropriate, stain the background;
> Mount in a medium miscible with water.

A positive result of the reaction is shown by a brilliant red precipitate.

Techniques involving indoxyl acetates

Methods which use indoxyl have been developed for the detection of carboxylic esterases and their application to the detection of other kinds of enzymatic activity seems to be highly promising. We owe to Barrnett and Seligman (1951) and to Holt (1952) the first attempts to demonstrate non-specific esterases using indoxyl acetate. The principle of the method is simple, the indoxyl liberated by the primary reaction being oxidised by atmospheric oxygen to indigo blue, a dye which is strictly insoluble in water. Improvements of the technique have involved acceleration of the oxidation using catalysts added to the incubating bath, on the one hand, and on the other hand modifications of the indoxyl molecule so as to increase its substantivity and to diminish the tendency for the indigoid to crystallise, as well as the solubility in lipids. Modern authors consider that 5-bromo-4-chlor-indoxyl acetate is the best substrate of this group.

Holt's technique using halogenated indoxyl acetates. — The method was conceived for work using frozen sections taken from material fixed in the cold for at least 24 hours in formaldehyde-calcium or in neutralised 10% formalin. Washing the tissue blocks in water prior to sectioning them should be avoided. The frozen sections are directly collected in the incubating medium which should be prepared *immediately* prior to use in the following way

> dissolve 1.5 mg of *o*-acetyl-5-bromo-indoxyl acetate or, better, 5-bromo-4-chloro-indoxyl acetate in 0.1 ml of absolute alcohol; add 2 ml of the 0.1 M of the tris-hydrochloric acid buffer, pH 8.5, 1 ml of 0.05 M solution of potassium ferricyanide, 1 ml of 0.05 M potassium ferrocyanide, 0.1 ml of a M solution of calcium chloride and 5 ml of 2 M solution of sodium chloride; make up to 10 ml with distilled water (the addition of potassium ferro- and ferricyanide is intended to accelerate the oxidation of the indoxyl liberated by the primary reaction); The incubation may take place at laboratory temperatures or at 37°C for a period ranging from a few moments to 15 hours; the margin of tolerance in this procedure is very great and the sections may be examined under the microscope during the reaction;
> Rinse in tap water;
> Where appropriate, stain the nuclei using carmalum or the aluminium lake of fast nuclear red;
> Wash in tap water;
> Mount in a medium miscible with water.

A positfve result of the reaction is shown by a blue colour, often quite intense, of structures endowed with esterase activity. Diffusion artefacts are reduced to their simplest expression through the perfectioning of the substrata and the technique may be considered as one of the best for histochemical tests for non-specific esterases were its use not limited by the high cost and the poor keeping qualities of 5-bromo-4-chlor-indoxyl acetate.

LIPASES

As Desnuelle (1961) has commented, the term "lipase" is somewhat lacking in precision the eserine-resistant carboxylic esterases designated by this name being capable of hydrolysing mono- or polyesters which are soluble or insoluble in water, the acyl group being either aliphatic or aromatic; alcohols or phenols may ensure esterification. In consequence the terms "lipase" and "esterase" when given their ordinary meanings are not essentially different from one another.

However imprecise it may be for the biochemist, the boundary between non-specific esterases and lipases is still hazier for the histochemist. Most authors attach a great deal of importance to the activation of true lipases with solutions of sodium taurocholate; in the histochemical field such activation was known to Gomori (1952) and to Wachstein and his colleagues (1961) so far as pancreatic lipase was concerned. The concentrations used vary from 0.05 M (0.22% approximately) to 0.1 M (about 0.54%). All other non-specific esterases, in these conditions, undergo inhibition to a greater or lesser extent but some doubt has recently been cast on this fact.

The technique using thioacetic acid and those involving indoxyl acetates or naphthyl acetates may be used to detect lipases. Moreover, Gomori's classical method (1945) using "Tweens" detects lipases and Pearse (1960) considers that the hydrolysis of "unsaturated Tweens" is the best, so far as we can tell at present, of the techniques for detecting true lipases.

The compounds which serve as substrates are esters of sorbitane or mannitane with a fairly long chain; substances other than those which are sold under the name of Tweens may be used but the common practice involves the latter. Tween 20 (laurate), Tween 40 (palmitate) and Tween 60 (stearate) are saturated whereas Tween 80 (oleate) is not. Experience shows that the extent of the hydrolysis decreases as the chain length is increased and from this standpoint the laurates seem to be the most advantageous, however in practice this advantage is counterbalanced by the bulky nature of the precipitate obtained so that its localising value is much diminished.

The technique may be applied to paraffin wax sections taken from material treated with chilled acetone; it is in fact most advantageous to use frozen sections cut after a short fixation in chilled calcium-formaldehyde or in 10% formalin or in glutaraldehyde or sections made in a cryostat, fixed in chilled formalin, or, yet again, paraffin wax sections taken from material treated by freeze-drying. In certain cases, the lipase withstands treatment with ethyl alcohol but it is better to avoid contact of the sections with this fluid.

Gomori's technique using Tweens:

Incubate the sections for 8 to 24 hours, at 37°C, in the following medium
    a 5% aqueous solution of the chosen tween .... 1 ml
    a 0.05 to 0.1 M tris- or sodium veronal buffer, pH 7–7.4 .. 45 ml
    a 2% calcium chloride solution .... 3 ml
Wash for 5 to 10 minutes in distilled water which should be renewed several times;
Treat for 10 minutes with a 2% solution of lead nitrate in distilled water;
Rinse carefully several times in distilled water;
Treat for 2 minutes with the dilute solution of ammonium sulphide;
Wash for 2 to 3 minutes in running water;
Where appropriate, stain the background with haemalum;
Wash in running water (1 to 3 minutes);
Dehydrate rapidly in absolute alcohol or acetone, clear and mount in a synthetic resin, avoiding benzenoid hydrocarbons as clearing agents or as solvents for the resin (dichlorethylene or ligroin are quite suitable); *in practice, mounting in a medium miscible with water is preferable.*

A positive result of the reaction is shown by a colour varying between yellow and golden brown; naturally any pre-existing calciferous inclusion is shown up with the same colour and any inclusions containing a metal which has a black sulphide would appear on the preparations. The inactivation of control sections may be obtained using heat treatment (10 minutes in water at 90–100°C) or by Lugol's fluid (for one minute at laboratory temperatures) or in 5% phenol (one minute at laboratory temperatures).

C. — SULPHATASES

Among the four types of sulphatase known to biochemists, glucosulphatases and chondrosulphatases have not yet been discovered in animal tissues and attempts to demonstrate myrosulphatases have not yet succeeded. Only the arylsulphatases are therefore mentioned here.

Several types of arylsulphatases have been described in a variety of vertebrate tissues during the last fifteen years; the extent to which our knowledge has been added to since the classical review of Fromageot is substantial but the functional significance of these enzymes which are defined by their capacity to catalyse the hydrolysis of arylsulphates is as yet unknown.

Among the methods for demonstrating their existence that due to Rutenburg and his colleagues is the most used. It depends on the decomposition of the sulphuric ester of 6-benzoyl-2-naphthol under the influence of the enzyme, the benzoyl-naphthol liberated by the primary reaction being coupled with the diazo salt of o-dianisidine.

The technique of Rutenburg and co-workers. — The preparation of the tissues must take into account the great variation depending on the origin of the material. The enzymes of rat tissues are preserved after fixing for several days or several weeks in 10% neutralised and chilled formalin. In primate tissue enzymes can only be detected on sections of fresh tissue cut in a cryostat and dried in air, so that it is necessary to treat unfixed sections in an incubating medium rendered hypertonic by the addition of sodium chloride.

The normal substrate is prepared by dissolving 25 mg of potassium 6-benzoyl-2-napthyl-sulphate in 80 ml of a 0.85% sodium chloride solution; it is generally necessary to warm in order to dissolve; 20 ml of Walpole's buffer, 0.5 M, of pH 6.1, is added.

For the treatment of fresh tissue 2.6 g of sodium chloride is dissolved in the substrate as defined above.

Working technique. — Wash the sections taken from fresh tissue in three baths of 0.85%, 1%, and 2% sodium chloride and incubate them in the hypertonic substrate; incubate sections taken from formalin-treated material in the normal substrate. Only sections taken from one and the same organ should be incubated in any given bath.

The incubation takes place at 37°C, the duration being from 2 to 16 hours according to the activity of the tissues.

Sections of fresh tissue are washed with the three saline solutions in the decreasing order of their concentration, the sections of formalin-treated tissue are washed in water prior to undergoing post-coupling for 5 minutes in a 0.1% solution of fast blue B salt dissolved in 0.05 M Sörensen buffer of pH 7.6; naturally the fluid should be chilled to about 4°C.

The preparations are then washed in a chilled solution of 0.85% sodium chloride (3 baths of about one minute) and mounted in a medium miscible with water.

The strongest arylsulphatase activity is shown by a blue colour and the weakest by a colour varying from purple to red.

As Lillie (1965) has commented, a technique involving simultaneous coupling would be more satisfactory from the theoretical standpoint but the solubility of 6-benzoyl-2-naphthol seems to be sufficiently slight for diffusion artefacts not to give rise to serious disquiet, on the scale of the light microscope.

D. — GLUCOSIDASES (GLYCOSIDASES)

This group incorporates β-glucuronidases and β-glucosidases, α-glucosidase, the galactosidases, N-acetyl-β-glucosaminidase and many other enzymes which cannot be detected histochemically. Only tests for β-glucuronidase are mentioned here.

The β-glucuronidases which are widely distributed in animal tissues specifically catalyse the hydrolysis of the β-glucoside link in a large number of natural or synthetic glucuronides. Among their inhibitors we may mention organic acids (citric, mucic, saccharic and ascorbic) and heparin.

Since the first attempts at detecting the histochemical activity of such enzymes, due to Friedenwald and Becker (1948), the technique for demonstrating them has been improved several times. The original method of Friedenwald and Becker consisted of incubating the sections in a substrate containing the glucuronide of o-hydroxyphenylazo-2-naphthol, so that a coloured azo-dyestuff is precipitated as a result of the enzymatic reaction; this method has been abandoned: it so happens that the hydrolysis of the substrate is very slow and the product of the primary reaction is highly soluble in lipids so that serious diffusion artefacts are likely. The second method due to Friedenwald and Becker consisted of incubating in a substrate containing the glucuronide of 8-hydroxyquinoline and detecting the 8-hydroxyquinolein liberated by the primary reaction by chelating it with iron followed by a histochemical detection of this latter cation; this method has been improved by several authors, the most important variations being those of Billet and McGee Russel (1955), and Fishman and Baker (1956). Pearse (1960) was originally strongly in favour of the last of these variations but later (Janigan and Pearse, 1962) considered that it was devoid of all meaning, positive results being obtained either following inhibition by copper ions or after incubation in a substrate devoid of glucuronide. On the contrary, Fishman (1964) defends the validity of the method.

Whilst we await the results of further studies capable of resolving the problem just mentioned, it seems reasonable to call into play another reaction for the demonstration of β-glucuronidase; the validity of this other reaction is generally agreed and it only involves compounds whose synthesis can be carried out in the laboratory whereas 8-hydroxyquinoline glucuronide must be obtained by biosynthesis through the administration of 8-hydroxyquinoline to rabbits and the collection of their urine. This method, the technique of Seligman and his colleagues (1954), depends on the enzymatic hydrolysis of 6-bromo-2-napthyl-β-D-glucopyruronoside, demonstrating the 6-bromo-2-naphthol by post-coupling with the diazo salt of *o*-dianisidine.

The technique of Seligman and co-workers. — These authors recommend working with sections of fresh tissue cut on a cryostat, the sections being fixed for about twelve minutes, at approximately 4°C, in 10% neutralised and chilled formalin, and then washed for 15 minutes in cold water to remove the formalin. Experience shows that the enzymatic activity is preserved in a large number of instances by a short fixation in 10% neutral and chilled formalin, the sections being cut on a freezing microtome and washed.

> Incubate for 4 to 6 hours, at 37°C, in the substrate prepared in the following way— dissolve 30 mg of 6-bromo-2-naphthyl-β-D-glucopyruronoside in 5 ml of absolute methyl alcohol, add 20 ml of McIlvaine's buffer (pH 4.95), and 75 ml of distilled water;
> Wash in distilled water (for about one minute);
> Couple for 2 minutes in a 0.1% solution of fast blue B salt prepared in 0.02 M Sörensen buffer of pH 7.5 (chill before dissolving the salt);
> Wash in two baths of chilled distilled water (for a few seconds);
> Wash in 0.1% acetic acid (for a few seconds);
> Mount in a medium miscible with water.

β-glucuronidases are indicated by a blue colour, free lipases being stained red. Wolfgram (1961) suggests that the sections should be extracted with chloroform prior to incubation to avoid this red staining of the lipids but he mentions that the reaction becomes negative when practised under these conditions on sections of nerve tissue.

E. — CARBONIC ANHYDRASE

Since its discovery by Meldrum and Roughton (1932, 1933) this enzyme, which is defined by its ability to catalyse the cleavage of carbonic acid and carbonates with the liberation of CO_2, has been the subject of many biochemical investigations and its intervention in many of the essential functions of the vertebrate organism is well known.

We must emphasize, with all possible clarity, that the histoenzymological data relating to this enzyme are nowhere near as good as is our biochemical knowledge; *in actual fact no attempt to detect them histochemically has given results in which confidence can be placed.*

The principle of Kurata's (1953) method, which is carried out, as a first stage, on thin slices of tissue and, in a second stage, on sections of fresh tissue after fixing in acetone or after short fixation in chilled formalin, is simple. The material is incubated in a bath the substrate of which is represented by sodium bicarbonate; the carbonate ions formed during the primary reaction are precipitated *in situ* through the addition of salts of manganese, calcium, nickel or cobalt to the incubating bath, the reaction being completed by the histochemical detection of the precipitates so formed. It is the variation using cobalt which has been adopted by most of those who have followed Kurata (see Arvy 1963 for a list of the principal investigations).

The results so obtained seem to be satisfactory at least so far as the optical qualities of the preparations are concerned but when the data so obtained are compared with those derived from biochemical studies all illusions are dispelled. In fact, the systematic studies of Lutwak-Mann (1955), Böving (1959), and Fand and his colleagues (1959) clearly show that the reactions are either false positives or false negatives. At the present time, workers are unanimous in commenting that Kurata's technique can in no way be considered as a reaction for the detection of carbo-anhydrases (see in particular Pearse, 1960; Arvy, 1963; Barka and Anderson, 1963; and Lillie, 1965). It seems logical to attribute the failure of the method to a weakness in the capture reaction; in all probability the —HCO_3 ions are liberated very rapidly, their solubility in the lipids and in water as well as their mobility serving to explain their failure to be precipitated *in situ*. It therefore seems useless to me to describe the technique in question here.

F. — PEPTIDASES

The group of enzymes which irreversibly hydrolyse the acid —CO—NH— link are obviously of the first importance but only one representative, namely leucine-aminopeptidase, is directly accessible to histochemical detection.

Since Gomori's (1954) original work devoted to the demonstration of this enzyme, the principle of the method has for all practical purposes remained unmodified, but numerous developments have taken place concerning the choice of substrates and the way in which the product of the primary reaction is detected. Gomori, in effect, incubated the sections in a bath containing glycyl- or alanylnaphthylamides and demonstrated the naphthylamine liberated by the primary reaction through simultaneous coupling with fast garnet GBC salt. In addition to alanyl-β-naphthylamide and leucyl-β-naphthylamide Nachlas and his colleagues introduced the chlorhydrate of L-leucyl-4-methoxy-2-naphthylamide, the aryl group of which couples more rapidly than does 2-naphthylamine with diazonium salts. As for these latter, some authors have remained faithful to fast garnet GBC salt whereas others prefer fast blue B salt, despite its inhibiting action on amino-peptidase, because the coloured azo-dyestuff formed by the capture reaction is capable of fixing copper ions by chelation which intensifies its colour and suppresses its solubility in alcohol and in benzenoid hydrocarbons so that it is possible to mount in Canada balsam or in equivalent resins. The inhibition of control sections may be obtained by the use of versene or of 10^{-2} M sodium citrate.

Preparation of the tissues. — Workers belonging to Seligman's school work with sections of fresh tissue cut on a cryostat and stuck on to slides, adhesion being ensured by drying in air; Burstone prefers freeze-dried material embedded in paraffin, all contact of the sections with alcohol and with benzenoid hydrocarbons being avoided. Short fixation with 10% formalin, chilled to 4°C, is possible in certain cases, the frozen sections being washed so as to eliminate all traces of the fixative and stuck to slides or treated in baths. Ackerman (1960) recommends that blood smears in which this enzyme is to be tested should be fixed in a 1% solution of osmium tetroxide in dimethylformamide, the liquid being chilled to $-10°C$; the fixation, which lasts for 2 minutes, is followed by washing in water in order to eliminate all trace of the fixative.

Ackerman's technique:

Incubate the smear for 4 to 6 hours, at 20-25°C, in a medium containing—
  alanyl-β-naphthylamide .... 40 mg
  distilled water .... 50 ml
  0.1 M Sörensen buffer, pH 6.7 .... 50 ml
  magnesium sulphate .... 5 mg
  fast garnet GBC salt .... 50 mg
Wash for one to two minutes in running water;
Mount in a medium miscible with water.

A positive result of the reaction is shown by a red precipitate which often has a characteristic appearance; it is this granular, even crystalline, appearance of the precipitate which is the major disadvantage of fast garnet GBC salt as a coupling agent.

The technique of Nachlas et al. (1957) using leucyl-β-naphthylamide:

Incubate the sections for 20 minutes to 4 hours, at 37°C, in the following bath
  0.1 M Walpole's buffer, pH 6.5 .... 50 ml
  0.8% sodium chloride solution .... 40 ml
  2.10^{-2} M (1.3 g/l) potassium cyanide solution .... 5 ml
  a solution of 8 mg/ml of leucyl-β-naphthylamide in distilled
    water .... 5 ml
  the diazo salt of o-dianisidine (fast blue B salt) .... 50 mg
Wash for 2 minutes with a 0.8% solution of sodium chloride;
Treat for 2 minutes with a 0.1 M aqueous solution of copper sulphate;
Wash in the 0.8% sodium chloride solution;
Fix for 2 to 4 hours, at about 4°C, in 10% formalin;
Dehydrate in absolute alcohol, clear in a benzenoid hydrocarbon and mount in a synthetic resin or in Canada balsam.

A positive result of this reaction is shown by an intense blue or purple colour. The potassium cyanide plays the part of an activator of the enzyme in this reaction.

The technique of Nachlas et al. (1960) using the chlorhydrate of L leucyl 4 methoxy-2-naphthylamide.

Incubate the sections for 30 minutes to 4 hours, at 37°C, in the following medium
0.1 M Walpole's buffer, pH 6.5 .... 10 ml
a 0.85% aqueous solution of sodium chloride .... 50 ml
a 2.10^{-2} M aqueous solution of potassium cyanide .... 35 ml
a solution of 4 mg/ml of the substrate in distilled water ... 5 ml
the diazo salt of o-dianisidine .... 50 mg
Complete the reaction as in the preceding variation;
The positive result of the reaction is shown by a red colour with purplish tones.

G. — DEOXYRIBONUCLEASE

This enzyme, which is characterised by its ability to split deoxyribonucleates with the formation of purine- and pyrimidine-nucleotides, has been known to biochemists since the beginning of the 20th century, as has ribonuclease. It has been obtained in the crystalline condition and serves as a control reagent during the histochemical detection of deoxyribonucleic acid.

The detection of deoxyribonuclease on sections of tissue has been attempted by two methods, the first of which cannot possibly be called histochemical as it does not allow us to undertake a true histological study at the level of the cell. This is the method of Daoust (1955, 1957, 1961) which is very ingenious and suitable as a qualitative test with a rapid and clear response; only its principle is mentioned below. The second method, due to Aronson and his colleagues (1958) and to Vorbrodt (1961), discloses only the deoxyribonuclease II of the biochemists, characterised by having an optimum pH between 4.5 and 6, whereas that of deoxyribonuclease I is of the order of 7 to 8; it is also characterised by its insensitivity to magnesium ions which, on the contrary, activate deoxyribonuclease I.

Daoust's technique depends on the following principle. Two slides, one of which bears the section under investigation and the other a thin film of gelatin in which deoxyribonucleic acid has been incorporated, are pressed against one another so that the section is in contact with the gelatin layer. After incubation, the two slides are separated, fixed in dilute formalin, washed and stained. The presence in the section of deoxyribonuclease is disclosed by a clear zone on the slide carrying the gelatin layer corresponding to the enzymatic digestion of the deoxyribonucleic acid. A similar procedure has been applied by Daoust and Amano (1960) to the demonstration of ribonuclease and by Tremblay (1963) to that of amylase, as well as by Adams and Tuqan (1961) to that of proteases in general.

The technique of Aronson (1958) and Vorbrodt (1961) can be applied to sections cut from fresh material in a cryostat with fixation of the sections adhering to slides by a mixture of formaldehyde, water and acetone (10/40/50) for 5 minutes at $-10°C$, the fixative being removed by washing in equal parts of acetone and water and then in water. It is also possible to fix for a short time in diluted and chilled formalin, followed by the preparation of frozen sections.

> The incubation takes place at 37°C for from 30 minutes to three hours in the substrate:—
>
> deoxyribonucleic acid from Herring sperm .... 5 mg
>
> or
>
> deoxyribonucleic acid from the calf thymus .... 1 mg
> acid phosphatase (commercial preparation) .... 2.5 mg
> 0.2 M Walpole's buffer, pH 5.9 or 5.2 .... 6.2 ml
> a 3.31% lead nitrate solution (0.1 M) .... 0.5 ml
> distilled water to make up to .... 25 ml
>
> The sections are then washed carefully in distilled water, rinsed in 1% acetic acid and treated for 2 minutes with a dilute solution of ammonium sulphide, then washed in water and mounted in balsam, with or without a background stain.

A positive result of the reaction is disclosed by a black precipitate of lead sulphide whose appearance is a consequence of the following mechanism. The nucleotides formed during the primary reaction from the deoxyribonucleic acid of the medium play the part of the substrate and are hydrolysed by the acid phosphatase added to the incubating bath, so that phosphate ions are liberated; these are precipitated by the lead present in the incubating medium in the form of lead phosphate which is then detected by means of the ammonium sulphide; that is to say, the technique, the primary reaction apart, amounts to the detection of acid phosphomonoesterase using Gomori's lead technique, the product of the primary reaction subsequently playing the part of the substrate. It is the "doubly" indirect nature of the reaction which should lead us to regard it with the greatest circumspection when interpreting its results. At the tissue level, the method gives results which agree strictly with those given by Daoust's technique. At the level of the organelle, incubating in a medium of pH 5.9 serves particularly to localise lysosomes, that at pH 5.2 for nuclear localisation.

HISTOCHEMICAL DETECTION OF TRANSFERASES

The enzymes corresponding to this class in Hofmann-Ostenhof's (1954) table catalyse chemical reactions whose general sequence is

$$R{-}A + R'{-}B \rightleftharpoons R{-}B + R'{-}A.$$

Only the histochemical detection of phosphorylase and of amylo-1,4,1,6-transglucosidase are mentioned here.

As the names indicate, we have to deal with enzymes which reversibly catalyse the transformation of glucose-1-phosphate (Cori's ester) into glycogen. The phosphorylase establishes 1.4 links between molecules of glucose and thus builds linear chains of amylose, amylo-1.4,1.6-transglucosidase forming the 1.6 links needed for the branched molecular chains of glycogen (*branching enzyme*).

The first attempt at the histochemical identification of phosphorylase was due to Yin and Sun (1947) and related to plant tissues, the incubation being undertaken in a solution of glucose-1-phosphate; the starch formed during the reaction was detected by the iodine technique. Among the improvements to which this method has been subjected the most important, namely the introduction of activating agents, are due to Takeuchi and his colleagues (1955 to 1958).

Takeuchi's technique for the detection of phosphorylase and of amylo-1,4,1.6-transglucosidase. — The technique is only applicable to sections of fresh tissue cut on a cryostat or on a microtome with a chilled blade; their thickness may be as great as 40 μ; it is advantageous to avoid sticking them to slides unless the tissue is extremely friable. In the latter case, the sections should be placed in the incubation bath before they are completely dry.

The incubation bath is prepared in the following way

potassium glucose-1-phosphate	50 mg
muscle adenylic acid	10 mg
glycogen (optional)	2 mg
distilled water	15 ml
0.1 to 0.5 M Walpole's buffer, pH 5.8	10 ml
insulin	10 units

The incubation takes place at 37°C; it lasts for 1 to 3 hours. When taken out of the incubating bath the sections are rapidly rinsed in 40% alcohol and stuck to slides (unless this process was carried out prior to incubation), and fixed for 2 to 4 minutes in absolute alcohol, then treated with Gram's iodine-iodide solution (distilled water 300 ml; iodine 1 g; potassium iodide 2 g) diluted 10 times. The mounting takes place in glycerine or in iodated glycerine (glycerine 9 volumes, Gram's solution 1 volume) after 5 to 10 minutes passage through the iodine-iodide solution; the preparations are sealed with paraffin wax or with a cellulose varnish.

A positive result is shown by the appearance of a blue colour in structures which are simply endowed with phosphorylase activity (synthesis of amylose), whereas this tint varies from purple to mahogany wherever both enzymes are to be found (synthesis of glycogen). Evidently other histochemical reactions for neutral polysaccharides may also be applied; the PAS technique is particularly indicated when it is desired to obtain permanent preparations because the stains obtained with the iodine reaction keep very poorly. Controls using α-amylase or β-amylase may be conducted prior to the histochemical detection of the polysaccharides formed during the reaction (prior to staining with iodine).

The criteria which permit us to distinguish between the two enzymes discussed here are summarised in Table 22, constructed from the data provided by Takeuchi's school.

Table 22. — DISTINCTION BETWEEN PHOSPHORYLASE AND AMYLO-1.4, 1.6-TRANSGLUCOSIDASE

Reaction	Phosphorylase	Amylo-1.4, 1.6-transglucosidase
Iodine	blue	mahogany
PAS	red magenta	red magenta
Polysaccharide synthesised	amylose	glycogen
α-amylase	fully digested	fully digested
β-amylase	fully digested	not attacked
Ethanol (20%)	inhibition weak or none	inhibition strong
Mercuric chloride (10^{-4}M)	moderate inhibition	complete inhibition

From the practical standpoint the ethanol is added to the incubating medium so as to produce a final concentration of 20% (5 ml of absolute alcohol for 25 ml of substrate); in the same way, the mercuric chloride is incorporated in the incubating medium. The enzymatic attack takes place, as I remarked above, at the end of the enzymatic reaction prior to the detection of the polysaccharides so formed.

Polysaccharides which pre-existed must obviously be detected on control sections; these latter are obtained by incubating in a bath which differs from that of the reaction properly so called in the absence of glucose-1-phosphate or of adenylic acid. Experience shows that pre-existing glycogen generally disappears during the incubation of the sections.

All authors emphasize the reliability of the method and the excellent quality of the results which it provides. For the PAS reaction it is advisable to use an alcoholic solution of periodic acid prepared according to Hotchkiss' (1948) formula by dissolving 0.4 g of periodic acid in 35 ml of absolute alcohol; 5 ml of sodium acetate in 0.2 M aqueous solution (27.2 g of the crystalline salt in 1 litre of water) and 10 ml of distilled water are added. This solution should be kept in the cold and rejected as soon as it becomes brownish. The other stages of the reaction take place as usual; I might remind the reader that the reducing rinses of Hotchkiss' technique are of no value.

THE HISTOCHEMICAL DETECTION OF OXYDO-REDUCTASES

As Lison (1960, p. 579) quite rightly remarked, the nomenclature of the enzymes corresponding to this class in the Hoffmann-Ostenhof system is of the greatest complexity; difficulties and misunderstandings may therefore result. We should also recognise that the histochemistry of the compounds in question has not reached the high degree of development attained by their biochemical study. It would be dangerous to hide from ourselves, indeed, that a large number of the procedures described in original works and in specialised accounts are not of sufficiently reliable value to justify their entry into current practice.

We adopt here the nomenclature of Baldwin (1957), following in this respect Lison (1960), and so we are led to distinguish the following categories.

The *oxidases* specifically catalyse the transfer of hydrogen to molecular oxygen; *peroxidases* catalyse the transfer of hydrogen either to hydrogen peroxide or to organic peroxides. The *aerobic dehydrogenases* catalyse the transfer of hydrogen to molecular oxygen (in an aerobic medium) or to another acceptor (methylene blue, tetrazolium salt, etc...), whereas the *anaerobic dehydrogenases* catalyse this transfer to an acceptor which is never molecular oxygen.

The methodological difference between tests for oxydases and that for dehydrogenases has been most appropriately stressed by Lison (1960); although it is true that both types of enzyme catalyse hydrogen transfer, it is the *hydrogen donor* which originates the colour reaction when we are dealing with the *detection of oxidases, its oxidation product being coloured*, whereas it is the *hydrogen acceptor* which in the great majority of cases is the product of the *histochemical reaction of dehydrogenases, its reaction product being coloured*.

A. — OXIDASES

Among the oxydases (aerobic transelectronases of Hoffmann-Ostenhof), cytochrome-oxydase, tyrosinase and the phenoloxydases are accessible to histochemical detection using reactions which are sufficiently well tested to be included here.

CYTOCHROME-OXIDASE

Cytochrome-oxydase, which has been known since the beginning of the 20th century (indophenoloxydase, the respiratory ferment) is a metalloprotein which contains iron and perhaps copper. The development of the biochemical data concerning this substance has been summarised in a masterly fashion by Keilin and Slater (1953). Its function in the organism consists in oxidising cytochrome c.

The principal histochemical technique allowing us to localise cytochrome-oxydase was in fact developed by Ehrlich (1885) but used by this author solely for macroscopical observations (the blue tint of certain mammalian organs after the injection of a mixture of α-naphthol and dimethylpara phenylenediamine solutions). Winckler was the first to use it in histology, and Gierke (1911) codified the experimental conditions for the reaction and until recently histologists used the technique in the way recommended by this latter author; the names of Moog (1943), Nachlas and his colleagues (1958) and Burstone (1959, 1960, 1961) are associated with recent developments of the nadireaction whose name evokes the initials of the reagents.

The principle of the nadireaction is simple. A mixture of α-naphthol and dimethylparaphenylenediamine gives a blue coloured condensation product by oxidation, indophenol blue, whose stability is not very great. When carried out on fresh tissue and without the addition of alkalis this reaction detects the cytochrome-oxydase, the mixture playing that role of hydrogen donor which, *in vivo*, is played by the cytochrome (*G-Nadioxydasereaktion, labile Oxydasereaktion, Gewebsoxydasereaktion* of German authors). It is appropriate to mention at this point that the same reagent when rendered alkaline and acting on tissues fixed in formalin detects verdoperoxidase (*M-Nadioxydasereaktion, stabile Oxydasereaktion, Myelooxydasereaktion*).

The classical technique whose principles have just been mentioned has certain disadvantages which modern modifications to some extent diminish. The reduction of indophenol blue by dehydrogenases may evidently lead to false negatives; it may be avoided by inactivating these enzymes with a pre-treatment using a 0.003 M solution of phenylurethane (Moog, 1943). The indophenol blue is soluble in lipids and authors from 1910 to 1930 feared that it might behave as a lysochrome demonstrating not oxidases but free lipids; this does in fact happen but the stains obtained are too distinct for there to be any confusion. The solubility of the stain in water and its non-affinity for structures containing cytochrome-oxidase, its instability and its tendency to crystallise are, on the other hand, serious disadvantages. The optical qualities of the preparations are improved by replacing the dimethylparaphenylenediamine in the reagent with 4-amino-1-N-N'-dimethylnaphthylamine (Nachlas and his colleagues, 1958); moreover, α-naphthol increases the toxicity of the reagent for the enzymatic system to be detected and its replacement by other substances has been suggested by Burstone (1959). Besides the technique of Moog (1943), the two most recent methods which have just been mentioned are discussed here.

The preparation of the tissues in all cases includes the cutting of sections from fresh tissue, the use of dissociating techniques or the treatment of tissue blocks of rather small size. The old practice of free-hand sections may be replaced by cutting in a cryostat or in a microtome with a chilled blade (see also p. 124 and 261); it is advantageous to cut rather thick sections. *No fixation is possible without considerable losses, or even the complete inactivation of the enzyme.*

Moog's technique:

Incubate the sections, at 37°C, for 3 to 5 minutes or at laboratory temperatures for 10 minutes to 1 hour, with the following medium prepared at the time of use:—

Sörensen's buffer, pH 7.2 to 7.6 .... 25 ml
1% solution of α-naphthol in 40% ethanol .... 1 to 2 ml
1% aqueous solution of dimethyl-para-phenylenediamine chlorhydrate .... 1 to 2 ml

Follow the progress of the reaction with the naked eye or under the microscope, stopping it when the blue colour seems to be sufficiently intense;

Wash in saline water (0.85% for tissues of homeotherm vertebrates);

Mount in a medium miscible with water; Moog (1943) recommends a 5% solution of potassium acetate, the preparations to be sealed; in any case the blue stain, diagnostic of a positive result, very rapidly fades;

Treat control sections with a 0.003 M solution of sodium azide (NaN_3), incubate them in the medium indicated above but with the addition of 0.003 M sodium azide so as to verify the negative result following the action of this specific inhibitor;

Treat control sections with a 0.003 M solution of phenylurethane and incubate them in the substrate indicated to which 0.003 M phenylurethane has been added so as to verify that the negative results are not due to the destaining of the indophenol blue by dehydrogenases.

This work should be carried out on fresh tissue, the sodium azide and the phenylurethane should be dissolved in "physiological" solution, isotonic with the body fluids of the animal whose tissues are being examined.

The technique of Nachlas and his colleagues:

Incubate the sections for 10 to 30 minutes, at laboratory temperatures, in the following medium prepared immediately prior to use

0.1 M Sörensen buffer, pH 7.4 .... 3 ml
α-naphthol (an aqueous solution of 1mg/ml) .... 4 ml
catalase (commercial preparation) at 30 mg/ml............ 1 ml
cytochrome C (an aqueous solution of 5 mg/ml) .... 3 ml
4-amino-1-N,N'-dimethylnaphthylamine chlorhydrate or oxalate (an aqueous solution of 2 mg/ml) .... 4 ml

The addition of cytochrome C which is particularly costly may be omitted when the tissues are known to contain an active cytochrome-oxidase;

Wash rapidly in physiological saline;

Mount in a medium miscible with water.

A positive result of the reaction is shown by a purple stain; the affinity of the stain and its stability are much better than those of indophenol blue.

Burstone's technique:

Incubate the sections in the following medium prepared at the time of use
N-phenyl-p-phenylenediamine (the *base* and not the chlorhydrate) .... 10 ml
1-hydroxy-2-naphthanilide .... 10 ml
absolute ethanol .... 0.5 ml
distilled water .... 35 ml
the tris-hydrochloric acid buffer, pH 7.4 .... 15 ml
stir and filter.
The incubation may last for 10 minutes to 1 hour or even longer; it takes place at laboratory temperatures;
Treat the sections, without washing by the mixture
10% formalin (not neutralised) .... 100 ml
cobalt acetate .... 10 g
0.2 M Walpole's buffer, pH 5.2 .... 5 ml
The treatment with this mixture, which ensures chelation and fixation, may last for an hour or more;
Wash in running water for about 10 minutes;
Mount in a medium miscible with water.

The 1-hydroxy-2-naphthanilide of the incubating medium may be replaced by other compounds (10 mg of 2-cyano-acetylcoumarone, 1-phenyl-3-methylpyrazolone, p-methoxy-p-aminodiphenylamine, 3-amino-9-ethylcarbazol, 1 drop of 8-amino-1,2,3,4-tetrahydroquinoline). A positive result of the reaction is shown by a red stain with all compounds, with the exception of the last which gives blue stains. Control reactions using inhibitors (potassium cyanide) are to be recommended. The preparations are stable.

TYROSINASE AND DOPA-OXIDASE

Following the work of Lerner's (1949) school it is agreed that the oxidation of tyrosine to dihydroxyphenylalanine (DOPA) and the oxidation of this latter compound, an essential stage in melanogenesis, is in fact associated with a single enzyme whose constitution is highly complicated, a metalloprotein containing copper being associated with an *o*-diphenol and with metallic ions (Kertesz, 1952).

The histochemical detection of DOPA-oxidase dates from the time of Bloch (1917), its principle consists in incubating slices of tissue cut from fresh material with a solution of dihydroxyphenylalanine and then of examining under a microscope for the black precipitate diagnostic of the formation of melanin. Improvements in this technique are due to Laidlaw and Blackberg (1932), Gomori (1952), and Rappaport (1955).

At the time of writing we know that it is not essential to have recourse to sections of fresh tissue; tests for the enzymatic activity are also successful after a short fixation (less than 7 hours) in 10% neutralised and chilled formalin, the tissue blocks being sectioned on a freezing microtome. Paraffin wax sections taken from freeze-dried material also give good results.

Laidlaw and Blackberg's technique:

> Fix the tissue blocks for one hour, at laboratory temperatures, in 10% formalin;
> Cut the material into slices whose dimensions should not exceed 2 mm and wash them in running water for 3 minutes;
> Incubate the slices for one hour, at 37°C, in the medium
> 0.1 M Sörensen buffer, pH 7.4 .... 100 ml
> dihydroxyphenylalanine .... 0.1 g
> Change the liquid, continuing the incubation for 12 to 15 hours;
> Wash for about 12 minutes in running water;
> Refix in Bouin's fluid for 24 hours;
> Dehydrate, embed in paraffin wax, section and stick the sections to slides, practising a background stain where appropriate and then mount in Canada balsam or in a commercial synthetic resin.

A positive result of the reaction is shown by the appearance of granules whose colour varies between brown and black; the preparations are permanent.

Gomori's technique:

> Fix for several hours in 10% neutralised and chilled formalin;
> Section on a freezing microtome;
> Rinse the sections rapidly in distilled water and incubate them at laboratory temperatures or at 37°C in Laidlaw and Blackberg's substrate; change the bath once or twice if the duration of incubation exceeds one hour; do not incubate for more than 5 hours;
> Wash the sections in tap water, stain the background where appropriate, cause the sections to adhere to slides, dehydrate, clear and mount in Canada balsam or in a synthetic resin.

A positive result of the reaction results in a stain varying between grey-brown and black.

POLYPHENOLOXIDASES

These enzymes, which were confused by older authors with tyrosinase and with DOPA-oxidase, catalyse the transformation of *o*- and *p*-diphenols and aminophenols into quinones or quinone-imines. Their influence on quinonoid tannins which results in the hardening of certain cuticular secretions or of structural material in the invertebrates is well known; recent publications devoted to the arthropod integument and the general survey of Arvy (1957/58) give much data on this topic.

The demonstration of polyphenoloxidases has been successful on fresh tissue blocks or after short fixation with formalin or alcohol; embedding in paraffin wax seems only to have been used after freeze-drying. A positive reaction has also been obtained on tissue blocks after fixing in 70% alcohol, followed by washing in water (for about 30 minutes).

The demonstration technique (Brunet, 1951; Smith, 1954) consists of incubating the tissue blocks or fixed sections, cut free-hand, in a 0.2% aqueous solution of catechol (pyrocatechol). The excess reagent is removed by washing in tap water (for about 30 minutes). Background staining may be undertaken; mounting in Canada balsam or in a synthetic resin of the same kind is possible.

The brown or red stain which indicates a positive result of the reaction is in most cases destroyed by dilute solutions of sodium hypochlorite. Inhibition of the reaction can be obtained using 0.002 M potassium cyanide but sodium azide, which inhibits cytochrome oxidase, is without effect on polyphenoloxidases.

B. — PEROXIDASES

These enzymes catalyse the transfer of hydrogen from a donor to peroxides (hydrogen peroxide or monosubstituted peroxide). The hydrogen donors activated by the peroxide-peroxidase system are rather numerous; Lison (1960, p. 589) gives a list in which are to be found, in particular, hydroiodic acid, polyphenols such as hydroquinone and gaiacol, aromatic amines such as o-phenylenediamine and benzidine, various aromatic compounds such as vanillin, and lastly leucoderivatives of quinonoid stains (expecially the zinc-leucobases).

Apart from the detection of pigments of the haemoglobin type, the essential application of tests for peroxidase activity is the demonstration of blood cells of the myeloid series of vertebrates, characterised by the presence of verdoperoxidase (Agner, 1941).

Among the numerous techniques suggested those involving a gaiacol, pyrogallol, or orthophenylenediamine have no more than historical interest. The benzidine reaction still enjoys a certain favour and one of the most recent of its variations, that of Gomori (1952), is described below. The α-naphthol reaction introduced into histological technique by Loele (1926) is generally carried out on blocks; Ritter and Oleson's formula (1947) is a variant of this. The zinc-leucobases, applied in the way described in relation to the histochemical detection of haemoglobin (p. 569), give striking preparations which keep very well; this is probably the method of choice not only for blocks of small size and for sections but also for smears; for these latter the reagent, to which an equal volume of hydrogen peroxide has been added, is then diluted with 9 volumes of distilled water. The nadireaction undertaken in alkaline media and after formalin fixation also detects the peroxidase activity of cells of the myeloid series (the M-nadireaction of Graeff).

The benzidine reaction (Gomori's technique). — The technique may be applied to small tissue blocks, to sections or to smears; fixing may be carried out in acetone, ethanol or formalin-alcohol; it is better to avoid embedding in paraffin wax but to cut frozen sections.

> Treat the sections or smears for about 5 minutes with the mixture stock solution of benzidine (dissolve 0.2 to 0.3 g of benzidine in 100 ml of 95% alcohol and add 0.5 g of sodium nitro-prusside dissolved in several ml of distilled water) mixed with equal volumes of 10 volume hydrogen peroxide (3%) diluted 50 fold;
> The duration of action may be prolonged for small tissue blocks;
> Wash rapidly in tap water;
> Where appropriate, use a nuclear red stain;
> Dehydrate in absolute alcohol, clear in a benzenoid hydrocarbon and mount in Canada balsam or in a synthetic resin.

A positive result of the reaction is shown by a blue stain which tends to turn brown; the preparations are not very stable.

The α-naphthol reaction (Ritter and Oleson's technique):

> Fix the tissue blocks whose dimensions should not be greater than 4 mm for 24 hours with the mixture
>
> | | |
> |---|---|
> | 95% alcohol | 90 ml |
> | commercial formalin | 10 ml |
> | 0.1 N soda | 1 ml |
>
> Wash for 30 minutes in running water and then for 2 hours in tap water which should not be renewed;
> Treat the tissue blocks for 24 hours with the mixture
>
> | | |
> |---|---|
> | 40% alcohol | 100 ml |
> | α-naphthol | 1 g |
> | 30% hydrogen peroxide (105 volumes) | 0.2 ml |
>
> *freshly prepared*;
> Wash for 10 minutes in running water;
> Treat for 3 to 24 hours with the solution
>
> | | |
> |---|---|
> | 40% alcohol | 96 ml |
> | pyronine | 0.1 g |
> | aniline | 4 ml |
>
> Wash for 1 hour in 80% alcohol;
> Dehydrate in absolute alcohol, clear in a benzenoid hydrocarbon and embed in paraffin wax;
> Mount the sections in Canada balsam or in a synthetic resin after dewaxing, or hydrate them and carry out a nuclear staining with haemalum, dehydrate, clear and mount.

A positive result of the reaction is shown by an intense red colour due to the fact that the granules which have reacted with α-naphthol have acquired a strong affinity for pyronine which is a basic dyestuff.

The M-nadireaction. — This technique may be applied to frozen sections taken from formalin treated material or to smears fixed for at the most two hours in formalin-alcohol (95% alcohol 40 volumes; formalin 10 volumes). Rapid embedding in paraffin wax is possible according to certain authors but it is better avoided

> The reagent must be prepared *immediately* prior to use by mixing the following two solutions
>
> *a) α-naphthol*. Boil 1 g of this compound with 100 ml of distilled water; the molten naphthol is dissolved by adding, drop by drop, 25% potash; it is allowed to cool; when kept in darkness this solution keeps for about one month.
>
> *b) dimethyl-p-phenylenediamine*. Dissolve 1 g of this compound (or, better, of its more stable chlorhydrate) in 100 ml of boiled distilled water; when kept in the dark this soluion keeps for two to three weeks.
>
> Treat the sections or the smears for 1 to 5 minutes at laboratory temperatures with a mixture of equal parts of the solutions a and b;
>
> Stabilise the dye using a treatment lasting for 2 to 3 minutes with Lugol's fluid diluted to one third; the granulations which were blue on being removed from the reagent become brown;
>
> Wash in water rendered alkaline with lithium carbonate until the blue colour of the granulations reappears;
>
> Stain the background with a nuclear red stain;
>
> Mount in a medium miscible with water.

A positive result of the reaction is shown by a blue colour.

C. — AEROBIC DEHYDROGENASES

In addition to xanthine-oxidase whose histochemical detection has been attempted by Bourne (1953) in work which has not been taken up by more recent authors, this group of enzymes includes, among its histochemically detectable representatives, the amine-oxidases, compounds whose chemical constitution corresponds to that of the flavoproteins and which catalyse the oxidative deamination of certain enzymes with the formation of aldehydes. When the reaction takes place under aerobic conditions it does indeed result in the formation of hydrogen peroxide, the hydrogen acceptor being molecular oxygen.

It is classical to distinguish a monoamine-oxidase which is active towards tyramine, adrenaline and 5-hydroxytryptamine (serotonin) as well as a diamine-oxidase which acts on histamine and on related diamines (putrescine and cadaverine).

Most attempts at histochemical detection have dealt with the monoamine-oxidases, these techniques depending either on the detection of aldehydes arising during deamination (the technique of Oster and Schlossman, 1942, using Schiff's reagent; the technique of Koelle and Valk, 1954 using 2-hydroxy-3-naphthoic hydrazide) or on the reduction of tetrazolium salts (Francis, 1953; Glenner, Burtner and Brown, 1957; Shimizu, Morikawa and Okada, 1959).

Amongst the inhibitors, the most widely used is isonicotinic 2-isopropyl-hydrazide (Marsilid) with 0.01 M solutions of which the material should be preincubated.

The technique of Koelle and Valk. — This technique requires frozen sections taken from fresh material, sectioned on a cryostat or on a microtome with a chilled blade and adherent to slides.

Incubate for 2 hours, at 37°C, in the following substrate
- distilled water .... 1.5 ml
- a 0.1 M aqueous solution of tryptamine chlorhydrate .... 0.1 ml
- a 0.005 M aqueous solution of 2-hydroxy-3-naphthoic hydrazide .... 3 ml
- N soda .... 0.15 ml
- a 0.2 M solution of disodium phosphate .... 15 ml
- a 40% solution of sodium sulphate .... 7.5 ml

Rinse in distilled water;
Couple for 5 minutes with a solution of fast blue B salt (about 0.1%) in Sörensen buffer of pH 7.4;
Rinse in distilled water;
Fix in 10% formalin;
Rinse in tap water;
Mount in a medium miscible with water.

A positive result of the reaction is shown by a blue or purple colour. Control sections are subjected to a pre-incubation bath containing Marsilid and are treated with an incubating medium to which this latter compound has been added (0.15 ml for the size of bath indicated in the formula).

The technique of Glenner and his colleagues. — As in the technique of Koelle and Valk, that of Glenner and his colleagues requires the use of sections taken from fresh tissue, adherent to slides.

Incubate, at 37°C, for 30 to 45 minutes in the following bath
- tryptamine chlorhydrate .... 25 mg
- sodium sulphate (optional) .... 4 mg
- nitro-blue tetrazolium .... 4 mg
- 0.1 M Sörensen's buffer, pH 7.6 .... 5 ml
- distilled water .... 15 ml

Wash in running water for 10 minutes;
Fix for about 12 hours in 10% formalin;
Mount in a medium miscible with water.

A positive result is shown by a red, purple or blue colour; the first two colours are extractable by dehydration in acetone and clearing in benzenoid hydrocarbons, as is recommended by Glenner et al. for mounting in a synthetic resin; moreover, Pearse (1960) recommends the mounting system given here which respects all the stains given by the reaction.

Data concerning the histochemical detection of diamine-oxidases are much more summary. The adaptation of the technique due to Oster and Schlossman for this purpose has been attempted by Valette and Cohen (1952) who replaced the tyramine by histamine in the incubating medium. The staining reactions obtained are fugitive and their localising value is quite as weak as in Oster and Schlossman's technique which was criticised by Gomori (1952) because of the risks of diffusion artefacts. Arvy (1957) uses a method involving tetrazolium salts and modifies Francis's incubating medium for the detection of monoamine-oxidase by introducing histamine in place of tyramine. The results are controlled by the addition to the incubating bath of amino-guanidine which is a specific inhibitor of the enzyme under test; the results are only satisfactory after the incubation of small pieces of tissue for one hour in the substrate which had been previously warmed to 37°C.

D. — ANAEROBIC DEHYDROGENASES

Enzymes of this group catalyse the transfer of hydrogen from a specific donor to an acceptor which is necessarily distinct from molecular oxygen. Their histochemical demonstration thus requires the presence in the incubating medium of a specific substrate and of adjuvants intended to keep the pH at the required level and also of the acceptor whose transformation indicates that the reaction is positive. It follows that the acceptor must fulfil two conditions other than the requirements of a suitable oxidation-reduction potential, namely that of changing its colour and that of being insoluble when it passes into the reduced conditions.

The development of compounds capable of satisfying these requirements is the essential element in modern progress in the histochemical study of dehydrogenases, progress whose extent has been emphasized many times (see in particular Pearse, 1958, 1960; Burstone, 1962; Lillie, 1965). Methylene blue, the classical hydrogen acceptor of biochemical research, was put forward by Semenoff (1935), the author of the first technique for demonstrating dehydrogenases but its disadvantages are such that this course has not been followed. The tetrazolium salts, whose essential characters have already been mentioned in relation to the histochemical detection of reducing compounds (p. 329), are far more suitable and represent the hydrogen acceptors in all modern techniques aiming at the demonstration of dehydrogenases. It is appropriate to recall, as did Lison (1960), that methylene blue may serve as an intermediary between the hydrogen donor and the tetrazolium salt; a technique developed by Farber and Louvière (1956) for the demonstration of succino-dehydrogenase is based on a reaction of this type.

The theoretical bases of the histo-enzymology of dehydrogenases are set out in masterly fashion by Pearse (1960) and a reading of the corresponding chapters of his work is cordially recommended to all those who desire information on this subject. It scarcely seems useful to mention the facts in question again here and this section is voluntarily limited to the essential technical concepts relating to the detection of the succino-dehydrogenase system and those concerning NAD- and NADP-dehydrogenase-diaphorases. The Δ^5-3-β-hydroxy-steroido-dehydrogenase is discussed elsewhere.

THE SUCCINO-DEHYDROGENASE SYSTEM

The hydrogen donor upon which this very widespread enzyme acts is succinic acid which is oxidised by the enzyme to fumaric acid. The physiological acceptor is ferrocytochrome C. The succino-dehydrogenase is firmly linked to cytoplasmic particles and there need be no concern about its diffusion in the course of the histochemical detection, so long as these manoeuvres do not entrain gross phenomena such as cytolysis, but any kind of fixation results in a loss of its activity so that *it is absolutely essential to work with sections of fresh tissue* cut free-hand on a cryostat or on a microtome with a chilled blade (see also p. 261).

In addition to Semenoff's technique mentioned above and a method due to Wachstein (1949), modified by Gomori (1952), which depends on the reduction of sodium tellurite, a method abandoned because of its low localising value, all the other techniques of histochemical detection use tetrazolium salts, in particular blue tetrazolium and nitro-blue tetrazolium; the second of these compounds is much more suitable but its cost is very high and many authors recommend that it should be reserved for cases where the enzymatic activity under investigation is weak. Moreover, the technique of Farber and Louvière (1956) is mentioned in addition to the more recent procedures of Nachlas and his colleagues using nitro-BT, and of Pearse (1957) using MTT-cobalt.

The technique of Farber and Louvière:

Frozen section of fresh tissue collected in 0.1 M Sorensen buffer, pH 7.4, chilled to the temperature of melting ice.
Incubate for 10 minutes, at 37°C, in the following medium
    0.5 M solution of sodium succinate .... 0.3 ml
    0.1 M Sörensen buffer, pH 7.4 .... 1 ml
    0.004 M solution of calcium chloride .... 0.3 ml
    0.6 M solution of sodium bicarbonate .... 0.15 ml
    0.1% solution of blue tetrazolium .... 0.7 ml
    0.1% solution of methylene blue .... 0.05 ml
    distilled water .... 0.5 ml
blowing the air out of the receptacle with a current of nitrogen;
Rinse rapidly in distilled water, fix for about 30 minutes in 10% formalin;
Wash in tap water and mount in a medium miscible with water.

A blue precipitate of formazan shows that the reaction is positive. The methylene blue serves as an intermediary in this reaction for the transport of hydrogen the effect of which is to increase considerably the sensitivity of the method; when used without this precaution, tetrazolium blue is only suitable as a hydrogen acceptor in instances where the succino-dehydrogenase activity is very strong.

The technique of Nachlas and co-workers:

Frozen sections from fresh tissue mounted on slides or on coverslips and used immediately after cutting;
Incubate for 5 to 20 minutes, at 37°C and without removing the air from the receptacle, in the medium—

0.1% solution of nitro-BT	10 ml
0.2 M solution of sodium succinate	5 ml
0.2 M Sorensen buffer, pH 7.6	5 ml

Wash in physiological saline;
Fix in 10% formalin for 10 minutes;
Wash and mount in a medium miscible with water or dehydrate in absolute alcohol, clear in a benzenoid hydrocarbon and mount in Canada balsam or in a synthetic resin; the first of these procedures is preferable.

A positive result of the reaction is shown by a blue precipitate of diformazan; the fineness of this precipitate accounts for the localising value of the technique whose sensitivity is much greater than is that of the preceding variation.

Pearse's technique. — This technique differs from the preceding ones in using as a tetrazolium salt the bromide of 3-(4,5-dimethyl-thiazolyl-2)-2,5-diphenyltetrazolium (MTT), the optical qualities of the preparations being increased through the chelation of cobalt so that a black precipitate is formed. Pearse (1960) recommends two ways of preparing the incubating medium, the first being advisable for very precise studies and the second for routine work.

a) Add 0.3 ml of a 0.5 M aqueous solution of cobalt chloride ($CoCl_2$) to 2.5 ml of 0.06 M Sörensen buffer of pH 7.4; add to the filtrate 2.5 ml of MTT solution of a concentration of 1 mg/ml and 3 ml of a sodium succinate solution of a concentration of 0.57 g/ml; adjust the pH to 7 with the solution of trihydroxymethylaminomethane which was used to prepare the tris-hydrochloric acid buffer; make up to 10 ml with distilled water and add 0.75 g of polyvinylpyrrolidone.

b) Add to 2.5 ml of the tris-hydrochloric acid buffer of pH 7.1 to 7.2, 0.3 ml of 0.5 M cobalt chloride, 2.5 ml of the MTT solution of concentration 1 mg/ml, 3 ml of the sodium succinate solution of concentration 0.54 g/10 ml and 1.7 ml of distilled water; stir and dissolve 0.75 g of polyvinylpyrrolidone in the mixture.

Working technique.—Sections of fresh tissue, cut on a cryostat or on a microtome with a chilled blade, and adhering to slides or coverslips.

Incubate for 5 to 30 minutes, at 37°C, covering the sections with one of the two media indicated above;
Rinse rapidly with 1% hydrochloric acid if the incubation has been carried out using a medium containing Sörensen's buffer; with the other media pass directly to the following stage;

Fix for about 12 minutes in calcium-formaldehyde or in 10% formalin;
Mount in a medium miscible with water to which a small quantity of cobalt acetate has been added;
A positive result of the reaction is shown by a black deposit.

THE NAD—DEHYDROGENASES—NAD—DIAPHORASES AND NADP—DEHYDROGENASES—NADP—DIAPHORASES SYSTEM

These systems include dehydrogenases which are not only specific so far as the hydrogen donor is concerned but also in respect of its acceptor, the latter being either diphosphopyridine-nucleotide (coenzyme I, DNP in the old nomenclature, now NAD) or triphosphopyridine-nucleotide (coenzyme II, TNP or NADP). These cofactors become reduced because of the enzymatic reaction (NADH or NADPH).

The ensemble of the substrate and the NAD or NADP dehydrogenase function in a manner closely linked with that of another enzyme system which transfers the hydrogen of the reduced substrate to another acceptor, the second enzyme being designated by the name of diaphorase.

Histochemical studies on enzymes of this group date back about 12 years; following the original work of Farber and his colleagues (1952 to 1956) all authors have used techniques involving tetrazolium salts. We now know that the study of the enzyme systems may bear upon one or other of the two reactions mentioned, that is to say that it is possible to localise either diaphorases or dehydrogenases provided that the diaphorases are associated with these latter enzymes.

The histochemical localisation of dehydrogenases and diaphorases was carried out until recently on sections of fresh tissue cut in a cryostat, incubation directly following section cutting. Recent authors in most cases prefer to submit the sections to a short fixation in acetone (15 minutes at 3°C) this procedure having the advantage of extracting the free lipids and in this way of avoiding certain artefacts without notably altering the enzymatic activity. Fixing in calcium-formaldehyde under the same conditions of temperature and the same duration of fixation may also be practised without destroying the enzymes but the free lipids are obviously preserved. The acetone is removed from the sections by air drying, the formalin by washing in distilled water (see, in particular, Hitzeman, 1962; Lillie, 1965).

Modern techniques for the detection of diaphorases

These techniques depend on two different principles. Some authors practise incubation in a medium the substrate of which is represented by the reduced form of the coenzymes (NADH, NADPH); this is the reaction adopted by

Scarpelli, Hess and Pearse (1958) which uses MTT as a tetrazolium salt and also practises chelation with cobalt. Other authors incubate the sections in a medium containing one of the cofactors in the oxidised condition as well as a commercial preparation of the specific dehydrogenase, the true substrate of the reaction catalysed by the diaphorase being "manufactured" during the incubation; this second principle has been adopted by Farber et al. (1956), and by Nachlas et al. (1958).

The technique of Scarpelli, Hess and Pearse. — The **solvent** needed to prepare the incubating bath is prepared in the following way—

> mix 2.5 ml of 0.06 M Sörensen buffer, pH 8.2, with 0.3 ml of a 0.5 M solution of cobalt chloride; stir and filter; add to the filtrate 2.5 ml of MTT solution of concentration 1 mg/ml, 4.1 ml of distilled water, and dissolve in it 75 mg of polyvinylpyrrolidone adjusting the pH to 7.2 with 0.2 M tris buffer, using a glass electrode pH meter to regulate the process. Store the bath at 0–4°C; the mixture will keep for about a month.

Working technique.

> Frozen sections of fresh tissue, adherent to cover-slips, the tissue may or may not have received a short fixation as described above;
> Incubate at 37°C, for 5 to 30 minutes, in the medium prepared in the following way:
> solvent .... 1 ml
> NADH or NADPH .... 1 mg
> stir until dissolved, adjust the pH to 7.2 with one or two drops of tris-hydrochloric acid buffer, pH 8.5; this medium will only keep for about 90 minutes;
> Rinse rapidly in 1% hydrochloric acid;
> Fix in calcium-formaldehyde for 5 to 30 minutes;
> Where appropriate, carry out a very light nuclear stain (a diluted solution of methyl green or of Mayer's carmalum diluted with 9 volumes of water);
> Mount in a medium miscible with water.

A positive result of the reaction which discloses the presence of NAD- or NADP-diaphorase, according to the substrate utilised, is shown by a black deposit of formazan-cobalt.

The technique of Nachlas and co-workers. — The composition of the medium differs according to whether we are testing for NAD- or NADP-diaphorase, the working technique being the same in the two cases.

> *a)* Incubating medium for detecting NAD-diaphorase.
> 0.5 M solution of sodium lactate .... 0.6 ml
> 1.5% solution of lactic dehydrogenase .... 0.2 ml
> NAD solution of concentration 5 mg/ml .... 0.3 ml
> solution of nitro-BT of concentration 5 mg/ml .... 0.3 ml
> 0.2 M Sörensen buffer, pH 7.4 .... 1.0 ml
> distilled water .... 0.6 ml

The solutions of NAD and of dehydrogenase are prepared in distilled water without adjustment of the pH; they are preserved at —20°C; the solutions of sodium lactate and nitro-BT are adjusted to pH 7.4 and preserved at 4-6°C.

b) Incubating medium for detecting NADP-diaphorase.

1.1 M solution of sodium isocitrate (racemic)	0.6 ml
2.5 M solution of sodium L-malate	0.5 ml
0.005 M solution of manganese chloride	0.3 ml
NADP solution of concentration 5 mg/ml	0.2 ml
nitro-BT solution of concentration 5 mg/ml	0.3 ml
0.05 M veronal-acetate buffer, pH 7.4	1.1 ml

The NADP solution, made up without adjusting its pH, is preserved at —20°C; the other solutions should have their pH adjusted to 7.4 and are preserved at 4-6°C.

Working technique.

Sections of fresh tissue which may or may not have been fixed for a short time as described above;
Incubate at laboratory temperatures for 5 to 30 minutes in the medium chosen in the light of the enzyme which is to be detected;
Rinse rapidly in physiological saline;
Fix in saline formalin for about 12 minutes;
Mount in a medium miscible with water;
A positive result of the reaction is shown by a blue precipitate of diformazan.

Modern techniques for the detection of NAD- and NADP-dehydrogenase

These techniques involve reactions which use either MTT or nitro-BT as a tetrazolium salt. The substrate and the cofactor obviously vary in the light of the enzyme sought, one or other of the two tetrazolium salts being particularly recommended according to the circumstances; Table 23, taken from Pearse (1960) sets out this choice.

Table 23. — TETRAZOLIUM SALTS USED IN THE DETECTION OF SPECIFIC DEHYDROGENASES
(after PEARSE, 1960, complete with indication of cofactors)

MTT	*Nitro-BT*
Glucose-6-phosphate-dehydrogenase (NAD) 6-phosphogluconate-dehydrogenase (NADP) β-hydroxybutyrate-dehydrogenase (NADP)	alcohol-dehydrogenase (NAD) lactate-dehydrogenase (NAD) isocitrate-dehydrogenase (NAD or NADP) glutamate-dehydrogenase (NAD or NADP) α-glycerophosphate-dehydrogenase (NAD) malate-dehydrogenase (NAD or NADP)

Table 24, due to Lillie (1965), indicates the composition of the incubating media as they were proposed by Pearse (1960), or by Hitzeman (1963) as well as suggesting a standard substrate (Lillie, 1964).

Table 24. — FORMULAS OF SUBSTRATES FOR DEHYDROGENASE RESEARCH
(after LILLIE, 1964, simplified)

	PEARSE, 1960	HITZEMAN, 1963	LILLIE, 1964
Specific substrate	3 ml M	15 ml 0.1M	15 ml 0.1M
Cofactor	3 ml 0.1M	0.2ml 0.1M	0.3ml 0.1M
Cyanide or amytal	3 ml 0.1M	1.5ml 0.1M	
Sörensen buffer pH 6.8 —7	—	13.5ml 60M	9 ml 0.1M
Tris-HCl buffer pH 7	7.5ml 0.1M	—	
Nitro-BT		2.5mg	5 mg
MTT	0.25 mg		
Cobalt chloride	1.5ml 0.5M		
Polyvinylpyrrolidone	2.25 mg		
Distilled water to make up to	30 ml	30 ml	30 ml

We need hardly add that the preparation of 30 ml lots of a costly material which keeps badly is only to be recommended for mass production work; simple division provides the composition of smaller amounts. I might mention, whilst we are on the subject, the widespread practice of preparing the incubating medium in amounts of 1 or 2 ml and of conducting the incubations by simply covering the sections when the slides are placed horizontally.

Table 25. — MOLECULAR WEIGHTS OF SUBSTRATES AND COFACTORS USED IN DEHYDROGENASE RESEARCH
(after LILLIE, 1965. simplified)

Substrate	Salt		Acid
	Cation	Mol. wt.	Mol. wt.
Ethanol	—	46.07	—
Glucose-6-phosphate	K_2	336.32	—
Glutamate	Na	187.14	147.13
α-glycerophosphate	Na	216.05	—
β-hydroxybutyrate	Na	126.09	104.10
Isocitrate	Na_3	276.08	192.12
Lactate	Na	112.06	90.08
L-malate	Na_2	187.07	134.09
Pyruvate	Na	110.05	88.06
6-phosphogluconate	Ba	409.47	—
Succinate	Na_2	270.16	118.01
NAD	—	663.4	
NADH	Na_2	763	
NADP	Na	801	
NADPH	Na	834	

Table 25 which is also due to Lillie indicates the molecular weights of the principal compounds used in these reactions.

Working technique:

Frozen sections taken from fresh tissue adherent to slides or to coverslips which may or may not have undergone fixation of short duration in acetone as noted above;
Incubate for 5 to 30 minutes, at 37°, in the substrate made up according to the directions of Table 24;
Rinse very rapidly in 1% hydrochloric acid in cases where the incubation has been conducted in a medium containing cobalt chloride;
Fix for 10 minutes in calcium formaldehyde;
Mount in a medium miscible with water.

The deposit which indicates a positive reaction is black when MTT is used and purple when nitro-BT is employed; with this latter method certain structures take on a red tint, devoid of significance, which may be greatly weakened by washing in 15% alcohol prior to mounting. Pearse (1960) emphasizes the intramitochondrial localisation of deposits indicative of the presence of dehydrogenases.

We may mention, in connection with tests for dehydrogenases linked to NAD or to NADP, one of Zimmermann and Pearse's (1959) findings, namely the reduction of tetrazolium salts which is particularly clear at pH values above 8 and which occurs in the absence of the substrate but is suppressed when the cofactor is not added to the medium. This effect ("the nothing-dehydrogenase" of Racker, 1955) is due to a non-enzymatic reduction of the cofactors associated with sulphydrylated compounds present in the tissues.

Δ^5-3-β-HYDROXYSTEROIDODEHYDROGENASE

The cofactor for this dehydrogenase is diphosphopyridine-nucleotide (NAD) whose physiological interest is widely illustrated by recent work. In fact, it intervenes, not only in the respiratory metabolism of tissues in general, but in steroidogenesis by oxidising the 5-hydroxy groups of pregnenolone or of dehydroepiandrosterone to carbonyl groups. This enzymatic reaction can be coupled with NAD-diaphorase, the result being the reduction of the tetrazolium salt to formazan. This is the principle of Wattenberg's (1958) method; most recent authors prefer the working technique recommended by Levy, Deane and Rubin (1959).

The method is carried out on frozen sections taken from fresh tissue; the sections may undergo a fixation of short duration in cold calcium formaldehyde; experience shows (Arvy, 1962) that frozen sections cut after fixation for a few hours in 10% formalin which has been chilled to 4°C may be used.

Working technique:

Frozen sections obtained under the experimental conditions defined above, free or adherent to slides;
Wash in modified Krebs solution (for about 10 minutes)

0.21 M solution of sodium chloride	1000 ml
0.21 M solution of potassium chloride	40 ml
0.21 M solution of magnesium chloride	10 ml
0.12 M Sörensen buffer, pH 8	360 ml

Incubate for 20 to 30 minutes, at 37°C, in the medium:—

dehydroepiandrosterone	4 mg
propylene glycol	10 ml
solution of nitro-BT of concentration 1 mg/ml	20 ml
solution of nicotinamide of concentration 1.6 mg/ml	14 ml
solution of NAD of concentration 3 mg/ml	16 ml
0.05 M Sörensen buffer, pH 7.4	80 ml

Wash in Krebs solution; where appropriate, fix in 10% formalin for 10 minutes;
Mount in a medium miscible with water;
A blue deposit of diformazan shows that the reaction is positive.

APPENDIX

Among the tables included in this appendix, only the last one is partially the result of my personal experience. The others cannot claim the least originality and their source is explicitly indicated.

1° Table of atomic weights (after TIAN and ROCHE, 1956)

Names of the elements	Symbol	Atomic weights	Names of the elements	Symbol	Atomic weights
Actinium	Ac	227	Molybdenum	Mo	96.0
Aluminium	Al	26.97	Neodymium	Nd	144.27
Antimony	Sb	121.77	Neon	Ne	20.2
Argon	A	39.94	Nickel	Ni	58.69
Arsenic	As	74.96	Niobium	Nb	93.3
Barium	Ba	137.37	Nitrogen	N	14.008
Beryllium	Be	9.2	Osmium	Os	190.8
Bismuth	Bi	209.00	Oxygen	O	16.00
Bromine	Br	79.916	Palladium	Pd	106.7
Boron	B	10.82	Phosphorus	P	31.027
Cadmium	Cd	112.41	Platinum	Pt	195.23
Caesium	Cs	132.81	Polonium	Po	210.0
Calcium	Ca	40.07	Potassium	K	39.096
Carbon	C	12.000	Praseodymium	Pr	140.92
Cerium	Ce	140.13	Radium	Ra	225.95
Chlorine	Cl	35.457	Radon	Rn	222.0
Chromium	Cr	52.01	Rhodium	Rh	102.91
Cobalt	Co	58.94	Rubidium	Rb	85.44
Copper	Cu	63.57	Ruthenium	Ru	101.7
Dysprosium	Dy	162.46	Samarium	Sm	150.43
Erbium	Er	167.7	Scandium	Sc	45.10
Europium	Eu	152.0	Selenium	Se	79.2
Fluorine	F	19.00	Silicon	Si	28.06
Gadolinium	Gd	157.26	Silver	Ag	107.88
Gallium	Ga	69.72	Sodium	Na	22.997
Germanium	Ge	72.60	Strontium	Sr	87.63
Gold	Au	197.2	Sulphur	S	32.064
Hafnium	Hf	178.6	Tantalum	Ta	181.4
Helium	He	4.00	Tellurium	Te	127.5
Holmium	Ho	163.4	Terbium	Tb	159.2
Hydrogen	H	1.008	Thallium	Tl	204.39
Indium	In	114.8	Thorium	Th	232.15
Iodine	I	126.932	Thulium	Tu	169.4
Iridium	Ir	193.1	Tin	Sn	118.70
Iron	Fe	55.84	Tungsten	W	184.0
Krypton	Kr	83.7	Uranium	Ur	238.14
Lanthanum	La	138.90	Uranium X2	UrX_2	234
Lead	Pb	207.20	Vanadium	V	50.96
Lithium	Li	6.94	Xenon	X	130.2
Lutecium	Lu	175.0	Ytterbium	Yb	173.6
Magnesium	Mg	24.32	Yttrium	Y	88.99
Manganese	Mn	54.93	Zinc	Zn	65.38
Mercury	Hg	200.61	Zirconium	Zr	91.2

2° Formulae and molecular weights of the principal chemicals used in the preparation of the buffer solutions indicated below

(after LILLIE, 1965).

Compound	Formula	Molecular weight
Acetic acid	CH_3COOH	60.05
Ammonia	NH_3	17.032
Boric acid	$B(OH)_3$	61.84
Citric acid, anhydrous	$C_3H_4OH(COOH)_3$	192.12
Citric acid, crystalline	$C_3H_4OH(COOH)_3, H_2O$	210.14
Disodium phosphate	Na_2PHO_4	141.98
Ferric chloride, anhydrous	$FeCl_3$	162.22
Ferric chloride, crystalline	$FeCl_3, 6H_2O$	270.32
Formic acid	$HCOOH$	46.03
Glycine (glycocoll)	H_2NCH_2COOH	75.07
Hydrochloric acid	HCl	36.465
Maleic acid	$HOOCCH=CHCOOH$	116.07
Monopotassium phosphate	KH_2PO_4	212.275
Monosodium phosphate	NaH_2PO_4, H_2O	138.01
Nitric acid	HNO_3	63.016
Oxalic acid	$(COOH)_2$	90.038
Potassium chloride	KCl	74.553
Potassium hydroxide	KOH	56.104
Sodium acetate, anhydrous	CH_3COONa	82.04
Sodium acetate, crystalline	$CH_3COONa, 3H_2O$	136.09
Sodium barbitone (veronal)	$C_8H_{11}O_3N_2Na$	206.18
Sodium borate (borax)	$Na_2B_4O_7, 10\ H_2O$	381.43
Sodium chloride	$NaCl$	58.448
Sodium citrate, crystalline	$C_3H_4OH(COONa)_3, 5H_2O$	357.17
Sodium citrate, granular	$C_3H_4OH(COONa)_3, 2H_2O$	294.12
Sodium hydroxide	$NaOH$	40.005
Sodium oxalate	$Na_2C_2O_4$	134.004
Sulphuric acid	H_2SO_4	98.082
Trihydroxymethylaminomethane (tris)	$H_2NC(CH_2OH_3)$	121.14
Tripotassium phosphate	K_3PO_4	212.275

3° Preparation of normal solutions of hydrochloric acid, nitric acid, and sulphuric acid from commercial concentrated acids

(after LILLIE, 1965)

The demands of histological work are less rigorous than those of chemical analysis; it is sufficient therefore to put, in a 1000 ml volumetric flask, the quantity of concentrated acid indicated in the last column of the table and make up to 1,000 ml. further adjustment by means of the classical acidimetric titration is not needed in the case of quantitative work.

HYDROCHLORIC ACID

Density	% HCl (weight)	HCl (g/l)	Normality	ml for 1 l, 1 N
1.178 9	36	424.4	11.64	86
1.183 7	37	438.0	12.01	83.3
1.188 5	38	451.6	12.38	80.8
1.193 2	39	465.4	12.75	78.4
1.198 0	40	479.2	13.14	76.2

NITRIC ACID

Density	% HNO_3 (weight)	HNO_3 (g/l)	Normality	ml for 1 l, 1 N
1.404 8	68	955.3	15.16	66.0
1.409 1	69	972.3	15.43	64.9
1.413 4	70	989.4	15.70	63.8
1.417 6	71	1 006.0	15.96	62.6
1.421 8	72	1 024.0	16.25	61.6

SULPHURIC ACID

Density	% H_2SO_4 (weight)	H_2SO_4 (g/l)	Normality	ml for 1 l, 1 N
1.833 7	95	1 742	35.31	28.2
1.835 5	96	1 762	35.93	27 86
1.836 4	97	1 781	36.31	27,6
1.846 1	98	1 799	36.68	27.3

4° *Buffers*

As in the case of the dilution of mineral acids (preceding table), the demands of histology in the preparation of buffer solutions are less rigorous than they are in chemical research. Verification with a pH meter is only rarely required, and boiled distilled water is sufficient for the preparation of the solutions. The reagents ought to be pure, certified for analysis by the supplier; it is desirable to use the samples specially prepared for making buffers in all cases where the choice is available. It goes without saying that the indications concerning the molecular weight and the degree of hydration of the chemicals, as shown on the label, must also be taken into consideration. It appears to me useless to dwell on the subject of general precautions (choice of balance, graduated glassware, etc...) which are self-evident.

It is, on the contrary, reasonable to recall that many buffers require a "stabilisation time" before taking up the specific pH for their formula and their keeping qualities are often mediocre. The addition of several drops of chloroform prevents the development of moulds without introducing a cause of appreciable error on the scale of the histologist's work.

a) **Hydrochloric acid — monosodium phosphate** (after Lillie, 1965). — Prepare the N and 0.1 N solution of hydrochloric acid, M and 0.1 M solution of monopotassium phosphate. The table indicates the quantities to mix to obtain a buffer of the desired pH.

HCl ml	KH_2PO_4 ml	pH		HCl ml	KH_2PO_4 ml	pH	
		1 M	0.1 M			1 M	0.1 M
30	20	0.69	1.53	15	35	1.92	2.27
29	21	0.75	1.56	14	36	2.02	2.31
28	22	0.81	1.63	13	37	2.11	2.38
27	23	0.90	1.66	12	38	2.20	2.44
26	24	0.98	1.71	11	39	2.29	2.50
25	25	1.05	1.77	10	40	2.38	2.56
24	26	1.12	1.80	9	41	2.45	2.63
23	27	1.23	1.84	8	42	2.52	2.70
22	28	1.35	1.89	7	43	2.62	2.79
21	29	1.43	1.94	6	44	2.72	2.89
20	30	1.52	2.00	5	45	2.85	3.02
19	31	1.61	2.05	4	46	3.00	3.14
18	32	1.70	2.10	3	47	3.17	3.23
17	33	1.76	2.15	2	48	3.32	3.44
16	34	1.83	2.23				

b) **Hydrochloric acid — sodium citrate buffer** (after Lillie, 1965). — The solutions are prepared taking into consideration the degree of hydration of the sodium citrate and the density of the hydrochloric acid; the quantities of the solutions to mix to obtain the desired pH and the molarity of the solutions are shown in the table.

HCl ml	Na citrate ml	pH 1M	pH 0.1M	pH 0.01M	HCl ml	Na citrate ml	pH 1M	pH 0.1M	pH 0.01M
50	0	0,25	1.11	2.10	24	26	4.78	5.20	5.52
49	1	0.27	1.14	2.15	23	27	4.85	5.28	5.61
48	2	0.30	1.19	2.20	22	28	4.92	5.35	5.70
47	3	0.35	1.24	2.25	21	29	5.00	5.41	5.79
46	4	0.40	1.29	2.30	20	30	5.05	5.48	5.87
45	5	0.45	1.34	2.35	19	31	5.10	5.54	5.93
44	6	0.51	1.38	2.40	18	32	5.17	5.60	5.97
43	7	0.58	1.42	2.45	17	33	5.22	5.65	6.01
42	8	0.67	1.50	2.50	16	34	5.28	5.70	6.06
41	9	0.80	1.65	2.60	15	35	5.33	5.75	6.10
40	10	0.97	1.85	2.70	14	36	5.37	5.79	6.14
39	11	1.30	2.12	2.85	13	37	5.42	5.83	6.19
38	12	2.00	2.52	3.02	12	38	5.49	5.87	6.25
37	13	2.60	2.90	3.24	11	39	5.56	5.93	6.31
36	14	2.95	3.24	3.50	10	40	5.63	6.00	6.36
35	15	3.25	3.58	3.80	9	41	5.70	6.06	6.42
34	16	3.50	3.82	4.03	8	42	5.79	6.14	6.50
33	17	3.67	4.00	4.22	7	43	5.88	6.21	6.60
32	18	3.84	4.18	4.40	6	44	5.97	6.30	6.69
31	19	4.01	4.36	4.60	5	45	6.06	6.39	6.78
30	20	4.18	4.52	4.75	4	46	6.16	6.48	6.88
29	21	4.30	4.67	4.91	3	47	6.27	6.57	6.98
28	22	4.40	4.79	5.05	2	48	6.42	6.73	7.11
27	23	4.50	4.90	5.20	1	49	6.66	6.97	7.25
26	24	4.59	5.00	5.31	0	50	7.17	7.51	7.82
25	25	4.69	5.10	5.42					

c) **Laskey's N maleic acid −0.1 N sodium hydroxide buffer** (after Lillie, 1965). — The two reagents are mixed according to the table, *the total volume, in all cases, being made up to 50 ml by the addition of distilled water.*

Maleic acid N, ml	Sodium hydroxide 0.1 N, ml	Distilled water ml	pH	Maleic acid N, ml	Sodium hydroxide 0.1N, ml	Distilled water ml	pH
5	6	39	1.83	5	26	19	2.70
5	7	38	1.87	5	27	18	2.75
5	8	37	1.89	5	28	17	3.05
5	9	36	1.90	5	29	16	3.31
5	10	35	1.94	5	30	15	3.62
5	11	34	1.98	5	31	14	4.40
5	12	33	2.00	5	32	13	4.71
5	13	32	2.02	5	33	12	4.91
5	14	31	2.08	5	34	11	5.00
5	15	30	2.10	5	35	10	5.15
5	16	29	2.15	5	36	9	5.27
5	17	28	2.20	5	37	8	5.34
5	18	27	2.22	5	38	7	5.45
5	19	26	2.28	5	39	6	5.50
5	20	25	2.30	5	40	5	5.59
5	21	24	2.38	5	41	4	5.62
5	22	23	2.42	5	42	3	5.68
5	23	22	2.49	5	43	2	5.73
5	24	21	2.55	5	44	1	5.75
5	25	20	2.62	5	45	0	5.83

d) **Walpole's hydrochloric acid—sodium acetate buffer, modified by Pearse (1960) and Lillie (1965).** — 1 N hydrochloric acid and 1 M sodium acetate are mixed according to the table, the total volume being brought up to 50 ml with distilled water or *other reagents*; it is essential to heed this condition.

HCl 1 N ml	Acetate 1 M ml	H_2O ml	pH	HCl 1 N ml	Acetate 1 M ml	H_2O ml	pH
20	10	20	0.65	9.7	10	30.3	3.09
18	10	22	0.75	9.5	10	30.5	3.29
16	10	24	0.91	9.25	10	30.75	3.49
14	10	26	1.07	9.0	10	31	3.61
13	10	27	1.24	8.5	10	31.5	3.79
12	10	28	1.42	8	10	32	3.95
11	10	29	1.71	7	10	33	4.19
10.7	10	29.3	1.85	6	10	34	4.39
10.5	10	29.5	1.99	5	10	35	4.58
10.2	10	29.8	2.32	4	10	36	4.76
10.0	10	30	2.64	3	10	37	4.92
9.95	10	30.05	2.72	2	10	38	5.20

e) **Walpole's acetic acid — sodium acetate buffer** (after Lillie, 1965). — For the required molarity, the two solutions are mixed according to the table.

Acetic acid ml	Sodium acetate ml	0.2 M pH	0.01 M pH	Acetic acid ml	Sodium acetate ml	0.2 M pH	0.01 M pH
20.0	0.0	2.696	3.373	13.0	7.0	4.360	4.473
19.9	0.1	2.804	3.420	12.0	8.0	4.454	4.527
19.8	0.2	2.913	3.477	11.0	9.0	4.530	4.600
19.7	0.3	2.994	3.503	10.0	10.0	4.626	4.717
19.6	0.4	3.081	3.523	9.0	11.0	4.710	4.807
19.5	0.5	3.147	3.543	8.0	12.0	4.802	4.910
19.4	0.6	3.202	3.590	7.0	13.0	4.900	5.000
19.2	0.8	3.315	3.593	6.0	14.0	4.990	5.077
19.0	1.0	3.416	3.647	5.0	15.0	5.110	5.183
18.5	1.5	3.592	3.737	4.0	16.0	5.227	5.373
18.0	2.0	3.723	3.863	3.0	17.0	5.380	5.500
17.0	3.0	3.900	3.980	2.0	18.0	5.574	5.713
16.0	4.0	4.047	4.110	1.0	19.0	5.894	6.003
15.0	5.0	4.160	4.223	0.5	19.5	6.211	6.227
14.0	6.0	4.270	4.337	0.0	20.0	6.518	6.777

f) McIlvaine's citric acid—dibasic sodium phosphate buffer, modified by Lillie (1965). — This buffer, specially designed to maintain the pH of various stains, is prepared from stock solutions (0.1 M for the citric acid, 0.2 M for the dibasic sodium phosphate) dissolving each in 750 ml of distilled water and then mahing up to 1000 ml with methyl alcohol. To obtain the desired pH, 20 ml of the mixtures indicated in the table are brought up to 50 ml with distilled water or with the stain one wants to buffer. Because of the addition of methyl alcohol, the solutions keep well.

pH	Citric acid ml	Dibasic sodium phosphate ml	pH	Citric acid ml	Dibasic sodium phosphate ml
2.5	20.0	0	5.3	9.5	10.5
2.6	19.5	0.5	5.5	9.0	11.0
2.65	19.0	1.0	5.7	8.5	11.5
2.7	18.5	1.5	6.0	8.0	12.0
2.75	18.0	2.0	6.1	7.5	12.5
2.8	17.5	2.5	6.3	7.0	13.0
2,9	17.0	3.0	6.4	6.5	13.5
3.0	16.5	3.5	6.5	6.0	14.0
3.05	16.0	4.0	6.6	5.5	14.5
3.1	15.5	4.5	6.8	5.0	15.0
3.2	15.0	5.0	6.9	4.5	15.5
3.3	14.5	5.5	7.0	4.0	16.0
3.45	14.0	6.0	7.1	3.5	16.5
3.6	13.5	6.5	7.2	3.0	17.0
3.75	13.0	7.0	7.3	2.5	17.5
3.95	12.5	7.5	7.4	2.0	18.0
4.1	12.0	8.0	7.5	1.5	18.5
4.3	11.5	8.5	7.7	1.0	19.0
4.5	11.0	9.0	8.0	0.5	19.5
4.75	10.5	9.5	8.3	0	20.0
4.95	10.0	10.0			

g) Sörensen's phosphate buffers. — Solutions of monobasic potassium (or sodium) phosphate and dibasic sodium phosphate, prepared to the desired molarity, are mixed according to the table. It is as well to point out that the dibasic sodium phosphate is particularly prone to the development of microorganisms (keep in the cold, add a small quantity of chloroform).

KH_2PO_4Na H_2PO_4 H_2O ml	Na_2H PO_4 ml	pH			KH_2PO_4Na H_2PO_4 H_2O ml	Na_2H PO_4 ml	pH		
		0.1 M	0,067 M	5 mM			0.1 M	0,067 M	5 mM
50	0	4.41	4.47	4.77	24	26	6.81	6.86	7.09
48	2	5.31	5.42	5.63	23	27	6.84	6.91	7.13
47	3	5.53	5.60	5.81	22	28	6.87	6.94	7.16
46	4	5.67	5.74	5.95	21	29	6.89	6.96	7.18
45	5	5.78	5.83	6.06	20	30	6.91	6.98	7.20
44	6	5.86	5.91	6.14	19	31	6.94	7.01	7.22
43	7	5.94	5.99	6.22	18	32	6.97	7.03	7.25
42	8	6.02	6.07	6.30	17	33	7.00	7.05	7.28
41	9	6.08	6.14	6.36	16	34	7.02	7.07	7.31
40	10	6.12	6.19	6.42	15	35	7.06	7.11	7.34
39	11	6.17	6.24	6.47	14	36	7.10	7.15	7.38
38	12	6.23	6.28	6.51	13	37	7.14	7.20	7.41
37	13	6.28	6.32	6.56	12	38	7.19	7.24	7.45
36	14	6.33	6.37	6.61	11	39	7.24	7.28	7.51
35	15	6.37	6.41	6.65	10	40	7.30	7.33	7.59
34	16	6.41	6.45	6.68	9	41	7.36	7.40	7.65
33	17	6.45	6.49	6.72	8	42	7.42	7.47	7.70
32	18	6.49	6.53	6.75	7	43	7.49	7.54	7.75
31	19	6.53	6.56	6.79	6	44	7.57	7.61	7.80
30	20	6.55	6.59	6.82	5	45	7.65	7.69	7.87
29	21	6.58	6.63	6.86	4	46	7.73	7.77	7.96
28	22	6.61	6.68	6.91	3	47	7.81	7.85	8.05
27	23	6.65	6.72	6.95	2	48	7.92	7.97	8.15
26	24	6.70	6.76	7.00	0	50	8.98	8.93	8.73
25	25	6.76	6.81	7.05					

h) Glycine—hydrochloric acid buffer (after Burstone, 1962). — 0.2 M solutions of glycine and hydrochloric acid are prepared; 50 ml of the glycine solution plus x ml of hydrochloric acid are diluted to 200 ml to obtain the pH buffer indicated in the table.

pH	x	pH	x
3.6	5.0	2,8	16.8
3.4	6.4	2.6	24.2
3.2	8.2	2.4	32.4
3.0	11.4	2.2	44.0

i) Glycine—sodium hydroxide buffer (after Burstone, 1962). — 0.2 M solutions of glycine and sodium hydroxide are prepared; 50 ml of the glycine solution plus x ml of sodium hydroxide are diluted to 200 ml to obtain the pH buffer indicated in the table.

pH	x	pH	x
8.6	4.0	9.6	22.4
8.8	6.0	9.8	27.2
9.0	8.8	10.0	32.0
9.2	12.0	10.4	38.6
9.4	16.8	10.6	45.5

j) Oxalic acid—sodium oxalate buffer (after Lillie, 1965). — The 0.1 M solutions of oxalic acid and sodium oxalate are mixed as shown in the table.

Oxalic acid 0.1 M ml	Sodium oxalate 0.1 M ml	pH	Oxalic acid 0.1 M ml	Sodium oxalate 0.1 M ml	pH
25	0	1.34			
24	1	1.40	9	16	3.51
23	2	1.45	8	17	3.61
22	3	1.50	7	18	3.73
21	4	1.55	6	19	3.92
20	5	1.65	5	20	4.05
19	6	1.71	4	21	4.18
18	7	1.80	3	22	4.37
17	8	1.89	2	23	4.58
16	9	1.99	1	24	4.95
15	10	2.12	0	25	7.02
14	11	2.36			
13	12	2.59			
12	13	2.88			
11	14	3.22			
10	15	3.35			

k) Holmes' borax - boric acid buffer (after Lillie, 1965). — This buffer is particularly recommended to maintain the pH of reagents containing silver salts. The quantities of 0.05 M sodium borate (19 g/litre) and 0.2 M boric acid (12.4 g/litre) to be mixed are shown in the table.

pH	H_3BO_2 0.2 M ml	$Na_2B_4O_7$ $10 H_2O$ 0.05 M ml
7.4	18	2
7.6	17	3
7.8	16	4
8.0	14	6
8.2	13	7
8.4	11	9
8.7	8	12
9.0	4	16

*l) **Sodium oxalate - ferric chloride** (after Lillie, 1965). — 0.1 M solutions of the two salts are mixed according to the table.

Sodium oxalate 0.1 M ml	Ferric chloride 0.1 M ml	pH	Sodium oxalate 0.1 M ml	Ferric chloride 0.1 M ml	pH
25	0	7.0			
24	1	4.92	9	16	1.48
23	2	4.6	8	17	1.44
22	3	4.27	7	18	1.40
21	4	3.7	6	19	1.38
20	5	2.3	5	20	1.36
19	6	1.9	4	21	1.33
18	7	1.88	3	22	1.32
17	8	1.80	2	23	1.30
16	9	1.75	1	24	1.28
15	10	1.70	0	25	1.24
14	11	1.60			
13	12	1.59			
12	13	1.55			
11	14	1.51			
10	15	1.49			

*m) **Michaelis' hydrochloric acid - sodium veronal buffer** (after Lillie, 1965). — The quantities of 0.1 N hydrochloric acid and 0.1 M sodium veronal to mix to make up 40 ml of buffer of the desired pH are shown in the table.

pH	HCl 0.1 N ml	Sodium veronal 0.1 M ml	pH	HCl 0.1 N ml	Sodium veronal 0.1 M ml
6.4	19.6	20.4	8.1	10.3	29.7
6.5	19.5	20.5	8.2	9.2	30.8
6.6	19.4	20.6	8.3	8.2	31.8
6.7	19.3	20.7	8.4	7.1	32.9
6.8	19.1	20.9	8.5	6.1	33.9
6.9	18.8	21.2	8.6	5.2	34.8
7.0	18.6	21.4	8.7	4.4	35.6
7.1	18.2	21.8	8.8	3.7	36.3
7.2	17.8	22.2	8.9	3.1	36.9
7.3	17.3	22.7	9.0	2.6	37.4
7.4	16.8	23.2	9.1	2.2	37.8
7.5	16.1	23.9	9.2	1.9	38.1
7.6	15.4	24.6	9.3	1.5	38.5
7.7	14.5	25.5	9.4	1.0	39.0
7.8	13.5	26.5	9.5	0.8	39.2
7.9	12.4	27.6	9.6	0.6	39.4
8.0	11.4	28.6	9.7	0.4	39.6

n) Gomori's tris-maleate buffer (1948). — Molar solutions of maleic acid (116.07 g/l), trihydroxymethylaminomethane (121.14 g/l) and 0.5 N sodium hydroxide (20 g/l) are mixed in the proportions shown in the table, the volume being made up to 50 ml with distilled water.

Maleic acid M ml	Tris M ml	Sodium hydroxide 0.5 M ml	Distilled water ml	pH
5	5	1	39	5.08
5	5	2	38	5.30
5	5	3	37	5.52
5	5	4	36	5.70
5	5	5	35	5.88
5	5	6	34	6.05
5	5	7	33	6.27
5	5	8	32	6.50
5	5	9	31	6.86
5	5	10	30	7.20
5	5	11	29	7.50
5	5	12	28	7.75
5	5	13	27	7.97
5	5	14	26	8.15
5	5	15	25	8.30
5	5	16	24	8.45

o) Gomori's tris-hydrochloric acid buffer (after Lillie, 1965). — One mixes, according to the table, 0.2 M solution of tris, 0.1 N hydrochloric acid and distilled water; the quantities are calculated for a total volume of 50 ml.

pH	Tris 0.2 M ml	HCl 0.1 N ml	Distilled water ml	pH	Tris 0.2 M ml	HCl 0.1 N ml	Distilled water ml
7.19	10	18	12	8.23	10	9	21
7.36	10	17	13	8.32	10	8	22
7.54	10	16	14	8.41	10	7	23
7.66	10	15	15	8.51	10	6	24
7.77	10	14	16	8.62	10	5	25
7.87	10	13	17	8.74	10	4	26
7.96	10	12	18	8.92	10	3	27
8.05	10	11	19	9.10	10	2	28
8.14	10	10	20				

p) Michaelis' universal sodium veronal-sodium acetate buffer (1931). — The main interest of this buffer is the invariability of the strength of the salts, the absence of ions of a valency greater than 1 and the absence of precipitation of calcium.

The stock solution contains M/7 sodium acetate (9.714 g/500 ml) and M/7 sodium veronal (14.714 g/500 ml). 5 ml of the stock solution are added to n ml of 0.1 N hydrochloric acid and where isotonic solutions are needed 2 ml of 8.5% sodium chloride; the volume is made up in this case to 25 ml with boiled distilled water. The values for 'n' are indicated in the table.

pH	n ml HCl 0.1 N	pH	n ml HCl 0.1 N	pH	n ml HCl 0.1 N
9.16	0.25	7.42	5.0	4.66	10.0
8.90	0.5	7.25	5.5	4.33	11.0
8.68	0.75	6.99	6.0	4.13	12.0
8.55	1	6.75	6.5	3.88	13.0
8.18	2	6.12	7	3.62	13.0
7.90	3	5.32	8	3.20	15.0
7.66	4	4.93	9	2.62	16.0

The intermediate values, between those which appear in the table, may be determined by linear interpolation. The pH of 5 ml of the stock solution, diluted with or without the addition of sodium chloride, but without the addition of the hydrochloric acid, at 25 ml is 9.64, but the buffering capacity of this liquid is obviously weak.

5° Equivalents between the Fahrenheit and centigrade thermometric scales
(after LANGERON, 1949).

F	C	F	C	F	C	F	C
+212	+100	+154	+67.78	+96	+35.55	+38	+3.33
211	99.44	153	67.22	95	35.00	37	2.78
210	98,89	152	66.67	94	34.44	36	2.22
209	98.33	151	66.11	93	33.89	35	1.67
208	97 78	150	65.55	92	33.33	34	1.11
207	97.22	149	65.00	91	32.78	33	0.55
206	96.67	148	64.44	90	32.22	32	0.00
205	96.11	147	63.89	89	31,67	31	—0,55
204	85.55	146	63.33	88	31.11	30	1.11
203	95,00	145	62.78	87	30.55	29	1.67
202	94.44	144	62.22	86	30.00	28	2.22
201	93.89	143	61.67	85	29.44	27	2.78
200	93.33	142	61.11	84	28.89	26	3.33
199	92.78	141	60.55	83	28.33	25	3.89
198	92.22	140	60.00	82	27.78	24	4.44
197	91.67	139	59.44	81	27.22	23	5.00
196	91.11	138	58.89	80	26.67	22	5.55
195	90.55	137	58.33	79	26.11	21	6.11
194	90.00	136	57.78	78	25.55	20	6.67
193	89.44	135	57.22	77	25.00	19	7.22
192	88.89	134	56.67	76	24.44	18	7.78
191	88.33	133	56.11	75	23.89	17	8.33
190	87.78	132	55.55	74	23.33	16	8.89
189	87.22	131	55.00	73	22.78	15	9.44
188	86.67	130	54.44	72	22.22	14	10.00
187	86.11	129	53.89	71	21.67	13	10.55

F	G	F	G	F	G	F	G
186	85.55	128	53.33	70	21.44	12	11.11
185	85.00	127	52.78	69	20.55	11	11.67
184	84.44	126	52.22	68	20.00	10	12.22
183	83.89	125	51.67	67	19.44	9	12.78
182	83.33	124	51.11	66	18.89	8	13.33
181	82.78	123	50.55	65	18.33	7	13.89
180	82.22	122	50.00	64	17.78	6	14.44
179	81.67	121	49.44	63	17.22	5	15.00
178	81.11	120	48.89	62	16.67	4	15.55
177	80.55	119	48.33	61	16.11	3	16.11
176	80.00	118	47.78	60	15.50	2	16.67
175	79.44	117	47.22	59	15.00	1	17.22
174	78.89	116	46.67	58	14.44	0	17.78
173	78.33	115	46.11	57	13.89	−1	18.33
172	77.78	114	45.55	56	13.33	2	18.89
171	77.22	113	45.00	55	12.78	3	19.44
170	76.67	112	44.44	54	12.22	4	20.00
169	76.11	111	43.89	53	11.67	5	20.55
168	75.55	110	43.33	52	11.11	6	21.11
167	75.00	109	42.78	51	10.55	7	21.67
166	74.44	108	42.22	50	10.00	8	22.22
165	73.89	107	41.67	49	9.44	9	22.78
164	73.33	106	41.11	48	8.89	10	23.33
163	72.78	105	40.55	47	8.33	11	23.89
162	72.22	104	40.00	46	7.78	12	24.44
161	71.67	103	39.44	45	7.22	13	25.00
160	71.11	102	38.89	44	6.67	14	25.55
159	70.55	101	38.33	43	6.11	15	26.11
158	70.00	100	37.78	42	5.55	16	26.67
157	69.44	99	37.22	41	5.00	17	27.22
156	68.89	98	36.67	40	4.44	18	27.78
155	68.33	97	36.11	39	3.89		

6° *Number of drops to a gram of several usual reagents*

(after LANGERON, 1949).

It stands to reason that these instructions are only rigorously valid at 20°C for the normal dropper of the Pharmacopoeia (exterior diameter 3 mm, lumen 0.6 mm).

Reagents	Number of drops per gram	Reagents	Number of drops per gram
Absolute alcohol	68	Ferric chloride	19
95% alcohol	64	Hydrochloric acid	21
90% alcohol	61	Iodine	61
80% alcohol	57	Lactic acid	39
70% alcohol	56	Methyl salicylate	37
60% alcohol	53	Nitric acid	24
Acetic acid (glacial)	56	Pyridine	41
Ammonia	25	Sulphuric acid	26
Chloroform	59	Sulphuric ether	93
Distilled water	20	Turpentine	56

7° Metric equivalents of the english (Imperial) system of measures of weight and capacity

(after LANGERON, 1949).

1 grain =	....	0.065 g
2 —	....	0.130 g
3 —	....	0.194 g
4 —	....	0.259 g
5 —	....	0.324 g
6 —	....	0.389 g
7 —	....	0.454 g
8 —	....	0.518 g
9 —	....	0.583 g
10 —	....	0.648 g
20 —	= 1 scruple ..	1.296 g
30 —	....	1.944 g
40 —	....	2.592 g
50 —	....	3.240 g
1/4 ounce	....	7.087 g
1/2 ounce	....	14.175 g
1 ounce	....	28.350 g
16 ounces = 1 pound		453.592 g

1 minim	....	0.06 cm³
2 —	....	0.12 cm³
5 —	....	0.30 cm³
10 —	....	0.59 cm³
20 —	....	1.18 cm³
30 —	....	1.8 cm³
40 —	....	2.4 cm³
50 —	....	3 cm³
60 — = 1 fluid dram		3.5 cm³
120 — 2 —	.....	7 cm³
150 — 2½ —	.....	9 cm³
180 — 3 —	.....	10.5 cm³
248 — 4 —	......	14 cm³
480 — 1 fluid ounce ..		28 cm³
2 fluid ounces	......	57 cm³
3 —	....	85 cm³
3½ —	....	99 cm³
4 —	....	113.6 cm³
20 — = 1 pint	.....	568 cm³
35 —	....	1 l
160 — = 8 pints = .. 1 gallon ...		4.5 l

8° Suggestions for a histochemical nomenclature of tissue carbohydrates

by S. S. SPICER, T. J. LEPPI and P. J. STOWARD (1965).

Because of the difficulties that arise, in most cases, when one endeavours to collate the biochemical data and the results of histochemical techniques for the identification of carbohydrates, the authors suggest a nomenclature which does not entirely prejudge the chemical nature of compounds found in sections, while being sufficiently evocative from the histochemical point of view. The term 'mucopolysaccharides' is reserved for mucosubstances of connective tissue, 'mucins' for mucosubstances of epithelial origin.

The criteria of classification are, moreover, derived from histochemical reactions and marker stains (Periodic acid—Schiff reaction, metachromasia, presence or absence of sulphate radical, behaviour in relation to various enzymatic preparations, etc....)

The American authors end with the following table.

I. Neutral PAS-positive mucosubstances   *mucosubstance G*

II. Acid mucosubstances

A. SULPHATED

1) *PAS-negative connective tissue mucopolysaccharides*

    a) not affected by testicular hyaluronidase
— takes up Alcian blue in the presence of 1 M $MgCl_2$ *S-mucopolysaccharides*

    b) affected by testicular hyaluronidase
— alcohol resistant metachromasia at pH 2   *S-mucopolysaccharides B2*

— alcohol resistant metachromasia at pH 4   *S-mucopolysaccharides B4*

2) *Epithelial sulphomucins, not affected by testicular hyaluronidase*

    a) PAS-negative
sulphate esters carried by vic-glycol   *mucins GS*
sulphate esters carried by groups other than vic-glycol   *mucins S*
— alcohol resistant metachromasia at pH 2   *S-mucins B2*
— alcohol resistant metachromasia at pH 4.5   *S-mucins B4.5*

    b) PAS-positive (acid glycoproteins?)
— alcohol resistant metachromasia at pH 2   *SG-mucins B2*

— alcohol resistant metachromasia at pH 4.5   *SG-mucins B4.5*

B. NON SULPHATED

1) *Rich in uronic acids*   *U-mucopolysaccharides*

2) *Rich in sialic acid*

    a) Connective tissue sialomucopolysaccharides   *C-mucopolysaccharides*

    b) Epithelial sialomucins (acid glycoproteins)
' Very labile to sialidase, PAS-positive, metachromatic
     CG-mucins BS

" Slightly labile to sialidase
— PAS-positive   *CG-mucins S+*
— PAS-negative   *C-mucins S+*

"' Stable to sialidase
Rendered labile and metachromatic by saponification
     S-mucins (Sap) BS

Stable to sialidase after saponification
— PAS-positive   *GC-mucins*
— PAS-negative   *C-mucins*

In the table, the letter U indicates the presence of hexuronic acid, C carboxyls, S sulphates, G vic-glycol. B indicates basophilia, A affinity for Alcian blue, T labile to testicular hyaluronidase; S labile to sialidase; these qualifications being placed after the terms -mucin, mucosubstance or mucopolysaccharide.

9° List of recommended material used in tests for the main compounds mentioned in the third part of this book

The list given below is intended to facilitate the use, on suitable material, of the main histochemical reactions mentioned in this part of the book, and also the verification of techniques by workers already familiar with such methods. It is, evidently, neither exhaustive nor limiting. It shows a preference for tissues easily obtained from animals whose capture and maintenance in the laboratory do not present any difficulties; material which results in particularly spectacular preparations, but is derived from rare animals, is set in parentheses.

The so-called general reactions for proteins are not included, as these give positive reactions in all animal tissue; we only give the greater or lesser abundances of reactive compounds which are of real interest. In the same way, we exclude a list of metals only met with in experimental investigations.

Compound	*Suitable material*
Calcium	Mantle rim, *Helix pomatia*, *Helix aspersa*. Digestive gland, same species, and most Stenoglossan Gastropods of the family Muricidae. Left collaterial gland, Blattidae. Digestive gland, Decapod Crustaceans.
Zinc	Prostate, bone marrow, pancreas of mammals.
Ionic iron	Spleen of mammals, particularly after increased haemolysis (injection of phenylhydrazine chlorohydrate, etc...) Macrophages of the liver, reptiles and batrachia, (if necessary after oxidative depigmentation). (Pigmented macrophages of the perirenal tissue of *Protopterus annectens*) Digestive gland of *Nassarius reticulatus*, Prosobranch gastropods of the family Trochidae; connective tissue of the same species.
Glucose	Liver, kidney of mammals.
Ascorbic acid	Adrenal cortex of mammals.
Glycogen	Liver of mammals, autopsy during the period after a good meal. Glycogen body (lumbar swelling) of the spinal chord of birds. Connective tissue (Leydig cells) of most gastropods and lamellibranchs. Fat body, Insects. Connective tissue, Decapod crustaceans (at certain periods of the intermoult).
Galactogen	Albumin gland, Stylommatophore Gastropods.
Tunicin	Tunic of Ascidians.
Neutral mucosubstances	Covering epithelium, stomach of mammals. Thyroid colloid. Coagulant glands of the male genitalia, Mouse and Rat. 'Serous' cells of the salivary glands, Rat and Mouse.

Compound	Suitable material
Sulphomucopolysaccharides (very acid)	Ground substance of cartilage, young Mammals. Mast cells (basophilic tissue). Colic goblet cells, small Rodents (Muridae). Pedal gland, Gastropods. Mantle rim, Helicid Gastropods.
Sulphomucopolysaccharides (weakly acid)	Pyloric glands, Rat and Mouse. Goblet cells, duodenum and jejunum, Rat and Mouse. Brunner's glands, duodenum, Guinea pig and Pig.
Sialomucins	Sublingual and submaxillary glands, Rat and Mouse. Vagina of Rat or Mouse (dioestrus, gravid).
Glycerides	Adipose tissue, mammals. Liver, mammals (particularly in the case of 'fatty degeneration'). Kidney of certain mammals (particularly in the rat during alloxanic diabetes). Adipose tissue, Insects. Connective tissue, digestive gland, Stenoglossan gastropods.
Phospholipids	Nervous tissue, Mammals.
Sphingolipids	Nervous tissue, Mammals.
Steroids	Adrenal cortex, mammals. Ovary, mammals (theca interna of developing follicles and the corpus luteum as they form). Leydig cells of testes, mammals.
Chromolipids (ceroid, lipofuchsins, etc...)	Adrenal cortex of mammals (zona reticularis); macrophages of the liver, reptiles and Batrachia; pathological human material.
Arginine	Tissues full of nuclei (thymus, lymphatic nodes, spleen of mammals.
Tyrosine	Secretory granules, exocrine pancreatic cells, chief cells of the fundus, parotid of Rodents. Vitelline plaques, oocytes of gastropods and insects. Soft keratin, cortex of hair of mammals.
Indolic compounds	Chief cells, fundic glands of mammals; exocrine pancreatic cells; A cells, islets of Langerhans. (Perirenal zone of *Protopterus annectens*). (Venom gland, *Conus mediterraneus*).
Thiol groups	Soft keratin. Secretory granules, "serous" glands of mammals. Striated muscle of Mammals. Red blood corpuscless.
Disulphur groups	Hypothalamic neurosecretory products (neurohypophysis of Mammals, Birds, and anuran Batrachia). Stratum corneum of the epidermis of Mammals. B cells of the endocrine pancreas.
Deoxyribonucleic acid	Tissues full of nuclei.
Ribonucleic acid	"Serous" glands of Mammals (pancreas, fundic region of the stomach, parotid). Nerve cells. Ovaries of molluscs, insects, and Crustaceans. Silk glands, Lepidoptera. Tegumentary glands, Crustaceans.
Haemoglobin	Blood and haematopoietic organs of Mammals.

Compound	Suitable material
Catecholamines	Adrenal medulla of mammals, chromaffin tissue of other Vertebrates.
Melanin	Skin of mammals and snakes.
	Macrophages of the liver, Batrachia and certain reptiles.
	(Perirenal zone, *Protopterus annectens*).
	Skin of decapod cephalopods *(Sepia, Sepiola)*.
	Skin and connective tissue of certain Prosobranch Gastropods (Trochidae, *Pisania maculosa*, etc...).
	Skin and connective tissue of decapod Crustaceans.
Haemosiderins	Spleen of mammals.
Bile pigments	Liver of mammals.
Urates	Pathological human material.
	Kidney (organ of Bojanus) of the Snail.
	Fat body, Insects.
	Malpighian tubes, dipneumone Araneids.
Guanine	Skin of Snakes and Batrachia.
	Skin and connective tissue of Spiders *(Epeira, Tegenaria)*.
Alkaline phosphomonoesterase (non-specific)	Brush border, duodenum of mammals.
	Brush border, proximal convoluted tubule of the kidney of Vertebrates.
	Capillary endothelium, mammals.
Adenosine-triphosphate	Striated muscle, myocardium of mammals; liver of mammals
5-nucleotidase	Neurohypophysis, kidney, testes of mammals.
Acid phosphomonoesterases (non specific)	Prostate, kidney, liver of mammals.
Phosphamidase	Nervous tissue, hair follicles of mammals.
Glucose-6-phosphatase	Kidney, liver, small intestine of young mammals (Mouse, Rat).
Cholinesterases	Striated muscle of mammals (myoneural junctions); nervous tissue.
Non-specific esterases	Kidney, liver, intestine of Mammals.
Lipases	Pancreas of mammals.
Arylsulphatases	Liver, parathyroid of mammals (great specific variations).
β-glucuronidase	Liver, kidney, pancreas, lung, adrenal cortex of Mammals.
	Digestive gland, Snail.
	Malpighian tubes, Insects.
Aminopeptidases	Liver, kidney, intestine of mammals.
Phosporylase and amylo-1, 4, 1,6 transferase	Liver, striated muscle of mammals.
Cytochromeoxidase	Kidney, liver, intestine, stomach, striated muscle and myocardium of mammals.
Tyrosinase, dopa-oxidase	Skin of mammals (non-albino)
Polyphenoloxidase	Colleterial glands, *Blatta*.
	Vitelline glands, Trematodes and Cestodes.
	Byssus gland, Lamellibranchs.
Peroxidases	Blood and haematopoietic organs, Vertebrates.

Compound	Suitable meterial
Monoamine-oxidase	Skin of mammals (sweat glands); kidney of mammals.
Succinic dehydrogenase	Kidney, striated muscle, liver of mammals; nerve cells.
NAD and NADP-dehydrogenases and diaphorases	Striated muscle and myocardium, kidney, liver and nervous tissue of mammals.
Δ^5-3-β-hydroxysteroidodehydrogenase	Adrenal gland, ovary, testes of Vertebrates.

PART FOUR

THE METHODS OF GENERAL CYTOLOGY

> The cytologist is customarily thought of as a morphologist, and this point of view is still a legitimate one.
> C. P. SWANSON (1957).

CHAPTER 23

INTRODUCTION TO THE TECHNIQUES OF GENERAL CYTOLOGY

When defining the techniques of general cytology and distinguishing them from those of the other branches of histological research, one encounters as much difficulty as in the case of the so-called general methods that I mentioned previously. The very field of general cytology is not easy to define and the particular orientation of a worker is clearly tributary to the sense that he accords to the term.

Etymologically, the term "general cytology" denotes a study of the general characteristics of the cell irrespective of the techniques involved. Though at first purely morphological, general cytology is increasingly based on biophysics and biochemistry. Today it may still be regarded as a morphological discipline but it will surely not be so for long.

Even those who accept its morphological connotation do not always give it its true meaning For the cytogeneticist, cytology is the determination of the caryotype and its anomalies; for the school of Parat it signified the demonstration of the chondriome and the "vacuome" of the animal cell, by means of predisposed techniques intended to be convergent, all other constituents being contemptuously left aside; in clinical language and in that of hospital administrations this term applies to an activity that is indeed far removed from true cytology.

In practice, cytology may be conveniently distinguished from other branches of histology by the scale on which the study is effected. Thus, when the study can no longer be considered as microscopic anatomy, or when the state of the cells and their organelles is the preponderant concern of the author, one may speak of cytological research whatever the techniques employed. In other words, general methods or histochemical reactions can be very useful, and even indispensable, for true cytological work.

It is thus, following an arbitrary convention, that works on histological techniques include certain methods for the study of the fundamental organelles of the cell under "general cytological techniques". I shall therefore conform myself to this usage and group, in the following pages, those techniques used in the study of the nucleus and the cytoplasmic organelles in all or most types of Metazoan cells. The fundamental principles of cytological technique are the same as those of microscopic anatomy and histochemistry; however, the scale on which it is practised implies particular precautions, especially in fixing the material. Furthermore, certain staining techniques, whose specificity depends more on the pretreatment of the material than on the actual stains used, play such an important role in cytological technique that their discussion in the introductory chapter seems justified to me.

THE PROBLEM OF CYTOLOGICAL FIXATION

It would be a hardly excessive generalization to affirm that the exigencies of cytological fixation are quite the opposite of those demanded by certain aspects of histology, especially histo-enzymology. I have recalled in a previous chapter that the preservation of the chemical state, that is, the preservation of enzymatic activity, is the dominant concern in histo-enzymology. In cytology, it is the morphological state, namely the preservation of structure, which imposes itself and the investigator learns to accept extreme chemical transformation of the cell constituents provided they maintain an aspect in permanent preparations as close as possible to that observed vitally.

The comparison of fixed preparations with the living object is useful in all branches of histology and is of primordial importance in cytology. It is by such a comparison and by using particularly favorable material that the cytologist chooses reliable techniques of fixation and staining. In order to satisfy all the guarantees, exigible vital examination can require equipment that is not normally available in histological laboratories and can call for a certain level of technical competence that all cytologists do not possess. Thus, only specialized workers practice it, but every cytologist should be familiar with their results and take them into account in choosing his techniques.

The requirements of a cytological fixative differ in some points from those of a topographic fixative (p. 177). *Penetration* need not be as great since in most cases very small pieces suffice for cytological examination. *Uniformity of fixation* over the whole thickness of the piece is likewise of less importance. A minimum of *shrinking* is, of course, desirable, but the cytologist is often forced to sacrifice this quality. The period of *fixation* and the *delay before subsequent treatment* of the sample can be more critical than in microscopic anatomy. On the contrary, a good preparation for inclusion in paraffin is absolutely necessary in all cases where the material is to be sectioned. The *range of staining* procedures feasible after a given fixation, which should be as wide as possible for topographic fixatives, may be restricted with cytological fixatives since the particular staining technique is usually decided at the time of choosing the fixative. The *cost* of the fixative is also less important, since the small size of the pieces usually allows the habitual use of an expensive fixative without undue concern for laboratory budgets.

Two types of fixation by *physical agents* should be mentioned among cytological techniques, namely, the desiccation of smears at room temperature and freezing-drying. The drying of smears is important in haematological technique; it can also be used in other cases but necessitates the later use of a chemical fixing agent as well. Freezing-drying *can* ensure the preservation of organelles as well as the best of cytological fixatives, but this does not necessarily follow automatically. The success of the remarkable fixations referred to is of considerable doctrinal importance and demonstrates the validity of good chemical fixation. The latter, however, is preferable for routine work, and it seems to me that freezing-drying, for the cytologist, is not as important as it justly is for histochemical research.

Among the *chemical fixing agents*, osmium tetroxyde is the only one used in cytology without any adjuvant. All other fixatives are used in mixtures.

Osmium tetroxyde, whose general properties have already been described under histological fixatives, is perhaps the most "loyal" of all fixatives, one that best spares cellular structures and preserves them really close to their living state. All authorities properly emphasize this fundamental feature, but several do not insist sufficiently on the fact that osmium tetroxyde can deploy its qualities only under certain conditions, namely, as its vapour, acting on cells that are isolated or at the most in double layers and which should not be embedded subsequently. Fixation becomes very irregular when the solution of osmium tetroxyde has more than 100 μ of tissue to penetrate and admirably fixed cells may be observed side by side with coarse artefacts. Moreover, osmium tetroxyde used alone is quite unsuitable before embedding in paraffin and its adjuvants in chromo-osmic fixatives diminish some of its qualities. It is therefore best confined to the treatment of smears and imprints, at least in light microscopy. The relevant techniques will be described when dealing with the nucleus and the chondriome.

Fixatives used in cytological technique may be classified into four groups, namely, chromo-osmic mixtures, chromic mixtures without osmium tetroxyde, mixtures based on heavy metals other than chromium and osmium and, finally, chromoacetic mixtures. There are valid grounds for including chloroplatinic fixatives among the chromo-osmic mixtures. The above list is evidently not limiting; several fixatives already referred to under General Methods can be of great use in cytological research.

CHROMO-OSMIC SOLUTIONS

The number of these mixtures, to which those containing chloroplatinic acid may be added, is indeed great, but the majority of formulae are quite redundant. In this respect, Table 26, which indicates the ingredients of certain fixatives of this group, serves more to inform the reader of the type of fixatives used in cytology than to provide a list of indispensable ones.

Table 26. — Composition of the principal chromo-osmic and chloroplatinic solutions

Compound (% solution)	Osmium tetroxyde (2)	Chromium trioxyde (0.5) (1)	Acetic acid	Potassium dichromate (5) (3) (2.5)	Chloro-platinic acid (1)	Mercuric chloride (5)	Uranyl nitrate (4)
Flemming...	4	—	15	1	— — —	—	—	—
Hermann...	4	—	—	1	— — —	15	—	—
Lindsay-Johnson...	10	—	—	5	— — 70	15	—	—
Benda...	4	—	15	III	— — —	—	—	—
Meves...	4	15	—	III	— — —	—	—	—
Bensley...	4	—	—	II	— — 16	—	—	—
Laguesse...	4	—	8	II	— — —	—	—	—
Heitz...	4	—	15	—	— — —	—	—	—
Altmann...	10	—	—	—	10 — —	—	—	—
Hirschler (a)...	1	—	3	—	— 3 —	—	—	—
Hirschler (b)...	8	—	4	—	— 4 —	—	—	—
Champy...	4	—	7	—	— 7 —	—	—	—
Nassonov...	4	—	8	—	— 8 —	—	—	—
Benoit...	5	—	—	—	6 — —	—	5	4

All substances are used as solutions in distilled water, except acetic acid, which is pure, and mercuric chloride, which is dissolved in a "physiological" solution isotonic with the internal medium of the animal. Arabic numerals indicate millilitres and Roman numerals indicate drops. All the above fixatives are preferably prepared just before use; the stock solutions are however quite stable.

The first three fixatives contain a far from negligible quantity of acetic acid. Baker (1958) rightly observes that the level of acetic acid (5%) in Flemming's fluid usually adopted is a maximum, Flemming himself having insisted on the possibility of reducing this dose. The presence of chromium trioxyde and acetic acid explains why none of these three fixatives preserves the chondriome. On the other hand, nuclear structures, the centrosomes and the spindle, cytological differentiations such as brush borders and striated borders, and cilia are remarkably well fixed. Osmiophilic lipids are well conserved. All three may be used with thin membranes (such as the tails of Batracian larvae) to be mounted in *toto* or to be sectioned. Fixation should range from 12 to 24 hours; longer periods are hardly profitable. The chromium trioxide should be removed by careful washing (for at least 24 hours) in running water. Inclusion in celloidin is possible but pointless since the usual staining methods involved require thin sections. I particularly recommend Cedarwood oil as an intermediary between dehydration in absolute alcohol and paraffin. Shrinking is much less with these fixatives than with those of the two following groups. Apart from the staining methods discussed in this part of the book, the nucleal reaction of Feulgen and Rossenbeck as well as safranin-light green may also be adopted.

Fixatives of the second group contain a quantity of acetic acid sufficient to improve the preparation for embedding in paraffin but insufficient to destroy the majority of the chondriome; but this is not an absolute rule and it is preferable to use those of the third group for particularly fragile objects. Among the four fixatives of the second group I prefer that of Bensley which is more rational than the others since it contains no chromium trioxide and very little acetic acid. The time of fixation in all four cases lasts 24 hours, and rinsing and inclusion are as for those of the first group.

Those of the third group are the best chromo-osmic fixatives of the chondriome. All give excellent results; my personal preference is for those of Altmann and of Benoit since they contain no chromium trioxide so that the potassium dichromate can freely exercise its properties as a cytoplasmic fixative (p.49). The most frequently used is that of Champy. Nassonov's solution has been simplified by the omission of pyrogallol which is entirely inoperative. Samples are fixed for 24 hours, followed by the usual rinsing in running water and osmic impregnation for Golgi bodies, or rehydration. The use of Cedarwood oil before embedding is strongly recommended.

The technical conditions governing the use of chromo-osmic fixatives follow from their properties. They penetrate badly, fix irregularly, harden the pieces and are not suitable before embedding in paraffin especially when they contain little or no acetic acid. But they conserve organelles remarkably well and are an excellent prelude to cytological stains. Only very small pieces, not exceeding 2 mm in one dimension and obtained from perfectly fresh material, may be fixed by these solutions. Fixation is carried out *at room temperature*; none of the chromo-osmic or platinic fixatives gives good results for light microscopy when the temperature of fixation is less than 12°C. Storage of pieces in 70% alcohol should be avoided. My personal experience is that storage in 10% formalin is possible with proper rinsing. Cedarwood oil is the best preservative for pieces fixed in chromo-osmic mixtures. No particular precaution need be observed at the time of embedding. Sections should be thin.

In short, these fixatives are to be used under precise circumstances. Their use for anatomical studies, or when the material is not perfectly fresh from all points of view, only betrays a deplorable lack of critical sense in the user.

CHROMIC FLUIDS WITHOUT OSMIUM TETROXYDE AND ACETIC ACID

The solutions of this group are typical of the fixatives to be used in research on the chondriome. As in the case of the chromo-osmic fixatives, a considerable number of formulae burdens histological literature, and only the most important ones have been retained in Table 27.

Table 27. — COMPOSITION OF THE PRINCIPAL CHROMIC FIXATIVES WITHOUT OSMIUM TETROXYDE AND ACETIC ACID

Solution (%)	Müller	Zenker	Potassium dichromate (3)	(3.5)	(5)	Formalin	Chrome alum
ORTH	9	—	—	—	—	1	—
KOPSCH	—	—	—	4	—	1	—
REGAUD	—	—	4	—	—	1	—
KOLSTER	—	—	—	—	4	2	4
HELLY	—	9.5	—	—	—	0.5	—
MAXIMOW	—	9	—	—	—	1	—

Müller's solution is prepared by dissolving 2.5 g of potassium dichromate and 1 g of sodium sulphate in 100 ml of distilled water. Zenker's solution contains, in addition to the above, 5 g/100 ml of mercuric chloride (see p. 184). Formalin should be neutralized and added only just before use. None of these fixatives may be kept for more than 24 hours.

Among these six fixatives, two contain mercuric chloride while four do not. The latter allow the osmic impregnation of the Golgi apparatus which is otherwise quite mediocre following Helly's or Maximow's fluids.

As a whole the preservation of cytoplasmic structures by these solutions is not as good as that obtained with a successful chromo-osmic fixation, but they have other advantages. They penetrate much better and pieces of up to 3 mm in one direction may be fixed. Fixation is much more regular and the danger of peripheral overfixation and inner autolysis is less. They permit the choice of a wide range of stains and histochemical reactions. From the technical point of view treatment with them is good before embedding in paraffin and shrinkage is less than with osmic solutions without acetic acid. Consequently, I tend to consider fixatives of this group as expedient for routine work on cytoplasmic structures, the more so as their cost is moderate.

The choice between fixatives with mercuric chloride and those without depends not only on the customary practice of the investigator but also on the object studied. Experience has shown that the preservation of cells rich in secretory granules is better after fixation in Helly's fluid, or even more with Maximow's fluid, than after the others. Furthermore, both of the above fixatives are particularly recommendable before Pappenheim's panoptic staining with its variants and they are indispensable in studies on haematopoietic organs and certain connective cells. In spite of the great similarity between the two formulae that of Maximow gives better results and I find it preferable to that of Helly.

Among fixatives based on formalin and potassium dichromate those of Orth, Kopsch and of Regaud yield strictly equivalent results and any discrimination among them can only be dictated by the individual practice of an investigator or the tradition of a laboratory.

Kolster's solution merits special mention; although its present fashion is not very great, it is certainly the best non-osmic mitochondrial fixative. I recommend it in all cases where a demonstration of the chondriomes is the chief object of the study, especially as the usual mitochondrial stains applied after this fixative are effective without post-chromatization, which is a considerable saving of time.

The *technical conditions of fixation* entailed by the above solutions differ in some respects from those described for osmic fixatives. Freshness of the material is equally important but the dimensions may be greater (up to 3 or 4 mm). It is good practice to cool the fixative in an ice-bath before introducing the pieces and to maintain them at less than 10°C for the first few hours of fixation, although good results may also be obtained at room temperature. The period of fixation is rigorously limited, never exceeding 6 hours with Helly's or Maximow's fluids and 24 hours with the others. A modification of Maximow's fluid (see Table 27) that contains, in addition 10% of a 20% solution of osmium tetroxyde allows fixation for up to 24 hours. After fixation, pieces treated with Kolster's solution are washed until all excess of fixative is removed, dehydrated and embedded in paraffin. Other solutions may be followed, according to the aim of the study, either by a rapid rinse in tap-water and post-chromatization (for demonstrating chondriomes), by careful washing for 24 hours in running water before dehydration and inclusion or, as when following the solutions of Orth, of Kopsch and of Regaud, by careful washing for 24 hours in running water and osmic impregnation of the Golgi apparatus.

FLUIDS BASED ON HEAVY METALS OTHER THAN CHROMIUM AND OSMIUM

The three fixatives included in this group, namely that of Ramon y Cajal with uranyl nitrate, that of da Fano with cobalt nitrate and that of Aoyama with cadmium chloride preserve the chondriome and are highly suitable before silver impregnation of the Golgi apparatus. In fact, their range of use is not very great, being principally conceived for the demonstration of the Golgi apparatus by the above technique. Their compositions are given in Table 28.

Table 28. — Cytological fixatives based on heavy metals other than chromium and osmium

Compound (% solution)	Uranyl nitrate (1)	Cobalt nitrate (1)	Cadmium chloride (1)	Formalin
Ramon y Cajal	85	—	—	15
Da Fano	—	85	—	15
Aoyama	—	—	85	15

The numbers are volumetric units. Stock solutions are stable. Most authors recommend that formalin be added just before use, although no chemical reason exists for this. It however goes without saying that the formalin should be neutralized.

CHROMO-ACETIC FLUIDS

These solutions preserve neither chondriomes nor Golgi bodies. They are meant for studies on secretory granules, ergastoplasm, ciliated structures and for caryology. Their penetration is sufficiently rapid for them to be considered as topographic fixatives. Thus the fluids of von Telliesniczky, of Zenker, of Kolmer, which is a prototype of all "kaformacet" solutions, and that of Sanfelice have already been described in the chapter devoted to topographic fixation and will not be discussed here.

In addition to the above fixatives, Baker's formaldehyde-calcium is excellent for chondriome and the Golgi apparatus. On the contrary, its use is quite undesirable for caryological studies. Both the fluids of Clarke and of Carnoy, topographic fixatives described earlier, are suitable for caryology and observation of the ergastoplasm. Bouin's fluid, Heidenhain's Susa and Halmi's fluid are useful for secretory products, while solutions containing corrosive sublimate and formalin or acetic acid can be helpful not only for secretory granules but also for studying the centrosome, the fusorial apparatus and ciliary structures. These details are given in the chapters concerning the particular organelles.

As a rule, cytological fixation demands an even more rapid removal of samples than topographic fixation. It should be recalled that the removal of material for cytological examination is not to be compared to dissection as understood by anatomists, during which the tissues are scrupulously stretched and distorted. Above all, the rapid immersion of a particular tissue in the chosen fixative is aimed at, and one should not hesitate to remove it by sacrificing all its surroundings. Perfusion is necessary in all cases where the tissue cannot be brought into contact with the fixative within three minutes of the death of the animal. Instances of these are the internal ear, the brain, the hypophysis of large animals etc.

No cytological fixative is universal. In most cases the investigator should bear in mind the chief objective of the study and have consequently chosen the fixative at the time of removing samples. Chromo-osmic solutions are not necessarily the most suitable. The possibility of adopting histochemical techniques and the difficulty of dividing the tissue into sufficiently small pieces can lead to a preference for fixatives that are normally less advantageous but otherwise more penetrant and of regular efficacity.

REGRESSIVE STAINING WITH HAEMATOXYLIN LAKES

Regressive stainings with haematoxylin lakes play the same role in cytology as that of the corresponding progressive lakes in topographic histology. In spite of the empiricism of their invention and the impossibility of explaining the mechanism of their affinity for a given structure or of attributing any chemical significance to their results, their adaptability and the optical quality of the preparations are such that no cytologist can reasonably do without them. It is besides reciprocally true that the manner in which one practises methods like that of iron-haematoxylin is often an excellent criterion of one's mastery of cytological technique.

Present conceptions of the mechanism of regressive staining in general and of the mode of action of differentiators have been briefly described in the paragraph devoted to histological staining. It may be pointed out here that a careful study made by Wigglesworth (1952) shows that mordanting with iron-alum fixes iron on to the acidic groups of tissue structures, especially the phosphate groups of nucleic acids and the carboxyls of amino acids, and that metal can be detected by methods other than the treatment of sections with haematein in solutions. Under these conditions there is a clear relation between the abundance of acidic groups in tissue proteins and the degree of siderophily. Furthermore, methylation greatly decreases the siderophily of tissues, whereas deamination is without effect. As noted by Baker (1958) this mechanism explains the siderophily of phospholipids, provided that the above compounds have been retained in the sections. However, this simple phenomenon cannot explain all the results obtained on regressive staining with haematoxylin lakes. In fact, Puchtler and Sweat (1964) have pointed out that these lakes deeply stain muscle fibers and terminal bars that are not particularly renowned for their siderophily. They also suggest that hydrogen bonds can connect the haematein molecule to certain tissue structures instead of the chelation of ferric ions hitherto considered as the only link between the stain and its target.

Aluminium and chromium lakes of haematoxylin are of subsidiary interest in cytological technique where iron and copper lakes preponderate.

FERRIC LAKES

Although the first technique of regressive staining with a ferric lakes of haematoxylin is due to Benda (1886), it is the process invented by M. Heidenhain (1894) that has gained deserved popularity and stands even today as one of the fundamental techniques of cytology. Regaud's technique (1910), which gives identical results, differs only in details of the composition of the staining solution. A technique due to Hirschler (1927), derived from an earlier one of Dobell (1914), does not involve a solution of haematoxylin matured so as to obtain haematein but a solution of the latter itself. Other techniques of regressive staining with the ferric lakes of haematoxylin do not possess any noteworthy practical advantages over those mentioned above.

1° *Heidenhain's haematoxylin and its variants*

The principle of this method is very simple. Thin sections (those of more than 5 μ stain so heavily that a detailed examination is difficult in spite of proper differentiation) are mordanted in a solution of iron alum, treated with an aqueous solution of haematoxylin that has been matured to obtain a partial transformation of haematoxylin into haematin, and then differentiated in a solution of iron-alum under the microscope so as to terminate differentiation as soon as the desired structures appear to be sufficiently clear against the background of the preparation. Pretreatment of the tissues, preparation of the reagents and the technique itself call for a certain number of comments.

a) **The pretreatment of tissues** evidently conditions the final result of the staining. Only structures well conserved in sections can be stained. Their degree of siderophily varies considerably according to the fixation, postchromatization or their mordanting, treatment by oxidizing agents and even stainings effected prior to that by the ferric lakes of haematoxylin. The relevant technical details are given in the chapters concerning the different organelles of the animal cell.

b) Certain precautions have to be observed in **the preparation of reagents**. The solution of iron-alum used for mordanting deteriorates easily, and I advise that it be prepared immediately before use from *chemically pure* iron-alum. Early histologists paid much attention to the size of the crystals and their violet colour. In fact quite satisfactory material is now available from manufacturers as a white micro-crystalline powder hardly tinged with violet. The solubility of this compound is however essential and provides the histologist with a simple test of its quality. Any sample that does not dissolve *completely* at 5% in distilled water should be rejected. As a solid it shows a strong tendency to decompose on contact with air, especially in a humid atmosphere. It is therefore safer to provide it in small quantities and to see that the bottles are well stoppered after use. Different authors propose widely varying concentrations of mordant; I suggest a fresh solution at 5% in distilled water. The solution of haematoxylin (*) is prepared, according to the formula of Heidenhain as well as that of Regaud, from a stock solution of 10% in 96° alcohol matured over several months or even years. Every histologist worthy of his name should have such a solution at hand. It is certainly not indispensable for regressive iron- haematoxylin staining since the solution can be immediately matured with various oxidizers (see p. 195). However, this procedure cannot be adopted for copper lakes and for certain neurohistological techniques. Alcoholic solutions at 10% keep very well (from 10 to 20 years) provided they are protected from direct sunlight and stored in good quality glassware from which no alkali leaches out. Heidenhain's solution is prepared by mixing 5 ml of the stock solution with 95 ml of distilled water, whereas that of Regaud contains 10 ml of the stock solution, 10 ml of glycerol and 80 ml of water. Both may be kept and used for several years if they are filtered from time to time.

My personal experience, which agrees with that generally reported in the literature, is that solutions matured at short notice by the addition of an oxidizer (usually sodium or potassium iodate; see p. 195 for the proportions) are as satisfactory as those matured by ageing. However, they do not keep as well, especially when the suggestion of Baker and Jordan (1953) of reducing the quantity of oxidizer by a third, or even by half, is not followed.

*c) **The procedure** consists of the following steps, each of which is commented upon.*

> Deparaffin sections, include in collodion if required and hydrate them.
> Mordant for 24 hours at room temperature in a fresh 5% solution of iron-alum in distilled water.
> Rinse carefully in distilled water (3 to 4 rinses of one minute each).
> Treat for 24 hours, at room temperature, with a solution of haematoxylin (according to Heidenhain, Regaud or after maturing with oxidizers).
> Rinse for 3 to 5 minutes in tap water.
> Differentiate, under the microscope, in a 5% aqueous solution of iron-alum (the solution used as mordant is quite suitable for this purpose).
> Terminate differentiation, as soon as the desired result is obtained, by a vigorous rinse in tap water.
> Rinse at length (at least 30 minutes) in running water. Apply, if necessary, a background stain.
> Dehydrate in absolute alcohol, clear in benzene hydrocarbon and mount in Canada balsam or even better, in a commercial synthetic resin.

Mordanting is practised differently by various authors with respect to the concentration of iron-alum as well as the temperature and duration. Certain authors specify 3 to 12 hours, while others extend it up to 36 hours; the level of iron-alum can vary from 2.5 to 7.5%; the temperature is raised to 37°, or even

---

(*) I have indicated, on p.194, the faulty usage of referring to haematoxylin when the actual stain is haematen.

60°, in an effort to shorten the treatment. In fact mordanting at high temperatures causes the lakes to hold badly during differentiation. The times given above have always given me satisfaction.

Rinsing in distilled water between mordanting and staining is an important step; it partly governs the ease of differentiation and the specificity of staining. The rinse in tap water before differentiation in iron-alum is not less important.

The concentration of iron-alum that I have suggested for differentiation will surely be judged excessive by some readers. I admit that several classical authors advise solutions of 1 or even 0.5%, but experience has shown that much more regular results are obtained at higher levels because the threshold of local concentration is attained more evenly at the beginning of treatment.

Prolonged rinsing after differentiation is also essential. It is during this step that the stain is rendered permanent and the conservation of preparations ensured by the removal of the last traces of iron-alum. Stains sometimes brighten during this rinse and the experienced worker allows for this by extending the destaining in iron-alum to a little beyond the desired result.

By observing the above precautions and by mounting under coverslips that spread over a much wider area than that of the sections, so that oxydation by the diffusion of air is prevented, the preparations keep better than after the great majority of other methods. I have had the privilege of examining, in 1959, preparations made by M. Heidenhain in 1899 which had lost none of their sparkle. It is fairly certain that mounting in synthetic resins will preserve iron-haematoxylin stains even longer.

The intensity and precision of staining are equalled only by certain silver impregnations. No background stain is necessary when this method is adopted for cytological study. As for the nature of the stained structures, many of the organelles and inclusions of the cell can be siderophilous according to the circumstances. So that iron-haematoxylin is a suitable means of depicting but never a sure test of identification. After "topographic" fixation in acetic acid solutions this method stains nuclei, ergastoplasms, secretory granules retained by fixation, ciliatures, brush borders and striated plateaux, centrosomes and the spindle. Postchromatization applied after a fixation that conserves the chondriomes renders them highly siderophilous, which offers a means of their specific detection. Collagen fibers stain with troublesome intensity, and the structural details of striated muscle fibers are well brought out. All inclusions containing metals that can form lakes with haematoxylin are disclosed, this being independent of the use of the iron-alum mordant. Highly acid mucosubstances show themselves sufficiently siderophilous to be detected.

The substitution of ferric chloride for iron-alum as a mordant as well as for differentiation (Mallory 1900) does not procure any practical advantage. Differentiation in picric acid has been advised by P. Masson when regressive staining with iron-haematoxylin is the first step of the triple stain referred to on p. 214;

in which case mordanting in iron-alum and staining with Regaud's haematoxylin are effected with heating (30 minutes in a paraffin oven) and the slides differentiated under the microscope in alcohol-picric acid. (1 volume of 96° alcohol saturated with picric acid and 2 volumes of 96° alcohol). Under these conditions the destaining of collagen fibers is faster than that of the nuclei so that, in spite of an intense nuclear stain persisting, the collagen tissue is sufficiently stripped to make way for the rest of Masson's triple stain. As I have remarked on p. 213, this method is outmoded since progressive iron-haematoxylin lakes ensure a more rapid and, as it were, automatic staining of the nuclei of a quality that amply suffices for topographic histology.

Yet another way of reducing the affinity of collagen fibers for iron-haematoxylin lakes, that of staining with certain acid stains *before mordanting in iron-alum*, is of undoubted interest. Bordeaux R and eosin have been used to this effect. The technical details differ in both cases.

*d) **Heidenhain's Bordeaux R and iron haematoxylin.*** — This technique is based on the reduced siderophily, after prior staining in dilute Bordeaux R, of all structures except the centrosome, and hence facilitates demonstration of the latter. The method is as follows.

> Paraffin sections, preferably of material fixed in a liquid containing corrosive sublimate, are deparaffined, collodioned if desired and hydrated.
> Stain for about 10 minutes in a 0.1% aqueous solution of Bordeaux R (other Bordeaux are equally suitable).
> Rinse rapidly in distilled water.
> Mordant for 24 hours at room temperature in a 5% solution of iron-alum.
> Rinse carefully in distilled water.
> Stain for 24 hours with haematoxylin (Heidenhain's or Regaud's solution, or one matured at short notice).
> Wash thoroughly in tap water.
> Differentiate under the microscope in the same solution of iron-alum used as mordant.
> Wash at length in running water.
> Dehydrate in absolute alcohol, clear with a benzenic hydrocarbon and mount in a synthetic resin or Canada balsam.

The prior staining with Bordeaux R causes the siderophily of the centrosome to surpass that of all other structures so that it easily shows up in black on a red background. With care the black stain of the nucleus can be maintained while collagen fibers and striated muscle destain from the outset of differentiation.

*e) **A. Prenant's triple stain.*** — As mentioned on p. 209, this technique, wrongly held to be a topographic one, is in fact a very valuable cytological method provided the stipulations of the author are met with *by treating the sections with eosin before proceeding to stain with iron-haematoxylin*. The prior staining considerably reduces the siderophily of collagen fibers and basement membranes, whereas the fundamental organelles of the cell remain unmodified. Well stripped preparations, ready to be stained with light green, are thus easily obtained if the material is accordingly fixed and postchromatized, without having to pursue differentiation up to a point where nuclear structures, ciliary corpuscles and chondriomes fade. The original technique consists of the following steps.

> Paraffin sections are deparaffined, collodioned if desired and hydrated.
> Stain for about 10 minutes in a 1% aqueous solution of eosin or erythrosin.
> Rinse rapidly in distilled water.
> Mordant for 24 hours at room temperature in a 5% aqueous solution of iron-alum.
> Rinse thoroughly in distilled water.
> Treat for 24 hours at room temperature with haematoxylin (Heidenhain's or Regaud's solution or one matured at short notice).
> Wash carefully in tap water.
> Differentiate under the microscope in the solution of iron-alum used as mordant.
> Wash very carefully in running water.
> Stain rapidly on slides with a dilute solution (0.5%) of light green in 50° or 70° alcohol; follow the progress of staining through the thin layer of stain that has been poured over the sections and terminate when the overall colour turns greyish.
> Dehydrate directly in absolute alcohol, clear in a benzenic hydrocarbon and mount in a synthetic resin or, if it cannot be helped, in Canada balsam.

Collagen fibers, mucins and certain secretory granules take a more or less deep green, while siderophilous structures stand out intensely black on the red background of the preparation.

One of the practical inconveniences of the method, namely the poor persistence of light green, will probably disappear with the use of synthetic resins that do not oxidize. The delicate step of the technique, which is the staining with light green (there is no suitable means of rectifying overstaining with green) is rendered entirely automatic by replacing the alcoholic solution of light green with the mixture described on p. 216 in connection with my variant of Gomori's trichrome. Staining for 5 to 10 minutes with the eosin-fast green F C F-phosphotungstic acid mixture followed by dehydration in absolute alcohol and mounting yields preparations that are equal in all respects to those obtained by the classical method without the slightest risk of overstaining. I therefore recommend the practice of A. Prenant's triple stain in this form.

2° *Dobell—Hirschler haematoxylin*

The essential feature of this method, all the steps of which are carried out in an alcoholic medium, lies in that staining is not effected by a solution of haematoxylin matured naturally or by the addition of an oxydant, but by means of a solution of haematein. Success therefore depends on the quality of the sample of haematein at one's disposal. The results can be remarkable, with less time consumed than in the regressive staining of Heidenhain, but the solutions keep badly and haematein is definitely costlier than haematoxylin. The technique consists of the following steps.

> Sections are deparaffined, collodioned and brought to 70° alcohol.
> Mordant at room temperature in a 1% solution of iron-alum in 70° alcohol that is prepared by dissolving a gram of iron-alum in 23 ml of water and, when fully dissolved, adding 77 ml of 96° alcohol. A ten minute mordant is enough for the selective staining of nuclear structures, whereas the demonstration of chondriomes requires two to three hours.
> Rinse rapidly in distilled water.
> Stain, for the same time given to the mordant, in a 1% solution of haematein in 70° alcohol.
> Rinse in 70° alcohol.
> Wash for 30 seconds in one or two changes of distilled water.
> Differentiate under the microscope in a 2 or 2.5% aqueous solution of iron-alum. Hirschler recommends placing the slide in a Petri dish, covering it with the differentiator and following the process under the microscope which generally requires about 2 minutes. Dehydrate in absolute alcohol, clear in a benzenic hydrocarbon and mount in Canada balsam or a synthetic resin.

The result are comparable to those with Heidenhain's technique.

CUPRIC LAKES

The cupric lakes of haematoxylin are much less favoured by histologists than the ferric lakes. Such disdain is not justifiable. The blue tint of the cupric lakes is perhaps less marked than the black of ferric lakes, but the precision of staining is the same in both cases and results obtained much more rapidly than by the method of Heidenhain.

The introduction of cupric lakes in histological technique is due to Bensley (1911–1912), and from my own experience his method is preferable to that of Cowdry (1913).

Reagents:

> Saturated aqueous solution of copper acetate. 5% aqueous solution of potassium chromate (not to be confounded with the bichromate!)
> 0.5 or 1% solution of haematoxylin, prepared by a fresh dilution in distilled water of a well-matured stock solution at 10% in 96° alcohol.
> Borax-ferricyanide: Dissolve 4 g of borax and 5 g of potassium ferricyanide in 600 ml of water and store in a refrigerator.

Technique:

> Paraffin sections are deparaffined, collodioned and hydrated.
> Mordant for 5 minutes in the solution of copper acetate.
> Rinse in distilled water.

Treat for about one minute in the solution of potassium chromate.
Rinse in distilled water.
Treat for one minute in the solution of haematoxylin.
Rinse in distilled water.
Return for a few seconds to the copper acetate solution.
Differentiate prudently under the microscope with the borax-ferricyanide; differentiation is very rapid and the solution indicated above may diluted to half in distilled water with advantage.
Wash at length (at least one hour) in running water. Dehydrate in absolute alcohol, clear in a benzenic hydrocarbon and mount in a synthetic resin or Canada balsam.

The results are the same as those given by the ferric lakes of haematoxylin except that structures are stained blue instead of black. In Cowdry's variant treatment with potassium chromate follows staining with haematoxylin; its duration is the same as that in the technique of Bensley and all other steps are identical.

CHAPTER 24

TECHNIQUES FOR STUDYING THE NUCLEUS

The morphology of the nucleus may be studied under quite different circumstances, and the techniques employed can differ widely according to the case. Sometimes a very good demonstration of the structural details of the nucleus is required without, for that matter, sacrifying the cytoplasmic organelles; such an orientation being arbitrarily designed as the general study of nuclear structure. In other cases, as in the study of caryotype, the enumeration of the chromosomes and the analysis of their morphological structure are the sole aims, while the cytoplasmic structures are deliberately sacrificed and destroyed during preparation. A particular example is the study of the sex-chromatin; or else it may be the nucleolus and the different intra-nuclear inclusions that are of prime concern to the investigator. The different sections of the chapter are accordingly defined.

THE GENERAL STUDY OF NUCLEAR STRUCTURES

All the general methods of histological examination, from vital observation to histochemical reactions, can serve in the study of nuclear structures. Evidently only the most important techniques are retained here.

VITAL OBSERVATION

The progress of microscopy has enabled nuclear structures to be conveniently observed *in vivo*, the limits to the technique not being inherent in the means of observation but in the possibility of obtaining really vital conditions of examination.

In fact the phase contrast and inteferential microscopes have remarkable successes to their credit in the study of nuclear structures. The events of mitosis have been cinematographed in divers material (seminal cells of Invertebrates, fibroblast cultures etc). A detailed analysis of the interphase nucleus can also be based on vital preparations if the object lends itself to the purpose. I further recall that, before the advent of phase-contrast microscopy, ultra-violet photography enabled us to rectify the error of interpreting the nucleolus as the only structured element of the interphase nucleus by showing that the apparent homogeneity under a light field microscope was solely due to the similar refractive indices of structures that really exist *in vivo* and whose appearance after fixation is not at all an artifact.

But the restrictions enounced in the first part of this book concerning the general limitations of vital examination hold entirely for the nucleus as well. There is no question of adapting this method to the observation of any object whatever, and on the contrary it is the object that has to be chosen as a function of the technique adopted. I might mention that the salivary glands of Molluscs, the so-called salivary glands of Dipteran larvae and the male gonads of many Invertebrates are particularly favorable material. The technical advantages of tissue cultures should also not be neglected.

Properly speaking, the technique calls for no particular comment. The chosen object is removed as rapidly as possible and placed under a coverslip in a medium propitious for survival, the best of such media being evidently the blood of the animal. Short-term observation does not necessitate any precautions concerning temperature or oxygen supply. Special contrivances (hot plate, hanging drop etc.) are useful only for prolonged examination or when a phenomenon is cinematographed.

VITAL STAINS

The advent of phase contrast and interferential microscopy has rendered the vital staining of nuclei with dilute neutral red, methylene blue and other stains somewhat obsolete. However, fluoroscopic examination after treatment with very dilute acridine orange has retained its interest since the tint of secondary fluorescence is a valuable indication of the vitality of cells. Bukatsch and Haitinger (1940) and Strugger (1942, 1950) use a 0.01% solution of acridine orange in Sörensen's buffer (pH 7.7) for 3 to 4 minutes. After both washing and observation in a physiological solution the cells appear green if living or a copper red otherwise.

NUCLEAR STRUCTURES IN SMEARS

The analysis of nuclear structures in smears offers the advantage of examining entire cells, of applying osmic fixative under the best conditions and of rapid preparation. It can be effected only in cases where the cells are normally isolated or loosely held.

It seems to me opportune at this point to recall the exact connotation of the terms smear, imprint and squash, since they are often used indiscriminately. A *smear* (*frottis, Ausstrich*) is made by sprending isolated cells in their liquid medium between slide and coverslip, or dissociating easily separable cells. In an *imprint* (*empreinte, Abklatsch*) a slice of organ is pressed against a slide or coverslip taking care not to impart any lateral displacement; this is repeated several times on the same slide so that as many cells are detached from the organ as possible. A *squash* (*écrasement, Quetschpraparat*) is made by crushing a suitably treated piece of organ between slide and coverslip. This implies that in smears and imprints the flattening of cells is the result of their drying, either before or after fixation, while in the case of squashes it is obtained by exerting pressure—often very firmly—perpendicular to the slide.

Squashes are suitable only for the study of the caryotype since cytoplasmic structures are almost entirely destroyed in the course of the preparation described below. Smears and imprints, on the other hand, conserve cytoplasmic structures as well as nuclear structures other than chromosomes.

Smears and imprints followed by immediate air drying are properly indicated only for Pappenheim's panoptic staining or similar procedures. They will hence be described in the chapter on haematological techniques. All other staining techniques, especially those meant for nuclear structures may be practised after fixation in osmic vapours. An essential condition for success is the rapidity of manipulation, since the osmium tetroxyde vapours should act before drying. The following technique gives satisfactory results.

A 2% aqueous solution of osmium tetroxyde is kept covered in a suitable vessel, such as a small Petri dish, whose height is such that the smears can be held in very close proximity to the fixative. The smear or imprint is made as rapidly as possible, but without brusqueness; liquids containing a suspension of cells may be smeared with a ground slide as described for the preparation of blood samples; often a drop may be sufficiently spread with a lancet; imprints are made by quickly applying the cut surface of an organ. Immediately, *and before any drying*, the vessel containing the fixative is uncovered and the slide held inverted over it so that not more than 1 or 2 mm separate the preparation from the surface of the liquid. The whole may be covered by a bell-jar. Fixation time, from 10 seconds to 2 or 3 minutes depending on the object, is determined by trial and error. If the cells are very fragile it is preferable to smear properly only after fixation; they may be only lightly spread at first with a needle to hasten contact of the cells with the osmium tetroxyde vapour.

In protistological work it can be useful to cover the slide with a very thin layer of Mayer's albumin to help adherence; this precaution is generally unnecessary for Metazoan cells.

The fixation with osmic vapours described above usually suffices before staining smears. However, the techniques destined for caryology give better results after an additional short fixation in Benda's solution, Bensley's solution or a mixture of equal parts of 6% mercuric chloride and 1% osmium tetroxyde (Apathy's solution). This treatment evidently in well-stoppered vessels, is carried out for a few minutes (10 at the most). The slides are then washed for ten minutes in several changes of distilled water followed by a period of about 30 minutes in 70° alcohol before staining.

Not all techniques of staining may be applied to smears treated in the above manner. In particular, aluminium lakes of haematin fare badly after treatment with osmic vapours. Among those that I suggest are staining with haematoxylin lakes as described in the previous chapter, the nucleal reaction of Feulgen and Rossenbeck with the hydrolysis time indicated on p. 553 for Flemming's solution, azur eosinates as described for haematological techniques, safranin-light green and gentian violet.

1° Staining of smears with safranin light green after Geitler (1940)

This technique differs slightly from that described for general methods and the reagents are the same as those for Benda's technique (p. 230).

Stain for 10 minutes on slides or in tubes, with the aqueous alcoholic solution of safranin.
Rinse rapidly in distilled water.
Rinse rapidly in 96° alcohol.
Differentiate and stain the background with a 1% alcoholic solution of light green (from 15 seconds to one minute).
Dehydrate in absolute alcohol, clear in a benzenic hydrocarbon and mount in a synthetic resin or Canada balsam.

Chromatin and the nucleoli stain red, the centrosome and fusorial spindle dark green and the cytoplasm a light green.

2° Staining of osmic smears with Gentian violet after Geitler (1940)

Stain for 10 minutes in a solution of gentian violet
    according to Gram: Distilled water saturated with anilin   100 ml
    Saturated solution of gentian violet in 96° alcohol ....   11 ml
Rinse in distilled water.
Treat for a few minutes in an iodine-iodide solution:
    Potassium iodide .... 2 g
    Iodine .... 1 g
    Distilled water .... 300 ml.
wash in 96° alcohol to remove all excess violet (about one or two minutes).
Dehydrate in absolute alcohol, clear in a benzenic hydrocarbon and mount in a synthetic resin or Canada balsam.

Chromatin takes an intense violet, nucleoli pale violet and the cytoplasm is much paler or even uncoloured.

NUCLEAR STRUCTURES IN SECTIONS

The importance of a clear demonstration of nuclei in any histological examination is such that the majority of the so-called topographic techniques have been devised with this requirement in view. All the methods described in the second part of this book will therefore serve this purpose. Some fixations and stains are nevertheles preferable to others.

Fixation may be carried out in alcoholic solutions; Clarke's and Carnoy's liquids generally give satisfactory results. However, aqueous liquids are to be preferred for fragile objects. Bouin's fluid is often suitable though Allen's modification of it, designated B15, is preferable in all cases destined for the nucleal stain of Feulgen and Rossenbeck. This liquid is prepared by fully dissolving 1,5 g of chromium trioxide in 100 ml of Bouin's fluid at 37°C followed by the addition of 2 g of urea. At least one dimension of the piece should be less than 3 mm and the period of fixation, effected at 37°C, should not exceed 2 hours. Pieces are then washed in 70° alcohol before dehydration and embedding. Sanfelice's fluid (p. 183) is also an excellent fixative for caryology. This is equally true for the fixations based on potassium dichromate mentioned in the table. Post-chromatization is obviously unnecessary. The superiority of chromo-osmic fixatives containing acetic acid (Table 26) is shown in studies of cell division where the faultless fixation of the cytoplasmic structures surrounding the chromosomes is of greater importance than in studies of the interphase nucleus. For this reason several authors advise the use of chromo-osmic fixations, even without acetic acid, particularly Champy's fluid. In this respect I should not fail to mention that chromo-osmic fixations ensure an excellent preparation of tissues for the nucleal stain of Feulgen and Rossenbeck.

Dehydration and embedding in paraffin does not call for any particular remark. Embedding in celloidin is rarely needed (very heterogeneous objects into which paraffin penetrates badly). Finesse is less exacting for sections than for the study of cytoplasmic structures.

Histochemical reactions can be very useful in caryological studies, with the nucleal *reaction* of Feulgen and Rossenbeck evidently heading the list. As practised according to the instructions given on p. 556 it ensures an excellent demonstration of chromatin and, furthermore, offers the advantage of a precise chemical signification for the shades obtained. Among the fixatives mentioned here Bouin's is the only one that is unsuitable for preparing tissues for this reaction. In addition quite mediocre results follow fixation in alcohol, acetone or formalin; but the use of these liquids is, in any case, not advised for caryological reserch. Staining with the chromic lake of gallocyanin also provides an excellent demonstration of nuclear structures in all cases when fixation has not been done in chromo-osmic liquids. The basic blues of the thiazine group (toluidine, azur etc.) are also recommended. The methyl-green-pyronin technique, whose advantages in the analysis of nuclear structures have been described on p. 547, can be adopted only after fixation in Clarke's or Carnoy's liquids, or after chromic fixatives without osmium tetroxyde.

Besides these histochemical reactions and indicative stains, regressive staining with haematoxylin lakes, especially the ferric ones, yields remarkably clear preparations that may be applied after all fixatives; Heidenhain's azan may however be practised only on sections of material that has neither been osmified nor post-chromatized. Safranin light green, according to the instructions on p. 230 and Ramon y Cajal's trichrome (p. 202) are also recommended. An excellent demonstration of nuclear structures is ensured by Flemming's triple stain described in the study of the centrosome.

PREPARATIONS FOR THE STUDY OF CARYOTYPE

Classical cytogenetic research has been carried out on preparations made in he manner just described and they remain useful in certain cases; besides them he study of tissue cultures, suitably fixed and treated by a nucleal reaction, is deal for the caryotype. But most of modern research involves different techniques where all cytoplasmic detail is deliberately sacrificed at the outset since the preparation of tissues is meant to dispose the chromosomes in an optical plane or even to swell them to facilitate their counting. This technique of preparing squashes consists of three stages, namely, the pretreatment of tissues, their proper preparation and the rendering of preparations permanent

Pretreatment of tissues varies according to the case, certain operations being principally aimed at increasing the number of cells in mitosis at the time of preparation. The recent work of Sharma and Sharma (1965) is amply documented on this subject which will not be envisaged here. Other procedures, meant to facilitate the separation of cells from each other, are left out as they are really useful only for plant cells. There remain finally the means of obtaining clearer images particularly by the destruction of cytoplasmic structures and the swelling of chromosomes. Among them, the treatment of fresh pieces in distilled water (Makino and Ishimara 1954) or in hypotonic sodium citrate (0,37%) is counselled by recent authors in all cases where chromosomes are numerous and small.

Fixation is effected by certain authors before preparing the squashes, others make both the operations coincide by squashing the fresh tissues in the fixative. Clarke's liquid or that of Carnoy can serve to fix tissues before squashing, but most authors prefer immersing in aceto-carmin or aceto-orcein for 10 minutes to several hours depending on the optimum time determined by trial and error for each object.

Of the formulae for aceto-carmin, that of Belling (1921) is the most employed. It consists of boiling a gram of carmin in 100 ml of 45% acetic for 30 minutes. to one hour in a pyrex flask to which a condenser or a long glass tube is atached. After cooling, the supernatant is decanted and filtered. This solution keeps very well. The aceto-carmin of Schneider (1930) differs from the above only by the use of more carmin (5 g) and one casts doubts on the need for this modification since the greater part of the solid remains undissolved in the flask.

Aceto-carmin is prepared by dissolving one or two grams of stain in 45 ml of acetic acid previously warmed to 60° and making up to 100 ml with distilled water after cooling. According to La Cour (1941), to whom the introduction of orcein in caryological technique is due, the strength of acetic acid can be increased up to 70%.

The actual *execution* of squashes consists in placing a morsel of tissue, either fresh or pretreated, in a drop of aceto-carmin or aceto-orcein on a slide very thinly coated with Mayer's albumin. A very lightly greased coverslip (by passing a finger on the forehead and smearing the little sebum thus removed on the lower surface of the coverslip) is laid over. The slide is placed on a pad of filter paper resting on a perfectly plane surface. A sheet of filter paper is placed on the coverslip and pressure is exerted across this with the inside of the thumb. The pressure varies according to the object and should often be quite strong, avoiding with great care the slightest lateral shear of the coverslip. The preparation may be examined under the microscope after brief cleaning of any overflow. Though it can be photographed there and then, it is preferable to render it permanent. Professor H. J. Guénin (Laboratory of Zoology, University of Lausanne), who has kindly taught me some of the tricks described above, suggests detaching the coverslip by holding the slide vertically in 70° alcohol followed by nuclear staining with haemalum or the reaction of Feulgen and Rossenbeck, the optimum time of hydrolysis being the same as that after fixation in Clarke's fluid. Obviously other nuclear stains can also be used. After staining the preparation is dehydrated in absolute alcohol, cleared in a benzenic hydrocarbon and mounted in Canada balsam or a synthetic resin.

The chromosomes are well spread in a plane and can be singled out in a successful preparation. Their details appear much more clearly than in sections. The photography of preparations of this type is very easy. It enables the measurement of the chromosomes and their alignment after cutting them out from prints.

PREPARATIONS FOR STUDYING THE SEX CHROMATIN

The studies of Barr and Bertram (1949) on the sex chromatin of the cat's neurone have led to considerable research which will not be discussed here; but from the methodological point of view it should be noted that the demonstration of the sex chromatin in human cells is now current practice and it plays a certain rôle in histopathological routine.

As Barr (1966) observes in a well documented review, the sex chromatin of the mammalian female is heteropycnotic (X-chromosome) and consequently all the techniques for staining chromatin and the histochemical reactions for deoxyribonucleic acid can be used for its detection. It may be aptly recalled that the discovery of the sex chromatin was made on preparations treated with cresyl violet to show nuclei and Nissl bodies.

The sex chromatin may be studied in smears, squashes or sections. Smears of the buccal or vaginal mucosa, of blood (for detecting "drumsticks" in neutrophil granulocytes), cutaneous biopsies and teased out amniotic membranes are commonly employed objects.

It is evident that fixation with osmic vapours, for smears, and with chromoosmic fixatives, for pieces, is quite unnecessary. Blood smears should be treated according to the technique of Pappenheim (panoptic staining of dry smears). Smears of buccal or vaginal mucous, made by scraping with the ground-glass tip of a rod or slide and spreading the sample on a slide, are usually fixed in a mixture of equal volumes of ethanol and ether for several hours, a period of fixation that would appear to be definitely too long. Davidson has proposed a fixative containing 30 ml of 96° alcohol, 20 ml of commercial formalin, 10 ml of acetic acid and 30 ml of distilled water, intended for pieces. It is obvious that all topographic fixatives are suitable and the opportuneness of inventing this mixture is questionable.

As for staining, the nucleal stain of Feulgen and Rossenbeck, gallocyanin, toluidine blue buffered at about pH 4.2 and azur A are advocated according to the procedures outlined in the other chapters of this book. I am including the description of a technique due to Klinger and Ludwig (1957) for the sake of information; but I must add that its results are not better than those given by the classical variants to the nucleal reaction of Feulgen and Rossenbeck.

> Fix in 96° alcohol for 30 minutes to 3 hours in the case of smears and thin embryonal membranes. Pieces are fixed in Davidson's fluid (see above) for 3 to 24 hours, dehydrated, embedded in paraffin without any special precaution and sectioned as usual. Smears, or paraffin sections duly deparaffined, collodioned and hydrated are treated as follows:
>
> Hydrolyse for 20 minutes in 5 N hydrochloric acid at room temperature.

Rinse carefully in distilled water.
Stain for 15 to 60 minutes in the following mixture:
>   Saturated solution of thionine in 50° alcohol .... 40 ml
>   Michaelis' buffer (sodium veronal, sodium acetate and hydrochloric acid) at pH 5.7 .... 60 ml

Wash in several changes of distilled water and then in 50° alcohol.
Extract excess of stain in 70° alcohol (until the emission of blue cloudiness in the alcohol bath ceases).
Dehydrate in absolute alcohol, clear in a benzenic hydrocarbon and mount in a synthetic resin or Canada balsam.

The sex chromatin appears a deep blue, and other chromosomes a light blue. The cytoplasm is usually uncoloured while fibrin and the metachromatic mucins range from red to violet.

MORPHOLOGICAL STUDY OF THE NUCLEOLUS

The vital examination of the nucleolus presents no technical difficulty. It is one of the easiest to observe among the fundamental organelles of the cell, and even the light field microscope often permits quite a detailed study if the cells chosen for examination in the fresh state are not too voluminous or not too rich in inclusions.

The demonstration of the nucleolus in permanent *preparations* is equally easy. All the fixatives reviewed elsewhere in this book and, *a fortiori* those intended for cytology fix this organelle and all stains allow, as it were, not only a study of its size and shape but also the observation of certain intranucleolar structures (vesicles, condensations) which can be of cytological interest. The high level of ribonucleic acid explains its strong basophily and hence the excellent demonstration by basic blues of the group of thiazines, gallocyanin, pyronin etc. But the associated basic proteins exhibit a strong affinity for acid stains and consequently most nucleoli take acid fuchsin whether anilinic or not, ponceau and azocarmine.

The real problem that arises in the study of the nucleolus has to do with the distinction between this organelle and the masses of chromatin (caryosomes, chromocentres etc.) endowed with the same basophilia. Under these conditions, the wealth of ribonucleoproteins in the nucleolus furnishes an excellent means of discrimination. Methyl-green-pyronin staining, applied after suitable fixation (p. 546), yields the most spectacular preparations conferring a red tint on the nucleoli which appears strikingly against the green of the chromatin. When the fixation stipulated for this staining, particularly that with Carnoy's fluid, has not been or cannot be applied then extraction of the ribonucleic acid with ribonuclease or by acid hydrolysis (p. 560–565) clears the doubt. In fact these tests suppress the basophilia of the nucleolus without interfering with that of the chromatin since deoxyribonucleic acid is not affected by ribonuclease and its depolymerization after short acid hydrolysis is insufficient for removal. Gallocyanin or toluidine blue stain only desoxyribonucleic acid under these conditions, while the basic proteins associated with the ribonucleic acid of the nucleolus can be stained red with eosin. It goes without saying that the nucleal reaction of Feulgen and Rossenbeck removes the last doubt in this respect, since the chromatin is red while the nucleolus takes the background stain (light green, the picric acid of picro-indigocarmine etc.)

Certain histochemical reactions can be useful in the cytological study of the nucleolus. Its reactivity to PAS has been reported as well as the high level of sulphydrylated proteins that it contains. Reactions that detect arginine and tyrosine often show nucleoli very clearly.

Filamentous structures called nucleolonema, described by Estable and Sotelo (1951, 1952), can be selectively demonstrated by the technique of silver impregnation and staining with iron-alum pyrogallol given below.

Silver impregnation of the nucleolonema.

Fix for 4 to 24 hours in the following mixture
- 96° alcohol .... 60 ml
- Distilled water .... 30 ml
- Formalin .... 5 ml
- Ether .... 5 ml
- Uranyl nitrate .... 1 g

The optimum time of fixation is determined by trial and error; it is usually less then 6 hours for animal tissues, and about 24 hours for plant tissues.

Rinse very rapidly in distilled water or merely wipe with a piece of filter paper.

Impregnate at 37° for 36 to 48 hours in the dark with a 1.5 to 2% aqueous solution of silver nitrate.

Wash for 3 to 5 minutes in 50° alcohol.

Reduce for 5 to 10 hours in the dark with the following mixture:
- Pyrogallol .... 1 g
- Commercial formalin .... 10 ml
- 96° alcohol .... 20 ml
- Distilled water .... 70 ml

Wash in two or three changes of distilled water for 10 minutes. Section in a freezing microtome or dehydrate and embed in paraffin (embedding in celloidin is possible but paraffin is required for the study of thin sections). Tone the colour (after deparaffining and hydration in the case of paraffin sections) with a 0.2% aqueous solution of gold chloride.

Rinse in distilled water.

Fix for about 10 minutes in a 3 or 5% aqueous solution of sodium thiosulfate (hyposulfite).

Dehydrate in absolute alcohol, clear in a benzenic hydrocarbon (adding a little creosote to the first bath if necessary) and mount in a synthetic resin or Canada balsam.

When the technical conditions have been suitably adopted to the material the result represents a very pure impregnation of the nucleolonema in black on a clear yellow background. As the authors of this technique have noted the change of colour with gold is not indispensable and can lead to attenuated impregnation. It is therefore advisable to follow it under the microscope and terminate as soon as the desired colour is attained by washing in distilled water.

As in most silver impregnations the outcome of the method is largely conditioned by the fixation. Estable and Sotelo report that the presence of ether and the maintenance of alcohol above 50° in the fixative have the effect of preventing the simultaneous impregnation of nucleolonema and the Golgi apparatus. When the ether is omitted from the mixture and the quantity of alcohol reduced to 30 ml with a corresponding increase of water to maintain the total volume constant, simultaneous impregnation is obtained in all cases, which is advantageous for certain investigations. Simultaneous impregnation of the nucleolonema and neurofibrils can be obtained in favourable cases by omitting ether and increasing alcohol.

Staining of nucleolonema by the pyrogallol—iron method (Estable and Soleto). — This technique is based on the fact that in the presence of a ferric salt pyrogallol gives a blue—black precipitate on the addition of a ferrous salt to the medium.

> Paraffin sections of material fixed in formalin, Sanfelice's fluid or any other fixative based on chromium trioxide, are deparaffined and hydrated.
> Immerse sections for at least 10 minutes in a 3% aqueous solution of iron alum.
> Rinse rapidly in distilled water.
> Immerse sections in an aqueous solution of potassium ferricyanide (the concentration of this solution is not indicated in the original description; I have obtained good results with a 1% solution).
> After a lapse of 30 seconds a few drops of a 2% aqueous solution of pyrogallol are added (8 to 10 drops per Borrel cylinder); staining is almost instantaneous).
> Wash in tap water.
> Dehydrate in absolute alcohol, clear in a benzenic hydrocarbon and mount in a syntheic resin or Canada balsam.
> The nucleolonema appears a very dark blue that is almost black.

DEMONSTRATION OF INTRANUCLEAR INCLUSIONS DIFFERENT FROM THE NUCLEOLE

"Intranuclear" inclusions that differ both from the chromatin and the nucleolus have been described in a great variety of normal and pathological cells. But no study of these structures as a whole has been made by classical authors, and modern work with histochemical techniques and infrastructural cytology has led to the negation of the truly intranuclear character of several of these inclusions.

The disparate nature of the cytological studies with the light microscope concerning the intranuclear inclusions treated in this paragraph renders the codification of the procedures of detection very difficult. Two cases may be distinguished schematically, namely the spherical, ellipsoïdal or irregular inclusions and the erythrophilous crystalloids.

Non-cristalloid inclusions have been described from preparations obtained after topographic or cytological fixation and a wide variety of stains and histochemical reactions. One of their essential traits is the great similarity of their behaviour towards histological reagents with that of the perinuclear regions of the cytoplasm or of the perinuclear granules. This fact suffices to cast doubt on the truly intranuclear nature of these formations, the more so as they are often observed in pleomorphic nuclei with very irregular contours. When the study bears on objects particularly favoured by their size and cytological peculiarities, the light microscope is sufficient to show that the structures at issue are really cytoplasmic invaginations. The electron microscope has provided proof in other cases up to now. In other words, the study of this type of apparently intranuclear inclusion does not raise any real technical problem.

Erythrophilous crystalloids have been described in a few objects of remarkable zoological diversity ranging from Mammals to Protists. They represent an entity characterized by the geometrical shape of the inclusions, whose truly intranuclear localization has never been disproved, their tinctorial affinities and their histochemical features.

These formations may be conserved by the so-called topographic fixatives, but it is the cytological fixations reviewed in chapter 23 that afford the best prelude to embedding in paraffin. Chromo-osmic fluids are not indispensable; quite satisfactory results are obtained with fixatives based on potassium dichromate and lacking acetic acid. Even those containing the latter acid can conserve intranuclear crystalloids but with considerable deformation.

As their name indicates, these inclusions strongly take certain red stains such as eosin and erythrosin, ponceau and aqueous or anilin acid fuchsin. Basic fuchsin and azocarmine also stain them. Intranuclear crystalloids are highly siderophilous and stain well with iron—haematoxylin. Good detection is afforded by azan, Heidenhain's haematoxylin, the trichrome of Ramon y Cajal, methyl-blue-eosin according to Mann, Altmann's fuchsin and by the trichromes of Masson and of Gomori. Safranin—light-green shows them up in red.

As for their histochemical characteristics certain methods of amino-acid detection such as the alloxan—Schiff reactions, the coupled tetrazonium reaction of Danielli and the detection of sulfhydrylated proteins with DDD according to Barrnett and Seligman yield results with a precision that is not less than that of the stainings enumerated above (Arvy, Bassot and Gabe, 1963).

CHAPTER 25

TECHNIQUES FOR DEMONSTRATING THE GOLGI APPARATUS

Of all the fundamental organelles of the cell it is probably the Golgi apparatus (Golgi bodies, dictyosomes) that has nourished the most passionate discussion, but these controversion were principally over the interpretation of preparations. The technique of demonstrating this particular organelle has been masterly codified by Bowen (1928) and since then there have been few examples of technical advance destined for light microscopy (silver impregnation according to Aoyama (1941), Sudan black according to Baker (1941), direct silver impregnation following Elftman (1952). The advent of the electron microscope brought to an end the sterile discussions concerning the very existence of the Golgi apparatus, of its relation to the "vacuome" etc. From the technical point of view the electron microscope has deprived detection of the Golgi apparatus in paraffin sections of almost all interest.

In fact the methods of detecting the Golgi apparatus under the light microscope are based on metal impregnations whose capriciousness should be emphasized. No worker is sure of succeeding at the first attempt even with material of his own choice, and the most experienced cytologist can give up before one that is imposed. The techniques that I am referring to are devoid of any specificity and can impregnate other organelles, metalliferous inclusion and metabolic products. The interpretation of preparations requires great experience and a solid knowledge of the other organelles of the cell. Under the electron microscope, however, the unambiguous identification of the ultrastructural equivalents of the Golgi apparatus is disarmingly easy. The number of cytological studies devoted to this organelle before and after the introduction of ultrastructural techniques is eloquent testimony of this. What is more, experience has shown that the analysis of a single optical plane, such as is seen under the electron microscope, usually suffices for the study of the morphological features of the Golgi apparatus, so that the examination of thicker sections as practised in light microscopy offers no further advantage.

Consequently the role of metal impregnation of the Golgi apparatus in modern cytological technique is quite restricted. Apart from particular cases such as when preparing material for teaching or in the event of the practical impossibility of electron microscopy, the techniques described in this chapter should be considered as musical "scales"; they are part of the education of every genuine cytologist, but are hardly ever needed in research.

Vital observation of the Golgi apparatus is easy even without resorting to the phase—contrast or interferential microscope if favorable objects are chosen such as the cells of the germinal line of the snail, its salivary glands or multifid gland, the mammalian pancreas etc. Dahlia, neutral red and methylene blue have had a certain amount of success among the *vital stains*; they were either injected into the animal or as in the case of aquatic animals added to the external medium or in low concentrations to the physiological solution used for mounting preparations. It should be noted that none of these vital stains is "specific" for the Golgi apparatus and the results obtained with neutral red have led to sharp controversy and it is now only of historical interest.

Fixation of the Golgi apparatus is easier than that of the other organelles, especially the chondriome. The usual precautions concerning the freshness of the material remain valid, but are less exacting than during the preparation of tissues for mitochondrial stains. Pieces should be quite small not exceeding 3 mm in at least one side. As for the choice of fixatives all solutions containing neither alcohol nor acetic acid conserve the Golgi apparatus, but metal impregnation requires certain fixatives rather than others. I might point out that "negative" images of the Golgi apparatus are often obtained after cytological fixation with stains that impart very intense colours to the cytoplasm.

OSMIC IMPREGNATION

Osmic impregnation of the Golgi apparatus is usually considered as the best of the metallic impregnations not only because of the optical quality of the demonstration but especially because it may be adopted after the best cytological fixations.

As noted by Bowen (1928) osmic impregnation was first used by A. Prenant (1888) for studying the Golgian structures in the parasomes of snail gonocytes. But it was Kopsch (1902) who codified this technique and showed its equivalence with the silver impregnation practised by Golgi (1898). Kopsch used the formalin dichromate fixative named after him (Table 27). The advantages of chromo-osmic fixation have been recognised by Weigl (1910) whose method includes fixation in Mann's fluid (a mixture of equal parts of saturated mercuric chloride and 1% osmium tetroxide). In this connection, Bowen rightly points out the unfairness, widespread among American authors, of designations of this technique as the Mann-Kopsch method. Following the work of Kolatschew (1916) and of Nassonov (1923) it is Champy's fluid (or Nassonov's modification of it) that has been adopted by almost all cytologists.

Its practice consists of the following steps:

Fix fresh pieces of very small dimensions in Champy's or Nassonov's fluid at room temperature. The classical authors allow a fixation time of up to a week, but nothing at all is gained after the first 24 hours, and I do not advise it unless in case of absolute necessity.

Wash thoroughly in running water. This is one of the essential steps of the technique since the persistence of the slightest trace of potassium dichromate or chromium trioxide is a sure cause of failure. The advice given in the first part of this book applies particularly to the osmic impregnation of the Golgi apparatus. It consists in leaving the washed pieces covered with tap water which should remain colourless at the end of two to three hours.

Impregnate with a 1% aqueous solution of osmium tetroxide in an oven at 37°. The condition of the pieces is verified every day and the solution renewed if it darkens before the fourth day. The optimal period of impregnation cannot be foreseen and should be adjusted in all cases according to the indications given in the following paragraphs.

Wash for a few hours in running water.

Dehydrate rapidly, impregnate with Cedarwood oil and embed in paraffin.

Make thin sections and mount after deparaffining or hydrate, bleach if desired, give a background stain and mount in Canada balsam or a synthetic resin.

In successful preparations mounted without background stain the Golgi apparatus is seen in black against pale yellow or grey. Osmophilic lipids that darken during the early stages of impregnation often lose their colour after the fifth day in the oven. Other cell organelles are conserved and may be seen in preparations mounted without background stain. They may obviously be stained.

Apart from the thorough removal of the last traces of potassium dichromate and chromium trioxide success of impregnation depends on the length of stay in the solution of osmium tetroxide. Some authors suggest the daily removal, from the fourth day onwards, of a very small fragment which is squashed in a drop of glycerol and examined under the microscope to check the blackening of the Golgi apparatus while the background should not be too dark. Others prefer to impregnate concomitantly a number of pieces and to remove an entire piece every day after the fifth day. One rarely needs to go beyond the ninth day of impregnation.

I must not fail to mention that pieces submitted to the above treatment become very brittle. They should be handled with care, and Cedarwood oil is an indispensable step between dehydrations in alcohol and embedding in paraffin. The cutting of sections is difficult and softening the paraffin blocks by soaking in water is often necessary.

There is no means of rectifying an insufficient impregnation on sections, but the type of fixation usually renders them suitable for demonstrating other fundamental organelles. Excessive impregnation either obscures the background or produces troublesome black precipitates. Such excess may be repaired by **bleaching** which is, in fact, oxidation of the sections. Three agents have been used to this effect; turpentine, hydrogen peroxide and potassium permanganate.

Bleaching with turpentine is intended for destaining structural lipids blackened by a deposit of osmium. The deparaffined slide is transferred from the benzene hydrocarbon solvent to turpentine and left for 15 minutes to 24 or even 48 hours. It is periodically examined under the microscope and the process terminated by washing in the solvent as soon as the desired degree of bleaching is attained. Slides may then be mounted directly or submitted to background staining. Priority for this technique, highly recommended by Cramer (1919), Gatenby (1921) and Ludford (1921), should be accorded to Bergen (1904).

Bleaching with hydrogen peroxide suggested by Kopsch (1925, 1926) is very rapid and its execution requires constant attention. After deparaffining and hydration the slides are dipped in a very dilute solution of hydrogen peroxide which is prepared by adding a few drops of peroxide at 10 volumes (usually 4 or 5 drops) to 100 ml of distilled water. In the majority of cases the desired result is obtained in 15 seconds to one minute. Washing in tap water stops bleaching and the sections can be either dehydrated, cleared and mounted, or submitted to background staining.

Bleaching with potassium permanganate, which is the cytological application of a technique destined for other purposes by Lustgarten (1884) is highly recommended by Bowen (1928). Deparaffined and hydrated sections are treated with a 0.1% aqueous solution of potassium permanganate. They take a brownish yellow tint and the result is almost as rapid as with hydrogen peroxide. Washing in distilled water stops the process and the slides are passed, until destaining (for a few seconds to one minute) through a 0.1% solution of oxalic acid or a 2% solution of sodium metabisulfite. Thorough washing in tap water eliminates all traces of these reagents and the slides may then be dehydrated and mounted or further stained.

I must remark here that bleaching as described above plays a certain role in the demonstration of chondriome. It is besides useful in all cases where the overall staining of sections fixed in chromo-osmic fixatives is too dark (especially with caryological stains).

Among the possible background stains after osmic impregnation of the Golgi apparatus I particularly suggest the nucleal reaction of Feulgen and Rossenbeck (hydrolysis time as after a simple fixation in Champy's fluid), safranin light green (p. 230) and the mitochondrial stains according to Nassonov, Benoît or Kull (p. 730). The black colour of the Golgi apparatus explains why staining with ferric haematoxylin, though technically possible, is not quite indicated.

The practical advantages of the osmic impregnation of the Golgi apparatus thus lie in the quality of the fixation which enables sections to be recuperated from material whose impregnation has failed as well as the possibility of rectifying excessive impregnation. The conservation of the other organelles allows this technique in conjunction with other stains or histochemical reactions which finally provide very demonstrative synthetic preparations. As for its disadvantages, the chief one is that of its irregularity. In the best of cases impregnation succeeds only in a narrow band of tissue, the periphery being overfixed and overimpregnated with the center underfixed and unimpregnated. The requirement of a very small size of pieces is more exacting than with silver impregnations and the cost of preparations is greater.

SILVER IMPREGNATION

Silver impregnation is in fact at the origin of the discovery of the "apparato reticolare interno" as a fundamental organelle of the animal cell. It was by means of the silver chromate method (*reazione nera*) that Golgi (1898) obtained the very first pictures. But this technique gives very variable results just as a silver impregnation after fixation with arsenious anhydride, also due to Golgi. The most frequently practised of the silver impregnation techniques are those of Ramon y Cajal (1915) with uranyl nitrate, of Da Fano (1920) with cobalt nitrate, of Aoyama (1929) with cadmium chloride and of Elftman (1952) with silver nitrate.

All these processes are bulk impregnations, which is also the case for osmic impregnations, but the latter is preceded by an excellent cytological fixation and the deposits of osmium are easy to remove from the sections, silver impregnations on the other hand require fixatives that conserve other organelles badly and it is difficult to get rid of silver nitrate deposits. Moreover they leave the tissue badly fixed with their histochemical properties and affinities for stains considerably altered. These drawbacks are countered by the greater rapidity and cheaper cost of the method. In practice the technique of Ramon y Cajal and that of Da Fano differ only in the composition of the fixative; both can thus be described together.

Techniques of Ramon y Cajal (uranyl nitrate) and of Da Fano (cobalt nitrate).

Pieces not exceeding 2 to 3 mm in one dimension are fixed in Ramon y Cajal's fluid containing uranyl nitrate or Da Fano's fluid containing cobalt nitrate (Table 28); the period of fixation suggested by different authors varies from 6 to 24 hours, and all insist on the need for adjusting this by trial and error according to the material. The simplest procedure is to fix several pieces at a time for different periods. Fixing at 37°C is deplored and the majority of authors fix at room temperature; from my experience fixing at about 10°C gives very good results.

Rinse rapidly for a few seconds in distilled water.

Impregnate for at least 24 hours, or 48 hours at the most, in the dark in a 0.75–1.5% aqueous solution of silver nitrate. The use of a 1% solution may be adopted as standard procedure. As in the case of fixation I advise a temperature of about 10°C rather than room temperature.

Wash thoroughly in distilled water. Opinions differ as to the period of washing, and the majority of handbooks propose a rapid one of a few seconds to a minute. However following Gatenby (1919) and Brambell (1925) I advise 15 to 45 minutes in distilled water changed three or four times. It is useful to check that the last wash no longer precipitates with the reducing agent.

Reduce for at least 8 hours with the following solution that should be freshly prepared:

Distilled water .... 85 ml
Formalin (neutralized) .... 15 ml
Hydroquinone .... 1 g

Anhydrous sodium sulfite (added sufficiently to give a light yellow colour).

Pieces may be left in the fluid for longer. The presence of formalin helps conservation and the silver nitrate that has not been reduced in the first eight hours does not risk being reduced in three or four days.

Remove excess of reducing agent by washing in running water.

Dehydrate, embed in paraffin and make thin sections of not more than 5 μ.

Deparaffin, collodion if necessary and hydrate the sections.

The success of impregnation may be judged by observation at this stage.

Tone for one or two minutes (until disappearance of the brownish background) with a 0.2% aqueous solution of gold chloride.

Rinse in distilled water.

Fix for 30 seconds to a minute in a 1% aqueous solution of sodium thiosulfate.

Wash for two to five minutes in running water.

Stain the background or dehydrate, clear and mount in Canada balsam or a commercial synthetic resin.

In successful preparations only the Golgi apparatus appears black against a background that is yellowish before toning or colourless to pale grey after toning.

Among background stains I especially recommend Ramon y Cajal's trichrome, safranin-light green, hemalum-picro-indigocarmin and azan. The nucleal reaction of Feulgen and Rossenbeck is technically possible but it should be confined only to well fixed pieces. The chondriomes are, as a rule, well conserved and they may be stained with Altmann's fuchsin if impregnation of the Golgi apparatus is very pure. The majority of secretory granules are equally well conserved and may also be stained, but it should not be forgotten that the above treatment considerably modifies the usual tinctorial affinities of the organelles.

There is no convenient means of rectifying excessive impregnation. Bleaching with permanganate or with Farmer's mixture though theoretically feasible, are in fact methods that do not discriminate between undesirable precipitates and the deposit of metallic silver that demonstrates the Golgi apparatus. The risk of diffuse precipitation is a major drawback and such precipitates obviously indicate failure of the silver impregnations described here. In any case, only a strip of tissue flanked by an outer over-impregnated shell and a central poorly impregnated, or even unimpregnated, core is fit for examination.

The best way to avoid such precipitates is to carefully adjust the periods of fixation and washing before and after impregnation with silver nitrate. I must recall that even the greatest care in these steps will not prevent the blackening of calcium phosphate and carbonate deposits found in sections. This is of no consequence if the deposits are intercellular but can be very troublesome if intracellular. Similarly a slight blackening or granular precipitation in collagen fibres can hardly be avoided.

Technique of Aoyama (Cadmium chloride). — Aoyama has suggested replacing uranyl or cobalt nitrate with cadmium chloride for its better penetration and greater stability in the solid state which enables the preparation of well-defined fixatives. The inclusion of chloride ions in the fixative evidently requires that impregnation be preceded by thorough washing in distilled water; this simple precaution seems to have been overlooked by the author of the method and by others who have described the technique.

> Fix pieces of small dimensions at room temperature for three to four hours in the solution given in Table 28.
> Wash thoroughly for three to five minutes in several changes of distilled water.
> Impregnate in the dark at room temperature in a 1% solution of silver nitrate for up to 10 or 15 hours.
> Wash thoroughly in many changes of distilled water. Aoyama suggests a rapid wash in two changes of distilled water, but the earlier remarks concerning other silver impregnation techniques of the Golgi apparatus are evidently applicable to the present case.
> Reduce for five to ten hours, at room temperature, with the agent as described in the techniques of Ramon y Cajal or of da Fano. Wash in tap water and proceed as in the techniques of Ramon y Cajal or of da Fano.
> The preparations cannot be distinguished from those provided by other techniques of silver impregnation of the Golgi apparatus. In my experience the method gives very satisfactory results but I am not convinced of its superiority over that of da Fano which I recommend whenever small quantities of the analytical grade of cobalt nitrate are available.

Technique of Elftman (Silver nitrate). — The originality of this technique, pleasing in its simplicity, lies in the use of a fixative based on silver nitrate so that its capacity to denature tissue proteins and its affinity for the Golgi apparatus are availed of concomitantly. This method has given me very satisfactory results with the tissues of the rat and albino mice, but it does not yet seem to have been applied to Invertebrates.

> Fix small pieces, for two to three hours, at room temperature in the dark in the following solution:
>   Neutralized formalin .... 10 ml
>   distilled water .... 90 ml
>   silver nitrate .... 2 g
> Rinse *rapidly* in distilled water.
> Reduce for two hours at room temperature in the following mixture:
>   neutralized formalin .... 15 ml
>   distilled water .... 85 ml
>   hydroquinone .... 2 g
> Wash in tap water.
> Refix if necessary for about ten hours in 10% formalin.
> Dehydrate, embed in paraffin and proceed as for the other silver impregnation techniques of the Golgi apparatus. In successful preparations the Golgi apparatus appears black on the pale yellow background.

CHOICE BETWEEN OSMIC AND SILVER IMPREGNATIONS

Silver impregnation is well adapted for mammalian tissues and is excellent for certain tissues of air-breathing gasteropods, but unsuitable for marine Invertebrates. Osmic impregnation has no such limitations. Silver techniques are rapid and cheaper than osmic ones; they are hence convenient for teaching purposes, where the quality of fixation is of less importance since preparations showing several organelles are not really desirable. In all cases of rare material the osmic techniques should be preferred since unsuccessful impregnation does not necessarily mean loss of the piece which can be bleached if overimpregnated. Complete decoloration by other means can be easily achieved on osmic preparations, while they are laborious and unsuitable for silver impregnated pieces.

DEMONSTRATION OF THE GOLGI APPARATUS BY STAINING OR HISTOCHEMICAL REACTIONS

A classical example of the demonstration of the Golgi apparatus is the staining of the acroblast of spermatids with light green and related stains. A PAS positive reaction has been reported for the Golgi apparatus of intestinal cells, and they have also been demonstrated by reduction of the silver alkaline complex after chromic or periodate oxydation (Arzac and Flores, 1951). The Golgi apparatus of the sympathetic ganglional cells of the rabbit and of intestinal cells may be detected in frozen sections by staining with black Sudan B (Baker 1941). But these are special cases and the methods have not been extended to other material so that it is difficult to afford any opinion as to its generalization.

CHAPTER 26

TECHNIQUES FOR DEMONSTRATING THE CHONDRIOME

Of all the fundamental organelles of the animal cell it is probably the chondriome that raises the most difficult problems with respect to fixation and staining for light microscopy. Mitochondrial fixation is indeed the most exacting as to the freshness of samples and tolerates the least delay between removal and the time of contact between fixative and organelle. Mitochondrial staining also, though not really difficult, requires that a certain number of precautions be taken. This explains why investigations involving the demonstration of the chondriome have been relatively rare before the advent of the electron microscope.

In fact, if the technical difficulty of demonstrating the chondriome for the light microscope were to be compared to that for the electron microscope the former is equalled only by that encountered with the Golgi apparatus. This is clearly illustrated by the recent proliferation of studies on the chondriome carried out solely by means of electron micrographs.

However, the demonstration of the chondriome by classical techniques still carries a certain interest which is no longer so for the Golgi apparatus. In fact only the electron microscope provides information about the internal structure of the chondriomes; even modern histoenzymological techniques, especially the demonstration of dehydrogenases and specific diaphorases mostly localized in these organelles, do not seem to have borne out the expectations of Pearse (1960, p. 572–573). However, the general arrangement of the chondriome within the cell is even now of considerable importance for certain histophysiological studies and this disposition appears much better in preparations for light microscopy than in electron micrographs. Mitochondrial techniques therefore continue to be an important means of research and the cytologist finds occasion to apply them more often than the metal impregnations of the Golgi apparatus.

I must recall, to avoid possible confusion, that the classical terminology is adopted here; the term *chondriome* collectively designates all the *chondriosomes* of the cell, these chondriosomes being either the elongated *chondrioconts* or the spherical *mitochondria*. To my mind there is no valid reason for attributing a generic meaning to the term "mitochondrion" that was never implied in the ideas of its creator, Benda (1901, 1903). Indeed the term was invented with a precise morphological acceptation.

Vital observation of the chondriome, practised long since by classical authors on the elements of the amphibian and gastropod seminal lines, and on chondroblasts has been rendered much easier by the progress of phase contrast and interferential microscopy. Fibroblast cultures are particularly suited and the excellent cinematographic records made by Chèvremont and Frederic (1952) and Frederic and Chèvremont (1952) clearly illustrate the scope of the method when it is applied to favorable material.

Vital staining of the chondriome has also played an important role in gaining knowledge of this organelle; it still can be of great help in such studies. Early authors suggested Dahlia violet for this purpose, but the investigations of Michaelis (1900) have shown that Janus green (diazine green) is much better and indeed heads the list of all vital stains for chondriosomes; demonstration of affinity for the latter stain, *under vital conditions*, amounts in practice to formal proof of the mitochondrial nature of the stained organelle. Only the detection in electron micrographs of the ultrastructural characteristics of chondriosomes is superior to a demonstration by vital staining with Janus green.

The striking specificity of vital staining with Janus green for chondriosomes has led to several attempts at interpretation. Most modern authors admit the hypothesis of Lazarow and Cooperstein (1953) according to whom this selectivity is really due to the living processes that occur in the cell. Indeed, Janus green shows no affinity whatever for fixed chondriosomes while it stains, in sections, a wide range of cell constituents which are rich in proteins. Lazarow and Cooperstein thus admit, basing themselves on the findings of Michaelis (1900, 1901, 1903) and of Fischer (1927) as well as on their own data, that the Janus green absorbed by all cell constituents is rapidly reduced to the colourless leucobase except in the chondriosomes where the cytochrome-oxidase/cytochrome C system maintains it in the oxidized state.

In practice Janus green can be used in various ways. Freshly removed tissues are placed on slides and brought into contact with a very dilute solution of the dyestuff (0,005 to 0,01%) in a physiological liquid, left in a moist chamber for 10 to 20 minutes, and then covered with a coverslip which is sealed with vaseline before examining under the microscope. A technique that has been devised for hematological use often gives very good results on isolated cells or loose tissue. Slides are coated with a very thin layer of the following solution.

```
Absolute or 96% alcohol ........................................ 2 ml
0.1–0.5% solution of Janus green in absolute or 96% alcohol ..... 1 ml
0.5% solution of neutral red in absolute or 96% alcohol .......... 1 ml
```

A drop of this mixture is spread in the manner of a blood smear (see p. 788); slides thus prepared may be stored after drying. For vital examination the cells to be studied are placed in the observation medium (blood of the animal, physiological liquid etc...) on a coverslip and the coverslip inverted over the layer of dyestuff and sealed to the slide. This procedure invented for hematology (Sabin and Doan 1929, Seeberg 1930) gives excellent results not only with blood but also with all tissues whose cells can be easily dissociated (e. g. Invertebrate gonads).

As I have remarked in the first part of this book, the pancreas of the mouse is an exceptionally favorable material for vital observation and for vital staining of the chondriome since it can be studied while all the vascular and nervous connections of the gland are maintained. Covell (1926) and Hirsch (1931 to 1933) have codified the technique following the works of Kühne and Lea (1889). The animal, anaesthetized under ether or a barbiturate, is placed on an upper stage carrying a glass window about 1 mm thick and placed to coincide with the window of the actual stage of the microscope. The spleen is extruded through a left sub-costal incision; its ablation, after ligaturing the splenic vessels, greatly facilitates the rest of the operation. The tail of the pancreas is spread with the greatest care using a strip of filter-paper moistened with physiological liquid. A solution of Janus green in physiological liquid, whose concentration may be as much as 0.1%, is placed with the help of a drop-bottle over the stretched pancreas. After five or ten minutes of exposure to air a ring of vaseline is laid over the preparation which is then covered with a coverslip. The height of the observation chamber can be adjusted by exerting very mild pressure on the coverslip, and a small quantity of physiological liquid may be added to make up for loss by evaporation. Under proper anaesthesia observation may be prolonged for hours, and photomicrographs taken in selected thin zones do not differ in sharpness from those of classical mitochondrial stains. This experiment is obviously of considerable value in teaching.

Making permanent mitochondrial preparations includes three steps, namely, fixation which is meant to conserve the chondriome as close to the living state, treatment aimed at imparting tinctorial affinities to the chondriosomes and, finally, the mitochondrial staining itself.

MITOCHONDRIAL FIXATIONS

A large body of research involving various techniques has shown that the chondriome is the most fragile of all the fundamental organelles of the cell. Its morphology is altered when the cell is placed under abnormal conditions, although under the same conditions the morphological features of other cell organelles remain quite normal. This extreme fragility of the chondriosomes bears on the procedure of fixation meant to demonstrate this particular organelle in tissues.

The greatest possible rapidity is required in removing samples. It is indeed better to abandon any morphological study of the chondriome if the delay between death and removal of the sample exceeds about ten minutes, especially in the case of homeothermic animals. Thus it is practically impossible for a histologist to successfully remove single-handed all the organs of a mammal larger than, for instance, an albino rat. Several persons would have to share the task of removing the various organs, according to a plan laid beforehand, of a medium sized dog if it is intended to fix for demonstrating chondriome. Such an operation cannot therefore be easily carried out in a slaughterhouse, and I do not think myself rash in venturing that the pancreatic chondriome of the blue whale will never be properly demonstrated.

If the organs are to be sliced it should be done with a sharp blade, without any undue force and rather by a sawing-movement than by pressure on the piece. In the case of fixation without osmium tetroxyde one dimension of the piece should not exceed 3 mm; with fixatives containing this compound even pieces of 2 mm thickness show mediocre fixation in the centre.

It has been classically maintained that acidity of the fixative brings about destruction of the chondriome, but recent experimental data casts doubt on this axiom. Indeed the classical work of Zirkle (1928) recalled in the general comments on fixation, indicates the part played by the anion of the fixative agent in the conservation of organelles. Following this, Casselman and Gordan (1954) were able to show that *certain* chondriomes can be conserved and stained properly after fixing tissues in 0.1 N hydrochloric acid; other acids are less suitable, while yet others destroy all chondriomes even though the pH of the "fixative" liquid is clearly higher than that of one-tenth normal hydrochloric acid. This confirms an old fact well established from experiences, namely, that acetic acid is more harmful to chondriomes than trichloracetic acid. From the practical point of view the deleterious affect of acetic acid, which according to the above notion should be attributed to the acetyl ion rather than to the final pH of the fixative, should be stressed, and no liquid containing acetic acid should be used if mitochondrial staining is envisaged.

Ethyl alcohol, methyl alcohol and acetone are also equally harmful; only fixation by chemical agents in an aqueous medium ensure proper conservation of chondriomes.

These factors guide the operator in the choice of fixative mixtures; of the chromo-osmic mixtures (Table 26) those that contain appreciable quantities of acetic acid are to be peremptorily eliminated, and it is better to avoid even the ones that contain small quantities although most chondriomes do withstand their action. The best fixatives of this class are those that do not contain any acetic acid at all. In the relevant paragraph of chapter 23 I have expressed my personal preference for the liquids of Altmann and of Benoît which do not contain chromium trioxyde and hence allow the potassium dichromate to manifest all its qualities as a cytoplasmic fixative.

Fixatives based on potassium dichromate and formalin, with or without mercuric chloride, are quite suitable. They penetrate much better than the chromo-osmic liquids, produce more homogeneous fixation and enable better embedding in paraffin.

In addition to their intrinsic qualities, their cheaper cost renders them preferable to chromo-osmic mixtures in all cases where abundant lipid structures in the cell would otherwise favour the use of the latter. I have already noted that the liquids of Orth, of Kopsch and of Regaud give strictly equivalent results, that Kolster's liquid is a remarkable fixative for chondriomes and that, to me, Helly's or Maximow's liquids can be recommended specially for cells very rich in secretory granules, which are always better conserved by fixatives containing mercuric chloride.

Fixatives which are specially meant for demonstrating the Golgi apparatus by silver impregnation also conserve the chondriomes, but their use gives no particular advantage over the mixtures mentioned above.

Saline formalin and formaldehyde-calcium are excellent fixatives of the chondriome and can be used to this effect, but their disadvantage lies in a mediocre fixation of nuclear structures and a poor preparation for paraffin embedding.

They are evidently required before the silver impregnation of chondriomes in frozen sections. The formalin which is to be diluted to prepare these solutions should obviously be neutralized with care as formic acid is almost as harmful as acetic acid to the chondriomes. The good quality of fixation of the chondriomes by formalin does necessarily mean that mitochondrial staining can be carried out on formalin-treated material under the technical conditions of pathological practice; all the precautions concerning the rapidity of removing pieces and their dimensions should be observed even with formalin fixation when the aim of the study is to demonstrate the chondriomes.

It should be added that freezing-drying *can* ensure impeccable conservation of the chondriomes, although it does not follow automatically and it is in no way superior to the very good fixations by chemical agents. Similarly, sections of fresh tissue made in a cryostat and fixed for a short time in formaldehyde-calcium give a good demonstration of chondriomes if the precautions concerning the dimensions of pieces and the rapidity of cooling mentioned in the relevant chapter of the first part of this book are observed; it need hardly be remarked that this is, however, a rather rare eventuality.

Chromo-osmic fixations for mitochondrial staining should be carried out at room temperature. Other fixative mixtures discussed here may be advantageously, though not necessarily, cooled to about 4°C and maintained at this temperature during the first hours of fixation.

On the whole, fixation at room temperature in a chromo-osmic mixture without acetic acid is recommended when the piece can be easily cut into thin slices and when one seeks faultless conservation of all cell organelles but is prepared to pay the price of some irregularity in fixation. Kolster's liquid or that of Regaud and its equivalents are normally chosen when the study is mainly directed to the chondriome, while saline-formalin or formaldehyde calcium can be used with good effect in all cases where a demonstration of the chondriome is the only concern since caryological techniques may not be applied to such material.

I might note in passing that glutaraldehyde fixation is of not negligible interest in preparing for mitochondrial staining. This compound, introduced into electron microscopy by Sabatini and co-workers (1963), enjoys a well merited vogue in this field. Unpublished trials, carried out in collaboration with J. M. Bassot, have shown that glutaraldehyde possesses the same advantages and disadvantages as osmium tetroxyde for investigations in classical cytology; association with formalin and with mercuric acetate has shown itself to be particularly advantageous for mitochondrial fixation.

PREPARATION OF PIECES FOR MITOCHONDRIAL STAINING

The operations to which pieces meant for mitochondrial staining are to be submitted vary according to the fixative used and hence it is necessary to consider successively different particular cases.

Formalin-treated pieces meant for silver impregnation on frozen sections may be conserved in the fixative. I must recall that formaldehyde penetrates quickly but fixes slowly; a minimum of 48 hours must lapse before cutting sections and there is no harm in extending this delay considerably. The advisability of storing all pieces in formalin in darkness has already been pointed out several times.

Material fixed in chromo-osmic mixtures or in Kolster's liquid should be washed after 24 hours of fixation; certain authors admit to the possibility of a longer stay of pieces in fixatives containing osmium tetroxyde but I advise against it in all cases.

The washing in running water or frequently renewed tap-water after fixation should be thorough; it is of great importance to get rid of all trace of fixative before starting to dehydrate pieces; washing in running water is hence preferably followed by leaving pieces in a vessel full of tap-water in order to ensure that the last wash remains uncoloured.

It is common to recall that pieces meant for mitochondrial staining should be rapidly dehydrated; the precaution is useful but not imperative, especially with absolute alcohol, and the quality of dehydration should never be sacrificed in favour of rapidity. In any case, a reduced thickness of pieces allows one or two hours off each bath of alcohol.

I strongly advise adopting cedar-wood oil as an intermediate between the dehydrating alcohol and paraffin, and in which pieces can stay for a very long time.

Restriction to a very short stay in warm paraffin is a legend that is obligingly admitted but unfortunate; in fact *properly fixed chondriomes withstand warm paraffin for periods amounting to weeks* and I advise against any shortening of the period that has been indicated in the general remark on embedding.

Material fixed in these liquids is evidently best stored embedded in paraffin; if this cannot be done immediately pieces may be kept in cedar-wood oil where they run no risk of deterioration. I formally advise against conservation in alcohol of whatever strength; it is not harmful to chondriomes, especially if they have been well fixed, but pieces fixed in liquids containing potassium dichromate acquire a consistency after long exposure to alcohol that is quite unsuitable for cutting sections. If one is not sure of pursuing dehydration up to the cedar-wood oil stage one should rather leave pieces in 10% formalin after ensuring that all trace of such fixative liquids has been removed by thorough washing.

Material fixed in liquids containing potassium dichromate, but no osmium tetroxyde, and formalin-fixed material meant for paraffin sections should be treated, prior to dehydration, in order to complete fixation of chondriomes and particularly to impart tinctorial affinities that will be brought into play during mitochondrial staining. It should be remenbered that this treatment is unnecessary after fixation in a chromo-osmic mixture or Kolster's liquid.

The desired result can be obtained by two operations, namely postchromatization and mordanting with mercuric acetate.

Postchromatization, which may as well be applied to formalin treated material as to that fixed in mixtures containing potassium dichromate, consists in treating with an aqueous solution of the latter salt following fixation but without any particular washing; pieces may be at the most summarily rinsed in tap-water to remove any precipitate formed during the last hours of fixation in the formalin and potassium dichromate mixtures.

The technical details of postchromatization vary considerably according to authors; some (Parat, Baker, Elftman) recommend warm postchromatization in a 5% (Baker, Elftman) or saturated (Parat) solution of potassium dichromate (56°C for the 5% solution and 37°C when it is saturated). I do not advise such a procedure when preparing for mitochondrial staining, although it can be excellent for studying phospholopids. In fact my personal experience has entirely corroborated the opinion of certain authors like Hirschler who hold that warm postchromatization can result in the fragmentation of chondrioconts; the beaded appearance of mitochondria (the chondriomites of early authors) is quite frequent in pieces which are fixed in this manner. Furthermore, the duration of postchromatization is one of the critical steps of mitochondrial staining; any excess increases the difficulty of the actual staining and the determination of the optimal time is clearly easier at normal temperature, when it can last from three to nine days, than with warming, when it takes 12 to 48 hours. It is therefore for practical reasons that I recommend postchromatization at room temperature in a 3% solution of potassium dichromate in distilled water.

The optimal period of postchromatization is more or less constant for a given organ, but quite variable among the organs of the same animal species and, *a fortiori*, from one species to another. It is therefore advisable, when embarking upon a study of new material, to provide for a sufficient number of pieces to allow for preliminary trials; when for instance, postchromatization is carried out at room temperature, pieces may be taken out of the potassium dichromate bath at the end of three, five, seven and nine days; it is very rarely that longer times prove to be really useful and the postchromatizations lasting for weeks suggested by Regaud's school appear quite superfluous to me. During warm poschromatization pieces may be removed from the dichromate bath every twelve hours, and even then the chances of exceeding the limit are far from negligible.

Postchromatized material should evidently be submitted to the same thorough washing as that after chromo-osmic fixation; the procedure for dehydration is the same in both cases and all the remarks concerning it hold true for postchromatized material as well. Embedding can be carried out after passing through cedar-wood oil, butyl alcohol or methyl benzoate with clearing in benzene. No particular precaution need be observed about the period of embedding and assertions to the contrary, so frequent in works before 1940, pertain to superstition rather than to methodical trials.

As for osmified material embedding in paraffin is the best form of storage, failing which pieces may be left in cedar-wood oil, butyl alcohol or methyl benzoate; I strongly advise against keeping in ethyl alcohol. Formalin at 10% is a good storage medium for postchromatized and washed material which has not yet been dehydrated.

It cannot be denied that postchromatization hardens pieces, renders them brittle and favours shrinkage during dehydration and embedding. These are unavoidable, since mordanting in mercuric acetate, although less harmful in this respect, can be applied only after formalin fixation.

Mordanting in mercuric acetate, proposed by Gough and Fulton (1927) is an excellent prelude to mitochondrial staining and it is indeed a pity that the original description was greeted by almost all cytologists with complete indifference.

In fact, hardening and shrinkage is much less than in postchromotized material; mitochondrial staining with Altmann's fuchsin and iron hematoxylin succeeds as well as after postchromatization and the duration of the mercuric acetate bath is besides, shorter than that of potassium dichromate. But the method works really satisfactorily only after formalin fixation and that is perharps the reason why most cytologists disdain it.

The operating procedure is most simple. Pieces, fixed in saline formalin or formaldehyde-calcium for at least 48 hours are left for 48 hours in the following liquid:

Distilled water	100 ml
Acetic acid	0.1 ml
Mercuric acetate	3 g.

In practice the small quantity of acetic acid added to prevent the formation of basic mercury salts, which precipitate in the pieces, does not alter fixed chondriomes. The treatment is carried out at room temperature and is followed by thorough washing in running water (24 hours), dehydration and embedding in paraffin as with postchromatized material. Obviously, mercuric precipitates in sections should be removed by a bath in Lugol's liquid followed by treatment with sodium hyposulphite.

Decalcifying pieces meant for studying the chondriome does not afford any particular problem if the decalcifying agent is allowed to act only *after postchromatization* and washing or even after treating with 96% alcohol. I have observed from trials that the 5% trichloroacetic acid treatment even prolonged for 5 to 10 days does not result in any alteration of the chondriomes. Pieces which contain only few calcium deposits can be decalcified with a 2 or 3% solution of chromium trioxyde acting after the wash that terminates postchromatization, followed by renewed washing in running water. It may be observed that still lesser calcium deposits are dissolved during postchromatization and further remembered that no fixative containing potassium dichromate is suitable for the histochemical study of calcium.

None of the methods proposed for softening cuticular structures is compatible with the conservation of chondriomes.

In section cutting it is important to bear in mind the finesse and uniformity required of the procedures to be described in the following section. All mitochondrial stains are regressive and consequently all the sections on a slide should be, as far as possible, of the same thickness; they give very bright tints and therefore faults in sections show very clearly. In no case should the thickness exceed 5 μ and even this is a maximum which is better not attained. Furthermore, several mitochondrial stains involve abrupt changes in the surface tension of the medium and very vigorous washing; sections should therefore be perfectly well fixed and dried on slides following the indications found in the first part of this work. Collodioning is indispensable for all procedures of staining.

Clearly, the required thinness of sections does not allow mitochondrial staining after embedding in celloidin. Frozen sections for silver impregnation should be as thin as possible; I recommend lowering the thickness to below 10 μ whenever the nature of the material renders it possible.

MITOCHONDRIAL STAINS

The procedures described in the preceding section give chondriosomes a strong acidophily so that, theoretically, all acid stains may be used to show the chondriome in paraffin sections. Certain histochemical reactions, especially those indicating protein-bound sulphydryles also give positive results with the chondriome; this is also true for certain enzymatic activities such as those of cytochrome-oxydase and the dehydrogenases. In fact, however, acid fuchsin, the ferric, phosphotungstic, and cupric lakes of hematoxylin as well as crystal violet are the only stains of the chondriome which are of any real practical use.

A. — STAINING WITH ACID FUCHSIN

Acid fuchsin (rubin S, fuchsin S, acid magenta) is the earliest known of the stains for the chondriome, that which Altmann (1889) used in discovering this organelle. Chemically, it is a sulfonated derivative of basic fuchsin.

Commercial samples are always more or less complex mixtures since basic fuchsin is itself a mixture of pararosanilin and its mono- di- and trimethyl derivatives, so that each one of them can yield by sulfonation at least three different compounds. This notion is of considerable practical importance in cytological technique since all commercial samples of acid fuchsin are suitable for staining the cytoplasm or collagen fibres envisaged in Masson's trichrome and Van Gieson's method, but only certain samples give good mitochondrial staining. Rosanilin-sulfonic acid exists in commercial preparations of acid fuchsin as the disodium salt.

The solution of acid fuchsin used for staining chondriomes is called Altmann's fuchsin and it is still prepared according to the formula proposed by its author. It is a saturated (20%) solution of the dyestuff in ripened anilin water. The latter is obtained by leaving at rest an excess of anilin (about 3%) in distilled water; the solubility of anilin in distilled water being very weak and slow the anilin water requires to be "matured" over several weeks or even months. Anilin water may be stored in the dark indefinitely if closed with ground-glass stoppers or plastic caps; cork stoppers are rapidly attacked. Contrary to a widespread prejudice, acid fuchsin dissolves well and quickly in anilin water at a concentration of 20% and practice shows that the more concentrated solutions stain better. These solutions of acid fuchsin do not keep well; from the third month after their preparation onwards they gradually lose their staining capacity if stored in the dark and much more rapidly if left exposed to light. Large quantities of Altmann's fuchsin need not therefore be prepared beforehand.

Solutions of acid fuchsin are very sensitive to alkalinity; this is equally true for the stained preparation as well, so that any washing is tap-water after staining with Altmann's should be avoided. Distilled water is used instead and washing is, besides, done rapidly. Leaving sections in tap-water or water rendered alkaline by adding lithium carbonate or ammonia is indeed the best means of destaining tissues of acid fuchsin.

The purpose of adding anilin to Altmann's fuchsin is quite easy to understand its presence has the effect of reducing the size of the particle of dyestuff and facilitating their penetration into the chondriosomes which have a very dense texture. In confirmation of this classical viewpoint Seki (1933) showed that phenol can play the same role and proposed the use of a 5% solution of acid fuchsin in water containing 3 to 5% phenol. From my personal experience the results of this method, with the samples of acid fuchsin available nowadays, are inferior to those given by Altmann's formula.

Staining chondriomes with Altmann's fuchsin is obtained with warming. The result is a diffuse overstaining of tissues and the background should therefore be cleared by differentiation. The regressive nature of the method is evidently a source of difficulty.

The interpretation of the Altmann stain has been resumed by Baker (1958) as follows. Most dyestuffs penetrate with difficulty because of the texture of the chondriosomes, and hence it is necessary to use very concentrated solutions of acid fuchsin with warming. However, it also follows that once it has penetrated the dyestuff is more difficult to be extracted from the chondriome than from any other structure, and this enables efficient differentiation.

Though to my knowledge the phenomenon cannot be interpreted in chemical terms, experience has shown that the "fastness" of the fixation of Altmann's fuchsin on the chondriosomes closely depends on the length of postchromatization. Weak or none at all at first, the stain takes on more and more strongly and resists differentiation as the stay in the potassium dichromate bath is prolonged; but if it lasts too long the selective affinity of the chondriome for acid fuchsin is gradually lost and sections can no longer be stained by this method. The primordial importance of a correctly determined postchromatization period can thus be appreciated.

Altmann's stain consists of the following steps:

> Thin and perfectly well attached paraffin sections are dewaxed, collodioned and hydrated.
>
> Stain with warming in freshly prepared Altmann's fuchsin; the classical procedure consists in warming the slide covered with dye-stuff thrice until vapours evolve and then cooling. Equally good results can be obtained by leaving the slide covered with dye-stuff on a hot plate set at a suitable temperature (50° to 60°) until it takes on a syrupy consistency (in about 5 minutes). Warming until dry, according to Nassonov (1923) seems unnecessary to me. In any case the boiling temperature should never be attained. Allow to cool. Any attempt at washing slides while they are still warm only increases the chances of detaching sections. Wash vigorously, but quickly, with a jet of distilled water to remove all excess of stain around sections; any deposit of acid fuchsin which persists outside sections will appear as precipitates during the later stages of staining.
>
> Continue the procedure according to any one of the variants indicated below.

Obviously Altmann's fuchsin cannot be re-used; the reagent keeps badly if warmed and this prevents it from being used in Borrel tubes or dishes placed in an oven at the right temperature although it may appear to be logical in itself.

The difficulty of differentiation, a crucial step in Altmann's technique, probably explains the several variants proposed. I shall briefly mention the principle of all those with which I am acquainted and give the operating procedure in detail only for those which appear to me really useful. These variants are classified quite naturally according to whether the differentiation is followed or not by another stain. It should, however, be remembered that all differentiators are themselves stains and impart a tint to the background; thus dichromic and polychromic methods may be distinguished.

DICHROMIC TECHNIQUES

The differentiator, in these techniques, gives quite a pale background stain and organelles other than the chondriome are not in any way demonstrated selectively.

Altmann's technique. — The preparations are stained with the solution of acid fuchsin in anilin water, washed, then differentiated *with warming* in a saturated solution of picric acid in 96% alcohol, washed in 96% alcohol, dehydrated and mounted. This method is now abandoned because of its very uneven results.

Metzner's technique. — It differs from Altmann's technique only in that differentiation in alcoholic picric acid is carried out at *room temperature*, which facilitates control under the microscope.

Galeotti's technique. — Preparations, stained with Altmann's fuchsin are washed, differentiated in a saturated solution (about 0.5%) of aurantia in 70% alcohol, washed in 96% alcohol dehydrated and mounted.

A. Prenant's technique. — Preparations, stained with Altmann's fuchsin and washed, are differentiated in picro-indigocarmine (p. 201) dehydrated and mounted.

None of these techniques can, however, rival the polychromic methods in the final results; they are mentioned here only for their historical interest.

POLYCHROMIC TECHNIQUES

What is common to these methods, apart from the demonstration of the chondriome, is that they include a stain that increases contrast and shows other organelles. Differentiation may, according to the case, precede the staining of other structures, follow it or be carried out concomitantly. It can be effected in an aqueous or alcoholic medium. The following variants are given chronologically.

Altmann's fuchsin—methyl green (Bensley 1910; Cowdry 1913, 1918). — Sections, stained in Altmann's fuchsin and washed, are differentiated *and* stained by an aqueous 1% solution of methyl green, dehydrated and mounted.

Altmann's fuchsin—toluidine blue—aurantia (Kull 1913). — Sections, stained with Altmann's fuchsin and washed, are stained with an aqueous 0,5% solution of toluidine blue, then differentiated with an alcoholic solution of aurantia following Galeotti, rinsed with distilled water, dehydrated and mounted.

Altmann's fuchsin—picric acid—light green (Benoît 1925). — The sections are stained with acid fuchsin, washed, differentiated at room temperature in picric acid and briefly rinsed in 70% alcohol before being submitted to background staining with a diluted (about 0.2%) aqueous solution of light green; they are then dehydrated and mounted.

Althmann's fuchsin—aurantia—phosphomolybdic acid—polychrome blue—tannin—orange (Volkonsky 1927). — Sections, stained with Altmann's fuchsin and washed, are differentiated in aurantia as in the technique of Galeotti (or in a 0.5% solution of orange G in 70% alcohol) washed in distilled water, treated with a 1% aqueous solution of phosphomolybdic acid neutralized with normal sodium hydroxide, rinsed in distilled water, stained with a polychrome blue without methylene violet and differentiated in the tannin—orange of Unna (p. 803) before dehydrating and mounting.

Altmann's fuchsin—phosphomolybdic acid—methyl blue—orange (Hollande 1930). — Sections, stained with Altmann's fuchsin and washed, are treated for 5 minutes with a 1% aqueous solution of phosphomolybdic acid, washed in distilled water, stained for about 10 minutes in a 1% aqueous solution of methyl blue and finally differentiated in a saturated aqueous solution of orange G in 80% alcohol before dehydration and mounting.

Altmann's fuchsin—methyl green picrate (Gabe 1947). — Sections stained with Altmann's fuchsin and washed, are dehydrated with absolute alcohol and treated with a saturated solution of methyl green picrate in methyl alcohol; a small quantity of distilled water is added to the slide and left for 30 seconds; the slides are then rinsed in distilled water, dehydrated and mounted.

Each of these variants can give spectacular preparations under optimal conditions of postchromatization and none of them should be rejected at the outset.

All do not, however, have the same use. Benoît's technique is admirably suited to osmified pieces and it was perfected on material fixed in the author's own fixative; it is less useful for postchromatized material fixed without osmium tetroxyde. The chief advantage of Kull's method is that the background is stained *before* any differentiation. Indeed it is known from experience that treatment with picric acid, aurantia or orange G, used as differentiators, considerably modifies the tinctorial affinities of tissue and cell constituents, and it is just this disadvantage that is avoided by following Kull. Its drawback lies in the impossibility of really checking the progress of differentiation under the microscope. The aurantia is meant to differentiate the fuchsin and start differentiating the toluidine blue which continues during dehydration in alcohol so that the final tint becomes apparent only at the time of mounting. Hollande's technique duplicates that of Kull and does not seem to have imposed itself. That of Volkonsky, which has enjoyed some vogue, has the disadvantage of differentiation with aurantia before any staining of the other organelles; the actual need for the phosphomolybdic acid treatment does not appear at all clear to me and the high level of glycerine in the background stain implies a serious risk of smudged preparations; in any case the results are not any better than those given by Kull's method. The Bensley-Cowdry technique is attractive in its simplicity, and of all the techniques mentioned here it demands the most rigor in adjusting the time of postchromatization. It is besides quite noteworthy, that Bensley (1910) has provided, in connection with this stain, the means to rectify a lack or excess of postchromatization. The technique using methyl green picrate calls for the preparation of a differentiator which cannot be obtained commercially. In spite of the repugnance I feel in praising a procedure of which I am the author, I feel it difficult to avoid admitting, after twenty years of experience, that this technique excels all other mitochondrial stains in flexibility and dependability. I am therefore sure of not being partial or sectarian in retaining, for detailed description, the technique of Benoît, that of Kull and that with methyl green picrate.

Benoît's technique

Sections, preferably of chromo-osmic fixed material, are dewaxed collodioned and hydrated.
Stain with Altmann's fuchsin.
Rinse vigorously and rapidly in distilled water.
Differentiate, under the microscope, in a saturated solution of picric acid in 96% alcohol; if differentiation occurs too soon a mixture of one volume of alcoholic picric acid and two volumes of alcohol may be used
Terminate differentiation by a rapid rinse in 70% alcohol.
Counterstain with a dilute aqueous solution of light green (the original text does not specify the concentration; I suggest 0.1 to 0.2%).
Dehydrate directly in absolute alcohol, clear in a benzenic hydrocarbon and mount in a synthetic resin or, if unavoidable, in balsam.

When successful the chondriosomes show a very bright red in striking contrast to the background; their outlines should be perfectly sharp; cytoplasm appears grey, yellow or light green; the green stain of the nuclei is also sufficiently intense for them to be seen clearly against the background; osmiophilous lipids appear black and the Golgi apparatus can be localized as a "negative image".

Kull's technique

Often wrongly designated the Champy-Kull technique, this method can be used after chromo-osmic fixation, chromic fixation with postchromatization or fixation with Kolster's liquid without postchromatization.

I advise against its use after formalin fixation and mordanting in mercuric acetate since formalin prepares badly for staining with the basic blues of the thiazine group such as toluidine blue.

> Paraffin sections are dewaxed, collodioned and hydrated.
> Stain with Altmann's fuchsin.
> Rinse vigorously and quickly in distilled water.
> Stain for 30 seconds to two minutes, or a slide or in a Borrel cylinder, with an aqueous 0,5% solution of toluidine blue; prolong the staining beyond if the sections do not take a definite blue shade as seen under the microscope.
> Rinse in distilled water and wipe the slides around the sections.
> Cover the slide quickly with a saturated solution of aurantia in 70% alcohol, lay it flat and follow the progress of differentiation as viewed by transparence across the layer of solution; terminate the process by washing in distilled water when the general shade turns grey.
> Dehydrate in absolute alcohol (a little toluidine blue is extracted during this operation) clear in a benzenic hydrocarbon and mount in a synthetic resin or in Canada balsam.

Successful preparations show chondriomes red tending towards violet at times, with their shapes absolutely well delineated; erythrophil secretory granules also stain red, but differ from the chondriome especially after fixation in a chromo-osmic liquid; the chromatin of the nuclei is coloured blue and the nucleoli stain red or blue according to the duration of postchromatization and differentiation; the cytoplasm is bluish, grey or yellow; Vertebrate erythrocytes retain a bright red or turn yellow; the metachromatic reaction of acidic mucosubstances is often maintained. In other words, successful preparations are really striking, and in particular the demonstration of nuclear structures is of the very best quality.

The methyl green picrate technique

Instigated by the desire to blend the qualities of the Bensley-Cowdry technique using methyl green with the advantages of differentiating Altmann's fuchsin in an alcoholic medium, this technique adopts the same trick as in the staining of blood smears with methylene blue eosinate (the May-Grünwald stain). Following Altmann's fuchsin the sections are treated with a saturated solution of methyl green picrate in methyl alcohol, a neutral stain that is stable in alcohol and which effects differentiation. Distilled water is then added to bring about the dissociation of the methyl green picrate whose moieties stain both basophil and acidophil structures.

Preparation of methyl green picrate:

Mix equal parts of an aqueous saturated solution of picric acid and aqueous 1% solution of methyl green; a dense and bulky precipitate forms immediately.
Separate the precipitate by filtration and wash it several times with distilled water.
Dry in an oven at 37° or 56° (in the latter case the precipitate often conglomerates into dense masses).
Dissolve to saturation in methyl alcohol.

Both the powder as well as the methanolic solution may be conserved almost indefinitely.

Operating procedure. — This technique may be applied to osmified material (if necessary, after bleaching) to pieces fixed in Kolster's liquid or to chromated material fixed in other non osmified liquids. It is well suited for staining pieces mordanted in mercuric acetate.

Paraffin sections are dewaxed, collodioned and hydrated.
Stain with Altmann's fuchsin.
Rinse very vigorously and rapidly in distilled water.
Dehydrate in absolute alcohol.
Cover the slide with the solution of methyl green picrate in methanol and allow it to act for 10 seconds to three minutes according to the type of the piece.
Add a little distilled water (about the same quantity as the alcoholic solution of methyl green picrate) incline the slide in all directions so as to mix the two liquids and leave them in contact for about 30 seconds.
Rinse in distilled water.
Dehydrate with absolute alcohol, clear in a benzenic hydrocarbon and mount in a synthetic resin or Canada balsam.
The progress of differentiation may be followed under the microscope by discarding the solution of methyl green picrate and renewing it after examination. The final result of the combined differentiation and background stain may also be verified before the dehydration that precedes mounting by taking into account the fact that absolute alcohol extracts some methyl green. In case of insufficient differentiation the slide is dehydrated, covered with the methanolic solution of methyl green picrate and differentiation recommenced.

Chondriosomes appear deep red, the chromatin of the nuclei green and nucleoli red or green according to the length of postchromatization and the way differentiation has been carried out. Basophilic cytoplasm is green or grey and very acidophilic cytoplasm yellow; mucosubstances are often stained by methyl green, especially when they are very acid (granules of mast cells, ground substance of the cartilage etc...). Erythrocytes appear red or yellow and secretory granules range from red to green.

RECTIFYING ERRORS OF POSTCHROMATIZATION ON SLIDES

The outcome of Altmann's stain may be improved, in case of insufficient or excessive postchromatization, by means of what is called postchromatization on slides and bleaching, introduced by Bensley (1910).

Postchromatization on slides is recommended in all cases when differentiation occurs too rapidly, premature destaining of chondriomes before the normal time taken for differentiation indicating that the stay of pieces in potassium dichromate has been insufficient. The operation may, theoretically, be carried out at room temperature, but it is more efficacious with warming. The following procedure has given me satisfactory results.

> Place dewaxed, collodioned and hydrated sections in a 3 or 5% solution of potassium dichromate in an oven at 37°.
> Remove the slides five minutes, ten minutes, half an hour and one hour after their immersion in the warm potassium dichromate, wash in tap-water until the yellow tint disappears and apply the particular variant of Altmann's stain chosen.
> Experience has shown that postchromatization on slides for more than an hour is of no use; continuing treatment with potassium dichromate up to 24 hours does not improve the result any more.

Bleaching, practised as in the osmic impregnation of the Golgi apparatus, is, on the contrary, aimed at attenuating excessive postchromatization. Among the three methods indicated on p. 712 that with the essence of turpentine is not particularly recommended. The method with hydrogen peroxide may be applied, but it is the one using potassium permanganate that most authors prefer. Oxydation can require from 10 seconds to one minute and is generally of no use beyond since the excess of postchromatization is too much to be rectified. Sections are bleached with oxalic acid or with sodium metabisulfite and washed *at length* in running water before staining with Altmann's fuchsin.

My personal experience has shown that a spectacular improvement of Altmann's stain results if dewaxed, collodioned and hydrated sections are left for about twelve hours in tap-water before staining with acid fuchsin. I do not possess the facts necessary to interpret the mechanism of this improvement in chemical terms; the washing could act by removing traces of chromic salts that remain in the tissues or by a phenomenon similar to the alkaline detersive action (*Entschlackung*) suggested by Schultze for certain neurofibrillar impregnations. The operation is surprisingly efficacious and I advise its systematic use in all cases where a preliminary trial leads one to expect some difficulty in obtaining satisfactory preparations.

THE SIGNIFICANCE OF ALTMANN'S STAIN

It should be strongly emphasized that Altmann's stain is not "specific" for the chondriome. The binding of acid fuchsin is characteristic of chondriosomes as well as a great many other structures under the technical conditions just defined. All erythrophilic secretory granules, lysosomes, tonofibrils, ciliary bodies, metalliferous inclusions and those rich in chromolipoids take Altmann's fuchsin as intensely as do the chondriosomes. This fact explains the difficulty of demonstrating the chondriome by Altmann's stain in cells which are rich in secretory products. In any case properly fixed and postchromatized chondriosomes always take Altmann's fuchsin, which, therefore, is of some value in demonstrating these organelles, but the affinity of the stain is surely no proof at all of the mitochondrial nature of a stained structure; in this respect crystal violet is much more significant.

B. — STAINING WITH CRYSTAL VIOLET

Most authors admit that crystal violet is the most selective of the mitochondrial stains, but what has been noted for acid fuchsin is also true for this stain. The affinity for crystal violet is in no way confined to the chondriosomes and staining with this substance does not necessarily follow automatically; indeed the technical difficulties are even greater than with acid fuchsin. But the optical qualities of successful preparations are such that it is a pity most modern cytologists do not practise Benda's stain (1900, 1901) any longer.

The author of the method has suggested, in a methodological study (1926), that positive results may be had after all mitochondrial fixations or even after simple formalin fixation; in fact, however, fixing objects in a chromo-osmic mixture seems to be an essential element of success. The method of embedding also is of primordial importance; concurring with Benda (1926) I consider that adopting cedarwood oil as an intermediary between the dehydrating alcohol and paraffin is almost compulsory.

Apart from the technique of Benda (1901), that of Nassonov (1923) also uses crystal violet for staining the chondriome, with Altmann's fuchsin for secretory granules. Both techniques are described below.

BENDA'S METHOD

The difficulty of the technique explains the modifications in the details of operating procedure, particularly those proposed by Meves and Duesberg (1908) and Watanabe (1923). From my personal experience it is the last among the publications of Benda (1926) which describes the surest procedure. It is indicated below:

> Paraffin sections, not more than 5 μ thick, made from material fixed in a chromo-osmic liquid containing little or no acetic acid and embedded after cedarwood oil, are dewaxed, collodioned and hydrated.
> Mordant for 24 hours at room temperature in a freshly prepared 4% aqueous solution of iron alum.
> Rinse rapidly in distilled water.
> Stain for 24 hours at room temperature in the following solution:
> > Distilled water .... 100 ml.
> > Aqueous saturated solution of sodium alizarin-sulfonate ... 1 ml.
>
> Rinse rapidly in distilled water.
> Place slides, face upwards, in a glass vessel such as a Petri dish, containing a sufficiently deep layer of the following *freshly prepared* mixture:
> > 3% solution of crystal violet in 96% alcohol } in equal parts
> > Ripened anilin water (see p. 726)
>
> Place the whole on a hot-plate and warm until vapours are given out, remove and allow to cool for about 5 minutes.
> Rinse rapidly in distilled water.
> Differentiate under the microscope with approximately 30% acetic acid (1 volume glacial acetic acid and 2 volumes distilled water) differentiation is usually accomplished in one or two minutes, though at times it can take more or less.
> Terminate differentiation by washing in tap-water as soon as the desired shades are obtained. Prolong washing in running or frequently renewed water for at least ten minutes so that all traces of acetic acid are removed.
> Blot slides with filter paper.
> Dehydrate in acetone, clear with a benzenic hydrocarbon and mount under Canada balsam or a commercial synthetic resin.

The original operating procedure included a very rapid dehydration in absolute alcohol, but this was later abandoned by Benda himself because of the very great risk of tints being considerably weakened during dehydration.

In a successful preparation the cytoplasm is stained a very light pink by the ferric lake of alizarin; the chondriosomes, stained a deep reddish violet, appear with extraordinary clearness. I have no hesitation in affirming that no other mitochondrial stain gives such contrasted preparations. Secretory granules, just as basement membranes, stain violet or blue; fibrillar differentiations of the cytoplasm take a darker red than the background, while ciliary bodies appear blue. Particulate lipids, which are blackened by osmium tetroxyde in the fixative, retain their tint.

NASSONOV'S METHOD

This method, based on the mitochondrial technique of Kull, may be applied to material fixed in a chromo-osmic liquid, either with or without osmic impregnation of the Golgi apparatus. It gives really synthetic preparations where the nucleus, Golgi apparatus, chondriome and secretory granules all appear with different tints. Nassonov has used it as the basis of a key to distinguish among the various cell organelles. Its use is considerably less since the advent of the electron microscope, but I am giving the original operating procedure for its documentary interest.

Operating procedure:

> Very thin sections (2 to 3 μ) of material fixed in a chromo-osmic liquid, with or without osmic impregnation of the Golgi apparatus, are dewaxed, collodioned and hydrated.
> Stain with Altmann's fuchsin (p. 726).
> Rinse vigorously and rapidly in distilled water.
> Stain for three to ten minutes with a saturated solution of crystal violet in 70% alcohol.
> Rinse vigorously in distilled water.
> Differentiate in a 0.5% solution of aurantia in 70% alcohol. (this solution is close to saturation, and the saturated solution recommended by Galeotti for differentiating Altmann's fuchsin can be used instead). Its period of action can last from five seconds to a minute or more according to the case.
> Rinse rapidly in 96% alcohol, dehydrate in absolute alcohol, clear in a benzenic hydrocarbon and mount in Canada balsam or a commercial synthetic resin.

In a successful preparation the Golgi apparatus appears black if the technique has been applied to sections of pieces impregnated with osmium; the chondriome comes out as deep violet and the specificity of staining is greater than that of Benda's method. Secretory granules are brick red and can be immediately distinguished from chondriosomes. Chromatin appears a pale violet, nucleoli red and the cytoplasm a background of varying shades of yellow. Vertebrate erythrocytes are stained red or yellow.

But this result is not obtained automatically. The major disadvantage of the method is that it is carried out "blindly" since no checking is possible under the microscope during the procedure. Sections take their final tints only after dehydration in absolute alcohol is completed, and one should not hope for success as described above from the very first section of a given block. As in Kull's method the aurantia is supposed to completely differentiate Altmann's fuchsin and commence differentiating crystal violet which is pursued during dehydration. It follows that staining with Altmann's fuchsin and with crystal violet should be carefully adjusted by varying the time of exposure to each. If staining with Altmann's fuchsin is too intense it results in smudgy secretory granules which can be stripped with aurantia only at the risk of destaining the chondriomes which then turn red. Insufficient staining with Altmann's fuchsin gives, on the other hand, violet secretory granules. On the whole one gains by laying emphasis on staining with crystal violet, a dye-stuff which is extracted by both aurantia and the dehydrating absolute alcohol, while acid fuchsin is quite insoluble in the latter.

Distinguishing the fundamental organelles of the cell. — Nassonov (1923) has suggested comparing various preparations made under the following technical conditions.

> Fixation in Champy's liquid, embedding without osmic impregnation, and mounting dewaxed unstained sections: secretory granules should be light yellow while chondriomes and the Golgi apparatus are invisible.
> Fixation in Champy's liquid, embedding without osmic impregnation and staining with Altmann's fuchsin-crystal-violet-aurantia: chondriomes stain violet and secretory granules red, while the Golgi apparatus is either invisible or appears negatively contrasted.
> Fixation in Champy's liquid followed by osmic impregnation and mounting dewaxed, unstained sections: the Golgi apparatus should be black and secretory granules yellow.
> Fixation in Champy's liquid, osmic impregnation and staining with Altmann's fuchsin-crystal violet- aurantia; the Golgi apparatus stains black, chondriomes violet and secretory granules red. Fixation in Zenker's or Carnoy's liquid, paraffin embedding and staining with Heidenhain's hematoxylin: chondriomes and the Golgi apparatus are invisible, secretory granules may or may not be conserved, while nuclei, ciliary bodies, the ergastoplasm and related structures are well demonstrated.

RECTIFICATION OF MITOCHONDRIAL STAINING BY CRYSTAL VIOLET

It has been noted earlier that mitochondrial staining with crystal violet following either Benda or Nassonov gives satisfactory results only on sections of material fixed in a chromo-osmic liquid. Experience has shown that the period of exposure of the material to the potassium dichromate is much less exacting than in the case of Altmann's fuchsin or the hematoxylin lakes. Consequently, postchromatization on slides according to Bensley is never really useful. The inverse operation, namely, the bleaching of preparations, can, on the other hand be very useful since it facilitates the binding of dye-stuffs especially when the piece has been submitted to osmic impregnation of the Golgi apparatus. As in the case of mitochondrial staining with Altmann's fuchsin, bleaching with potassium permanganate is quite suitable. When pieces have been impregnated with osmium for demonstrating the Golgi apparatus, bleaching with hydrogen peroxide and checking under the microscope can be recommended. In both cases, thorough washing in running water (15 to 30 minutes) should precede the staining of bleached sections.

C. — *REGRESSIVE STAINING OF THE CHONDRIOSOMES WITH THE HEMATOXYLIN LAKES*

Ever since its introduction into mitochondrial technique by Regaud (1910), regressive staining by the hematoxylin lakes has been widely adopted in all countries. A systematic search of all investigations in cytology carried out with the light microscope during the last fifty years will probably show that these lakes are the most used among the mitochondrial stains. Their practical advantages are great; in fact, the staining solution keeps very well, it can be used for other purposes, and the operating procedure itself does not differ from that used to demonstrate other organelles; all the steps of staining can be carried out at room temperature; with but one exception all the others can be practised on a large number of slides at a time and ferric hematoxylin is indeed the ideal method for the serial staining of many sections. Preparations are remarkably well conserved, far better than those with Altmann's fuchsin or even crystal violet. I may add that reversing the procedure is easier with ferric hematoxylin than with any of the other mitochondrial stains.

> Besides these practical advantages, mitochondrial staining by the hematoxylin lakes also presents considerable interest. They provide evidence for the essential role of pretreating pieces, especially postchromatization, in the successful staining of the chondriome.
> Indeed, the careful comparison of fragments of the same piece, fixed in a chromic mixture without osmic acid, and then submitted to increasing periods of postchromatization or none at all, will lead to the following observations.
> When applied to pieces after cytological fixation, but not postchromatized, regressive staining by the ferric lake of hematoxylin gives a remarkable demonstration of nuclear structures, the ergastoplasm and related formations (ergastoplasmic parasomes, yolk bodies etc...) tonofibrils, ciliary bodies and secretory granules. Chondriosomes do not show any particular siderophily; they destain immediately on differentiation with iron alum and negative images are obtained. Fairly short postchromatization is enough to suppress any real siderophily of the ergastoplasm without significantly attenuating that of the chromatin. As for the chondriosomes they acquire a siderophily that is often insufficient for their demonstration since it cannot withstand the proper stripping of the background. By prolonging the period of postchromatization the siderophily of the chondriome increases while that of other structures decreases; in this case only nuclei and chondriosomes retain the ferric lake of hematoxylin strongly enough to withstand suitable differentiation. Even further postchromatization results in a lowering of nuclear siderophily; first the chromatin and then the nucleoli destain during the early part of differentiation, while the chondriome remains as the only organelle to be stained an intense black against a background which may be colourless, light grey or yellowish according to the extent of ripening of the hematoxylin solution used. This indeed is the result aimed at by classical authors, particularly by Regaud and his school, and it explains their practice of very long postchromatization.

I personally do not advise carrying out postchromatization to the extent of obtaining the above result. From the methodological point of view the possibility of confusing chondriosomes with secretory granules or tonofibrils is quite frequent, especially when only iron-hematoxylin stained sections are examined, but the chances of confusion with nuclear structures are evidently not to be feared and hence very long postchromatization is unnecessary. Furthermore, the difficulty of cutting sections and the tendency of pieces to shrink during dehydration and embedding evidently increases with longer postchromatization. Sections of such material are also unsuitable for all mitochondrial stains other the hematoxylin lakes and most general techniques give very poor results or none at all. Clearly, they are of no use in histochemistry either. Finally, there is also a danger of overshooting the limit set by Regaud and his school; overchromatized material is characterized by a loss of siderophily in all organelles, including the chondriome; cells appear glassy in sections and refuse to take most stains. No amount of bleaching can improve the condition of these spoilt pieces. In short, I would recommend the same average postchromatization period (three to nine days according to the object) for the regressive hematoxylin lakes as for the variants of Altmann's fuchsin.

The *operating procedure* need not be described again. The Heidenhain-Regaud technique, that of Dobell-Hirschler and that of Bensley with cupric hematoxylin are all used for demonstrating the chondriome in the same manner as for detecting the other fundamental organelles of the cell; it is the pretreatment that ensures the specificity of mitochondrial staining, and all the practical details indicated on pages 689-695 apply here as well. After differentiation with iron alum and washing, sections can evidently be submitted to a counterstain as certain authors do; others recommend mounting without counterstaining, which I prefer personally.

Both postchromatization on slides and bleaching are suitable *rectifying procedures* as in the case of Altmann's stain; the detersive action of a stay in tap-water, mentioned in this connection is evidently of no purpose when staining with the ferric lake of hematoxylin since sections are left for 24 hours in a solution of iron alum; it may, however, be used before staining with copper lacques.

D. — SILVER IMPREGNATION OF THE CHONDRIOME

Techniques derived from the tannin-silver impregnation of connective fibres following Achucarro (1911) give excellent impregnation of the chondriomes in frozen sections of formalin-treated material. The original procedure has been greatly improved and adapted for the present purpose by Del Rio Hortega (1916); among the four variants proposed by this author the first will be described here, the second and third being meant for connective fibres and the fourth for neuroglia.

THE TANNIN-SILVER VARIANT OF DEL RIO HORTEGA

The first tannin-silver variant of del Rio Hortega demonstrates nuclear structures, the centrosome and spindle, epithelial fibrils and myofibrils, and the chondriome and secretory granules. Among the fibrous structures of connective tissue, the elastic fibres and fibrin are impregnated, while reticulin fibres and collagenous tissue are not. Preparations show admirable optical qualities, but the large number of structures which get impregnated require that thin sections be used. Technically, sections undergo mordanting with tannin followed by treatment with a silver-ammonium complex.

Preparation of the silver ammonium complex. — All the usual precautions concerning the use of silver complexes, described for neurofibrillar impregnation, should evidently be observed for the ammonium complex used here.

XL drops of 40% caustic soda solution are added to 30 ml of a 10% aqueous solution of silver nitrate; a heavy brownish precipitate forms immediately. The supernatant is decanted off and the precipitate washed by decanting about ten times in distilled water; from 1000 to 1500 ml of distilled water may be used for this purpose. After the last wash the precipitate is suspended in 50 ml of distilled water and dissolved by the gradual addition of ammonia. It is essential not to add any more than is strictly necessary for dissolving; in other words, the last portion of ammoniac should be added dropwise with constant agitation. It is then made up to a final volume of 150 ml with distilled water and stored in a brown bottle in the dark. The reagent keeps for a long time, even at room temperature.

Operating procedure. — Frozen sections are made from material fixed for ten days or longer in 10% neutralised formalin, saline formalin or formaldehyde-calcium. Sections should be as thin as possible and be collected in distilled water.

Mordant for five minutes at about 50° C with an aqueous 3% solution of tannin.
Wash in the following mixture until sections regain transparency and suppleness:
    distilled water .... 20 ml
    ammonia .... 4 ml
(Progress of the operation may be followed by observing against a dark background)
Sections are transferred successively into three dishes placed on a white background and containing the following mixture:
    distilled water .... 10 ml
    ammonium-silver complex .... 1 ml
Sections are transferred using glass rods which are changed every time. The transfer from the first to the second dish is made when sections begin to turn yellow, and from the second to the third when they are definitely yellow; they are left in the third until the shade does not deepen any more.
Wash thoroughly in distilled water (four or five baths, agitating sections with a clean glass rod).
Tone for 20 to 30 minutes, at 40-45°C, with a 0.2% aqueous solution of gold chloride; sections should take a mauve tint.
Wash carefully in distilled water.
Treat for about one minute with a 5% aqueous solution of sodium hyposulfite.
Wash at length in several changes of tap-water.
Stick sections to slides, dehydrate in absolute alcohol, clear in a benzenic hydrocarbon and mount in Canada balsam or a synthetic resin.

TECHNIQUE OF FERNANDEZ-GALIANO (1934)

This technique, which is derived from the one just described, is more specific for the chondriome. It involves the reduction, with formalin, of sections which have undergone mordanting with tannin and treatment with the ammonium-silver complex.

> Frozen sections are prepared as in del Rio Hortega's technique and washed in distilled water.
> Treat for ten minutes at room temperature with a 0.5% aqueous solution of tannin.
> Wash thoroughly in distilled water.
> Transfer sections to a vessel containing the following mixture and leave until they take a yellow tint:
>
> distilled water .... 10 ml
> Ammonium complex of del Rio Hortega III to VIII drops
> Transfer sections to distilled water in which the shade should intensify; watch this evolution (using a glass dish on a white background is advantageous) and pass to the next step when there is no more intensification of colour.
> Reduce for one or two minutes with 20% formalin (1 volume of commercial formalin and 4 volumes of tap-water).
> Wash thoroughly in tap-water, stick on slides, dehydrate, clear and mount after impregnation according to del Rio Hortega.

According to Valmitjana-Rovira (1948) the 20% formalin used for reducing may be better replaced by a 5, 10 or 20% solution of glucose.

Clearly, minor modifications in the period of stay in the various reagents, in the level of the ammonium-silver complex for impregnating according to Fernandez-Galiano and mordanting with tannin at temperatures different from those indicated permit adapting these techniques for demonstrating chondriosomes in particular objects.

E. — CHOICE OF MITOCHONDRIAL TECHNIQUES

Apart from the above techniques, others enable demonstrating the chondriome in particular cases. The high level of protein-bound sulphydryls in this organelle has already been noted. Chondriosomes can be stained, in frozen sections of formalin-treated material, by all lysochromes and especially by Sudan black H. They also give positive results with the acid hematein method of Baker and with that of Elftman; both techniques are described with reference to the histochemical detection of lipids. A selective staining of the chondriome of the Rat kidney by naphthol black B (amido black 10 B) in paraffin sections of formalin-treated material has been suggested by Geyer (1960) and explained in terms of the protein content of the organelle. But none of these stains or histochemical reactions is meant to be a general method; they do not have the morphological advantages of the procedures described in this chapter.

As regards the choice between the different staining techniques and silver impregnation it should be noted that the latter, in spite of its great adaptability and the possibility of using only pieces merely fixed in formalin, is also as exacting with respect to the speed of fixation and the size of pieces as the other staining methods. As I have already mentioned there is no question of applying it to material fixed according to the traditional methods of human pathology. It should not be forgotten that the specificity of demonstrating the chondriome by silver impregnation is not as great as that given by either Altmann's fuchsin or, *a fortiori*, crystal violet. In fact, silver impregnation of the chondriome is chiefly practised by those who otherwise specialize in silver methods.

Stainings with crystal violet after chromo-osmic fixation are methods of investigation which have lost much of their practical importance since the advent of the elctron microscope. In spite of the admirable optical qualities of preparations, these techniques have always remained the speciality of but a minority of cytologists, and such a state of affairs will only be accentuated in the future.

Altmann's fuchsin and the hematoxylin lakes are procedures generally used by histophysiologists to demonstrate chondriosomes. The choice between the two techniques is in no way a crucial one. As I have already noted, prolonged postchromatization meant to suppress the siderophily of all organelles other than the chondriome surely renders the material unfit for Altmann's stain but is of no use. It is very easy to keep the delay of postchromatization to within reasonable limits so that sections lend themselves to both Altmann's fuchsin as well as iron hematoxylin, and I strongly advise that both techniques be practised concomitantly. Altmann's fuchsin gives a fascinating polychromy to preparations, while those of ferric or cupric hematoxylin conserve better; a comparison of the results given by both results can be very useful.

CHAPTER 27

TECHNIQUES FOR DEMONSTRATING THE ERGASTOPLASM AND RELATED STRUCTURES

Even since the classical descriptions of Solger (1894) and of Bensley (1899) and the general studies of A. Prenant (1899/1900) and his pupil Garnier (1900), the ergastoplasm has been the matter of a very large number of publications after a period of misunderstanding and indifference. The histophysical investigations of Caspersson (1936–1939) and the histochemical studies of J. Brachet (1940) were a turning point in the evolution of our knowledge of this organelle and the beginning of a long series of studies which contribute to present conceptions of the mechanism of the transfer of genetic information. Electron microscopy has also contributed greatly to our knowledge of the ergastoplasm. As a whole, our knowledge of the biochemistry of ribonucleic acid and its role in the working of the cell has progressed at such a pace that the revelatory findings of hardly twenty five years ago appear to be ancestral knowledge today.

It is especially in histophysiological research that the study of the ergastoplasm and related structures with the light microscope continues to carry undoubted interest. Electron micrographs permit judging the quantity of ribonucleic acid which would otherwise be lost in applying even the most sensitive of histochemical techniques for light microscopy; they also reveal, with greater precision, the relation between the ergastoplasm and other organelles of the animal cell. However, classical techniques retain all their value in the preliminary exploration of objects studied for the first time and when the morphological analysis of the ergastoplasm was not intended at the time of fixation. Furthermore they are much more rapid and less expensive than the techniques of electron microscopy, and are hence undoubtedly superior in all cases where the presence of an ergastoplasm and related structures is already known and their evolution has to be followed under defined conditions.

The procedures used for detecting ergastoplasmic parasomes should quite naturally be included along with those meant for the ergastoplasm, while the same methods apply to mitochondrial and Golgian parasomes as well. I have furthermore included the proven techniques for the morphological study of yolk nuclei in this chapter to avoid an undue dispersion of this subject matter.

TECHNIQUES FOR DEMONSTRATING THE ERGASTOPLASM AND ERGASTOPLASMIC PARASOMES

Vital examination under the light microscope is of no avail in study the ergastoplasm since this organelle is a masked structure in the sense of Peterfi (1929); similarly, *vital staining* has practically not played any role in advancing our knowledge of the subject. However, ultraviolet photomicrography gives an excellent demonstration of the ergastoplasm or its equivalents in living cells.

In practice, a study of the ergastoplasm almost always involves permanent preparations.

Fixation of the ergastoplasm and ergastoplasmic parasomes is very easy. Apart from osmium tetroxyde used without adjuvant, which is very bad when embedding in paraffin is envisaged, or formalin without adjuvant, which does not suit later staining with the basic blues of the thiazin group, all other liquids described in this book, including ethyl and methyl alcohols, can be used in principle. However this wide possibility can be limited by two considerations, namely, the need to conserve structures well so that the cell is not deformed, and the aptitude for certain stains.

Resorting to chromo-osmic fixation is evidently of no use. Chromic fixatives with or without acetic acid but without osmium, Bouin's liquid, and Susa and similar mixtures are very well suited. Clarke's liquid and that of Carnoy are very useful in all cases where the subsequent staining of sections with methyl-green-pyronin is envisaged. Although not a really satisfactory fixative ethyl alcohol is often used to demonstrate Nissl bodies in nerve cells, which are in fact equivalent to an ergastoplasm. Obviously, freezing-drying followed by paraffin embedding gives suitable sections. Sections of fresh tissue made in a cryostat and fixed for few minutes in ethyl alcohol, methyl alcohol or any of the other fixatives mentioned above may also be used.

Operations preceding section-cutting and section-cutting itself call for few comments. The structures dealt with here can be demonstrated in paraffin sections, nitrocellulose (celloidin) sections or frozen sections. The techniques of dehydration, embedding and cutting can be applied in the usual manner. One should, however, insist on rapid embedding as a prolonged stay in liquids other than cedarwood oil, methyl benzoate or methyl salicylate can result in the depolymerisation and partial loss of ribonucleic acid.

None of the procedures recommended for softening cuticular structures is compatible with a protection of the basophily of the ergastoplasm or its equivalents; the same is also unfortunately true for the usual decalcifying techniques. Staining with the basic blues of the thiazin group or by gallocyanin often provides a poor demonstration or none at all when pieces have been decalcified with nitric acid, formic acid or trichloroacetic acid; this is even more so for staining with methyl-green-pyronin. The best practical solution consists in abandoning these methods and reducing the size of pieces so that a 24-hour stay at room temperature in Bouin's or Halmi's liquids would sufficiently decalcify objects to allow paraffin sections. If one desires to complete decalcifying in a bath of an aqueous solution of trichloroacetic acid it is best to practise it on pieces which have already been partially dehydrated in 96% alcohol. Ribonucleic acid withstands decalcifying with chromium trioxyde solutions relatively well, but the decalcifying action is not strong and several structures acquire a basophily, due to the oxidising action of the compound, that has nothing to do with the presence of ribonucleic acid.

The stains now used for demonstrating the ergastoplasm and ergastoplasmic parasomes are based on the basophily of ribonucleic acid which is a characteristic constituent of these particular structures.

Of the so-called general methods hemalum picro-indigocarmine stains them brown while Ramon y Cajal's trichrome and Krause's variant of it with safranin impart a red tint. The Mann-Dominici method shows them up in blue as indeed do all stains with the azur eosinates; gentian violet, crystal violet and cresyl violet stain a deep violet, but these procedures are useful only as an indication.

In the truly modern techniques of staining the ergastoplasm, which involve the histochemical detection of ribonucleic acid, the effect of toluidine blue, azur A, thionin or gallocyanin is verified in control sections with a preparation of commercial crystallised ribonuclease or, failing which, a short acid hydrolysis. The operating procedure has been described in all necessary detail under the histochemical detection of ribonucleic acid (p. 541–549).

The same chapter in the third part of this book also carries a description of the methyl-green pyronin stain which furnishes by far the most spectacular preparations of the ergastoplasm but which gives good results only if the material has been fixed with a view to this procedure.

Loss of basophily of the ergastoplasm or the ergastoplasmic parasomes after ribonuclease treatment or acid hydrolysis, just as in the case of nucleoli, does not imply that these structures have been "dissolved" away; they remain receptive to acid stains, this acidophily corresponding to the presence of the basic proteins normally associated with ribonucleic acid. Their presence explains the possibility of demonstrating the ergastoplasm, and especially ergastoplasmic parasomes, by certain reactions for proteins, in particular those based on the detection of tyrosine, of arginine and of cystine.

TECHNIQUES FOR DEMONSTRATING YOLK NUCLEI

Thanks to the investigations of Jacquiert (1936) and of Urbani (1949 to 1955) we know that the yolk nuclei of the 19th century authors are in fact of two sorts. In some cases they are merely simple cytoplasmic condensations (the "deutoplasme d'attente" of Jacquiert) that differ from the fundamental cytoplasm only in a greater affinity for all the usual stains; in other cases they are complex structures containing a central mass, a series of concentric stratifications like an onion bulb, and a light peripheral halo. These latter are the true yolk nuclei a classical example of which is seen in the oöcyte of certain Araneids.

Obviously the demonstration of deutoplasm spheres does not raise any technical problem; these cytoplasmic condensations are conserved by all fixatives and appear with a deeper shade of the same type as the fundamental cytoplasm after all stains. None of the organelles such as the chondriome or the Golgi apparatus go to form part of them. The level of ribonucleoprotein is high if the cytoplasm contains any and it can be nil in the opposite case.

True yolk nuclei are very easy to identify in vital preparations because of their higher birefringence than that of the cytoplasm. They may be fixed satisfactorily with all the usual fixatives. Among the topographical stains, azan, the one-step trichrome, Mann's method with methyl-blue eosin, the Mann-Dominici stain and Millot's triple stain provide particularly striking preparations. Histochemical reactions such as the PAS method, the Morel-Sisley reaction for tyrosine, that of McLeish and his co-workers for detecting arginine as well as the techniques for demonstrating sulfhydrylated proteins give spectacular preparations. This is equally true for Altmann's fuchsin and ferric or cupric hematoxylin; postchromatization is obviously required in all cases where it is desired to demonstrate chondriomes at the same time.

CHAPTER 28

TECHNIQUES FOR STUDYING THE CENTROSOME AND FIBRILLAR DIFFERENTIATION OF THE CYTOPLASM

The desire to avoid an excessive dispersion of matter in this part of the book has let me to group, in a single chapter, the techniques for demonstrating the centrosome along with those for detecting fibrillar or lamellar differentiations of the cytoplasm such as the tonofibrils and terminal bars, brush borders and striated borders and, finally, all those used in studying ciliary structures. This is partly justifiable from the technical point of view since, as opposed to the chondriome and the Golgi apparatus, all the above mentioned structures can withstand fixation in liquids containing acetic acid or alcohol although the presence of these two substances may not actually be indispensable. Understanding of the morphology of all these structures has been entirely revised thanks to the resolving power of the electron microscope, and the share of fibrillar and lamellar formations in their constitution can afford a further apparent justification for such a grouping.

Vital observation of these structures is very easy, even under a light-field microscope, if favourable objects are chosen. The spermatocytes of Lepidoptera and the gonocytes of certain Turbellaria and certain leeches are classical objects for the vital study of the centrosome. Tonofibrils can be conveniently studied in vital preparations of the tegument of small decapod Crustaceans. Dissociation of the intestinal mucosa affords the possibility of examining striated borders, for which it is evidently preferable to choose poikilothermic animals. The Malpighian tubules of insects are suitable for the vital examination of brush borders; lesser precautions can be taken than in the case of studying the kidney of Amphibians (Ghiron 1919) or even Mammals (Edwards 1928). As for cilia, the branchial epithelium of Prosobranch Gasteropods and Lamellibranchs and the oesophageal epithelium of the frog are classical material for manipulating by students, while many more do exist.

The fixation of these structures is, in certain respects, clearly easier than that of the chondriome or the Golgi apparatus. Saline formalin or formaldehyde-calcium is indicated in cases where the silver impregnation of frozen sections is intended. Chromo-osmic fixatives even when rich in acetic acid, give admirable fixation. All liquids based on mercuric chloride are particularly suitable for the study of centrosomes. Mixtures containing potassium dichromate and formalin, Bouin's fluid and its derivatives, and Heidenhain's Susa are also convenient; even liquids rich in acetic acid and in alcohol such as those of Clarke and of Carnoy, can be used. This resistance to fixatives is, besides, one of the distinguishing features between chondrioconts and tonofibrils.

The wide choice of possible fixatives should not lead to a neglect of the other precautions to be observed in cytological fixation, particularly the rapid removal of samples. Structures such as the tonofibrils evidently show some resistance to autolysis upon death of the tissues, but cilia undergo *post mortem* agglutination very easily while brush borders, striated borders, centrosomes and the fusorial spindle can be subject to drastic alterations under these conditions.

No particular precaution needs be observed before section cutting; formalin treated material is cut in a freezing microtome, while other fixatives may be followed by paraffin embedding. Obviously, postchromatization of material fixed in mixtures which conserve the chondriome is called for only if a study of this particular organelle is intended. Embedding in celloidin is of no use since thin sections are required. All the usual techniques for decalcifying may be practised without affecting the morphological characteristics of these organelles, though their histochemical properties may be considerably modified.

TECHNIQUES FOR DEMONSTRATING THE CENTROSOME

Demonstrating the centrosome in frozen sections of formalin treated material succeeds very well by the first tannin-silver variant of Del Rio Hortega described on p. 739 along with mitochondrial stains.

With paraffin sections the chief topographical techniques, particularly the method of Mann with methyl blue and eosin, the Mann-Dominici stain, the azur eosinate stains and Ramon y Cajal's trichrome show up the centrosome, although the actual identification of the organelle is based more on the theoretical knowledge of the observer rather than on any special affinity for a given stain. The regressive stains using hematoxylin lakes are more selective; the Dobell-Hirschler technique and that of Bensley with cupric hematoxylin give excellent results, but I suggest, in the first place, Heidenhain's Bordeaux R ferric hematoxylin stain specially devised for the purpose.

Spectacular results are given by Flemming's triple stain using safranin, gentian violet and Orange G, a method somewhat neglected as a caryological technique since the advent of squash preparations but which can be credited with some remarkable success. The original operating procedure of Flemming (1891) has now been given up, and several variants have been proposed in an effort to adapt the technique to fluctuations in the quality of commercial samples of the various dye-stuffs, especially of safranin. Two of these variants, namely that of de Winiwarter (1923) and that of Matthey (1947) are given below.

In any case the technique gives good results only with sections of material fixed in Flemming's liquid. A long storage of pieces in paraffin blocks is better avoided, and once sections are fixed to slides they should be stained within a few weeks. If the technique is to be applied to sections from blocks that have been kept for several years the tinctorial affinities of the tissue constituents should be re-established by treating dewaxed, collodioned and hydrated sections for 24 hours in Flemming's liquid, which may have served already, and washing in running water until the yellow tint disappears before staining.

Flemming's triple stain (variant of de Winiwarter):

Paraffin sections, 5 to 10 μ thick, are prepared as indicated above.
Stain for 24 hours at room temperature in a water-alcohol solution of safranin which is the same as that given for the safranin light-green technique (p. 230); at the end of the bath sections should be a deep red, but transparent, and should not tend to be brown; in the latter case it would mean that the solution is too concentrated for the material (dilute with 50% alcohol) or that the commercial sample of safranin is not suitable.
Wash for about 30 seconds in distilled water.
Stain for 24 hours in a 1% aqueous solution of gentian violet.
Wash for about 20 seconds in one or two changes of distilled water.
Treat for exactly 30 seconds with a 1/2000 solution of orange G, which is prepared by diluting 10 times a 0.5% solution of this dye-stuff in distilled water.
Pass through the following mixture for not more than 2 or 3 seconds:
  Absolute alcohol .... 100 ml
  Hydrochloric acid .... III drops
Rinse immediately and abundantly in absolute alcohol so that all trace of hydrochloric acid is removed.
Differentiate in the following mixture:
  Clove oil .... 50 ml
  Absolute alcohol .... 5 ml
Differentiation may be followed under the microscope, or with the naked eye if the preparation shows contrasting zones that are relatively rich and poor in nuclei; the former should take a blue tint and the latter orange.
Terminate differentiation in a bath of pure clove oil.
Drain off the clove oil by placing the slide vertically in a Borrel tube or Coplin jar; the vessel should be covered.
Remove the clove oil completely in a benzenic hydrocarbon and mount in Canada balsam or a commercial synthetic resin.

In a successful preparation the cytoplasm should take on a brownish yellow shade; fibrillar differentiations, centrosomes and the fusorial spindle appear very clearly; interphase chromatin is stained deep blue, chromosomes deep red, and degenerating chromatin shows a more or less deep brown or violet; nucleoli are red as are the erythrocytes; osmiophilic lipids retain their black tint.

The brief passage of slides in the dilute solution of orange G is an essential step, and the proper concentration of this solution should be readjusted after a trial slide; it is increased if the cytoplasmic yellow is too light and decreased if it tends to be too brown. It is the duration of treatment in the alcoholic hydrochloric acid that governs the intensity of the blue tint of interphase nuclei; it may be lengthened if necessary, but if too much blue has been extracted it is better to reduce the level of hydrochloric acid rather than to shorten the period spent by sections in the reagent. The uneven quality of samples of commercial dyestuffs explains the variability of results and necessitates the above adjustments.

Flemming's triple stain (variant of Matthey). — This technique is derived from an earlier variant of Margolena (1938). In contrast to that of de Winiwarter it includes several very convenient modifications especially for caryological use. The gentian violet, a chemically ill-defined dyestuff that varies much from batch to batch, is replaced by crystal violet. Mordanting with a solution of lugol in an alcoholic medium helps stabilizing the violet stain. The orange G is dissolved in clove oil and the passage in alcoholic hydrochloric acid is omitted.

Stain in the water-alcohol solution of safranin for two-and-a-half hours.
Rinse in three baths of distilled water.
Treat for five minutes with the following solution:

Potassium iodide	2 g
70 or 80% alcohol	300 ml
iodine	1 g

Stain for 15 minutes in a 1% aqueous solution of crystal violet.
Wash and, if necessary, leave in distilled water.
Treat for 20 seconds in the alcoholic iodine-iodide solution.
Treat in two baths of absolute alcohol for 10 seconds each. Differentiate, if necessary under the microscope, in clove oil saturated with orange G.
Remove excess of differentiator in several baths of a benzenic hydrocarbon and mount under Canada balsam or a synthetic resin.

The results concerning nuclear structures are similar to those given by de Winiwarter's variant, and they are much more easily obtained; cytoplasmic tints are however quite often less intense, which is why I have indicated both techniques.

TECHNIQUES FOR DEMONSTRATING TONOFIBRILS

Structures designated as tonofibrils by Heidenhain (1894) and as epitheliofibrils by Del Rio Hortega (1916) are found in various epithelial cells. Having been considered by early authors as representing a "cytoskeleton" or even a means of uniting adjacent cells, they are now correctly interpreted from data obtained with the electron microscope. The same is true for the desmosomes, thickenings of the cell membrane at the points of contact between neighbouring cells. In certain cases such contact gives rise to the formation of cell frames or terminal bars (*Kittleisten* of german authors).

The above structures are conserved by fixatives based on alcohol or acetic acid, withstand the operations that prepare for embedding in paraffin, celloidin or other embedding mass, and persist after pieces are decalcified.

They are easily stained; the so-called general methods show their presence since all these structures are acidophilic. In most cases iron hematoxylin followwing the technique of Heidenhain or of Regaud is used to demonstrate them selectively in paraffin sections. Heidenhain's technique with Bordeaux R and ferric hematoxylin (p. 693) is not advisable since the pretreatment of sections with the acid dyestuff favours destaining of the tonofibrils and related structures at the beginning of differentiation in iron alum. A. Prenant's triple stain (p. 694) is on the other hand admirably suited. All these structures are also stainable with Bensley's cupric haematoxylin, even in material that is not postchromatized.

Tonofibrils, cell frames and desmosomes exhibit a strong affinity for acid fuchsin. This explains why they appear an intense red with all the variants of Altmann's stain, so that confusion with chondrioconts is sometimes possible. In fact, however, the two organelles are easily distinguished. Tonofibrils may be conserved by fixation based on alcohol or acetic acid, which is not the case with the chondriosomes. Besides, their general morphological features resemble those of the chondrioconts quite remotely, and only a superficial examination of sections can lead to error. Histochemical characteristics and affinities for descriptive stains also render the identification of tonofibrils very easy; they are indeed highly PAS-positive, unlike the chondriosomes. Periodate or permanganate oxydation in an acid medium (p. 759) and performate or peracetate oxydation give them strong affinity for fuchsin-paraldehyde, when practised following the instructions on p. 467, as well as for alcian blue. Chondriosomes do not show any such histochemical character.

The first tannin-silver variant of Del Rio Hortega (1916) ensures a remarkable demonstration of tonofibrils in frozen sections of formalin treated material; chondriosomes are also shown if pieces have been fixed to that effect.

TECHNIQUES FOR DEMONSTRATING BRUSH BORDERS AND STRIATED BORDERS

Striated and brush borders were considered by early authors as ciliary derivatives and compared to immobilized cilia. The correct interpretation of these structures made through the electron microscope, however, shows them to represent in fact microvilli of the cell membrane pressed against each other.

The demonstration of these borders is of considerable histophysiological importance since numerous cases prove that such formations signify an active exchange of substances between the particular cell and the medium in which its differentiated apex is bathed.

The details concerning the *fixation* of all the other organelles discussed in this chapter are also valid for striated and brush borders. Mixtures containing alcohol or acetic acid conserve them well; all topographical fixatives can therefore be used for their study. Clearly, cytological fixations can also be applied. Furthermore, the demonstration of an enzymatic activity that is easily conserved and detected, namely non-specific alkaline phosphomonoesterase, plays an important role in the study of these formations. Experience has shown, in fact, that all the striated borders and brush borders examined up till now possess very strong alkaline phosphatase activity, and this serves as an excellent means of detecting these structures. Fixation with chilled acetone, saline formalin, formaldehyde-calcium or any one of the other methods recommended for conserving alkaline phosphomonoesterase activity must therefore be applied in all cases where the object shows the type of differentiation discussed here.

Pieces meant for morphological study may be cut with freezing or embedded either in paraffin or celloidin; evidently the rules stated in the chapter devoted to the demonstration of enzymatic activity in general should also be observed when investigating that of alkaline phosphatase.

With regard to the stains for demonstrating brush and striated borders it should be noted that most topographical stains show their presence. These differentiations of the apex have no particular affinity for Altmann's fuchsin, they do not take crystal violet neither do they appear siderophilous; but the excellent conservation of cellular structures in general resulting from the treatment of preparations by mitochondrial techniques greatly facilitates their study.

It is by their histochemical features that brush and striated borders may be specifically demonstrated. They are known to be strongly PAS-positive and the procedure described on p. 400 shows them up most clearly. Furthermore, periodate oxydation gives them a strong affinity for paraldehyde-fuchsin (Scott and Clayton, 1953); this oxydation is carried out as in the PAS reaction, but the subsequent treatment of sections follows the procedure indicated on p. 352;

brush borders should appear a deep violet. Permanganate oxydation in a sulfuric acid medium may be substituted for periodate oxydation. It should be noted that esterification with sulfuric acid renders these borders very strongly metachromatic, but the specificity of demonstration by this procedure is less than that of the other techniques described above. Among the techniques for showing proteins, those that detect cysteine and cystine give the most contrasting preparations.

The ferric-ferricyanide reaction, DDD and all other methods for detecting protein-bound sulphydryls give satisfactory preparations. The specific demonstration of striated and brush borders by their alkaline phosphomonoesterase activity has already been mentioned; I particularly recommend Gomori's technique with sodium α-naphthylphosphate and those of Burstone using AS naphthol phosphates.

TECHNIQUES FOR DEMONSTRATING CILIA

As I have remarked at the beginning of this chapter, all the usual fixatives are suitable for conserving cilia; but proper fixation, where the cilia are not agglutinated, often requires very early fixation. Ciliary bodies and roots are also fixed by topographical fixatives, but the advantages of cytological fixation lie in the better conservation of cellular structures as a whole. All chromoosmic fixatives are well suited, as are those containing potassium dichromate and formalin, with or without mercuric chloride.

Embedding and cutting call for no particular remark.

As for stains, the mitochondrial techniques, Flemming's triple stain, the method of Pasini (p. 849) that of Unna with orcein and water blue, and even topographical stains which give deep tints to sections clearly show ciliary bodies, roots and the cilia themselves. These structures appear very clearly in preparations treated with Danielli's coupled tetrazonium and after demonstration of protein-bound sulfhydryl.

One should not hide the fact that very short and sparse cilia are difficult to see under the light microscope; none of the classical techniques gives them a particularly deep stain so that they easily escape observation. Electron micrographs have shown the presence of cilia in a far from negligible number of cases where the light microscope would not have led to any suspicion of their existence.

CHAPTER 29

TECHNIQUES FOR DEMONSTRATING SECRETORY GRANULES

The presence of secretory granules in the cytoplasm is not a feature common to all Metazoan cells and the techniques for their detection should, properly speaking, be described elsewhere than in this part of the book. However, the importance of demonstrating secretory granules in histophysiological research on glandular cells and the need to distinguish these structures from elements of the chondriome are such that I feel it suitable to group the relevant techniques in a single chapter.

The term "secretory product" is used here in its histological sense and denotes the structured products of glandular activity. I refer the reader to recent publications (Junqueira and Hirsch, 1956; Palay, 1958; Gabe and Arvy, 1961; Gabe, 1964) for the definition of glandular activity and a description of the process.

A fundamental precept, which can be illustrated by several examples, dominates the morphological study of secretory products; it is that in all cases where a secretory product can be detected both by staining or by a histochemical reaction the latter should be preferred. In fact the colour produced by a positive result in the case of a histochemical reaction can be interpreted in chemical terms while even the most investigated of stains are to some extent empirical. A histochemical reaction is always easier to standardize than a staining technique, and it is particularly important that the identical technical conditions of a previous study be reproduced in histophysiological research involving the detection of secretory products. A positive histochemical reaction can, furthermore, indicate the function of active principles elaborated by the glandular cells in question, while a tinctorial affinity by itself allows no such interpretation.

Consequently, the techniques for the histochemical detection of sugars, lipids, proteins and their derivatives, and inorganic substances, described in the third part of this book turn out to be ideal methods for studying secretory products once the presence of such substances and the feasibility of their detection by these techniques has been shown. The spectacular progress made in the cytology of the adenohypophysis with the help of the PAS reaction clearly illustrates my point. In fact the demonstration of "secretory granules" by staining is only a temporary solution, whose histophysiological value can be great but whose substitution by a histochemical reaction is always preferable, of course on condition that the chosen reaction is sufficiently reliable and that the morphological features, especially the integrity of structures, are maintained.

Vital observation of secretory granules is generally easy. The procedure described for the vital study of the pancreatic chondriome of the mouse permits a detailed analysis and even the cinematographic recording of the secretory cycle. In most cases the difference in the refractive index between secretory granules and the hyaloplasm is sufficient for even detailed light-field observation.

Fixation of secretory granules is on the whole much easier than that of the chondriome and the Golgi apparatus. Rapid removal and the fixation of thin slices is, however, imperative, especially when the cells produce proteolytic enzymes. The so-called topographical fixatives conserve several secretory products so that liquids such as that of Bouin and its variants, that of Zenker, Heidenhain's Susa, and even those of Clarke and of Carnoy can be very useful in this type of work. It is none the less true that only the concomitant use of a series of fixative liquids including aqueous and alcoholic mixtures, both with and without acetic acid, and potassium dichromate and chromo-osmic liquids, allows one to conclude, from negative results, that secretory granules detectable under the light microscope are indeed absent.

There are cases where secretory granules rich in lipids are lost in the course of the operations preceding paraffin embedding. Apart from this routine method for studying secretory granules, it can be useful to examine frozen sections of formalin-treated material, or even sections of fresh tissue. Celloidin embedding which inherently prevents shrinkage can be advantageous in certain cases, but this advantage is barely enough to compensate for the time spent in this type of embedding and section cutting.

Almost all the techniques described in this book can show the presence of secretory granules, and this is true for stains as well as histochemical reactions. Their description would amount to a mere enumeration of a long series of special cases and such an enterprise cannot anyway be really complete. Only the more important ones are therefore retained and I shall not attempt to deny the somewhat arbitrary classification adopted.

TOPOGRAPHICAL STAINS

Some of the topographical stains already described in the second part of this book can be of great use in the study of secretory granules. Heidenhain's azan and Mann's method with methyl blue and eosin head the list in this respect.

Masson's trichrome and its variants, the one-step trichrome, and more generally all techniques involving several acidic stains are also very useful.

Two categories of secretory granules can be distinguished by these methods; the first, erythrophilous, take the xanthenes of the eosin family (erythrosin, phloxine, etc..) acid fuchsin and ponceau, and sometimes basic fuchsin and safranin; the others are cyanophilous and stain with dyestuffs of the anilin blue family, light green and fast green.

I must point out that referring to this second category as "basophil granules", often done by cytologists specializing in the adenohypophysis, is a misuse of the term that should by strictly forbidden. The mechanism of erythrophily and cyanophily under the technical conditions of the methods described here has been discussed on p. 137. It is worth recalling that these differences in tinctorial affinity do not necessarily depend on differences in the chemical composition of the stained structures.

CYTOLOGICAL TECHNIQUES

Some cytological techniques, especially staining by Altmann's fuchsin and by the hematoxylin lakes, are very good methods for demonstrating secretory granules. All erythrophilous granules strongly fix Altmann's fuchsin, and postchromatization of pieces is not strictly necessary for demonstrating this staining affinity although, at the most, differentiation may be facilitated by it. Similarly, erythrophilous secretory granules are siderophilous under the technical conditions of the Heidenhain-Regaud method and often take Bensley's cupric hematoxylin. The yellow tint that most secretory grains take after chromo-osmic fixation enables their identification in unstained sections mounted after simple dewaxing (see p. 736).

STAINING WITH NEUTRAL DYES

A very selective demonstration of certain secretory granules may be obtained by *staining with neutral gentian violet according to Bensley or by ethyl violet and orange G following Bailey* (1926). These methods, originally applied by their authors to show the types of cells in the endocrine pancreas, can be useful in many other cases as well.

Preparations of stains. — Both are instances of neutral stains prepared by precipitating an aqueous saturated solution of gentian violet or ethyl violet by the gradual addition of an aqueous saturated solution of orange G; any excess of the latter should be avoided since the precipitate is soluble in a dilute solution of the acidic dye. The progress of precipitation may be checked by spotting. (Place a drop of the liquid, taken after agitation, on a filter paper and allow it to spread before estimating the quantity of precipitate accumulated at the centre of the spot. The intensity of colour of the peripheral halo formed by the liquid also gives some indication). When precipitation has been judged to be complete the precipitate is recovered by filtration, dried, and dissolved to saturation in absolute alcohol. Some suppliers of products for microscopy offer both neutral dyes as powders which can be dissolved directly. The alcoholic stock solution may be stored indefinitely.

Operating procedure. — In theory, the technique may be applied to sections of pieces fixed in any of the mixtures that ensure the conservation of secretory granules, but experience has shown that the best results are obtained with material fixed in Helly's liquid or that of Maximow. Sections should be thin and they may be collodioned.

> Stain for 24 hours with a solution of neutral gentian violet or ethyl violet and orange G, prepared by adding one volume of the alcoholic stock solution to nine volumes of distilled water or ethyl alcohol at 20, 30, or 70%.
> The choice of the optimum level of alcohol for a given material is made by trial and error.
> Blot the slide with filter paper.
> Dehydrate in two baths of acetone (10 to 20 seconds each).
> Clear in a benzenic hydrocarbon and check under the microscope taking care to avoid drying.
> If necessary differentiate under the microscope with the mixture:
> Clove oil .... 3 volumes
> Absolute alcohol .... 1 volume
> This may be applied directly on removal from the benzenic hydrocarbon without any intermediate.
> Remove excess of differentiator by thorough washing in the chosen benzenic hydrocarbon, and mount in a synthetic rezin or Canada balsam.

Secretory granules take a blue or red tint according to the case; their selectivity is perfect.

A whole series of other neutral stains can be prepared and used following the same procedure. According to Bensley (1911) and Bensley and Bensley (1938), the precipitation of a solution of crystal violet by a solution of acid fuchsin, and that of a solution of safranin by acid violet (eriocyanin) provide very useful neutral stains.

GOMORI'S METHOD AND ITS VARIANTS

The staining techniques whose principle is based on the investigations of Gomori (1939, 1941, 1950) on the demonstration of the cellular types of the endocrine pancreas have gained first-rate importance not only in the histophysiological study of this organ but also in research on neurosecretion and the cytology of the adenohypophysis. In fact these methods cover a much more extensive field and their application forms part of any work on secretory granules whose tinctorial affinities and histochemical features are being explored for the first time.

All these procedures depend on the fact that certain secretory products acquire a strong basophily following extended oxydation either by potassium permanganate in the presence of sulfuric acid or by performic or peracetic acids. Periodic and chromic oxydations are not suitable.

A large number of basic dyes may be used, according to theory, to reveal the basophily that appears after oxydation, but in practice some are more suitable that others. Gomori (1939, 1941) has used a chromic lake of hematoxylin that corresponds in some measure to the chromic dioxyhematein of Hansen (1926) whose formula is given in the second part of this book. Toluidine blue and the Mann-Dominici technique give excellent results (Gabe 1950). Paraldehyde-fuchsin and paraldehyde-thionin are applied following the procedure for staining indicative of anions (p. 349). Phthalocyanins of the alcian blue group are used according to the method of Adams and Sloper (1955) for detecting protein-bound sulfhydryls, oxydation being affected by a peracid or potassium permanganate with sulfuric acid.

A histochemical interpretation of the result of these methods has been attempted repeatedly; the essential facts are given on p. 353. The oxydation of cystine and cystein into cysteic acid very probably plays an important part in the appearance of anionic radicals which are responsible for the affinity towards the dyestuffs given above, but other acidic groups could be involved (see also p. 353 and p. 524).

From a practical point of view the association of a basic stain with an acidic counterstain increases the sharpness of preparations and is advisable in all cases where the technique is not adopted with a histochemical aim.

Some of the practical associations that have been described are the stain with chromic hematoxylin and phloxine following Gomori (1941) that of Mann-Dominici after permanganate oxydation (Gabe 1950), that with paraldehyde-fuchsin, Groat's hematoxylin and picro-indigocarmine (Gabe 1953) and the technique of Adams and Sloper (1955) indicated on p. 524.

The chromic hematoxylin and phloxine technique is the only one of those discussed here which calls for a refixation of dewaxed collodioned and hydrated sections for 24 hours at 37°C in Bouin's fluid to which 3% chrome alum has been added. The addition of chrome alum generally produces an abundant precipitate which completely redissolves on warming. The mixture of Bouin's fluid and chrome alum may be prepared beforehand and reused several times.

Although not strictly indispensable such refixation can be useful in the Mann-Dominici stain; it is most often of no use when sections are to be stained by paraldehyde-fuchsin, paraldehyde-thionin or alcian blue, though it might improve the results even in these cases.

1° Chromic hematoxylin phloxine

Preparation of the stain. — Gomori's chromic lake is prepared as follows:

> Mix 50 ml of a freshly prepared 1% aqueous solution of hematoxylin and 50 ml of a 3% aqueous solution of chrome alum. Add 2 ml of a 5% aqueous solution of potassium dichromate and 1 ml of 5% sulfuric acid. Allow it to mature for 48 hours at room temperature and store in the cold in a waxed bottle. Filter before each use.

The staining capacity of the lake alters even if all the above precautions are scrupulously observed; it can hardly be kept beyond a month and a half. As I have noted, Hansen's chromic hematoxylin (p. 197) can be used instead of Gomori's.

Operating procedure:

> Dewaxed sections are collodioned and hydrated.
> Refix for 24 hours at 37°C with Bouin's fluid adding 3 g/100 ml of chrome alum.
> Oxydise until a shade of tobacco is obtained (from 30 seconds to a few minutes) with the following mixture:
>
> | | |
> |---|---|
> | 2.5% solution of potassium permanganate | 1 volume |
> | 5% sulfuric acid | 1 volume |
> | Distilled water | 6 to 8 volumes. |
>
> Rinse briefly in tap-water.
> Destain with a 2-5% solution of sodium metabisulfite or a 2-4% solution of oxalic acid.
> Wash for 5 minutes in running water.
> Stain for 10 minutes with freshly filtered chromic hematoxylin.
> Rinse in tap water.
> Differentiate if necessary (this step is very often unnecessary) in absolute alcohol containing 0.5 to 1% hydrochloric acid; in some cases sections should be rewashed in tap-water until a blue shade is obtained.
> Stain for one to five minutes in a 0.5% to 1% aqueous solution of phloxine.
> Rinse in tap-water.
> Treat for one minute in an aqueous 5% solution of phosphotungstic acid.
> Wash for 5 minutes in tap-water.
> Dehydrate in absolute alcohol, clear in a benzenic hydrocarbon and mount in a synthetic resin or Canada balsam.

Certain secretory products take an intense blue stain, while others are red. Nuclei lose their affinity for chromic hematoxylin under the above technical conditions, but the latter evidently stains all structures carrying anionic groups, especially mucins, elastic fibres, chromolipoids etc...

The removal of excess phloxine by 70% alcohol, often recommended in descriptions of the technique, is only rarely useful; a brief examination of sections before dehydration will show whether it is necessary. A critical step of the method, as seen from experience, is the length of the permanganate oxydation. In this respect chromic hematoxylin is less suitable than the other stains described below.

2° *The Mann-Dominici stain after permanganate oxydation*

Dewaxed sections are collodioned and hydrated, fixed in Bouin's fluid containing chrome alum, and then washed as in Gomori's method.

Oxydise with potassium permanganate in the presence of sulfuric acid (same formula as for chromic hematoxylin-phloxine) for one minute.

Rinse briefly in tap-water.

Destain in sodium bisulfite or oxalic acid.

Wash at length (for at least 10 minutes) in running water.

Stain for one or two minutes in the solution of erythrosin and orange G (p. 234).

Rinse briefly in tap-water.

Stain for one to three minutes in a 0.5% aqueous solution of toluidine blue; if necessary prolong the stay until a very deep uniform blue shade is obtained.

Rinse briefly in tap-water.

Commence differentiation by leaving sections in water containing 0.2% acetic acid; the shade should turn reddish violet.

Terminate differentiation by leaving in 96% alcohol; the general shade of the sections should turn definitely blue, while acidophilic zones show a contrasting bright pink.

Dehydrate with absolute alcohol, clear in a benzenic hydrocarbon and mount under Canada balsam or a synthetic resin.

As in the case of the chromic hematoxylin-phloxine stain, basophilic structures, whether their basophily follows permanganate oxydation or not, take a blue colour but the shade can range from a deep blue, almost black, to a light blue tending towards green. I do not know what these differences signify, although they are often useful in discriminating between secretory products and other structures. Structures which retain their acidophily in spite of permanganate oxydation are stained red, pink, or yellow. This variant of the Mann-Dominici method, while giving results which correspond to those of the chromic hematoxylin-phloxine method, has the added advantage of using stain solutions that can be stored almost indefinitely. The optical quality of preparations is excellent and there is less risk of smudging than with chromic hematoxylin. Differentiation should evidently be followed very closely if it is desired to obtain tints that are strictly comparable from section to section.

3° *The paraldehyde-fuchsin Groat's hematoxylin and picro-indigocarmine stain*

The variant, as indeed all others, of the paraldehyde-fuchsin stain has the advantage over the two previous methods of not imperatively requiring refixation of sections and hence results in appreciable time-saving. Refixation in Bouin's fluid containing chrome alum is useful, as shown by experience, only in very rare cases, especially when the original fixation of the material has been imperfect. Refixed sections withstand permanganate oxydation better and greatly increase the contrast of preparations.

Dewaxed sections are collodioned, hydrated and refixed if necessary.
Oxydise with potassium permanganate in the presence of sulfuric acid (as for chromic hematoxylin-phloxine); the period of oxydation is not critical since a length of 30 seconds to 3 minutes gives apparently equivalent results.
Rinse briefly in tap-water or distilled water.
Destain in a 2 or 5% solution of sodium metabisulfite.
Rinse briefly in tap-water (the prolonged washing indicated for the two previous methods is unnecessary here).
Stain for about three minutes with a solution of paraldehyde-fuchsin prepared by diluting a stock solution or directly from the powder (p. 350).
Rinse in tap-water.
Remove excess of paraldehyde-fuchsin by leaving sections in 96% alcohol containing 0.5% concentrated hydrochloric acid.
Wash for a few seconds in tap-water.
Stain nuclei with Groat's hematoxylin (p. 198).
Wash for two to five minutes in running water.
Treat sections for 10 to 20 seconds with picro-indigocarmine (p. 201).
Dehydrate with absolute alcohol, clear in a benzenic hydrocarbon and mount in Canada balsam or a synthetic resin.

Those structures which show an affinity for fuchsin-paraldehyde, either due to oxydation or otherwise, appear deep violet. Nuclei are stained black, basophilic cytoplasm light grey, acidophilic structures yellow and collagen fibres blue. This variant of the paraldehyde-fuchsin stain gives greater contrast than any of the others, especially the one-step trichrome (p. 821). It is recommended in cases where preparations are to be photographed in black and white.

METHOD OF SOLCIA, VASSALLO AND CAPELLA

This technique was invented in 1968 during the course of investigations on the endocrine cells of the gastro-intestinal mucosa and the islets of Langerhans of the pancreas. It gives excellent results to demonstrate a whole series of endocrine cells in Mammals, especially those that are known to produce polypeptide hormones and which belong to the APUD series of Pearse. The procedure does not seem to have been applied as yet methodically in investigations on Invertebrate tissues or exocrine glandular cells, but such applications look to be quite promising.

The principle of the method is very simple. It consists in detecting the appearance of an orthochromatic or metachromatic basophily, following hydrolysis with hydrochloric acid, in structures which are quite devoid of the slightest basophily before such pretreatment.

Fixation of pieces meant for this method is preferably carried out in Bouin's or Helly's fluid, or better still in a mixture containing glutaraldehyde. That which Solcia and co-workers have denoted by the abbreviation GPA is particularly suitable. It contains one volume of a 25% commercial solution of glutaraldehyde, three volumes of a saturated aqueous solution of picric acid and enough acetic acid or sodium acetate to give a final concentration of 1%. From my personal experience sodium acetate is preferable to acetic acid Pieces, one of whose dimensions should not exceed 3 to 5 mm, are fixed for 24 hours, dehydrated in 96% alcohol and from then on treated as material fixed in Bouin's fluid.

As far as I know, only paraffin sections have been submitted to this procedure. No particular precaution needs to be taken in embedding; the thickness of sections should remain less than 10 μ, and they may be stuck with albumin or gelatine in the usual manner.

In the actual method hydrolysis in hydrochloric acid is followed by staining with a basic dye.

The trials of Solcia and co-workers have shown that the best temperature for this hydrolysis varies between 60 and 70°C; temperatures below 50° are not suitable and serious artifacts are produced above 80°. The optimal molarity of the hydrochloric acid seems to be 0.2 N, though the range of tolerance is quite wide (0.1 to 0.4 N). With respect to the time of hydrolysis, actual trials are necessary to determine the optimum. It is generally better not to exceed three hours when the material has been fixed in Bouin's fluid. The optimum is nearer to 8 hours after fixation in a glutaraldehyde mixture, but quite satisfactory staining can be obtained in many cases with shorter hydrolysis.

For the staining itself thiazins (toluidine blue, azur A, methylene blue) safranin, pseudo-isocyanin and phthalocyanins can be used.

Toluidine blue should be preferred to all other stains in cases where a distinction between orthochromatic and metachromatic products is sought. Azur A also gives very satisfactory stains. The authors of the method consider staining with the thiazins as unstable; in fact, however, stability can be gained by the classic bath in 5% ammonium molybdate, which thus renders mounting in Canada balsam or a synthetic resin possible. From my personal experience clear staining cannot be obtained with the samples of alcian blue that are now available, but it succeeds with some batches of astra blue. The use of pseudo-isocyanin is justifiable only when it is desired to examine preparations under a fluorescence microscope.

The pH of the staining solution is very important. Experience has shown that the most satisfactory results are obtained at a pH from 6 to 5 (Mc Ilvaine – Lillie or Walpole buffers). Extinction is situated between pH 3.8 and 5 for the types of endocrine cells examined by Solcia and co-workers.

Obviously the hydrolysis results in the extraction of nucleic acids and certain acid mucins, but others persist; thus mast cells remain perfectly recognizable.

From the practical point of view I specially recommend staining by toluidine blue with stabilization in ammonium molybdate, by astra blue and by pseudo-isocyanin.

1° Staining with toluidine blue

Its advantage over the other variants lies in the very clear distinction between ortho- and metachromatic products. The operating procedure given here differs from that of the authors of the technique only in the inclusion of stabilization by ammonium molybdate, which enables obtaining permanent preparations.

Reagents:

> 0.2 N hydrochloric acid
> 0.05% solution of toluidine blue in Walpole's or McIlvaine's buffer, pH 5-6
> 5% aqueous solution of ammonium molybdate

Operating procedure:

> Paraffin sections of material fixed in an aqueous liquid are dewaxed, collodioned if necessary and hydrated.
> Hydrolyse for 3 (Bouin) to 8 (glutaraldehyde) hours at 60°C with 0.2 N hydrochloric acid.
> Rinse thoroughly in tap-water (several baths rather than in running water in order to avoid any risk of detaching sections).
> Stain for 5 to 10 minutes with the solution of toluidine blue.
> Rinse in distilled water; sections may be mounted in distilled water and examined under the microscope after this step.
> Treat for 5 minutes with the ammonium molybdate solution.
> Wash thoroughly in tap-water.
> Blot with filter paper, dehydrate in absolute alcohol, clear in a benzenic hydrocarbon and mount in a commercial synthetic resin.

The secretory product of certain endocrine cells (D cells of the endocrine pancreas, gastrin cells of the stomach, calcitonin cells of the thyroid) is strongly metachromatic; that of other endocrine cells (A cells of the endocrine pancreas, gastro-intestinal enterochromaffin cells) is orthochromatically stained.

2° Staining with astra blue

When compared to the method using toluidine blue, this variant has the disadvantage of giving a uniform stain to the different secretory products, but the preparations are perhaps better conserved.

Reagents:

> 0.2 N hydrochloric acid
> 0.5% solution of astra blue in Walpole's buffer, pH 5. Aluminium lake of nuclear fast red.

Operating procedure:

> Paraffin sections are prepared and hydrolysed as for the toluidine blue variant.
> Rinse thoroughly in tap-water.
> Stain for 3 to 5 minutes with the aluminium lake of nuclear fast red.
> Wash in tap-water.
> Stain for 15 minutes with the solution of astra blue.
> Rinse in tap-water.
> Dehydrate in absolute alcohol, clear with a benzenic hydrocarbon and mount in Canada balsam or a commercial synthetic resin.

A positive result of the method is shown by a strong blue-green shade. From my personal experience a previous counterstain greatly increases the selectivity and precision while decreasing the diffusion of astra-blue in the background which is no longer negligible at a high pH.

3° *Staining with pseudo-isocyanin*

Because of the instability of preparations this method should be utilized only when photography under the fluorescence microscope is intended. Contrast is much stronger than with other variants, but morphological analysis is less easy.

Reagents:

> 0.2 N hydrochloric acid.
> 0.02% solution of pseudo-isocyanin in distilled water.

Operating procedure:

> Sections are prepared and hydrolysed as in the other variants of the method.
> Rinse thoroughly in distilled water.
> Treat for about ten minutes in the pseudo-isocyanin solution.
> Rinse thoroughly in distilled water.
> Mount in distilled water, examine and photograph immediately under a fluorescence microscope.

Cell types that are metachromatic after toluidine blue (D cells of the endocrine pancreas, gastrin cells of the stomach, calcitonin cells of the thyroid gland) show a bright yellow fluorescence that is characteristic of polymerized pseudo-isocyanin. Preparations are highly labile.

The chemical interpretation of the method of Solcia and co-workers is still open to discussion. All authors however agree that there is a relation between a positive result and the presence of anionic groups in the stained structures. According to the authors of the method an essential factor of a positive result is the presence of a relative large number of carboxyl side chains in the proteins that are detected. A clustering of carboxyls would explain the metachromasy. Pearse (1969) admits that a positive result with the method of Solcia and co-workers indicates the presence of carboxyl or carboxamide groups in the side chains but insists that the chief factor of metachromasy is rather the predominance of a random-coil configuration in the proteins.

SILVER IMPREGNATION TECHNIQUES

Silver impregnation techniques enable a very selective demonstration of certain secretory products. These methods, to be distinguished from the argentaffin reaction (p. 328) are of no histochemical significance. They derive from neurofibrillar techniques and are generally adapted by their authors for use under well defined circumstances; some particularly important examples are reported in the following section of this book.

I must also recall that the first tannin-silver variant of del Rio Hortega (1916) enables the impregnation of various secretory products in frozen sections of formalin-treated material.

DISTINCTION BETWEEN SECRETORY GRANULES AND LYSOSOMES

The distinction between secretory granules and lysosomes can be impossible at the level of the light microscope.

The latter structures have been studied particularly by biochemical techniques and with the electron microscope. Most investigators prefer to explore in fine detail widely studied objects that are easily obtained rather than to embark on comparative studies which might perhaps reveal the true general characters of lysosomes. I should point out that the form of lysosomes and their general morphological features do not provide any formal criterion of identification under the light microscope, while ultrastructural features are more characteristic. Lysosomes are PAS—positive but this is so for a great many secretory granules as well. Both types of structures can be strongly acidophilic, and both are conserved by topographical fixatives. Even the enzymatic complement of lysosomes, primarily made up of hydrolases, is not always enough to distinguish between the two organelles since secretory granules can show up when testing for the same enzymatic activites.

The establishment of reliable distinguishing criteria, valid for many cases, is thus left to future research.

PART FIVE

HISTOLOGICAL EXAMINATION OF THE PRINCIPAL TISSUES AND ORGANS

> On peut dire que l'histologie, sans cesser d'agrandir le champ de ses investigations morphologiques, doit chercher à devenir histophysiologique, en s'attachant à l'étude des variations fonctionnelles des éléments et des tissus. La morphologie ne doit être qu'une étape dans la connaissance, dont le but est la physiologie.
>
> A. PRENANT (1899).

Any of the topographical, cytological and histochemical techniques dealt with in the earlier parts of this book can evidently be applied to the study of all the tissues and organs of any of the Metazoa. As I noted in the introduction, research histology evades codification, and the usefulness of an initial application of a technique on material not yet studied by this means cannot generally be predicted with any certainty.

It is nevertheless true that the information accumulated during a century of histological research allows us to suggest, for each tissue or organ, techniques particularly suitable for demonstrating such and such a structure. Such suggestions are particularly valuable in histophysiological research because they permit one to go straight to the objective without spending time on preliminary experiments of what strictly speaking are a technical nature, such as are inevitable in investigations relating to research histology.

It is the setting out of the procedures to which I have just referred that is the objective of the last part of the present work. To an extent which is even greater than for the other parts, techniques serving more than one purpose have had to be omitted in order to allow me to give the essential information without expanding the whole beyond measure. In no way have I the foolish pretension of being complete; in addition to deliberate omissions, relating to techniques which are out of date or devoid of real interest, numerous lacunae no doubt show up the inadequacies of my literature survey or of my experience; apologies are due to the authors of the methods in question.

One of the most fruitful orientations of histological research is defined by comments on which little emphasis has been placed; the microtome and the microscope can be the physiologist's tools just as much as the smoked drum, the oscillograph, the balance and the burette. No structural detail is accidental, no morphological change is a random event; in every case there is a functional reason for them, one of the tasks of the histologist being to bring them to light. In addition to techniques which allow us to demonstrate the details of classical structures, those which permit us easily to detect functional changes must find a place in the following chapters. Certainly, it would have been tempting to set out simultaneously the criteria which need to be considered when assessing the functional state of tissues or organs, criteria a knowledge of which does in fact form part of histological methodology. Such was my initial intention, which I renounced solely in order not to lengthen the text unreasonably.

It goes without saying that the suggestions given, in relation to the various tissues and organs, are in no way limiting. I might once again comment that major discoveries have been due to the sometimes fortuitous application of a well-known technique to material not yet investigated in this way.

CHAPTER 30

TECHNIQUES FOR ISOLATION AND MACERATION AND THE DEMONSTRATION OF CELL BOUNDARIES

Most topographical and cytological techniques as well as many of the histochemical methods show up the cell boundaries very clearly thus facilitating the study of their form; the same remark holds good for the constituent parts of various organs (secretory canals, excretory canals etc.) the morphological study of such formations being greatly aided by graphical or plastic reconstruction.

It is nevertheless true that the techniques for graphical reconstruction and, *a fortiori*, of plastic reconstruction are long and laborious; the mental reconstruction after examination of serial sections necessitates much background experience and necessarily remains as a very first approximation, no measurements being possible. This state of affairs allows us to see the advantages which even at the present day are still presented by techniques for the isolation of cells by maceration and dissociation which were much in favour amongst histologists of the nineteenth century. Certainly the modern investigator can go through the successive stages of a long and brilliant career as a histologist without once having to utilise the procedures to which I allude; it is nevertheless true that their application by those who know what they are doing can lead to a very real advance in their knowledge; I might mention as an example the histopathological studies of Oliver's school which constitute an application of the classical investigations of Huber and of Peter on the structure of the normal nephron.

In addition to a summary description of the procedures in question, this chapter contains technical details relevant to several methods particularly suitable for the demonstration of cell boundaries, certain of these techniques being reserved for thin membranes, others for blocks of material destined ultimately to be sectioned, and yet others intended for sections prepared according to the usual routines.

MACERATION TECHNIQUES

The isolation of tissues and of cells for histochemical study has different requirements from those of cellular isolation by enzymatic action which are familiar to embryologists. In practice, the latter try to preserve at all costs the vitality of the isolated cells, possible modifications of the form of the element being accepted from the beginning. The preservation of the normal form of the isolated elements is the essential requirement of the histologist's work, the vitality of the elements being sacrified from the beginning.

All the maceration media put forward by histologists are liquids containing fixative agents, but their concentration is much lower than that which is used for histological fixatives properly speaking.

30% alcohol, introduced by Ranvier (1874), remains one of the best maceration media; it involves a mixture of 30 ml of 96% alcohol and 60 ml of distilled water, the optimal duration of action varying from 12 to 24 hours. Ewald (1897) followed this treatment with a bath of short duration (1–2 hours) in a 0.5% solution of osmium tetroxide and with washing in water before proceeding to what, properly speaking, was the isolation.

0.1% osmium tetroxide has the advantage that it preserves the form of the cells very well, but its feeble penetrative properties limit its use to pieces of material of very small size; the duration of action is of the order of 24 hours, dissociation being preceded with washing in distilled water.

The iodated serum of Schultze (1864) is prepared by dissolving 0.1 g of chemically pure iodine in 700 ml of amniotic fluid; the replacement of this latter by a physiological saline seems not to have been attempted but should be possible; the duration of action is also on an average 24 hours.

Sodium fluoride in a 1 or 2% aqueous solution acts more rapidly than the preceding liquids; the optimal treatment for tissues such as the epidermis or smooth muscle is from 3 to 4 hours (G. Levi, 1904).

Chromium trioxide in a 0.1% aqueous solution, *potassium bichromate, or ammonia*, in the same concentrations, *Müller's liquid* (p. 686) diluted to one part in a hundred may, on the other hand, act for several weeks.

Dilute acetic acid (0.25–2% according to circumstances) is particularly indicated for the isolation of the epidermis of vertebrates; it can be used at laboratory temperatures or at 30°C; the duration of action varies according to the material investigated and may be determined by trial and error.

Concentrated hydrochloric acid acting for a short period is principally used for the isolation of the nephron of mammals.

Technical details of maceration and the isolation of cells. — The fluids which have just been mentioned can be used on either fresh or fixed material, the best course to follow varying with the circumstances; it is the treatment of fresh material which gives the most satisfactory results when we primarily wish to isolate the cells, the dissociation of the constituent parts of an organ being easier when fixed material is macerated.

In any case, the amount of liquid to be used should be small; this rule is diametrically opposite to that which histological fixation requires. Most authors advise an amount which is twice or thrice the volume of the material treated. As I have indicated, the optimal duration of action varies according to the fluid utilised and according to the material subjected to its action.

Washing, after maceration in 30% alcohol, is not useful; washing in distilled water is recommended after all the other fluids mentioned above.

The practice of isolation itself varies according to the circumstances; the epidermis and the mucosa which require to be flattened are detached from the underlying tissue by prudent traction by means of fine forceps; the dissociation of the organs with the object of isolating their constituent segments is triggered off by agitating the macerated material and finished off by means of glass needles, where appropriate using a binocular microscope to assist in the process; the isolation of the cells can be obtained by agitation or by *controlled* pressure exercised by little taps of a needle on the cover slip which has been placed over a small fragment of the tissue under investigation placed on the slide.

In certain cases, the material is stained in bulk before isolation, but after maceration; the techniques indicated in chapter 9 are wholly suitable for this purpose.

When isolation has been carried out in a liquid medium, and taken as far as the separation of the isolated cells, the washing needed before and after staining can be undertaken in a centrifuge by sedimentation followed by resuspension in the new reagent or by centrifugation at low speeds. The spreading of the sediment can take place just before mounting. This latter operation calls for no special commentary.

DEMONSTRATION OF CELL BOUNDARIES ON SPREAD MEMBRANES

The classical method of Ranvier (1868) for the silver impregnation of cell boundaries is only applicable to fresh material; it is a preimpregnation in the sense of Apathy (1897). A wash in distilled water, which should be as rapid as possible, but sufficiently careful to eliminate the blood with which the material may be contaminated is indicated for material taken from terrestrial or fresh water animals; it should be replaced for material from marine animals by washing with a 5% solution of potassium nitrate.

The treated membrane should not be folded; it is best to keep it under tension from the washing stage onwards, fixing it with hedgehog quills or with glass needles (drawn from a rod) on a support of paraffin wax or of dental wax; Hoggan's rings (histological sleeves), conical pieces one of which fits inside the other, specially devised with this operation in mind, are no longer commercially available.

The impregnation itself is carried out in an aqueous solution of silver nitrate, whose concentration varies from 0.5 to 0.2% (Ranvier, 1868, 1872); Hertwig advises that the silver nitrate should be dissolved in a 0.5% solution of osmium tetroxide, but this precaution is only worth while if good fixation of the cellular organelles is also required. It is essential to undertake the impregnation in full daylight, in sunshine, and to terminate the action of the silver nitrate solution as soon as the tissue has taken on an opaque whitish tint (in general 5 minutes). The material is then transferred to a large quantity of distilled water and kept under full illumination up to the point at which it begins to become brown. It is then carefully rinsed in distilled water and can be examined immediately after mounting in glycerine. It is often advisable to dehydrate it progressively (50%, 70%, and 96% alcohol), stretching it over a support if the impregnation is being carried out without this precaution, and to use nuclear staining (haemalum or the aluminium lake of nuclear fast red) on the partially dehydrated material (return this to water after treatment with 70% alcohol), and then to wash it and dehydrate it completely before clearing it in a benzenoid hydrocarbon and mounting it in Canada balsam or in a synthetic resin. We need hardly add that stretching it out before dehydration greatly aids the dissection into fragments of membranes which are too large to be mounted as a whole; this dissection should be made after complete dehydration, the fragments being cleared on slides.

DEMONSTRATION OF CELL BOUNDARIES BY BULK STAINING

Bulk staining in osmic haematoxylin using Schultze's technique (1910) very clearly demonstrates the cell boundaries, closing bands and tonofibrils; it also shows up the chondriome; from my personal experience, it is a good preparation for staining with Best's carmine. This technique has the following stages.

> Fix very small blocks of material (of a dimension which should be less than, or at the most equal to, 1 mm) with a 1 or 2% aqueous solution of osmium tetroxide; the fixation takes place at laboratory temperatures and lasts for from 24-48 hours;
> Wash in distilled water, several times renewed, for 30 minutes to 24 hours (a duration which should not be exceeded);
> Treat with a 0.5% solution of haematoxylin in 70% alcohol, prepared two or three days beforehand and allowed to mature, in an open receptacle, at 35–40°C; the liquid rapidly blackens and should be renewed when it is on the point of losing its brown colour (generally after two occasions of use); allow it to act for 48 hours;
> Replace the haematoxylin solution by 70% alcohol renewing this until the last bath remains substantially colourless; allow this to act for 24 hours;
> Dehydrate, embed in paraffin wax passing through cedar wood oil;
> Cut into thin sections (2 or 3 μ);
> Mount without staining after dewaxing, or stain the glycogen with Best's carmine (p. 411) but obviously omitting any nuclear stain.

The structures enumerated above stain in black; glycogen is stained in red if the sections have been treated with Best's carmine. Preparations which are too dark can be bleached; I advise bleaching in hydrogen peroxide (p. 712) in preference to the use of other methods.

DEMONSTRATION OF CELL BOUNDARIES ON PARAFFIN WAX SECTIONS

Topographical stains which confer sufficiently intense colours on the cytoplasm generally show up the cell boundaries well; the same is true of reverse staining using haematoxylin lakes, and of mitochondrial techniques, and of Flemming's triple stain and that of neutral gentian violet using Bensley's technique. A staining technique using orcein-water blue-eosin, which was developed by Unna (1894) is particularly suited to the selective staining of cell boundaries, of ciliations and of tonofibrils. Sections taken from material fixed in Helly's liquid are advocated by the author of the technique, but material fixed in Regaud's fluid or its equivalents, that of Bouin, formalinated alcohol or formalin are also suitable.

Technique using orcein-water blue-eosin

This method calls into play two staining solutions, the first of which is stable, the second (orcein-water blue-eosin) being prepared immediately prior to use by mixing two solutions, each of which keeps well.

a) **Safranin solution.**—Dissolve 1 g of safranin 0 (a mixture of tolu- and phenosafranin) in the warm in 30 ml of 96% alcohol (*warm on a water bath and not with a flame*), allow it to cool and add 70 ml of distilled water, and filter.

b) **Solution of orcein-water blue.**—Dissolve 1 g of water blue (aniline blue) in 100 ml of distilled water and 1 g of orcein in 50 ml of 96% alcohol. Mix the two solutions when their contents have completely dissolved and add 20 ml of glycerine and 5 ml of acetic acid.

c) **Solution of eosin.**—Dissolve one g of alcohol soluble eosin in 80 ml of absolute alcohol.

Method of use:

Dewaxed sections, treated with collodion where appropriate, and hydrated;
Stain for 10 minutes with the mixture
    solution of orcein-water blue .... 10 volumes
    solution of eosin .... 3 volumes
    The mixture keeps poorly; it is preferable not to prepare more than the amount needed for each working session;
Rinse in distilled water;
Stain for 10 minutes with a safranin solution;
Rinse in distilled water;
Treat for from 10–15 seconds with a 0.5% aqueous solution of potassium bichromate;
Rinse in distilled water;
Dehydrate in absolute alcohol, clear in a benzenoid hydrocarbon, mount in Canada balsam or in a synthetic resin.

Chromatin is stained in reddish-violet, the nucleoli in a bright red, cytoplasm becoming violet and the cell boundaries showing up very clearly, the epitheliofibrils taking on a reddish tint; among the fibrous structures of the connective tissue the collagen fibres are blue, the elastic fibres brown.

CHAPTER 31

TECHNIQUES FOR THE HISTOLOGICAL STUDY OF THE INTEGUMENT AND OF ITS OUTGROWTHS

The techniques which should be used for the histological examination of the integument obviously depend on its constitution; apart from certain very special cases, the possible variations can be grouped schematically into three fundamental types, namely the integument of *Tetrapod vertebrates*, characterised by the evolution of the epidermal cell in the direction of holocrine keratinisation, that of *Arthropods*, characterised by the production of a cuticle sustained by the apical pole of the cells as a result of the secretory activity of the epidermis, and lastly that of *Molluscs* which are often ciliated and rich in unicellular glands. These three types will be discussed separately.

THE INTEGUMENT OF VERTEBRATES AND ITS OUTGROWTHS

The classical distinction, in the integument of vertebrates, of an epidermis of ectodermal origin and of a dermis of mesodermal origin is too well known for it to be necessary for us to lay stress on it here. The methods for the histochemical examination of fibrous structures and of the cells of the dermis are identical to those used for the study of connective tissue discussed in one of the following chapters. Only the techniques required for the study of the ectodermal parts are, therefore, mentioned here.

VITAL EXAMINATION

Vital observation of suitably chosen regions is an excellent way of studying the vascularisation of the mammalian integument; capillaroscopy is now part of the routine of physiological research into cutaneous capillaries, but vital examination can provide only slight morphological information where the other constituents of the integument are concerned.

PREPARATIONS IN TOTO

Preparations involving maceration play a far from negligible part in investigations of the superficial relief of the integument, of the dermal crests, and of the distribution of tactile receptors, not only in the integument but in the ectodermal parts of the digestive mucosa.

Dry preparations suitable for the study of epidermal relief and of dermal crests may be obtained, according to Horstmann (1952), in the following way.

> Stretch the fragment of skin with the dermal face downwards using hedgehog quills on a piece of cork;
> To macerate, keep the preparation in 0.25 or 0.5% acetic acid, until the epidermis can be detached by slight traction with forceps without tearing it;
> Stretch the detached epidermis on another cork plate, rinse with tap water, and dehydrate with 50, 70 and 96% alcohol and finally with absolute alcohol;
> Treat with two baths of turpentine spirits;
> Allow to dry slowly (desiccation may require one to two weeks);
> Cut the tissue into suitably sized fragments, stick them to slides using a mixture of a rather thick celloidin solution (5% for example) in a mixture of equal parts of absolute alcohol and ether.

The tissue should be white and rather stiff; its examination should take place under oblique illumination; Horstmann (1952) notes that it is advantageous to study slightly enlarged photographs rather than the preparations themselves.

Preparations stained in bulk are better suited to the study of the foetal integument and are indispensable for topographical investigations of the sensory receptors. Fleischhauer (1953) and Kaplick (1953) recommend the following working technique.

> Immerse tissue, obtained as fresh as possible, in 1% acetic acid; macerate it at 30°C to the point where the epidermis can be detached without tearing;
> Wash in tap water so as to eliminate the excess of acetic acid;
> Stretch on a block of paraffin wax or dental wax;
> Stain for about one minute with haemalum;
> Wash in tap water until the tissue becomes blue;
> Cut into fragments, dehydrate with absolute alcohol, clear in a benzenoid hydrocarbon and mount in Canada balsam or in a commercial synthetic resin.

Obviously the epidermal face that one needs to study should be turned upwards; the examination of both faces is nevertheless possible except when using objective lenses of very short focal length, by reversing the slide.

EXAMINATION OF THE SECTIONS

The examination of the sections is undoubtedly of most importance in histological work on the vertebrate integument.

Topographical study

Topographical studies involve the fixatives described in relation to so-called general methods; there is no reason for preferring alcohol and this bad habit of dermatologists should certainly not be recommended. Bouin's fluid and its variations, Heidenhain's susa and formalin-alcohol are all quite suitable, as is Carnoy's fluid; fixatives with a potassium bichromate base should only be used with small tissue blocks because penetration is particularly slow in the case of avascular tissue such as the epidermis. Material intended to be sectioned whilst frozen can be fixed in dilute formalin, whether saline or not, or in formaldehyde calcium.

The preparation of the tissue blocks for embedding requires only one comment, namely the major disadvantage arising from the practice of leaving the fragments of skin for a long time in ethyl alcohol prior to embedding them in paraffin wax. When this latter technique for embedding is adopted everything should be done so that the tissue, once correctly dehydrated, is moved as quickly as possible into methyl benzoate or salicylate, or into cedarwood oil or butanol. This need to shorten the dehydrating time does not obtain for embedding in celloidin. It is appropriate to mention that this latter embedding technique avoids any shrinkage; its use is, therefore, to be recommended in all cases where the thickness of the horny layer, or the size of the tissue block, might lead one to fear an excessive hardening during passage into hot paraffin wax. In the same way, sectioning on a freezing microtome, which is also a way of avoiding this disadvantage, is recommended when the nature of the work does not involve the need for thin or serial sections. Whilst on the subject I might remark that the prolonged passage of the tissue blocks through hot paraffin wax is highly advantageous because the epidermis is difficult to penetrate.

Among the stains, techniques for the selective demonstration of collagen fibres, described in the chapter dealing with topographical stains give excellent results. I would particularly recommend azan, one-step trichrome, that of Ramon y Cajal, and the methods of Van Gieson and Heidenhain using naphthol blue-black as well as Masson's trichrome and its variations. The PAS reaction, together with, in suitable cases, alcian blue staining using Mowry's technique (p. 413) also gives very clear preparations.

Morphological details of the epidermal cells

Such details usually appear very clearly on preparations treated using topographical techniques but their very selective demonstration may require the methods set out here.

The fibrillar structures of the epidermal cells show up clearly when examined under polarised light in sections cut on a freezing microtome. They are preserved by all the usual fixatives and are acidophilic when trichrome stains are used. The technique of Unna (p. 774) involving orcein-water blue-eosin, is particularly suitable for demonstrating them as is the PAS reaction followed by a background stain with Groat's haematoxylin or picro-indigocarmine (p. 400); staining with fuchsin-paraldehyde-one-step trichrome, as described in relation to the demonstration of the hypothalamic neurosecretory product (p. 965), also allows a sound morphological study. Regressive staining using the ferric and cupric lakes of haematoxylin, as well as those which involve phosphotungstic lakes, can also be used for the study of the fine details of the structure as can the first tanno-argentic variant of del Rio Hortega's method, when practised on frozen sections taken from formalin treated material.

Keratohyalin may be shown up through its basophilia; I might recall that this dyestuff affinity is only partially due to the presence of ribonucleic acid. Haem-alum-picro-indigocarmine (p. 201) gives particularly clear images, the flecks and grains of keratohyalin stand out as a deep brown colour; experience shows that affinity for the progressive ferric lakes of haematoxylin is less than it is for the aluminium or chromic lakes. Ramon y Cajal's trichrome and staining with toluidine blue are also recommended for the detection of keratohyalin grains.

Eleidin is well preserved on preparations fixed with topographical stains not containing corrosive sublimate. A stain involving picro-nigrosine, due to Unna (1928) also ensures highly selective demonstrations.

> Paraffin wax sections, taken from material fixed in a fluid which does not contain mercuric chloride, dewaxed, treated with collodion and hydrated;
> Stain for 5 minutes with a saturated aqueous solution of picric acid;
> Rinse in tap water;
> Stain for one minute with a 1% aqueous solution of nigrosine;
> Rinse in tap water;
> Dehydrate with absolute alcohol, clear in a benzenoid hydrocarbon, and mount in Canada balsam or in a synthetic resin.

The keratinised zones take on a striking yellow colour, eleidin becomes blue-black.

Keratin can be identified, on preparations treated with topographical stains, through its strong acidophilia. During the action of the usual trichromes it takes up those acid stains whose diffusion coefficient is highest and whose particle size is least. We might mention that very dense keratin cannot be penetrated, even on thin sections, by any of the normal histological stains and so it keeps its yellowish tint. Numerous stains were recommended by the classical authors (see in particular Martinotti, 1924, and Unna, 1928) for the highly selective staining of keratin; only one is mentioned here, namely staining with haemalum-Congo red.

> Paraffin wax sections, dewaxed, treated with collodion and hydrated;
> Stain the nuclei with haemalum;
> Wash for 3 to 5 minutes in running water;
> Stain for 5 to 10 minutes with a saturated aqueous solution of Congo red;
> Rinse carefully in tap water;
> Extract the excess stain and dehydrate with absolute alcohol, clear in a benzenoid hydrocarbon and mount in Canada balsam or in a synthetic resin.

The nuclei and the keratohyalin show up blue, the keratin in deep red.

In fact, all the older methods have been surpassed, so far as the demonstration of keratin is concerned, by techniques for the detection of protein-bound sulphydrils and disulphide links; in addition to these reactions, which are discussed in the following section and described in Chapter 18, staining with paraldehyde-fuchsin allows us to identify the keratinised structures of the integument quite well but its histochemical significance is not as clear cut as is that of the true reactions; the advantages of the method for studying mammalian tissue have been well set out by Braun-Falco (1952); I recommend that it should be associated with one-step trichrome using the working technique described in relation to the hypothalamic neurosecretory product (p. 965).

The dermal membrane, whose ultrastructural peculiarities do not correspond to those of normal basement membranes, is endowed with all the histochemical characteristics and dyestuff affinities of collagen tissue. These are, then, the techniques for studying such tissue which will serve for its demonstration.

The chondriome and the Golgi bodies of the epidermal cells are difficult to detect using light microscopic techniques; their study is of no diagnostic interest.

Histochemical characteristics

The histological characteristics of the epidermal cells may be studied using the techniques described in the third part of this work; all the procedures mentioned there can be applied and their use calls for no particular technical commentary. It is only necessary to comment that the demonstration of PAS-positive carbohydrates, ribonucleins, and, in particular, proteins rich in cystein and cystine are of the greatest interest when studying the integument of mammals, birds and reptiles. Among the methods for studying the protein-bound sulphydrils and disulphide bonds, techniques such as that of Adams and Sloper, using performic acid-alcian blue, and of Pearse, using performic acid-Schiff reagent, give a very clear demonstration of keratin and allow us to appreciate the amount of total protein-bound sulphydrils present, but the analysis of preparations subjected to the DDD reaction, with or without preliminary reduction of the disulphide bonds, allows us to make an inventory of the true amino acids just mentioned and should be used in all cases where the histochemistry of a vertebrate integument is the objective of the work. No less interesting is the histo-enzymological inventory; the review of Montagna and Ellis (in Graumann and Neumann, 1962) gives a detailed description of the results obtained using different techniques and the application of the latter to the integument calls for no particular comment.

Cutaneous blood vessels

Cutaneous blood vessels can be studied on preparations obtained by vascular injection, using techniques mentioned in one of the following chapters, after demonstrating the erythrocytes using the peroxidase activity of haemoglobin and following the detection of alkaline phosphomonoesterase activity; this latter method, widely used by Montagna's school (see 1962, 1963) gives truly spectacular results; from my own experience the demonstrative value of the preparations can be still further increased by staining the free fats with a blue or red lysochrome. I would therefore recommend the following operational technique.

> Fix in saline formalin or in formaldehyde-calcium, at about 4°C, for 12 to 16 hours;
> Cut on a freezing microtome into sections 20 to 40 μ thick (the topographical analysis of cutaneous capillaries is easier when the sections are not too thin);
> Rinse the sections, collected in tap water, in distilled water;
> Treat them for about a dozen minutes with Gomori's medium for the detection of alkaline naphthylphosphatase activity (p. 607);
> Follow the progress of the reaction under the microscope and keep the sections for 24 hours in saline formalin or formaldehyde-calcium at about 4°C; as Montagna remarks, this precaution avoids the production of numerous bubbles of gas in the period following mounting;
> Stain the free fats with BZL blue (p. 452) or oil red (p. 453);
> Wash in distilled water, stick to slides, and mount in a medium miscible with water·

The cutaneous capillaries are shown up through the alkaline phosphatase activity of the endothelium, with striking selectivity, in black on a clear yellow background; free fats are stained red or blue. If one refrains from staining the lipids, the sections can be stuck to slides, dehydrated in absolute alcohol, cleared in a benzenoid hydrocarbon and mounted in a commercial synthetic resin or in Canada balsam. The transparency of the preparations is in this way further increased, which may be an advantage during the examination of fixed sections.

Cutaneous nerves and tactile receptors

The cutaneous nerves and tactile receptors whose topographical study calls for no particular comment may be studied using general neurohistological techniques, as set out in the appropriate chapter. The method using methylene blue can give excellent results; among the silver impregnations, that of Gros-Schultze, devised for frozen sections, and those of Bodian and of Palmgren for paraffin wax sections allow us to obtain highly demonstrative preparations.

Skin and hair follicles

The skin and hair follicles can be studied by the same techniques as for the integument. It is often advantageous to shorten the hairs at the time of fixation by cutting them with scissors to within one to two mm of the epidermal surface (never shave the integument intended for histological studies). Tissue blocks may be sectioned whilst frozen or after embedding in celloidin or paraffin wax; they may be oriented in all cases so as to ensure that the razor first sections the hair follicles and then the skin. We should not lose sight of the fact that serial sections may be useful during a detailed study of hair follicles. I might mention that the dyestuff affinities of trichohyalin are different from those of keratohyalin and that staining with haemalum does not show it up. Unna (1928) recommends the following technique for the selective staining of trichohyalin.

> Paraffin wax sections, dewaxed, treated with collodion where appropriate and hydrated;
> Stain for 30 seconds to one minute with a 1% aqueous solution of Bordeaux R;
> Rinse in tap water;
> Stain the nuclei with haemalum;
> Wash for 3 to 5 minutes in running water;
> Treat for 30 seconds with absolute alcohol to which a very small quantity of ammonia has been added (3 drops per 100 ml);
> Dehydrate in absolute alcohol, clear in a benzenoid hydrocarbon, mount in Canada balsam or in a synthetic resin.
> The nuclei are stained blue (the principal objective of the treatment with ammoniacal alcohol is to obtain this colour), the trichohyalin in red.

We may mention that preparations using PAS-Groat's haematoxylin-picro-indigocarmine are particularly advantageous for the morphological study of hair follicles.

Horny excrescences (nails, horns)

Horny excrescences can pose practically insoluble problems so far as the preparation of sections is concerned; their texture may be studied on sections obtained by grinding and polishing in cases where microtome sectioning is quite impossible. Softening using chlorine dioxide, in acetic acid (diaphanol) or, better, nitric or sulphuric acids (see p. 248) allows us in principle to section the tissue, even of the consistency of a horse's hoof (Drahn, 1926), but this result is obtained at the cost of substantial chemical changes in the tissue and certain structures (secretory granules, etc...) suffer a great deal; it should therefore be kept for what are, properly speaking, anatomical studies. Bird feathers may be treated in the same way; we should not lose sight of the fact that chlorine dioxide decolourises melanins. The working technique is described in Chapter 10.

Cutaneous glands

The cutaneous glands may be studied, from the topographical standpoint, by the same techniques as for the integument. The use of frozen sections taken from material fixed in saline formalin or formaldehyde-calcium is indispensable since the detection of free fats is one of the essential steps in the examination of sebaceous glands; staining with lysochromes and any of the histochemical reactions of lipids give interesting results; staining with Nile blue, in particular, allows us to follow the maturation of the sebum. The development of the cells of sebaceous glands during holocrine secretion is well illustrated by tests for ribonucleins (methyl green-pyronine after fixing in Carnoy's fluid, gallocyanine after other fixatives). Contrary to what happens in the case of epidermal cells, the demonstration of the chondriomes of sebaceous cells is easy, any of the classical mitochondrial stains giving satisfactory results.

The examination of frozen sections, treated as for the detection of free fats, is also indispensable when examining sweat glands or mammary glands; for these organs it is desirable, moreover, to apply a large number of cytological and histochemical techniques, in particular tests for glycogen, nucleic acids, and chondriomes (Altmann's fuchsin or ferric haematoxylin); there is much specific variation in their content of enzymes (see Montagna and Ellis, 1962).

The myo-epithelial cells of the apocrine sweat glands may be demonstrated with great selectivity using Heidenhain-Regaud's ferric haematoxylin stain or phospho-tungstic haematoxylin, the material having been treated with any topographic fixative; Masson's trichrome and its variations confer an intense red stain on the elements in question.

Whole preparations of cutaneous glands can be obtained by mass staining using boracic carmine or carmalum (p. 239–240).

Tissue blocks containing fragments of bone

Tissue blocks containing bony fragments (teleostian scales, the osteoderms of reptiles, claws, etc...) should be decalcified as indicated in Chapter 10. The unequal consistency of the tissues may give rise to serious difficulties during section cutting. An excellent technique, due to Petersen (1929), specially developed for the preparation of topographical sections using rather large blocks of tissue, is indicated here.

> Fix in a fluid not containing picric acid, if possible by perfusion;
> Decalcify where appropriate, and soften the strongly keratinised blocks of tissue;
> Dehydrate, embed in 8% celloidin, thickening the embedding material as required by the addition of pellets of celloidin;
> Harden the tissue block in chloroform vapour and then in 70% alcohol; preserve in this latter liquid;
> Wash in running water for 24 hours;
> Cut on a freezing microtome and treat the sections as if they were frozen sections taken from formalin treated material.

THE INTEGUMENT OF ARTHROPODS AND OF OTHER ANIMALS HAVING AN EPIDERMIS COVERED WITH A CUTICLE

The essential problems which arise during the examination of the arthropod integument and that of other animals having an even slightly rigid or thick epicuticle lie in the difficulties of obtaining satisfactory fixation of the epidermis whilst avoiding any tendency for the sections to come unstuck, and that of preparing sections which can be used for the cytological and histochemical study of the epidermal cells, without having recourse to softening the cuticle with too drastic chemical agents.

Fixing the animals to be studied as a whole only rarely gives satisfactory results and as far as possible one should assist the penetration of the fixative by cutting into slices, and by making incisions (these should be made systematically when the visceral mass of the animal is very soft fluid); injection of the fixative into the body cavity may be helpful.

Decalcification (the integument of crustaceans, and of diplopods, etc..) should be carried out as recommended in Chapter 10; the embedding in celloidin prior to treatment with a decalcifying agent can be helpful (p. 246). Procedures allowing the cuticular structures to be softened (diaphanol, etc...) should only be used as a last resort. Butanol is the intermediate liquid of choice between the dehydrating alcohol and the paraffin wax; softening the tissue by keeping the cut block under water is very beneficial.

Any cytological and histochemical technique can be applied to the study of epidermal cells; tonofibrillae and tendons are clearly demonstrated by the PAS reaction followed by staining with Groat's haematoxylin-picro-indigocarmine or by permanganate oxidation in an acid medium followed by staining with paraldehyde-fuchsin-one-step trichrome. Regional differences in the cuticle can generally be followed when it is stained with trichromes in terms of erythrophilic and cyanophilic zones. The behaviour of chitin towards the PAS reaction was discussed on p. 433; the demonstration of this compound by Schultze's technique plays only a minor part in the examination of the integument of arthropods and of related animals. The detection of polyphenols (p. 372) and of polyphenol oxidase (p. 647) may be helpful during studies on sclerotisation.

Details of the structure of the cuticle itself are clearly shown after staining with PAS or with paraldehyde-fuchsin; in large animals with a strongly sclerotised or calcified integument, the preparation of thin sections by grinding and polishing may be rewarding.

Sub-cuticular layers interposed between what is, properly speaking, the cuticle and the epidermal cells, can be shown up by techniques for the detection of acid mucosubstances.

THE INTEGUMENT OF MOLLUSCS AND OF OTHER ANIMALS WITH A CILIATED EPIDERMIS ON WHICH GLANDULAR CELLS ARE SCATTERED

The absence of a cuticular exoskeleton greatly assists the proper fixation of the integument of these animals but the rather frequent presence of glandular cells, whether isolated or in groups, requires great speed in the dissection and in immersion in the fixative so as to avoid abnormal appearances caused by the emptying of all the glandular cells of the tissue (in particular the mucosal cells) under the effect of shock. Moreover, the ciliature often borne on the epidermal cells may be very fragile and only its rapid immersion in a large volume of fixative may serve to avoid agglutination of the cilia. Deposits of mucus formed during dissection on the surface of the tissue represent a considerable handicap to the penetration of the fixative and should either be removed while the tissue is fresh or soon after their coagulation by the fixative.

The choice of fixatives depends on the objective of the work; when we have to deal with an as yet unexplored tissue, it is very useful to consider, from the outset, fixing in an alcoholic medium (Clarke's or Carnoy's fluid) in addition to fixation in an aqueous medium; I might mention that many secretory products are well fixed only by mixtures with a potassium bichromate base and that tests for free calcium may be useful, hence the necessity for fixing the tissue in alcohol or, better, by an alcohol-chloroform mixture (p. 306).

No particular comment is called for in relation to the embedding of the tissue and its cutting into sections.

Topographical stains are advisable when orienting the tissue and studying it anatomically; any cytological and histochemical technique can, according to circumstances, give useful data. This is particularly true for tests for mucosubstances and for secretory products rich in proteins.

CHAPTER 32

TECHNIQUES OF THE HISTOLOGICAL STUDY OF BLOOD AND OF HAEMATOPOIETIC ORGANS

The morphological study of the blood is indissolubly linked with that of the haematopoietic organs. In fact, the circulating blood only contains the late stages of maturation of the different lineages of cells in vertebrates and in those invertebrates which have haematopoietic organs, so that only the study of the sites of formation can provide information on stages earlier than that of maturity. Even in cases where the "globuligenic" organs are not anatomically identifiable, the formation of blood cells from fixed cells of the connective tissue is the most likely hypothesis, that which first comes to mind.

From the strictly technical point of view, the morphological examination of the circulating blood calls into play special methods, this state of affairs being due in the first place to the existence of a liquid intercellular substance in between the cells to be studied. Vital examination is much facilitated by this, the preparation of permanent specimens involving, above all, the technique of making smears; it is also true that quantitative and semi-quantitative procedures have entered into haematological technique well ahead of the first attempts to apply them to other tissues and organs. The importance of the haemogram in human and veterinary medicine explains the high degree of refinement of certain staining techniques; we should mention that clinically oriented haematologists have, on the contrary, neglected the application of general histological techniques to their material, so that the link between what are properly speaking the haematological details on the one hand, and those of general cytology on the other, may be difficult to discern. It did indeed require the development of histochemistry and of the electron microscope for the haematologists whom I have just mentioned to admit the advantages of using, on blood cells, procedures which had proved their merit in the study of other objects.

It is the examination of smears which plays the primary role in the morphological study of blood cells; the study of sections is, nevertheless, the essential stage in the study of haematopoietic organs.

HISTOLOGICAL EXAMINATION OF THE CIRCULATING BLOOD

The morphological study of the blood cells can be carried out *in vivo* by vital examination, of animals of sufficiently small size which are also sufficiently transparent, or that of flattened organs; such observations are highly instructive so far as the general appearance of the blood cells is concerned and also provide information about their changes of shape during the passage through the capillaries or in very narrow spaces, but it hardly needs to be said that such methods do not permit of a detailed analysis of the morphological features of elements which, because of their mobility within the preparation, cannot be examined under high-power magnification. The taking of blood samples, therefore, represents the first stage in its morphological study.

BLOOD SAMPLING

The most satisfactory way to sample blood destined for morphological analysis, especially if quantitative techniques need to be used, consists of piercing a blood vessel in those animals with a closed circulatory system or, in those which have an open circulating system, by penetrating a major blood vessel or the general body cavity. The addition of an anticoagulant is to be recommended in all cases in which the mechanism of blood coagulation is known; in vertebrates, blood can be sampled using heparin or using an isotonic solution of trisodium citrate; the amount of the fluid added and the total volume of the sample should be measured as precisely as possible so as to take into account this volume during any counts of the free elements which become necessary. The choice of anticoagulants is much more difficult to make in the case of invertebrates. Sampling by pricking the finger pad or the edge of the nail, the ear lobe, the comb of gallinaceous birds, etc... is sanctioned by custom but may result in a mixture of blood and of interstitial fluid; this source of error is even greater when the blood is taken by sectioning the end of the tail (mouse, rat) or the extremity of a finger (frog) or through the amputation of an invertebrate leg, all being manoeuvres which should be avoided as far as possible. Naturally the method of sampling, the nature of the blood vessel pierced, etc... should be specified carefully in all cases where counts are to be made. Even where the study is qualitative, sampling should be carried out without exercising even the slightest pressure on the area of skin near the puncture because a manipulation of the integument as is often practised may mobilise the connective cells and introduce foreign bodies into the blood sampled.

VITAL EXAMINATION

Examination between the slide and coverslip, without vital staining, calls for no particular comment; precautions intended to avoid variation in the osmotic concentration (sealing with vaseline) are useful only when the observations are prolonged; it is only necessary to use a hot-plate, under such conditions, when examining the blood of homeotherms. The use of a phase contrast or interference microscope is cordially to be recommended and the use of dark ground illumination may be helpful in the examination of very thin cellular prolongations.

Among the vital stains, the neutral red-janus green stain was described in the section devoted to the chondriome; many other stains can be used in the same way. I might mention that the demonstration of the reticulocytes of vertebrates can be obtained by vital staining, but the result is independent of whether the cells examined are still alive or not; the description of the working technique is given in a later section.

PERMANENT PREPARATIONS

Blood cells can be studied using dry smears or wet smears, each of these two methods having its own very special requirements. Dry smears are very suitable for the majority of what, properly speaking, are haematological stains, especially the panoptic stain, for demonstrating reticulocytes, when testing for peroxidase activity, and wet smears are indicated for the application of classical cytological techniques and for most histochemical reactions.

Dry smears can be prepared on slides or on coverslips, this last way of proceeding being of material use only when extremely costly reagents are to be used.

The preparation of dry smears on slides involves the following stages:

- Place a properly calibrated drop of blood at approximately 1 cm from the end of a clean slide which has been carefully degreased (where necessary, washed in alcohol to which a small quantity of hydrochloric acid has been added, thoroughly rinsed, further rinsed in distilled water and dried);
- Offer up to the drop of blood a slide whose edges have been ground down and one corner of which has been broken off so as to reduce its size; touch the drop of blood with the edge of the ground slide so as to spread the drop linearly, whilst it is held in the acute angle formed by the two slides;
- Slide the ground glass slide uniformly and fairly rapidly along the greatest dimension of the other slide taking care that the edges of the two slides remain parallel; the drop of blood, which should be stretched out into a fold by the earlier stage, should then spread into a uniform layer whose thickness is regulated by the angle between

the two slides (the film becomes thinner as the ground glass slide approaches the horizontal position); the "tail" of the smear should reach the carrier slide and the "head" of the smear should not be too thick;

Dry immediately, by waving the slide bearing the smear in a series of rapid fan-shaped movements, the axis of these movements being the manipulator's wrist and not his elbow.

A successful smear should be thin, without inequalities or "scratch marks", the whole drop of blood being spread out and accessible to microscopic examination. The technique described, which amounts to "smearing" the drop of blood along the carrier slide, is only applicable when the relative number of free elements exceeds a certain threshold; it is perfectly suitable for the blood of normal vertebrates but should be replaced when preparing smears of highly anaemic blood or that normally impoverished in free elements, by procedures which are explicitly disavowed in normal haematological practice, which consist of "pushing" the drop of blood stretched out into a thread; the ground slide is then placed between the drop of blood and the extremity of the slide close to it and then brought up towards the drop so as to form an acute angle open towards that part of the slide where the blood is to be spread out.

The preparation of a dry smear on a coverslip is obtained in the following way:

Place a small drop of blood in the center of a coverslip cleaned as described above;

Place a second coverslip on the first, the second being turned through 45° with respect to the first so as to free the lower left corner of the coverslip bearing the blood droplet from the upper right-hand corner of the top coverslip; allow the blood droplet to spread without exercising even the slightest pressure; its dimensions should be such that all the blood is retained between the two coverslips without any spilling over the edges;

Separate the two coverslips from one another with a fairly rapid and uniform withdrawal movement by pulling on the corners freed from one another in the preceding stage, then dry the two coverslips immediately using fan shaped movements.

Wet smears can be prepared on slides or on coverslips but drying should be avoided; as soon as it is made the smear should be immersed in liquid fixative or subjected to fixative vapours.

Any chemical fixatives mentioned in the other parts of this book can be applied to blood smears; it is the fixative agent or mixture particularly recommended for such purposes which should be used for histochemical purposes; the procedures described for the study of nuclear structures are entirely suitable for the analysis of the general morphological characteristics of the elements of the blood. Fixing using osmic vapours gives very good results. When the smears need to be stained using azur eosinates Weidenreich (1909) advises that several drops of acetic acid should be added to the osmium tetroxide solution and that the slide should be exposed to the vapours of this mixture for one minute at the most and then bleached gently in potassium permanganate (using a very dilute aqueous solution) prior to staining.

The technique recommended by Grassé (1926), for the cytological study of flagellates, gives excellent results with invertebrate blood; its application to that of vertebrates may be impeded by the abundance of erythrocytes but the results are very satisfactory when working with suspensions of leucocytes obtained by controlled centrifugation or by spontaneous sedimentation of blood to which an anticoagulant has been added; I might remark in passing that constricted tubes and other equipment have been manufactured with this end in view (see Bessis, 1954). Grassé's technique involves the following stages.

Fix a very small droplet in osmium vapour; the time for this fixation varies between 5 and 20 seconds, the optimum, which varies according to the material, should be determined by trial and error;

Spread on a slide and stir until half-dried; the optimum amount of drying varies according to the amount of fixation and should be determined by trial and error;

Wash for 10 to 30 minutes in tap water which is either running or frequently renewed;

Mordant for 10 to 15 minutes using a 3% aqueous solution of iron alum which has been freshly prepared;

Rinse rapidly in distilled water;

Stain for 10 to 15 minutes with a 1% solution of haematoxylin prepared by diluting a suitably matured 10% alcoholic solution with distilled water;

Rinse in distilled water;

Differentiate under the microscope using an iron alum solution; the solution used for mordanting is suitable, less concentrated solutions should only be used when the differentiation is particularly rapid;

Wash at length in running water;

Dehydrate in absolute alcohol, clear in a benzenoid hydrocarbon, and mount in a synthetic resin or in Canada balsam.

The siderophilic organelles (the chondriome, various granules, etc...) stand out intensely black on a grey or yellow background.

It may happen that the intercellular liquid takes on too intense a grey colour which hinders the examination of the preparations. Grassé (1926) advises that the duration of mordanting with iron alum should be prolonged in such cases (4 to 24 hours) using a more dilute solution (0.5 to 1%) followed by prolonged washing in distilled water and staining, for 10 minutes to 1 hour, in a more dilute solution of haematoxylin (0.1 to 1%). Differentiation is then carried out using a dilute solution of iron alum.

The working technique for stains and histochemical reactions applied to wet fixed blood smears calls for no particular comment; the time spent in the chosen fixative may be much reduced compared with that for tissue blocks intended for embedding; there is only rarely any advantage in exceeding 10 minutes. The techniques are carried out in the same way as for the treatment of paraffin wax sections.

HAEMATOLOGICAL STAINS

This designation is used arbitrarily for methods particularly recommended for the identification of the various categories of cell in the circulating blood. Among the older methods, the triacid technique (Ehrlich, 1876), which consists of treating dry smears fixed by heat (for several seconds at about 90°C) in the mixture described on p. 231 for 5 to 10 minutes, and then washing in distilled water until all excess of the stain has been extracted followed by drying, is now only of historical interest and the same remark holds good for techniques put forward for the selective demonstration of one or other of the categories of blood granulocytes. In fact, the whole of modern diagnostic haematology depends on the examination of dry smears stained with eosinates of azur, preferably after staining with the eosinate of methylene blue. This particular association which was designated by its inventor, A. Pappenheim (1910, 1911), under the name of the panoptic method is universally adopted in European countries.

Its principle is simple and ingeneous. The dry smears are covered with a solution of the eosinate of methylene blue, a neutral stain, in methyl alcohol, this latter fluid completing the "fixation" begun by the desiccation; a small quantity of water is added, the eosinate of methylene blue dissociates into its two constituents so that both acidophilic and basophilic structures are stained. This first stain is followed by treatment with a dilute solution of eosinate of azur. Washing with distilled water is followed by drying at laboratory temperatures (*never warm*) and the smears are ready for examination.

The eosinate of methylene blue (May-Grünwald's stain, Jenner's stain) is commercially available either in the form of a powder, 0.25 g of which should be dissolved in each 100 ml of pure methyl alcohol (for analysis), or in the form of a solution ready for use. The intensive employment of this stain in clinical haematology provides the industry with a turnover sufficient to make its careful manufacture a paying proposition and almost all commercial samples are quite suitable. Purchase of the powder is only to be recommended when one wishes to avoid transporting the liquid.

Among the commercial preparations of eosinate of azur, Giemsa's stain is that most used in European countries; its Anglo-Saxon equivalents are Wright's stain and Leishman's stain. In all three cases we have to deal with complex mixtures containing yellowish eosin, methylene blue, azur A and azur B, together with methylene violet. As in the case of the eosinate of methylene blue the stains which have just been mentioned are available in powder form or in that of solutions which are ready for use. Giemsa's stain in powder form is dissolved to the extent of 0.8 or 1% in a mixture of equal parts of methanol and glycerine, the stains of Leishman and Wright to the extent of 0.5% in pure methyl alcohol. Almost all the samples on the market provided by European manufacturers give very good results; the purchase of the stains in powder form, followed by laboratory preparation of the solutions, is indicated under the same conditions as for the eosinate of methylene blue.

The pH of the distilled water used for diluting the stains and for washing is one of the essential factors in the success of the stain. The use of a Sörensen phosphate buffer or of that of McIlvaine-Lillie (p. 667) in place of distilled water is cordially recommended. As for the pH to be chosen we need to take into account the fact that low pH values favour reddish tints whereas high pH values favour blue ones. Lillie (1965) recommends a pH value around 6 for bone marrow smears, from 6.5 to 6.8 for blood smears and 7 for slides intended for examination of blood parasites. In practise, the use of pH values between 6.5 and 6.8 gives satisfactory results for the great majority of objects.

Pappenheim's panoptic stain:

> Dry smears, less than one week old;
> Cover the smears with 10 to 20 drops of May-Grünwald's stain allowing this to act for two to three minutes;
> Add 10 to 20 drops of distilled water or of buffer, stirring to ensure the mixture of the two liquids and allow to stand for 3 minutes;
> Rinse rapidly in distilled water or in the chosen buffer;
> Cover the slide with a dilute solution of Giemsa's stain, containing one drop per ml of distilled water or of buffer; prepare this solution just before use by allowing the stain to fall drop by drop into the distilled water or the buffer; reject the mixture if a precipitate should form; the duration of the staining is from 10 to 20 minutes;
> Wash vigorously in distilled water or in buffer and allow to dry at laboratory temperatures (blotting with tissue paper is possible);
> The smears so stained may be examined without mounting using an oil immersion objective; to explore them at lower magnifications they should be covered with a coverslip previously treated, on the face in contact with the smear, with a drop of immersion oil or of vaseline oil. The smear can be washed in a benzenoid hydrocarbon but all washing in alcohol should be avoided. The principal misadventure likely during the method, namely the precipitation of eosinate of azur on the smear, may undoubtedly be avoided by working with chemically clean glassware, particularly free from acids, and by preparing the dilute Giemsa stain immediately prior to each use; the dilute solution does not keep for more than an hour.

The nuclei take on a violet red tint, this dyestuff affinity being directly conditioned by the staining with the eosinate of methylene blue which was undertaken in the first stage of the method; basophilic cytoplasm is blue, acidophilic cytoplasm is red and mixed colours (polychromatophily) is diagnostic of the intermediate stages in the maturation of the erythrocytes; the azur granules of lymphoid cells stain purple, those of myeloid cells stain violet; neutrophil grains are brownish or bluish, eosinophil grains are brick red, whereas basophilic grains stain ultra-marine blue.

Wright's stain. — The original working technique is based on that used for May-Grünwald's stain, the first stage of the panoptic method.

Dry smears, less than one week old;
Cover the smears with about 0.5 ml of the stock alcoholic solution of Wright's stain and allow this to act for 2 minutes;
Add 1.5 ml of distilled water or of the chosen buffer, inclining the slide in all directions to accelerate the mixture of the two liquids and allow to stand for 3 to 5 minutes;
Rinse vigorously in distilled water, blot with tissue paper and allow to dry.

A variation put forward by Lillie (1954, 1965) gives better results and allows us to use the same quantity of diluted stain at least twice; the stock solution is prepared by dissolving the commercially available powder in a mixture of equal parts of methanol and glycerine to the extent of 0.5 g per 100 ml of the mixture.

Dry smears prepared for not longer than one week;
Fix for 2 to 3 minutes in methyl alcohol;
Stain for 5 minutes in Borrel tubes or in Coplin jars, using the mixture stock solution of Wright's stain
> (methanol-glycerine) .... 4 ml
> acetone .... 3 ml
> M/15 Sörensen buffer, pH 6.5 .... 2 ml
> distilled water .... 31 ml

Rinse vigorously in distilled water, blot with tissue paper, and allow to dry;
The results correspond substantially to those obtained by the panoptic method;
Giemsa's stain can be substituted in this formula for that of Wright.

Numerous variations derived from these techniques offer no practical advantages over those which have been described here; the substitution of Pappenheim's panchrome for Giemsa's stain, which is of no great interest when staining smears, is on the contrary of advantage when staining sections and I would cordially recommend it (see p. 802).

When followed to the letter, these techniques give preparations which allow us to identify the cellular categories of circulating blood, of bone marrow, of the spleen and of the lymph nodes of vertebrates, imprints of squash preparations of these organs being treated as if they were dry smears. Naturally, an account of the characteristics of the various cell types would exceed the scope of a work concerned with technique (see, on this topic, Bessis, 1948, 1954 and other haematological texts). It is nevertheless appropriate to stress the fact that "equivalent images" in Nissl's sense are obtained by this means. The nuclear structures, whose essential role in the identification of blood cells is too well known to require me to restate them here, are not identical on smears or on sections; the dyestuff affinities of the cytoplasmic granulations, mentioned above as available when smears are used, are almost impossible to obtain with the same degree of detail when using sections.

The staining of the reticulocytes, an account of which is of some interest for diagnostic haematologists, may be obtained *in vivo* but it is not a vital stain.

The "granulo-filamentous" substance of older authors corresponds to a precipitation of ribonucleins under the effect of the dyestuff, the homogeneous distribution of ribosomes in the cytoplasm, which is well shown up by electron microscopy, being destroyed.

The reticulocytes can be demonstrated by any basic stain but the ones to be used for preference are brilliant cresyl blue and methylene blue.

> **Pappenheim's technique** involves the following stages;
> Spread out into a thin layer a 1% alcoholic solution of brilliant cresyl blue on a carefully cleaned carrier slide; allow to dry; the slides so prepared may be set aside;
> Place a droplet of the blood to be examined in the middle of a coverslip and then place it on the prepared slide so that the blood, as it spreads, will cover the layer of dry stain;
> Examine under the microscope and count the percentage of reticulocytes.
>
> **A technique recommended by Bessis** (1948) involves staining prior to spreading;
> Mix equal parts, in a small tube (a haemolysis tube), of blood sampled without an anticoagulant and a 1% solution of brilliant cresyl blue in a physiological fluid isotonic with the blood of the animal;
> Allow to stand for 20 to 30 minutes;
> Make dry smears and examine under oil immersion.
>
> **Sabrazès' technique** consists of placing a small droplet of a 2% aqueous solution of methylene blue on a coverslip and reversing this coverslip on to a dry smear. The preparation may be examined immediately.

In all cases the "granulo-filamentous substance", once demonstrated, may be stained by the panoptic method, in blue; it is therefore sufficient to subject the preparations, after examination, to the May-Grünwald-Giemsa stain to render them permanent.

ENUMERATION OF THE FREE ELEMENTS OF THE BLOOD

As I remarked in the introduction to this chapter, the liquid condition of the intercellular substance of the blood greatly assists the use of quantitative techniques; their importance in clinical haematology is well known to everyone.

The principle of all the counting techniques is simple; a given quantity of blood is diluted with some preserving fluid, an aliquot of this fluid is sampled and the elements are counted in an exactly calibrated volume of the fluid; the rule of three allows us to calculate the number of free elements per cubic mm of blood. We may need to consider separately a count of erythrocytes (red blood cells, haematic cells), that of leucocytes (white blood cells) and that of blood platelets; a few words about the establishment of the leucocyte formula should also play a part in this section.

1° *Enumeration of the erythrocytes of vertebrates*

The traditional technique consists of sampling a very small quantity of blood, exactly measured using a specially calibrated pipette, which is widened so as to include the glass bead intended to facilitate mixing, and then making up the volume using a diluting fluid, and lastly placing a drop of the mixture in a counting cell and counting the number of the elements in a known volume of liquid.

Diluting pipettes (Potain's mixer, Thoma's pipette, etc...) allow us to obtain dilutions of 1/100 to 1/500; it is helpful to use an average dilution so as not to increase too much the error stemming from the measurement of the blood volume and so as not to increase excessively the counting error. Naturally, the pipettes should be carefully maintained, washed in water, alcohol and ether, and then dried with care after each use, and cleaned with dilute warm alkali if deposits form within them. They may be calibrated by weighing after filling with mercury up to the mark.

Two diluting fluids enjoy great favour with haematologists, these are Marcano's fluid

sodium sulphate	5 g
commercial formalin	1 ml
methylene blue	0.01 g
distilled water	to make up to 100 ml

and Hayem's fluid

mercuric chloride	0.5 g
sodium chloride	1 g
sodium sulphate	5 g
distilled water	200 ml

but naturally any other liquid isotonic with the blood to be sampled will serve. Dacie (1950) particularly recommends a mixture of 1 ml of formalin and 99 ml of a 3% solution of trisodium citrate.

Blood is, then, drawn into the pipette up to the required mark (1/200, 1/300 for the mammals normally used in physiological experiments, 1:100 for anaemic blood, etc...); the volume is immediately made up to the division labelled 101 on the pipette, situated above the neck, by sucking in the diluting liquid; it is advisable to rotate the pipette during aspiration with a movement of two fingers of the right hand so as to improve the homogeneity of the mixture. Once filled, the pipette is laid on a horizontal surface; what is, properly speaking, the enumeration should be made in the hour following the sampling, after careful shaking of the pipette.

All counting cells include a glass base carrying a type of graduation which varies according to the manufacture (squares and rectangles of exactly known dimensions) as well as a permanent arrangement for siting the carrier coverslip at an exact distance from the base so that a knowledge of the volume of the liquid can be found from the graduation on the bottom of the cell. In some models the coverslip is set in place after dropping a droplet of the blood-dilution liquid on the base of the cell (the Malassez cell). In others (those of Thoma, Bürker, Levy-Hauser, etc...) the coverslip is placed in position from the outset on blocks of carefully calibrated and scrupulously cleaned glass, the correct position being indicated by the formation of Newton's rings. The blood-dilution liquid mixture is introduced from the pipette to the edge of the carrier coverslip and sucked in by capillarity to the interior of the cell. Each of these principles evidently entrains a source of error. In the Malassez cell the definitive volume which forms the basis of the enumeration is only reached after the introduction of the drop of diluted blood so that some error from excess, all the greater when the delay elapsing between the two manoeuvres is prolonged, must be accepted by the experimenter; moreover, the correct position of the coverslip cannot by regulated in advance. In the other types of counting cells, which have just been mentioned, filling by capillarity obviously introduces a distributional error, the regions which are far away from the edge of the coverslip on which the drop of diluted blood has been placed being poorer in the free elements.

Enumeration itself is greatly facilitated by waiting until the cells to be counted have had time to fall to the bottom of the cell. The condenser and the diaphragm of the microscope are suitably adjusted and the enumeration is carried out with a dry objective of moderate magnification. The number of squares or rectangles in which the cells should be counted depends on the type of cell that is used and on the dilution practised; the literature which accompanies the haematometers provides all necessary information in this respect. All the cells contained within the squares or rectangles should be counted; so far as those elements which overlap the lines delimiting the divisions of the cell are concerned, one possible convention consists of counting half of them, another consists of counting all those which overlap two of the edges and not counting those on the other two.

Naturally, the leucocytes should not be included in the enumerations; it is easy to distinguish them by their refringence; the same remark holds good for the thrombocytes of vertebrates other than mammals.

Once the counting has been completed the rule of three provides the content of the erythrocytes for each cubic mm, as a function of the dilution and the volume of the liquid which has served for the enumeration.

Some authors have suggested the use of phase contrast objectives for counting; others recommend the taking of photographs since the work of counting is easier on prints than it is under the microscope. So far as I am aware none of the attempts to replace visual counting by a simple automatic counter have given truly satisfactory results. Equipment using electronic integration, which is very effective, is obviously restricted to laboratories with a high level and a substantial budget.

As Dacie (1950) has quite rightly commented there is no reason to reduce the sample of blood to such minute quantities as the traditional method has used. Dilution in a counting pipette may, therefore, by replaced by sampling using precision pipettes of a greater quantity of blood and of dilution liquid, the mixture being made in a small glass tube (haemolysis tube) together with, where necessary, the addition of a solid anticoagulant (heparin, sulpharsenol).

A detailed discussion of the sources of error in counting blood cells and the statistical validity of the results stemming from these counts would obviously exceed the scope of this work; the various manuals and treatises of haematology include sections or chapters devoted to the question. Nevertheless, it seems to me useful to comment that the counting of blood cells represents an approximate way of estimating them, the presentation of the results showing dozens, hundreds, thousands, or even dozens of thousands being entirely inappropriate in the case of mammalian blood; it is in millions that the numbers of red blood cells should be expressed, since in this way the author respects the convention according to which the penultimate figure is certain and the last one dubious; from this point of view writing 5.40 millions or 5 400 000 in no way carries the same significance.

2° *Enumeration of the nucleated elements in the blood of mammals*

As Bessis (1948, 1954) has quite rightly commented, the traditional technique of counting leucocytes in mammals does in fact consist of counting all nucleated elements, any erythroblasts which may possibly be present in the circulating blood being counted as leucocytes. It so happens that dilution is carried out using 1% acetic acid to which, subsequently, is added a small quantity of a basic stain (1 ml of a solution of 1% gentian violet or methylene blue for every 100 ml of dilute acetic acid). Under these conditions, the red blood corpuscles are destroyed by haemolysis. Because of the small number of leucocytes per mm^3 of blood, dilution is carried out to the extent of one tenth or one twentieth using a suitably graduated pipette; the technique of counting, properly speaking, does not differ from that which has been described for red blood cells.

Another way of conducting the enumeration, less precise but generally adequate to give an order of magnitude, consists of counting the leucocytes, which have been identified through their special refringence, in the diluted blood used for the enumeration of red blood corpuscles, but counting over the whole field of the cell; the calculations are made taking into account the dilution and the volume of the liquid in which the enumeration has been completed.

3° Enumeration of leucocytes and thrombocytes in the blood of Sauropsida and Anamniota

The technique of enumeration which consists of haemolysing the red blood corpuscles patently cannot be applied to the blood of these animals; the dilute acetic acid would preserve all the nuclei of the erythrocytes and their enumeration would be practically impossible. The only practical solution, therefore, consists in enumerating all the different elements of the sample taken for counting the erythrocytes and calculating the number of the leucocytes and that of the thrombocytes according to the results obtained from the leucocyte formula. An experienced manipulator will, moreover, recognise the thrombocytes in the counting cell as their form is very characteristic and their refringence different from that of the leucocytes.

4° Enumeration of blood platelets of mammals

The enumeration of the thrombocytes is rendered difficult by their strong tendency to agglutinate; in consequence, the counting of these elements on smears of blood stained using the panoptic method, followed by the establishment of their relative number in relation to the red blood cells and to the leucocytes, represents only a rough approximation. In the same way, counting in a haematometer using a blood sample intended for counting the red blood cells gives highly approximate results which should be regarded with some suspicion.

Techniques of direct counting use very diluted blood either mixed with Marcano's fluid or with that of Achard and Aynaud

sodium tricitrate	10 g
sodium chloride	5 g
commercial formalin	10 ml
distilled water	to make up to 500 ml

A small quantity of blood taken by piercing a blood vessel is diluted in this liquid, the red blood cells and the thrombocytes are counted throughout the whole extent of the haematometer; counting the red blood cells under normal conditions gives the comparative information which allows us to calculate, using the rule of three, the number of the platelets per mm^3 of blood.

5° Enumeration of the blood cells of invertebrates

The principle of the method is the same as for counts of the blood cells of vertebrates, but the much smaller number of these free elements generally makes any dilution unnecessary. We take, therefore, freshly sampled blood which is placed as rapidly as possible in the counting cell, counting following this sampling process. In the rare cases where dilution is shown to be necessary, a fluid isotonic with the blood of the animal is used (a solution of 0.6% sodium chloride or Tyrode's fluid for invertebrates in the case of terrestrial animals, filtered sea water for marine animals). There may be a strong tendency to agglutinate; the coagulation of the blood may also introduce a serious artefact into the work.

6° The leucocyte formula

The examination of a dry smear stained by the panoptic method obviously allows us to count the different types of leucocytes met with and to calculate their percentage (a leucogram); the same manoeuvre applied to smears or to squash preparations of bone marrow, of spleen or of lymph nodes allows us to establish respectively the myelogram, the splenogram, and the adenogram.

The distribution of the cells in a smear of blood is not random; generally speaking, the cells of small size tend to cluster in the center, the more voluminous elements predominating at the edges and particularly at the tail of the smear. It is therefore essential to explore the various regions and in particular to include trajectories across the edges in the counts and also to include the tail of the smear in the percentage sampled and to verify that particular elements have not been held up in the head of the smear. The same precautions should be observed for smears of the bone marrow, of the spleen, and of the lymph nodes. In the case of imprint preparations we should not forget that the first prints are particularly rich in blood cells and the last ones particularly rich in the elements of the connective network; it is on the intermediate prints that we should undertake counting with classification into categories.

Only percentages with a relative value can be established during the examination of smears and *a fortiori* of prints of the bone marrow, spleen, or lymph nodes, the pulp so spread out being, in all cases, mixed with blood in proportions which are variable and impossible to determine. In the case of blood smears, counts made at the same time will indicate the overall number of leucocytes and allow us to express the abundance per mm^3 of the various leucocyte categories; only absolute numbers have real significance. It is indeed according to the data derived from the leucocyte formula that we can determine the number of erythroblasts and that of thrombocytes in the blood of Sauropsida and Anamniota.

The remarks formulated in relation to the way of expressing the results of overall counts obviously hold good here; it would be dangerous to forget that all the methods of counting mentioned here are rather rough approximations and that the presentation of their results with an excess of rigour serves only to illustrate the lack of numeracy and of good sense of the experimenter.

HISTOLOGICAL EXAMINATION OF THE HAEMATOPOIETIC ORGANS

As I have commented, the identification of cells corresponding to the various haematopoietic lineages is much easier on smears stained using the panoptic technique than on sections, so that the preparation and staining of smears or of prints plays an important part in the study of haematopoietic organs; it is nevertheless true that certain elements of the morphology of haematopoietic organs cannot be studied on smears and even that the cells of the connective network show up very poorly on the latter, that smears do, moreover, furnish no true quantitative data and that the architecture of the sites of blood formation is not necessarily visible on them. The examination of sections therefore plays an essential part in the study of the haematopoietic organs and even clinical haematologists, for whom examination of the bone marrow could at one time be summarised in the preparation of smears stained using the panoptic method, now advise, to an ever increasing extent, the embedding and cutting of sections of small fragments of the marrow removed by the needle during puncture of a bone like the sternum.

The general direction of histological examination is the same for all haematopoietic organs but certain special requirements exist for each one of them, requirements which it is appropriate to review in succession.

TECHNIQUES SPECIALLY REQUIRED FOR THE STUDY OF HAEMATOPOIETIC ORGANS

Any of the methods mentioned in the preceding parts of this work can evidently be applied to the haematopoietic organs, but the study of these benefits primarily from the use of certain topographical and histochemical techniques; among the classical cytological techniques the demonstration of the chondriome and of the Golgi bodies is not, in this case, of the same importance as it is for other tissues, but variations of Altmann's fuchsin give spectacular preparations in which certain types of granulocytes show up particularly well.

Fixation in Maximow's fluid (p. 686) with or without osmium tetroxide plays a particularly important role in the study of haematopoietic organs;

this is the method which gives the best preliminary treatment prior to panoptic staining, and is virtually indispensable for the examination of the sites of blood formation in vertebrates. I might recall that the size of the tissue pieces should be kept as small as possible, one of their dimensions being less than 2–3 mm; the time spent in the fixative should not exceed 6 hours for the mixture without osmium tetroxide; it may extend to 18 hours for the formula which does contain this compound. When embedding has to be undertaken in paraffin wax cedar-wood oil is the intermediate which it is most advantageous to use in between the alcohol used for dehydration and the embedding material; embedding in celloidin is conducted in the usual way. From this point of view I might mention that a virtually exclusive recourse to celloidin sections, as advocated by Maximow, is not wholly justified. When paraffin wax embedding is conducted with all the necessary precautions it does result in preparations which are almost as good as those provided by celloidin embedding even though the time and effort expended may be much less.

Naturally, any one of many stains can give valuable information about the structure of haematopoietic organs; the essential information is summarised below. Two techniques which are particularly useful in the circumstances we have to deal with at this point require description, these are the panoptic stain applied to sections and staining with polychrome blue (blue polychrome) as used by Unna.

Panoptic staining on sections:

Paraffin wax sections, dewaxed, treated with collodion and hydrated, or celloidin sections adherent to slides with the embedding material removed;
Stain for 20 minutes, at 37°C, with the freshly prepared mixture
  May-Grünwald's solution .... 1 volume
  distilled water or Sörensen buffer, pH 6.8 .... 8 volumes
Rinse rapidly in distilled water or in the buffer used for dilution;
Stain for 40 minutes at 37°C with the mixture prepared at the moment of use
  Giemsa's solution or Pappenheim's panchrome .... 1 volume
  distilled water or Sörensen buffer, pH 6.8 .... 75 volumes
Rinse in distilled water or in the buffer;
Differentiate rapidly (10 to 25 seconds according to circumstances) in 0.15% acetic acid;
Wash carefully in distilled water;
Blot with tissue paper;
Dehydrate with 2 baths of pure acetone;
Clear in a benzenoid hydrocarbon and mount in a synthetic resin.

The dilute stains are placed in an oven about 10 minutes prior to use in order to take up the appropriate temperature; each bath should be used only once; care should be taken with the cleanliness of the glass-ware in order to avoid the formation of precipitates. The slides should be placed vertically in the tubes or jars used for the stain-baths and it is best to orient them obliquely, the face carrying the preparations being turned downwards to avoid any possibility of precipitates depositing on the sections. The working technique described above differs from the original formula by the introduction of rinsing in distilled water after the action of each stain and in the suppression of the mixture of equal parts of absolute alcohol and acetone recommended by Pappenheim for the dehydration of the sections. Given these precautions, the method virtually always succeeds and can be applied to material fixed in a whole series of fixatives; nevertheless it is after fixing in Maximow's or Helly's fluids that the most striking stains are obtained. Mounting in a synthetic resin is by far preferable to that in Canada balsam, the keeping qualities of the preparations being much better.

The stains obtained closely approximate to those mentioned in relation to the staining of dry smears using this technique; it is appropriate to mention, moreover, the demonstration of collagen fibres in a clear blue colour and of mucins in a blue or violet one; muscles take on a pink colour, cartilage is blue, the various types of secretory granules stain red, pink, violet or blue. The preparations are truly spectacular and the usefulness of this stain certainly exceeds the limited field of haematopoietic organs.

Contrary to what was observed in the case of smears, it may be advisable to replace the Giemsa stain by Pappenheim's panchrome. This latter stain, which was developed in 1912, has the following composition:

methylene blue	1 g
toluidine blue	0.5 g
azur A	1 g
methylene violet	0.5 g
yellow eosin	0.75 g
methyl alcohol	250 ml
glycerine	250 ml
acetone	50 ml

It is sold in the form of a powder and also as a solution which is ready for use; most commercial samples are quite suitable and I would recommend the purchase of the solution ready to be diluted at the moment of use in all cases where the avoidance of transporting bulk liquids is not a paramount requirement.

From my own experience, the technique which has just been described gives results far superior to those obtained using the older methods which consisted of staining simply by the use of methylene blue eosinate or with an eosinate of azur, or alternatively by using a mixture of the solutions of methylene blue eosinate and eosin. Despite the very considerable success of these methods, it does not seem to me worthwhile describing them, because Pappenheim's technique, as set out here, can replace them to advantage not only so far as the ease of use is concerned but also in respect of the striking qualities of the results.

Staining with blue polychrome. — As I have had occasion to remark, the polychrome methylene blue and blue polychrome (the usual French term «*bleu polychrome*» is a false translation from the German name *Blaues Polychrom* hallowed by long usage) introduced into histological technique by Unna, are prepared by boiling solutions of methylene blue or of mixtures of that substance and of toluidine blue in the presence of potassium carbonate. In addition to these compounds which are introduced at the beginning the two solutions contain azur A and methylene violet. Their preparation in the laboratory confers no advantages by comparison with the purchase of the ready-to-use solution supplied commercially.

The two stains have no advantages over toluidine blue and azur A when used as indicators of basophilia for histochemical purposes; the lack of precision in the chemical composition of commercial samples does indeed lead me to refrain from recommending their use when the objective of the study is the rigorous definition of basophilia or metachromasia. Nevertheless, experience shows that stains obtained through their use have advantages from the purely morphological standpoint over those given by the thiazines mentioned above and it is solely for the study of haematopoietic organs and connective cells that their use seems to me truly advantageous.

Paraffin wax or celloidin sections, taken from material fixed in Maximow's, Helly's Carnoy's or Bouin's fluids; I would not recommend the use of this technique with sections taken from blocks fixed in formalin. The paraffin wax sections are dewaxed, treated with collodion and hydrated, celloidin sections are stuck to slides, the embedding material being dissolved;

Stain for about 12 minutes in a commercial solution of polychrome blue (blue polychrome, Unna's blue);

Rinse in distilled water;

Differentiate carefully (for, at the most, one minute) using Unna's "glycerol ether" diluted with 10 to 20 volumes of distilled water;

Wash in distilled water or in tap water so as to remove the last traces of the differentiating agent (3 to 4 minutes);

Blot with tissue paper;

Dehydrate in acetone, clear in a benzenoid hydrocarbon and mount in a synthetic resin or in Canada balsam.

The "glycerol ether" of Unna, a compound which is poorly defined from the chemical standpoint, is prepared by distilling glycerine in the presence of calcium chloride; as in the case of the stain itself its preparation in the laboratory has no advantages over direct purchase from firms which furnish products for microscopical work, the commercially available liquid being ready for dilution. Masson (1923) recognised the possibility of replacing this differentiater with a dilute solution (0.2%) of acetic acid. Another way of differentiating, recommended by Unna, consists of using tannin-orange (a 25% aqueous solution of tannin to which 2 g of orange G have been added to each 100 ml); cytoplasm stains yellow but the blue stain is less fine than after differentiation in "glycerol ether" or in acetic acid. Tannin-orange is commercially available in a form ready for use.

In addition to the excellent staining of basophilic structures the polychrome blue method causes all metachromatic structures to appear red or purple; in the particular case of haematopoietic organs it is particularly to be recommended for the demonstration of stem cells, whose cytoplasm is rich in ribonucleins and for that of blood basophils such as the mast cells (tissue basophils).

THE HISTOLOGICAL EXAMINATION OF BONE MARROW

The exploration of smears and of sections is necessary for the study of any of the morphological characteristics of bone marrow.

Smears can be prepared, in the case of homeotherm vertebrates, by puncture of a long bone which is not filled with air, a mixture of blood and of the medullary pulp being aspirated using a syringe with a metal piston, and then spread on slides, following the technique described on p. 788. Such slides are stained by the panoptic technique and allow us to construct a myelogram. Among the histochemical techniques the test for peroxidases on smears and the test for M-nadi-oxidase (p. 648 and 649) can be useful in doubtful cases when identifying cells belonging to the myeloid series; the demonstration of haemoglobin through its peroxidase properties (p. 567) is only rarely useful; tests for free iron using the reactions of Perls or of Tirmann and Schmelzer may be of far from negligible interest.

Samples intended for the study of sections should be taken as far as possible by dissociating the marrow from the bony tissue which surrounds it or, at least, by making large enough holes for there to be rapid contact of the fixatives with the cells. It is Maximow's fluid which should be used in the first place in any case where its use is not contra-indicated for reasons such as the size of the tissue blocks or the need to use certain histochemical reactions. The tissue blocks can be decalcified in nitric or trichloracetic acids, but it is better to avoid this process since the extraction of the ribonucleins seriously modifies the dyestuff affinities of the stem cells. In addition to panoptic staining and staining with polychrome blue, Lillie's technique using eosinates of azur (p. 235) and the Mann-Dominici technique (p. 233) give most instructive preparations in so far as the details of the cell structure are concerned. The connective web may be studied by techniques involving silver impregnation of the reticulin described in the following chapter. The distribution of haematopoietic parenchyme and of adipose tissue within the bone marrow shows up clearly on sections treated by topographical stains. Among the histochemical techniques, tests for free iron, peroxidase activity, and the PAS reaction are those most used when the bone marrow is examined for diagnostic purposes.

HISTOLOGICAL EXAMINATION OF THE SPLEEN

The cellular composition of this organ is easy to study on dried prints stained by the panoptic method; it may be difficult to obtain suitable smears and spleenic puncture, which gives a mixture of blood and pulp, which is easy to spread, has its own dangers.

The choice of techniques to be used on sections should take account of the need for an anatomical study, which is much more important than it is in the case of the bone marrow, as well as the possibilities presented by the use of what are, properly speaking, haematological stains.

Fixation of the entire organ can only be done when the animal is of small size and even then highly penetrating fluids should be used. In all cases where the smallest dimension of the organ reaches or exceeds one centimetre, cutting into slices is obligatory and requires the use of extremely sharp instruments. The microscopic anatomy and the connective-muscular web of the spleen may be studied after fixing in Bouin's fluid, in formalin alcohol, or in Zenker's fluid; fixation in formalin is necessary when impregnation by tannin-silver techniques needs to be employed; it is also useful as a preparatory stage in tests for haemoglobin; when carried out in the cold and followed by a very rapid passage on a freezing microtome, the same fixation is valuable as a preparation for histo-enzymological techniques; thin slices, may, moreover, be fixed in Maximow's or Helly's fluids.

Topographical stains, amongst which I would particularly recommend azan, the Mann-Dominici method and that of Lillie involving eosinates of azur are suitable for anatomical studies and, where required, for the determination of the relative volumes of white and red pulp, involving sketching, cutting out and weighing; procedures involving linear integration, as mentioned in the first part of this work, usually give results which are sufficiently precise and represent a substantial gain of time over the older methods. The same stains very clearly show muscle fibres.

Techniques for the selective demonstration of collagen fibres, of reticulin, and of elastic tissue are indispensable for the morphological analysis of the connective web; the first of these methods was described in relation to topographical stains, the others are mentioned in the chapter which deals with connective tissue. I would like to stress the need to call into play silver impregnation for the reticulin, no staining technique giving a sufficiently complete demonstration of these fibres.

Among ***the histochemical reactions***, the test for free iron and, where appropriate, for total iron by micro-incineration is often needed. The PAS technique gives topographical preparations of high quality and allows us to localise carbohydrates bearing *vic*-glycol groups; tests for free lipids and those for the breakdown products of their metabolism and for melanin pigments are required during the study of spleen macrophages.

What are, properly speaking, ***haematological techniques*** serve to complement the information available from the study of smears and of prints.

HISTOLOGICAL EXAMINATION OF THE THYMUS

The types of cell in this organ are much less numerous than are those of the bone marrow or of the spleen; as a result, the examination of prints or of smears is less important; the study of suitably stained sections will suffice to show any of the morphological peculiarities of this organ.

Fixation of the thymus as a whole can be carried out when the species involved is of small size; in practice, cutting into slices is only needed for the thymus of large mammals, especially if we refrain from using chromic-osmic fluids, Helly's or Maximow's fluids. Fixing in Bouin's, Stieve's, or Halmi's fluids or in Heidenhain's Susa will serve very well for a general morphological study; the use of Carnoy's fluid may be advantageous as a preparation for silver staining of the reticulin and for the nucleal reaction of Feulgen and Rossenbeck. Naturally, cytological fixatives are required for a study of the structural details and in addition any histochemical techniques can be used.

Embedding in celloidin is only truly of use for slices of large size; paraffin wax is suitable in all other cases.

Topographical stains give a good general study of the organ; I would in particular recommend the Mann-Dominici technique, azan, one-step trichrome, all procedures which give an excellent contrast between the cortex and the medullary of the thymus lobes. The quantitative study of this organ has been codified in detail by Hammar (1914, 1926); it depends on the evaluation of the relative surface of the different constituents (cortex, medullary, interstitial connectives) by weighing or planimetry on four transverse sections of the entire organ. The expression of the results in grams may be secured by taking into consideration the total fresh weight, the specific weight of the constituents and of their coefficients of shrinkage during embedding, all these being experimentally determined.

The same stains clearly show structural alterations characteristic of the general syndrome of adaptation and of normal involution of the thymus; the detailed study of the phenomena of pycnosis and of phagocytosis of the nuclear remnants obviously benefits from being supplemented by the examination of sections treated with Feulgen and Rossenbeck's nucleal reaction or by staining with methyl green-pyronine. The general characters of the Hassall bodies also show up on the sections.

Among *the histochemical techniques,* the PAS reaction and methods for demonstrating protein-bound sulphydryls are particularly useful when studying the Hassall bodies.

The selective staining of collagen fibres, silver impregnations of the reticulin, and the so-called haematological stains allow us to analyse the connective web and the various cell categories of the thymus; I might mention that it is of considerable interest to show up the mast cells.

HISTOLOGICAL EXAMINATION OF THE LYMPH NODES AND RELATED STRUCTURES (TONSILS, PEYER'S PATCHES IN THE INTESTINE, ETC...)

As in the case of the thymus, the examination of sections usually suffices, lymph node puncture with a view to the preparation of smears or the printing technique being of real value only when the cellular composition has been seriously altered by a spontaneous disease or through an experimental treatment.

All the information given with respect to the thymus holds good for the lymphoid structures enumerated above. The quantitative study was set out in detail by Hammar (1932); it depends on the same principles as for the thymus; the study of the connective web is as important as it is for the latter organ; moreover, the test for free iron should always be carried out and other techniques mentioned in relation to the spleen macrophages may also be useful.

I might mention, whilst on the subject of lymphoid organs, that the histological study of the peripheral lymphoid layer of the Urodel Batracian liver and that of the cranial part of the Teleostean kidney form an integral part of the exploration of the haematopoietic organs of these animals.

HISTOLOGICAL EXAMINATION OF THE HAEMATOPOIETIC ORGANS OF INVERTEBRATES

The diversity of these organs and the paucity of modern investigations dealing with a sufficiently large number of species prevents us from codifying the techques for their examination. Many authors have contented themselves, in the course of their studies, with the results given by so-called general histological techniques. It does indeed seem legitimate to specify the following essential requirements, from the technical point of view, when studying the organs in question: these are tests for dividing cells, the demonstration of any morphological similarity between certain stages of the cells and of the free elements of the circulating blood, and any possible means of detecting the connective web.

It seems, therefore, justified to recommend fixation in fluids which form a suitable preparation for stains such as the Mann-Dominici method or Mann's method using methyl blue-eosin, azan, or even possibly the nucleal reaction of Feulgen and Rossenbeck, and of the so-called haematological stains, in particular Pappenheim's panchrome and silver impregnation of the reticulin.

CHAPTER 33

TECHNIQUES OF THE HISTOLOGICAL STUDY OF THE CONNECTIVE TISSUE

In addition to its intrinsic interest, the morphological study of the connective tissue has a substantial bearing on the histological examination of most of the tissues and organs of metazoans, since the fibrous structures and connective cells play a part in their structure which may be greater or lesser in individual instances but which is never negligible.

As in the case of other tissues and organs any of the topographical, cytological or histochemical techniques can be called into play during the study of the three fundamental constituents of the connective tissue, namely the ground substance, the fibres and the cells; the account of the most interesting methods, given in this chapter, is therefore in no way limiting.

THE HISTOLOGICAL STUDY OF THE GROUND SUBSTANCE

The histological study of the ground substance of the connective tissue primarily depends on the demonstration of its carbohydrate constituents, in particular of the acid mucopolysaccharides. Such a study should, therefore, involve techniques for the detection and identification of acid mucosubstances as studied in the third part of the present work (Chapter 17) and there is clearly no point in redescribing the working techniques of the reactions in question. It is sufficient to recall the importance presented in such a study by techniques permitting us to discriminate between sulphomucopolysaccharides and other acid mucosubstances as well as the tests involving enzymatic digestion which ensure the identification of hyaluronic acid and of sialomucins. Only the detection of the amyloid substance needs to be mentioned here.

The amyloid substance is considered by the majority of modern authors (see Arvy and Sors, 1958; Pearse, 1960; Lillie, 1965) as being a complex of acid mucopolysaccharides of the chondroitin-sulphuric acid type and of proteins.

Insoluble in water, alcohol and dilute acids, it is well preserved by most of the usual fixatives; its demonstration can be carried out on frozen sections or on paraffin wax or celloidin ones.

Among the stains for the amyloid substance, the classical iodine reaction which consists in treating the sections with the iodine-iodide solution of Gram, then in rinsing in water and mounting in iodide glycerine as recommended by Takeuchi (p. 641) confers a mahogany stain on the deposits but the preparations keep rather poorly and Bennhold's (1922) technique using Congo red seems to be preferable. The most constant results are given by Puchtler's (1962) variant.

Staining the amyloid substance with Congo red after Puchtler:

Paraffin wax sections, dewaxed and treated with collodion where appropriate, and then hydrated;
Stain the nuclei with haemalum;
Wash in running water until the sections take on a blue tint;
Treat for 20 minutes with the freshly prepared mixture
    saturated solution of sodium chloride
        in 80% alcohol .... 40 ml
        1% soda .... 0.4 ml
Stain for 20 minutes with the freshly prepared mixture
    saturated solution of Congo red in 80% alcohol .... 40 ml
    1% soda saturated with sodium chloride .... 0.4 ml
Dehydrate in absolute alcohol, clear in a benzenoid hydrocarbon and mount in a synthetic resin.

The amyloid substance is stained red or pink, the elastic tissue in a clear pink, and the nuclei blue.

Among the histochemical characteristics of the amyloid substance we may mention in particular the positive result of applying the PAS reaction and the feebly positive or negative results of the majority of the general reactions for proteins as well as a clear metachromasia after staining with gentian violet, methyl violet or crystal violet. Lillie (1965) recommends the following working technique for this stain.

Staining with crystal violet-methyl violet following Lillie:

Frozen or paraffin wax sections, brought into water;
Stain for 3 to 5 minutes in the solution
    crystal violet .... 1 g
    methyl violet 2B .... 0.5 g
    absolute alcohol .... 10 ml
    distilled water .... 90 ml
Rinse in 1% acetic acid;
Wash carefully in tap water;
Mount in water, in glycerine or in any other medium miscible with water.

The nuclei and the cytoplasm stain bluish-violet, the amyloid and the fibrinoid substances stain purplish red; the preparations are unstable.

The metachromasia of the amyloid substance is much clearer after staining with the triphenylmethanes mentioned here than when the thiazines are used.

HISTOLOGICAL STUDY OF THE CONNECTIVE FIBRES

The general morphological characteristics, the dyestuff affinities and the histochemical peculiarities of the collagen fibres, the elastic fibres, and the reticulin fibres (precollagen fibres) allow us to distinguish them among the fibrous structures of the connective tissue; the techniques for demonstrating these formations and for demonstrating fibrin are mentioned successively in what follows.

COLLAGEN FIBRES

The techniques for demonstrating collagen tissue through its dyestuff affinities have already been dealt with in relation to topographical stains, since the selective staining of this tissue greatly aids the morphological analysis of most organs. The dyestuff affinities so described hold good for the entirety of the metazoa and virtually always allow us to identify collagen with certainty; we may add to this that the fibres in question are PAS positive and that this method shows them up in a red colour in all cases where the technique does not involve the use of a background stain conferring a different colour on them. The techniques for silver impregnation of the reticulin, as described in the following section, also show up the collagen fibres with a different tint from those of the precollagen; a technique for selective impregnation of the collagen fibres, due to del Rio Hortega (1916) is described here.

Selective impregnation of collagen fibre by Del Rio Hortega's technique (the 3rd tanno-argentic variation):

Frozen sections taken from formalin treated or alcohol fixed material and washed in water prior to freezing;
Treat for 5 minutes, at 50–55°C, with a 1% solution of tannin in 96% alcohol;
Rinse rapidly in distilled water;
Treat with 3 baths of ammoniacal silver complex (p. 740), one ml of which is diluted with 10 ml of distilled water; keep the sections in the silver complex until they become brownish-yellow in colour;
Wash carefully in frequently renewed distilled water;
Tone with a 0.2% solution of gold chloride, at 40–45°C; keep the sections in this bath until they become violet in colour;
Rinse in distilled water;

Treat for 1 minute with a 5% aqueous solution of sodium thiosulphite (hyposulphite); Wash at length in tap water, mount on slides, dehydrate with absolute alcohol, clear in a benzenoid hydrocarbon and mount in Canada balsam or in a synthetic resin; The collagen fibres take on a fairly deep violet colour, sometimes with a reddish tint; the reticulin is not shown up.

I might mention in addition that the collagen fibres are endowed with a uniaxial birefringence of the crystalline type; examination under polarised light will therefore disclose them with great clarity in all cases in which the preparations have not been treated with compounds which suppress the birefringence (for example, phenol). The dyestuff affinities and histochemical characteristics of the *basement membranes* are identical with those of collagen tissue.

RETICULIN FIBRES

Reticulin fibres are isotropic and therefore do not appear when the sections are examined under the polarising microscope; most of the stains for collagen fibres, which involve aniline blue or light green, do not completely reveal them; they are PAS positive and therefore show up on preparations treated with this reaction. Their true detection however depends on their argyrophilia; techniques for silver impregnation give results which are incomparable from the point of view of their clarity and of the homogeneity of the results, so that no other method can rival them.

These techniques for silver impregnation are of two types; some intended exclusively for demonstrating reticulin—and collagen tissue—on frozen sections, stem from the tanno-argentic method of Achucarro (1911); the remainder, which may be applied either to frozen sections or to paraffin wax sections, are modifications of the technique for impregnating neurofibrils developed by Bielschowsky (1904).

A substantial number of variations have been suggested to simplify the original techniques or to improve their efficacy. Amongst those derived from Achucarro's technique, the best, from my own experience, is the second tanno-argentic variation of Del Rio Hortega (1916) which we deal with here; I might mention that the first variation is intended for the impregnation of the intracellular structures (p. 739), the third for the selective demonstration of collagen fibres (see the preceding section), the fourth being a technique for the impregnation of the neuroglia.

As for variations of Bielschowsky's technique, their use on frozen sections has, in my opinion, only minor interest, the technique of Del Rio Hortega being much quicker and more practical; they are, on the other hand, the method of choice so far as paraffin wax sections are concerned. The number of procedures described since 1904 is substantial and there is no point in my enumerating them, all the more so because Lillie's book (1965) includes a comparative study which is remarkably complete and precise. We mention here, therefore, only the two techniques which seem to me to be the best and which render all the others obsolete, namely those of Gomori (1937) and Oliveira (1936) whose recommendations are slightly different.

1° Selective impregnation of reticulin according to Del Rio Hortega (2nd tanno-argentic variation)

Frozen sections, taken from material fixed in dilute formalin, formaldehyde calcium, or in alcohol (hydrate blocks of tissue fixed in the latter liquid prior to microtome sectioning);

Treat for 5 minutes, at 50–55°C, with a 1% solution of tannin in 96% alcohol;

Wash very rapidly (prior to the complete chilling of the sections) in distilled water;

Impregnate using 3 baths of ammoniacal silver complex (p. 740) diluted with 10 volumes of distilled water; leave the sections in the impregnation bath, without agitating them, until a pale yellow colour appears;

Transfer the sections to distilled water and leave them there without disturbing them until a homogeneous and rather deeper tint has been obtained;

Rinse *very rapidly* in a new bath of distilled water;

Transfer immediately into neutralised formalin diluted with 5 volumes of tap water, leaving the sections there for about 30 seconds;

Wash for a long time in tap water, dehydrate, clear and mount in Canada balsam or in a commercial synthetic resin;

The critical stages of the method are the washing which precedes reduction and the duration of this latter process; too prolonged a washing results in incomplete impregnation, too short a reduction results in too pale a colour.

Reticulin fibres appear intensely black, collagen fibres being either unstained or a pale brown colour.

2° Silver impregnation of reticulin fibres according to Gomori

This method which is derived from Bielschowsky's technique includes a permanganate oxidation of the sections intended to prevent any neurofibrillar impregnation, a mordanting with iron alum and impregnation by an ammoniacal silver complex, followed by reduction in formalin and toning with gold chloride. Remarkably good results can be obtained after the use of any of the usual fixatives; Carnoy's, Bouin's, or Halmi's fluids or Heidenhain's Susa seem particularly suitable; good results can be obtained after formalin fixation and even after a short fixation using mixtures with a potassium bichromate base. When reticulin needs to be impregnated in material which has been post chromated or fixed with a chromic osmic mixture, Oliveira's technique is preferable to that of Gomori.

Reagents:

- a 1% aqueous solution of potassium permanganate;
- a 1–3% aqueous solution of sodium metabisulphite;
- a 2% aqueous solution of iron alum, *prepared the very same day*;
- ammoniacal silver complex: mix 10 ml of a 10% aqueous solution of silver nitrate and 2 ml of 10% potassium hydroxide (free from carbonate); stir; redissolve the precipitate by adding, drop by drop, ammonia, stirring with each addition so as not to exceed the end-point; add further, drop by drop, the 10% aqueous solution of silver nitrate, stirring until the precipitate which forms after each addition dissolves slowly and with difficulty; dilute the liquid so obtained with an equal volume of distilled water;
- 10% formalin (diluted with 9 parts of tap water);
- a 0.1 or 0.2% aqueous solution of gold chloride.

Working technique:

- Paraffin wax sections, well stuck to slides, dewaxed, not treated with collodion, and hydrated;
- Oxidise for 1 to 2 minutes with the potassium permanganate solution;
- Wash for 5 minutes in running water;
- Decolourise in sodium bisulphite;
- Wash for 5 to 10 minutes in running water;
- Mordant for one minute with the iron alum solution;
- Wash for three to five minutes in running water;
- Wash in 2 baths of distilled water, each lasting for 2 minutes;
- Impregnate on slides or in tubes using the ammoniacal silver complex for one minute;
- Rinse *very rapidly (at the most for 10 seconds)* in distilled water;
- Reduce in diluted formalin for 5 minutes;
- Wash for 5 minutes in running water;
- Tone for 10 minutes with gold chloride;
- Rinse in distilled water;
- Reduce for one minute with the sodium metabisulphite solution;
- Treat for one minute at the most with a 1% aqueous solution of sodium hyposulphite (this step in the method seems to me of the most dubious utility and its duration should be very brief);
- Wash at length in running water;
- Dehydrate in absolute alcohol, clear in a benzenoid hydrocarbon, and mount in Canada balsam or in a synthetic resin.

The critical stages of the method are the preparation of the ammoniacal silver complex and the duration of the washing process intercalated between the action of the ammoniacal silver complex and the reduction stage. The presence of an excess of ammonia in the silver complex results in incomplete impregnation of the reticulin; an insufficient amount of ammonia results in a dark and irregular background stain. Insufficient washing results in the formation of precipitates, whereas too prolonged a washing stage results in incomplete and granular impregnation of the reticulin.

In practice, the acquisition of suitable control over the two critical stages, which have just been mentioned, is easy and the quality of the preparations represents an adequate recompense for any histologist who loves his work. The reticulin fibres show up black, the precision with which they are demonstrated exceeds that with any other type of stain; the collagen fibres take on a stain which varies between red and purple and the distinction between the two types of fibre is instantaneous; the nuclei are stained black, all the details of their structure being clearly visible; according to circumstances the cytoplasm takes on a stain varying between yellow and grey; it may remain unstained.

3° *Silver impregnation of reticulin fibres according to Oliveira*

This technique which represents a combination of Wilder's (1935) method and a second impregnation using silver chromate, succeeds even on post-chromated material and this is when it is most valuable, since the method of Gomori gives the same results after topographical fixatives have been used, and this with less effort.

Reagents:

a 10% aqueous solution of phosphomolybdic acid;
a 1% aqueous solution of uranyl nitrate;
Foot's fluid: add ammonia, drop by drop, to 5 ml of a 10% aqueous solution of silver nitrate until the precipitate formed just redissolves; once this stage has been reached add 5 ml of 3% sodium hydroxide (free from carbonate) and redissolve the new precipitate by the addition of ammonia;
make up to 50 ml with distilled water;
this ammoniacal silver complex should be prepared immediately prior to each use;
first reducing solution:

    neutralised commercial formalin .... 3 ml
    1% solution of uranyl nitrate .... 1 drop
    distilled water .... 100 ml

silver chromate: mix 10 ml of a 5% solution of potassium bichromate and 5 ml of a 10% solution of silver nitrate; wash the precipitate with distilled water, allow to settle and decant, repeating the process until the last wash-liquid remains uncoloured; suspend the precipitate in 40 ml of distilled water, and dissolve it by the careful addition of ammonia (do not exceed the end-point), make up to 85 ml with distilled water; this solution should be prepared immediately prior to each usage;
second reducing solution:

    neutralised commercial formalin .... 30 ml
    hydroquinone .... 0.3 g
    distilled water .... 70 ml

0.2% aqueous solution of gold chloride;
5% aqueous solution of sodium thiosulphate (hyposulphite).

Working technique:

> Paraffin wax sections, dewaxed, *not treated with collodion*, and hydrated;
> Mordant with phosphomolybdic acid for one minute;
> Rinse for 10 to 20 seconds in distilled water;
> Mordant for 5 seconds with uranyl nitrate;
> Rinse for 5 seconds in distilled water;
> Treat for one minute with Foot's fluid;
> Rinse for 5 seconds in 96% alcohol;
> Reduce for one minute with the first reducing solution; the sections take on a yellow tint;
> Wash for 3 to 5 minutes in distilled water;
> Treat for 15 to 20 minutes at 56°C with silver chromate previously brought to this temperature; the sections turn brownish-red;
> Wash for 3 to 5 minutes in distilled water;
> Treat for one minute with a second reducing solution; the sections turn deep brown in colour;
> Wash for 3 to 5 minutes in tap water;
> Tone for 5 to 10 minutes, at 56°C, with the gold chloride solution previously brought to this temperature;
> Fix for 5 minutes at laboratory temperatures with the sodium hyposulphite solution.
> Wash at length in tap water;
> Dehydrate in absolute alcohol, clear in a benzenoid hydrocarbon, and mount in Canada balsam or in a synthetic resin.

The reticulin fibres stain intensely black, the collagen fibres stain a violet red colour; the nuclei show up black, the cytoplasm grey or yellow.

ELASTIC FIBRES

In addition to the morphological characteristics which it would obviously be inappropriate to set out at length in a manual on histological technique, the elastic fibres are endowed with a range of histochemical characteristics and dyestuff affinities which greatly facilitate their selective demonstration. Most of the methods requiring mention here were developed on mammalian tissues and the older histologists considered that the elastic tissue was restricted to vertebrates; this prejudice should be abandoned as recent research has shown that structures endowed with the morphological characteristics of elastic fibres exist in invertebrates; it is nevertheless true that such results are not yet sufficiently numerous for the histological peculiarities of the elastic tissue of invertebrates to be discussed on the basis of any wide range of material.

The elastic fibres of vertebrates are isotropic; they do not appear when the sections are examined under polarised light. They are more or less acidophilic according to the circumstances and become erythrophilic after the use of the usual trichrome stains, but the stains so obtained are not always sufficiently intense or sufficiently precise to allow of satisfactory study. Vigorous chromic oxidation and, in particular, permanganate oxidation in the presence of sulphuric acid (p. 759) transform this acidophilia into a strong basophilia so that it becomes possible to stain the elastic fibres, after this pretreatment, with chromic haematoxylin as in Gomori's method, or by toluidine blue using the Mann-Dominici technique and, more generally, by most basic dyestuffs. The presence of free aldehydes which have not so far been identified with any degree of certainty explains the red stain that the elastic fibres take on, in most cases, after the use of any technique involving the Schiff reagent, pretreatment of the sections (oxidation, hydrolysis, oxidative deamination, etc...) in no way interfering with the conditioning of this reactivity. In the same way, general techniques for demonstrating reducing compounds (the ferric ferricyanide reaction, or the tetrazolium salt reaction) stain elastic fibres. Moreover, they take on a characteristic stain after most histochemical reactions have been applied which include coupling with a diazonium salt.

In addition to the older staining technique of Verhoeff using haematoxylin, which depends on overstaining the sections with a mixture of Lugol's solution, ferric chloride solution and haematoxylin solution, with differentiation using ferric chloride, the techniques for staining elastic fibres may involve either orcein or derivatives of basic fuchsin.

Staining with orcein

This amphoteric stain is used in the form of an aqueous solution acidified with a strong mineral acid and, according to the mechanism set out on p. 137, it is taken up by the elastic fibres and confers a deep brown colour on them which is optically advantageous; when fixed in Bouin's or Halmi's fluids the nuclei are also stained. The keeping quality of the preparations is good, the selectivity of the demonstration of elastic tissue satisfactory. The major disadvantage of the process is the variability of commercial samples of orcein which is an expensive natural dyestuff; synthetic orcein which has been commercially available for about fifteen years, gives results distinctly less good than does natural orcein.

The classical stain of Taenzer-Unna (1894) involves the use of a 1% solution of orcein in 70% alcohol, acidified by the addition of 0.7 ml of concentrated hydrochloric acid; the staining of the elastic fibres (and of the nuclei after fixing in Bouin's fluid) that is obtained through alcoholic differentiation can be combined with the demonstration of the collagen fibres by van Gieson's picro-fuchsin or picro-indigocarmine; it is in this form that the technique gives the most advantageous preparations. Another combination, due to Kornhauser (1945), consists in associating the nitric orcein stain with a minor modification of Petersen's method (p. 224).

Staining with hydrochloric orcein-picrofuchsin or picro-indigocarmine:

Paraffin wax sections, dewaxed, treated with collodion, and hydrated;
Stain for 30 minutes or more (according to the quality of the commercial sample of orcein) using the solution

70% alcohol	100 ml
orcein	1 g
concentrated hydrochloric acid	0.7 ml

Rinse in distilled water;
Treat for 10 to 20 seconds with van Gieson's picrofuchsin (p. 204) or picro-indigocarmine (p. 201);
Extract the excess of orcein and dehydrate by treating the sections with absolute alcohol, a treatment which should be continued until the background is clear;
this stage is not critical because the staining of the elastic fibres well withstands alcoholic treatment;
Clear in a benzenoid hydrocarbon, mount in Canada balsam or in a synthetic resin.

In cases where orcein does not stain the nuclei, staining with a progressive ferric lake of haematoxylin (Weigert, Hansen or Groat, p. 197) should be inserted between the orcein and the picrofuchsin or picro-indigocarmine; it is only rarely useful to take this precaution.

The elastic fibres and the nuclei are stained deep brown, acidophil cytoplasm stains yellow, collagen fibres red or blue, according to whether picrofuchsin or picro-indigocarmine has been used; this second way of working gives preparations which are easier to photograph in black and white than does the first.

Staining with Kornhausser's quad:

Paraffin wax sections, treated with collodion and hydrated;
Stain for one to 24 hours with the solution

96% alcohol	100 ml
orcein	1 g
concentrated nitric acid	0.4 ml

Wash in 85% alcohol until all excess of orcein is extracted;
Wash in distilled water;
Stain for 5 to 10 minutes with the solution

Acid alizarin blue (*and not alizarin S blue*)	0.35 g
Aluminium sulphate	10 g
Distilled water	100 ml

Boil for 10 minutes, allow to cool, add several drops of a concentrated solution of ferric chloride; keeps well;
Rinse in distilled water;
Treat for 10 to 30 minutes (according to the fixative) with an aqueous 5% solution of phosphomolybdic acid;
Rinse in distilled water;
Stain for 10 minutes with the solution

orange G	2 g
light green	0.2 g
distilled water	100 ml
acetic acid	2 ml

Dehydrate in absolute alcohol, clear in a benzenoid hydrocarbon and mount in a synthetic resin or in Canada balsam.

The elastic fibres stain a reddish-brown, the nuclei and the other basophil structures stain blue-purple, the muscular fibres and the cytoplasm stain violet, the collagen and reticulin (only partially shown up) green, the erythrocytes, the myelin and the erythrophilic secretory granules stain orange.

The technique using orcein-water blue-eosin developed by Unna (p. 774) also confers a brownish-red stain on the elastic fibres.

Staining with resorcinol-fuchsin

Resorcinol-fuchsin (cresofuchsin, fuchselin) was introduced into histological practice by Weigert (1898) and gives excellent results with elastic fibres but it has the disadvantage that the solution keeps poorly. The stain is available commercially in powder form, the preparation of the solution from this powder varying according to the suppliers; each bottle carries instructions. It is often adviseable to prepare the solution in the laboratory, the best of the formulae being that of Romeis (1948):

> Dissolve 0.5 g of basic fuchsin and 1 g of chemically pure resorcinol in 50 ml of distilled water, warming where necessary; dissolve 2 g of chemically pure ferric chloride in 10 ml of distilled water; warm the resorcinol-fuchsin solution until it begins to boil and add the ferric chloride solution maintaining the whole at simmering point for 5 minutes; allow to cool, collect the precipitate on a filter paper and allow it to drain; place the filter paper containing the precipitate in an Erlenmeyer flask of suitable size, cover it with 100 ml of 96% alcohol, warm on an electric hotplate or on an electrically heated water-bath (*never boil an alcoholic liquid on a gas jet*) until it begins to boil and keep it in this condition until the precipitate has dissolved; allow to cool, acidify with 0.7 ml of concentrated hydrochloric acid.

As was noted by Lillie (1954, 1965) the basic fuchsin can be replaced by crystal violet in this formula; 0.5 to 2 g of dextrin should be added over and above the resorcinol, the preparative technique otherwise undergoing no change; the material so obtained stains elastic fibres a deep green colour.

An intense staining of the elastic fibres (blue-black with resorcinol-fuchsin, green with resorcinol-violet crystal is obtained by treating the sections after they have been dewaxed, treated with collodion and hydrated, with the solution whose mode of use has just been described, for 10 to 30 minutes, at laboratory temperatures. They are then washed for about one minute in running water and differentiated in 96% alcohol, where necessary the process may be regulated by inspection under the microscope, until the background is completely clear, only the elastic fibres and certain secretory products remaining stained.

Evidently, this stain for elastic fibres benefits greatly from being associated with other techniques; we can use silver impregnation of the reticulin, *which should be undertaken prior to the demonstration of the elastic tissue*; Lillie (1954, 1965) recommends the variation using crystal violet (giving a green colour to the elastic tissue). Combination with the Masson-Goldner trichrome (p. 214) gives very good results, the resorcinol-fuchsin staining being carried out first; the results correspond to those set out on p. 214, with the additional feature that the elastic fibres are stained a deep blue-black. Combination with azan stain (Romeis' Kresazan, 1940) gives particularly striking results; the working technique is described in relation to techniques for the histological study of the hypophysis.

Staining with Gallego's ferric fuchsin

This technique which was described by Gallego in 1919 puts to good use the fact that basic fuchsin stains turn an intense violet colour when the preparations are treated with a mixture of formalin and ferric chloride (Biot, 1902). Among the various formulae derived from the original working technique the most precise is that of Lillie (1954) which is given here.

Paraffin wax sections, dewaxed, treated with collodion and hydrated;
Stain the nuclei with a progressive ferric lake of haematoxylin;
Wash in running water;
Mordant for 30 seconds with the *freshly prepared* mixture
    distilled water .... 200 ml
    concentrated nitric acid .... 1.5 ml
    commercial formalin .... 1 ml
    ferric chloride solution B.P. (25 to 29%) ...... 1.5 ml
(it is adviseable to dilute each of the reagents with equal volumes of distilled water and to prepare the mixture in the order indicated), it keeps badly;
Rinse rapidly in tap water;
Stain for 5 minutes with the mixture
    Ziehl's fuchsin (p. 202) .... 3 ml
    0.2% acetic acid .... 50 ml
Rinse rapidly in tap water;
Treat for 2 minutes with the mordant;
Rinse in tap water;
Stain for one minute with the solution
    saturated aqueous solution of picric acid ...... 100 ml
    aniline blue .... 0.1 g
Rinse in 0.2% acetic acid;
Dehydrate in acetone, clear in a benzenoid hydrocarbon and mount in Canada balsam or in a synthetic resin.

The nuclei are stained black or grey, the collagen and reticulin fibres blue, the muscles are stained orange or a greenish tint, and the elastic fibres are stained reddish-violet, the cytoplasm becomes brown or a greenish-olive, and the massed cell granulations an intense red colour, the ground substance of the cartilage and the mucins stain blue or violet.

Staining with paraldehyde fuchsin

Gomori (1950) introduced this technique in his original work on paraldehyde-fuchsin and it is certainly the best and the simplest of the various ways of demonstrating elastic fibres. The affinity of these structures for the stain in question is very strong and does not depend on any pretreatment. The working technique recommended here consists of associating the stain, used in the way described on p. 352, but without pretreatment, with one-step trichrome (Gabe and Martoja, 1957).

> Paraffin wax sections, treated with collodion, and hydrated;
> Stain for about 3 minutes with the customary paraldehyde-fuchsin solution, prepared from a stock solution in 70% alcohol or from the powder (p. 351);
> Rinse in tap water;
> Eliminate the excess stain using alcohol acidified with hydrochloric acid; this stage is not critical since treatment lasting for several hours does not destain the elastic fibres;
> Rinse in tap water;
> Stain for 10 minutes with one-step trichrome (p. 217);
> Wash for about 20 seconds in distilled water;
> Dehydrate in absolute alcohol, clear in a benzenoid hydrocarbon, and mount in Canada balsam or in a synthetic resin.

Over and above the results given by one-step trichrome, when used alone (p. 218), notably the intense green stain of the collagen fibres, is the fact that the elastic fibres and structures rich in acid mucosubstances (mast cell granules, the ground substance of the cartilage, and certain mucins) are stained an intense violet colour.

FIBRIN

Fibrin, which is derived by coagulation from the fibrinogen contained in blood plasma, is characterised by a series of histochemical characteristics which distinguish it clearly from other fibrous substances of vertebrate tissue. It has no metachromasia, is PAS positive which may be due to substances fixed at the moment of coagulation, and is rich in indol groups corresponding to the presence of tryptophane, and is strongly acidophilic after staining with anionic dyestuffs, whereas it is cyanophilic after the use of the usual trichrome stains; fibrin may therefore be detected with great selectivity on paraffin wax sections either by the classical *Weigert's technique* (1887) using methyl violet, or using Mallory's (1900) phosphotungstic haematoxylin.

> Paraffin wax sections, dewaxed, treated with collodion and hydrated;
> Bleach the sections taken from material fixed in a chromic fixative by treating them for about 12 minutes with a 0.33% aqueous solution of potassium permanganate, this treatment being followed by rinsing with water, a passage of several hours through an aqueous solution of oxalic acid (3 to 5%) and then a further washing with water; this stage is superflous after other types of fixative;

Stain the nuclei with alum carmine (p. 570), carmalum (p. 239) or the aluminium lake of nuclear fast red (p. 203);

Rinse in tap water;

Stain the slides for about 15 seconds with an aniline treated solution of methyl violet prepared immediately prior to use by mixing 27 ml of a saturated aqueous solution of this stain and 3 ml of a saturated solution of the same stain in a mixture of 33 ml of absolute alcohol and 9 ml of aniline; each of these solutions keeps well but the mixture has poor keeping qualities;

Throw away the stain, blot with tissue paper and cover the sections with an iodine iodide solution—

potassium iodide	2 g
iodine	1 g
distilled water	100 ml

and allow this to act for about 15 seconds;

Blot with tissue paper and differentiate under microscopic control with a mixture of equal parts of xylene and aniline until the background clears, the fibrin remaining stained an intense violet colour;

Wash carefully several times with a benzenoid hydrocarbon to eliminate the last traces of aniline, mount in Canada balsam or in a commercial synthetic resin.

The nuclei show up red, the fibrin violet, the cytoplasm becomes greyish or a pale violet colour when differentiation has not been carried to the point of its complete destaining.

As Lillie (1954, 1965) has remarked, the methyl violet solution used by Weigert can be replaced to advantage with a crystal violet solution, the two best formulae being those of Stirling (1925) (crystal violet 5 g; absolute alcohol 10 ml; aniline 2 ml; distilled water 88 ml), and of Hucker and Conn (1928) (dissolve 2 g of crystal violet in 20 ml of 96% alcohol, dissolve 0.8 g of ammonium oxalate in 80 ml of distilled water, mixing the two solutions). The two formulae give very stable dye baths which keep for years.

We might mention whilst on the subject that all attempts at a histochemical interpretation of "Gram's reaction" (the process of rendering insoluble, using an iodine iodide liquid treatment, the stain produced by gentian violet, methyl violet or crystal violet) have so far failed so that no general explanation for it can be given at present (see, in this respect, Pearse, 1960, pp. 215–223).

Staining with phosphotungstic haematoxylin

This technique, which gives highly polychromatic preparations and does not involve any differentiation, was developed for paraffin wax sections taken from material treated with Zenker's fixative; sections taken from formalin treated material are also suitable some authors advising, in this latter instance, mordanting of the dewaxed and hydrated sections for three hours at 56°C with a saturated aqueous solution of corrosive sublimate. Masson (1923) obtained excellent results with sections taken from material fixed in Bouin's fluid, provided that the dewaxed sections were treated with Lugol's fluid for three to 24 hours and then destained with a 5% solution of sodium hyposulphite which it is necessary to remove by careful washing prior to proceeding to what is, properly speaking, the staining process.

The original formula for preparing the stain involved the solution of 1 g of haematoxylin and 20 g of phosphotungstic acid in 1,000 ml of distilled water; the stain takes several weeks to mature. Its maturation may be obtained immediately by the addition of 177 mg of potassium permanganate or 2 ml of 10 volume hydrogen peroxide (see p. 195 on this topic), but many authors have stressed the superiority of solutions which have matured spontaneously.

Two other formulae have been put forward recently for the preparation of the phosphotungstic lake of haematoxylin; from my own experience both give very good results.

The formula of Levene and Feng (1964) differs from the original working technique indicated above only in respect of a 48 hour maturation period after the addition of potassium permanganate. It consists of dissolving 0.1 g of crystalline haematoxylin in 100 ml of warm distilled water and allowing this solution to cool, adding 2.0 g of phosphotungstic acid after chilling. When complete dissolution of this latter reagent has been obtained 2.5 ml of a 1% solution of potassium permanganate is added and the whole is allowed to stand for 48 hours. Occasional filtration of the dyestuff solution is advantageous and it keeps for one to two years.

The formula of Terner, Gurland and Gaer (1964) has the special feature of commencing the preparation of the lake from commercial samples of haematein and not from haematoxylin. The preparation, which is very simple, consists of dissolving 12 g of phosphotungstic acid and 1.2 g of haematein in 1,000 ml of distilled water. The staining bath is ready for use as soon as the ingredients have dissolved and keeps for several years. Its staining power is greater than that of the two formulae given above and I would recommend that the duration of staining be reduced systematically as compared with the times generally recommended for lakes prepared according to the other formulae. The 24 hour duration of staining, at laboratory temperatures, which was recommended by Terner et al. to obtain the most intense stains may, from my own experience, be reduced to three hours, but obviously there is nothing absolute about this recommendation because the staining capacity of the lake will evidently vary with the commercial sample of haematein used for its preparation.

The working technique is of the simplest.

> Paraffin wax sections, dewaxed, treated with collodion, hydrated and where appropriate having undergone one of the pretreatments mentioned above;
> Stain for 12 to 24 hours with phosphotungstic haematoxylin;
> Rinse *rapidly* in distilled water;
> Dehydrate rapidly in absolute alcohol or acetone, clear in a benzenoid hydrocarbon, and mount in a commercial synthetic resin (the stains keep rather poorly in Canada balsam).

The nuclei, centrosomes, the spindle and chondriome, the fibrin and neuroglial fibres take on a blue stain, the collagen fibres, reticulin, and elastic fibres as well as the cartilage and the bony matrix stain a yellow or brownish-red colour.

FIBRINOID

As Lillie (1952, 1954, 1965) and Pearse (1960) have both remarked, this term has been used, since it was coined by Neumann (1880), by pathologists to designate pathological material whose chemical constitution varies substantially according to the circumstances and whose definition by means of histochemical criteria is impossible in the present state of our knowledge.

Fibrinoid deposits are acidophilic when topographical techniques are used and may be either metachromatic or not; they are cyanophilic or erythrophilic after staining with azan and its variations, Masson's trichrome and methods derived from it and they stain blue or yellow with Mallory's phosphotungstic haematoxylin. They may react very strongly to PAS, the affinity for paraldehyde fuchsin being always absent. Weigert's technique using methyl violet stains fibrinoid in some cases, the results being negative in others; many authors have mentioned a certain degree of argyrophilia.

OXYTALAN FIBRES

These fibres which were characterised by Fullmer (1958) and Fullmer and Lillie (1958) are known only from mammals; they are morphologically identical with elastic fibres but only have their dyestuff affinities after peracetic oxidation. They withstand the action of elastase and of hot formic acid, this last characteristic being shared with oxytalan and elastic fibres; alkalis, however, destroy them without attacking other connective fibres. The demonstration of these fibres therefore depends on the comparison of two neighbouring sections, one of which is stained to show up the elastic fibres, the other undergoing the same stain after peracetic oxidation; the oxytalan fibres remain unstained on the first slide but are stained on the second (see p. 467 for the technique of peracetic oxidation).

THE USE OF ENZYMATIC PREPARATIONS FOR THE IDENTIFICATION OF CONNECTIVE FIBRES

The working technique for the use of enzymatic preparations to identify proteins was described on p. 535 and will serve for our present purposes. It is simply necessary to remember that the collagen fibres and reticulin are digested by pepsin, the elastic fibres withstanding this enzymatic attack very well. Trypsin only modifies collagen fibres when the digestion is prolonged but it rapidly attacks elastic fibres. These latter are selectively attacked by elastase. The oxytalan fibres are not attacked by this enzyme but become sensitive to its action if the sections have undergone peracetic oxidation.

HISTOLOGICAL STUDY OF THE CONNECTIVE CELLS

The histological study of the connective cells involves the same techniques as does that of the haematopoietic organs. The examination of smears here plays only a diminished role, methods such as the classical "oedematous ball" of Ranvier giving preparations whose usefulness is limited in general to elementary histological teaching. It is the examination of sections which is the essential stage in the morphological study of connective cells.

Topographical fixatives, followed by staining with so-called general methods give highly instructive preparations from this point of view; the identification of the various categories of connective cells is yet easier after the use of the Mann-Dominici technique or of that of Lillie using eosinates of azur and especially after the panoptic technique has been used; fixing in Maximow's fluid represents the best preparatory treatment for these stains, whose working technique is described in relation to the general techniques and to the study of haematopoietic organs. Evidently a list of the morphological characteristics which allow us to identify the categories of connective tissues cells would be out of place here. Techniques for the histochemical study of lipids obviously play an essential part in the histological examination of adipose tissue.

The demonstration of mast cells (tissue basophils, heparinocytes) depends on the presence of sulphomucopolysaccharides in the granulations of these elements; notable among these are heparin and its precursors. Since the discovery of the metachromatic reaction by Ehrlich (1877), staining with thiazins or with triphenylmethanes which give rise to the phenomenon in question represents the method of choice for the selective staining of mast cells. The procedures are very numerous and there is not much point in enumerating them. In practice, the Mann-Dominici staining technique and all the techniques which involve thiazins such as toluidine blue or azur, as well as the eosinates, confer a very characteristic metachromatic stain on the mast cell granulations. The toluidine blue stains, when used according to the working techniques recommended for studies of basophilia (p. 339), show up the mast cells quite selectively as do polychrome blue stains. The abundance of sulphomucopolysaccharides in the specific granulations explains the strong affinity for paraldehyde-fuchsin observable without any pretreatment of the sections; the working technique described for the demonstration of elastic fibres serves well for this purpose. Mowry's method for the detection of acid mucosubstances (p. 413) allows us to assess the degree of sulphuric esterification of the compounds of the heparin group fixed within the granulations of these cells, some of which still give the PAS reaction and become red, others only taking up alcian blue (Arvy and Rancurel, 1958). A combination of stains for the mast cells using cresyl violet and the demonstration of collagen fibres using van Gieson's picrofuchsin (Arvy and Gabe, 1950) gives preparations which are full of contrast and in which the mast cells are easy to count. This technique involves the following stages.

Paraffin wax sections, dewaxed, treated with collodion and hydrated;
Stain for 3 to 5 minutes with a 1% aqueous solution of cresyl violet;
Rinse in distilled water;
Treat for 5 to 10 seconds with van Gieson's picrofuchsin (p. 204);
Dehydrate in absolute alcohol stirring the fluid until all excess of the cresyl violet has been extracted, clear in a benzenoid hydrocarbon and mount in Canada balsam or in a synthetic resin.

The picrofuchsin causes the staining of the nuclei to turn black and that of the basophilic cytoplasm to turn grey when cresyl violet has been used; acidophilic cytoplasm is stained yellow and the granulations of the highly acid mucosubstances in the mast cells keep the violet stain which greatly assists their identification.

I might mention that the histochemical detection of histamine gives positive results on mast cells (p. 586); this is obviously not a routine method to be recommended for the identification of the cells in question(*).

Histiocytary elements can only be identified unambiguously through their ability to fix particles vitally, especially electronegative colloids, an ability known as athrocytosis. It is the detection of compounds injected *intra vitam* which gives preparations in which the histiocytes stand out clearly against the background; this process has, moreover, substantial experimental value. Indian ink (avoid modern sketching inks which are based on aniline dyes), or lithium carmine, trypan blue or trypan red are the most used of the numerous

---

(*) I have avoided the use of the term "mastocytes" so often used to designate mast cells. This word is ridiculous; to those who naively suppose it to be the translation of the German word *Mastzellen*, created by Ehrlich for the cells in question, I might mention that the German word *Mast* (fattening) cannot serve as the root *masto-* and that the latter, which is derived from the Greek μαστός, can only mean a mound, protuberance or udder. The use of the term mastocytes is therefore a blunder much worse than the barbarism of associating German and Greek roots.

possible compounds; ferric salts, in particular iron saccharate, are also entirely suitable.

The best samples of Indian ink are those provided by the pharmaceutical industry for ophthalmological usage; solutions of trypan blue and trypan red should be prepared immediately prior to use, at concentrations of 0.5%, in distilled water or in physiological saline, because if they are kept, even at low temperatures, they acquire a toxicity whose mechanism is still unknown. Lithium carmine is supplied in the form of a powder by certain manufacturers of products for microscopy but it is better prepared in the laboratory by boiling 2.5 g of carmine in 100 ml of a solution of lithium carbonate in distilled water, saturated when cold. Saturated aqueous solutions of lithium carbonate are of approximately 1% concentration. The solution when boiled for 10 to 16 minutes is chilled and filtered prior to use.

The technique for the administration and the doses to be injected vary according to the objectives of the work. When these objectives are the demonstration of histiocytes in subcutaneous areas the injection by this route is suitable; the histiocytary elements of the viscera may be reached rapidly by intravenous injection or intraperitoneal injection, and more slowly by repeated subcutaneous injections, the migratory histiocytes then coming into play whilst the substance is being transported. Most authors recommend subcutaneous injections of from 0.2 to 0.5 ml in the mouse, of from 1 to 3 ml in the rat, and 10 to 15 ml in the rabbit; these doses should be reduced when administration is intraperitoneal or intravenous. The repetition of the injections is particularly to be recommended when subcutaneous injections are used.

The preservation of the carbon or lithium carmine particles at the moment of fixation poses no problems and any of the normal fixatives will serve; in the case of trypan blue or trypan red the best results are obtained by fixing in Bouin's, Romeis, or Halmi's fluids or in Heidenhain's Susa. The tissue blocks may be cut whilst frozen or embedded either in paraffin wax or in celloidin; the stains should be chosen having regard to the colour of the injected particles. When the animal has received injections of iron saccharate or any other iron compound fixing in Bouin's fluid followed by the demonstration of free iron using Perls' or Tirmann and Schmelzer's techniques is obviously the method of choice; it is appropriate to mention that the demonstration of free iron allows us to identify the histiocytary elements in cases of endogenous deposition of iron (haemolytic anaemia, etc....).

Naturally many histochemical techniques can be used for the identification of histiocytary cells, in particular of macrophages; their choice depends on the nature of the particles present in the cytoplasm, these being very variable according to circumstances.

CHAPTER 34

TECHNIQUES FOR THE HISTOLOGICAL STUDY OF CARTILAGINOUS, BONY AND DENTAL TISSUE

Because of the mineralisation of the ground substance bony and dental tissue need to be studied by techniques which differ in certain respects from those used for the histological examination of other types of connective tissue. It is moreover legitimate to place the study of cartilage and that of bony tissue in the same general category. The old and rather restrictive idea according to which cartilage is confined to the vertebrates and true cartilage is always a precursor of bony tissue, the normal developmental sequence of cartilage being ossification, has indeed become untenable, but it is nevertheless true that ossification is the most frequently met with of the transformations undergone by cartilaginous tissue so that it is appropriate to discuss the techniques required for the histological study of these three tissues in one and the same chapter.

The vital examination of cartilage and of bony tissue was widely undertaken by the classical authors; it is even true that this method has recently given spectacular results particularly in the study of osteoclasts; however, the training of the operator and the amount of equipment involved are such that it is impossible to consider this technique as being of sufficiently general application to be described here.

Permanent preparations of cartilage and of bony and dental tissue can be obtained by staining *in toto*, followed by mounting, as well as by the technique of sectioning. The first of these procedures is described here before we go on to other methods.

SELECTIVE STAINING OF CARTILAGE AND OF BONE ON WHOLE MOUNTS

Lundvall's technique, developed in 1904, has been much used in research on the embryonic skeleton; it was improved and rearranged several times by its author; the variation described here (1927) is the last to be described.

Fixation should be carried out using the mixture

    commercial formalin .... 10 ml
    a 30% solution of oxalic acid in
        96% alcohol .... 10–20 ml
    96% alcohol .... 70-80 ml

a mixture which penetrates rapidly and, in addition to fixing the tissues, ensures controlled depigmentation. The tissues should be inspected every day, the fixative being renewed as soon as it becomes cloudy; it is advisable to continue the action of the fixative until depigmentation is complete or, at least, highly advanced.

Pieces of tissue which contain only cartilage should be transferred directly into 96% alcohol, renewed several times, and may be allowed to stand in that fluid. Tissue containing bony material may be treated for at least 24 hours with 1% ammonia and then with 10% formalin for a time as long as that spent in the alkaline solution; it may then be washed in water and dehydrated in 96% alcohol. In cases where depigmentation is to be completed a small quantity of hydrogen peroxide (1 ml of 110 volume hydrogen peroxide for every 100 ml of fluid) should be added to the ammonia or to the first bath of 96% alcohol. The air bubbles which accumulate in the tissue may be removed under moderate vacuum (water pump).

Staining of cartilage:

    Treat the tissue for several days at 40°C with the solution
        70% alcohol .... 100 ml
        toluidine blue .... 0.25 ml
        concentrated hydrochloric acid .... 1 ml
    or
        70% alcohol .... 100 ml
        methyl green .... 0.1 g
        acetic acid .... 0.5 ml
    Rinse in 70% alcohol;
    Differentiate for several days at 40°C using the mixture
        70% alcohol .... 100 ml
        concentrated hydrochloric acid .... 0.25 ml
    if staining has been carried out with toluidine blue, but use 70% or 96% alcohol if the staining has been carried out using methyl green;
    Wash in 96% alcohol;
    Dehydrate in absolute alcohol, clear in a benzenoid hydrocarbon and mount in Canada balsam if the size of the tissue permits this or else preserve in a mixture of 1 volume of benzene and two volumes of benzyl benzoate.

Combined staining of cartilage and bone:

    Treat the tissue for several days at 40°C with a mixture prepared immediately prior to use of 1 volume of a 0.1% solution of toluidine blue in 96% alcohol and 4 volumes of a solution of sodium alizarine sulphonate in acetic alcohol (a saturated solution of sodium alizarin sulphonate in 10 ml of 96% alcohol together with 90 ml of 70% alcohol containing 1% acetic acid);

Differentiate by passing the tissue alternately through very dilute acetic acid (0.5% at the most) and through 70% alcohol until all excess of the stain has been removed; Dehydrate and clear as above.

Staining of bony tissue:

Treat the bony tissue for several days at 40°C or at laboratory temperatures using the mixture

96% alcohol .... 95 ml
a saturated solution of sodium alizarin sulphonate in
96% alcohol .... 5 ml

Differentiate by keeping the tissue in 96% alcohol to which one may or may not wish to add a small quantity of acetic acid;
Dehydrate and clear as above.

The cartilaginous tissue shows up blue or deep green according to whether the stain used was toluidine blue or methyl green; the combined stain turns cartilaginous tissue blue and bony tissue red; only this last stain is obtained when the alizarin is not used.

HISTOLOGICAL EXAMINATION OF CARTILAGE

It is evident that any topographical, cytological or histochemical technique may be applied to cartilage; the general morphological characteristics of this tissue appear clearly in preparations stained by topographical techniques; it is only necessary to mention here a few precautions concerning the preparation of the tissue and the principal techniques used for the selective demonstration of the various constituents of cartilage.

Fixation may be carried out with any topographical mixture; chromoosmic fluids should be reserved for very small blocks of tissue; Flemming's liquid gives particularly spectacular preparations showing the nuclear characteristics of chondrocytes and the general disposition of the intercellular substance. The special requirements of fixation prior to the application of different histochemical reactions should evidently be respected when such methods are subsequently needed. In the course of dissection the size of the tissue block should be chosen so as to take into account the slow penetration of fixatives within cartilage.

Manipulation preparatory to embedding calls for only one remark, namely the possibility that the ground substance may have been calcified especially when the tissue has been removed from adult mammals; it is therefore necessary for the experimenter to reassure himself that the preparation of paraffin wax sections will not be rendered impossible by the presence of calcified zones; he should do this by cutting sufficiently thin slices of material fixed in a non-decalcifying liquid. Methyl benzoate (or salicylate) and butanol are equally suitable as intermediates between the dehydrating alcohol and the paraffin wax. Embedding in celloidin requires no special precautions; in the same way no technical problems are posed by the cutting of sections on a freezing microtome.

The embedding time in warm paraffin should be lengthy because cartilaginous tissue is often difficult to penetrate using this embedding material. The sections should be spread out on Ruyter's fluid (p. 113); it is particularly helpful to blot them with absorbent paper before drying.

TECHNIQUES SPECIALLY RECOMMENDED FOR THE STUDY OF CHONDROCYTES

The general morphological characteristics of these elements appear clearly on preparations stained using topographical methods as described in the second part of this work. The demonstration of chondriomes is generally easy if fixation has been correctly undertaken, both Altmann's fuchsin and iron haematoxylin giving equally satisfactory results; it is generally unnecessary to have recourse to crystal violet for the selective staining of the chondriosomes in the chondrocytes since these elements do not contain granules of acidophilic secretion. The nuclear reactions and gallocyanin stains show up the nuclear structures clearly, the same remark holding good for Flemming's triple stain. Among the histochemical techniques, tests for glycogen and for ribonucleins, as well as the demonstration of free lipids, are particularly valuable; the detection of acid and alkaline phosphatase, phosphorylase, succinodehydrogenase. and cytochrome-oxidase activity also affords highly informative preparations.

TECHNIQUES PARTICULARLY RECOMMENDED FOR A STUDY OF THE GROUND SUBSTANCE

In most cases, topographical stains permit a simple distinction between the fibrous structures of the connective tissue (perichondrium, etc...) and the ground substance of the cartilage. A technique specially developed by Romeis (1911, 1948) gives very clear preparations.

> Paraffin wax sections, taken for preference from material fixed in Helly's fluid; from my own experience, topographical fixatives give equally satisfactory results;
> Stain the nuclei using carmalum (p. 240) or the aluminium lake of nuclear fast red (p. 203);

Stain for 12 to 24 hours using the mixture
  distilled water .... 100 ml
  a saturated aqueous solution of methylene blue .... 3 drops
  a 0.5% solution of hydrochloric acid .... 20 drops
Rinse in distilled water;
Treat for 2 to 3 hours with a 5% aqueous solution of ammonium molybdate;
Wash for several minutes in running water;
Stain for 1 to 3 minutes using a saturated solution of chromotrope 2 R in 96% alcohol;
Dehydrate in absolute alcohol, clear in a benzenoid hydrocarbon and mount in Canada balsam or in a synthetic resin.

The cartilage becomes blue, the nuclei take on a red or violet colour, the collagen tissue, the muscles, and the bundles of fibrils together with the osteogenic tissue become red.

The older stains suggested for the demonstration of the enclosures in which the chondrocytes and the capsules which surround them are to be found, are now only of historical interest (see Schaffer, 1926, 1930 for a bibliography of this topic); they may be advantageously replaced by histochemical techniques, especially those which enable us to detect acid mucosubstances. Mowry's method using alcian blue-PAS, reactions involving the capture of ferric ions, and Ravetto's method using alcian blue-alcian yellow together with the different variations of the metachromatic reaction give preparations which are much easier to interpret than those given by the older procedures. The working technique of the histochemical reactions and diagnostic stains which have just been mentioned is described in Chapter 17.

The metachromasia of the ground substance of cartilage which is associated with the presence of chondroitine-sulphates is strong enough to show up clearly even after certain topographical stains have been used. We find, in this way, that Ramon y Cajal's trichrome generally confers a violet colour on the ground substance of cartilage, a colour very different from the red of the nuclei; the same remark holds good for safranine stains. Trichromes which involve the use of aniline blue, of light green or of stains belonging to the same families show that the ground substance of cartilage is strongly cyanophil. A very clear yellow metachromasia appears after staining with good commercial samples of pyronine.

We may remark, moreover, that dilute solutions of haemalum, when allowed to act for notably longer than is appropriate for nuclear staining using concentrated solutions, confers on the ground substance of cartilage a very intense blue-violet colour which may be highly advantageous from a morphological point of view. Even the common haemalum stain, when carried out as the first stage of a topographical method, succeeds in demonstrating the ground substance of the cartilage if the lake has been prepared using a good sample of commercial haematin. During staining by haemalum-picro-indigocarmine the blue colour of the nuclei and the ergastoplasm turns brown under the action of the picric acid of the picro-indigocarmine whereas the ground substance of the cartilage remains stained a bluish-violet.

Tests for certain enzymatic activities, especially acid and alkaline phosphomonoesterase and phosphorylase, can give very interesting information; such enzymatic activity is in effect very clearly represented in the ground substance of cartilage at certain stages of osteogenesis.

We need hardly add that histochemical tests for calcium are much to be recommended during a study of cartilage, of its calcification, and of its transformation at the moment of osteogenesis; one should obviously use nondecalcifying fixatives and allow for the capture of metallic ions by the acid mucosubstances of the cartilaginous matrix when interpreting the results of von Kossa's reaction or of that of Stoeltzner; we can arrive at such interpretations by comparing our material with preparations in which the calcium has been demonstrated by chelation with dyestuffs or by comparison with control sections decalcified by a short passage (a dozen minutes or so) through a dilute mineral acid bath.

TECHNIQUES SPECIALLY RECOMMENDED FOR THE STUDY OF FIBRILLAR STRUCTURES

The collagen fibrils of the *so-called hyaline cartilage* are easy to detect because they are birefringent when paraffin wax sections are examined under the polarising microscope. The same remark holds good for sections embedded in celloidin, or for frozen sections of cartilaginous tissue; naturally one should avoid any contact with substances which destroy the birefringence (for example phenol).

These fibrils are often difficult to detect by staining or by silver impregnation, a fact which was explained by Hansen (1905) in terms of the presence of a coating of ground substance. The dissolution of this ground substance may be ensured by treating the dewaxed sections, treated with collodion and hydrated, for 1 to 2 hours with 0.5% potash solution; it is also possible to apply the same treatment to free floating sections on the surface of the alkaline solution. Sections whose fibrils have thus been "decoated" are treated for 1 to 3 hours in a solution of formalin in alcohol (Schaffer's formula, p. 186), washed with care and stuck to slides if they were treated with the potash solution in the free floating condition, and then subjected to one of the staining or silver impregnation techniques suitable for collagen fibres.

Digestion with trypsin also results in a satisfactory removal of the coating in the sections, especially in cases where the tissue was fixed in Carnoy's fluid, and in such cases any method for demonstrating collagen fibres will then give good results.

The bundles of collagen fibres of the *fibrocartilage* are obviously much more abundant than are those of the hyaline cartilage so that the detection of collagen tissue necessitates no pre-treatment; the same is true of the elastic fibres of the *elastic cartilage* which are easy to demonstrate by any of the stains described for the study of elastic tissue.

HISTOLOGICAL EXAMINATION OF BONY TISSUE

The calcification of the intercellular substance of bony tissue complicates, to a quite remarkable extent, the technical problems arising during its histological examination. The calcium phosphates and carbonates with which the organic matrix is encrusted are indeed easy to dissolve using mineral or organic acids or chelating agents, but such dissolution can only be carried out, without changing the structures, after fixation so that the rapidity of penetration of the fixatives within the bony fragments is considerably slower than in blocks of tissue of the same size but which contain only soft material. Moreover, the very consistency of fresh bony tissue makes the cutting of sections rather difficult for pieces of a suitable size without creating more-or-less severe artifacts. We might add that even the most gentle of the techniques for decalcification substantially modify the chemical constitution of the tissue in any case where the dimensions of the tissue blocks make it necessary to use a decalcifying time which is in any way prolonged. We might further add that the most interesting problem posed by the histochemical analysis of the movements of calcium during osteogenesis is in any case hard to study because the act of decalcification, which is practically indispensable for the preparation of sufficiently thin sections, requires the extraction from the tissue of precisely that chemical compound which we are seeking to localise.

The vital staining of bone by oral administration of garence or alizarin enabled substantial advances to be made in our knowledge of the growth of bony tissue but it is not a histological technique in the strict sense of the term and the working technique is not described here.

Certain details of the structure of bony tissue and of the organs which we call bones may be studied in section by grinding and polishing material taken from tissue which is unfixed and either fresh or dry; such techniques will be dealt with first before we set out those which depend on traditional histological methods.

STUDY OF SECTIONS OF BONY TISSUE
PREPARED BY GRINDING AND POLISHING

Sections prepared by grinding and polishing are particularly suitable for the study of the texture of bony tissue and for demonstrating the canalicular system characteristic of bony tissue (the cavities corresponding to osteocytes and the canaliculi which link them, the canals of Havers and Volkmann). Either fresh or dried bone may be used for their preparation.

Sections prepared by polishing fresh bone allow us to demonstrate osteocytes and their prolongations very clearly; the lamella formations are easily visible by examination under polarised light. Ruppricht's (1913) technique for the preparation of sections of this kind was simplified and developed by Krompecher (1937) whose working technique is adopted here.

Immerse thin material (slivers obtained by fracture or slices cut as thinly as possible using a metal saw) taken from *fresh* bone in a saturated solution of basic fuchsin in 50% acohol; allow them to remain there for 2 to 3 days;

Transfer the tissue to a saturated solution of basic fuchsin in 96% alcohol leaving it to stand for 2 to 3 days;

Transfer the tissue into absolute alcohol saturated with basic fuchsin, leaving it there for 2 to 3 days;

Transfer the tissue after wiping it rapidly (avoiding any desiccation) into xylene where it can be allowed to stand;

Grind down the sections using a file or a grindstone by polishing with pumicestone or on a glass plate sprinkled with powdered pumice, *taking the utmost care to avoid desiccation*; the material should be damped down continually with xylene in preference to any other benzenoid hydrocarbon since it is less volatile than they are;

When the section has been reduced to the required thickness, rinse it carefully in several baths of xylene, cleaning the surfaces with a camel hair brush where necessary and mount in a synthetic resin or in Canada balsam.

The osteocytes and their prolongations show up as intensely red without any retraction being visible, the background remaining practically unstained; the nuclei often take on a more intense red colour which allows us to recognise them.

This method, which only gives of its best when used on fresh tissue, renders the experimenter liable to inhale a far from negligible amount of xylene vapour; the precautions which should normally be taken to obviate the inhalation of the vapours of benzenoid hydrocarbons should not be forgotten.

Sections prepared by grinding dried bone allow us to study the canalicular system and the lamella formations. Their preparation is greatly facilitated by appropriate maceration of the bony tissue. The fresh bone from which the soft parts have been removed is kept for several months in tap water in a warm environment. The bony tissue is energetically brushed, washed in water and dried in air, and then immersed for several days in petroleum spirit or in trichlorethylene in order to extract the lipids as completely as possible.

When macerated in this way the bone is cut into thin slices using a very fine metal saw (a watchmaker's saw) or with a diamond toothed wheel as is used in dental surgery. The slices are then ground down either using a mineralogist's grindstone or by rubbing between two pieces of pumice-stone, or else by grinding on a glass plate sprinkled with powdered pumice-stone and water. The amount of water should be slight at the beginning of the polishing and become greater as the sliver of bony tissue is reduced in thickness. The sliver is applied to the glass plate and moved about with the smooth surface of a suitably sized cork on which the manipulator exercises quite considerable pressure perpendicular to the surface of the glass. The risk that the bony sliver will fragment obviously increases as its thickness decreases. Slices cut from very spongy bone may be dried and stuck on to slides with Canada balsam or with Dammar resin applied in blobs and melted by warming over a Bunsen flame. This procedure has the disadvantage that it is often difficult to dissolve the last traces of the resin after the polishing.

Once polished, the section is carefully washed in water, a rather stiff camel hair brush being used where necessary, and dehydrated in absolute alcohol, cleared in benzene and dried in air.

The lamella formations are easy to see during examination in ordinary light or in phase contrast or polarised light, the birefringence of bony sections mounted in water, glycerine or any other medium being in no way diminished; the study of the canalicular systems is greatly facilitated by filling the system of cavities either with air or with a coloured substance.

Demonstration of the cavities by filling with air. — The classical technique of mounting in dry balsam involves the following stages.

> Melt a blob of Canada balsam or of Dammar resin of suitable size on to a slide; eliminate the bubbles of air using a hot needle and stand the slide on hot plate, brought to an appropriate temperature;
> Place the bony section, dried according to the instructions given above, in the droplet of balsam or of resin and cover it immediately with a slightly warmed coverslip and then remove it from the hotplate.

The success of this manoeuvre depends on the speed with which the manipulation is carried out; the mounting medium must be prevented from entering the canaliculi and replacing the air and the accumulation of air bubbles in the preparation must also be avoided. Very rapid chilling is thus an essential condition for success.

An unpublished technique due to B. Schramm (private communication) represents a substantial simplification of the working technique; it is carried out in the following way.

Place the bony section, polished and dried according to the instructions given above, on a clean slide; cover both faces with a cellulose varnish (colourless nail varnish); where necessary, accelerate the drying of the varnish by using a draught;

Mount in Canada balsam or in a synthetic resin in the usual way.

The layer of cellulose varnish impedes the penetration of the mounting medium into the canaliculi; it becomes easy to remove the air bubbles.

The preparations so obtained show the system of canaliculi in black on a slightly yellowish background if the bony section is rather thin. The lamellar and fibrillar structures show up well; examination under polarised light is possible as is a study under phase contrast provided that the polishing has been well done.

Demonstration of the cavities by filling with a coloured substance. — This is Ranvier's (1875) classical technique which can be undertaken in two different ways.

a) **A variation using aniline blue**:

Place a sliver of dried bone, cut with a saw and ground down using pumice-stone, in a 1% solution of aniline blue soluble in alcohol and prepared with either 96% or absolute alcohol; avoid any confusion with aniline blue soluble in water (methyl blue or cotton blue); allow to stand for several hours and then evaporate on a hotplate;

Complete the polishing of the bony slivers on a pumice-stone, and then on Arkansas stone, moistening it with a 2% aqueous solution of sodium chloride;

Wash *rapidly* in distilled water; allow to dry;

Mount in Canada balsam or in a commercial synthetic resin.

The cavities, which are filled with aniline blue, stand out very distinctly against the almost uncoloured background of the preparation.

b) **A variation using acid fuchsin:**

Immerse a bony sliver, which has been cut off by a saw and thinned by polishing, in a saturated aqueous solution (about 20%) of acid fuchsin, contained in a watch-glass or in a small crystallising dish; place the recipient in a vacuum desiccator attached to a water-pump, keep the pump running for about an hour, shut off the desiccator, and wait until the preparation has become completely dry.

Complete the polishing of the bony sliver on pumice-stone and then on Arkansas stone moistening it with *absolute* alcohol and dehydrating it in this latter liquid, clearing it in a benzenoid hydrocarbon and mounting in Canada balsam or in a commercial synthetic resin.

The cavities, which are filled with acid fuchsin, appear red; because of the dehydration and the clearing the lamellar structures when examined normally under a microscope show up less clearly than they do using the aniline blue variation but the background is much more transparent and the morphological study of the cavities and the canaliculi is greatly facilitated.

STUDY OF BONY TISSUE ON SECTIONS TAKEN FROM FIXED MATERIAL

All topographical, cytological and histochemical techniques can in principle be applied to bony tissue, but the presence of a mineralised ground substance in most cases implies the need for decalcification and strictly limits the possibilities of bringing histochemical techniques into play.

A suitable way of **cutting non-decalcified bony tissue into sections** for the histochemical study of the calcareous deposits has been set out by Bloom and Bloom (1939); this technique, which may be applied to the long bones (tibia, femur) of small mammals, includes the following stages.

Fix in absolute alcohol; dehydrate in this liquid and impregnate with alcohol-ether and then embed in celloidin using the alcohol procedure and taking the greatest possible care over the hardening of the tissue block (a viscous solution with a high nitrocellulose content to which, where necessary, fragments of nitrocellulose have been added to the last impregnation bath, prolonged dehydration in a desiccator over sulphuric acid, etc...); cut the celloidin sections on a microtome using a hollow ground razor (profile C) or a bevel edged hollow ground razor (profile D).

Stick the sections on to slides and dissolve the embedding medium according to the instructions given on page 121; apply von Kossa's reaction, followed by a background stain of haemalum or, better, of the aluminium lake of nuclear fast red, passing the sections through picro-indigocarmine (p. 201), then dehydrate using absolute alcohol, clear in a benzenoid hydrocarbon and mount in Canada balsam or in a commercial synthetic resin.

Stoeltzner's method using cobalt nitrate may be substituted for that of von Kossá. In both cases, the calcified zones appear black or deep brown. The preparations so obtained show, with a remarkable clarity, the development of calcification during the formation and growth of the long bones, but the difficulty of cutting very fine sections from material embedded in celloidin makes it hard to examine the sections at the level of the individual cell.

I might note that microtomes specially designed for the cutting of non-decalcified bony tissue are supplied by certain manufacturers.

Bony tissue which contains only a little calcium (the bones of young rats or mice) can be sectioned after embedding in paraffin wax or, for preference, in celloidin-paraffin wax using Apathy's technique (p. 96), provided that very thorough penetration of the embedding medium is secured.

Tissue intended for decalcification may be fixed, according to the objective of the work, in so-called topographical mixtures, in cytological fixatives or in fixatives particularly recommended for the several histochemical methods.

Fluids with a picric acid base (Bouin, Hollande, etc...) are quite suitable for a topographical study as is Heidenhain's Susa and Romeis' and Halmi's fluids; all these fixatives act as decalcifying agents and small blocks of material containing but little bony tissue may be embedded and sectioned after their use without any special decalcification. Mixtures of formalin and alcohol or of formalin and mercuric chloride require a special decalcifying medium to be applied after a dehydration which has proceded as far as 96% alcohol. Fixatives with a potassium bichromate or chromium trioxide base are also decalcifying but their action should be completed by a special decalcification in all cases where the tissue contains even a moderately important amount of bony tissue; such decalcification can be carried out using trichloracetic acid or chromic acid when the demonstration of chondriomes features in the programme of study.

The general progress of decalcification was described in Chapter 10; I might recall the practically inevitable chemical modification of the tissue entrained by a prolonged action of a strong acid for several days, in particular the removal of glycogen and of nucleic acids; a substantially satisfactory preservation of these compounds can be obtained by reducing the size of the tissue blocks to an extent that would permit the application of a decalcifying fixative (Bouin's fluid for example) to ensure the satisfactory preparation of the sections.

The decalcification of tissue intended for histo-enzymological research evidently poses special problems; techniques which enable us to preserve alkaline phosphatase activity are mentioned on p. 610 to 611; according to Cabrini (1961) decalcification by buffers of a pH bordering on 4 may be possible when tests for acid phosphatase activity are envisaged; β-glucuronidase activity often withstands the action of buffers of pH 5; it is obvious that phosphorylase and any oxidase or dehydrogenase activity will be lost after decalcification.

Various precautions should be applied to the *embedding* of decalcified material; small tissue blocks fixed in a decalcifying mixture may obviously be embedded in paraffin without any particular precautions but blocks containing bony tissue of a certain size will harden considerably whilst passing through benzenoid hydrocarbons and hot paraffin wax even if the extraction of calcium salts has been complete. Butanol and cedar-wood oil then represent the best intermediate substances. Embedding in celloidin allows us to obtain blocks of tissue which are easier to cut and should be employed in all cases where the volume of the tissue blocks may give rise to disquiet about the difficulties of section cutting. Even tissue which has been incompletely decalcified is easy to cut on a freezing microtome and we would emphatically advise the reader to have recourse to this technique when the preparation of serial sections is not necessary.

The spreading of the sections should be carried out on Ruyter's fluid (p. 113); the free floating sections have an annoying tendency to harden and to become fragile under the influence of absolute alcohol and benzenoid hydrocarbons; it is best to replace these fluids during the mounting process by terpineol or to mount the sections in euparal.

Staining techniques should be chosen with the objectives of the study in view and also taking into account modifications which the tissue may undergo during decalcification.

Any topographical technique can be applied to decalcified tissue provided that the passage through the decalcifying agent has not been too prolonged; sections intended for staining with Heidenhain's azan should be treated prior to the staining process for a few hours with aniline in alcohol (use the same formula as for differentiation) in order to render them alkaline because azocarmine is taken up very poorly on sections which contain the slightest trace of acid. Techniques for the selective demonstration of collagen fibres, described as part of the so-called general techniques, give very distinct preparations.

Details of the structure of the bony tissue (canaliculi, lamellae, etc...) are often well demonstrated by haemalum staining especially if the action of the staining bath is prolonged beyond the stage of simple nuclear staining; Hansen's haemalum (p. 195) is particularly suitable for this purpose. Even clearer preparations may be obtained by the use of thionine-picric acid or thionine-phosphotungstic acid using Schmorl's technique (1904).

The thionine-picric acid technique:

Fix the material in a mixture which contains formalin but which does not contain corrosive sublimate; fluids with a picric acid or potassium bichromate base are suitable;

Decalcify in nitric acid (p. 244) using Müller's fluid to which 3% of concentrated nitric acid or 1 to 3% of hydrochloric acid diluted with a saturated aqueous solution of sodium chloride has been added; this latter decalcifying fluid, recommended by Ebner (1875), is admirably suited for the preservation of the fibrillar and lamellar structures of the bony tissue but gives disastrous results so far as the cells are concerned; from my own experience decalcification using trichloracetic acid can also be used provided that the eventual swelling of the collagen tissue has been forestalled by a 24 hour bath in a 5% aqueous solution of sodium sulphate;

Embed in celloidin or section on a freezing microtome;

Wash the celloidin or frozen sections for about 12 minutes in tap water;

Stain for about 12 minutes in Nicolle's phenolic thionine
  phenol-water (2.5% phenol in 100 ml of water) .... 100 ml
  a saturated solution of thionine in 50% alcohol .... 10 ml
or in a water-alcohol solution of thionine without phenol, the proportions being the same as in Nicolle's formula;

Rinse in distilled water;

Treat for about 1 minute with a saturated aqueous solution of picric acid;

Rinse in tap water;

Extract the excessive thionine using 70% alcohol (for 5 to 10 minutes);

Dehydrate in 96% alcohol, clear in a benzene-phenol mixture or in terpineol, and mount in Canada balsam or in a synthetic resin.

The cavities of the bony tissue (canaliculi or Havers' canals etc...) appear deep brown on a yellow or very light brown background, the cellular structures being coloured red.

The thionine-phosphotungstic acid technique:

Fix, decalcify and prepare the sections as for the preceding technique;
Stain in Nicolle's phenolic thionine or with the water-alcohol solution of thionine of the preceding technique, to which one drop of ammonia has been added for every 50 ml of the staining solution; the optimum duration of staining is about 12 minutes;
Rinse in distilled water;
Transfer the sections for about a minute in a saturated aqueous solution of phosphotungstic acid (avoid any contact of this solution with metallic instruments, manipulate the sections using glass rods);
Wash in tap water until the sections have become a clear blue colour (in general 5 to 10 minutes);
Treat for 1 to 2 hours in commercial formalin, diluted to 50% with tap water, or for 5 minutes using ammonia diluted with 9 volumes of distilled water;
Wash in 2 baths of 90% alcohol;
Begin dehydration using 96% alcohol, complete it and clear with the benzene-phenol mixture (p. 74), passing through a benzenoid hydrocarbon, and mount in Canada balsam or in a synthetic resin.

The cavities and the canaliculi become bluish black, the cellular structures become a clear blue and the ground substance becomes sky blue, red or purple (this latter colour is obtained after fixation and decalcification in fluids containing potassium bichromate); the boundaries of the lamellar formations are shown up with the greatest clarity. In cases where the ground substance is too intensely stained the sections may be differentiated using 90% alcohol acidified with 1% of concentrated hydrochloric acid after they have been treated with formalin or ammonia and passed through 90% alcohol; the differentiation may be stopped by washing in tap water and further passage of the sections through 90% alcohol before they are dehydrated and mounted.

One of the best among the techniques for staining the lamellar and fibrillar structures of the bony tissue on paraffin wax sections is that of Weidenreich (1923) using gentian violet-aniline. The working technique is similar to that described for the demonstration of fibrin (p. 821).

Paraffin wax sections, dewaxed, treated with collodion and hydrated, bleached using potassium permanganate and destained with oxalic acid if fixation has been carried out using a fluid with a potassium bichromate base;
Stain the nuclei using carmalum or with the aluminium lake of fast nuclear red;
Rinse in tap water;
Stain for 10 to 15 minutes using an aniline-treated solution of gentian violet, methyl violet or the crystal violet-ammonium oxalate solution (p. 822);
Remove the stain and blot with absorbent paper;
Treat for 5 to 10 minutes using the iodine-iodate solution of Weigert;

Blot with absorbent paper, differentiate under microscopic inspection using a mixture of aniline and xylene (1 volume of aniline for three of xylene if destaining is very rapid, one of xylene to one of aniline if it is slow); it may be helpful to finish the differentiation in pure aniline;

Wash several times, with great care, in a benzenoid hydrocarbon in order to eliminate the last traces of aniline, and mount in Canada balsam or in a synthetic resin.

The fibrillar and lamellar structures become violet, the ground substance being stained pale violet or a clear grey colour according to the amount of differentiation; the nuclei are red.

The distinction between uncalcified bony tissue (osteoid tissue) ***and calcified bony tissue*** plays an important part in research on osteogenesis. The most uniquivocal results are obtained by histochemical tests for calcium, the embryonic bony tissue being fixed in a non-decalcifying fluid; it is generally unnecessary to resort to the technique for embedding and section cutting developed by Bloom and Bloom (p. 838) since the material can be embedded in paraffin wax and sectioned without any special precautions. The methods of von Kossa and Stoeltzner give equally satisfactory results, any of the background stains mentioned in relation to the histochemical tests for calcium using these methods being suitable for use.

When calcification is too advanced for the methods noted above to be used and Bloom and Bloom's technique cannot be used, it is best to fix the tissue in a fluid with a potassium bichromate base, decalcifying in nitric acid, using Müller's fluid to which nitric or trichloracetic acid has been added, the sections being cut after embedding in paraffin wax and staining using Schaffer's haemaum-Congo red (1926).

The haemalum-Congo red technique.

Fix in Helly's or Regaud's fluid or their equivalents;
Decalcify in nitric acid, with or without the addition of Müller's fluid or trichloracetic acid;
Wash for several hours in a 5% aqueous solution of sodium sulphate renewed once or twice;
Wash in running water until all excessive potassium bichromate has been removed;
Dehydrate, clear and embed in paraffin wax, cutting the sections in the usual way;
Dewax the sections, treat them with collodion and hydrate;
Stain strongly with haemalum (Schaffer advises the use of Delafield's haematoxylin, but any other aluminium lake will serve equally well);
Wash in running water;
Stain for 1 to 5 minutes with a 0.3% aqueous solution of Congo red;
Rinse in 96% alcohol;
Dehydrate in absolute alcohol, clear in a benzenoid hydrocarbon and mount in Canada balsam or in a synthetic resin.

The nuclei and the cartilage become blue, the calcified bony tissue pink, whereas the bony tissue which is not yet calcified becomes brick red.

The application of cytological and histochemical techniques mentioned in other parts of this work to decalcified bony tissue calls for no particular comment.

THE HISTOLOGICAL EXAMINATION OF DENTAL TISSUE

All the recommendations given for the study of bony tissue are valid in the case of the teeth, but the histologist's task is further complicated because of the paucity of organic material in enamel, so that it is difficult to preserve it on decalcified sections; moreover, the difference of consistency between the mineralised parts of the teeth and the pulp is such that to obtain sections in which the two tissues are equally well preserved can be genuinely difficult.

The preparation of sections by grinding and polishing poses no special problems when the soft parts can be sacrificed, the preservation of these latter being rendered possible by Koch's technique (1878) which can be of the greatest value during the study of ground sections of a wide range of material (corals, etc...). The material is fixed and washed and, where appropriate, bulk-stained and then dehydrated and impregnated with chloroform; it is then placed in Canada balsam dissolved in chloroform. The solvent is *very slowly* evaporated and the tissue subsequently hardened by keeping it at a rather high temperature (50°C) for several months. Sections prepared by grinding and polishing can then be made in the usual way.

Tissue intended to be decalcified can be fixed in any of the fluids recommended for bony tissue; when the maxillary is fixed as a whole, truly satisfactory penetration is only obtained by perfusion through the primitive carotid artery. In cases where this procedure cannot be used it is best to make a substantial openning in the pulp using a dentist's drill or to cut into the tooth in the neighbourhood of the pulp using a diamond edged wheel.

Decalcification of dental tissue uses the same fluids as are used for bony tissue; it is highly desirable to use Burket's method (p. 246) especially where one wants to preserve the enamel.

Any topographical technique and any method described for the histological examination of bony tissue may be applied to sections of teeth; details of the structure of the enamel and of the dentine show up well when the usual trichrome stains have been used, in particular one-step trichrome and Heidenhain's azan; Weidenreich's technique using aniline-gentian violet also gives very clear preparations.

We know from recent work (see Weill, 1963, 1965 for a detailed exposition of the results) that histochemical techniques show up very clearly most of those details of the structure which were once studied by staining reactions alone. Some of the histochemical techniques in question may be applied as a routine measure; this is true of the PAS technique whether or not it is associated with alcian blue staining or with the metachromatic reaction, or with reactions which demonstrate amino acids, as described in the third part of this work. The association of alcian blue staining and Danielli's coupled tetrazonium reaction or the DDD reaction of Barrnett and Seligman (1952) may be used to particularly good effect; the working technique as set out by Weill and Tassin (1961) includes the following stages.

Wax sections, taken from material fixed and decalcified by the usual techniques.

> Carry out either Danielli's coupled tetrazonium reaction (p. 509) or the test for protein bond sulphydryls using DDD with or without a reduction of the disulphide linkages (p. 518);
> Wash for about 12 minutes in water containing 1% acetic acid;
> Stain for about 15 minutes with a solution of alcian blue in 3% acetic acid as recommended by Mowry (p. 413);
> Rinse in tap water;
> Dehydrate in absolute alcohol, clear in a benzenoid hydrocarbon and mount in Canada balsam or in a synthetic resin if the sections have undergone the tetrazoreaction and staining with alcian blue; those sections which have been treated with the DDD reaction prior to staining with alcian blue should be mounted in a medium miscible with water.

Methodological studies prove that the histochemical reactions mentioned as well as alcian blue staining preserve all their validity when used in association.

The demonstration of *nerve fibres* within the dental tissue, especially within the dentine, presents considerable difficulties which are partly associated with the abundance of collagen fibres and of reticulin. In addition to the usual neurofibrillar techniques, as mentioned in another chapter of this book, the technique advocated by De Castro (1926) for the impregnation of neurofibrils in calcified tissues may give good results.

> Fix for 1 to 4 days (until decalcification is complete) by one of the following fluids: chloral hydrate 2.5 g; distilled water 50 ml; absolute alcohol 50 ml; nitric acid 3.4 ml;
> ethylurethane 1 to 2 g; distilled water 40 ml; absolute alcohol 60 ml; nitric acid 3.4 ml;
> 2 to 4 ml of a 20% solution of *Somniphen*; absolute alcohol 60 ml; distilled water 40 ml; nitric acid 3.4 ml;
> renew the fluid 2 or 3 times and also cut up those pieces of tissue which are too bulky into slices 4 to 5 ml in thickness, after 24 hours;
> Wash in frequently renewed distilled water for 24 to 36 hours;
> Treat for several hours with 96% alcohol to which 4 drops of ammonia have been added for every 50 ml; allow this latter quantity for 3 to 4 tissue blocks of average dimensions (with sides 4–5 ml);
> Wash in distilled water (3 baths of 5 to 10 minutes);

Impregnate for 5 to 7 days (until the tissue blocks become brown or grey), at 37°C, with a 1.5 to 2% aqueous solution of silver nitrate;
Rinse rapidly in distilled water;
Reduce for 24 hours in the following fluid prepared immediately prior to use
- pyrogallic acid .... 1 g
- commercial formalin .... 10 ml
- distilled water .... 90 ml

Wash in running water (several minutes to 1 hour), dehydrate in alcohol, embed in paraffin wax or in celloidin and cut into sections.

The neurofibrils stand out black or dark brown on a yellow background when the sections are mounted without any treatment beyond dewaxing (for paraffin wax sections) or dehydration and clearing (celloidin sections). A black colour of the neurofibrils on a clear grey background may be obtained by toning with gold, using the working technique described in relation to neurofibrillar techniques.

CHAPTER 35

TECHNIQUES FOR THE HISTOLOGICAL STUDY OF MUSCLES AND TENDONS

The histological study of muscle fibre, of muscles and of tendons does not call into play a great many of those "special" procedures which serve only for the histological study of these structures. Most of the topographical, cytological and histochemical data which need to be collected during a study of the muscle tissue can be obtained by means of techniques already described, so that the present chapter is primarily devoted to setting out particular points of interest rather than to the description of methods which have not yet been discussed.

Vital examination and ***vital staining*** of the muscle tissue have great successes to their credit, but all the classical morphological data, established by means of these techniques, can to-day be obtained by means of the study of permanent preparations as their manipulation is much easier to codify.

The dissection of blocks of tissue intended for histological examination should be done with care avoiding any crushing or attrition of the tissue; the state of contraction at the moment of fixation should be taken into consideration, and it is often advisable to fix the bundles of striated muscle fibres whilst their attachment to the bones is still preserved, at least in so far as the dimensions of the pieces allow one to do so; the reduction into fragments of smaller size can be carried out in the course of fixation.

No special points of interest arise so far as the choice of *fixatives* is concerned; topographical or cytological fixatives or fluids which are of particular use in the various histochemical reactions should be used according to the objective of the study.

Manipulations prior to the preparation of the sections should be carried out with care, particularly in cases where the measurement of the fibres or bundles of muscle fibres form part of the programme of study; a considerable retraction may be difficult to avoid during embedding in paraffin, particularly when the blocks are embedded passing directly from the dehydrating alcohols to the benzenoid hydrocarbon chosen as the intermediate between alcohol and paraffin. It is good practice to pass through methyl benzoate or methyl salicylate, butanol or cedar wood oil. The retractions are evidently less when embedding in celloidin is adopted but the delay in obtaining these preparations is considerably increased and the preparation of serial sections becomes much more laborious. From this point of view embedding in gelatine using Apathy's technique (p. 91) gives results which are still better than when embedding in celloidin is used but the procedure is equally long and laborious. A simpler solution, which can be used in cases where the preparation of serial sections is not indispensable but where retraction of the tissue should be avoided come what may, consists in cutting up the blocks on a freezing microtome, if necessary after inclusion in gelatine using Baker's technique (p. 92).

All the **staining techniques** and **histochemical reactions** can be used for the morphological study of muscular tissue. The essential features are set out in the paragraphs below according to the objective of the work.

IDENTIFICATION OF MUSCLE FIBRES AS SUCH

It is not easy to confuse bundles of grouped muscle fibres even when seen anatomically as individual muscles, with other structures; the morphological characters suffice for an immediate distinction. The same is not true when isolated muscle fibres are surrounded with other fibres, in particular those of collagen tissue, so that selective staining may be of some interest.

This objective is easy to attain; all the selective stains for collagen fibres, set out on pages 200 to 227, confer on muscular tissue a colour which is quite different from that of the collagen tissue; azan, single stage trichrome, Masson's trichrome and its variants give preparations which are particularly easy to analyse and also show the connective constituents of the muscle bundles. The method of van Gieson and its variant using thiazine red are equally appropriate as are the techniques using naphthol black (Curtis, Heidenhain).

A very selective blue stain for the muscle fibres can be obtained using the technique of Becher (1924) which uses gallamine blue. The stages of this very simple technique are as follows.

Sections in paraffin, dewaxed, treated with collodion if appropriate, hydrated;
Stain progressively, examining the section from time to time under the microscope, using the following solution:
gallamine blue .... 0.1 g
distilled water .... 100 ml
This solution should be prepared by boiling, chilled and filtered;
Wash for several minutes in tap water until the muscle fibres have taken up a sufficiently intense blue colour, the background being practically unstained;

> Where appropriate, stain the nucleus with the aluminium lake of nuclear fast red;
> Dehydrate in absolute alcohol, clear in a benzenoid hydrocarbon, mount in Canada balsam or in a synthetic resin.

Even better are the results obtained by a technique recommended by Neubert (1940).

> Sections in paraffin, dewaxed, treated with collodion and hydrated;
> Stain from 5 to 30 minutes using the aluminium lake of alizarin acid blue, prepared according to Petersen's method (p. 225);
> Rinse in distilled water;
> Treat for 30 minutes with a 5% aqueous solution of phospho-tungstic acid;
> Rinse in distilled water;
> Treat for from 5 to 30 minutes with a 5% aqueous solution of copper acetate;
> Wash for about 12 minutes in running water;
> Dehydrate in absolute alcohol, clear in a benzenoid hydrocarbon, mount in Canada balsam or in a synthetic resin.

The staining of the muscle fibres, which are red at the moment of differentiation by phosphotungstic acid, becomes intensely blue during treatment with copper acetate. The preparations obtained are clear. The aluminium lake of alizarin acid blue can be diluted with distilled water when the sections to be stained are very thick; in the same way, the concentration of the solution of copper acetate may be reduced; another way of adjusting the staining according to the nature of the subject and the thickness of the sections consists in varying the time of treatment using alizarin acid blue lake and the solution of copper acetate.

DEMONSTRATION OF THE STRUCTURAL DETAILS OF STRIATED MUSCLE FIBRES

The myofibrils and their striation show up very well on preparations stained using topographical techniques, but not all the stains described in Chapter 9 are equivalent from this point of view. As Gomori (1950) has very justly remarked, azan and its variants are not very suitable; a differentiation which is sufficient to be satisfactory so far as the nuclear structures are concerned ends up by staining the muscle fibres yellow; the selectivity of their demonstration is perfect but the detail of the structure of the myofibrils does not appear too well, the stain which orange G confers on them not being particularly advantageous from the optical point of view. Masson's trichrome and its variants (p. 213–215), Gomori's trichrome (p. 215) and one-step trichrome (p. 217) are better in this respect, the muscle fibres being stained in red.

Preparations which are particularly suitable for the study of myofibrils can be obtained by staining with thiazine red-methylene blue using the method of

Heidenhain (1903), with the ferric haematoxylin-thiazine red technique of Peterfi, with Unna's method using orcein-water blue-eosin (p. 774) or that of Pasini (1904); staining with haematoxylin-phosphotungstic acid is also to be commended.

Staining with thiazine red-methylene blue:

> Sections in paraffin, for preference coming from material fixed using a fluid with a base of trichloracetic acid, dewaxed, treated with collodion and hydrated;
> Stain, inspecting the section from time to time, with a 0.5% or 1% aqueous solution of thiazine red; when examined by transmitted light on a white background, the sections should be strongly coloured without being quite opaque;
> Rinse rapidly in distilled water;
> Stain for about 12 hours with a 1% aqueous solution of methylene blue or of thionine;
> Rinse in distilled water;
> Differentiate in 96% alcohol to the point where all excess basic stain has been removed;
> Dehydrate in absolute alcohol, clear in a benzenoid hydrocarbon, mount in Canada balsam or in a synthetic resin.

The Q bands remain unstained. The bands Z, M, I and h are very clearly shown up; Heidenhain recommends differentiation in methyl alcohol in cases where the extraction of the basic dye by 96% alcohol is too slow; according to my personal experience, very good results can be obtained when one shortens the differentiation as in the Mann-Dominici technique (p. 233) by a rapid passage of the stained and rinsed sections through a solution of 0.2–0.5% acetic acid.

Staining with ferric haematoxylin thiazine red:

> Secitons in paraffin, treated with collodion and hydrated;
> Stain with ferric haematoxylin lake using the technique of Heidenhain-Regaud (p. 691);
> Wash carefully in running water;
> Stain the background with a 0.5% aqueous solution of thiazine red;
> Rinse in distilled water;
> Dehydrate in absolute alcohol, clear in a benzenoid hydrocarbon, mount in Canada balsam or in a synthetic resin.

The connective tissue and the sarcolemma are stained red, the myofibrils blue-black or black, the Q bands being particularly clear.

Pasini's Stain. — This method, which may be applied to sections in wax or in celloidin, gives preparations where the details of the structure of the myofibrils, of the collagen tissue, the epithelio-fibrils, the ciliatures and the secretory grains show up very clearly.

Reagents:

Water blue-orcein. Dissolve a gram of water blue (water soluble aniline blue) in a 100 ml of water, a gram of orcein in 50 ml of absolute alcohol, adding to the second solution 5 ml of acetic acid and 20 ml of glycerine and then mixing the two solutions; this formula is different from that used in staining with orcein-water blue-eosin (p. 774);
A 2% solution in 50% alcohol of bluish eosin soluble in alcohol;
A saturated aqueous solution of acid fuchsin;
A 2% aqueous solution of phosphotungstic acid.

Procedure:

Sections in celloidin or sections in paraffin, dewaxed, treated with collodion and hydrated;
Treat for 20 minutes with the phosphotungstic acid solution;
Rinse rapidly in distilled water;
Stain for 15-20 minutes using the mixture

water blue-orcein	30 ml
eosin	30 ml
acid fuchsin	4 ml
neutral glycerine	25 ml

Wash in distilled water;
Differentiate in absolute alcohol, examining, as far as is necessary, the section under the microscope;
Wash for several seconds in a solution of phosphotungstic acid;
Dehydrate directly in absolute alcohol, clear in a benzenoid hydrocarbon, mount in Canada balsam or in a synthetic resin.

The nuclei, the epitheliofibrils, the myofibrils and the keratohyaline are stained red, the keratin is stained a yellowish red, the cytoplasm being stained a clear blue and the collagen fibres an intense blue; the secretory grains stain in red, in yellow or in blue, intermediate colours being possible.

A variant of this technique, due to Walter (1929), is longer but simpler in execution.

Paraffin sections, treated with collodion, and hydrated;
Treat for 24 hours with an aqueous mordant consisting of a 2.5% aqueous solution of iron alum to be prepared just before it is used;
Rinse carefully in distilled water;
Stain for 24 hours in Pasini's fluid;
Rinse in tap water;
Wash in 96% alcohol to the point where any release of coloured clouds has ceased;
Dehydrate in absolute alcohol, clear in a benzenoid hydrocarbon, mount in Canada balsam or in a synthetic resin.

With this technique, the nuclei and the cytoplasm are coloured in red, the remaining stains corresponding to those which were noted above in relation to the original technique.

An excellent demonstration of the structural details of the myofibrils is obtained after mitochondrial fixation and reverse staining using the ferric or cupric lakes of haematoxylin as well as using Altmann's fuchsin; moreover, these methods provide us with preparations which allow us to study the sarcosomes under the best technical conditions.

Among the histochemical techniques, the PAS reduction and the tetrazo-reaction of Danielli give particularly good preparations for the study of the details of the myofibril structure. A further advantage worthy of mention is the demonstration of oxydo-reductases.

DEMONSTRATION OF THE STRUCTURAL DETAILS OF SMOOTH MUSCLE FIBRES

The myofibrils of the smooth muscle fibres appear very clearly during examination in polarised light; they are birefringent throughout their length whereas those of the striated muscle fibres show the classic alternation between isotropic and anisotropic zones. The techniques mentioned in relation to the striated muscle fibres show up the structure very clearly; iron haematoxylin and Pasini's method are very suitable for selectively demonstrating the contractile nodes.

The disposition in the form of a network, which so frequently happens in the case of smooth muscle fibres, explains the importance of a very clear demonstration of collagen fibres and of reticulin during the histochemical examination of smooth muscle tissue, the connective web being quite often less well developed than in the case of striated muscles. Azan, Masson–Goldner's trichrome and single stage trichrome are most appropriate for this purpose, but silver impregnation of the reticulin fibres following Gomori's technique (p. 813) or that of Oliveira (p. 815) can also be useful.

The features of those techniques which are, strictly speaking, cytological and histochemical are the same as for striated muscle fibres; the demonstration of smooth muscle fibres by the histochemical detection of potassium using aurantia, as in the method of Carere-Comes (p. 297), has been suggested by some authors but the chemical significance of this technique is, to say the least, dubious.

DEMONSTRATION OF THE INNERVATION OF MUSCLE FIBRES

The selective staining of nerve fibres within the muscle mass as well as that of the nerve endings is obtained by the general methods used for the examination of the peripheral nervous system; these procedures are described in a later chapter. I only wish to comment here on the special usefulness of post-vital staining using methylene blue and of silver impregnation, especially the technique of Gros-Schultze for frozen sections, as well as those of Tinel, Bodian, and Palmgren for wax sections.

The myoneural synapses can be studied by techniques which are, strictly speaking, cytological, by neurofibrillar impregnations as have just been mentioned, and ultimately by histochemical techniques. The demonstration of the sub-neural apparatus by post-vital staining using janus green led to the discovery of this organelle (Couteaux, 1945), but this is not a method for routine use. The histochemical detection of cholinesterase activity allows one to obtain highly revealing preparations far more easily. Among the variants of Koelle's method, that of Coers (p. 624) is particularly suitable for this purpose; the technique using thiolacetic acid (p. 625) is less specific from the chemical point of view but less costly and gives preparations which are just as clear.

DEMONSTRATION OF THE FIBRES OF TENDONS

The tendons stain by all the techniques for demonstrating collagen fibres and are thus easy to distinguish from muscle fibres. Silver impregnations of the tissue collagen and of reticulin show up better than do simple stains the relations of the tendon fibres with the muscle fibres on the one hand and with the periostium or perichondrium on the other hand; examination under polarised light shows that the tendon fibres are birefringent.

The only comment we need to make relating to the techniques for the histological study of the tendons concerns the preparation of the sections; this poses no particular problem in small animals but the process of obtaining correct sections of voluminous tendons can be of the very greatest difficulty even after embedding in celloidin or in frozen sections. Heidenhain (1913) notes the possibility of making freehand sections after complete desiccation of the tendon and of causing the sections to swell by hydrating them, the tendon fibres thus taking up their normal volume, followed by staining in ruthenium red, but this is a somewhat summary technique appropriate to the preparation of material for teaching and not as a means of research.

CHAPTER 36

TECHNIQUES FOR THE HISTOLOGICAL STUDY OF THE CIRCULATORY APPARATUS

The histological study of the circulatory apparatus brings into play the topographical, cytological and histochemical techniques already mentioned; one objective of this chapter is to show how preparations can be made by vascular injection, another is to explain how techniques already described in the earlier chapters can appropriately be applied rather than to set out new procedures.

TECHNIQUES FOR THE HISTOLOGICAL STUDY OF THE HEART

The topographical study of the organ may be conducted by so-called general methods, in particular those which give a clear demonstration of the collagen tissue. Fixation of the whole heart can only be carried out in small species; the experimenter should try to remove blood clots which may accumulate during dissection in the lumen of the auricles and ventricles of the heart. Embedding requires no special precautions; it should be undertaken in celloidin for large-sized pieces of tissue. Cutting on a freezing microtome may also be advantageous.

The pericardium and *the endocardium* may be nitrated using Ranvier's technique (p. 772); the membrane is then detached with forceps and mounted, if necessary, after staining the nuclei and showing up the free fats with a lysochrome.

The histological study of the myocardium may be assisted by any of the techniques suggested in the preceding chapter for the study of striated muscle fibres.

The valve apparatus should be studied by the techniques advocated for the histological examination of the connective tissue; the presence of calcified zones, especially in large mammals, may necessitate the decalcification of the tissue.

The simplest of the methods for selectively demonstrating the nodal tissue is the histochemical detection of glycogen; this polysaccharide is so abundantly present in this tissue that even the usual topographic fixatives will prepare the tissue adequately for the PAS reaction or for staining with Best's carmine; this latter stain may be used to advantage because of the narrower range of positive results which it shows. The isolation of the Purkinje fibres is facilitated by the following technique which is due to Ranvier (1875).

> Macerate thin slices of tissue, including the endocardium and the underlying zones of the myocardium, in a small amount of 30% alcohol or in a 5% solution of ammonium chromate;
> After 24 hours detach the endocardium and examine the slice of tissue under the binocular microscope;
> Dissect out the Purkinje fibres with needles; these fibres appear clearly and should be detached from the tissue and mounted in glycerine with or without a stain.

Ranvier (1875) particularly advocated the use of the interventricular wall of the horse, the goat or of sheep; the manipulation above gives only mediocre results when practised on the human heart.

TECHNIQUES FOR THE HISTOLOGICAL STUDY OF BLOOD VESSELS

The vital examination of special cutaneous regions, such as external intestinal folds, the tongue of batracians, etc..., allows us to observe *in vivo* the structure and function of the capillary blood vessels; in the same way the vital study of the retinal blood vessels forms part of current ophthalmological practice. Such methods have greatly enriched our morphological and physiological knowledge but do not form part of current histological practice because their use requires special equipment and a certain degree of training of the manipulator; moreover, the number of favourable subjects is limited; the description of such methods would thus be out of place here.

The fixation of the tissue for an examination of the blood vessels, and their subsequent treatment, pose no particular technical problem apart from the necessity of introducing decalcification in certain cases and the advantageous use of cutting frozen sections or of embedding in celloidin for the larger vessels.

The cutting of sections can present serious difficulties especially if blocks rich in elastic tissue have been embedded in paraffin without introducing one of two stages between the dehydrating alcohol and the benzenoid hydrocarbon; these stages are a prolonged submersion in methyl benzoate and the use of butanol as an intermediate between the 96% alcohol bath and the process of embedding. Softening the blocks of tissue by soaking them in water greatly facilitates the cutting procedure; there is nevertheless a considerable tendency for the sections to pucker when they are being spread out and to become detached during staining. It may be helpful to stain the sections in paraffin wax before causing them to adhere to slides by floating them on the surface of the staining bath. Good results can be obtained using material fixed in Bouin's fluid with orcein and picro-indigocarmine, the working technique being as follows.

Paraffin wax sections, spread on the surface of a petri dish, filled with hot water and placed on a hot-plate (p. 114);

With the aid of a metallic spatula or a carrying slide transfer the sections to a petri dish containing the solution of orcein hydrochloride as used by Taenzer-Unna (p. 817); allow them to float on the surface of the liquid for about 20 to 30 minutes;

Transfer the section to the surface of a petri dish containing distilled water and allow it to remain there for a few seconds;

Transfer the section to the surface of a petri dish containing absolute alcohol, allowing it to remain there until all excessive stain is removed;

Transfer the section to the surface of a petri dish containing distilled water, allowing it to remain there for several seconds;

Transfer the section to the surface of a petri dish containing picro-indigocarmine, allowing it to remain there from 10 to 20 seconds;

Transfer the section to the surface of a petri dish containing absolute alcohol, which should be slightly warmed (tepid), if folds tend to form during the staining;

Float the section onto a lightly albumenised slide, blot it with absorbent paper and dry it in an embedding oven;

Dewax in a benzenoid hydrocarbon and mount in Canada balsam or in a synthetic resin.

The results are in every way the same as those already described on p. 818.

Any other technique for the study of collagen, reticulin and elastic fibres as well as the other general methods can be of considerable service during the morphological analysis of the vascular walls and the working technique calls for no particular comment. Among histochemical techniques, the PAS method with the various background stains (p. 398–402), the techniques for the detection of free lipids, and those for demonstrating calcium, as well as tests for alkaline phosphatase activity are the most rewarding tests for lipids and that for calcium being, obviously, only required for the study of pathological tissue.

The epithelioid pads of the arterio-veinous anastomoses show up very clearly on preparations stained with azan, one-step trichrome and the Masson–Goldner trichrome.

The pericytes (Rouget cells) can be identified by their morphological characteristics in preparations treated by so-called general techniques; I would just mention that their vital examination is possible in certain favourable subjects (the meso-appendix of the rabbit); Zimmermann (1923) and Plenk (1929) advocate an impregnation technique derived from Golgi's method using silver chromate for the selective demonstration of the pericytes but I have no personal experience of this technique; the working technique given below follows to the letter the publications quoted.

> Fix cubes of tissue of side approximately 1 cm in Kopsch's fluid (p. 686);
> Treat for 3 to 7 days with a 3.5% aqueous solution of potassium bichromate;
> Treat for 5 to 8 days with an 8% aqueous solution (Zimmermann) or a 1% aqueous solution (Plenk) of silver nitrate;
> Embed in paraffin (Zimmermann) or dehydrate and impregnate rapidly in celloidin and then harden in chloroform and finally in alcohol (Plenk);
> Cut into sections of 25 to 30 μ, dewaxing where appropriate;
> Treat the sections for several days with the following freshly prepared mixture;
>
> > commercial formalin .... 10 ml
> > a saturated solution of sodium carbonate in 50% alcohol .... 20 ml
>
> (change the liquid once in the course of the treatment);
> Wash the sections in 50% alcohol to which sufficient 5% aqueous solution of iron alum has been added to obtain a clear yellow colour; follow the destaining of the background under the microscope;
> Stop the differentiation by careful washing in tap water as soon as the background is sufficiently clear;
> Where appropriate stain the background with haemalum;
> Dehydrate in absolute alcohol, clear in a benzenoid hydrocarbon and mount in Canada balsam or in a synthetic resin.

In successful preparations the intensely black pericytes stand out; the authors of this technique remark on its capricious character.

The cellular boundaries of the small blood vessels can be nitrated using the technique described on p. 772 or by injecting a solution of silver nitrate into blood vessels which have been previously washed with a 3.3% solution of sodium sulphate or with any other isotonic fluid which does not contain chloride ions.

METHODS OF FOLLOWING THE FLOW OF BLOOD IN THE TISSUES AND ORGANS

The methods described in this paragraph are intended to enable one to study the distribution of blood vessels in a tissue or in an organ without showing up the details of the structure of the vascular walls. We should distinguish between techniques which depend on the staining of the vascular contents or wall on the one hand and those which involve filling the circulatory system on the other. The latter techniques do not necessarily form part of the range of histological techniques; in fact, the selective demonstration of the blood vessels is obtained in some of these methods by the use of procedures which result either in the destruction of the tissues (corrosive methods) or in severe changes of the structures. The techniques in question are mentioned here only summarily because they belong to anatomy rather than to histology.

TECHNIQUES WHICH DEPEND ON STAINING THE NORMAL CONTENT OF BLOOD VESSELS

These methods are particularly intended for vertebrate tissues but can be applied in any case where the blood of the animal studied contains haemoglobin; they depend either on staining this metalloprotein or on the demonstration of its peroxidase activity.

The dissection of the organ to be examined requires special precautions; it is in fact necessary to have the blood vessels as full as possible. The animal should not be killed by bleeding but by the inhalation of an anaesthetic or of coal gas; it is helpful to place the body of the dying animal in a position which will cause its blood to accumulate in the organ being studied; the afferent and efferent blood vessels should be ligatured at the time of dissection, section cutting not taking place until after a greater or shorter length of time in a fixative.

The choice of *fixative* depends to a large extent on the technique adopted; topographic fixatives and fluids with a potassium bichromate base, but not containing acetic acid, are suitable in cases where only the staining of the vascular contents forms part of the programme of work; neutralised and diluted formalin or formaldehyde-calcium should be adopted for the demonstration of haemoglobin using the zinc-leucobases, formalin-potassium ferricyanide (p. 567) or formalin—lead acetate are suitable fixatives for its detection using benzidine. The material may be sectioned on a freezing microtome or embedded in paraffin wax, the first process being much the more preferable when the consistency of the tissues permits its use for thick sections which are particularly valuable in investigations of the blood flow.

Among *the stains*, the Mann–Dominici method and Mann's method using methyl blue-eosin, as well as techniques using the azur eosinates, confer a very intense stain on the erythrocytes which stand out very clearly against the background of the preparation; the same remark holds good for the mitochondrial techniques but not all such methods are suitable for the study of thin sections. When the thickness of the sections substantially exceeds 5 μ the best solution lies in the use of Fautrez and Lambert's method using cyanol (p. 570).

The peroxidase reactions of haemoglobin give very clear preparations even when they are applied to thick sections or even to small pieces of tissue. The method of Fautrez using the zinc-leucobase of patent blue (p. 569) and that of Dunn using the zinc-leucobase of cyanol (p. 569) give excellent results not only on frozen sections but on those in paraffin wax; the working technique was described in chapter 20; it should be applied with no modifications.

Reactions with benzidine once enjoyed considerable prestige; in fact, the stains obtained are less agreeable to the eye and less stable than those given by the zinc-leucobase methods; moreover, they require the use of a special fixative which renders the tissue unsuitable for certain purposes whereas the techniques involving zinc-leucobases are quite successful when applied to material treated with formalin; among the various formulae that of Slonimsky and Lapinsky (p. 568) is the one I would personally recommend, the fixative being either the one used by those authors (p. 568) or the one recommended by Slonimsky and Conge (1932) which is prepared by dissolvoing 10 g of sodium chloride and 4 g of potassium ferricyanide in 250 ml of water with 25 ml of commercial formalin being added after dissolution is complete; this fixative should be prepared immediately prior to use.

TECHNIQUES DEPENDING ON THE SELECTIVE STAINING OF THE VASCULAR WALLS

The principal method falling into this group is the histochemical detection of alkaline phosphomonoesterase activity whose wide distribution in the vascular endothelium of vertebrates is well known. In all those organs which are not particularly rich in alkaline phosphatase activity the demonstration of this activity gives preparations whose clarity scarcely yields to the results of good vascular injections and exceeds that of preparations obtained by the detection of haemoglobin.

Another advantage of this technique over certain methods remarked upon in the preceding paragraph rests in the fact that it can be carried out after fixation in saline formalin or in formaldehyde calcium provided that the fixative has been chilled to about 4°C and that the pieces of tissue are kept at this temperature prior to their sectioning on a freezing microtome; it follows from this that a large number of histo-enzymological techniques can be carried out on sections which are near neighbours of those which have been used to demonstrate the capillary vessels provided that in the course of section cutting one alternates thick sections intended for the detection of alkaline phosphomonoesterases and thinner sections to be used for other histo-enzymological techniques; these latter sections may also be useful for tests for free lipids, for silver impregnation using silver carbonate as in del Rio Hortega's method (p. 205), conducted with a topographical study in mind, and many other methods, in short the large number of uses to which the technique can be put, whereas those involving the formalin-ferricyanide fixative are suitable for no other histo-enzymological investigation than tests for the pseudo-peroxidase activity of haemoglobin.

The working technique was described in relation to the demonstration of the cutaneous capillaries and should be followed to the letter whatever the tissue involved (p. 780); the results are excellent in all cases where the alkaline phosphatase activity of the vascular walls is sufficiently strong to provide a substantial degree of contrast in the preparations.

TECHNIQUES OF VASCULAR INJECTION

The technique of vascular injection has given rise to numerous investigations since its invention by the seventeenth century anatomists (De Graaf, 1668; Swammerdam, 1672; Nuck, 1692) and its introduction into histological practice (Liberkühn, 1748); the equipment and the materials to be injected have undergone development such that the method has currently become the prerogative of specialised laboratories equiped for this purpose. Naturally, a detailed account of the techniques of vascular injection would exceed the limits of the present work; a fully documented review of work prior to 1926 is given by Hoyer (*in* Krause, 1926); modern techniques intended particularly for the vascular injection of the organs of large mammals have been described in publications by Trueta and his co-workers (1947).

Some techniques of vascular injection have as their objective the filling of the vascular system as completely as possible, the tissue being then immersed in a concentrated acid so as to leave only casts of the blood vessels (preparation by corrosion); obviously, such methods do not require discussion here. In other cases the tissues which surround the injected blood vessels are not destroyed, the tissue being cleared as a whole or fixed and cut into more or less thick sections.

Any technique for vascular injection necessitates the preliminary washing of the blood vessels to be injected in order that the injected material shall fill them homogeneously. The animal should be sacrificed by the inhalation of in anaesthetic, the blood vessels to be injected are laid bare as quickly as possible, a glass or metal cannula is placed in the afferent artery of the area under nivestigation and the organ is perfused using an isotonic solution which has been warmed to the body temperature if the work is being carried out on a homeothermic animal. The addition of an anticoagulant and a vasodilating agent (for example, amyl nitrite) to the perfusion liquid has been recommended. The efferent vein of the area under investigation should be widely opened so as to allow the blood to flow. The duration of the perfusion varies from case to case; it is highly desirable to work quickly when the injected tissues are to be studied in sections since prolonged perfusion may result in perivascular oedemas which seriously disturb the anatomical relationships; this precaution is less imperative when the vascular injection is to be followed by corrosion.

The injection itself is undertaken as soon as the blood has been eliminated by washing as just described. Some of the materials to be injected are liquid at laboratory temperatures and may be used as they are, others require to be maintained throughout the apparatus at a temperature close to 40°C.

Small pieces of tissue can be washed and injected with a syringe; the use of a reservoir and a perfusion flask is recommended in all other cases, the difference in level between the flask and the reservoir allowing one to regulate the pressure. In any case the chances of success of the injection are all the greater if the area to be injected is rather limited; when the injection is undertaken through the aorta all the arteries which lead to the organ to be injected are ligatured so as to avoid incomplete results.

Once the injection is complete ligatures are placed on the afferent and efferent blood vessels of the organ to prevent the material injected from flowing out; the tissue is immersed in the fixative and rapidly chilled in all cases where the injection has been carried out with material which is solid at ordinary temperatures.

Subsequent treatment includes the depigmentation of the tissue in hydrogen peroxide followed by clearing in a mixture of equal parts of methyl benzoate or methyl salicylate and of benzyl benzoate (Spalteholz's method) in cases where the study has to be carried out on the tissue as a whole, embedding and section cutting, followed by staining by techniques chosen appropriately with respect to the colour of the injected material when the circulation of the blood is to be studied in sections.

The choice of material to be injected depends on the subsequent treatment of the tissue. Resins with a base consisting of vinyl salts have supplanted all the older injectable material recommended for preparations by corrosion; some authors recommend the injection of the monomer followed by polymerisation within the injected blood vessels themselves, others inject solutions of the polymer in acetone, hardening being obtained by diffusion and evaporation of the solvent; different stains can be added to the synthetic resin. The need to work under a rather high pressure generally involves the use of special apparatus, injection through a syringe being unsuitable; the work of Trueta and his co-workers (1947) includes a detailed description of the technique.

Preparations intended to be cleared and then examined macroscopically or under a relatively slight magnification can be injected with synthetic resins, as has just been stated, but the older materials using gelatin can also be of value provided that the injection of the previously washed blood vessels takes place at about 40°C. The very numerous formulae given by the various authors are extremely vague so far as the concentrations are concerned, the amounts of gelatin to be used having only rarely been set out; Hoyer (1926) remarks that it is better to be guided by the consistency of the tepid material rather than by recipes on a weight for weight basis; on the whole the gelatin concentration remains below 5%. When it is desirable that the injected material should be opaque, insoluble dyestuffs ground into as fine a powder as possible are intimately mixed with the gelatin solution. The organ whose blood vessels are to be injected is placed in a water bath at about 40°C, the material to be injected, which is warmed to the same temperature, should also be kept in a water bath in all cases where the size of the tissue makes it likely that penetration will be slow. Concentrated solutions of gelatin do not penetrate the capillaries, so that it is possible to have tricoloured injections, the arteries and the veins being filled with material of different colours whereas the capillaries remain unstained.

Preparations intended to be cut into sections can be injected using gelatinised material, stained but transparent, or using Indian ink.

It is injection by Indian ink which is the simplest technique; it requires no warming of the material to be injected, the only really important precaution being an extremely careful filtration so as to avoid the presence in the liquid injected of particles capable of blocking the smaller blood vessels. Generally, commercial Indian ink is used, diluted with two or three volumes of a physiological saline; it is indispensable to filter the liquid several times before use and Spanner (1931) advises its centrifugation after the last filtration. The liquid when diluted and freed from suspended particles easily penetrates into the finest capillaries and it is easy to follow the progress of the injection; even the preliminary washing of the vascular system may not be required, the blood being first of all displaced by Indian ink through the efferent vein, this latter being then closed or ligatured for the final filling of the blood vessels. Once the injection is complete the tissue is fixed in any one of the topographical mixtures, embedded and cut into sections.

Gelatinised material for injection is generally stained with carmine or with Prussian blue.

Carminised gelatin is still prepared using the classical formula of Ranvier (1875).

> Dissolve 1 g of carmine in 2 ml of commercial ammonia and 6 to 8 ml of water; warm in an Erlenmeyer flask, on a sand bath, until the excess ammonia has evaporated, the colour of the liquid changing from deep red to clear red; filter after chilling;
> Prepare an approximately 3% solution of gelatin, taking care not to warm the previously soaked gelatin above 60°C;
> Stain this solution with ammoniacal carmine, adding an amount sufficient to obtain an intense colour; maintain at 60°C until a clear red colour is attained;
> Add 5 to 10% (by volume) of glycerine and 2% (by weight) of chloralhydrate to the stained material, filter it warm through a very porous paper or a very fine cloth and keep in an open vessel covered with a belljar;
> For use, melt in a water-bath at 40°C.

The essential stage in the preparation of this material for injection is the elimination of the excessive ammonia; if the injected fluid contains an excess of it the colour will diffuse out from the blood vessels; on the other hand, if too great a quantity is removed granular precipitates may block the capillaries; we should aim at obtaining a colloidal solution of sufficiently fine particles.

Gelatin stained with Prussian blue:

> It is obtained by colouring a 2 to 5% solution of gelatin prepared as in the preceding formula by means of a concentrated solution of water soluble Prussian blue, as commercially available. The two solutions are kept in a water-bath at 60°C, that containing the Prussian blue is added to the gelatin until the desired tint is obtained; the solutions are mixed with great care using a glass rod until a macroscopic examination of the rod when taken out of the liquid reveals no sticky deposit of the stain. The processes of filtration, the addition of glycerine and of chloral hydrate take place as in Ranvier's formula for carminised gelatin.
> The material for injection should be melted on a water-bath at 40°C prior to use.

Tandler (1901) remarked that the effect of adding potassium iodide at a concentration of 5% (5 g for every 100 g of material to be injected) to the gelatin stained with Prussian blue, as described above, is to lower the melting point to 17°C so that it is possible to carry out the injection at laboratory temperatures.

Certain precautions are common to all the techniques for injection. It is essential to avoid any entry of air into the blood vessels being filled so that some authors advise that the dissection and introduction of the catheter should take place under water. The pressure used for the injection should be very slight at the beginning and thereafter progressively increasing; it should never be increased to the point at which the blood vessels burst.

The fixation of tissue into which Indian ink has been injected can be carried out using any of the topographical fluids; formalin, alcohol and mixtures of these two liquids are generally advised after the injection of carminised gelatin; even fixatives containing potassium bichromate can be used subsequent to the injection of gelatin stained with Prussian blue. It happens in some cases that the tissue or the sections which have been injected by this latter material become pale during the histological manipulations; the original colour can be reestablished by treatment with clove oil; Romeis (1948) remarks on the advisability of adding a small quantity of ferric chloride to the alcohol used for dehydration in order to avoid such an occurrence.

The injection of lymphatic vessels for their histological examination should be undertaken through an interstitial route. Hoyer (1926) recommends the following variant of Gerota's technique.

> Prepare the material to be injected by grinding 2 g of Prussian blue and 3 g of turpentine in a mortar for five minutes; add 15 g of ether and filter through a chamois leather moistened with turpentine;
> Draw the material to be injected into a Record syringe provided with a needle for intradermal injection or with a very fine glass cannula;

Insert the cannula or the needle practically tangentially with respect to the surface of the body or the organ and inject under rather slight pressure; continue the process, advancing the cannula progressively whilst continuing to press slowly on the plunger;

Remove the blobs of stain on the surface of the organ with a ball of cotton wool soaked in turpentine; the slight massage which results from this process facilitates the penetration of the stain into the lymphatic vessels;

Let the tissue stand for from one to several hours and then fix it using diluted formalin or formaldehyde calcium;

Cut on a freezing microtome into sections of about 50 μ thickness, mount in a medium miscible with water or dehydrate in alcohol, clear in a benzenoid hydrocarbon and mount in Canada balsam or in a synthetic resin.

In cases where it is desired to combine this technique with a nuclear stain, the thickness of the sections obviously makes it necessary to use very dilute solutions of haemalum or of the aluminium lake of nuclear fast red, the latter being preferable because of the blue tint of the injected lymphatic system. Naturally the delay which occurs between injection and fixation renders the tissue unsuitable for the study of its cytological details.

CHAPTER 37

TECHNIQUES FOR THE HISTOLOGICAL STUDY OF THE DIGESTIVE APPARATUS

The structural diversity of the segments of the digestive tract and of the glands attached to it accounts for the substantial number of techniques which need to be used in the course of its histological study; much morphological and histophysiological information can be obtained by means of topographical techniques, but cytological and histochemical methods play an essential part in the histological examination of the digestive apparatus especially in that of the invertebrates.

Physiologists who specialize in the study of mammals do, in fact, have great difficulty in realizing how little we know of the physiology of digestion in many invertebrates. Even the site of digestive absorption is known with certainty only in the insects and in some molluscs. The functional significance of many of the glands attached to the digestive tract of several invertebrates remains to be discovered and the difficulties which arise during their study by classical physiological techniques throw into relief the considerable advantages to be gained from the use of histological techniques which are much easier to use in the case of these animals.

The vital examination of the digestive tract and of its annectant glands can be undertaken without difficulty in animals which are transparent and of sufficiently small size; in the case of the vertebrates it requires the dissecting out of the segment to be studied and thus implies equipment and operating techniques designed specially for each case. The vital study of fragments which are dissected and placed between a slide and coverslip is of only minor interest.

The technical requirements for the production of permanent preparations differ considerably according to the part of the digestive apparatus under study. For this reason we need to consider them segment by segment.

HISTOLOGICAL EXAMINATION OF THE ANTERIOR PART OF THE DIGESTIVE TRACT

The tissues of the buccal cavity, of the pharynx and of the oesophagus of vertebrates should be examined by the techniques described in relation to the study of the integument. The so-called general methods give instructive preparations; selective staining of the keratin and histochemical tests for protein-bound sulphydril allow us to delimit the extent of the keratinised zones. In this respect I might mention that a true malpighian epithelium extends as far as the stomach in the Muridae. The dermal relief of the buccal and pharyngeal mucosa should be analysed using *in toto* preparations, prepared according to the recommendations given in Chapter 31. The method of choice in studies of the intra-epithelial mucocytes, which often occur in the buccal mucosa of Anamniota and Sauropsida, is Mowry's technique using alcian blue-PAS (p. 413). Obviously any cytological and histochemical technique may be applied to the detailed study of the glands and glandular cells enclosed within the buccal epithelium, the techniques described in relation to the study of the connective tissue being used for the analysis of the sub-epithelial layers of the bucco-pharyngeal mucosa.

In the same way, the study of the anterior parts of the digestive tract of the arthropods brings into play the techniques recommended for the morphological study of the integument of these animals. The existence of particularly hard parts of the cuticle or of other masticatory structures in some arthropods and in molluscs and annelids necessitates special precautions during the handling of the fragments of organs which contain them; embedding through the use of butanol as an intermediate stage, decalcification, and softening of the cuticular structures using chlorine dioxide (p. 248) may be necessary; it is always helpful to assist the preparation of paraffin wax sections by soaking the cut block in water (p. 107) and it may be necessary to have recourse to embedding in celloidin.

The taste buds of the bucco-pharyngeal mucosa of the vertebrates and the isolated or clustered sensory cells of the anterior part of the digestive tract of the invertebrates may be studied by the techniques described for the histological examination of the peripheral nervous system. The various tissues which go to make up the tongue of vertebrates require the procedures set out in the relevant chapters of this work.

HISTOLOGICAL EXAMINATION OF THE STOMACH

Proteolytic pro-enzymes occur in the glandular cells of the gastric mucosa; they pour into the lumen of the organ at the same time as they are activated, and in consequence, tissue intended for histological examination needs to be dissected very rapidly. The same observation holds good for the intestine and for certain glands attached to the digestive tract. A complete autopsy of a small animal, when undertaken by a single experimenter, should begin with the organs which have just been mentioned. When the size of the animal exceeds that of the rabbit or cat, team work, in which one person takes charge of the dissection of the digestive apparatus, is essential.

One should take account of the different regions of the mucosa in the course of *dissecting the stomach of vertebrates;* whenever the size of the animal permits, a piece of tissue which includes all the zones from the oesophageal orifice down to the pylorus should be fixed in a moderately extended condition, pinned on to a plate of dental wax and held in place by hedgehog quills or by glass needles. Fixation as a whole, after injection of the fixative into the gastric cavity, should only be used for animals of small size. Obviously, there should be no scraping of the mucosa, the remains of the gastric contents which adhere to it being removed during dehydration by means of a jet of alcohol. For animals of large size, fragments which are dissected so as to be able easily to discover their orientation with respect to the organ as a whole should be fixed after pinning carried out as described above; obviously, the serous face of the gastric wall should be applied to the wax plate.

The choice of fixative depends to a large extent on the objective of the work. Carnoy's fluid, Heidenhain's Susa, Halmi's fluid and that of Bouin are quite suitable for topographical studies and for showing up the types of cell in the gastric mucosa, but Regaud's fluid or those of Helly or Maximow are much superior for the preservation of the details of the structure of the glandular cells. It is best to use both types of fixative in all cases where the conditions under which the dissection is carried out permit it. Diluted formalin, whether saline or not, is the fixative of choice for tissue intended for neurofibrillar impregnation of frozen sections. When special cytological or histochemical techniques are to be used any special requirements during fixation should obviously be used where appropriate.

The preparation of tissue for the cutting of sections only requires special precautions when the muscular layer is strongly developed; it is advantageous to embed in paraffin wax, passing through methyl benzoate (or salicylate) or through butanol; embedding in celloidin is only necessary for very large pieces of tissue.

Among the *staining techniques,* the so-called general methods are suitable for anatomical study and generally suffice to distinguish the different regions of the mucosa. The keratinized zones (the rumen of the rodent stomach) should be studied by the same techniques as for the integument (Chapter 31). The fundic region was studied by the classical authors using methods for staining the "mucoid" secretory products; all the older techniques (mucicarmine and mucihaematin, molybdic haematoxylin, Best's carmine, etc.) have been rendered obsolete by the PAS technique. This latter technique gives the clearest preparations for distinguishing the types of glandular cell (surface epithelium, neck glands, principal cells and parietal cells of the fundic glands). One of the most useful of the combinations of stains is that of Marks and Drysdale (1957) which derives from a technique due to Zimmermann (1925), PAS being used in place of mucicarmine.

Staining of the fundic mucosa of the stomach using Marks and Drysdale's technique:

Dewaxed sections, treated where appropriate with collodion and hydrated;
Oxidise for 2 to 5 minutes with 0.5% periodic acid;
Wash in running water for 2 minutes;
Treat for 5 to 15 minutes with Schiff's reagent;
Wash very energetically in distilled water;
Wash for 5 minutes in running water;
Stain the nuclei vigorously with haemalum;
Wash in running water until the sections become bluish;
Treat for about 10 seconds with a 0.5% solution of aurantia in 50% alcohol;
Rinse in 96% alcohol;
Dehydrate in absolute alcohol, clear in a benzenoid hydrocarbon and mount in Canada balsam or in a synthetic resin.

The nuclei appear deep blue, the secretory granules of the principal cells in a very clear blue or red according to the animal species concerned, the parietal cells become intensely yellow, the secretory product of the mucous neck glands and the surface epithelium are stained red; the erythrocytes become yellow.

The secretory products of the cardiac and pyloric glands of the surface epithelium and of the neck glands of the fundic region should be studied by techniques for the histochemical demonstration of carbohydrates; the acidity of the mucins in question varies according to the species, the PAS method, that of Ravetto, and staining by paraldehyde-fuchsin after periodic or permanganate oxidation giving the best preparations from a morphological point of view. The metachromatic reaction is also useful.

An excellent demonstration of the secretory product of the principal cells of the fundic mucosa can be obtained by staining with Altmann's fuchsin or with ferric haematoxylin, the material having been fixed and postchromated as for the staining of the chondriomes. Neutral gentian violet also gives very good results. Among the histochemical reactions Danielli's coupled tetrazonium reaction, the methods for demonstrating protein-bound sulphydrils and those for detecting indole groups confer a particularly intense colour on the secretory granules of the fundic cells, so that preparations obtained in this way are as good as those given by cytological techniques. In addition to the presence of characteristic secretory granules we may ensure the identification of the fundic cells and distinguish them from the parietal cells by demonstrating the presence of ribonucleins; under the light microscope these compounds exist only in the principal cells, so that the parietal cells remain unstained in preparations which have taken up toluidine blue, gallocyanine, or methyl green-pyronine.

The essential staining affinity of the parietal cells consists of a marked acidophilia of its cytoplasm. It enables us to identify the elements in question when any topographic stain has been used. Mann's method using methyl blue-eosin, that of Mann-Dominici and stains using the eosinate of azur are, from this point of view, more advantageous than either azan or Masson's trichrome or variations on these themes. Particularly clear contrasts between the parietal cells and the other constituents of the fundic mucosa of mammals are given by the following technique which was much employed by the classical authors.

Staining of the parietal cells using Congo red:

> Paraffin wax sections, for preference taken from material fixed in Carnoy's fluid, dewaxed, treated with collodion where appropriate and hydrated;
> Stain the nuclei with haemalum;
> Wash for 2 to 3 minutes in running water;
> Stain for 2 to 5 minutes in the mixture
>
> distilled water .... 100 ml
> a saturated aqueous solution of Congo red .... 3 ml
>
> Rinse in distilled water;
> Remove the excess of Congo red by keeping the sections in 50% alcohol (where necessary inspecting under the microscope);
> Dehydrate in absolute alcohol, clear in a benzenoid hydrocarbon and mount in Canada balsam or in a synthetic resin.

The parietal cells and the eosinophil granulocytes become red varying to brown, the other structures are stained with the haemalum. As Romeis (1948) has remarked, if any preparation stained with Congo red comes into contact with an acid the effect is to turn the stain blue with a consequent loss of selectivity in the staining technique which has just been described.

Mitochondrial stains show the parietal cells with great clarity; the abundance of chondriosomes in these cells accounts for the intense red colour when any variation of Altmann's fuchsin has been used, and the black or blue colour after staining with the ferric or cupric lakes of haematoxylin, or the violet colour after staining with crystal violet.

The inter- or intracellular canaliculi of the parietal cells (Golgi corbs) may be shown up by impregnation using silver chromate, using the technique described in relation to the study of the nerve cells. These structures are also stained after periodic oxidation with paraldehyde-fuchsin. Naturally a study of the electron micrographs is the method of choice for a morphological analysis.

Kultschitzky's cells (argentaffin cells) and other types of endocrine cell in the stomach may be demonstrated by the techniques described in one of the following paragraphs.

The chorion and the other layers of the gastric wall may be studied by techniques for the histological examination of the connective and muscular tissue.

The diversity of that segment of the digestive apparatus which, in the **invertebrates,** is called the stomach obviously prevents us from codifying the techniques to be used for its histological study. At the most it is possible to draw attention to the frequent occurrence of structures which allow food to be ground up (calcareous plates, or cuticular structures) or of filtering apparatus requiring special precautions during the preparation of tissue for section cutting. Among staining techniques those which will show up the secretory product are particularly indicated since isolated or clustered glandular cells are very often enclosed within the gastric epithelium. Cilia play an essential part in the movement of food along the gastric cavity of a large number of molluscs; the *in vivo* study of the ciliary movements may be supplemented by using techniques for the study of these structures on sections. The clearest preparations of the crystalline stylet of the stomach of Lamellibranchs and certain Gastropods are obtained using techniques for the histochemical detection of mucins.

HISTOLOGICAL EXAMINATION OF THE INTESTINE

As in the case of the stomach, the designation "intestine" is applied to segments of the digestive tract of representatives of different branches of the Metazoa, even when the functional similarity (analogy) of these segments has not always been demonstrated, and their structural diversity may be very substantial. In all cases which have been sufficiently studied from this point of view, the intestine or some part of it is the principal site of digestive absorption, the essential morphological characteristics of this zone being the presence of a striated plateau with a clear alkaline phosphomonoesterase activity at the apical pole of the cells and the existence of a special type of chondriome made up of basal chondrioconts, of mitochondria and of apical chondrioconts; a cytoplasmic zone which is clear under the conditions of the light microscope (the terminal web of Leblond's school) is intercollated between the apical chondriome and the striated plateau. The techniques set out in the third and fourth part of this work for demonstrating the special features which have just been set out thus represent an essential stage in the histological study of the intestine.

The intestinal epithelium may, according to circumstances, be made up of one or of several categories of cell; the secretion of substances rich in mucins by the glandular cells is of particularly frequent occurrence. Connective and muscular tissue, nerves and blood vessels participate in the make-up of the intestinal wall; glands may be included in it as well as lymphoid follicles.

Dissection of the intestine should be done as quickly as possible, the reasons for this speed being the same as in the case of the stomach. In vertebrates, another source of artefacts stems from the violent contraction of the smooth muscle tissue which occurs even during the very rapid dissection of a deeply anaesthetized animal and which may result in the extensive detachment of the mucosa and even of tears in the sub-mucosa. A rather complicated technique which was developed by Wolf-Heidegger (1939) is much to be commended in any case where the dissection precedes an anatomical study. It consists of perfusing the circulatory system of the animal under anaesthesia through the inhalation of ether or chloroform using the following solution.

> Bring 250 ml of Ringer's solution to a temperature approximating to 80°C and suspend in it 15 g of kava-kava powder (the *radix kava-kava subtilis* of the German and Swiss pharmacopoeias) allowing it to cool to 37°C; add a pinch of malt diastase dissolved in several ml of Ringer's solution and allow it to stand for about 2 hours at 37°C, filter and use immediately.

The intestine should be removed as soon as the perfusion is complete (allow about 500 ml of solution for a cat), incised along the mesenteric attachment and fixed immediately or kept for about a quarter of an hour in the kava-kava extract chilled to the temperature of melting ice before being fixed. Naturally the method is only applicable when the sole reason for the autopsy of the animal is the anatomical examination of its intestine; it is also true that the delays involved may compromise the results of most cytological techniques.

The choice of fixatives obviously depends on the object of the work. In the case of vertebrate intestine a topographical study, the selective demonstration of the striated border, and the detection of mucins and of alkaline phosphatase activity should be undertaken in all cases; the selective staining of the chondriomes may also be very useful. It is thus appropriate to fix fragments of the intestine, opened along the mesenteric attachment, in Bouin's fluid, Heidenhain's Susa or Halmi's fluid or in saline formalin or formaldehyde calcium, these two fixatives being chilled to the temperature of melting ice, or one may use Maximow's or Regaud's fluid with postchromatisation, or Kolster's fluid, this last fixative allowing the chondriomes to be demonstrated without postchromatisation. Any other fixative described in the corresponding chapters of this work can be used for cytological or histochemical research.

The same fixative mixtures are indicated for the study of the intestine of invertebrates; the small size of the pieces of tissue often makes it necessary to fix in acetone, followed by paraffin wax embedding for tests for alkaline phosphomonoesterase activity; moreover, tests for calcium and for metallic iron are often notably of value during the histological examination of the invertebrate intestine, whereas its usefulness is much less in the histological study of the normal vertebrate intestine. Fixing in Carnoy's fluid is often useful.

The preparation of the tissues for section cutting and the section cutting itself call for the same comments as in the case of the stomach (p. 866).

Among the *stains,* methods for selectively demonstrating the collagen fibres afford a clear distinction of the different layers of the intestinal wall and show the relationships of the epithelium to the basement membrane, often giving an indication of the number of types of cell in the epithelial coating. In the case of vertebrate intestine they may be supplemented by silver impregnation of the reticulin fibres, the demonstration of these latter greatly facilitating a study of the connective axis of the villi. Staining with gallocyanin or with methyl green-pyronine often affords very clear contrasts between the regeneration crypts of the intestinal epithelium of arthropods and the functional enterocytes.

The demonstration of the cytological details of the enterocytes should be undertaken using the techniques described in the fourth part of this work. I might mention the usefulness of caryological stains, of the detection of the chondriome and of the striated border and of the study of the ciliatures which are so frequent in the intestinal epithelium of animals other than vertebrates or arthropods.

The glandular cells of the invertebrate intestine may in particular be studied by techniques for demonstrating secretory granules and by the histochemical reactions of the carbohydrates and of the proteins. We have remarked above on the usefulness of tests for calcium and for metallic iron.

In the intestinal epithelium of vertebrates the types of cell other than the enterocytes (goblet cells, Paneth cells, Kultschitzky cells) may be identified on preparations treated by topographical techniques through their general morphological charachteristics but their detailed study greatly benefits from the methods set out below.

a) **Goblet cells.**—The secretory product of the elements in question is a mucin which is to a greater or lesser extent acid according to the animal species involved; that is to say that the PAS technique, that of Mowry using alcian blue-PAS or that of Ravetto as well as the metachromatic reaction are the techniques of choice for their histological examination. The procedures which have just been mentioned make it unnecessary to use the older formulae which include staining with the aluminium lakes of haematoxylin, mucicarmine or mucihaematin, etc. The enumeration of the goblet cells should be carried out according to Moe (1952, 1953, 1955, 1963) using whole mounts of the villi and of the intestinal crypts after fixation in 2/1 alcohol formalin and treatment of blocks of tissue with the PAS technique.

b) **Paneth cells.**—The secretory granules characteristic of these cells may be preserved in fixative mixtures not containing alcohol; the presence of acetic acid does not compromise their fixation but the best results are obtained using mixtures with a potassium bichromate and formalin base, with or without corrosive sublimate (Regaud or its equivalents, Kolster, Helly or Maximow). The acidophilia of the secretory granules explains the clear demonstration of the Paneth cells using Mann's technique or that of Mann-Dominici or the panoptic stain of Pappenheim; the most spectacular results are obtained after mitochondrial fixation and staining with Altmann's fuchsin or with ferric haematoxylin.

GASTRO-INTESTINAL ENDOCRINE CELLS OF THE VERTEBRATES

This group which until recently was represented solely by the enterochromaffin cells (argentaffin cells, basal granulated cells, Kultschitzky cells, etc...) has had a certain number of types of cell added to it. The publications of Pearse's school (see in particular Pearse 1969; Pearse et al., 1970) and of Rouiller (see in particular Forci et al., 1969) and of Solcia (see in particular Solcia et al., 1968, 1969, 1970; Vassallo et al., 1971) as well as the reviews of Pentilla (1966), Vialli (1966), Dawson (1970) and Lefranc and Pradal (1971) provide an excellent source of information concerning the literature on the types of cell, some of which can only be identified by ultrastructural peculiarities and which in consequence do not require mention here.

In conformity with the excellent suggestion of Dawson (1970), the first group of these elements should be designated by the name of enterochromaffin cells; it corresponds to the former group of argentaffin cells and has all the characteristics discussed in relation to the histochemistry of the products of proteinaceous metabolism. It is more difficult to put forward a satisfactory name for the second group of gastro-intestinal endocrine cells. These elements are not argentaffin; nevertheless as Dawson (1970) has remarked, the term "argentaffin" has been so often used in a sense which differs from its accepted histochemical meaning that it would undoubtedly be preferable to give up its use entirely. There can be no question of utilizing, as was once done, the term "argyrophilic cells" since certain types in this group are not argyrophilic. The most satisfactory nomenclature, that based on the hormone which is secreted, can only be applied, in the present state of our knowledge, to the gastrin cells. All these elements belong to the APUD series of Pearse (1969) and Dawson (1970) has put forward the term "APUD cells" to designate them; in using this nomenclature we run the risk of forgetting that the gastrointestinal mucosa is not the only site of cells of the series in question and that enterochromaffin cells also possess certain characteristics of the APUD series. These nomenclatorial difficulties deserve to be mentioned here but they pose no problems at the level of a discussion of the techniques because only the enterochromaffin cells and the enterochromaffin-like cells (cellules de type enterochromaffine) and the gastrin cells need to be considered here. Pancreatic cells of types A and D also occur in the gastro-intestinal mucosa; they may be shown up by the methods described in relation to techniques for the study of the islets of Langerhans.

1° Demonstration of all types of endocrine cells by staining with lead haematoxylin (Solcia et al., 1969).

We know from the work of Solcia's school that staining with lead haematoxylin, using a formula which differs slightly from that of McConaill which was included in the techniques for the study of the nervous system, shows up very clearly all types of endocrine cells in the gastro-duodenal mucosa. Fixatives with a formalin or glutaraldehyde base are quite suitable; it is better to avoid fixatives containing picric acid. Helly's fluid may be used to advantage when a clear discrimination between the enterochromaffin cells and the other types is desired since the stainability of the enterochromaffin cells undergoes a highly selective weakening after such fixation.

The lake used for staining is prepared in the following way:

Mix equal parts of a 5% aqueous solution of lead nitrate and a saturated aqueous solution of ammonium acetate;
After filtration, add 2 ml of commercial formalin for every 100 ml of mixture; this "stabilised lead solution" of McConail keeps for several days or weeks;
Just before use, mix
  the stabilised lead solution .... 10 ml
  distilled water .... 10 ml
  haematoxylin dissolved in 1.5 ml of 95% alcohol .... 0.2 g
and stir several times; allow to stand for 30 minutes, filter and make up to 75 ml with distilled water and then use immediately.

Working technique:

Dewaxed sections, treated where appropriate with collodion (ensure that the nitrocellulose skin is kept thin) and hydrated;
Stain for 2 to 3 hours at 37°C or 1 to 2 hours at 45°C in the freshly prepared lake in which the sections should have been placed before being taken to the incubator;
Wash for 1 to 2 minutes in tap water;
Dehydrate in absolute alcohol, clear in a benzenoid hydrocarbon, mount in a synthetic resin or in Canada balsam.

The staining solution blackens spontaneously during incubation; it is obviously desirable to arrest the staining before this change of colour takes place since it heralds the onset of precipitation. In practice, it is rarely useful to keep the sections in the stain for more than 60 to 80 minutes at 45°C.

The reactive structures become intensely bluish black. It may be useful to mention that the results vary somewhat according to the species of animal involved.

2° Methods for selectively demonstrating endocrine cells using silver impregnation (Grimelius, 1968)

A technique for silver impregnation using a dilute solution of silver nitrate, acting at pH 5.6, was developed by Grimelius (1968) for the selective impregnation of the A cells of the endocrine pancreas. According to Solcia et al. (1969,

1970) and Bussolati and Pearse (1970) this method clearly shows up the gastrointestinal endocrine cells of mammals as well as the other types of endocrine cell, in particular the calcitonin cells. The enterochromaffin cells, the enterochromaffin-like cells and the gastrin cells are also impregnated.

Fixing by formalin, glutaraldehyde, Solcia et al.'s GPA (1968) and Bouin's fluid will work equally well.

Dewaxed sections, treated where appropriate with collodion (take great care to ensure the thinness of the nitrocellulose film) and hydrated;
Impregnate for 24 hours at 37°C or 3 hours at 60°C in the mixture.
Walpole's buffer using 0.2 M acetic
    acid-sodium acetate at pH 5.6 .... 10 ml
    Doubly distilled water .... 87 ml
    A 1% aqueous solution of silver nitrate .... 3 ml
Wipe the slide around the sections (do not rinse) and reduce for 1 minute, at 40 to 45°C, in the mixture —
    distilled water .... 100 ml
    hydroquinone .... 1 g
    crystalline sodium sulphite .... 5 g
Rinse in distilled water;
Stain, where appropriate, using the aluminium lake of nuclear fast red;
Wash in tap water, dehydrate, clear and mount in a synthetic resin or in Canada balsam.

When the impregnation is too weak a double impregnation, practised *before background staining*, greatly improves the result; this manoeuvre involves the following stages.

Impregnated sections, reduced and quickly rinsed in tap water;
Treat for 2 minutes with a 5% aqueous solution fo sodium thiosulphate (hyposulphite);
Wash for 5 minutes in frequently renewed distilled water;
Impregnate, at laboratory temperatures, for 10 minutes in a fresh bath of the silver solution prepared as for the first impregnation;
Reduce for 1 minute as in the first impregnation at 40 to 45°;
Wash in tap water, stain the background, dehydrate, clear and mount.

From my own experience, the double impregnation, which is very easy and rapid, is useful in the majority of instances. The method confers on the gastrointestinal cells a colour which, according to the way in which the various stages have been conducted, varies from brown to black and the background is practically unstained. It is thus helpful to stain it in practically all cases and the topograhical value of the preparations is considerably improved supplement staining using nuclear fast red and picro-indigocarmine following the working technique set out in Chapter 9 (p. 203).

3° Methods for the selective demonstration of enterochromaffin cells

The secretory granules characteristic of the enterochromaffin cells are well preserved by most aqueous fixatives, in particular by dilute formalin, formaldehyde calcium, Bouin's fluid, and mixtures with a formalin and potassium bichromate base, for preference without corrosive sublimate. Modern research, in particular that of Solcia et al. (1966, 1967, 1969), proves that fixatives with a glutaraldehyde base are even more suitable so far as the majority of histochemical reactions is concerned.

These represent in fact the best techniques for the selective demonstration of enterochromaffin cells. An attentive study of preparations treated with topographic stains or by mitochondrial methods will certainly allow us to recognise the enterochromaffin elements, but silver impregnation, marker staining and histochemical reactions are obviously preferable by far.

Among the silver impregnations that of Grimelius using silver nitrate has just been described as a general method for demonstrating the gastro-intestinal endocrine cells. Most of the techniques stem from the method of Bielschowsky or that of Ramon y Cajal and give the same results when applied to sections. I might in particular mention Davenport's method which, when used according to the working techniques advocated by the Swedish school for the study of the islets of Langerhans, gives good results; the same remark holds good *with some samples of silver proteinate* for Grimelius' method using protargol (1964) which was also described in relation to techniques for the study of the endocrine pancreas. Naturally, these procedures show up the argyrophilic cells at the same time as they demonstrate the enterochromaffin cells which are argentaffin; they should not be considered therefore as techniques for the selective demonstration of this type of cell.

First place among the marker stains is held by the method of Solcia et al. (1968) described in relation to the study of secretory granules in general (Chapter 29). The basophilia which appears in the secretory product of the enterochromaffin cells following hydrochloric acid hydrolysis is orthochromatic; when this hydrolysis is followed by staining with toluidine blue the distinction between the enterochromaffin cells and the other gastro-duodenal endocrine cells is immediately apparent. Any of the fixatives described above may precede the application of this method.

So far as histochemical reactions are concerned some rest on the demonstration of the reducing nature of the compound which appears in the secretory product following fixation by mixtures which include formaldehyde or glutaraldehyde. Such a reducing capacity explains the excellent demonstration of the enterochromaffin cells using the ferric ferricyanide method (p. 322); Lillie

(1954, 1965) has quite rightly stressed the advantages of this method in routine work. The argentaffin reaction, whose use to show up the enterochromaffin cells is well known, also gives well-contrasted preparations; I would particularly recommend the working technique recommended by Gomori (1948, 1952) in which the silver content of the bath is less than it is in Fontana's liquid, which is used in the classical techniques of Masson and Hamperl; the technical details given in relation to the general discussion of the argentaffin reaction (p. 325) remain entirely valid when the object of the study is the demonstration of the enterochromaffin cells. A background stain using nuclear fast red-picro-indigo-carmine increases the topographical value of the preparations and does not change the contrasts involved.

The azo-reaction gives excellent results in showing up the enterochromaffin cells. I would particularly recommend the working technique of Gomori (1952) which includes the following stages.

> Dewaxed sections, treated where appropriate with collodion and hydrated;
> Treat for 1 to 5 minutes on slides with the reagent
> distilled water chilled to 4°C .... 10 ml
> the appropriate diazonium salt (see below) .... about 50 mg
> a saturated aqueous solution of borax .... 5–10 drops
> Wash in tap water;
> Where appropriate, stain the background using a dilute solution of toluidine blue, or iodine green, or the aluminium lake of nuclear fast red;
> Dehydrate in absolute alcohol, clear in a benzenoid hydrocarbon and mount in a synthetic resin or in Canada balsam.

The azo-dyestuff formed under these conditions is insoluble in alcohol so that it is possible to dehydrate the preparation. When the material has been fixed in Bouin's fluid, Fast red B salt, Fast garnet GBC salt and Fast black K salt give equally satisfactory stains veering from deep orange to brownish-black. After fixing with mixtures having a glutaraldehyde base, in particular the GPA of Solcia et al. (1968), Fast black K is much to be preferred to the other diazonium salts. The secretory product of the enterochromaffin cells takes on an intense black stain, the azo-reaction of the proteins is responsible for the yellow or pink colour of the background, no background stain being required. The amount of contrast is equivalent to that obtained with silver impregnation.

As I noted in relation to the histochemical detection of biogenic amines, the detection of indole groups, using the reaction with xanthydrol, shows up the enterochromaffin cells very clearly provided that the material has been fixed using glutaraldehyde based mixtures (Solcia and Sampietro, 1967; Solcia and Vassallo, 1966).

In this context the possibility of a fluoroscopic detection of the enterochromaffin cells may be mentioned. Unlike the histochemical demonstration of indole groups the appearance of this yellowish fluorescence is closely associated with formaldehyde fixation in a liquid medium or in the gas phase. Geyer's (1968) work, which was mentioned in Chapter 21, introduced the interpretation of this difference in reaction in terms of the fixative used.

We might mention that the histological characteristics of the enterochomaffin cells of vertebrates are highly uniform.

4° Demonstration of the enterochromaffin-like cells (Solcia et al., 1969) or histamine-storing cells (Hakanson et al., 1967, 1969, 1970)

These elements, whose presence in the stomach of eight mammalian species has just been established (Capella *et al.*, 1971), are argyrophilic and clearly shown up using Grimelius' method with silver nitrate; they do not give the argentaffin reaction and are demonstrated neither by the azo reaction nor by the method used by Solcia *et al.* (1968) involving toluidine blue after hydrochloric acid hydrolysis. The affinity for lead haematoxylin is variable. Moreover, a liability to accumulate and decarboxylate amine precursors is common to these elements and to other cell types of the APUD series. Tests for histamine give positive results in the stomach of the rat and mouse but not in that of the other mammals investigated from this point of view. We may add at this point that the elements in question have a violet metachromasia after staining with toluidine blue at pH values higher than 4.5 in certain species of animal (cat, rabbit) (Vassalo *et al.*, 1969) and that hydrochloric acid hydrolysis as used by Solcia *et al.* (1968) does not cause this metachromasia to disappear. Staining with phosphotungstic haematoxylin gives positive results in certain species. Evidently there is no case for spending time at this point on the morphological and ultrastructural characteristics of the cells in question.

5° Demonstration of the Gastrin cells

The endocrine significance of these elements has been shown by immunohistochemical methods in the stomach of mammals (McGuigan, 1968; Bussolati and Pearse, 1970). They have also been detected in the stomachs of Sauropsida and Batrachia (Gabe, 1969) as well as in that of a Teleost (Gabe and Mme. Martoja, 1971). As in the case of the enterochromaffin cells their histological nature seems to be very uniform.

All tests for polyphenols and indol compounds give negative results in these cells whose preservation is ensured by most aqueous fixatives; the GPA of Solcia *et al.* (1968) is particularly advantageous but Bouin's and Helly's fluids serve equally well. The argentaffin reaction, the azo-reaction and the xanthydrol method give negative results. Among the silver impregnations that of Grimelius using silver nitrate gives very strongly positive results in certain species but moderately positive or even negative ones in others. With Davenport's method, as modified by the Swedish school and applied according to the working technique set out in relation to the D cells of the endocrine pancreas, the results are positive in all cases. In the same way, Grimelius's technique using silver proteinate, using the samples of protargol which are currently available on the French market, ensures an excellent demonstration of the gastrin cells but their argyrophilia is of course shared with other endocrine cells of the gastro-intestinal mucosa. After hydrochloric acid hydrolysis using the technique of Solcia et al. (1968) the gastrin cells acquire a very strong metachromasia which immediately distinguishes them from the enterochromaffin cells which are orthochromatic. The enterochromaffin-like cells which are also metachromatic in certain species show such a metachromasia before any hydrolysis. Moreover, tests for α-glycerophosphate-dehydrogenases and acetyl or butyryl thiocholinesterases give intensely positive results in the gastrin cells (Carvalheira et al., 1968). We may remark that the gastrin cells possess one of the essential characteristics of the APUD series, that is to say their capacity for fixing amine precursors and for decarboxylating them, the amines so formed being capable of fluoroscopic detection.

HISTOLOGICAL EXAMINATION OF THE LYMPHOIDAL FORMATIONS OF THE DIGESTIVE TRACT OF VERTEBRATES

In addition to the so-called general methods, which suffice for the topographical examination of the lymphoid formations of the digestive tract (tonsils, closed follicles, Peyer's patches), the stains suggested for the study of the haematopoietic organs are obviously of the greatest value for their detailed study.

Fixing in Maximow's fluid, followed by panoptic staining, gives the most precise information about the cellular composition of the mass of lymphoidal tissue; silver impregnation of the reticulin and Pasini's stain show up the connective web clearly; the demonstration of metallic iron often allows us to identify the macrophages easily, the techniques mentioned on p. 825 being used for the study of mast cells.

A technique for the quantitative study of the lymphoid tissue of the intestine which was developed by Hellman (1922) includes the following stages.

Fix the intestine, which is opened along its mesenteric attachment, using dilute formalin or formalin-alcohol, keeping it tense on a cork sheet;
Wash for several days in running water;
Stretch the piece of tissue, cutting it up if necessary into long ribbons of 15–20 cm, on filter paper, immerse it for 2 to 5 days in 2 or 3% acetic acid; the pieces of tissue should become transparent;
Wash for several hours in running water;

Stain for 12 to 60 hours in haemalum diluted 1/100 with distilled water; Hellman advises the use of Harris' haemalum, but any other formula involving the aluminium lake of haematoxylin will serve equally well;

Differentiate for 12 to 24 hours in 2% acetic acid to the point where the lymphoidal formations stand out clearly from the background;

Wash for a long time in running water;

Use forceps to detach the mucosa from the underlying layers;

Preserve in Kaiserling's fluid (distilled water 1000 ml; potassium acetate 100 g; glycerine 200 ml) or in Jores' fluid (distilled water 100 ml; potassium acetate 300 g; glycerine 600 ml).

The surface occupied by the lymphoidal tissue can be evaluated by sketching, weighing and cutting out or by planimetry; the counting of the closed follicles is very easy.

DEMONSTRATION OF BLOOD VESSELS AND NERVES OF THE GASTRIC AND INTESTINAL WALLS

Any technique for the histological study of the lymphatic and blood vessels, as set out in Chapter 36, can be applied to the wall of the digestive tract of vertebrates; injection techniques give results which are particularly agreable to the eye so far as the intestinal villi are concerned, but they require a pretreatment of the tissue pieces which generally compromises the success of the majority of cytological techniques; the exigences of this pretreatment are slighter for the demonstration of the capillary walls because of their alkaline phosphatase activity and this latter method (p. 780) is particularly easy to apply to slices of the stomach or intestine of large mammals.

In the same way, the techniques recommended for the study of the peripheral nervous system (Chapter 41) will serve equally well to show up the nerves and their endings in the gastro-intestinal tract; the study of the ganglia of Auerbach's plexus and Meissner's plexus should be completed by the demonstration of the Nissl bodies for which purpose it is quite satisfactory to use gallocyanin staining and the Bielschowsky-Plien method.

HISTOLOGICAL EXAMINATION OF SALIVARY GLANDS

In addition to the general cytological techniques applied to the particular case of the salivary glands with no modification of the working technique, the histochemical identification of secretory products plays an essential part in the histological examination of these organs. The classical distinction into serous and mucous glands certainly does not retain the importance once accorded it; modern work has shown the existence of carbohydrate compounds in the secretory product of the "serous" glands of the most authentic kind and we know that the "mucous" and "serous" stages can follow one another in the secretory cycle of one and the same glandular cell. It is nevertheless true that mucins have an important role in the production of secretory material by the salivary glands of all the vertebrates and of that of the glands attached to the first part of the digestive tract of a large number of invertebrates, this state of affairs allowing us to understand the importance of histochemical reactions for polysaccharides in their study.

The demonstration of polysaccharides as well as of proteins is of some importance; in fact the secretory products of the salivary glands can contain proteins and polysaccharides at the same time, the nature of these two types of compound permitting a classification which has been put forward for the salivary glands of the lepidosaurians (Gabe and Saint Girons, 1969) but which can obviously be applied to any glandular cells. In the terms of this classification, the *mucous elements* contain only acid mucins, tests for proteins giving entirely negative results. The *muco-serous cells* contain more or less acid mucins as well as proteins. In the *sero-mucous cells* the tests for *acid* mucins are negative, but other carbohydrate compounds which are PAS positive co-exist with the proteins. Lastly, in the *serous cells* the secretory product is rich in proteins and devoid of histochemically detectable polysaccharides, that is to say it is PAS negative. A fifth type which is characterised by a secretory product which does not contain polysaccharides other than the acid mucins and is devoid of proteins is theoretically possible but no example seems to have been described so far.

All the rules discussed in relation to general cytological *fixation* are valid in the case of the salivary glands. The speed of dissection and the choice of suitable fixatives determines not only the preservation of the fundamental organelles *in situ* but also that of the secretory product. The topographical fixatives serve for an anatomical study, the demonstration of the myo-epithelial cells and even for the definition of the histochemical characteristics of some of the secretory products, but mixtures with a potassium bichromate and formalin base are much superior to them for the preservation of the secretory products within the cells. The unsuitability of fixatives with a corrosive sublimate base has been commented on by the classical authors, the presence of these compounds according to them inducing the swelling and the passage into solution of the "mucous" secretory granules; my personal experience does not allow me entirely to confirm this way of looking at the problem and modern publications include no particular warnings against liquid fixatives such as those of Helly or Maximow.

The preparation of the pieces of tissue for section cutting calls for no particular comment; a cytological study requires thin sections so that embedding in celloidin should be reserved for large pieces principally intended for anatomical study. Special manoeuvres such as decalcification or the softening of pieces of cuticle are useful only when the glands of small animals have been removed with the neighbouring tissue, or even in cases where the head has been fixed as a whole. Only the tests for ribonucleins and for glycogen can be harmed because of a decalcificatory process but the softening of pieces of cuticle (p. 247) is incompatible with the majority of cytological and histochemical techniques which it is obviously disadvantageous to avoid softening as far as is possible.

The stains required for an anatomical study call for no special comment; the methods for demonstrating collagen fibres serve well for an analysis at the level of microscopic anatomy disclosing the general architecture of the gland and giving information about the appearance of the glandular cells; those methods which depend on the demonstration of the staining affinities of the cytoplasm will help to characterise the secretory granules. Procedures such as the use of Heidenhain's azan, one-step trichrome, or Mann's method using methyl blue-eosin and the Mann-Dominici technique prepare the material for the studies to follow and help in choosing suitable histochemical reactions. In fact, secretory products which are rich in proteins and are devoid of any substantial amount of mucins will, under the technical conditions of these procedures, take up red or yellow stains; on the contrary, products rich in mucins become cyanophil or even metachromatic with the Mann-Dominici technique which also provides information on the distribution of ribonucleins. It is also very useful to employ the eosinates of azur as a stain.

The marker stains and the histochemical reactions of carbohydrates play an important part in the study of the salivary glands. The PAS method associated with staining by alcian blue allows us to identify the acid mucins and other polysaccharides; this technique, when supplemented by those mentioned in Chapter 17, enables us to classify the carbohydrate constituents of the gland under examination and I might mention how valuable it is, when setting out the results, to adopt the scheme put forward by Spicer and his collaborators (p. 674). I might also mention the possibility of a PAS reactivity of the secretory product of the "serous" glands, a secretory product which is erythrophil when the usual trichrome stains are used.

The histochemical reactions of proteins may be used according to the directions given in Chapter 19 to define the proteinaceous constituents of the secretory product of the glands being studied; the alloxane-Schiff method, the coupled tetrazonium reaction of Danielli and the techniques for demonstrating protein-bound sulphydryls and indole groups are particularly useful in this respect.

Naturally, **the histo-enzymological study** of the salivary glands can be very rewarding (see Arvy in Graumann and Neumann, 1962 for a survey of the principal results).

The fundamental organelles may be studied by general cytological techniques as described in the fourth part of this work. What is strictly speaking the cytological study may be augmented to great advantage by the nuclear staining reaction of Feulgen and Rossenbeck as well as by the demonstration of the ribonucleins, the analysis of the nuclear structures in the case of the salivary glands of certain invertebrates being liable to set the experimenter rather difficult problems; the abundance of cytoplasmic ribonucleins is moreover a piece of evidence in favour of the secretion of substances rich in proteins.

The canalicular system of the salivary glands may be studied on serial sections, if necessary followed by plastic or graphic reconstruction; the injection of a mass of coloured material through the insertion of a catheter into the principal excretory duct has also been practised.

Naturally all the technical details of the histological examination of the salivary glands will also hold good for the study of the Brunner glands of the duodenum.

HISTOLOGICAL EXAMINATION OF THE EXOCRINE PANCREAS

Of all the glands attached to the digestive tract of the vertebrates the exocrine pancreas is the one whose *vital examination* offers the greatest rewards from the general cytological point of view; the appropriate technique was described in relation to the demonstration of the chondriome. It is nevertheless true that the examination of permanent preparations plays an essential part in a histological study of this organ.

The secretion of proteolytic enzymes in the pancreatic cells explains why it is absolutely imperative *to dissect* the organ out with the greatest rapidity; at least one dimension of the pieces of tissue should be less than 0.5 cm.

Any topographical *fixative* is suitable for an anatomical study; the secretory granules of the exocrine pancreas of mammals and birds are only moderately preserved in Bouin's fluid, by Heidenhain's Susa or by Halmi's fluid; mixtures with a potassium bichromate and formalin base, with or without corrosive sublimate, serve much better for this purpose. Obviously, any fixative which has been particularly recommended for the various cytological and histochemical techniques should be used when these techniques form part of the experimenter's programme of work.

The preparation of the tissue for section cutting and the section cutting itself call for no special comment; embedding in celloidin is only justified when large pieces of tissue are used, intended for an anatomical study; the cutting of the pancreatic parenchyme on a freezing microtome may be difficult because of fragmentation into lobules and embedding in gelatin using Baker's technique (p. 92) may be useful when thin sections are needed.

Any topographical *stain* is suitable for an anatomical study, or for the analysis of the canalicular system or the delimitation of the lobules. Methods which demonstrate the cytoplasmic basophilia clearly are particularly needed in order to bring out the centro-acinous cells. The nuclear reaction of Feulgen and Rossenbeck and staining using methyl green-pyronine or by gallocyanine are useful for a detailed analysis of the nuclear structures; the first of these methods, when carried out after fixation using a mixture with a potassium bichromate and formalin base without postchromatisation, may be followed by mordanting with phosphotungstic acid and staining using Heidenhain's blue as with azan. This combination, recommended by Huber (1945), assists a parallel study of the nuclear structures and the secretory granules (see p. 555).

The chondriome may be studied by classical techniques; its demonstration is particularly easy, as is the metallic impregnation of the Golgi bodies; I might remark that the exocrine pancreatic cell is indeed one of the classical subjects for the demonstration of the ergastoplasm.

The secretory granules of the exocrine pancreatic cell are shown up very clearly by any of the stains which involve a red dyestuff of the eosin family or of acid fuchsin; they strongly take up the ferric and cupric lakes of haematoxylin; Altmann's fuchsin shows them up strikingly and the same remark holds good for neutral gentian violet. Permanganate oxidation in an acid medium causes the acidophilia to become a basophilia, as mentioned above, so that the secretory granules of the exocrine pancreatic cells may be stained using paraldehyde-fuchsin and chromic haematoxylin as in Gomori's method.

Among the histochemical reactions, Danielli's coupled tetrazonium reaction or Morel and Sisley's method for the detection of tyrosine, or any technique for demonstrating protein-bound sulphydryls and the indole groups would be suitable to discern the secretory granules of the exocrine pancreas, often with great selectivity; the extent of the **PAS** activity varies from species to species.

I might moreover remark that sound methods for demonstrating unspecific esterase activity, in particular the methods of Burstone using substituted naphthol AS acetates, will show up the secretory granules in question with a high degree of selectivity.

HISTOLOGICAL EXAMINATION OF THE LIVER

The anatomical complexity of the organ and the multiplicity of the functions of the hepatic cell account for the diversity of techniques which can be called into play for a complete histological study.

The essential requirements for a quick *dissection* and for rapid penetration by a fixative hold good as for the other segments of the digestive apparatus, especially in cases where the object of the work is other than microscopic anatomy.

The general topography of the organ may be studied after topographical methods have been used; Bouin's fluid, Halmi's fluid, and Heidenhain's Susa or formalin in alcohol are suitable, as is Carnoy's fluid. Heidenhain's azan, one-step trichrome, and that of Masson and its variations serve very well to demonstrate Glisson's capsule and its prolongations; van Gison's method or haemalum-picro-indigocarmine give very clear preparations in cases where the liver is rich in collagen fibres. We need hardly add that a study of the connective constituents of the organ should be supplemented by silver impregnation of the reticulin fibres; Gomori's technique (p. 813) serves very well to this end as do the second and third tanno-argentic variants of del Rio Hortega, all the more so because the hepatic parenchyme is particularly easy to cut on a freezing microtome.

Any cytological and histochemical technique may be applied to the study of the hepatic cells. The demonstration of the chondriome by staining with Altmann's fuchsin or with ferric haematoxylin, the demonstration of Berg's clumps, which are rich in ribonucleic acid, by staining with gallocyanine or with methyl green-pyronine, and the detection of glycogen using the PAS technique with a malt diastase control as well as tests for free lipids are all obligatory in any histophysiological work which includes a study of the liver.

The Kupffer cells of the sinusoids may be distinguished by means of their general morphological characteristics but the most spectacular preparations may be obtained after athrocytosis of indian ink particles or of lithium-carmine or of trypan blue. The intraperitoneal or intraveinous injection of these substances in the amounts which were defined in Chapter 33 should take place 24 to 48 hours before the autopsy of the animal.

The hepatic blood vessels may be shown up by detecting the pseudo-peroxidase activity of haemoglobin; I would in particular recommend the technique using the zinc-leucobase of patent blue or of cyanol which is much superior to methods using benzidine. Vascular injection should take place from the portal vein and the hepatic artery or, in small animals, from the abdominal aorta, with all the other branches of this latter blood vessel being ligatured; the injection of two lots of stain of different colours gives highly informative preparations.

The macrophages which occur so frequently in the hepatic parenchyme of the reptiles and all the Anamniota may be studied using techniques for demonstrating the particles which are contained in their cytoplasm; tests for free iron and for chromolipoids are particularly recommended; in a large number of cases, the melanic pigments which accumulate in the cells in question can be recognised from their natural colouration, and the distinction between melanins and chromolipoids is assured by the ease with which the former bleach under oxidation.

The identification and the histological study of the bile canals of a particular size as well as of the biliary vesicle apparently pose no particular problems; special methods are necessary for a clear demonstration of the biliary capillaries. Some of these techniques consist of injecting a concentrated solution of Prussian blue soluble in water or of some other injectable material into the common bile duct or into the biliary vesicle and then treating the tissue as after vascular injection (p. 860); the results are generally only satisfactory over quite limited areas. It is more worthwhile to use the techniques of vital injection with indigocarmine or scarlet R, staining with haematoxylin, Forsgren's (1928) method using barium chloride, or impregnation with silver chromate using Bohm's (1912) technique; certain histoenzymological techniques also serve very well.

Demonstration of the biliary capillaries using indigocarmine (Chrzonszezewsky, 1866):

At 30 minute intervals, make three intraveinous injections of a saturated aqueous solution of indigocarmine (a commercial sample certified for vital injection); the average doses are 50 ml for injection into a dog, 30 ml into a cat, 20 ml into an adult rabbit; an injection of 2 ml into the dorsal lymphatic sac will suffice for a frog or a toad;

Autopsy the animal in the 30 minute period following the last injection (wait 2 to 3 hours in the case of a frog) and fix the liver in absolute alcohol;

Embed in paraffin wax and cut without any special precautions;

Lay out the sections avoiding any contact with an aqueous fluid (p. 112), as indigocarmin is soluble in water;

Dewax in a benzenoid hydrocarbon and mount in Canada balsam or in a synthetic resin;

The biliary capillaries are filled with indigocarmine and clearly shown up provided that the moment for autopsy has been well chosen. Staining the nuclei using a solution of basic fuchsin or of safranin in absolute alcohol improves the legibility of the preparations although this possibility was not foreseen by the author of the method.

Demonstration of the biliary capillaries using scarlet R (Oppenheimer, 1923)

Administer a small quantity of olive oil saturated with scarlet R using a stomach pump (on an average 1 ml for an adult rat and 3 ml for a rabbit); it may be advantageous to include a small amount of cholesterol in the olive oil;

Autopsy the animal after three or four days of this treatment in the two hours which follow the last application of the stomach pump; fix the liver in dilute formalin whether saline or not;

Cut on a freezing microtome into sections of average thickness (10 to 20 μ);

Stain the nuclei with haemalum diluted with distilled water as was done after the staining of the lipids using a red lysochrome (p. 452);

Wash the sections in tap water so as to render the nuclear stain bluish;

Mount in a medium miscible with water.

The biliary capillaries, filled with lysochrome, appear reddish-orange; the stain extends down into the average sized bile ducts.

Staining of the biliary capillaries with haematoxylin (Otami, 1926):

> Paraffin wax sections, *taken from material fixed in a mixture which does not contain alcohol*, dewaxed, treated where appropriate with collodion and hydrated;
> Mordant for 1 to 2 hours, at 37°C, with a saturated aqueous solution of potassium bichromate;
> Rinse for 5 to 10 seconds in distilled water;
> Stain for 10 minutes to 1 hour (the optimal time varies according to the origin of the material and the way it has been fixed), at 37°C, using Kultschitzky's haematoxylin (p. 945).
> Rinse in tap water;
> Differentiate in Weigert's borax-ferricyanide (p. 947);
> Wash for a long time in tap water to eliminate all trace of the differentiating material; unless this is done the preparations will not keep;
> Dehydrate in absolute alcohol, clear in a benzenoid hydrocarbon and mount in Canada balsam or in a synthetic resin.

The biliary capillaries show up as a deep blue colour, the hepatic cells being a brownish-grey; from my own experience better results are obtained than with a method which is very close to that of Otami and is due to Holmer (1926).

Demonstration of the biliary capillaries by staining with acid fuchsin (Forsgren, 1928).

— This technique depends on the precipitation of the bile constituents *in situ* using barium chloride, the compounds so precipitated being demonstrated because of their affinity for acid fuchsin using Mallory's method; this method involves the following stages.

> Slices of the hepatic parenchyme should be freshly dissected and should not exceed 4 mm in thickness; these slices should be immersed in a large amount of a 3% aqueous solution of barium chloride and left there for 6 to 12 hours (allow 50 times the volume of the tissue);
> Transfer for 12 to 18 hours into saline formalin;
> Dehydrate rapidly, embed in paraffin wax, and cut into rather thin sections (5 μ);
> Dewax, treat with collodion where necessary and hydrate the sections;
> Stain for 1 to 3 minutes using a 0.1% aqueous solution of acid fuchsin (not all commercial samples are suitable);
> Rinse rapidly in distilled water;
> Treat for about 1 minute with a 1% aqueous solution of phosphomolybdic acid;
> Rinse carefully in distilled water;
> Stain for 3 to 5 minutes using the solution
>
> | | |
> |---|---|
> | distilled water | 100 ml |
> | aniline blue | 0.5 g |
> | orange G | 2 g |
> | oxalic acid | 2 g |
>
> (to be dissolved at boiling point, allowed to cool and filter);
> Rinse rapidly in distilled water;
> Dehydrate in absolute alcohol, clear in a benzenoid hydrocarbon and mount in Canada balsam or in a synthetic resin.

The nuclei of the hepatic cells show up blue or orange in colour, the intracytoplasmic granules which are stained a vivid red colour represent the bile constituents according to Forsgren; the Kupffer cells stain blue as does the epithelium of the bile ducts and the connective tissue; the erythrocytes stain orange, the biliary capillaries an intense red.

Impregnation of the biliary capillaries using silver bichromate. — This is a technique close to the variation of Ramon y Cajal for the impregnation of the nerve cells using silver chromate.

Fix pieces of tissue which do not exceed 1 cm^3 in volume for 3 days in the mixture
    a 3% aqueous solution of potassium
        bichromate .... 4 volumes
    a 1% aqueous solution of osmium
        tetroxide...................................... 1 volume
    changing the liquid fixative every 24 hours;
Transfer for 24 to 48 hours in a 0,75% aqueous solution of silver nitrate;
Rinse rapidly in distilled water;
Harden in alcohol and cut as for blocks impregnated by the Golgi technique or embed rapidly in paraffin wax and cut on a microtome;
The biliary capillaries stain brownish-black.

Among the *histo-enzymological techniques* described in the fourth part of this work, the tests for adenosine-triphosphatase activity will very clearly show up the biliary capillaries (Wachstein and Meisel, 1957; Arvy, 1959).

HISTOLOGICAL EXAMINATION OF THE DIGESTIVE GLANDS OF INVERTEBRATES

The term "digestive gland" (Verdauungsdrüse of German authors) is used to designate an organ which is attached to the endodermal part of the digestive tract of molluscs and of certain arthropods. This organ has often been considered to play a part in digestive absorption even though no real proof of this function has been provided and recent authors tend more and more to consider it as a source of digestive enzymes and a center for intermediate metabolism (see Urich, 1961; Martoja, 1964 on this subject). The name we use here has the advantage over the older names (the hepatopancreas of the molluscs, the digestive caeca in the Crustacea, the diverticular intestine of araneids, etc...) of not prejudging the functional significance whilst recalling the fact that the organ plays a part in digestion.

The morphological diversity of the glands collected under this heading is such that the establishment of any general scheme, valid for the histological examination of all the organs, can scarcely be contemplated; the fragmentary state of our knowledge also prevents us from codifying the histological examination of the digestive glands of molluscs and arthropods. Only a few general rules can be set out.

It should be unnecessary to stress the importance of a rapid dissection; embedding in paraffin wax can be used as a general method. It is only necessary to have recourse to celloidin embedding when the tissue is of large size or very heterogenous in its consistency. The fixatives required for the execution of the different cytological and histochemical techniques should be chosen bearing in mind the objectives of the study. Techniques which are particularly recommended are specified for the principal organs of this kind.

The digestive gland (hepatopancreas) of molluscs. — So-called general methods provide information about the topography of the organ, the distribution of the granular parenchyme and of the excretory ducts; azan, one-step trichrome, Mann-Dominici's technique and that of Mann using methyl blue-eosin as well as stains with an azur eosinate base allow us clearly to differentiate the three types of cell. The secretory products are well shown up by these procedures as they are by the PAS technique and by Danielli's tetrazoreaction. Tests for protein-bound sulphydryls and for indole groups are also worthwhile. The demonstration of glycogen, that of the free lipids, of iron and of calcium is indispensable. The "waiting cells" are characterised by their high content of cytoplasmic ribonucleins.

The digestive gland (hepatopancreas, digestive caeca) of the crustaceans. — The holocrine function of these organs accounts for the usefulness of a sound caryological study which should, in particular, include tests for the sites of mitosis. Topographical techniques will provide information on the types of cell and the information so obtained may be supplemented by cytological techniques on the one hand and tests for glycogen, for free fats and for chromolipoids, as well as for ribonucleins and protein-bound sulphydryls, together with reserves of calcium on the other.

The digestive gland (digestive caeca, the diverticulary intestine) of the Arachnida. — Usually the different types of cell appear as soon as the preparations are treated by topographical techniques; the so-called glandular cells are easy to characterise by techniques for demonstrating their secretory products. From the histochemical point of view, tests for glycogen and free fats, the detection of ribonucleins and protein-bound sulphydryls and ultimately an examination for the products of protein metabolism (melanic pigments, purine compounds) are those which are most usually found indispensable.

THE SECRETORY CYCLE OF THE GLANDULAR FORMATIONS OF THE DIGESTIVE APPARATUS

Most of the glandular cells which form part of the digestive apparatus function in rhythmic fashion and the same remark holds good on the scale of the whole organ in many cases. This fact implies that the histological examination of any given animal cannot give a complete picture of the glandular cells which form part of the digestive apparatus and this is true however carefully the preparations have been made and examined. To an extent which is even greater than for other organs a dynamic study is essential during histological studies of the digestive apparatus.

The demonstration of the histological criteria of the absorbant cell (striated border, alkaline phosphatase activity, characteristic chondriome) will at the best lead to presumptions about the site of digestive absorption, certainty in this matter being obtained through the administration of food which is easy to detect on the sections; radioactive tracers are highly advantageous from this point of view.

As for the digestive glandular cells, their study should include a morphological examination of all stages of the cycle, a series of preparations being made so as to correspond to the stages of the digestive cycle, since the administration of food represents the physiological stimulus which releases the secretory cycle in question in the great majority of cases. The enumeration of the cells, which are to be found in any given animal, at the different stages of this cycle, together with the preparation of graphs showing their development as a function of time (Stufenzählmethode, Hirsch, 1932), has been widely used by this author and his students. The initiation of this cycle by food is preferable to the administration of excitosecretory pharmacodynamic agents.

From the technical point of view, we may stress the usefulness of choosing a not too numerous selection of characteristic stages to define the secretory cycle of a cellular category; their identification should be based as far as possible on histochemical reactions rather than on staining reactions, since the first are much easier to standardize than the second. The counting should be carried out without allowing preconceived ideas to intervene, the serial nature of the stages being discovered from the figures obtained. Naturally, all the rules applicable to a statistical analysis of numerical data should be applied in the particular case with which we are concerned here.

CHAPTER 38

TECHNIQUES FOR THE HISTOLOGICAL STUDY OF THE RESPIRATORY SYSTEM

The histological examination of the respiratory system calls into play hardly any procedures restricted to this purpose; there is however great structural diversity in the arrangements for ensuring haematosis in the various branches, so that the technical details vary a great deal from one case to another.

HISTOLOGICAL EXAMINATION OF THE RESPIRATORY TRACT OF TETRAPODS

The respiratory mucosa of the nasal fossae may be fixed together with the underlying bony and cartilaginous tissue, but it is essential to ensure that the fixing agent penetrates thoroughly, as air bubbles can easily be trapped in the irregularities of this region so that a very annoying degree of unequal fixation may result. Perfusion from the ascending aorta or from the primitive carotid arteries is the method of choice for obtaining good fixation of the nasal fossae as a whole; good results are also obtained by opening the *cavum* along a parasagittal section parallel with the wall, followed by fixation in a moderate vacuum. Fragments of the mucosa should be removed together with the bony tissue from animals of large size.

The choice of fixatives calls for no particular comment. Very strongly penetrating and decalcifying fluids are to be recommended when it is necessary to cut the mucosa together with the hard tissue which carries it; Bouin's or Halmi's fluid or Heidenhain's Susa are very suitable for this purpose. The subsequent decalcification and embedding should be conducted in the usual way. Any other fixative may be used; when it is not possible to decalcify the tissue with the techniques required, the mucosa may be carefully detached from the underlying tissue by means of a very sharp knife after fixation.

In addition to topographical stains, the techniques for demonstrating the occurrence of polysaccharides are particularly useful for the detection of intra-epithelial mucocytes and the mucous areas of the nasal glands; procedures which allow us to demonstrate secretory granules serve for the identification of the "serous" parts of these glands. The chorion may be studied by techniques described in relation to the histological examination of connective tissue; the blood vessels may be traced by topographical techniques, by the pseudo-peroxidase reaction of haemoglobin or by tests for unspecific alkaline phospho-monoesterases; vascular injections, followed by clearing the tissue and mounting *in toto*, give very fine pictures of the vascular topography.

Naturally those techniques which are strictly speaking cytological, especially those which show up the ciliatures clearly, are most useful for the study of the respiratory mucosa.

The pharynx, the larynx and the tracheae can be fixed as a whole in small animals; dissection into fragments is essential in larger species, especially because calcified zones are a frequent occurrence. The choice of fixatives and the techniques to be used for the preparation of sections call for no special comment; embedding in celloidin is recommended for the preparation of sections of the larynx of large animals, especially if this organ has been fixed *in toto*.

The staining techniques mentioned for the nasal fossae are suitable in the case of the larynx and of the tracheae; in addition to these the study of the connective tissue, which underlies the epithelium, and of the cartilaginous tissue calls into play techniques described in Chapters 33 and 34; tests for elastic fibres are particularly important in the histological study of the larynx.

HISTOLOGICAL EXAMINATION OF THE PULMONARY PARENCHYME

The structure of the pulmonary parenchyme accounts for the difficulty with which it can be correctly fixed whilst at the same time preserving the anatomical relationships involved and ensuring a sufficiently rapid penetration of the fixative. Many authors consider that perfusion from the pulmonary artery or from one of its branches is the only truly satisfactory solution. The injection of the liquid fixative through the air ducts, the air already in the lung being removed by aspiration alternating with the injections, gives distinctly less good results. The two methods have a practical inconvenience, namely the need to fix the entire lung in a single fluid. When fixation is undertaken by the immersion of fragments of the parenchyme in the fixative, the air can be rapidly removed through the use of a moderate vacuum; fragments of the lung which float to the surface of the fixative will obviously be very poorly fixed.

The preparation of the tissue for section cutting calls for only a single comment, namely the possibility that bronchial or intraparenchymatous calcifications may occur in large animals, rendering decalcification necessary. Embedding in celloidin is only useful for truly voluminous blocks of tissue.

Fixation in Bouin's or Halmi's fluids, in Susa or in formalin-alcohol, followed by embedding in paraffin wax, serve well as a preparation for the use of topographical stains; techniques which confer a very intense colour on the collagen fibres and basement membranes are particularly recommended; most authors advise one to use Heidenhain's azan or Masson's trichrome. A clear distinction of the alveolar cells from the basement membrane of the capillaries may be obtained according to Clara (1936) by means of the following procedure.

Paraffin wax sections, dewaxed, treated with collodion and hydrated;
Mordant for 24 hours with 5% iron alum;
Rinse in tap water;
Stain for 24 hours using Heidenhain's or Regaud's haematoxylin;
Wash in tap water;
Differentiate with the solution of iron alum already used as a mordant, regulating the process by microscopic inspection;
Wash for a long time in tap water;
Stain for 5 minutes with a 0.1% aqueous solution of acid fuchsin;
Rinse rapidly in distilled water;
Treat for about 1 minute with a 1% aqueous solution of phospho-molybdic acid;
Rinse carefully in distilled water;
Stain for 3 to 5 minutes in aniline blue-orange G-oxalic acid, using Mallory's method (p. 212);
Rinse rapidly in distilled water;
Dehydrate in absolute alcohol, clear in a benzenoid hydrocarbon and mount in Canada balsam or in a synthetic resin.

The results correspond substantially to those obtained using the original technique with Masson's trichrome; the contrast between the red alveolar cells and the intensely blue basement membrane of the capillaries is particularly clear.

The techniques for staining collagen fibres, the silver impregnation of the reticulin and the demonstration of elastic fibres are particularly important in a study of the connective web of the lung; the bronchial cartilage and the musculature attached to it may be studied by the techniques set out in Chapters 34 and 35. The round cells (dust cells) which may be recognised on topographical preparations are relevant to techniques for the study of histiocytes; tests for free iron and those for other inclusions play an important part in the practice of pathological anatomy.

The older techniques for the silver impregnation of the cell boundaries in the alveolar epithelium have now only historical interest because of progress made in electron microscopy.

The pseudo-peroxidase reactions of haemoglobin, the tests for alkaline phosphatase activity and above all the techniques for vascular injection enable us to demonstrate the blood vascular network of the lung.

HISTOLOGICAL EXAMINATION OF THE SWIM BLADDER

The histological examination of the "swim" bladder and of the "gas gland" of teleosts call for only a few special comments.

Fixation may be carried out after incision and the flattening of the wall in cases where the objective of the work is the study of the connective and muscular layers of the wall; on the other hand, in cases where the investigator is interested in the cytology of the epithelium, in particular of that of the gas gland, it is desirable to carry out fixation without any substantial change of the pressure within the organ. The apparatus developed by Van de Kamer (1956) for fixing the parietal structures of cavities filled with liquid ought to be useful for this purpose.

Fixation in Bouin's fluid, Heidenhain's Susa or other topographical fixatives, followed by the application of selective stains for the collagen and elastic fibres, allows us to study the sub-epithelial layers of the wall; the same techniques show up the general characteristics of the epithelium, which may be pavimentous or prismatic according to circumstances.

Any cytological and histochemical technique may be adviseable for the study of the elements of the "gas gland".

The capillaries of the wall may be studied either in sections or by whole mounts of flattened fragments, after treatment with zinc-leucobases, the detection of alkaline phosphatase activity or vascular injection.

HISTOLOGICAL EXAMINATION OF GILLS

In most cases, the branchial lamellae or foliae are accessible to vital examination, observation between a slide and a coverslip allowing us to study the ciliary movements clearly when an apical ciliature exists.

Fixation does not involve the problems met with during the histological study of the respiratory tract of air-breathing animals; penetration by fixatives is easy to obtain. Any topographical, cytological or histochemical fixative can be used. It is imperative to fix the tissue rapidly and one should be careful, in appropriate cases, to clean the tissue of its superficial coating of mucus which may be secreted either by mucocytes buried in the branchial epithelium or by nearby mucous glands; the tendency of the branchial ciliatures to agglutinate is often very marked.

The preparation of the tissue for section cutting should take account of the texture of the gill flaps; the existence of calcified zones makes decalcification an evident necessity. Embedding in paraffin wax is suitable in most cases.

Bulk staining, followed by mounting *in toto*, may give good results; spectacular preparations of the gill lamellae of the larvae of batracians may be obtained after fixation in Flemming's fluid, washing in water and bulk staining in Flemming's triple stain (p. 749). In the same way, bulk staining with Apathy's haematein IA (p. 240), followed by embedding in paraffin and section cutting quite often gives very distinctive preparations, the staining of the cytoplasm being carried out on the sections.

The staining of the sections may call into play quite diverse procedures. Techniques for the study of connective tissue, of cartilage and of bone may be required, according to the circumstances, for the examination of the supports for the gill flaps. The epithelium itself may be investigated using topographical techniques, especially the trichrome methods which provide information about the presence or absence of ciliatures, of mucocytes and of glandular cells. The elements which have just been mentioned may then be analysed using the cytological and histochemical techniques set out in the third and fourth parts of this work. It is often useful to demonstrate the presence of tonofibrils.

HISTOLOGICAL EXAMINATION OF THE TRACHEA OF ARTHROPODS AND RELATED ANIMALS

There is no histological technique which is "specific" for the tracheae, enabling us to identify these formations automatically in the arthropods and Onychophora; the investigator's theoretical background and his training in histological examination are at least as important as the treatment to which the tissue under examination has been subjected.

The technical details, strictly speaking, are rather distinct according to whether we need to obtain preparations showing the whole of the tracheal network of tissue mounted *in toto* or whether we wish to study the tracheae and tracheoles on sections.

Simple mounting in glycerine, lactophenol or any other mounting medium miscible with water often gives preparations in which the tracheae of a certain size stand out very clearly against the background, the contrast being caused by the air which fills the tracheal lumen. Such preparations however will not keep indefinitely and the small tracheae, as well as the tracheoles, do not always show up satisfactorily.

Hagmann's technique (1940) depends on filling the tracheal system under a vacuum with a liquid stained by trypan blue, the tissue or the tracheae which have been so "injected" being fixed in a liquid containing barium chloride. The method involves the following stages.

Anaesthetize the animal with chloroform and place it in a small dish suspended in a flask within which a vacuum can be drawn;
Place the following solution in the bottom of the flask

    distilled water .... 90 ml
    acetic acid .... 10 ml
    trypan blue .... 2 g
    santomerse no. 3 .... 1 g

(santomerse no. 3 is a synthetic detergent supplied by the Monsato Chemical Co., St. Louis, U.S.A.);
Evacuate the flask using a mechanical pump and maintain the vacuum for about a quarter of an hour;
Tip the dish so as to throw the animal into the liquid, maintaining the vacuum for a further quarter of an hour;
Allow air to enter slowly until atmospheric pressure has been restored and transfer the animal into the following solution

    commercial formalin .... 15 ml
    acetic acid .... 10 ml
    a saturated aqueous solution of barium chloride .... 75 ml

and keep it there for 3 to 12 hours;
Transfer to 70% alcohol; the material may be allowed to stand in this last fluid if necessary;
Dehydrate, embed in paraffin wax and cut into sections;
Mount the sections after dewaxing or hydrate them, stain the background using the aluminium lake of nuclear fast red, wash, dehydrate and mount after clearing in a benzenoid hydrocarbon;
The tracheae and most of the tracheoles show up clearly because of their blue stain. The solubility of trypan blue in water may entrain losses when the sections are hydrated and stained using other techniques.

An excellent technique due to Wigglesworth (1959) involves filling the tracheal system with an unsaturated lipid and then staining the lipid by fixing in osmium tetroxide followed by treatment with ethyl gallate. The method involves the following stages.

Using the same procedure as in Hagmann's technique, fill the tracheal system with a mixture of equal parts of kerosine and olive oil;
Fix small tissue blocks with a 1% osmium tetroxide solution, buffered to pH 7.25, and containing sodium chloride (Palade's fluid)
stock-solution of Michaelis' buffer using sodium acetate-sodium

    veronal (p. 671) .... 10 ml
    8.5% sodium chloride solution .... 3.6 ml
    0.1 N hydrochloric acid .... 11 ml
    a 2% aqueous solution of osmium tetroxide .... 25 ml

the average duration of fixation is 4 hours;
Transfer the material for 24 hours into a saturated aqueous solution of ethyl gallate to which 0.5 g of cresol has been added as a preservative for every 100 ml of solution;
Mount in a medium miscible with water to which a small amount of ethyl gallate has been added or embed in agar-paraffin wax, using the technique described on p. 95, and cut into sections.

The tracheae and tracheoles take up an intense bluish-black colour which is very favourable for microscopic examination; on sufficiently fine sections the chondriomes are also clearly visible.

The observation of the larger tracheal trunks on sections poses no problems since their morphological characteristics are obvious after any topographical technique has been used, but the study of the tracheoles can be very difficult under such conditions. In addition to Wigglesworth's (1959) technique, described above, impregnation with silver chromate by the Golgi-Cajal technique, set out in the chapter devoted to the nervous system, gives highly instructive preparations but the technique is somewhat capricious. Generally speaking any technique of silver impregnation shows up the tracheae.

I might moreover mention that the tracheae of insects are often intensely stained after a paraldehyde-fuchsin stain has been used after permanganate oxidation in an acid medium; moreover, they give the reaction to ferric ferricyanide strongly and then appear intensely blue.

CHAPTER 39

TECHNIQUES FOR THE HISTOLOGICAL STUDY OF THE EXCRETORY SYSTEM

Modern research shows up the fundamental unity of the excretory system in all Metazoans studied with sufficient care, and underlines the opportunities which exist during their histological study for putting into effect techniques intended selectively to show up brush borders, chondriomes and alkaline phosphomonoesterase activities. In fact, experience shows that segments which have an apical differentiation, such as have just been mentioned, exist in practically every case in the urinary duct of the Metazoans; and it also shows that the structure in question is very often endowed with a histochemically detectable alkaline phosphomonoesterase activity and that the study of the chondriome can provide extremely useful information during the histophysiological interpretation. In the same way, the study of mucosubstances should never be omitted during the histological examination of the excretory system.

Nevertheless, the anatomical diversity of the excretory system explains why other histological techniques do not present the same general interest, so that a survey should be arranged according to the anatomical types and within the framework of the zoological order.

HISTOLOGICAL EXAMINATION OF THE KIDNEY OF VERTEBRATES

The vital examination of the kidney of suitable species is current practice in physiological laboratories oriented towards the study of excretion; the older techniques of Ghiron (1919), Ellinger and Hirt (1930, 1931) have been perfected and completed by the biopsy of various segments of the nephron, in order to analyse the chemical nature of the primary urine and of the liquids contained in the other parts of the urinary tract. The passage across the nephron of stains or coloured substances injected intravenously can be followed under the microscope. It is nevertheless true that the procedures to which I have just alluded do not form a part of histological practice and their detailed description would be out of place here.

The excision of the kidney for histological examination should be as rapid as possible. Numerous studies emphasise the sensitivity of the epithelial parts of the organ to ischemia and the rapidity of its post-mortem autolysis; we may remark that samples taken at autopsy, obtained under the conditions of anatomical—pathological practice, are quite unfitted for a true histological study of the kidney.

The size of the pieces should be chosen so as to facilitate on the one hand a rapid penetration of the fixative, and on the other hand the possibility of exploring, in a single section, all the segments of the nephron. The kidney of Batracians, that of the Teleostei and of reptiles of small size can be fixed as a whole, except when chromo-osmic fixatives are used; cutting the pieces up into fragments is indispensable even for small mammals. It is helpful to divide the organ up into sections by means of a razor blade so as to obtain fragments which include at one and the same time the cortex, the medulla and one of the papillae.

The choice of fixative depends evidently on the objectives of the work. Contrary to a rather widespread impression Bouin's fluid is suitable for anatomical studies, but Heidenhain's Susa, Halmi's liquid or that of Carnoy and that of Stieve are superior to it. A fixative which has a potassium bichromate and formalin base can also be used, mitochondrial techniques being in my opinion indispensable in the course of a correct histological study of the renal parenchyma; I particularly recommend the use of Kolster's fluid, but that of Regaud or of Helly with postchromatisation is also suitable. Moreover, fixation by dilute formalin, whether saline or not, with formaldehyde calcium in order to show up alkaline phosphomonoesterase activity is indispensable. Fixation by chilled acetone with embedding in paraffin can be substituted for this latter fixation if tests for other enzymatic activity do not figure in the programme of study. Otherwise, all the fixatives called for by the various cytological and histochemical techniques can be used.

Preparations made by maceration and isolation play a greater role in the study of the kidney of vertebrates than they do in the histological examination of most other organs; to illustrate this fact I would mention the morphological studies of Huber (1909), Peter (1927) and Sperber (1944), as well as the histopathological studies of Oliver and of his school. In addition to 30% alcohol (see Chapter 30), modern authors primarily utilise concentrated hydrochloric acid, the technique comprising the following stages.

- Treat slices of renal tissue, 1–1.5 mm. thick, for about 1 hour with concentrated hydrochloric acid (density 1.19);
- Wash with great care in distilled water which is frequently renewed;

Bulk stain in haemalum (it is sometimes necessary to keep the pieces in the stain for 24–48 hours);
Wash in tap water, taking care that the turbulence of the liquid does not tear the pieces of renal tissue;
Lay the piece on a slide and proceed to dissect it with needles using a binocular microscope;
Steadily replace the water, in which the fragments of nephron have thus been isolated, by glycerine, and mount in glycerine jelly.

Dissection at low temperatures may be rendered necessary by certain histochemical techniques which are incompatible with maceration; this procedure should also be carried out under a binocular microscope; we need hardly add that manipulation is very much more laborious than after maceration in hydrochloric acid.

The preparation of the pieces for sectioning and the cutting process itself cal for no special precautions. Frozen sections, coming from material fixed in dilute formalin, whether saline or not, with chilled formaldehyde calcium, are used to demonstrate alkaline phosphatase activity; formalated material is also employed, after cutting on a freezing microtome, for the study of dispersed lipids. Other material may be embedded in paraffin wax, always respecting the special features which stem from the choice of any particular fixative. Recourse to celloidin embedding need only be had for pieces of very large size intended for anatomical studies.

Topographical stains may be chosen to a certain extent to match the zoological origin of the material studied. In fact, the staining affinities of cytoplasm vary only a little from segment to segment in the case of the nephron of mammals, and secretory grains, some of which very probably correspond to lysosomes, are only poorly represented, so that priority may be given to techniques which ensure a clear demonstration of the connective fibres, in particular of collagen tissue and of reticulin. It is quite otherwise in the Anamniota and in the reptiles where secretory granules are, on the contrary, quite frequent in certain segments of the urinary tract and the stain affinities, moreover, vary from segment to segment. Techniques based on the demonstration of the stain affinities of cytoplasm are far more appropriate in the second case than in the first. In practice, azan, Masson's trichrome and its variants and single stage trichrome give very good results in all cases; the technique put forward by Clara (1936) for the study of the alveolar epithelium of the lung may be useful to distinguish the glomerular epicytes. Methods such as staining with eosinates of azur, the Mann-Dominici technique, and that of Mann are particularly useful in the study of the kidney of the Anamniota and of the Sauropsida.

Among **the histochemical techniques,** the PAS method, associated or not with alcian blue staining, is indispensable in the study of the nephron of vertebrates;

it shows up the connective web of the kidney very clearly and greatly facilitates study of the details of the structure of the glomerulus; the brush borders appear very clearly and attention is immediately attracted to the presence of carbohydrates, especially if the technique has been combined with alcian blue staining following the technique of Mowry (p. 413). The nature of these carbohydrates can be clarified by the other reactions and stains indicative of polysaccharides. This method when used together with that involving ferric iron capture (p. 409) affords preparations whose morphological value has been underlined by all recent authors. The detection of dispersed lipids and of chromolipoids is always useful, compounds of this type occurring frequently in the kidney of animals belonging to all the classes of vertebrates. Among the reactions of proteins the most useful are those of the sulphydril and disulphide groups which clearly show up the brush borders. The detection of urates presents considerable histopathological interest. The reducing and basophilic nature of these compounds, as set out in the third part of this book, accounts for their demonstration by the ferric ferricyanide technique; this is a convenient technique but far from unequivocal from the chemical point of view. The positive result of the argentaffin reaction and of staining by haematoxylin lakes is also explained by their reducing and basophilic nature. The method of de Galantha (1935), which is devoid of any formal chemical significance, is much in vogue among histopathologists; we give the processes involved below by way of completing our documentation as well as those involved in the methods of Schultz and Schmidt, which afford well contrasted preparations which are pleasant to look at without having the slightest chemical significance.

The authors of the majority of these techniques recommend fixation in absolute alcohol; as Gérard and Cordier (1932) remark and I can completely confirm their opinion, fixation in Carnoy's fluid is just as good so far as the preservation of urates is concerned and is at the same time clearly superior so far as the fixation of the brush borders and nuclei are concerned; it is thus the method which I would advise one to adopt in all cases.

Silver impregnation of urates by the method of Galantha:

Sections from material fixed in Carnoy's fluid or in absolute alcohol, dewaxed and passed into absolute alcohol; Lillie (1954) advises spreading in alcohol;

Transfer directly from absolute alcohol into an aqueous 20% silver nitrate solution exposed to full sunlight or to light from a source rich in ultraviolet for 1–4 hours; the crystals of urates take up a pink colour;

On removal from the silver nitrate, immerse the sections in the following freshly prepared solution.

An aqueous 3% solution of gelatine, warmed to 60°C ...... 10 ml
An aqueous 20% solution of silver nitrate .... 3 ml
An aqueous 2% solution of hydroquinone .... 2 ml

and allow them to remain to the point at which the urate crystals take up a blackish tint, the connective tissue remaining a clear yellow colour;

Wash freely in distilled water warmed to about 60°;
Dehydrate in absolute alcohol, clear in a benzenoid hydrocarbon, mount in Canada balsam or in a synthetic resin.

Staining of crystals and spheroliths of uric acid by carmine (Schultz and Schmidt):

Sections from material fixed in Carnoy's fluid or in absolute alcohol; dehydration of the material in acetone as advised by Schultz and Schmidt is useless; the sections are dewaxed and passed into absolute alcohol; it is possible to treat them with collodion but they must not be hydrated;

Stain the nuclei vigorously with haemalum without previous hydration of the sections;

Immerse the sections, when they have been taken out of the haemalum, with an ammoniacal solution of carmine (see below), allow this to act for about one minute whilst agitating the slide;

Dip the slide twice into absolute alcohol to which 0.5% of concentrated hydrochloric acid has been added and take it out immediately;

Treat with absolute alcohol to the point where the sections become bluish, this absolute alcohol having five drops of commercial ammonia added to it for every 50 ml of alcohol;

Wash in absolute alcohol, clear in a benzenoid hydrocarbon, mount in Canada balsam or in a synthetic resin;

Nuclei are stained blue, the uric acid deposits in red, the sodium urate remaining uncoloured; glycogen is only coloured by the carmine if the duration of action of the staining solution has been excessively prolonged;

The carmine solution, whose composition resembles that of Best's carmine (p. 411), should be prepared in the following way. Boil to dissolve 1 g of carmine, 2 g of ammonium chloride and 0.5 g of lithium carbonate in 50 ml of distilled water; after chilling add 20 ml of ammonia; when required for use, dilute 3 ml of this stock solution, which does not keep very well, with 1.5 ml of ammonia and 2.5 ml of methyl alcohol; the diluted solution will only keep for a few hours.

Staining of the crystals and spheroliths of uric acid by methylene blue (Schultz and Schmidt):

Sections coming from material fixed under the same conditions as above, dewaxed and passed into absolute alcohol and not hydrated; treatment with collodion is possible;

Treat for 5 minutes with the mixture
  methyl alcohol .... 8 volumes
  ammonia .... 2 volumes

Treat for about 30 seconds whilst maintaining the slides in motion with the following mixture:
  a saturated solution of methylene blue in 96% alcohol mixed with an equal volume
  of absolute alcohol.

Wash in absolute alcohol to the point where all excess of methylene blue has been extracted;

Treat for 15 seconds with the mixture:
  a saturated solution of picric acid in absolute alcohol .... 30 ml
  a saturated solution of acid fuchsin in 96% alcohol .... 10 drops

Wash in absolute alcohol, clear in a benzenoid hydrocarbon, mount in Canada balsam or in a synthetic resin.

The nuclei are stained bluish black, the tissue collagen is stained red, the crystals and spheroliths of uric acid take up a striking green tint.

Staining of uric acid crystals and of deposits of sodium urate (Schultz and Schmidt)

> Sections from material fixed in the same conditions as above, dewaxed and passed into absolute alcohol;
> On taking the sections out of absolute alcohol, stain them with the dilute ammoniacal solution of carmine;
> Rinse in absolute alcohol to which 0.5% hydrochloric acid has been added;
> Wash in absolute alcohol;
> Stain with an alcoholic solution half-saturated with methylene blue;
> Rinse in absolute alcohol;
> Treat for 15 seconds with the mixture: — aqueous saturated solution of
>   picric acid .... 9 volumes
>   aqueous saturated solution of sodium sulphate .... 1 volume
> Rinse and dehydrate in absolute alcohol, clear in a benzenoid hydrocarbon, mount in Canada balsam or in a synthetic resin.

The nuclei are stained greyish blue, the deposits of sodium urate in a striking green, and those of uric acid in a deep blue-green.

I may recall that the histochemical demonstration of urea and of chlorides using Leschke's technique (1914) does not meet the demands of histochemical methodology; the practice of these techniques should be discouraged.

We need hardly add that the histo-enzymological study of the nephron of the vertebrates is richly rewarding; the demonstration of alkaline phosphomonoesterase activity represents the indispensable minimum but many other enzymatic activities may be looked for, using the techniques indicated in Chapter 22, during the study of material which has not yet been exploited, or in the course of histophysiological studies.

Among the cytological techniques, it is the demonstration of the chondriomes which gives the most valuable information; the morphological differences between segments of the nephron are more marked after mitochondrial staining than after any other technique; on the scale of the light microscope, the modifications of the chondriome are the first indication of a change in the functional state. Ferric haematoxylin, cupric haematoxylin and all the variants of Altmann's fuchsin are equally suitable; it is generally useless to resort to crystal violet since the morphological characters are sufficient in the great majority of cases to distinguish the chondriosomes from the secretory granules or other acidophilic inclusions, which are particularly frequent in the Anamniota and the Reptilia. Methods for the detection of brush borders are evidently of interest and an examination for ciliatures is indicated during the study of the urinary tract of the lower vertebrates and of the reptiles.

The histological study of the elimination of trypan blue by the brush border tubes has had a certain vogue. A small quantity of a *freshly prepared* 0.5% solution of this stain is injected, subcutaneously in the mammals or in the dorsal lymphatic sac of the frog; Möllendorff (1915) advises the administration of 1 ml of this solution to the mouse or frog 48 hours before autopsy. Whole mounts can be obtained by maceration with concentrated hydrochloric acid which does not attack trypan blue but isolation has to be carried out without haemalum staining. Fixation in Bouin's fluid, by Heidenhain's Susa or by Halmi's fluid also preserves the stain and the material can then be cut into sections after paraffin embedding, without one having to take any particular precautions.

HISTOLOGICAL EXAMINATION OF THE URINARY TRACT OF THE VERTEBRATES

The histological study of the sub-epithelial layers of the bassinet, of the ureter, of the bladder and of the urethra call into play techniques described in relation to the histological examination of connective tissue and of muscles. The transitional epithelium itself may be used either to give squash preparations, the cellular limits being nitrated (p. 772), or to give sections. All the usual fixatives are quite suitable and the only recommendation we need to formulate here, so far as the preparation of the material for section cutting is concerned, is the need for a careful dehydration and a thorough embedding of the fragments of the bladder coming from animals of a certain size, since the vesical musculature hardens considerably during the passage into hot paraffin; the softening of the pieces by soaking the cut block in water is highly recommended.

All the topographical stains furnish preparations which clearly show the make-up of the wall of the urinary tract. Azan, single stage trichrome and that of Masson-Goldner are particularly useful. The PAS method also gives very distinct preparations; when the test with malt diastase is used as a control, it allows one to detect the sites of glycogen. The use of this technique in combination with alcian blue staining is very useful during studies of the urinary tracts of Anamniota and of Sauropsida.

We need hardly add that all the cytological and histochemical techniques should be brought into play to suit the particular objectives of the work.

HISTOLOGICAL EXAMINATION OF THE EXCRETORY SYSTEM OF INVERTEBRATES

Structural material plays a lesser part in the constitution of the excretory system of most invertebrates than it does in that of vertebrates, the connective fibres being generally represented only by basement membranes and by reticulin; thus we have not so much interest in calling into play selective stains for collagen tissue as we have in the case of vertebrates.

Vital observation and *vital staining* are easy to practice in the case of the malpighian tubules of insects and much more difficult in all those cases where the excision of an organ requires a laborious dissection.

Fixation is subject to the same requirements as for the kidney of vertebrates; the demonstration of chondriomes, examination for a brush border and tests for alkaline phosphomonoesterase activity represent from the histophysiological point of view the essential elements of a histological study, but it is appropriate to add to these a study of the filtering apparatus, which is capable of furnishing primary urine, and a study of the mechanisms of propulsion such as the ciliature, whose presence is frequent in animals other than the arthropods, and lastly the existence of folds in the membrane of the basal pole of certain segments of the urinary tract. These formations which correspond to the β-cytomembranes of electron microscopy are not visible under the light microscope in the nephron of vertebrates, but are often visible in the invertebrates.

The preparation of the material for section cutting and the sectioning process itself should be conducted according to the way in which the excision of the material has been made. Very often, pieces of cuticle which have been calcified or sclerotised cannot be removed during the dissection; in animals of very small size the studies are carried out on sections right across some part of the body and the way in which these pieces should be treated is evidently conditioned by the consistency of the tissues which surround the excretory apparatus. Decalcification is only a real problem when a detailed study of enzymatic activity figures on the schedule of study; the softening of cuticular structures in chlorine dioxide is to be avoided at any cost.

All **topographical stains** may give useful preparations; in addition to them, the PAS reaction, whether or not combined with alcian blue staining, generally gives a good demonstration of the basement membranes and the brush border and affords evidence of the presence of glycogen as well as that of mucosubstances. Among other histochemical techniques, tests for chromolipoids, for sulphydrilated proteins, for calcium and for dispersed iron as well as for urates should be practised in each case. The identification of the pigments contained in the epithelial cells of the excretory apparatus may pose very difficult problems especially as the chemical data which we have on this topic is often most fragmentary.

Among the *cytological techniques*, the demonstration of chondriomes and of brush borders is indispensable; that of the ciliature can be very useful; the methods for studying epithelio-fibrils can be extremely helpful. The folds of the membrane of the basal pole of the cells are generally acidophilic and show up after mitochondrial staining, even when the material has been fixed in a liquid containing acetic acid.

Caryological techniques and *tests for cytoplasmic ribonucleins*, which are always useful, become indispensable in cases where the excretory system is the site of the formation of secretory products rich in proteins; this is particularly the case in the malpighian tubules of certain insects.

CHAPTER 40

TECHNIQUES FOR THE HISTOLOGICAL STUDY OF THE NERVOUS SYSTEM

The place occupied in histological technique by methods for studying the nervous system is determined by the anatomical and functional peculiarities of the nerve-cell. From a morphological point of view, the neurone is essentially characterized by possessing prolongations, which may be very long, and by means of which contact is established with other cells which may or may not be nerve-cells; for many years the essential task of the neuro-histologist has been to show up these prolongations as selectively and as completely as possible, and to distinguish them clearly from other fibrous structures with which they are often associated. From a functional point of view the topography of these cellular prolongations, their grouping into bundles and the nature of their contacts with other cells are all of such importance that as a result the study of the cell-bodies themselves has long been neglected.

This specialization, the main reasons for which have just been mentioned, has led to the setting up of neurohistology as an autonomous domain. Techniques specially adapted to the above mentioned ends are employed by research workers, many of whom have resolutely turned their backs on general histology. The part played by empiricism in certain neurohistological techniques is probably even greater than in other histological techniques. In spite of the fundamental unity of the nerve-cell throughout the sub-kingdom of the Metazoa, the adaptation of certain neurohistological techniques to any particular material demands months or years of continuous effort, and this is another factor leading to specialization.

This evolution of neurohistology has certainly been fruitful; the spectacular strides made in our knowledge are due to the use of techniques which apply solely to nerve-tissue and which show up only certain aspects of it. But the dangers of an over-narrow specialization, which are evident in a great many cases, can be seen with the utmost clarity during the course of the evolution of neurohistology. After an extraordinarily fruitful period of pioneer work neurohistological techniques and in particular nerve-fibre impregnations have been applied, by some great neurohistological schools, under quite dubious methodological conditions. The results thus obtained have led some leading histologists to cast doubt on the validity of cell theory in the particular case of the neurone: a perusal of these works, which have been rendered completely obsolete by the advent of the electron microscope, clearly illustrates the danger of an over-narrow specialization, which is bound to lead one to over-estimate the value of certain techniques and neglect the possible contribution of other methods.

From a practical point of view the position of neurohistology among histochemical techniques, in some ways resembles that of histoenzymology. The need to give priority to the study of particular characteristics, which are peculiar to the nerve-cell, leaves its mark on the entire discipline; the methods of fixation and of staining, even the manner of preparing sections, all relate to a precise end. The whole treatment which the tissue blocks undergo has to be foreseen from the moment they are detached, and preservation of structures is often sacrificed to the technical success of a metallic impregnation. The need for a laborious and detailed perfection of techniques specially intended for a particular object results in a greater proliferation of "recipes" than is found in all probability in all the other sectors of histological research together.

Naturally, even an incomplete account of neurohistological techniques would be out of place here, and beyond my scope. Only essential techniques can be retained within the compass of a book devoted to histological technique in general. Apart from the manuals and treatises on histological technique already mentioned repeatedly, the works of Spielmeyer (1930), Bertrand (1930), Ramon y Cajal and de Castro (1933) and Davenport (1960) provide a rich source of documentation. In the pages which follow, strictly neurohistological techniques and those suitable for the study of neurosecretory cells are examined before a discussion of the directions for applying histological techniques to the study of the nervous system.

NEUROHISTOLOGICAL TECHNIQUES

Any cytological and histochemical technique can be applied to the study of the nervous system, and should be so applied to a greater extent than they are at present. The non-nervous components of the nerve-fibre of Vertebrates and of the central nervous system of Invertebrates may be studied by techniques for the examination of connective tissue, blood-vessels, etc. As for neurohistological techniques in the strict sense of the term, the following deserve special mention: techniques which detect Nissl bodies, staining of the ganglion cells, metallic impregnations of the same elements, nerve-fibre techniques, myelin methods and neuroglia methods.

A. — TECHNIQUES FOR THE DETECTION OF NISSL BODIES

All histophysiological, histochemical and ultrastructural research illustrates the importance of Nissl bodies in the functioning of the nerve-cell, and emphasizes the considerable significance of this author's master-work (1894); but the discovery that these structures are rich in ribonucleic acid leads to a rational explanation of their basophilia and makes their detection on sections much simpler.

Indeed, all fixatives which ensure the conservation *in situ* of ribonucleic acids can be used when tissue is being prepared for the detection of these acids.

Fixation in 95 per cent or absolute alcohol, recommended by Nissl, is still favoured by many neurohistologists, but fixation in Carnoy's fluid is just as suitable, and is preferable as far as the fixation of other structures is concerned. The practice of staining Nissl bodies in formalin-fixed material forms part of neurohistological routine, and even such fluids as Bouin, Halmi, etc., permit a good staining of the "tigroid bodies".

The same progress can be noticed in the preparation of blocks for section-making, and in the cutting of the sections. The practice of using sliding microtomes to cut blocks simply hardened by alcohol fixation and not embedded has long been abandoned. Frozen, celloidin, and paraffin wax sections are of equal usefulness; the use of these methods for the purpose now under consideration needs no special comment.

All techniques for detecting basophilia and all marker stainings of ribonucleic acids can, in principle, be used for the detection of Nissl bodies, the choice of method being primarily governed by tradition, by the size of the sections and by the fixation of the pieces. Nissl's original technique using methylene blue dissolved in a solution of Venice soap is hardly used at all. Of the many staining techniques which have been proposed we give here Laskey's technique (*in* Lillie, 1954) for frozen sections, Gothard's (1898) for celloidin sections and finally the techniques of Bielschowsky-Plien (1900) and Pischinger (1930) for paraffin wax sections. As well as these, staining with chromalum lake of gallocyanin ensures excellent detection of Nissl bodies on paraffin wax sections (Einarson, 1932) *and the mode of operation described on p. 542 for the staining of nucleic acids in general probably represents the best and most useful of the methods of detecting Nissl bodies.* Staining with methyl green-pyronin provides spectacular specimens, but gives only mediocre results on formalin-fixed material and the stains do not last as well as with the other techniques mentioned here.

Laskey's thionine technique for frozen sections:

Frozen sections from formalin-fixed material, cut at a thickness of 10 or 15 μ;
Wash the sections in distilled water;
Leave them for about 5 minutes in 70 per cent alcohol;
Wash in distilled water;
Stain for ten *seconds* in the solution

distilled water	95 ml
acetic acid M/5	4 ml
aqueous solution, M/5, of sodium acetate	1 ml
thionine	0.1 g

Rinse in distilled water;
Dehydrate with 96 per cent and absolute alcohol, clear in carbolic xylene (4 parts of xylene to one of phenol), mount in a synthetic resin.

This technique, which is, in short, a thionine staining in a pH 4 buffer medium, shows the Nissl bodies and the chromatin of the nuclei in deep blue on a practically colourless background.

Gothard's blue polychrome technique for celloidin sections:

>   Celloidin sections from alcohol-fixed material;
>   Stain for 24 hours, at laboratory temperature, in Unna's blue polychrome;
>   Rinse in 80 per cent alcohol;
>   Differentiate, controlling by microscope if convenient, with the mixture
>> creosote .... 50 ml
>> cajeput essence .... 40 ml
>> xylene .... 50 ml
>> absolute alcohol .... 160 ml
>
>   until all excess dye has been removed;
>   Wash in absolute alcohol;
>   Clear in cajeput essence, mount in Canada balsam or a synthetic resin.

The chromatin, the nucleoli and the Nissl bodies are stained deep blue: the colour of the background depends on the way the differentiation has been conducted. The speed of differentiation may be reduced by increasing the amount of xylene (80 ml instead of 50) without changing the proportion of the other ingredients of the mixture. Of course, the regressive character of the staining introduces a subjective element which is a nuisance compared with gallocyanin staining (p. 542) or with the Pischinger methylene blue method.

The Bielschowsky-Plien cresyl violet technique. — This technique, adopted as routine in great neurohistological institutes, can be applied to frozen, celloidin or paraffin sections, the slow mode of operation being more suitable for the paraffin wax, while the rapid variant is more suitable for the other sections.

>   Frozen, celloidin or paraffin wax sections from alcohol-fixed or formalin-fixed material;
>   Stain for 30 to 60 minutes in a 1 per cent aqueous solution of cresyl violet or for 24 hours in a very dilute solution of this stain (6 to 8 drops of saturated aqueous solution in 50 ml of distilled water);
>   Rinse in distilled water;
>   Dehydrate in 96 per cent (celloidin sections) and absolute alcohol, clear in cajeput essence, pass through a benzenoid hydrocarbon and mount in Canada balsam or a commercial synthetic resin.

The Nissl bodies, the chromatin and the nucleoli show up in violet against a very pale background. The reliability of the method is very satisfactory, but staining with gallocyanin and with Pischinger's methylene blue are superior to it in this respect.

Pischinger's methylene blue stain. — This technique, which is derived from the same author's method for estimating the zone of the isoelectric point of the constituents of tissues, uses methylene blue dissolved in a buffer of pH lower than the isoelectric point of most of the proteins of the tissues, giving great selectivity of staining with no need for any differentiation. The stain is rendered insoluble by treating with ammonium molybdate before dehydration.

Paraffin wax sections from material fixed in alcohol or Carnoy's fluid, dewaxed, treated with collodion and hydrated;
Stain for ten minutes in the mixture

Solution of N sodium acetate	1 ml
N acetic acid	1 ml
Distilled water	98 ml
Methylene blue	0.064 g

Rinse rapidly in the buffer without methylene blue (pH = 4.65);
Treat for five or six minutes with a 4 per cent aqueous solution of ammonium molybdate;
Wash well (for at least five minutes) in tap water;
Dehydrate with absolute alcohol, clear in a benzenoid hydrocarbon, mount in Canada balsam or a synthetic resin.

A very pure staining, in blue, of the Nissl bodies, the chromatin and the nucleoli is obtained in a strictly automatic manner.

B. — SELECTIVE STAINING OF THE GANGLION CELLS AND THEIR PROLONGATIONS

Many topographical stains ensure a good detection of the perikarya and of cellular projections of a certain calibre, but the selectivity of the stain is not usually sufficient for a detailed analysis of the specimens. The old stain with Gerlach's carmine (1871) gives splendid specimens, but does not show the very finest prolongations, needs frozen sections fixed for unforeseeable, often very lengthy, periods in Müller's fluid (p. 686) and makes use of a stain which is just as disadvantageous from an optical point of view as carmine. Apart from it, a very simple stain using a lead haematoxylin lake, developed by MacConaill (1947), ensures good staining of the nerve cells and their prolongations; the mode of operation is indicated below. But of all the methods in this group staining with methylene blue is obviously the most important.

MacConaill's stain with lead haematoxylin

The stain used for this method is prepared when required, by adding 10 ml of a 20 per cent haematoxylin solution in 96 per cent alcohol to 100 ml of "stabilized lead solution" and making up to 200 ml with tap water. This stabilized lead solution is prepared by mixing together equal parts of 5 per cent lead nitrate solution and of saturated ammonium acetate solution, both solutions being in tap water. The mixture is shaken and filtered and 2 ml of commercial formalin are added for every 100 ml of the filtered liquid. This solution keeps for several days, but the haematoxylin lake has to be prepared freshly each time it is used. Another way of preparing the solution is mentioned in relation to the gastrointestinal endocrine cells.

The working technique involves the following stages:

> Paraffin wax sections, from formalin-fixed material, dewaxed, treated with collodion if need be, hydrated;
> Leave the sections for about five hours in the lead haematoxylin lake whose preparation is described above;
> Wash in running water for several minutes;
> Dehydrate in absolute alcohol, clear in a benzenoid hydrocarbon, mount in a synthetic resin or, if necessary in Canada balsam.

The nerve-fibres are stained blue, their endings showing up clearly; in the perikarya the Nissl bodies are clearly visible; the cells of the neuroglia do not take up the lead haematoxylin lake.

Vital staining of cells and nerve-fibres with methylene blue

Since its invention by Ehrlich (1885), the staining of nerve-fibres with methylene blue has led to a considerable number of investigations. Dogiel and his school and Krause have adapted the method to very varied ends, but the most important improvements are due to Worobiew and his pupil Schabadasch. Among recent applications of the technique special mention should be made of the works of Hillarp (1946) and Taxi (1965) which show clearly how useful this method can be, provided one is prepared to deploy a quite considerable technical effort.

> The selective staining of the nerve-fibres and nerve-endings by methylene blue may be obtained, and observed, under truly vital conditions (study *in vivo* of the nerve-fibres of Rabbit cornea) but this is a rare eventuality. In fact, the staining obtained in most cases is produced only in fresh material, but the toxicity of the doses necessary to arrive at it prevents its being considered as vital (Schabadasch, 1925 to 1936). The hydrogen-accepting character of the dye plays, according to Schabadasch, an essential role in obtaining the stain, and the addition of organic reducing agents (pyrocatechin, resorcin, etc.) improves the result; the presence of glucose is very useful; so is the presence of chemical bodies which promote anaerobic glycolysis. Moreover, the optimum pH of the stain varies according to the organs and, for the same organ, according to the region within it; it is only exceptionally that it equals or exceeds 7.

Staining by perfusion through the aorta or through a large artery is the best method for vertebrates; naturally the liquid used should be isotonic and brought to body temperature when the perfusion is being carried out on a homeotherm. The quantity of liquid to be injected, the pH, the concentration of methylene blue (from 0.0037 to 0.5% according to Schabadasch) should be carefully adjusted. A detailed description of the mode of operation would be out of place here, and I refer the reader to the works cited.

Staining by sub-cutaneous injections are practised by injecting the animal, several times, with large doses of the stain, until the moment when death occurs from intoxication. The organ to be studied is then extracted as rapidly as possible and treated in accordance with the instructions given below.

Staining by interstitial injection or injection in a natural cavity is obtained, as with a sub-cutaneous injection, by means of isotonic solutions which are, however, richer in stain than in the case with perfusion (on an average, 0.5 per cent).

The same concentrations are used when fragments of organs are being **stained by immersion** in solutions of methylene blue, which should be isotonic and raised to body temperature for the tissues of homeotherms. It is useful to keep watch and see that the piece of tissue is covered by the smallest possible amount of liquid, but its desiccation should naturally be avoided. As in the case of perfusion, the optimum concentrations and the staining times should be adjusted by trial and error at each attempt.

The subsequent treatment of the pieces involves, in all cases, exposure to air for an optimum period of 10 to 30 minutes; during this exposure to the air the staining of the nerve-fibres deepens; stabilization (I prefer this term to the term "fixation" which, though correct insofar as the colour is fixed, is a cause of ambiguity) should be carried out at the requisite moment, lest the colours weaken.

This *stabilization* is carried out with a mixture of ammonium picrate and thiocyanide in Schabadasch's method when the pieces are destined to be mounted *in toto* and with ammonium molybdate or ammonium picrate when the programme of work involves cutting them into sections.

Schabadasch's technique consists of immersing the piece of tissue for 3 to 6 hours in a mixture prepared in the following manner.

> Saturate a 1.12 per cent aqueous solution of ammonium thiocyanide (a 2.11 per cent solution of ammonium iodide may be used instead), heated to 60°C, with ammonium picrate (orange crystals, not the microcrystalline yellow powder); leave undisturbed for several days; heat to 35°C in a *water-bath* before use. (*It should be borne in mind that dry ammonium picrate is explosive*).

This treatment causes the stain of the nerve-fibres to turn brownish violet. Mounting is done, without dehydration, in glycerine jelly prepared with ammonium picrate in the following manner:

> Saturate chemically pure glycerine with ammonium picrate, keeping it for at least six days, at 25°C, in contact with an excess of this salt;
> Allow 10 gm of good quality gelatine to swell in 50 ml of distilled water, add 50 ml of distilled water and dissolve over a water-bath, filter through a filter funnel maintained at a warm temperature.
> Mix the two solutions in equal parts, store in a flask of hard glass (pyrex, Jena).

Fairly small tissue pieces may be mounted, as in ordinary glycerine jelly, without further precautions. For more bulky pieces, a clearing bath in glycerine with ammonium picrate improves transparency and facilitates microscopic examination.

Stabilization with ammonium molybdate is obtained by immersing the pieces in a large quantity (50 to 100 times the volume of the piece) of a freshly prepared 5 or 8 per cent solution of ammonium molybdate, filtered before use. The addition of a small quantity of osmium tetroxide (about 5 drops of 1 per cent solution for 100 ml of liquid) is advised by some authors, but it seems to me permissible to doubt its efficacy as a fixative in the histological sense of the term. The pieces may remain for quite a long time in this liquid (24 hours or more). After that they are washed at length (for an hour or several hours) in tap water and can then be dehydrated. Romeis (1948) advises against the use of absolute alcohol and recommends passing the pieces rapidly through 96 per cent alcohol (about ten minutes for very thin pieces, 2 hours maximum for thicker ones, renewing the alcohol a certain number of times) followed by two baths of terpineol, a compound which completes dehydration and ensures clearing. To complete this last manoeuvre the pieces may be passed for more or less lengthy periods through a benzenoid hydrocarbon and can then be mounted in Canada balsam or a synthetic resin. Bethe (1895, 1896) to whom we owe the introduction of stabilization with ammonium molybdate, and Krause (1923) consider that pieces treated in this way and dehydrated could even undergo paraffin wax embedding, but this last operation results in many cases, in the extraction of all the stain, and it is decidedly better to cut any material that needs cutting by means of a freezing microtome, after washing with water and before dehydration; the use of the freezing microtome is all the more desirable when the sections should have a certain thickness.

Stabilization with ammonium picrate (Dogiel, 1900) is carried out by immersing the pieces, after the exposure to air intended to intensify their stain, in a saturated aqueous solution of this compound (about 1 per cent), adding 1 to 2 ml of a 2 per cent aqueous solution of osmium tetroxide to each 100 ml; the pieces should not be left in this liquid for more than 48 hours. They are then mounted (after cutting, if the need arises, with a razor, freehand, or by means of a freezing microtome) in a mixture of equal parts of glycerine and a saturated aqueous solution of ammonium picrate.

The combination of both stabilization techniques is advised by Romeis (1948) in cases where an attempt at paraffin embedding is desired. The operation involves the following stages.

Stain with methylene blue, intensify the stain by exposure to air;
Immerse the pieces in a saturated aqueous solution of ammonium picrate for 30 minutes to one hour;
Transfer, without washing, to the mixture
    5 per cent aqueous solution of ammonium molybdate ..... 100 ml
    0.5 per cent aqueous solution of osmium tetroxide .... 20 ml
and leave the pieces there for 12 to 24 hours;
Wash for 4 to 6 hours in frequent changes of distilled water;
Start dehydration by keeping the pieces a short while, first in 70 per cent alcohol, then in 96 per cent alcohol (for a maximum of two hours, renewing the liquid frequently); it is desirable to carry out this stage of the technique in the refrigerator, with alcohol previously cooled down to 4–5°C;
Complete the dehydration with several baths of terpineol; –
Clear rapidly in benzene, embed in paraffin; the use of a vacuum-oven is particularly advantageous, since it permits a noticeable shortening of the time needed for impregnation by the mass of embedding material;
Cut into sections, as far as possible avoid treating the sections with alcohol during the last manoeuvres.

The spectacular successes of the methylene blue method, especially in research on the peripheral nervous system, are too well known to be recalled here; nevertheless the very brief description of the mode of operation which has just been given shows up the major disadvantage of the technique—the mediocre preservation of cell and tissue structures. All details of the structure apart from the courses of the nerve-fibres need to be meticulously controlled on specimens made after carrying out a good chemical fixation. Besides, the method is capricious and it requires long development to perfect its application to a particular object. The reading of reports in which good results, obtained by means of this technique, were mentioned should not lead to its being considered as a universal panacea.

C. — SELECTIVE METALLIC IMPREGNATIONS OF THE GANGLION CELLS AND OF THEIR PROLONGATIONS

All the techniques in this group stem from the famous *reazione nera* of Golgi (1873), the impact of which on neurohistological research is too well known to need recalling here. The principle of the method is very simple; pieces of tissue fixed in a mixture of osmium tetroxide and of potassium bichromate are immersed in a solution of silver nitrate; a black precipitate of silver chromate forms in certain ganglion cells and in all their prolongations, so that the elements in question show up intensely black on a pale background. The mechanism of this impregnation has been studied at length by the classic authors; it is to Liesegang (1910) that we owe the most important attainments in this field.

The mixture, *in vitro*, of a solution of potassium bichromate and of a silver nitrate solution results in the formation of silver bichromate $Ag_2Cr_2O_7$, and also of silver chromate Ag_2CrO_4, the proportions of the two compounds being liable to vary according to the concentrations of silver nitrate and potassium bichromate, the temperature, and other factors; the same chemical reaction takes place when tissues impregnated with potassium bichromate are plunged in a solution of silver nitrate. But the first of these substances, as Liesegang has shown, displays an extraordinary mobility. When cubes of gelatine, impregnated with potassium bichromate, are plunged into a solution of silver nitrate, the reaction which has just been described takes place in the peripheral layers, while the centre of the cube loses some of its potassium bichromate. Furthermore, the silver chromate and bichromate do not first appear in a solid state; first of all super-saturated solutions form, precipitation taking place around 'seeds'. The result is that, during the course of impregnation certain regions become richer in both silver chromate and bichromate, obviously at the expense of other regions; this explains the partial and localized character of the precipitation, the places where the crystalline seeds begin to grow being determined by the physico-chemical and morphological characteristics of the impregnated zones.

The data existing at present do not allow for the unequivocal explanation of the physico-chemical mechanism which, in certain zones of the block of tissue, puts an end to the state of supersaturation of the silver chromate and bichromate solutions and promotes precipitation, but it is certain that the phenomenon is by no means confined to nerve-cells. The most varied structures may be impregnated by the silver chromate method; the inter- and intracellular canalicules, the excretory ducts of glands and the cell walls may be the seat of precipitation and so show up in intense black on a pale background. Golgi's method is used effectively to show up the structures which have just been listed. But the impregnation is non-specific to an extreme degree; Friedländer (1894, 1895) was able to obtain, in coagulated egg-white, cheese, celloidin moulded into blocks and in potatoes, precipitations whose form resembled quite closely that of nerve fibres. Naturally, this is not a reason for rejecting Golgi's argument *en bloc*, but I think it is useful to recall these old results as a clear illustration of the caution which is needed when studying specimens impregnated with silver chromate.

A simple statement of the principle of Golgi's method allows us to understand the danger of the silver nitrate being precipitated at the moment when the blocks are immersed in it; the surface region of these is, more often than not, unserviceable, and the interstices of the tissue provide an ideal site for meaningless precipitations. To Sehrwald (1889) we owe a technical contrivance which enables us to avoid superficial precipitations, but there is no remedy for the precipitations which take place deep inside the tissues.

The chief disadvantage of Golgi's method is its capriciousness; even in the hands of a highly skilled manipulator the result is literally unforeseeable. As Kallius points out (*in* Krause, 1926) an undertaking which sets out to obtain, in a single piece of tissue, the selective detection of a particular structure must be regarded as hopeless from the outset. It is only by multiplying the fixations and impregnations and carefully sifting out their favourable aspects that one can finally amalgamate the elements of the work, and anyone who has a certain experience in this field can understand what effort is represented by the monumental researches of Ramon y Cajal, carried out by means of Golgi's method.

Of the two fundamental methods (the quick and the slow), modified several times by Golgi (see 1894 for all the publications previous to this date), only the quick method, modified by Ramon y Cajal (1888), is given here; instructions are also given for the techniques of Bubenaite (1929), Cox (1891), and Fox (1951).

Silver chromate impregnation after Golgi-Cajal

Fix *fresh* tissue pieces, about 3 mm thick, in the mixture

    2.5 per cent aqueous solution (3.5 per cent according to Ramon y Cajal) of potassium bichromate .... 40 ml

    1 per cent aqueous solution of osmium tetroxide .... 10 ml

Fixation takes place at laboratory temperature; the amount of fixative given above is enough for 5 or 6 pieces measuring 1 mm along one side; it is as well to use brown, glass-stoppered bottles. *The optimum duration of the fixation is unforeseeable*; tests should be made between the 2nd and the 7th days, and it is rarely useful to go further than that:

Blot with blotting paper and rinse with a 0.75 per cent silver nitrate solution until all precipitation of silver chromate has ceased; immerse at this point in the silver nitrate solution, and keep the pieces there for 1 to 6 days: the operation takes place in darkness, at laboratory temperature or at 35°C, but never higher:

Wash for one to two hours in several changes of 40 per cent alcohol:

Harden first in 80 per cent then in 96 per cent alcohol:

Cut on a freezing microtome after returning to water, or cut free-hand, with a razor or roll in celloidin or paraffin to allow thick sections (30–100 μ) to be cut by microtome:

Collect the sections in 80 per cent alcohol, stick to cover-slips after renewing the alcohol several times to eliminate excess silver salts:

Dehydrate in absolute alcohol, clear in creosote and then in turpentine oil.

Cover with a layer of Canada balsam, Dammar resin or synthetic resin, protect from dust and leave to dry:

Stick the cover-slip, section side down, on a slide or staining-bath of the desired dimension, with a cavity at the centre so that the resin-covered section remains in contact with the air.

In successful cases, certain ganglion cells or other structures stand out in intense black on a fairly pale yellow background. The preparations do not keep very well.

The length of time the pieces are kept in the mixture of osmium tetroxide and potassium bichromate is one of the factors essential to success, and has to be determined empirically.

The blotting with tissue paper which precedes the immersion in silver nitrate can be supplemented very conveniently by *coating the tissue block in gelatine*; this trick, which we owe to Sehrwald (1889), is carried out by plunging the block which has been removed from the fixative and blotted, into a 10 per cent solution of gelatine melted in a water-bath, and letting it cool for a few minutes before immersing it in the bath of silver nitrate; the superficial precipitations form on the gelatine and can be very easily eliminated by removing the gelatine matrix with needles before dehydrating the impregnated piece.

Double or triple impregnation, recommended by Ramon y Cajal, is a considerable improvement on the original mode of operation; it consists of cutting a section when it has been removed from the silver nitrate and examining it, blotting the piece with tissue paper if the impregnation is inadequate and replacing it in the mixture of potassium bichromate and osmium tetroxide which was used for fixing; after 24 hours the block is blotted and transferred to the bath of silver nitrate which was used for the first impregnation, and is left there for 1 to 2 days. If the impregnation still appears inadequate, the operation can be repeated. The chances of the method being successful are thus greatly increased and a certain degree of control becomes possible during impregnation.

The impossibility of carrying out a true paraffin embedding, shocking at first sight, does not matter greatly in practice; frozen sections are very suitable, and there is not even any real difficulty in cutting pieces of tissue which are merely coated, on account of the thickness of the sections to be made. Bubenaite's variant, described below, permits rapid paraffin wax embedding.

The fact that the sections keep badly is a very serious disadvantage of the method; the best of the manoeuvres intended to counteract it is that of Kallius (1926) It involves the following stages.

> Use the technique which follows the working technique described above, with gelatine-coating and, where necessary, double or triple impregnation;
> Wash the sections in 80 per cent alcohol;
> Treat the sections with hydroquinone developer diluted with alcohol (see below) until a dark grey or black shade is obtained;
> Wash thoroughly in 70 per cent alcohol (at least 10 minutes);
> Treat for five minutes with a 20 per cent aqueous solution of sodium thiosulphate (hyposulphite);
> Wash thoroughly (for several hours) in frequent changes of tapwater; stick on to slides, dehydrate, clear, and mount in Canada balsam or a synthetic resin, without special precautions.

The mother-solution of the hydroquinone developer is made by dissolving 5 g of hydroquinone, 40 g of sodium sulphite and 75 g of potassium carbonate in 250 ml of distilled water; it keeps well, as long as it is protected from the light. For use, 20 ml are diluted with 250 ml of distilled water, one or two volumes of this solution being added to one volume of 96 per cent alcohol.

Some of the disadvantages of Golgi's method have been mentioned above; it is as well to add that the impregnation of the nerve endings is not necessarily complete, especially in the case of the post-ganglionic parts of the vegetative nervous system, when the stopping-point of the impregnation can simulate endings. A certain amount of experience and a great deal of prudence are therefore necessary in the interpretation of the sections. Furthermore, the impregnation *can* be obtained under conditions which are irreproachable from a cytological point of view, but this is not necessarily the case; contrary to what the composition of the fixing mixture might lead one to expect, the preservation of the cytological structures is often mediocre, the part of the tissue blocks where the osmium tetroxide can show off its paces being rendered useless by the silver chromate precipitation.

Bubenaite's impregnation with silver chromate

According to Romeis (1948) this method, derived from an older technique of Kopsch (1902), gives excellent results, being more regular than the technique of Golgi-Cajal. It involves the following stages.

> Fix in dilute formalin, saline or non-saline; one or two days fixation may suffice, but the results remain good even if the pieces remain in the fixative for years;
> Post-chrome, at 34°C, with a 2.5 per cent aqueous solution of potassium bichromate; the optimum period varies around 2 days;
> Blot with tissue paper, rinse rapidly with a 2.5 per cent aqueous solution of silver nitrate and impregnate with this solution, at 34°C, for two days;
> Wash in frequent changes of distilled water;
> Cut on a freezing microtome, or dehydrate rapidly and embed in paraffin, clearing in benzene, not taking more than two days over the entire operation;
> Treat the sections as in the original method.

Cox's impregnation with mercury

This technique, which many neurohistologists prefer to impregnation with silver nitrate, is particularly recommended for research on the central nervous system of mammals. It involves the following stages.

> Fix, at laboratory temperature or at 37°C, for one or two months, in the following mixture, prepared with scrupulous respect for the order of the instructions:
> 5 per cent aqueous solution of mercuric chloride .... 100 ml
> 5 per cent aqueous solution of potassium bichromate .... 100 ml
> distilled water .... 100 ml
> 5 per cent aqueous solution of potassium chromate ...... 80 ml
> the potassium chromate being diluted with the distilled water, then added to the mixture of the two other solutions.
> The fixative should be changed after 24 hours of contact with the tissue; the whole fixation is carried out in a well corked bottle, protected from light.
> Wash carefully in 96 per cent or 70 per cent alcohol to eliminate excess sublimate;
> Hydrate the pieces, cut on a freezing microtome;
> Wash the sections in distilled water, treat them for about an hour with a 5 per cent aqueous solution of sodium carbonate;
> Wash very carefully in frequent changes of tap water;
> Dehydrate, clear, and mount using the same precautions as with silver chromate impregnation.

The impregnated ganglion cells stand out in intense black on a very pale background; accidental precipitations are very much less frequent than with Golgi's method.

Fox's impregnation with zinc chromate-silver nitrate

Fix in dilute formalin (saline or non-saline); it is recommended that the tissue be kept in the fixing liquid for several months;
Cut the tissue into thin slices (about 3 mm thick);
Post-chrome for two days, at laboratory temperature, in the solution

    4 per cent formic acid .... 100 ml
    zinc chromate .... 6 g

Blot with tissue paper, rinse each slice with a 0.75 per cent aqueous solution of silver nitrate until the whole surface is a uniform red colour;
Suspend by threads in a large quantity of the same silver nitrate solution, leave to be impregnated for two days away from the light; the impregnation bath should be renewed after 24 hours, the surface of the pieces being brushed with a paint-brush to eliminate superficial precipitations of silver chromate;
Dehydrate, after the impregnation bath, by passing through 96 per cent alcohol for 15 minutes and passing twice through absolute alcohol, for 15 minutes each time;
Clear rapidly by leaving for ten minutes in a benzenoid hydrocarbon; coat the piece with paraffin by leaving it for about ten minutes, at 50°C, in a bath of soft paraffin wax, mould the block;
Cut with a Minot microtome in slices about 100 µ thick, collect the sections in 96 per cent alcohol; once cutting has been started a block should be divided completely into sections on the same occasion;
Dehydrate the sections in absolute alcohol, clear then in a benzenoid hydrocarbon, removing loose silver chromate crystals from the surface of the pieces;
Mount on slides, cover with a layer of synthetic resin, leave to dry for about a week protected from dust;
Cover with a new layer of synthetic resin, put the cover-slip in position.

The results agree with those of Golgi's original method, but there is greater regularity of impregnation.

According to Lillie (1954), a rapid embedding in celloidin would be possible, it being very much less harmful for the pieces to be kept in alcohol and an alcohol-ether mixture than to be passed through benzenoid hydrocarbons and, especially, hot paraffin.

D. — TECHNIQUES FOR NEUROFIBRILS

All techniques for neurofibrils are based on the affinity of these structures for metallic salts. The innumerable formulae proposed since the beginning of neurohistological research can be classified in the following manner:

a) The pieces are treated, after fixation, by a solution of ammonium molybdate, which is taken up selectively on the neurofibrils; excess of this compound is eliminated by an aqueous washing of the paraffin sections, dried on to the slides; this washing signifies a real differentiation and represents the crucial moment of the method; staining with thionine or toluidine blue leads to the selective detection of the nerve-fibres. The techniques of Donaggio (1896, 1904, 1906) and of Bethe (1900) which are based on this principle are used only exceptionally in current histological research; for a detailed description of them I refer the reader to specialized works.

b) Fresh or fixed pieces or paraffin wax sections are treated with an aqueous solution of gold chloride, then reduced by formic acid, in sunlight; introduced into histological technique by Ranvier (1892), this gold impregnation was perfected by Apathy (1897), to whom is due its application to fixed material. In fact these techniques—very capricious but, in successful cases, giving really spectacular preparations are little used by present-day neurohistologists. Only one recent variant, that of Carey (1942), is described here.

c) Blocks or sections are subjected, after "sensitization" by a bath of silver nitrate, first to the action of an alkaline compound of this metal, then to the action of an organic reducing agent. This is the principle of the classic method of Bielschowsky (1904), several variants of which play a leading role in neurohistological technique.

d) Blocks or sections undergo a bath of silver nitrate, followed by reduction by an organic reducing agent; introduced into histological technique in the form of a method for tissue blocks (Ramon y Cajal, 1903), this method is also represented by numerous processes which are indispensable in current neurohistological practice.

GOLD TECHNIQUES FOR NEUROFIBRILS

Apathy's (1897) "post-impregnation" (*Nachvergoldung*) technique for paraffin wax sections taken from material fixed by a mixture of osmium sublimate and osmium tetroxide no longer offer more than a historical interest, but the method of impregnation of fresh pieces ("*préimprégnation*", Apathy's *Vorvergoldung*) introduced into histological research by Ranvier (1872) can still be of use, especially in research on the peripheral nervous system and on the nerve centres of invertebrates. The most recent of the variants of the method is due to Carey (1942); it involves the following stages.

> Cut the fresh tissue into slices of about 3 mm thickness, immerse them in freshly squeezed and filtered lemon juice, leave it to take effect for five to fifteen minutes; the fragments should be manipulated with glass or plastic needles and spatulas, as no metal instrument should be allowed to come into contact with the reagents;
> Rinse in distilled water (Ranvier) or pass without rinsing to the next stage (Carey);
> Immerse the pieces in a 1 per cent aqueous solution of gold chloride; keep them away from direct sunlight while they are in this solution; the optimum duration of the immersion varies from 10 to 60 minutes according to the case;
> Treat, in darkness, for 8-12 hours, with 25 per cent formic acid (commercial concentrated formic acid diluted with 3 parts of distilled water); Ranvier's technique involves the same reduction; in Apathy's technique the pieces are left for 6 to 8 hours in bright light, in 1 per cent formic acid;
> Wash in distilled water, then in tap water, keep in a mixture of equal parts of 50 per cent alcohol and of glycerine;
> Dissociate in this mixture, mount in glycerine jelly

In successful specimens the nerve-fibres and nerve-endings take on an intense black shade, and stand out magnificently against the red or purple background; the extraordinary subtlety of the appearance of the sections should be emphasized.

TECHNIQUES FOR NEUROFIBRILS DERIVED FROM BIELSCHOWSKY'S METHOD

Of all the variants of Bielschowsky's technique which are intended for the impregnation of neurofibrils on frozen sections, the only one mentioned here is the technique of Schultze and Gros (1918), generally referred to as the Gros-Schultze method; remarkable for its suppleness and for the quality of its results, this technique can be applied generally. The techniques of Rogers (1931) and Tinel (1947) allow good impregnations of neurofibrils to be obtained on paraffin wax sections. Among the variants intended for the treatment of blocks the methods of Agduhr (1917) and Boecke (1916, 1917) are suitable for most objects.

Gros-Schultze's impregnation of neurofibrils

Reagents:

silver nitrate in 20 per cent aqueous solution;
formalin diluted with 4 parts of tap water;
ammonia diluted to 20 per cent with distilled water;
0.2 per cent aqueous solution of gold chloride;
5 per cent aqueous solution of sodium thiosulphate
ammoniacal silver nitrate prepared just prior to use:
   add, drop by drop, some ammonia (commercial concentrated solution) to a 20 per cent aqueous solution of silver nitrate; an abundant grey-brown precipitate forms immediately; continue adding the ammonia with extreme caution until it redissolves completely, without overshooting the mark; this liquid does not keep well and it is advisable not to prepare more than 10 ml at a time.

Working technique:

Fix in neutralized and diluted (1 in 3 or 1 in 10) formalin for at least ten days;
Wash the pieces in tap water (for about one hour);
Cut on a freezing microtome in sections from 20 to 30 μ thick;
Collect the sections in distilled water;
   treat for an hour, in darkness, with the 20 per cent silver nitrate solution; at this stage of the method shrinkage occurs in thin or weak sections;
Transfer directly into 20 per cent formalin, move the section around with a glass rod, transfer it into a new bath of formalin as soon as white precipitates begin to form, repeat the operation a few (4 to 6) times until the sections no longer give off any cloud (average length of time 4 to 7 minutes);

Transfer to the ammoniacal silver nitrate with the addition of one drop of ammonia to each ml of liquid, follow the progress of the impregnation attentively; it might be advisable to carry out the operation in small Petri dishes or watch-glasses and examine the sections in the ammoniacal silver nitrate with a microscope, using the low-power objective; a too-rapid impregnation, an excessive participation of the connective tissue and of the nuclei in the blackening process call for a stronger alkalinization of the compound; on the other hand an excessively slow impregnation calls for a reduction in the quantity of ammonia;

Transfer the section, as soon as the desired result is obtained, into the dilute ammonia, and leave it there for about a minute;

Transfer the section into distilled water or into very dilute acetic acid (2 to 3 drops for 20 ml of distilled water), and leave it there for about a minute;

Treat the sections with the gold chloride solution until a change of colour occurs (disappearance of the brownish yellow colour, change to grey);

Rinse rapidly in distilled water;

Treat rapidly with the 5 per cent sodium thiosulphate solution (a stage whose usefulness seems doubtful, but which all authors practise, and which does no harm).

Wash thoroughly in tap water;

Mount in a medium miscible with water or, after dehydration and clearing in a benzenoid hydrocarbon, in Canada balsam or a synthetic resin.

The neurofibrils appear intensely black against the background of the specimen; the colour of the other structures is conditioned by the way in which the technique has been carried out; in this way making the silver complex alkaline by means of ammonia, after the sections have been treated with the formalin, slows down reduction at the nuclei and collagen or reticulin fibres to such an extent that it can sometimes be useful to stain the nuclei with haemalum, carmalum, or with the alum lake of nuclear fast red; this staining is then carried out after the sections have been impregnated and washed with tap water. Among other factors liable to cause the result to vary, we should specially mention the duration of mordanting and the pH of the water used to dilute the formalin. It emerges from the research of Seki (1940) that the greatest selectivity of impregnation of neurofibrils is obtained when the sections mordanted with silver nitrate are passed through dilute formalin whose pH varies from 6.6 to 6.8; the lower pH resulting in feeble and incomplete impregnations, the higher pH resulting in an over-strong participation of the nuclei and connective tissue in the impregnation.

According to the general consensus of opinion, the Gros-Schultze technique is one of the best and most versatile of the methods for impregnating neurofibrils in frozen sections; it does not require any special precautions at the time of fixation, the sections adjoining those undergoing impregnation can be treated with other stains or histochemical reactions, the course of the impregnation can be followed through a microscope and the method can be easily adapted to particular cases.

The techniques of Rogers (1931) and of Tinel (1947) represent, in fact, an adaptation of the Gros-Schultze method to work on paraffin wax sections. The great interest of these methods lies in the possibility of carrying out impregnations of neurofibrils on sections taken from material fixed with mixtures as common as Bouin's or Carnoy's fluids; silver impregnations of the neurofibrils can thus be carried out on sections adjoining those which have undergone other stainings or histochemical reactions. Tinel's mode of operation has the advantage of being less costly and more flexible than that of Rogers; indeed Roger's technique involves a 40 per cent silver nitrate solution, while Tinel uses a solution with half that concentration; furthermore, adjustments to particular cases are easier with the second of the techniques. So it is Tinel's mode of operation which I have included here, incorporating in the description a certain number of unpublished technical details which the late Dr. J. Tinel taught me before the publication of the method.

Tinel's impregnation of neurofibrils

The technique of Tinel, like that of Rogers, gives the best results after fixation with Bouin's fluid; sections taken from material fixed by the Duboscq-Brazil or Carnoy's fluid are also suitable, but the impregnations are more "contrasty". Formalin-fixed material may also be used; even alcohol fixations may be suitable, but it is better to avoid the use of fixatives containing corrosive sublimate. In any case the material is embedded in paraffin wax without special precautions, the sections being stuck on the slides with albumen.

Reagents:

    20 per cent aqueous solution of silver nitrate;
    commercial formalin (not neutralized);
    ammonia water (ammonia diluted with nine parts of distilled water);
    0.2 per cent acetic water;
    ammoniacal silver nitrate, prepared as required, as in the Gros-Schultze technique;
    0.2 per cent aqueous solution of gold chloride;
    5 per cent aqueous solution of sodium thiosulphate;

Mode of operation:

    Paraffin wax sections, dewaxed, not treated with collodion, hydrated;
    Mordant for 6 to 24 hours, at 37°C and in darkness, with the 20 per cent silver nitrate solution;
    Blot the slide with tissue paper (*do not wash*);
    Cover the slide with commercial formalin, keep in contact for two to four seconds throw away excess formalin;
    Blot with tissue paper (*do not wash*);
    Cover the sections with several drops of ammoniacal silver nitrate, transfer the slide to the microscope stage, observe the progress of the impregnation, using a low power objective; impregnation should be very rapid (20 to 40 seconds);
    Rinse rapidly (several seconds) in dilute ammonia;
    Leave for two to three minutes in very dilute acetic acid;
    Wash in distilled water;
    Tone with gold chloride; (for a few seconds to several minutes);
    Rinse in distilled water;

> Rinse rapidly in sodium thiosulphate;
> Wash thoroughly in tap water; if need be stain the background;
> Dehydrate in absolute alcohol, clear in a benzenoid hydrocarbon, mount in Canada balsam or a synthetic resin.

The toning with gold may be omitted when one does not wish to carry out a background staining; in this case the sections are washed in tap water when they have been removed from the acetic water, then dehydrated and mounted in Canada balsam. Of the background stains, to be used in cases where impregnation has not been taken very far, I recommend especially Ramon y Cajal's trichrome (p. 202). The results are equivalent to those of the Gros-Schultze method.

Adaptation to special cases. — In most cases the working technique described above is suitable for the impregnation of the nerve-fibres and the spinal ganglia; for the peripheral nervous system it may be necessary to acidify the silver nitrate solution used for mordanting (2 to 4 drops of nitric acid for one Borrel tube of solution); the mordanting solution can be used two or three times. In any case, mordanting in a solution whose pH is too low causes impregnation on the nuclei to predominate, while an excessively high pH promotes the impregnation of the connective fibres.

The success of the impregnation is largely conditioned by an adequately rapid reduction of the ammonical silver nitrate; the reduction may be adjusted, as in the Gros-Schultze technique, by adding ammonia in cases where it is too rapid; a too-slow reduction means that, in the technical conditions of Tinel's method, "the mark was overshot" at the time of the redissolution of the ammoniacal silver precipitate when the ammoniacal silver nitrate was being prepared. An excessively massive and brutal impregnation can be corrected by adding 1 to 3 drops of pyridine to 4 ml of ammoniacal silver nitrate.

Experience shows that the activity of the ammoniacal silver nitrate begins to diminish about twenty minutes after it has been prepared; Tinel always advised against preparing more than 5 ml at a time.

When impregnation turns out to be very difficult, the results can be spectacularly improved by mordanting from 12 to 24 hours at laboratory temperature in one of the three following liquids, which should be tried out systematically.

```
a) 96 per cent alcohol .................................. 95 ml
   Ammonia ............................................   5 ml
b) Distilled water ...................................... 50 ml
   Commercial formalin ................................. 50 ml
   Concentrated nitric acid ............................  0.5 ml
c) Commercial formalin ................................. 50 ml
   Distilled water ..................................... 50 ml
   Anhydrous sodium sulphite ...........................  1 gm
```

The advisability of one or other of these mordants cannot be foreseen.

If the impregnation fails, the colour can be removed from the sections with Farmer's differentiating fluid

distilled water	100 ml
sodium thiosulphate	1 gm
potassium ferricyanide	5 gm

They are then washed in sodium thiosulphate (aqueous 10 per cent solution) and rinsed, first in distilled water and then in water acidified with a few drops of hydrochloric acid. Impregnation may be recommenced after mordanting with formalin-sodium sulphite (see above); according to unpublished information from J. Tinel, this de-staining followed by fresh impregnation is often advantageous in research on the peripheral nervous system. Derived from a technique of Bielschowsky (1911), which involves formalin fixation and passing through pyridine, the methods of Agduhr (1917) and Boeke (1916, 1917) involve impregnations of blocks of tissue. Their advantages over techniques applied to sections may be summed up as a greater uniformity in the results, which is why they are of interest for research whose essential aim is the detection of neurofibrils; on the other hand, failure of the impregnation obviously means the loss of the tissue, and the fixation of the structures in general is less good than with well-tried topographical fixatives or, *a fortiori*, cytological fixatives.

Agduhr's technique for bulk impregnation

Fix in neutralised formalin, diluted with an equal amount of tap water, for at least seven days;

If necessary, decalcify in nitric acid (p.244), treat the decalcified pieces for 48 hours with a 5 per cent aqueous solution of sodium sulphate, and fix again in formalin diluted with an equal amount of water for several days;

Treat for five to ten days, at laboratory temperature, with pure pyridine;

Wash for six to twenty days in distilled water, changed once a day; the length of time this washing lasts depends on the texture of the tissues;

Impregnate, for ten to twenty-five days, at laboratory temperatures and in darkness, with a 3 per cent aqueous solution of silver nitrate; it may be advisable to renew the solution once or twice during impregnation; embryos should be impregnated for longer periods (up to six weeks), but without changing the silver nitrate solution;

Rinse in distilled water;

Impregnate for one to three days, at laboratory temperatures, in the ammoniacal silver nitrate, prepared as follows
to 10 ml of a 10 per cent aqueous solution of silver nitrate add XX drops of 40 per cent caustic soda (not carbonate) and 400 ml of distilled water; redissolve the precipitate by adding ammonia with caution; it is better to leave a little precipitate remaining than to add too much ammonia;

Wash for 24 hours in 0.02 per cent acetic acid (this stage is unnecessary in the treatment of muscular tissue and embryonic material);

Reduce for four to six days in neutralized formalin, diluted with four times its volume of tap water; change the liquid until precipitation of the remnants of silver nitrate has ceased;

Wash in tap water, dehydrate, clear and embed in paraffin wax;
Cut the sections and stick them to slides without special precautions;
Dewax, treat with collodion if necessary, hydrate;
Treat with a dilute solution (coloured yellow very slightly) of gold chloride in distilled water until the connective tissue becomes discoloured (check through a microscope);
Rinse in sodium thiosulphate (0.5 per cent aqueous solution) for a few seconds;
Wash thoroughly in tap water, dehydrate, clear and mount in Canada balsam or a synthetic resin.

Boeke's technique for bulk impregnation

This impregnation, which differs in some details from that of Agduhr, is specially recommended by its author for research on the synapses and the peripheral nervous system.

Fix in the mixture
    neutralized formalin .... 12 ml
    distilled water .... 88 ml
fixation may take a long time;
Treat for three days with pure pyridine;
Wash for eight hours in frequent changes of distilled water;
Impregnate for five to six days, at 30–35°C, with a 3 per cent aqueous solution of silver nitrate;
Rinse quickly in distilled water or simply blot with tissue paper;
Treat for 24 hours with the ammoniacal silver nitrate, prepared as follows
    To 10 ml of a 10 per cent aqueous solution of silver nitrate add 5 drops of 40 per cent caustic soda (not carbonate);
    redissolve the brown precipitate of silver oxide by adding ammonia with caution, taking great care not to add too much;
    bring up to 100 ml with distilled water;
Wash for two hours in distilled water;
Reduce for 12 to 24 hours in neutralized formalin, diluted with four parts of distilled water;
Wash in tap water, embed in paraffin wax;
Treat the sections as in Agduhr's method or simply mount them, after dewaxing, in Canada balsam or a synthetic resin.

NERVE-FIBRE IMPREGNATIONS
DERIVED FROM THE SILVER REDUCTION METHOD

Ramon y Cajal's reduced silver method, derived from a method of Simarro (1900), is suitable for the impregnation of blocks. The pieces of tissue are treated with a dilute solution of silver nitrate, the argyrophilia of the neurofibrils being disclosed as a result of treating the tissue with an organic reducing agent. Apart from the original technique, of which about thirty variants have been suggested by its inventor, the methods of Foley (1939) and Favorsky (1930) give particularly satisfactory results.

But the same principle may be applied to frozen or paraffin wax sections; such important techniques as Schultze's soda technique and the methods of Davenport (1930), Bodian (1936), Holmes (1947) and Palmgren (1960) are connected with it.

Ramon y Cajal's silver reduction technique

The initial stage consisting of immersing fresh pieces of tissue in the silver nitrate solution, was soon abandoned by Ramon y Cajal himself, the preservation of the tissues being extremely poor. The other variants involve fixation, which varies according to the tissues and the aim of the work, the impregnation itself being identical in all cases. It would be out of place to give details here of the thirty or so variants recommended by the author of the method. Five of them are mentioned here, the rest falling within the scope of specialized works.

The precautions which are common to all silver impregnations, and which concern the choice of products and their use, are set out here in chronological order; they were in fact specified by Ramon y Cajal in connection with the impregnation mentioned in this section, but naturally they are valid for all the other methods.

The glassware used for silver impregnations should be cleaned meticulously, the requirements being the same as for quantitative chemical analysis; having been passed through a sulpho-chromic mixture it is washed thoroughly first in tap water then in distilled water, and finally dried, protected from dust; it is best to reserve a set of vessels specially for this purpose. All *the chemical products* used should be certified "for analysis"; an attempt at petty economies in this domain only leads to failures and to a waste of time out of proportion to any eventual saving. The instability of many of the reagents explains the necessity of keeping all the material away from *dust* and other organic matters; all *contact between the liquids and metallic instruments* should be avoided. It is not always necessary to keep the reagents in darkness, but the impregnations themselves should always, unless otherwise indicated, be carried out *away from the light*. The use of *bottles with ground glass stoppers* is not essential, but all contact between silver solutions and cork stoppers should be avoided.

The *pieces of tissue undergoing impregnation* should be dissected as rapidly as possible, and their size should take into account the peculiarities of the method; indeed there is a very great danger of over-impregnation of the superficial zones and an appreciable risk of a poor penetration of the silver nitrate and the reducing agent to the centre of the tissue block, which should, therefore, be neither too thin nor too thick.

It is in respect of *fixation* that the five variants of Ramon y Cajal's technique retained here differ from one another. The special requirements for each variant and the working technique are given in Table 29, numbered as in Ramon y Cajal.

Table 29. — Fixation and further treatment of the tissue in the variants of Ramon y Cajal's technique

Variant	II	III	IV	V	VI
Indications	Brain Cerebellum Motor and sense end-organs, regeneration	Medulla Spinal and sympathetic ganglions, general usage	Amyelinic fibres, cerebellum	Embryos	Motor plates, cerebellum
Fixative	96 per cent or absolute alcohol	96 per cent or absolute alcohol, with 1 to 12 drops of ammonia added to each 50 ml	Commercial formalin 15 ml, distilled water 85 ml	Pyridine 40 ml, 96 per cent alcohol 30 ml	Absolute alcohol 25 ml, distilled water 75 ml, chloral hydrate 5 g
Duration	24 hours	24 hours	24 hours	24 hours	24 hours
Treatment of fixed tissue before impregnation	Blot with tissue paper	Blot with tissue paper	Wash in running water (6 to 12 hours), treat for 24 h with alcohol containing ammonia (5 drops for 50 ml of 96 per cent alcohol), Blot with tissue paper	Wash in running water until all odour of pyridine disappears, treat for 6 to 12 h with 96 per cent alcohol, blot with tissue paper	Rinse in distilled water (1 minute), treat for 24 h with alcohol containing ammonia (4 drops for 50 ml of 96 per cent alcohol), wash in running water (12 to 24 hours), then in a change of distilled water (2 to 5 h)

The impregnation proper involves the following stages;
Material fixed and treated as indicated in the table;

> Impregnate for 5 to 7 days, at 30–35°C, in a 1 or 1.5 per cent aqueous solution of silver nitrate;
> Wash for about a minute in distilled water;
> Reduce for 24 hours, at laboratory temperatures, in the solution
> > hydroquinone or pyrogallol .... 1 to 2 g
> > neutralized formalin .... 5 ml
> > distilled water .... 100 ml
>
> Wash for about five minutes in distilled water;
> Dehydrate rapidly (if possible reduce the length of time the tissue remains in alcohol to a total of six hours), clear in benzene, embed in paraffin;
> Cut in sections of 10 to 15 µ, dewax and mount in Canada balsam or a synthetic resin; the sections may also be hydrated and their colour toned with gold as in the variants of Bielschowsky's method; background staining is generally unnecessary.

When the impregnation has succeeded the neurofibrils show up black against a yellow background; the other structural details of the slides show up more or less well.

Pieces which have been left for a long time in alcohol can be rendered suitable for silver impregnation by leaving them in 96 per cent alcohol, with about 2 g of chloral hydrate, veronal or somnifene added to each 100 ml of alcohol; this can be added systematically when Ramon y Cajal's variant II of the impregnation is being used; the rest of the treatment does not require any special precaution.

If it can be seen, when examining the sections before mounting, that the impregnation is too light, the results can be improved by treating the deparaffinated and hydrated sections for five to ten minutes with the mixture

distilled water	100 ml
ammonium thiocyanide	3 g
sodium thiosulphate	3 g
1 per cent aqueous solution of gold chloride several drops to	1 ml

The sections are then washed in tap water, dehydrated and mounted in Canada balsam or a synthetic resin after clearing in a benzenoid hydrocarbon.

FOLEY'S TECHNIQUE FOR IMPREGNATION

Fix, as far as possible by vascular perfusion, in the following liquid

3 per cent aqueous solution of potassium bichromate	49 ml
ammonia (28 per cent solution of NH_3)	1 ml
pyridine	15 ml
96 per cent alcohol	50 ml

and keep the tissue in this liquid, maintained at about 4°C, for 48 hours;

Wash the tissue blocks in baths of 50, 40, 30, 20 and 10 per cent alcohol, adding, at each bath, 15 ml of pyridine for 85 ml of alcohol; the object of this washing is to eliminate the potassium bichromate; the pieces are left for about an hour in each bath and the last bath should take on only a very faint yellow colour;

Treat for 24 hours with pure pyridine;

Bring to water, if necessary (delicate tissue) passing through mixtures of water and pyridine in constantly decreasing concentrations;

Wash for about 12 hours in tap water;

Wash for 24 hours in frequent changes of distilled water;

Impregnate for 5 to 7 days, at 37°C, in a 2 per cent aqueous solution of silver nitrate; change the bath on the third day;

Rinse rapidly in distilled water;

Reduce for 48 hours, at laboratory temperatures, in the mixture

distilled water	100 ml
pyrogallol	4 g
commercial formalin	5 ml

Dehydrate, impregnate with butanol, embed in paraffin wax;

Cut into sections and treat these as in Ramon y Cajal's technique or hydrate, tone with gold (a 0.2 per cent solution of gold chloride, with a few drops of acetic acid added) observing the operation through a microscope, carry out Feulgen and Rossenbeck's nucleal reaction (hydrolysis time about 20 minutes at 60°C), stain the background with phosphotungstic acid—Heidenhain's blue as in the azan technique of this author; the aniline blue of the latter stain may be replaced, in the case which interests us here, by light green which gives better contrasts between neurofibrils and collagen fibres.

Favorsky's technique for bulk impregnation

Fix for 24 hours in the following mixture
    50–80 per cent alcohol .... 100 ml
    acetic acid .... 0.5 to 5 ml
the alcohol content and the acetic acid content of the liquid being tentatively adjusted to suit the material being worked with;
Treat for a few hours with 50 per cent alcohol, changed once or twice;
Treat for 48 hours with the mixture
    96 per cent alcohol .... 100 ml
    ammonia .... 1 ml
Leave in distilled water, changed several times, until the tissue pieces remain at the bottom of the vessel, instead of floating to the surface;
Treat for one to two days with pure pyridine;
Wash for 12 to 24 hours in running water;
Wash for 2 to 3 hours in frequent changes of distilled water;
Impregnate for 4 to 10 days, at 37°C, in a 2 per cent aqueous solution of silver nitrate; the optimum impregnation time varies according to the size and texture of the pieces;
Blot with tissue paper or rinse very quickly in distilled water;
Reduce for 12 hours, at laboratory temperature, in the mixture
    distilled water .... 100 ml
    neutralized formalin .... 10 ml
    pyrogallol .... 1 to 2 g
Dehydrate, beginning with 96 per cent alcohol (alcohol of a lower degree is harmful to the impregnation), embed in paraffin or celloidin;
Cut in sections, mount with or without gold toning, as in the other techniques for silver impregnation of blocks;

Davenport's technique for impregnation of sections

This excellent method, whose application is not limited to the domain of neurohistology, since it has been used in recent researches of the school of Hellman on the cellular categories of the endocrine pancreas, may be used on celloidin or paraffin sections; it is one of the rare methods of silver impregnation where the treatment of the sections with collodion is expressly recommended. The layer of collodion, which should be fairly thick, is intended to be dissolved before mounting takes place; this eliminates all superficial silver precipitates which could hinder the examination of the specimens. The material can be fixed in dilute formalin, saline or non-saline, in acetic acid-formalin-water mixture (10 ml of formalin and 5 ml of acetic acid for 100 ml of fixative), or in Bouin's fluid; paraffin or celloidin embedding is carried out without special precautions. The impregnation proper involves the following stages.

    Paraffin or celloidin sections; celloidin sections are stuck on to slides, paraffin sections are set out in the usual manner; treatment with collodion is carried out by means of a 1 or 2 per cent solution (obtained by diluting the commercial 5 per cent collodion solution with a mixture of equal parts of absolute alcohol and ether);

after being immersed in the dilute collodion, the sections are exposed to air until they are half-dried, immersed in 80 per cent alcohol or in the 96 per cent alcohol-formalin mixture recommended on p. 141 for dewaxing, and finally hydrated;

Treat, in darkness and at 37°C, with the solution

silver nitrate	10 g
distilled water	10 ml
N nitric acid	0.5 ml
96 per cent alcohol	90 ml

dissolving the silver nitrate in the water and not adding the other ingredients until it is completely dissolved; the sections are left in this bath until they are a fairly light brown colour, which may take from one to 24 hours;

Rinse rapidly in 96 per cent alcohol;

Reduce, at laboratory temperature, in the mixture

96 per cent alcohol	100 ml
pyrogallic acid (pyrogallol)	5 g
commercial formalin	5 ml

keeping the slides in motion; the progress of the reduction can be observed by rapid examination through a microscope; it takes on an average two minutes; Lillie (1954) points out that the addition of 100 mg of glucose to the reducing agent prevents the formation of precipitates; 50 ml of reducing agent is enough to reduce about 20 slides;

Rinse in two or three baths of 96 per cent alcohol;

Dehydrate in absolute alcohol, dissolve the layer of collodion by bathing for a few minutes in a mixture of equal parts of absolute alcohol and ether;

Clear in a benzenoid hydrocarbon and mount in Canada balsam or a commercial synthetic resin; one can also hydrate the sections, tone with gold, and carry out a background staining.

The neurofibrils show up dark brown or black; the brown colours turn black if the sections are toned with gold.

Bodian's technique for impregnation of sections

Bodian's technique, which has enjoyed a considerable and justified popularity may be grouped with the silver reduction methods; but compared to the other methods considered in this paragraph it presents several peculiarities. Indeed, the source of silver is not the nitrate of this metal, but protargol (silver proteinate); copper, added to the impregnation bath, serves as an activator; gold-toning is obligatory and the tints are strengthened by treating the toned sections with oxalic acid, in order to complete the reduction.

The technique has numerous advantages; it can be practised after a great variety of fixations and has even been found to succeed after the use of liquids based on potassium bichromate and postchromisation; its selectivity of impregnation is greater than with a certain number of other techniques and a background stain, which makes it easier to distinguish the nerve fibres and the collagen tissue, may be carried out after gold toning. But the success of the impregnation is strictly conditioned by the quality of the commercial sample of protargol used and this is the chief disadvantage of the method, since this compound is poorly defined from a chemical point of view, and one cannot really guarantee success even by obtaining it from a reliable supplier.

The variants of Bodian's method chiefly concern the choice of reducing agent and the pretreatment of the sections. The variant of Fitzgerald (1964) is the one which gives the best results, and is the only one given here.

Fixation can be carried out by a whole series of mixtures; Bodian (1937) specially recommends a mixture of 90 ml of 80 per cent alcohol, 5 ml of acetic acid and 5 ml of commercial formalin, while noting that good impregnations can be obtained from sections taken from pieces fixed in Bouin's fluid, Carnoy's fluid, etc. Fitzgerald (1964) specifically advises a mixture of 70 ml of a saturated solution of picric acid in 90 per cent alcohol, 25 ml of commercial formalin and 5 ml of acetic acid, that is to say Bouin's fluid in which the water is replaced by 90 per cent alcohol. *Embedding* is done in paraffin, without any special precautions, and the sections are stuck with albumin. Impregnation by Fitzgerald's technique involves mordanting with silver nitrate, a procedure already suggested by Davenport and his collaborators, which greatly increases the chances of success; the addition of metallic copper to the impregnation bath has been abandoned.

Reagents:

10 per cent aqueous solution of silver nitrate (may be re-used a certain number of times);
reducing agent, prepared by dissolving *together* 10 g of anhydrous sodium sulphite and 1 g of hydroquinone in 100 ml of distilled water;
0.2 per cent solution of protargol in distilled water (to be prepared at the moment of using);
0.5 per cent aqueous solution of gold chloride, acidific by 1 drop of acetic acid to every 100 ml (may be re-used a certain number of times);
2 per cent aqueous solution of oxalic acid;
50 per cent alcohol, with 3 drops of aniline added to every 100 ml;
5 per cent aqueous solution of sodium thiosulphate.

Mode of operation:

Dewaxed sections not treated with collodion, but hydrated;
Wash for 20 to 30 minutes in several changes of distilled water;
Treat, in an embedding oven at 56°C, with the silver nitrate solution; the optimum length of time is about 2 hours for the peripheral nervous system, about 4 hours for the central nervous system, the sense organs and embryonic material;
Wash in three baths, each of 30 seconds duration, of distilled water;
Treat for 18 hours, at 37°C, with the protargol solution;
Rinse for 5 to 10 seconds in distilled water;
Reduce for 3 to 5 minutes with the hydroquinone—sodium sulphite;
Wash for 10 minutes and leave waiting where necessary in tap water;
Rinse quickly in distilled water;

Tone for about ten minutes with gold chloride;
Wash for two to three minutes in distilled water;
Treat for four to five minutes with oxalic acid (central nervous system, sense organs, embryonic material) or for 20 to 30 seconds with aniline-alcohol (peripheral nervous system);
Wash for about one minute in running tap water;
Fix for 5 to 10 minutes in sodium thiosulphate;
Wash thoroughly in running water;
Dehydrate in absolute alcohol, clear in a benzenoid hydrocarbon, mount in Canada balsam or a synthetic resin.

I strongly recommend, especially in the case of the organs of vertebrates, completing this impregnation by staining with van Gieson's picrofuchsin (p. 204), which imparts a yellow tint to the cytoplasm and shows the collagen tissue up in red. After they have been washed in running water the sections are treated with picrofuchsin for ten to twenty seconds, then immediately dehydrated, cleared and mounted.

Holmes's technique for impregnation on sections

The technique of impregnation on paraffin sections developed by Holmes (1947), like that of Bodian, allows very good preparations of neurofibrils to be obtained and has the further advantage of using compounds which are chemically well defined, so that its success does not depend on the quality of a commercial sample of a silver preparation which is not, in reality, a pure chemical compound.

The tissue may be fixed in dilute formalin, saline or non-saline, but the author specially recommends formalin-sublimate (10 ml of formalin and 90 ml of saturated aqueous solution of corrosive sublimate). Paraffin wax embedding is carried out without special precautions and the sections may be fairly thick (up to 25 μ); they are stuck on the slides with albumin.

Reagents:

20 per cent aqueous solution of silver nitrate;
impregnation bath, prepared as required as follows:
mix 55 ml of an aqueous solution of 12.4 g boric acid to the litre with 45 ml of an aqueous solution of 19.0 g of sodium tetraborate decahydrate (borax) to the litre; make up to 494 ml with distilled water, stir; add 1 ml of a 1 per cent aqueous solution of silver nitrate and 5 ml of a 10 per cent aqueous solution of pyridine; stir carefully;
reducing agent: dissolve 1 g of hydroquinone and 10 g of crystallized sodium sulphite in 100 ml of water;
0.2 per cent aqueous solution of gold chloride;
2 per cent aqueous solution of oxalic acid;
5 per cent aqueous solution of sodium thiosulphite.

Working technique:

> Dewaxed, hydrated sections not treated with collodion; crystals of sublimate should naturally be removed, following the technique described on p. 143, when the sections have been fixed in formalin-sublimate, and there is no harm in the slides taking several minutes to pass through the Lugol solution;
> Wash for ten minutes in running water, then in two baths of distilled water;
> Treat for two to twelve hours, at laboratory temperatures and in darkness, with the 20 per cent solution of silver nitrate; this solution may be re-used a few times;
> Wash for ten minutes altogether in three changes of distilled water;
> Impregnate for 12 to 36 hours, at 37°C, in the impregnation bath; allow about 20 ml of solution for each slide;
> Blot rapidly with tissue paper, reduce for two to five minutes in the reducing agent, which has been heated to 25–30°C before the slides are immersed in it;
> Wash carefully for five minutes in running water;
> Rinse, and leave waiting where necessary, in distilled water;
> Treat with the gold chloride solution until the brown shade of the sections turns to grey (3 minutes or more);
> Rinse in distilled water;
> Treat for two to ten minutes with oxalic acid solution; watch the process through the microscope and stop as soon as the axons become blue-black: leaving the sections too long in this bath can lead to a weakening of the impregnation;
> Rinse in distilled water;
> Treat for five minutes with the thiosulphate solution;
> Wash thoroughly in running water;
> Dehydrate in absolute alcohol, clear in a benzenoid hydrocarbon, mount in Canada balsam or a synthetic resin.

Palmgren's technique for impregnation of sections

Palmgren's technique, like that of Holmes, has an advantage over Bodian's method in that it uses only chemically well defined substances, whose purity may be verified, so that the user is freed from the risk to his work incurred when he uses products whose quality cannot be chemically controlled. Besides, the factors conditioning the success of the impregnation are analysed by the author of the method with praiseworthy care, and his very precise instructions make its adaptation to a particular material very much easier. So I feel myself entitled to predict that Palmgren's technique will occupy a foremost place in the neurohistologist's arsenal; it already has a great number of users.

As Palmgren quite rightly remarks, no rigid technique is suitable as it stands for nerve-fibre impregnation in all tissues; a process of adaptation is therefore necessary, and one of the essential qualities of Palmgren's memoir consists precisely in facilitating this work of adaptation; it seems to me therefore opportune to seek to retain this advantage by following the original text, in my account of the technique.

Fixation should be carried out, wherever the nature of the material allows it, in three fluids: Bouin's, Carnoy's and Bodian's no. 2 fixative (alcohol-formalin-acetic acid, see p. 932). Generally speaking fixation in Carnoy's fluid is advantageous for the central nervous system and suitable for the peripheral nervous system, while pieces of tissue fixed in Bouin's and Bodian's fluids are chiefly suited to the impregnation of the peripheral nerves. It is advantageous to fix for fairly long periods (48 hours).

The preparation of the pieces and the making of sections requires little special commentary; the pieces should not be left for too short a time in the dehydration alcohol as the extraction of the lipids should be as complete as possible when the material is intended for the impregnation of neurofibrils; one should however avoid leaving the tissue to stand in 96 per cent alcohol, and embedding should be carried out within a reasonably short space of time. The sections should be caused to adhere with albumin. When the technique is being adapted to a particular material the author recommends preparing about 15 trials slides, corresponding to the three fixatives mentioned above.

The preparation of the slides for impregnation naturally involves dewaxing, which should be carried out after 24 hours of drying in an oven, but without further delay; experience proves that prolonged storage of untreated sections adherent to slides, has a bad effect on the result of the impregnation. The sections can be treated with collodion, provided one is very careful to keep the layer of collodion thin. They are then hydrated. Sections taken from material fixed in Bouin's fluid are washed for a few minutes in 70% alcohol with about 1 ml of ammonia added to every 100 ml, in order to eliminate all the picric acid, and they are then washed in several changes of distilled water. After fixation in liquids which do not contain formalin it can be advantageous to treat the sections for 24 hours with a mixture of 5 ml of commercial formalin, 5 ml of acetic acid and 90 ml of water; this treatment has the effect of reducing the intensity of the non-specific colouring which the nuclei and other structures take on through silver impregnation.

The following *reagents* should be prepared for the impregnation of the sections

- N/10 and N/100 nitric acid;
- N/10 and N/20 sodium hydroxide;
- 0.02 per cent aqueous solution of pyridine;
- 2 per cent solution of borax in N/20 sodium hydroxide;
- 2 per cent solution of borax in distilled water;
- 0.5 per cent solution of gold chloride, acidified with 3 drops of acetic acid for every 100 ml;
- 0.5 per cent solution of oxalic acid in 50 per cent alcohol;
- 5 per cent aqueous solution of sodium thiosulphate.

All the solutions given above should be prepared using products certified "for analysis" with as much care as for chemical analysis (burettes, pipettes, graduated flasks, balances, etc.).

Before *impregnation,* material fixed in liquids containing formalin should be left for 24 hours in distilled water at 37°C; a small piece of camphor may be added to prevent the growth of microbes; the above-mentioned pre-treatment with acetic acid-formalin-distilled water should be carried out when the sections have been fixed in a mixture which does not contain formalin. The rest of the technique involves the following stages.

Rinse in three baths of distilled water;
Impregnate in one of three solutions
  10 per cent silver nitrate in N/1000 nitric acid ... about 12 hours
  10 per cent silver nitrate in distilled water ..... 15 minutes
  10 per cent silver nitrate in 0.02 per cent pyridine   2 to 20 minutes
   impregnation taking place in all cases at 37°C and away from the light: the solutions can be used daily for a fortnight;
Rinse in 5 baths of distilled water for a total of two minutes;
Treat for one minute, at laboratory temperatures, with the solvent of the chosen reducing reagent (solution of borax in soda or in distilled water);
Reduce for five to ten minutes, at 37°C, in one of the following solutions:
  1 g hydroquinone and 5 g sodium sulphite in 100 ml of solution of borax in N:20 sodium hydroxide
  1 g hydroquinone and 5 g sodium sulphite in 100 ml of solution of borax in distilled water;
  0.5, 0.1, 0.05 or 0.01 g hydroquinone and 5 g sodium sulphite in 100 ml of solution of borax in distilled water;
  each of these six reducing solutions will keep for about a week even if used daily;
Wash for 5 minutes (15 minutes if the sections have been treated with collodion) in 50 per cent alcohol, renewing the bath three times;
Tone, on slides, with the gold chloride solution until the brownish yellow shade disappears from the sections (generally 15–30 seconds);
Rinse rapidly in distilled water and strengthen the colour by leaving for two to three minutes, at 37°C, in the solution of oxalic acid (this solution keeps well);
Rinse in tap water, fix rapidly (15 seconds) in the 5 per cent solution of sodium thiosulphate
Wash in tap water, dehydrate, clear and mount in Canada balsam or a synthetic resin.
To sum up, the factors to be varied during the impregnation are:
  the pH of the silver nitrate solution;
  the time of impregnation;
  the choice of reagent.

Palmgren (1960) advises that attempts to adapt the technique to a particular material should be begun using the combinations set out in Table 30.

If an excessively purple stain of the neurofibrils is obtained in these conditions the impregnation time should be shortened; in certain cases impregnation need not last for more than two minutes.

In any case, one of the five variants mentioned in Table 30 usually turns out to be superior to the others: it serves as a base for the final refinement of the technique.

Table 30. — Types of experiment to be tried in adapting Palmgren's technique to a new material
(after the data of Palmgren, 1960)

Impregnation 10 per cent solvent of silver nitrate	Time at 37°C	Reducing agent
N/1000 Nitric acid	15 minutes	1 g hydroquinone, borax/soda
Distilled water	15 minutes	1 g hydroquinone, borax/soda
0.02 per cent pyridine	10 minutes	1 g hydroquinone, borax/soda
N/1000 Nitric acid	24 hours	1 g hydroquinone, borax/soda
Distilled water	24 hours	1 g hydroquinone, borax/soda

If the final colour of the neurofibrils is too purple and there is insufficient contrast, the other formulae for reducing agents are tried in place of the one shown in the table, which is suitable for the majority of cases.

Where the overall stain is too weak, while differentiation of the structures is satisfactory, double impregnation is called for; after being reduced and washed in alcohol, the sections are washed for 15 minutes in distilled water, then impregnated for 10 minutes in the silver nitrate solution chosen for the first impregnation, washed and reduced a second time in the same reducing agent.

When impregnation is being carried out on material fixed by Carnoy's fluid, and the sections have not been subjected to pre-treatment with formalin—acetic acid, it is very advisable to begin the experiments with long impregnation times (24 hours).

The experiments must naturally be carried out on sections taken from pieces fixed by the three mixtures given above. Once perfected, the method for any particular organ, gives more regular results than any other technique for impregnation of neurofibrils. It is applicable to frozen sections, whether adherent to slides or not, as well as to membranes spread out and fixed *in toto*.

Schultze's technique for impregnation on frozen sections

The technique of Schulze resembles that of Palmgren in that the impregnation can be widely adapted to different objects. The essential methodological peculiarity of this method — reserved for frozen sections of material which has been fixed in formalin for less than six months—is that it involves the treatment of the sections with an alkaline solution which acts as a detergent; the use of acids or water as detergents, originally proposed, is of less practical interest. This manoeuvre, whose true mechanism is still unknown, was referred to by Schultze (1918) under the term *Entschlackung* (*Schlacke* = slag), which is impossible to translate by a single word and does not occur in the classic vocabulary of German; the term "detersion" best expressed what Schultze had in mind: — that the treatment of the sections with dilute solutions of soda, acetic acid or water was intended to extract compounds which are harmful to silver impregnation. The general significance of this treatment is not limited to Schultze's method or even to nerve-fibre techniques in general; Palmgren (1960) mentions an improvement in the results of his impregnation technique when sections taken from material fixed in Bouin's fluid are subjected to a 24 hours' extraction in distilled water; I have referred (p. 733) to the favourable effect of a similar treatment when using Altmann's fuchsin as a stain, and it is likely that many other stains could benefit from this procedure. Schultze's technique was developed and recorded precisely by Stöhr (1922); it is on the procedure recommended by the latter author that the description given here is based.

Reagents:

N sodium hydroxide prepared with all the usual precautions, diluted more or less, according to the objects and the results desired;

10 per cent aqueous solution of silver nitrate, diluted according to the material, and used only once;

reducing agent: dissolve 2.5 g hydroquinone in 100 ml water, add 5 ml commercial formalin; this stock solution, which keeps for about three months, is diluted as required.

Mode of operation:

Frozen sections (average thickness 30 µ) taken from formalin-fixed material;

Treat for 24 hours, at laboratory temperatures, with dilute soda (see Table 31);

Wash very carefully indeed, for at least an hour, in several changes of distilled water; the last of these washing waters should not turn red on the addition of phenolphthalein, and no precipitate should appear when the sections pass through the silver nitrate;

Treat for 12 to 24 hours, at laboratory temperatures and in darkness, with the silver nitrate solution, diluted according to the material, (see Table 31); the sections should turn slightly brown;

Transfer directly to the reducing agent, diluted according to the material (see Table 31) and follow the progress of the reduction through a microscope; the best way is to place the section in a watch-glass or a little Petri dish, which can be placed in position on the microscope stage; the reduction should be interrupted as soon as the axons have turned black, the colour of the perikarya varying between fairly dark brown and black;

Wash in two baths of distilled water;

Dehydrate directly in 96 per cent alcohol and carbolic benzene, clear in benzene, mount in a synthetic resin or Canada balsam.

Several recent techniques for the silver impregnation of neurofibrils require mention here not merely because their results are satisfactory, but also because they are original in conception; these techniques are those of Romanes (1949), Samuels (1953) and Fraser-Rowell (1963).

Table 31. — Chronology of the stages in Schultze's technique and concentrations of the reagents

Material	24 hrs detersion in		Length of washing (hours)	24 hrs impregnation in silver nitrate	Dilution of reducing agent
	N soda (ml)	distilled water (ml)			
Telencephalon	6	50	1	2%	20 times
Cerebral trunk	10	50	1	10%	id.
Cerebellum	2	50	1	0.25%	id.
Bulb, medulla, ganglions	10	50	1	10%	id.
Peripheral nerves	10	50	2	10%	80—120 times
Cortical cells	0.5	50	1	0.5 %	20 times

Romanes' technique for neurofibril impregnation

This technique gives excellent results in most cases although it is sometimes contra-indicated, for as yet unexplained reasons, for use with olfactory fibres, and post-ganglion vegetative fibres. It includes a treatment with a silver chloride suspension at pH 7.8, followed by a reduction with a hydroquinone sodium sulphite mixture and gold toning. Wax sections, made adherent with albumen, and taken from material fixed in Bouin or Carnoy's fluids, formalin or the formalin-alcohol-acetic acid mixture serve very well, Subsequent decalcification with Bensley's fluid is required (a mixture of equal parts of 50% formic acid and a 20% solution of trisodium citrate).

Reagents:

   70% alcohol containing 2% of 0.880 ammonia;
   the impregnation bath: mix just prior to use and away from light: —
      0.1% aqueous solution of silve nitrate .... 3 ml
      distilled water .... 100 ml
      0.1% aqueous solution of sodium chloride .... 1 ml
   mix with care, adjusting the pH to 7.8 (with Johnston Comparator paper no. 6883) using very dilute ammonia.
   reducing agent:
      hydroquinone .... 1 g
      crystalline sodium sulphite .... 10 g
      distilled water, to make up to .... 100 ml
   2% aqueous solution of oxalic acid;
   5% aqueous solution of sodium thiosulphate.

Working technique:

   Dewaxed sections, not treated with collodion, hydrated and treated with several baths of 70% alcohol rendered alkaline with ammonia; these baths, the object of which is to remove the last traces of picric acid should the tissue have been fixed in Bouin's fluid, equally improves the results obtained with the other fixatives.

Impregnate for 16 h at 56°C in darkness using the impregnating bath which must be freshly prepared.
Place the sections directly in the reducing agent for 5 min and at laboratory temperatures.
Wash carefully in tap water;
Rinse in distilled water;
Tone with gold chloride for 10 min;
Wash for one min in distilled water, once renewed;
Reduce for 3 to 5 min (at the most) using the oxalic acid solution;
Wash in running water;
Fix for 3 to 5 min in sodium thiosulphate;
Wash in running water, dehydrate, clear and mount.

The nerve fibres and the intracellular neurofibrils are stained both purple and black, the nuclei are red, the keratin is yellow; the osteocytes are black.

Samuel's technique for neurofibril impregnation

This technique is particularly valued by research workers who study the nervous system of invertebrates. Its originality lies in removing all excess silver from the sections, after depositing 'seeds' responsible for the impregnation and prior to the reinforcement of the impregnation by physical development. All stages of the method are rigorously defined in terms of the physical conditions. Among fixatives, Samuel advises the use of formalin, the formalin-alcohol-acetic acid mixture of Bodian, or a modification of Bouin's fluid due to Adams, Thomas and Davenport (1948) (this is a saturated aqueous solution of 90 ml picric acid, 10 ml commercial formalin, and 2 ml of a 25% aqueous solution of trichloracetic acid); from personal experience, the classical formula of Bouin's fluid is just as good.

Reagents:

Sodium borate—boric acid buffer, pH = 6.8
    M/20 aqueous solution of sodium tetraborate .... 0.3 ml
    M/5 aqueous solution of boric acid .... 9.7 ml
    boiled distilled water .... 90 ml
1% aqueous solution of silver nitrate;
2.5% aqueous solution of sodium sulphite;

Physical developer:

    5.5% aqueous solution of silver nitrate .... 10 ml
    9% aqueous solution of crystalline sodium sulphite ...... 100 ml
    0.5% aqueous solution of hydroquinone .... 5 ml
Pour small quantities of the sulphite solution into that of silver nitrate, stir until the solution clears, adjust the temperature to 18–19°C and add the hydroquinone solution; the mixture, which does not keep, can be used only once and must be prepared immediately prior to use.

0.2% aqueous solution of gold chloride, acidified with 20 drops of acetic acid per 100 ml;
2% aqueous solution of oxalic acid;;
5% aqueous solution of sodium thiosulphate;

Working technique:

Dewaxed sections, treated with collodion, and hydrated;
Place in running water for 2 h;
Wash in 3 baths of distilled water;
Place the sections in the buffer and bring to 55°C in an oven; in the same oven, introduce a flask containing 99 ml of the buffer;
When the whole has attained 53.5°C pour 1 ml of the silver nitrate solution into the flask containing the buffer, stir, discard the buffer bathing the slides and replace it by that containing the silver nitrate; continue to keep the material in the oven as long as necessary, as determined by trial and error (see below);
Rinse in 3 baths of distilled water, and, where appropriate, allow to stand in distilled water at laboratory temperatures;
Wash for 2 min in the sodium sulphite solution;
Rinse vigorously in 3 baths of distilled water at 18°C, so as to avoid any sharp change of temperature when the physical developer is introduced;
Treat with the physical developer until an olive tint of the sections appears (on an average, after some 4 to 6 min);
Rinse in distilled water;
Wash in running water for about 20 min;
Rinse in distilled water;
Tone with gold chloride for 25 min (unlike the situation in other impregnation techniques, the time spent by the sections in the gold chloride is not critical);
Rinse in distilled water;
Where appropriate (particularly for sections of the central nervous system) treat for 3 min with the oxalic acid solution and rinse in distilled water;
Treat for about 5 min with the sodium thiosulphate solution;
Wash in running water, dehydrate, clear and mount in Canada balsam or in a synthetic resin.

The neurofibrils are impregnated black on a blue or grey background which is very pale.

Among the adjustments to be made in the course of this method, the most important is that of the "preimpregnation" time, at which stage the "seeds" of silver are deposited. Samuel advises that, when the experimenter is working on an as yet unknown tissue, he should stop the preimpregnation on one slide every hour, and on another every six hours. A duration of 4 to 5 min is set for the physical impregnation in such cases. When the optimum duration of preimpregnation has been determined in this way, experiments in which the development is stopped every minute can be carried out to discover the optimum for this second stage.

The technique can be applied to frozen sections.

Fraser Rowell's technique for neurofibril impregnation

This technique, which is particularly advantageous in studies of the nervous system of invertebrates, combines Holmes' (1947) impregnation and Samuel's (1953) physical developer.

Reagents:

20% aqueous solution of silver nitrate, which may be used several times;

Impregnating bath:

Holmes' borate/boric acid buffer, the pH of which should be adjusted by trial and error .... 20 ml
1% aqueous solution of silver nitrate .... 20 ml
2,6-dimethylpyridine (lutidine) .... 10 ml
distilled water .... 250 ml

2% aqueous solution of crystalline sodium sulphite;

Physical developer:

5% aqueous solution of silver nitrate .... 9 ml
9% aqueous solution of crystalline sodium sulphite ...... 300 ml
0.5% aqueous solution of hydroquinone .... 20 ml

0.2% aqueous solution of gold chloride acidified with several drops of acetic acid;
2% aqueous solution of oxalic acid;
5% aqueous solution of sodium thiosulphate.

Working technique:

Paraffin wax sections, taken from material fixed in Carnoy or Bouin's fluid, that of Duboscq, or in formalin; dewaxed, hydrated, rinsed in distilled water;
Mordant in 20% silver nitrate for 1 h in darkness;
Wash in distilled water;
Impregnate at a temperature of 30–70°C, to be adjusted as required in the impregnation bath, for 16 h;
Wash carefully in distilled water, which should be renewed several times;
Treat for two min with the sodium sulphite solution;
Allow the physical developer to act for 5 to 10 min at 20°C;
Rinse in distilled water;
Wash for 5 min in running water;
Rinse in distilled water;
Tone with gold chloride for 5 min;
Rinse rapidly in distilled water;
Reduce in oxalic acid for 5 min;
Rinse in distilled water;
Treat for 5 min with the sodium thiosulphate solution;
Wash in running water, dehydrate, clear and mount in a synthetic resin or in Canada Balsam;

The only stages that require adjustment are the impregnation and the physical development; the author of the technique specifies that the duration of 16 h is suitable in all cases, the temperature of impregnation and the pH of the buffer requiring to be adapted to the material impregnated. Generally speaking, raising the temperature from 30°C to 70°C and the pH from 7 to 9 intensifies the impregnation, but it also increases the risk that the sections will come unstuck and that silver nitrate will be precipitated.

Impregnation at 50°C with a bath buffered at pH 7.8 is a good starting point for trial runs. So far as the developer is concerned, its action should be checked as soon as the slide shows the first traces of a grey-green precipitate. Obviously, the development needs to be continued longer when the impregnation is less intense.

Nerve fibres are impregnated black on a greyish-purple background.

THE OSMIUM — IODIDE TECHNIQUE FOR STAINING NERVE-FIBRES AND NERVE ENDINGS

The osmium—iodide technique, of which I have no personal experience has been discussed from a histochemical viewpoint in connection with the detection of the catecholamines (p. 579); I have had occasion to remark, in this context, that recent research (Hillarp, 1959; Cruz, 1962) does not allow this procedure to be regarded as a histochemical reaction, but that its value as a morphological method of staining certain nerves is generally conceded, especially as the silver impregnation techniques for neurofibrils, Golgi's method and the methylene blue method, in the postganglionic parts of the autonomous nervous system, often lead to unaccountable failures. Recent authors (see especially Jabonero 1964; Taxi, 1965) stress the usefulness of the osmium—iodide method in such circumstances.

Apart from the original working technique described on p. 580, a variant due to Maillet (1959), which involves replacing the potassium iodide in the fixative by zinc iodide, is specially recommended by Jabonero (1964) and by Taxi (1965).

These two authors stress the advisability of preparing the zinc iodide solution as required to be used to fix the tissue, using the following very simple formula

> to 200 ml water add 15 to 20 g powdered zinc and 4 to 5 g iodine, shake and filter; the solution is ready to use.

Maillet's technique involves the following stages.

> Fix small-sized pieces for 18 to 20 hours, at laboratory temperatures, in the mixture
> 2 per cent aqueous solution of osmium tetroxide .... 2 ml
> zinc iodide solution (see above) .... 8 ml
> according to Taxi (1965) the tissue may be left in the fixative for up to 48 hours;
> Dehydrate rapidly, embed in paraffin wax.
> Cut into sections, dewax and mount in Canada balsam or a synthetic resin.

The nerve-fibres and nerve-endings show up black on a yellow background; the risk of diffuse osmic blackening of the superficial regions is much less than with the original technique of Champy (1913). Naturally, the result is a diffuse staining of the neuroplasma without the nerve-fibres showing up.

E. — MYELIN METHODS

Techniques for the detection of myelin play a certain part in research on the peripheral nervous system, but they principally apply to the systematisation of the central nervous system of vertebrates; taken together with cytoarchitectonics, based mainly upon the detection of Nissl bodies, myelotectonics represents one of the fundamental aspects of the microscopic study of the nerve centres of these animals. Myelin techniques also play a leading part in neuropathological research, whether it is a question of the precise localization of experimental lesions or of the histopathological study of morbid processes.

The myelin sheath of the peripheral nerves is easy to detect by osmic impregnation; the production of preparations containing osmium-treated nerves is described below. The classic myelin methods are all variants of Weigert's original procedure (1885) which depends upon rendering the myelin insoluble by postchromatization and then staining it with haematoxylin; the progress of histochemical research has greatly enriched the collection of techniques available—staining with Sudan black B, Feyrter's staining by mounting, Klüver and Barrera's staining with Luxol fast blue, and, finally, plasmal and pseudoplasmal reactions which ensure a very good detection of myelin. One should add to this list Marchi's standard method, intended to reveal changes in myelin during the process of degeneration.

PRODUCTION OF NERVES TREATED WITH OSMIUM TETROXIDE

Ranvier's standard technique (1872) is still used in the preparation of specimens for teaching purposes; fragments of osmium-treated nerves are, moreover, useful for reference, embedded in paraffin, concomitantly with tissue intended to be cut into serial sections for later reconstruction (p. 156). It involves the following stages.

Isolate, without damaging it, a nerve trunk (sciatic nerve of frog or mouse, etc...)
Place a fragment of glass rod of suitable size in contact with the nerve;
Join the nerve and the glass rod by binding in two places;
Excise both together rapidly, place them for 24 hours in a 0.5 per cent aqueous solution of osmium tetroxide;
Wash for about 30 minutes in distilled water;
Transfer for one to two hours into a mixture of equal parts of distilled water and glycerine, then for one hour into pure glycerine;

> Place on a slide in pure glycerine and dissociate with needles, tearing the perineurium and separating the fibres with "combing" movements of the needles, working in a lengthwise direction;
> Mount in glycerine jelly.

The myelin sheaths show up in black and Ranvier's nodes are clearly visible; the axons are stained light yellow, the nuclei and Schwann sheaths are also easy to perceive.

The fragments of osmium-treated nerve which have been prepared for reference during reconstruction are dehydrated, after the washing which follows the fixation in osmium tetroxide, and then set aside in cedar wood oil; they are rinsed briefly in benzene and embedded along with the pieces of tissue which they are to accompany.

In the working technique described above selective detection of Ranvier's crosses can be obtained by replacing the immersion in osmium tetroxide solution with a 24 hours' treatment with a 1 per cent aqueous solution of silver nitrate, followed by a washing in distilled water, and the specimens can be mounted after dissociation or embedded in paraffin and cut into sections lengthwise.

MYELIN METHODS DERIVED FROM WEIGERT'S METHOD

Weigert's classic technique involves four stages: primary mordanting, secondary mordanting, staining and differentiation. The very numerous modifications proposed by the author himself and later by his successors aim at reducing the disadvantages of the method, which are the very long mordanting times and the very unfavourable consistency of the pieces, which become brittle and poorly suited to the cutting of the flat and sizeable sections necessary for architectonic research. Among the variants which retain chromatisation of the pieces of tissue, as in the original method, those of Kultschitzky (1889), Pal (1886) and Wolters (1890), used in most neurohistological laboratories, are described below. Apart from these, the more recent techniques of Nageotte (1908), Loyez (1910), and Bacsich (1937), involving the mordanting of sections, play an important part in neurohistological research.

Kultschitzky's myelin method:

> Tissue fixed in dilute formalin, saline or non-saline.
> Mordant for three to six weeks in Müller's fluid (p. 686) or for four to five hours in Weigert's myelin mordant; dissolve at boiling point 5 g potassium bichromate and 2.5 g of chromium fluoride in 100 ml distilled water, cool and filter;
> Eliminate excess of mordant by washing repeatedly in 70 per cent alcohol;
> Dehydrate, embed in celloidin; wash the sections in distilled water;

Stain the sections for 12 to 24 hours in acetic haematoxylin
> *matured* 10 per cent alcoholic solution of haematoxylin ..... 10 ml
> distilled water .... 90 ml
> acetic acid .... 2 ml

Transfer directly to the differentiator
> saturated aqueous solution of lithium carbonate .... 100 ml
> 1 per cent aqueous solution of potassium ferricyanide .... 10 ml

Stop the differentiation when the white substance comes away cleanly, using a thorough washing in tap water;

Dehydrate in 96 per cent alcohol and carbolic benzene, clear and mount in Canada balsam or a synthetic resin.

The myelin sheaths show up black or blue-black, the grey matter is coloured pale yellow, the erythrocytes, fibrin and basal membranes also show up black.

Pal's myelin method:

Formalin-fixed pieces, mordanted in Müller's fluid or in Weigert's myelin mordant, embedded in celloidin as in the method already described;

Mordant the sections, where necessary, for several hours in a 3 per cent aqueous solution of potassium bichromate; the need for this mordanting is indicated by a greenish colour in the sections; when these are brown no mordanting is necessary;

Stain for 24 to 48 hours with Weigert's lithium carbonate haematoxylin
> matured 10 per cent alcoholic solution of haematoxylin .... 10 ml
> aqueous solution of lithium carbonate, prepared by
>> mixing .... 7 ml
>
> saturated aqueous solution and 93 ml distilled water ...... 90 ml

Wash carefully in tap water;

Treat for about 30 seconds with a 0.25 per cent solution of potassium permanganate;

Rinse in tap water and remove stain with the following solution, freshly prepared
> distilled water .... 200 ml
> oxalic acid .... 1 g
> potassium sulphite .... 1 g

The removal of the stain usually takes one to three minutes and can be controlled with the naked eye or through a microscope; if the grey matter retains too much haematoxylin, the sections are washed in tap water, and then treated a second time with the potassium permanganate and oxalic acid;

Wash very carefully in tap water, dehydrate and mount as before.

Wolter's myelin method:

Tissue treated as in Kultschitzky's technique, cut and stained with Kultschitzky's acetic haematoxylin;

Treat the haematoxylin-stained sections for a few seconds with Müller's fluid;

Differentiate with potassium permanganate and oxalic acid as in Pal's technique;

Wash thoroughly in tap water

Dehydrate and mount as in the preceding techniques.

Nageotte's myelin method. — This very simple technique has the considerable advantage of not requiring any pretreatment of the tissue blocks so that it can be used on frozen sections adjoining sections undergoing an impregnation of the neurofibrils, staining of the Nissl bodies by Laskey's technique, staining of the neuroglia, etc...

> Frozen sections taken from formalin-fixed material;
> Extract neutral fats by washing rapidly in absolute alcohol;
> Stain for about 30 minutes with haemalum (p. 195);
> Wash in tap water (one to two minutes);
> Differentiate in Weigert's borax—ferricyanide
>
> | | |
> |---|---|
> | borax | 2 g |
> | potassium ferricyanide | 2.5 g |
> | distilled water | 100 ml |
>
> watching the process with the naked eye or a low-power objective of the microscope.
> Wash in slightly alkaline tap water (lithium carbonate or ammonia);
> Dehydrate in absolute alcohol, clear in a benzenoid hydrocarbon, mount in Canada balsam or a synthetic resin.

When the staining is carried out on old formalin-fixed material, the haemalum often takes badly on the myelin sheaths; in these cases Nageotte advises mordanting with iron alum, in a 4 per cent aqueous solution for 24 hours followed by staining for 12 to 24 hours with Weigert's iron haematoxylin not containing lithium carbonate (p. 197); differentiation is done in the iron alum solution which was used for the mordanting.

The myelin sheaths show up violet-blue with haemalum, black with Weigert's haematoxylin, against a slightly yellow background.

Loyez's myelin method. — Applicable to celloidin sections taken even from old formalin-fixed material, this technique does not require any pretreatment of the blocks and differs from the previous techniques in having a double differentiation.

> Celloidin sections, washed in distilled water;
> Mordant for 24 hours, at laboratory temperatures, in a 4 per cent aqueous solution of iron alum;
> Wash quickly in distilled water;
> Stain for 24 hours, at 37°C., with Weigert's *lithium carbonate* haematoxylin (p. 946)
> Wash quickly in tap water;
> Differentiate, with the iron alum solution which was used for the mordanting, until the border between the grey matter and the white matter begins to be apparent;
> Wash carefully in tap water;
> Complete the differentiation in Weigert's borax—ferricyanide (p. 947);
> Wash carefully in tap water;
> Dip the sections for one or two minutes in water containing ammonia (1 ml ammonia to 100 ml water);
> Wash thoroughly in tap water;
> Dehydrate, clear and mount as in the techniques already described.

The myelin sheaths, the nuclei and the erythrocytes show up deep black on a light yellow background.

Bacsich's myelin method. — This method is especially interesting because of the perfect regularity of its results, the time gained through working with paraffin wax sections and the fact that pretreatment of the tissue is quite unnecessary; I consider it therefore the best method in all cases where the dimension of the tissue blocks being worked does not call for celloidin sections. It involves the following stages.

Fix in dilute formalin, saline or non-saline;
Wash for 24 hours in running water;
Dehydrate, treat with alcohol-ether mixture as for celloidin embedding, leave the tissue blocks for 48 hours in the 2 per cent celloidin solution used for this method of embedding;
Treat the tissue blocks with several baths of strictly anhydrous chloroform;
Clear in benzene, embed in paraffin;
Cut into sections of 15 to 30 μ; stick to the slide with albumen, without special precautions, dry;
Dewax, treat with collodion, hydrate the sections;
Mordant for two hours, at 37°C, in the mixture

distilled water	100 ml
chromium trioxide	1 g
chemically pure ferric chloride	1 g

(dissolve in the order given above)
Wash in distilled water, changed once or twice, until the sections are a pale yellow colour;
Stain for two hours, at 37°C, with lithium haematoxylin carbonate prepared in the following manner;

mature 10 per cent haematoxylin solution in 96 per cent alcohol	10 ml
distilled water	100 ml
saturated aqueous solution of lithium carbonate	10 ml;

Wash for two minutes in one or two changes of distilled water;
Wash in tap water to which has been added a few drops of saturated aqueous solution of lithium carbonate, until a clear difference is discernible between the grey substance and the white substance;
Rinse in distilled water;
Dehydrate in absolute alcohol, clear in a benzenoid hydrocarbon, mount in Canada balsam or a synthetic resin;

When complete elimination of the collodion film covering the sections is desired, these should be given a bath in a mixture of equal parts of absolute alcohol and ether between dehydration and clearing.

In the vast majority of cases no differentiation is necessary; the myelin sheaths are stained dark blue, the grey substance is stained red. In my own experience it is not essential to pass the tissue through alcohol-ether, 2 per cent celloidin and chloroform: results almost as satisfactory as those of the original method can be obtained after direct paraffin embedding.

A subsequent differentiation can be carried out with potassium permanganate-oxalic acid, following Pal's technique; when the result is rather mediocre this differentiation should be continued until the sections lose all their colour; they are then washed thoroughly in tap water and staining can be recommenced.

HISTOCHEMICAL REACTIONS AND DIAGNOSTIC STAININGS APPLICABLE TO THE DETECTION OF MYELIN SHEATHS

The techniques described in the third part of this work ensure excellent detection of myelin sheaths, and one may well wonder whether, in the future, they are not bound to supercede techniques deriving from Weigert's stain.

As Lison and Dagnelie (1935) pointed out after their work had introduced this lysochrome into histochemical technique, **Sudan black B stain** provides stains for myelin sheaths which are no less intense or precise than those of Weigert's method or of its variants. The technique is applicable to frozen sections taken from formalin-fixed material, and is the simplest way of adding a myelin method to work involving impregnations of neurofibrils or of the neuroglia in frozen sections; sections adjoining those used for other techniques may be used.

The working technique corresponds exactly with the directions given on p. 452, except that the sections may be left in the Sudan black B for as long as several hours. I would remind the reader of the advisability of using fairly fresh alcoholic solutions of this stain.

The metachromasia of myelin, which is very clear on frozen sections, may also be used profitably as a staining technique; apart from Feyrter's "staining by mounting" (p. 461) using thionine, very good results are given by staining with toluidine blue followed by washing in water and mounting in a medium which does not require dehydration; the only real disadvantage of the above-mentioned techniques is that the preparations do not keep well.

The plasmal reaction and pseudo-plasmal reactions, the PAS method and the peracid-Schiff method give a deep red colour to the myelin sheaths, especially when frozen sections are being used—a necessity for the first two techniques mentioned; the colours are usually fairly bright on paraffin wax sections taken from chromatised material and paler after fixation in liquids without potassium bichromate and paraffin wax embedding. The mode of operation is described in Chapters 17 and 18. Ashbel and Seligman's reaction (p. 368) also gives positive results on myelin sheaths and their optical anisotropy explains their easy identification with a polarizing microscope.

Staining with Luxol fast blue (p. 463), in spite of the uncertainty of its chemical signification, is of considerable practical benefit in detecting the myelin sheaths. The working technique described in Chapter 18 gives excellent results and may be applied to celloidin sections, whether adherent to slides or not; certain author advise a slight acidification of the Luxol fast blue solution (0.05 per cent acetic acid), but in my own experience this precaution is not indispensible. The blue staining of the myelin sheaths is fast enough for the technique to be combined with Bielschowsky and Plien's stain applied to the Nissl bodies or with the PAS method.

MARCHI'S METHOD

Unlike the techniques described above, which lead to the detection of normal myelin, Marchi's technique shows the transformation of myelin in the course of various stages of nervous degeneration.

The principle of the method has been evoked on p. 464; experience proves that normal myelin does not reduce osmium tetroxide in the presence of oxidizing agents such as chromium trioxide or potassium bichromate; the same applies to Golgi bodies and the necessity of a complete elimination of these oxidizing agents prior to impregnation with osmium tetroxide has been mentioned on p. 711. But the lipids which result from the degeneration of the myelin are osmiophilic even in the presence of potassium bichromate, so that it is easy to stain them black and distinguish them immediately from normal myelin.

The original working technique has undergone many modifications, and one of the essential preoccupations of the authors has been to prevent the deposits of osmium dissolving at the moment when the tissue is being prepared for paraffin or celloidin embedding. Here is the technique developed by Schmorl (1928), because of its simplicity.

Marchi's method (Schmorl's variant):

Fix for two days in Orth's or Regaud's fluid (change the fixative every 24 hours); formalin-fixed material may be used;

Mordant for seven days in a 2.5 per cent aqueous solution of potassium bichromate; change the liquid on the third and the fifth day;

Treat with osmium for fourteen days, changing the liquid on the seventh, using the mixture

    2.5 per cent aqueous solution of potassium bichromate ... 2 volumes
    1 per cent aqueous solution of osmium tetroxide .... 1 volume

placing the tissue blocks in a dark bottle with a ground glass stopper; the liquid should be changed when it ceases to emit the characteristic smell of osmium tetroxide; allow 100 ml for four to five blocks of average size;

Wash for 24 hours in running water;

Embed rapidly in paraffin (acetone may be used for dehydration; petroleum ether or cedar wood oil for impregnation; small sized tissue blocks are penetrated by the benzene so rapidly that there is no danger of the deposits of osmium dissolving).

Cut into sections, dewax and mount in Canada balsam or a synthetic resin.

The foci of degeneration stand out deep black on a yellow or brownish background.

Obviously, lipids resulting from the degeneration of myelin may be stained, on frozen sections, by any lysochromes; from a practical viewpoint it is of course advantageous to choose a lysochrome which does not stain the phospholipids, thus ruling out Sudan black B, BZL blue and, to some extent, Oil Red. Sudan II, Sudan III and scarlet R (Sudan IV) are perfectly suitable. The first of the three above-mentioned lysochromes is used in the excellent technique of Lillie (1954, 1965) which results in the concomitant detection of normal myelin and of the foci of degeneration.

Lillie's Sudan II-haematoxylin technique for the detection of myelin:

Fix in 10 per cent formalin, saline or non-saline.
Postchromatise for 2 to 4 days, at laboratory temperatures, in a 2.5 per cent aqueous solution of potassium bichromate;
Wash for several hours to one night in running water;
Cut with a freezing microtome;
Stain the sections for 45 minutes, at 55–60°C, in the mixture

    1 per cent aqueous solution haematoxylin, freshly prepared .... 5 ml
    4 per cent aqueous solution iron alum, freshly prepared .... 5 ml

using a stoppered container; it is as well to shake it from time to time;
Wash and put aside in tap water;
Differentiate in the mixture

    distilled water .... 100 ml
    borax .... 1 g
    potassium ferricyanide .... 2.5 g

watching the process as necessary through a microscope; the differentiation is very regular and the optimum time, determined for one section, is valid for all the other sections in the same lot;
Wash carefully in several changes of tap water, so as to eliminate all the differentiating agent;
Stain for 10 minutes in the following solution, prepared as required

    saturated stock solution of Sudan II in isopropylic alcohol   6 ml
    distilled water .... 4 ml

shake, leave undisturbed, for 7 to 10 minutes, filter;
Wash in tap water;
Stick on to slides, mount in a water-miscible medium.

The normal myelin is stained blue-black; the nerve-cells are light grey, the nuclei dark grey, the colour of the erythrocytes varies between yellow and black, according to the way in which the differentiation has been carried out; the free lipids of the foci of degeneration are stained yellow-orange.

The staining of normal myelin, indicated above, can of course be carried out on paraffin wax sections, the sections being left in the haematoxylin for one hour. Fixation and postchromatisation take place in the same way as above, and it is recommended that the material be passed through 2 per cent celloidin, as in Bacsich's technique, before the paraffin wax embedding.

F. — NEUROGLIA TECHNIQUES

The neuroglia can be identified on preparations treated by so-called general methods, and these are the only effective procedures for a large number of invertebrates. But the detailed study of the neuroglial elements of the central nervous system of vertebrates, especially of Man, depends on techniques specially conceived for this purpose, which can be classified in two groups—on the one hand are stains with Crystal Violet, Victoria Blue or haematoxylin, and, on the other hand, gold or silver impregnations.

It seems to me essential to point out that most of the techniques to be described in this section have been developed for the study of the human encephalon; some of them are successful only on this material, others give acceptable results on the central nervous system of the Mammals commonly used in research laboratories. A serious effort to adapt the techniques in question must be made whenever they are applied to other objects.

STAINS FOR THE NEUROGLIA

Techniques derived from Weigert's method and stains with Victoria Blue are, above all, methods for the detection of the fibrous neuroglia; the number of variants proposed is great, and illustrates the capricious nature of the methods in question; only Holzer's Crystal Violet technique and Anderson's Victoria Blue technique are mentioned here. Mallory's phosphotungstic haematoxylin gives preparations which allow a good general study of the neuroglia, but does not constitute a technique for the selective detection of this tissue.

Holzer's stain for the neuroglia

This technique, generally considered by neurohistologists as being the best stain for the fibrous neuroglia, differs from Weigert's method in suppressing the mordanting of the blocks with this author's neuroglia mordant (copper acetate 5 g, acetic acid 5 ml, chromium fluoride 2.5 g, distilled water to make up to 100 ml) and treating the sections instead with phosphomolybdic acid. Frozen, paraffin or celloidin sections, from formalin-fixed material, may be used. Celloidin sections are given a prolonged bath in methyl alcohol in order to dissolve the embedding mass, after they have been stuck on to slides; frozen sections are stuck on to slides, paraffin sections are deparaffinated and hydrated. Staining is carried out as follows:

Treat the sections, for about ten minutes, with 50 per cent alcohol;
Shake the following mixture for two to three minutes
    0.5 per cent aqueous solution of phosphomolybdic acid .... 1 volume
    96 per cent alcohol .... 3 volumes
Wipe the slide carefully all around the section and wipe the underside as well, to eliminate all trace of liquid;
Blot the section with a pad of tissue paper, impregnated with the mixture
    chloroform .... 8 ml
    absolute alcohol .... 2 ml
and sprinkle it with this mixture; at all costs avoid desiccation of the sections;
Pour just enough of the following mixture to cover the still damp section
    absolute alcohol .... 2 ml
    Chloroform .... 8 ml
    crystal violet .... 1 g
this mixture should be stored in a well corked bottle, and should be left for about five seconds to take effect;
Remove the stain by means of a 10 per cent aqueous solution of potassium bromide; the alkalinisation of the latter, prescribed in the original formula, has been abandoned by the author in later versions of his technique; it is essential completely to eliminate the film with greenish metallic glints, formed on the surface of the section during staining, and the specimen should be sprinkled with potassium bromide until it takes on a uniform velvety blue-black colour.
Blot with tissue paper;
Differentiate with the following mixture, freshly prepared
    aniline .... 4 ml
    chloroform .... 6 ml
    1 per cent acetic acid .... 1 drop
the optimum time varying, according to the nature of the objects and the relative humidity of the laboratory, from a few seconds to several minutes;
Wash carefully in a benzenoid hydrocarbon, mount in Canada balsam or a commercial synthetic resin.

In a successful preparation the nuclei and the fibroglia show up deep blue-violet against a pale background; the cytoplasm of the neuroglial cells is visible, but their fine prolongations are not very clear. Some connective fibres may be stained.

Anderson's neuroglia stain

Anderson's technique, applicable to frozen or paraffin sections from formalin-fixed material, is a Victoria Blue stain, with differentiation by Lugol's fluid, mordanted by a complex mixture, to be made up just before use, made by mixing together equal parts of a 5 per cent solution of ferric chloride and the following solution, which should be prepared in the order shown and stored in a well corked dark bottle.

    distilled water .... 100 ml
    crystallized sodium sulphite .... 5 g
    oxalic acid .... 2.5 g
    potassium iodide .... 5 g
    Iodine .... 2.5 g
    acetic acid (added after solution is complete) .... 5 ml

Working technique for frozen sections, about 20 μ thick.

Wash in several changes of distilled water, to eliminate all trace of formalin;
Leave the sections for 10 to 20 minutes in the neuroglia mordant described above, prepared by mixing the two solutions just before use;
Wash in distilled water;
Treat for about 5 minutes with a 0.25 per cent aqueous solution of potassium permanganate;
Treat directly, without washing, with Pal's oxalic acid-sodium sulphite mixture (p. 946), until all the colour is removed;
Wash in distilled water;
Stick the section to a clean albuminated slide, blot with a pad of tissue paper impregnated with absolute alcohol;
Dry with tissue paper;
Cover the slide with a 1.5 per cent aqueous solution of Victoria Blue heated to boiling point, and leave for about 2 minutes to take effect;
Discard the stain, cover the slide with Lugol's fluid (potassium iodide 2 g, iodine 1 g, distilled water 100 ml), leave for one minute to take effect;
Differentiate with a mixture of equal parts of aniline and xylene; interrupt this by washing in xylene and examining under a microscope; continue with another dose of the aniline/xylene mixture, watching the process through the microscope;
Wash in several baths of a benzenoid hydrocarbon, mount in Canada balsam or a synthetic resin.

Working technique for paraffin wax sections, of material fixed in formalin or Bouin's fluid.

Dewax, treat with collodion and hydrate the sections; where necessary remove picric acid by washing in hot water;
Treat for about twenty minutes with Anderson's neuroglia mordant;
Wash in distilled water;
Oxidize in 0.25 per cent potassium permanganate for 5 to 10 minutes;
De-stain, without an intervening wash, with Pal's liquid;
Wash rapidly in distilled water;
Dry with tissue paper;
Cover the slide with 1.5 per cent Victoria Blue solution heated to boiling point and leave for about 5 minutes to take effect;
Discard the stain, treat for one minute with Lugol's fluid;
Differentiate, clear and mount as in the variant for frozen sections.

In successful preparations the fibroglia appear deep blue on a pale background; the nuclei, erythrocytes and fibrin take on the same shade; the myelin sheaths and connective tissue remain colourless.

Staining of the neuroglia
with Mallory's phosphotungstic haematoxylin

Phosphotungstic haematoxylin, the preparation of which has been described in connection with the detection of fibrin (p. 822), permits a good detection of the fibroglia; the mode of operation given here is recommended by Bertrand (1930).

Fix in formalin or Bouin's fluid; treat the formalin-fixed material for one or two days with a saturated aqueous solution of picric acid;
Mordant for 4 to 6 days, at 37°C, in a 5 per cent aqueous solution of ammonium bichromate;
Dehydrate without aqueous washing, embed in celloidin;
Treat the sections for about 15 minutes with a 0.5 per cent aqueous solution of potassium permanganate;
Wash in distilled water;
De-stain with a 1 per cent aqueous solution of oxalic acid;
Wash very carefully in frequent changes of distilled water;
Stain for 24 hours in Mallory's phosphotungstic haematoxylin;
Rinse rapidly in distilled water;
Dehydrate in 96 per cent alcohol and origan essence, mount in Canada balsam or a synthetic resin.

The same process may be applied to paraffin wax sections; mordanting with ammonium bichromate is not necessary when fixation has been carried out in a liquid with a potassium bichromate base; needless to say, dehydration and clearing of paraffin sections can be done in the usual way.

The nuclei and neuroglia fibres show up blue, the neurones in pink and their prolongations likewise in pink, and the collagen is red. Lieb (1948) points out that the blue colour can be intensified by subjecting the sections, which have been oxidized in potassium permanganate and bleached, to an hour's mordanting in a 4 per cent aqueous solution of iron alum; the sections are then washed rapidly in tap water and stained with phosphotungstic haematoxylin.

METALLIC IMPREGNATIONS OF THE NEUROGLIA

Metallic impregnations of the neuroglia, developed by the school of Ramon y Cajal, provide spectacular specimens and their application has resulted in complete reconsideration of histological knowledge of this tissue; but it must not be forgotten that the techniques in question are subject to very strict requirements in regard to the fixing times of the tissues and the composition of the fixatives; moreover the mode of operation is chiefly ordered in terms of the impregnation of the neuroglia of the central nervous system of Man; acceptable results can still be obtained with so-called laboratory mammals, but the investigator who seeks to apply these methods to the impregnation of the neuroglia of lower vertebrates, let alone invertebrates, must expect much toil and many failures before they are perfected.

Only the most important of the techniques in question can be given here, namely Ramon y Cajal's gold sublimate method and Globus's variant of it, the fourth tannin-silver variant of del Rio Hortega, and the same author's silver carbonate techniques for astrocytes, the oligodendroglia and the microglia.

Ramon y Cajal's gold-sublimate method (1926)

This technique, specially developed for the study of the protoplasmic neuroglia of the human cerebral cortex, shows the protoplasmic neuroglia and the astrocytes with an extraordinary selectivity. In spite of its extreme simplicity, the method requires a great deal of care, and the instructions given below, which follow literally the dissertation of Ramon y Cajal, should be scrupulously respected.

Fix pieces, as fresh as possible and not more than 5 mm. thick, in brominated formalin
- distilled water .... 85 ml
- neutralized formalin .... 15 ml
- ammonium bromide .... 2 g

for about a fortnight (never more than a month);

Cut with freezing microtome in sections of 20 to 30 μ; gather these in the fixative;

Rinse for a few seconds (not more) in two baths of distilled water;

Impregnate for 4 to 8 hours, in darkness, in the bath of gold sublimate, prepared as follows:

dissolve 0.5 g of chemically pure mercuric chloride in 50 ml of twice distilled water, by heating it but without letting it boil; while the liquid is still hot add to it 6 ml of a 1 per cent aqueous solution of brown gold chloride (*never use yellow gold chloride which contains free hydrochloric acid and is suitable for toning silver-impregnated, sections but not for impregnation of the neuroglia*); leave to cool, filter; the mixture does not keep very well and it is as well to prepare it shortly before it is to be used, whereas the aqueous solution of brown gold chloride may be kept almost indefinitely in a brown glass-stoppered bottle;

35 ml of solution are usually allowed for 6 to 7 sections; these should be spread out flat on the bottom of the vessel, covered with a layer of liquid about 1.5 cm high; do not disturb in the course of impregnation;

From the 4th hour onwards examine a section through the microscope after rinsing it and placing it on a slide; repeat this examination every 30 minutes; exceeding the optimum length of time causes a rapid weakening of the colours;

When the neuroglia cells stand out clearly in purple stop the impregnation by washing carefully in several changes of distilled water;

Fix for 5 to 10 minutes in the mixture
- distilled water .... 70 ml
- 96 per cent alcohol .... 30 ml
- sodium thiosulphate .... 5 g
- commercial concentrated solution of sodium bisulphite .... 5 ml

or in a 5 per cent aqueous solution of sodium thiosulphate;

Wash thoroughly in 50 per cent alcohol, stick on to slides;

Blot with tissue paper, cover with absolute alcohol, pass through origan essence, complete the clearing in a benzenoid hydrocarbon, mount in Canada balsam or a synthetic resin.

The neuroglia cells and their prolongations stand out in purple against an almost colourless background; the perikarya are stained light pink, and the nerve-cells are colourless. The success of the method is determined by the extent to which the fixing times have been respected (short fixations favouring the staining of the astrocytes, long fixations favouring the staining of the fibres), the absolute chemical purity of the reagents used, which should never come in contact with metallic instruments, and finally the adjustment of the impregnation time and of the temperature. The latter should be from 18 to 22° for the cerebral cortex, from 25 to 28°C for the cerebral trunk, the cerebellum and the medulla and from 35 to 40°C for the olfactory lobe; the optimum temperature for material taken from lower vertebrates is between 25 and 35°C.

Gold sublimate method (Globus's variant, 1927)

The essential aim of this method is to avoid fixation in brominated formalin, so that material may be used which has been simply fixed in formalin for less than six weeks. The author does this by treating the sections with hydrobromic acid (hyperbromination). The technique gives excellent results on human material. It involves the following stages.

Frozen sections from material fixed in formalin for less than six weeks;

> Wash several times in distilled water;
> Leave for 24 hours at laboratory temperatures, in a covered vessel, in 10 per cent ammonia (concentrated commercial solution diluted with 9 volumes of distilled water);
> Rinse rapidly in two baths of distilled water;
> Treat for 2 to 4 hours, at laboratory temperatures, with a 10 per cent solution of concentrated commercial hydrobromic acid (d = 1.38), prepared with distilled water);
> Rinse rapidly in two baths of distilled water containing a few drops of ammonia;
> Rinse rapidly in distilled water;
> Treat with gold sublimate solution
>   1 per cent aqueous solution of brown gold chloride .... 10 ml
>   mercuric chloride .... 0.5 g
>   distilled water .... 60 ml
> until a purple shade is reached, which may take 15 to 18 hours;
> Rinse in distilled water;
> Fix and mount as in Ramon y Cajal's technique.

In successful cases the results are comparable with those of the original technique.

Fourth tannin-silver variant of del Rio Hortega (1917)

This tannin-silver method, specially intended for the study of the protoplasmic neuroglia, differs from the first three variants (see p. 739 and 811–813) in the composition of the tannin solution.

> Frozen sections taken from formalin-fixed material;
> Mordant at 40–50°C in the solution
>   tannin .... 3 g
>   ammonium bromide .... 1 g
>   distilled water .... 100 ml
>   for 5 to 8 minutes;

Wash until they are transparent, in water containing ammonia
   distilled water .... 30 ml
   ammonia .... 1 drop
Rinse very rapidly in distilled water;
Reduce for 30 seconds to 1 minute in neutralized formalin, diluted with 4 volumes of distilled or tap water (choose by trial and error);
Wash carefully in distilled water;
Tone with gold, fix in sodium thiosulphate and mount as in the third variant, intended for the impregnation of collagen tissue (p. 811).

The protoplasmic neuroglia shows up black.

del Rio Hortega's technique for astrocytes (1917)

This is a silver carbonate impregnation technique for frozen sections taken from material fixed in Ramon y Cajal's brominated formalin (p. 956). The duration of the fixing time is of prime importance; short fixations (2 to 10 days) are best for the impregnation of astrocytes, while much longer times are needed for the impregnation of the fibroglia. The technique involves the following stages.

Frozen sections, 20 to 30 µ thick, gathered in water containing a little ammonia;
Wash in four baths of distilled water;
Impregnate at 45–50°C, until the sections are a deep amber colour, in silver carbonate solution prepared as follows
   to 5 ml of a 10 per cent aqueous solution of silver nitrate add 20 ml of a saturated aqueous solution of lithium carbonate; dissolve the silver carbonate precipitate by a cautious addition of ammonia, being careful not to add too much, bring up to 75 ml with distilled water, filter, store in a dark bottle;
Rinse *rapidly* in distilled water;
Reduce for one minute in neutral formalin, diluted to 1 per cent with 99 volumes of distilled water;
Wash carefully in distilled water;
Tone with a 0.2 per cent aqueous solution of gold chloride until the sections are a grey colour; once this colour has been obtained, heat the bath to 40–50°C and keep the sections in it until they are a purple colour;
Rinse rapidly in distilled water;
Fix for one minute in a 5 per cent aqueous solution of sodium thiosulphate;
Wash thoroughly in running water;
Stick on to slides, dehydrate in 96 per cent alcohol and the following mixture
   benzene, toluene or xylene .... 80 ml
   beech creosote or benzyl benzoate .... 10 ml
   phenol .... 10 g
complete the clearing in a benzenoid hydrocarbon, mount in Canada balsam or a synthetic resin.

The astrocytes and their prolongations as well as the fibroglia stand out in black against an almost colourless background. It may be advantageous not to tone the specimens and to mount them after reduction in formalin when it is the cytoplasm of the neuroglia cells which is the main object of study (Romeis, 1948).

Technique of del Rio Hortega (1921) for the oligodendroglia

This technique ensures very good detection of the oligodendroglia, which shows up in black, but it often happens that the microglia is also impregnated; the astrocytes are not impregnated.

> Fix in brominated formalin for 12 to 48 hours at laboratory temperatures; one of the tissue blocks must be less than, or at the most equal to, 3 mm;
> Hyperbrominate the blocks by immersing them for 10 minutes in brominated formalin previously heated to 45–50°C;
> Cut with a freezing microtome into sections of 25 to 30 μ, gather them in distilled water;
> Wash in distilled water to which a few drops of ammonia have been added (10 for 70 ml);
> Wash in distilled water.
> Impregnate for 1 to 5 minutes at laboratory temperatures in silver carbonate solution (del Rio Hortega's "*plata fuerte*") prepared as follows:
> to 5 ml of a 10 per cent aqueous solution of silver nitrate add 20 ml of a 5 per cent aqueous solution of anhydrous sodium carbonate; redissolve the yellowish precipitate by adding ammonia prudently, avoiding an excess; make up to 45 ml with distilled water;
> Wash for 15 seconds in distilled water, keeping the section in motion;
> Reduce for one minute in 1 per cent formalin, as for the impregnation of astrocytes; put the section into the reducing agent and do not disturb during the reduction;
> Wash carefully in several changes of distilled water;
> Tone with 0.2 per cent gold chloride until a grey colour is obtained;
> Rinse rapidly in distilled water;
> Fix for one minute in a 5 per cent aqueous solution of sodium thiosulphate;
> Wash carefully in tap water;
> Dehydrate, clear and mount as in the technique for astrocytes.

del Rio Hortega's technique (1921) for the microglia and the perivascular neuroglia

The technique described here was used by del Rio Hortega (1921) in his basic thesis presenting the original description of the microglia; it differs from the technique for the impregnation of the oligodendroglia in the composition of the silver carbonate solution and in a few details of the working technique. One of the essential precautions is to respect the time of fixation in the brominated formalin, since the method loses all selectivity when the fixation has been over-prolonged.

> Fix for 1 to 3 days, according to the temperature of the laboratory, in brominated formalin (formula identical to that of Ramon y Cajal, (p. 956);
> Hyperbrominate for about ten minutes, at 45–50°C in a fresh bath of brominated formalin;
> Cut with freezing microtome in sections of 20 to 30 μ, gathering the sections into distilled water;

- Wash in three baths of distilled water, to the second of which 4 or 5 drops of ammonia have been added for each 70 ml of water;
- Impregnate for 20 seconds to 2 minutes, at laboratory temperatures in a silver carbonate solution prepared as follows:
  to 5 ml of a 10 per cent aqueous solution of silver nitrate add 20 ml of a 5 per cent aqueous solution of anhydrous sodium carbonate; redissolve the precipitate by adding ammonia prudently, without adding too much; make up to 75 ml with distilled water;
  the length of time the sections are left in the silver carbonate solution is one of the factors essential to success; Penfield (1924) recommends that the sections should be removed systematically, one section after 20 seconds, the second after 45 seconds, the third after two minutes, and that the results obtained in the three cases should be compared;
- Transfer directly, for one minute, to 1 per cent formalin, making the liquid move energetically (blow on it); the sections should take on a colour which is grey, not brown; they can be examined through a microscope, so that the times of impregnation and reduction may be adjusted; in fact, experience proves that it is often advantageous to leave the sections in the reducing agent for a longer period;
- Wash carefully in distilled water;
- Tone with 0.2 per cent gold chloride, watching the sections attentively; toning should be stopped before the colour has turned purple, for fear of excessive darkening;
- Rinse in distilled water, fix, wash and mount as in the preceding variants.

Successful specimens show the microglia in intense black; the astrocytes and the oligodendroglia, like the fibroglia, take on only a very pale grey colour.

Penfield's technique (1928) for the detection of the microglia and the oligodendroglia after fixation in formalin without bromide

The practical advantage of this technique lies in the possibility of using tissue simply fixed in formalin, as long as it has not been left in the formalin for longer than a week; it is therefore a very suitable method for routine work in neurohistopathological laboratories.

- Frozen sections, about 20 μ thick, gathered in distilled water;
- Wash in distilled water with a few drops of ammonia added; the sections may be left in this liquid all night;
- Brominate in a 5 per cent solution of hydrobromic acid in distilled water; the sections should be left in this liquid for one hour at 38°C.
- Pass through three baths of distilled water;
- Treat, for one to 5 hours, with a 5 per cent aqueous solution of sodium carbonate;
- Rinse briefly in distilled water (optional stage);
- Impregnate at laboratory temperature, for 3 to 5 minutes, in del Rio Hortega's weak silver carbonate solution (as for this author's impregnation of the microglia); the sections should acquire a fairly pale grey or brown colour;
- Reduce directly in 1 per cent formalin; Romeis (1948) stresses the advisability of concomitantly trying formalin diluted with tap water and formalin diluted with distilled water;
- Wash in several changes of distilled water;
- Tone with gold, fix, wash and mount as for other neuroglia impregnations on frozen sections.

Successful specimens show the microglia and the oligodendroglia at the same time; the astrocytes and fibrous neuroglia are not impregnated.

del Rio Hortega's technique (1927) for histiocytic elements, including the microglia

The scope of this technique exceeds the limits of neurohistology, since it permits the selective detection of histiocytic elements in a whole series of organs; a very reliable method, it is used on frozen sections taken from material fixed in brominated formalin in the case of the microglia, or in dilute saline or non-saline formalin in the case of other organs. Fixation may last from 2 to 8 days, no more. Hot bromination, as in the 1921 techniques, may be useful.

> Frozen sections, 20 to 30 μ thick; gelatine embedding is possible if the material is difficult to cut, but not indispensable for the success of the impregnation; the sections are gathered in distilled water;
>
> Treat the sections for at least 10 minutes with a mixture of equal parts of pyridine, ammonia and distilled water or with a 5 per cent aqueous solution of crystallized sodium sulphite;
>
> Rinse in distilled water (optional stage);
>
> Impregnate in three baths of silver carbonate solution, prepared as follows
>
> to 5 ml of a 10 per cent aqueous solution of silver nitrate add 20 ml of a 5 per cent aqueous solution of anhydrous sodium carbonate; redissolve the precipitate by a prudent addition of ammonia, avoiding even the slightest excess; *do not proceed to dilute this liquid*;
>
> the sections remain for about 30 seconds in the first bath, one minute in the second, one minute or more in the third;
>
> Rinse in distilled water or pass directly to the next stage (the best way of determining how to act is to proceed by trial and error);
>
> Reduce for one minute in 1 per cent formalin; according to the circumstances it is sometimes advantageous to keep the sections in motion or, as may be, to leave them undisturbed;
>
> Wash in one or two changes of distilled water;
>
> Tone with gold chloride in a 0.2 per cent aqueous solution; cold toning is sufficient in most cases, but it is often useful to intensify it by heating the solution slightly for the last few seconds that the sections remain in it;
>
> Wash in distilled water, fix and mount as in the other silver carbonate techniques.

TECHNIQUES FOR THE HISTOLOGICAL STUDY OF NEUROSECRETORY CELLS

In terms of the currently accepted definition, the neurosecretory cell is characterized by the existence, in the same protoplasm, of the morphological features of the neurone and those of the glandular cell. At the technical level the result of this is that methods intended for the study of these two cell types can and should be utilized in research on the neurosecretory cells.

The study of the neurone-like characteristics of the neurosecretory cell by means of the techniques of histology under the light microscope needs little commentary. The detection of the *Nissl bodies* is extremely easy; any of the methods set out in a previous paragraph of this chapter is perfectly suitable and the specimens thus obtained have, in some cases, great diagnostic value, as the marginal position of all the basophilic cytoplasmic substance of the neurosecretory perikarya has been observed in numerous vertebrates and invertebrates. The detection of the *neurofibrils* is much more difficult; all authors agree in considering that the neurosecretory perikarya represent, in the great majority of cases, unfavourable material for the silver impregnation of these structures. Among the techniques described in the paragraph corresponding to this chapter, Ramon y Cajal's alcohol technique (variant II, p. 928) gives satisfactory results in some cases; Favorsky's technique (p. 930) is strongly recommended by Goslar and Tischendorf (1955); most present-day authors also use the Gros-Schultze technique (p. 921) for frozen sections, and the techniques of Bodian (p. 931) and Palmgren (p. 934) for paraffin wax sections. It should be noted that, as Hagadorn (1958, 1962) pointed out, the nerve centres of Hirudineae are a particularly suitable material for silver impregnation of the neurofibrils in the perikarya and the neurosecretory axons. *Myelin methods* are of little use in histological research on the neurosecretory cells, since the prolongations issuing from these perikarya are, in the great majority of cases, of amyelinic type; the *tractus supraopticohypophysealis* of the horse represents an important exception (Brettschneider, 1955).

The study of the glandular characteristics of the neurosecretory cell, on the other hand, requires a longer discussion, since it involves the morphological criteria for distinguishing between the ordinary nerve-cell on the one hand and the "neuroglandular" cell on the other.

It seems to me essential to note that from a methodological point of view, the study of the neurosecretory cell presents, with a very special acuteness, the difficult problem of distinguishing in histological preparations between the secretory product characteristic of glandular activity and the intracytoplasmic inclusions which express the development of an ordinary metabolic phenomenon (energy reserves, waste pigments etc...). A static study of microscopic specimens by itself, no matter how modern the selective stains or histochemical reactions used to treat them, can in practice lead only to presumptions; the detection of a secretory cycle and, if possible, its connection with physiological phenomena represents a very valuable argument, but absolute certainty can only be obtained by means of physiological experimentation and biochemical study (see Bern, 1962, 1963; Gabe, 1966, for a detailed discussion of this question).

Vital examination, in light field, dark field or under phase contrast, often allows the identification of the product of neurosecretion inside the perikarya or the axons; a certain importance is usually attached to the bluish white colour of structures containing a neurosecretory product, a colour which shows up clearly in oblique lighting or dark field, but one cannot deny the fact that many mucosubstances present the same appearance. Generally speaking vital examination worthy of this name cannot be practised, as far as neurosecretory cells are concerned, except in a small number of favourable cases, and it would be disastrous to try to make it a routine method, to be applied indiscriminately to all objects.

The fixation of tissue intended for the study of neurosecretory cells can, in principle, be carried out by any of the fixatives envisaged in the preceding pages of this book; when the essential aim of the work is the detection of the product of secretion itself, the aqueous mixtures are most definitely preferable to the alcoholic mixtures, since the latter dissolve the product of neurosecretion in a great number of cases, or do not ensure a sufficient denaturation of it, which causes losses in later operations. Bouin's fluid, Halmi's fluid, Heidenhain's Susa, mixtures of sublimate and formalin, and those containing formalin and potassium bichromate are very suitable; because of their greater penetration Bouin's fluid, Susa, and Halmi's fluid are generally to be preferred to strictly cytological fixatives.

The preparation of tissue for sectioning and the cutting of sections does not need any special commentary; prolonged storage in dilute formalin or in 96 per cent alcohol is compatible with the conservation *in situ* of most of the products of neurosecretion, provided that the fixation was correct; needless to say, preservation in butyl alcohol, methyl salicylate, cedar wood oil or, better still, in block form is to be preferred. There is no real reason to prefer celloidin embedding, recommended in the first research on the neurosecretion of vertebrates; unless there is any contra-indication, where difficulties due to the size of the tissue blocks or the consistency of bony or cuticular parts have not been eliminated during dissection, paraffin embedding is very suitable. There is no advantage in cutting the tissue into sections which are over-fine or over-thick; except in special cases the optimum thickness for sections lies between 5 and 10 μ. The sections must be laid out strictly in order when the object of the work consists of the search for neurosecretory perikarya, the study of the course of axons or the detection of endings; the procedure given on p. 115 is to be used in all cases where sections which are adjacent to one another have to be treated with different stains or histochemical reactions.

All so-called general methods, all cytological techniques capable of detecting secretory particles and all histochemical reactions which can impart to them sufficient contrast in relation to the background can be applied to the search for neurosecretory products; a great number have in fact been used.

The behaviour of the neurosecretory products in regard to histological stains so far known provides the elements of a technical classification. In fact, *all* the neurosecretory products are more or less acidophilic on sections which have not received any special pre-treatment: this acidophilia can, after the use of the usual trichromes, manifest itself either as erythrophilia or as cyanophilia. But certain products retain this acidophilia even when the sections have undergone a strong permanganic oxidation in an acid medium, while others, under the same experimental conditions, acquire a marked basophilia.

NEUROSECRETORY PRODUCTS WHICH ARE ACIDOPHILIC IN SPITE OF PERMANGANIC OXIDATION OF THE SECTIONS

These acidophilic products of neurosecretion cannot be detected except by means of so-called general techniques and cytological stains specially adapted to the detection of acidophilic secretory products in general. Heidenhain's azan, Mann's methyl eosin blue method, the Mann-Dominici method, one step trichrome, and the azur eosinate methods are very suitable; Masson's trichrome and its variants can, in some cases, detect these secretory products clearly, but in other cases there is not sufficiently intense contrast in relation to the background. On the other hand, spectacular specimens are furnished by variants of Altmann's fuchsin, applied in the same experimental conditions as for the detection of the chondriomes, and also by regressive haematoxylin lake stains. Some of the techniques intended for the detection of the neurosecretory products of the second group make use, moreover, of acid-based stains which impart their colour to the products of the first group, which may also be present in the sections.

NEUROSECRETORY PRODUCTS WHICH ARE BASOPHILIC AFTER PERMANGANIC OXIDATION

These substances represent a very important category, since the hypothalamic neurosecretory product of vertebrates, that of the protocephalic neurosecretory duct of arthropods and some neurosecretory products of Annelida and Hirudinea are endowed with this characteristic. It was during work on the hypothalamo-hypophysial complex of mammals that Bargmann (1949) was able to detect this basophilia of the hypothalamic neurosecretory product and open up a line of research which has led to spectacular advances in our knowledge.

The characteristic certain products have of acquiring a strong basophilia after permanganic oxidation in an acid medium can be detected by staining with a large number of basic stains, but experience shows that certain combinations present sufficient practical advantages to justify their being adopteb as routine methods.

Staining with chromic haematoxylin-phloxin (Gomori 1939, 1941) should be used in accordance with the directions given on p. 759; it gives a very intense blue colour to the products of neurosecretion alluded to here; the acidophilic products, in spite of permanganic oxidation, are stained by the phloxin.

The Mann-Dominici stain used after permanganic oxidation (Gabe, 1950), which should be used following the directions given on p. 760, has the advantage of conserving the stains well; it affords preparations which are very pleasing to the eye and enables one to distinguish easily between structures which have become basophilic after oxidation and those which contain metachromatic compounds; it has the disadvantage that the slides need to be individually differentiated, which involves some loss of time when the work is on a large scale.

Staining with paraldehyde-fuchsin has occupied an important place in research on neurosecretion since it was first applied to the staining of the neurosecretory products which are basophilic after oxidation. The working technique described on p. 760 is perfectly suitable when what is mainly required is to show up the substance in question in great contrast; when the sections are needed for anatomical study or when there is an advantage in having simultaneous staining of several secretory products some of which remain acidophilic in spite of oxidation, it is useful to finish the staining with one step trichrome, (Gabe and Martoja, 1957) rather than with Groat's haematoxylin and picroindigocarmine. The stages of the method are as follows.

Dewaxed, collodion-treated, hydrated sections;
Refix in Bouin's fluid containing 3 per cent chrome alum only in cases where the fixation of the material has not been quite satisfactory; in all other cases pass on directly to the following stages;
Oxidize with potassium permanganate in the presence of sulphuric acid as in Gomori's haematoxylin chromic-phloxine method; the oxidation time has very much less importance than for the latter stain;
Rinse rapidly in tap water;
Bleach in 2–5 per cent sodium bisulphite;
Rinse in tap water;
Stain for 3 to 5 minutes in the usual acetified solution of paraldehyde-fuchsin (p. 352);
Rinse in tap water;
Lighten the background, where necessary, by treating briefly with absolute alcohol containing 1.5 per cent concentrated hydrochloric acid (experience proves that this is not a crucial stage).

Wash for a few seconds in tap water;

Stain for about ten minutes in one-step trichrome (p. 217);

Wash for about one minute in distilled water (experience proves that staining by paraldehyde-fuchsin is weakened in the presence of phosphomolybdic or phosphotungstic acid, and that the original colour returns after aqueous washing);

Dehydrate in absolute alcohol, clear in a benzenoid hydrocarbon, mount in Canada balsam or a synthetic resin.

The products of secretion which have, because of the permanganic oxidation, acquired an affinity for paraldehyde-fuchsin are stained a more or less intense violet; the other secretory products are stained red, green, or yellow; the nuclei are red or green, according to the intensity of the permanganic oxidation; the colours of the cytoplasm range from red to green, the collagen tissue is green and the elastic fibres, whose affinity for paraldehyde-fuchsin is independent of permanganic oxidation, are stained deep violet.

Staining by paraldehyde-thionin as advocated by Paget (1959) does not, in my own experience, offer any advantage over paraldehyde fuchsin and its use is limited by the impossibility of stabilizing the dye; on the other hand, one variant of this technique, that of Leray and Stahl (1961) deserves attention. After the paraldehyde-thionin staining these authors carry out a PAS reaction, followed by a background stain with a 1 per cent solution of naphthol yellow S in 1 per cent acetic acid. This background stain takes about ten minutes; the specimens are then dehydrated in absolute alcohol, cleared and mounted. The secretory product which has an affinity both for paraldehyde-thionin and for naphthol yellow (see p. 333 in this connection), is stained green; other secretory products which only take up the paraldehyde-thionin, notably the chromolipoids, retain their violet colour. In my own experience equally good results may be obtained by staining with paraldehyde-fuchsin as with paraldehyde-thionin.

Staining by pseudo-isocyanines, applied to sections oxidized with potassium permanganate in a sulphuric acid medium (Schiebler, 1958; Schiebler and Schiessler, 1960) gives very clear metachromatic staining of the hypothalamic neurosecretory product of vertebrates; the sections do not tolerate dehydration and keep rather badly, which detracts from the practical scope of the technique; but another way of using the same dyes, fluoroscopic examination, is of great interest (Sterba, 1961, 1963, 1964), the sensitivity of the method being much greater than that of other stains, so that otherwise undiscernable amounts of the neurosecretory product can be recognized through the secondary yellow fluorescence of the stain polymerized on the structures. But the very rapid depolymerization, accelerated by the examination in ultra-violet light, makes it necessary to photograph the specimens immediately; the weakening of the fluorescence can be very pronounced in less than a minute. Sterba's technique involves the following stages.

Paraffin wax sections, not more than 4 μ thick, taken from material fixed in an aqueous liquid, not containing trichloracetic acid (avoid Heidenhain's Susa and Halmi's fluid);
Oxidize in potassium permanganate in a sulphuric acid medium and bleach in sodium bisulphite as for the other stain envisaged here;
Wash carefully (for at least five minutes) in running water;
Treat for one to three minutes with the solution

N, N' — diethylpseudo-isocyanine chloride .... 14.5 mg
distilled water .... 100 ml

Rinse in faintly ammoniacal water (2 drops of ammonia for 100 ml distilled water), mount in the rinsing liquid, photograph immediately in ultraviolet light.

The performic acid-alcian blue technique (Adams and Sloper, 1955), already described on p. 523, detects the neurosecretory product clearly in all cases where permanganic oxidation in an acid medium brings about the basophilia of this substance; the working technique given on pp. 524 should be supplemented, when the aim of the method is morphological, by a background staining with the alum lake of nuclear fast red, followed by washing in water and mounting in balsam. All the remarks made about the histochemical significance of the technique as a reaction of protein-bound sulphydryls are naturally valid in the case of the products of neurosecretion; I would mention in particular that permanganic oxidation in an acid medium leads to results which are in every respect comparable to those of performic or peracetic oxidation, so far as the staining of the neurosecretory product itself is concerned.

A modification of Ravetto's method using alcian blue-alcian yellow (Peute, *in* van de Kamer, 1966; Peute and van de Kamer, 1968) represents a notable enrichment of the technical possibilities, since the method in question allows the subdivision of the neurosecretory products which have become basophilic after permanganic oxidation, in respect of the coefficient of dissociation of the anionic groupings formed after oxidation. The reagents used are those of Ravetto (p. 437), with the difference that the alcian yellow is dissolved in a buffer of pH around 1, the alcian blue in a buffer of pH 2.5. The technique described is based on Peute and van de Kamer (1968).

Reagents:

buffer of pH 1.1: mix 50 ml of N/1 aqueous solution of sodium acetate, 70 ml of N sulphuric acid and 130 ml of distilled water;
buffer of pH 2.5: mix 50 ml of N/1 solution of sodium acetate, 25 ml of N sulphuric acid and 175 ml distilled water;
0.4 per cent solution of alcian yellow, freshly prepared, in the buffer of pH 1.1;
0.05 per cent solution of alcian blue, freshly prepared, in the buffer of pH 2.5;
solutions of potassium permanganate, sodium bisulphite, sulphuric acid as for staining with paraldehyde-fuchsin.

Working technique:

Paraffin wax sections, dewaxed, treated with collodion and hydrated;
Oxidize with potassium permanganate in the presence of sulphuric acid, bleach in sodium bisulphite, rinse in water as for the other stains in this section;
Stain for 30 minutes, at laboratory temperatures, in the alcian yellow solution;
Rinse in the buffer of pH 1.1;
Stain for 3 minutes, at laboratory temperatures, in the alcian blue solution;
Rinse in the buffer of pH 2.5;
Dehydrate, clear, mount in Canada balsam or a synthetic resin.

Of the acid groups which form after permanganic oxidation, those which result from the chemical transformation of protein-bound sulphydryls ($-HSO_3$) and which are dissociated at a very low pH are stained yellow, while those which result from the oxidation of hydroxyl and carbonyl groups and which are dissociated at a higher pH are stained blue. Thus a very clear evolution of the neurosecretory product from the original perikarya to the neurohaemal organs can be detected in the frog (van de Kamer, 1966) and in the pterygote insects (Gabe, 1967). We should mention that the adoption of Ravetto's technique (alcian blue at a low pH, alcian yellow at a higher pH) is not possible for *Rana*, since the initial blue stain disappears when the sections are being passed through the alcian yellow solution (Peute and van de Kamer, 1968); this technique on the other hand, gives good results in the case of pterygote insects (Gabe, 1967), so that it is possible to control the results by reversing the stains.

From a practical point of view, I advise that the technique described above should be supplemented by a nuclear stain of the alum lake of nuclear fast red, followed by washing in water before dehydration.

It is, moreover, appropriate to remark that many commercial samples of alcian yellow are only soluble in water to the extent of some 0.1%; such saturated solutions nevertheless give satisfactory results.

Some of the staining techniques which have just been described, in particular the paraldehyde-fuchsin and paraldehyde-thionin techniques, can be applied to **bulk staining** of whole tissue blocks, which are then preserved in a clearing medium or mounted in a synthetic resin. The first application of the method was due to Braak (1962); the publications of Oksche, Mautner and Farner (1964), Mautner (1964) and Dogra and Tandan (1964) clearly show the services it is capable of rendering. The technique involves the following stages.

As meticulous a dissection as is possible of the fresh tissue, fixation in Bouin's fluid;
Wash for a long time in several baths of 70 per cent and then 90 per cent alcohol; complete the dissection;
Oxidize in performic acid (p. 467) for 5 minutes to 8 hours, according to the size of the tissue blocks;
Wash in several changes of distilled water;
Wash in several changes of 70 per cent alcohol;

Stain with paraldehyde-fuchsin (acetified normal solution, p. 532) paraldehyde-thionin, or with a solution of Victoria Blue 4B prepared as follows:
: boil 4 g resorcin, 2 g Victoria Blue 4B and 0.2 g dextrin in 200 ml distilled water, add 25 ml of a 29 per cent (B.P. or its equivalent) solution of ferric chloride and keep it boiling for 3 minutes; filter, dry the precipitate, dissolve it in 400 ml of 70 per cent alcohol, add 4 ml concentrated hydrochloric acid and 6 g phenol, leave to mature for about a fortnight; in my own experience this technique, which we owe to Humberstone, gives very beautiful stains, but its selectivity is not superior to that of the two other techniques which we have just mentioned; The optimum time ranges from 5 minutes to 24 hours, according to the size of the tissue blocks; on the whole, longer periods of staining are needed for Victoria Blue than for the two other stains;

Wash first in 70 per cent alcohol, then in 96 per cent alcohol after staining with Victoria Blue; where necessary differentiate in hydrochloric alcohol after staining with paraldehyde fuchsin or paraldehyde thionin, then wash in alcohol as after staining with Victoria Blue;

Dehydrate in absolute alcohol, clear and preserve in a mixture of 5 volumes of methyl salicylate and one volume of benzyl-benzoate; when the size of the tissue blocks permits, mounting between slide and cover-slip in Canada balsam or a synthetic resin is obviously the best solution.

Among *histochemical techniques*, the test for PAS-positive compounds, and protein-bound sulphydryls by means of true histochemical reactions, the detection of indole groups and of proteins rich in tyrosine and arginine all represent the indispensable minimum for histological research on a neurosecretory product still unexplored from this point of view. The search for free lipids is likewise very advisable, but technically less easy than the reactions enumerated, since it can involve the cutting of frozen serial sections of the piece of tissue under examination. In my own experience, staining with luxol fast blue also provides, in a great many cases, very informative preparations. Naturally, it is essential to identify compounds capable of simulating a product of secretion (metabolites, chromolipoids, melanic pigments, etc...)

Any of the cytological and histochemical techniques may be suggested as research methods when neurosecretory cells are being studied.

RECOMMENDATIONS CONCERNING HISTOLOGICAL TECHNIQUES APPLIED TO THE STUDY OF THE NERVOUS SYSTEM

The recommendations concerning histological techniques vary greatly according to the work being carried out on the nervous system.

In a great many cases, the aim of this work is very precisely defined at the outset, and the choice of techniques does not call for any special commentary; anyone who wishes to study the cytoarchitectonic characteristics of a particular region of the encephalon will mainly be led to use techniques for the detection of Nissl bodies and, subordinately, neurofibril impregnations of tissue blocks; staining with methylene blue, neuro-fibril impregnations, Golgi's method and its variants as well as the osmium-iodide method should be used in preference for research on the peripheral nervous system; myelin methods are foremost in investigations devoted to the systematic study of a segment of the central nervous system of a vertebrate.

It is the choice between similar procedures which, in the cases just mentioned, presents the greatest technical difficulty. The different techniques for detecting Nissl bodies are, indeed, equally good and reasons of a practical nature should lead one to prefer gallocyanine staining and also Pischinger's method using methylene blue buffered at pH 4.6; the state of fixation of the material helps one to choose from among the myelin methods and I might mention, in this connection, the outstanding advantage of staining with luxol fast blue and also that of those histochemical methods which are bound fairly soon to take the place of stains derived from Weigert's stain. But it is in connection with neurofibril techniques that the choice is really difficult, since many procedures have been specially adapted by their authors to a precise end, and it may require long labour to perfect their application to other material.

Generally speaking, impregnations of blocks are preferable to those of sections in all cases where the detection of neurofibrils is the essential aim of the work. In this connection, the selectivity of reduced silver procedures is greater than that of techniques deriving from Bielschowsky's method, but the latter give finer details. Techniques for the impregnation of sections are, on the other hand, the best procedure when a single piece of tissue must provide information as varied as the arrangement of Nissl bodies in the perikarya, myelotectonics and the morphology of neurofibrils, or even of the neuroglia. Among the techniques intended for frozen sections, the Gros-Schultze technique and Schultze's soda technique are foremost; they are easier to adapt to different objects than other impregnations of neurofibrils on frozen sections. Among the techniques for the impregnation of paraffin wax sections, those of Tinel, Bodian and Holmes give excellent results when they have been suitably adjusted to the particular material being studied, but Palmgren's technique is undeniably the easiest to adapt to very diverse objects.

It is in connection with the study of the peripheral nervous system that the greatest technical difficulties most often arise. All impregnations of neurofibrils can, when it comes to the point, display grave lapses, with incomplete impregnations simulating the existence of nerve-endings; it is by cross-checking with several methods that the research worker succeeds in taking into account the interruption of the impregnation in the terminal parts of the courses of the axons. Histochemical techniques, such as the tests for acetylcholinesterase activity and staining of the neuroplasma, not yet capable of interpretation in chemical terms like the osmium-iodide method can turn out to be of great assistance; the method of impregnation of the neurofibrils with gold should be tried in such a case, and also the methylene blue method.

When the research worker has only one piece of tissue at his disposal and wishes to make the best possible use of it, the best solution, in my opinion, consists of deliberately sacrificing the study of the neuroglia by selective impregnations and adopting fixation in Bouin's fluid, which is, at the same time, a good preparation for certain impregnations of the neurofibrils (Tinel, Palmgren, Bodian), for the detection of Nissl bodies and for staining the myelin with luxol fast blue; the search for neurosecretory cells is also possible on paraffin wax sections taken from material fixed in this way and the application of general histological techniques does not, of course, present any problem. Sections laid out according to the technique described on p. 115 can be used for different methods, with cells in very close proximity to one another, even successive slices of the same cell, undergoing varied techniques, thus giving a truly synthetic view of the tissue.

In cases where shortage of material is not so acute, and the particular aim of the work does not demand silver impregnation of blocks, the adoption of the three fixatives recommended by Palmgren (1960, see p. 934) seems to me to be the best approach. It is on the sections taken from the block fixed in Carnoy's fluid that the test for Nissl bodies will take place; sections from the same block and from the one fixed in Bouin's fluid will be used for general histological study; the second of the fixatives will provide material for staining the myelin with luxol fast blue, and for the test for possible neurosecretory cells; the whole of the material will be used for adjusting the impregnation of the neurofibrils according to the techniques of Palmgren, Bodian and Tinel. Naturally the addition of a fixative in formalin, with cutting done by a freezing microtome, greatly enlarges the technical possibilities, and fixatives specially adapted to the detection of the neuroglia will be needed for the central nervous system of vertebrates.

I think it is useful to recall, in conclusion, that the care needed to dissect tissue rapidly and gently as mentioned in connection with other parts of the anatomy, is just as necessary in the case of the nervous system. The "anatomoclinical method", consisting of carrying out formalin fixing *in toto* and hardening the mass of tissue in formalin—not really cutting off the blocks until weeks, even months, later—is tantamount, in Bertrand's own words (1930) to deliberately sacrificing the histological examination. In that case it is a question of a compromise made necessary by the demands of clinical neurology and the rules governing autopsies, but which has clearly no place in histological research. The method I have just mentioned can be replaced profitably by perfusion of the fixative through a vascular canal in all cases where tissue blocks of reasonable dimensions cannot be immediately removed, and in cases where the need to respect anatomical connections makes it necessary for blocks of a certain size to be cut off.

All general methods and all cytological and histochemical techniques have their place in the histological study of the nervous system; the sad fate of studies on structures situated at the limit of the resolving power of the light microscope, carried out, as their authors admit, by means of metallic impregnations which do not show the cell boundaries, should stimulate histologists to have as much recourse as possible to the general methods of this discipline even when it is a question of examining such specialized cells as neurones.

CHAPTER 41

TECHNIQUES FOR THE HISTOLOGICAL STUDY OF SENSE ORGANS

The technical requirements of a histological study of the sense organs vary a good deal from one case to another. In fact, most of the sense organs of the invertebrates have only been studied by so-called general histological techniques and by the neurofibrillar methods, the methylene blue technique playing an important part in the identification of the constituents of invertebrate nerves; the general cytological techniques are the methods of choice in an analysis of details of the structure of the sense cells. In the present state of our knowledge, it does not seem possible to me to codify these techniques. Among the sensory organs of the vertebrates some, such as the tactile corpuscles, the taste buds and the olfactory mucosa, do not require any "special" technique for their histological examination and the paragraphs which are devoted to them represent a statement of the special requirements and not a description of the particular techniques. Certain precautions which are required at the time of fixation should, on the contrary, occupy a prominent position in the examination of the stato-acoustic organ and of the visual apparatus.

HISTOLOGICAL EXAMINATION OF THE TACTILE CORPUSCLES

The dissection of those regions of the integument which contain the tactile corpuscles should be subject to the same rules as for the dissection of the integument in general (see Chapter 31). I might mention that Meissner's corpuscles are particularly abundant in the dermal crests of the chiridia of mammals, and in particular in the digital pulp; the corpuscles of Herbst and of Grandry are abundant in the waxy cuticle of the duck's beak and in the palatine crests of numerous birds. The mesocolon and the pancreatic peritoneum of the cat, as well as the skin of the palm of the primates, are rich in the corpuscles of Vater-Pacini; the groin of the pig is one of the classical subjects in which to study Krause's corpuscles.

Fixation should be carried out with one of the fluids indicated in relation to the study of the integument in general when only topographical techniques are required by the programme of work; the requirements of the different cytological and histochemical techniques should be taken into account whenever the techniques in question have to be applied. Frozen sections or sections in paraffin wax or celloidin should be used where appropriate; to obtain preparations using postvital staining with methylene blue it is best to mount thick sections taken freehand after stabilising them by the methods due to Schabadasch or Bethe-Dogiel (see p. 911 for the general technical requirements).

Among the ***topographic stains,*** azan, single stage trichrome, variations on Masson's trichrome and the trichrome used by Ramon y Cajal give very clear preparations entirely suitable for the study of the general characteristics of the tactile corpuscles and the selective demonstration of their connective constituents. Nervous structures should be studied on frozen sections, treated by the method of Gros-Schultze (p. 921) or by the soda method of Schultze (p. 937); impregnation using the techniques of Bodian, Holmes or Palmgren also give quite beautiful preparations but it is the methylene blue technique which gives the best results for the general study of the cutaneous innervation; researches of Weddel's school (see in particular 1945, 1954, 1956) and the review of Miller and his co-workers (1961) clearly show the potential usefulness of this technique when it is judiciously associated with general histological techniques and with silver impregnation. The same comments hold good for the study of the free nerve endings of the skin.

HISTOLOGICAL EXAMINATION OF THE PITUITARY MUCOSA

The dissection of the pituitary mucosa should be undertaken with the same precautions as for the respiratory mucosa of the nasal fossae (see Chapter 38), ensuring that the zones to be fixed come into rapid contact with the liquid fixative. So long as the size of the pieces of tissue is not too great, fixation should be carried out together with the underlying bony zones, the removal of these latter being undertaken where necessary, on pieces of tissue fixed and partly dehydrated, by means of a very sharp knife. It is obviously essential to cut at the level of the periosteum so as to conserve the sub-epithelial layers of the mucosa.

When the objective is a study of the whole organ, ***fixation*** should be carried out by one of the so-called topographical mixtures. Bouin's fixative, or that of Halmi, or Heidenhain's Susa are entirely suitable and, moreover, they initiate decalcification which can be an advantage in cases where the cutting of the bony tissue which supports the mucosa is required by the investigator. Carnoy's fluid also preserves the structures very well and is a suitable preliminary for the study of the ribonucleins as well as that of carbohydrates rendered insoluble by alcoholic fixatives. Mixtures having a base of potassium bichromate and formalin are indicated in particular for strictly cytological studies and for the study of the cellular categories of the sub-epithelial layers of the mucosa. Any other method of fixation may become suitable in the course of cytological or histochemical investigations of the pituitary mucosa. *The preparation of the tissue pieces for section cutting*, and this process itself, pose no particular problem; embedding in celloidin should be reserved for tissue pieces of very large size, containing decalcified bony material, otherwise, paraffin wax embedding should be used, frozen sections being employed where the staining techniques or histochemical reactions require them.

Any of the **topographical stains**, in particular those which ensure a clear demonstration of the collagen fibres, are suitable for a study of the organ as a whole. The details of the structure of the sense cells and of the tissue which supports them appear very clearly after regressive staining using the lakes of haematoxylin, in particular when the material has been fixed so as to allow the chondriomes to be demonstrated; Altmann's fuchsin also gives very handsome preparations and the same remark holds good for Flemming's triple stain.

Among the **histochemical reactions**, those which ensure the identification of carbohydrates are particularly appropriate because they show, better than the older stains, the presence of mucocytes and they also permit us to classify the sub-epithelial glands on a more solid foundation than the older distinction of serous and mucous cells. It is appropriate to remark that the PAS technique associated with alcian blue staining or with the reaction in which ferric ions are captured (p. 413 and 410) gives very fine topographical preparations.

The *fibrillar structures* of the supporting cells may be demonstrated by the techniques described in Chapter 28.

Neurofibrillar techniques are obviously of vital interest in studies of the pituitary mucosa. Impregnation by Gros–Schultze's technique using frozen sections gives excellent results; impregnation by Ramon y Cajal's technique, using blocks of tissue, is also suitable, as are the techniques of Bodian, Holmes, and Palmgren. The beautiful nature of preparations obtained using the methylene blue technique has been emphasized by Krause (1923); according to this author the head of the Ovidae constitutes a particularly favourable material. In this particular case the technique consists of perfusing a sheep's head taken at the time of slaughter (the freshness of the material is an essential feature) using Ringer's solution warmed to body temperature, by placing a cannula in the carotid artery and following this with about 500 ml of a 1% methylene blue solution and then ligaturing the blood vessels. About 30 minutes after the ending of the perfusion, the nasal fossae are opened by means of a parasagittal saw cut, the upper bones are cut out and stabilisation is effected with ammonium molybdate. Freehand sections are cut according to the techniques indicated in the relevant paragraph of Chapter 40; according to Krause, it is possible to embed in paraffin, the bony pieces requiring removal at the time that the piece of tissue is passed into absolute alcohol.

Preparations made by the maceration and isolation of the tissue give a good idea of the form of the sense cells; the older technique of Ranvier (1872) has maintained all its original value. Fragments of the olfactive epithelium, freshly dissected, are treated for from 1 to 3 hours using 30% alcohol (p. 770), and then, for about a quarter of an hour, with a 1% aqueous solution of osmium tetroxide; they are then rinsed in distilled water and dissected under a binocular microscope; mounting should be carried out in glycerine or in any other medium miscisble with water.

THE HISTOLOGICAL EXAMINATION OF TASTE BUDS

Apart from the application of neurofibrillary techniques, the histological examination of the taste buds calls into play the same techniques as does that of the anterior part of the digestive tract (Chapter 37).

The distribution of these structures can be studied on serial sections, but it il often advantageous to have recourse to whole mounts of the macerated bucca. mucosa which has been stained in bulk; the technique was described on page 776s

Fixation for topographical examination calls for no special commentary; I would just mention that the fungiform, caliciform, and foliated papillae of the tongue represent the material of choice for studying taste buds. Material intended for the demonstration of the neurofibrils should be fixed by fluids which best serve the chosen techniques, whereas material intended for histochemical reactions should be treated according to the needs of such methods. Flemming's fluid, that of Regaud and that of Kolster are particularly suitable for the manufacture of cytological preparations.

The preparation of the material for section cutting gives rise to no particular problem; frozen sections or those in paraffin wax or in celloidin can be used according to the circumstances.

The topographical stains recommended for the study of the buccal mucosa (p. 865) are perfectly suitable for the analysis of the general characteristics of the taste buds; the structural details of the sense cells and of the supporting cells appear very clearly on preparations stained using ferric haematoxylin or using Flemming's triple stain, the material thus having been fixed. The demonstration of neurofibrils should be carried out using Gros-Schultze's technique on frozen sections, or by the techniques of Bodian, Holmes or Palmgren using paraffin wax sections; the detection of acetylcholinesterase activity will also cause the innervation of the taste buds to appear very clearly.

HISTOLOGICAL EXAMINATION OF THE VISUAL APPARATUS

It is particularly striking to notice the contrast between the paucity of technical works concerned with the visual apparatus of the invertebrates and the multiplicity of the procedures put forward for the examination of that of the vertebrates. In addition to neurofibrillar techniques, the authors of works on the invertebrate eye have mainly employed the so-called general histological techniques; depigmentation by one of the procedures mentioned on page 581 is appropriate in many cases; according to my personal observations, made in the course of other work, the techniques using luxol fast blue, PAS, and paraldehyde-fuchsin-single stage trichrome, preceded by permanganate oxidation (p. 965), give particularly advantageous preparations for the study of the whole organ; but we need hardly add that any other staining technique may be used.

Some excellent general reviews have been devoted to the histological examination of the visual apparatus of vertebrates; in particular I would mention those of Herzog (in Krause, 1926), Kolmer and Lauber (1936) and Rohen (1963). Polyak (1956, 1961) also includes in his papers very valuable technical material. Only the essential data have been retained here.

VITAL EXAMINATION OF THE VERTEBRATE EYE

The introduction of the ophthalmoscope (Gullstrand) and the development of this instrument marked a real turning point in the morphological examination of the eye; the same remark holds good for the vital examination of the cornea, using a microscope specially devised for this purpose by Abbe and by Koeppe. Any account of the techniques for using this apparatus would obviously be outside the scope of this work and the reader is referred to ophthalmological texts; we might remark, nevertheless, that the apparatus just mentioned has permitted the true vital observation of the corneal nerves, stained with methylene blue (Knüsel, 1923, Vogt, 1930).

HISTOLOGICAL EXAMINATION OF THE EYE AS A WHOLE

The anatomical constitution of the vertebrate eye and the consistency of certain of its parts, in particular of the sclerotic and of the crystalline lens, account for the difficulties of this examination. Only perfusion through the vascular system will secure a truly irreproachable *fixation;* it should be undertaken using the internal carotid or the primitive carotid whilst the external carotid is ligatured. Fixation by immersion, after a very careful dissection, should be used when perfusion cannot be practised.

Among the *liquid fixatives*, many authors recommend Zenker's fluid (p. 184) or Heidenhain's Susa (p. 182); Bouin's fluid and that of Duboscq-Brazil are also widely used, as is Regaud's fluid and that of Orth (p. 686). We should mention here two formulae particularly adapted to the fixation of the entire eyeball, namely that of Verhoeff (1926) and ot Szent-Györgyi (1914).

Verhoeff's procedure involves fixation in a mixture of 10 ml of commercial formalin, 48 ml of 96% alcohol, 36 ml of water, and a gram of picric acid dissolved in this fluid. The entire eyeball is immersed in the fixative for 48 hours and then dehydrated without any special washing, beginning with 70% alcohol, and embedded in celloidin; the conservation of the shape is perfect and the retina shows no tendency to become detached.

In Szent-Györgyi's technique, the entire eyeball is fixed for from 2 to 7 days, according to its size, in a mixture of 100 ml of a 4% aqueous solution of mercuric chloride, 125 ml of acetone, 5 ml of acetic acid and 40 ml of formalin, prepared immediately prior to use; at the end of this period, acetone is added to the mixture to the extent of 50 ml for every 100 ml of fixative and the tissue is allowed to remain in this mixture for from 1 to 4 days according to its size; dehydration is then carried out in acetone with anhydrous calcium chloride placed at the bottom of the receptacle in which the pieces of tissue are suspended; the material is prepared for embedding in celloidin by the usual baths of alcohol/ether.

The embedding of eyeballs fixed as a whole should be undertaken in celloidin; the penetration of the embedded mass of tissue is greatly facilitated by cutting two small round tangential incisions laterally, using a *very sharp* blade.

Only *topographic stains* are to be used in the cases envisaged here. When sections which are not stuck to slides are to be treated it is advisable to choose techniques which do not stain the included mass; van Gieson's (p. 204) haematoxylin-picro-fuchsin method and the methods and their variations which use picro-blue (Curtis, p. 206) are particularly to be commended. Naturally, any other general technique can be applied to sections adherent to slides, the included mass having been dissolved; I would particularly advise the allochrome method of Lillie (p. 400).

METHODS PARTICULARLY RECOMMENDED FOR THE STUDY OF DIFFERENT PARTS OF THE VISUAL APPARATUS

The palpebral apparatus and the eyelashes, should be studied by the techniques set out in relation to the study of the integument and of its annectant processes as well as of the connective tissue; the same is true for the *lachrymatory canals*. The study of the *lachrymatory glands* and other glandular formations, attached to the eye socket, would profit from the use of techniques set out in relation to the salivary glands; naturally, any of the cytological or histochemical techniques may be used in the study of these organs whose comparative histology is very poorly understood.

The cornea is properly preserved during fixation if the eyeball as a whole and this is in fact the working technique which all authors advise, except when we face the problem of demonstrating the corneal cells by gold impregnation. Nitration of the superficial epithelium is easily carried out using the technique indicated on p. 772; the posterior epithelium (Descemet's epithelium) may be isolated by prudent dissection ofter removal of the cornea and a very short fixation (about 12 minutes) using acetic corrosive sublimate or Flemming's solution.

The corneal connective tissue is characterised by its intense metachromasia after staining with thionine; it is evident that any of the techniques for the study of such tissue may be used; the PAS technique gives particularly spectacular preparations. Cleavage into lamellae can easily be undertaken after maceration with one of the liquids mentioned in Chapter 30.

The corneal cells are very well demonstrated by staining with ferric haematoxylin, this technique being capable of application to the cornea fixed *in toto*, using Bouin's fluid (Krause, 1924); cleavage into lamellae can be carried out after staining, dehydration and clearing in a benzenoid hydrocarbon. The lamellae also show up well after gold impregnation; Romeis (1948) is a strong advocate of Lowitt's technique (1875), which comprises the following stages.

- Treat the fresh piece of tissue for from 10 to 20 minutes with a mixture of one part of formic acid and two parts of distilled water; it becomes transparent;
- Place, without washing, in a 1% aqueous solution of gold chloride and leave the piece of tissue for from 15 to 60 minutes; it takes on a yellowish tint;
- Replace the tissue in the formic acid solution which was used in the first stage of the method, and leave it there, in darkness, for 24 hours;
- Wash in distilled water which should be frequently renewed;
- Begin dehydration using 70% alcohol;
- Dissociate into the thinnest lamellae obtainable, complete the dehydration and clear in a benzenoid hydrocarbon, then mount in Canada balsam or in a commercial synthetic resin.

This technique shows up, in favourable cases, the nerves and their endings as well as the corneal cells; it is applicable to the study of nerve endings in other tissues.

Bielschowsky's technique and its variants, in particular that of Gros-Schultze, are also entirely suitable for the examination of the corneal nerves; I should like to mention the possibility of a truly vital demonstration of the structures in question.

The sclerotic may be studied by all the techniques described for the histological examination of the connective tissue; cutting it into sections may necessitate a decalcification process, particularly in the case of birds.

The histological study of **the iris** involves topographical techniques as well as those which are useful for studying connective tissue; depigmentation is often useful; in addition to the procedures set out on p. 581 I would mention Kopsch's method (1928) which involves treating the sections, after they have been dewaxed and hydrated, with a mixture, which should be *prepared on the spot*, of equal parts of a 5% aqueous solution of calcium hypochlorite and a 1% aqueous solution of chromium trioxide. Depigmentation is generally complete in from 10 to 20 minutes, and the staining affinities of the tissues are very well preserved.

The choroid should be examined in most cases after depigmentation, which may be undertaken as for the iris; in addition to the topographical techniques and those which can be used for the study of the connective tissue, vascular injection is obviously much to be commended; it is after fixation by perfusion that the microscopic anatomy of the choroid is most satisfactorily preserved.

The crystalline lens may be of a consistency such that cutting it into sections is quite impossible; Herzog (1926) remarks that this is often the case in old teleosts. Fixation should be carried out using Heidenhain's Susa or with a mixture of one part of a saturated aqueous solution of corrosive sublimate and one part of a 1% aqueous solution of chloroplatinic acid together with two parts of distilled water, specially devised for this purpose by Rabl (1894); the eye as a whole is immersed in this fluid, and after 30 minutes cut across the equator and immersed in the fixative for 24 hours. The tissue is then directly dehydrated and embedded in celloidin; embedding in paraffin wax is only possible with young animals.

Among the *topographic stains*, the clearest pictures are given by Heidenhain's azan; the PAS reaction, whether or not associated with alcian blue staining, and the allochrome method of Lillie also give preparations which are excellent from the morphological point of view.

The fibres of Zinn's zone are very well demonstrated by any stains suitable for elastic tissue, as well as by Held's molybdic haematoxylin (see below); they show up very well after the PAS reaction.

The vitreous body should be examined on thick sections taken from eyeballs fixed as a whole; the injection of liquid fixative, which is often practised in order to obtain a better preservation of the retinal structures, seriously alters the disposition of the fibrous network. This network shows up in red after the PAS reaction, and in blue on preparations treated by the allochrome technique of Lillie; it does not stain with basic thiazins of the thionine type. Lyon blue (alcohol blue) confers a very clear blue colour on it. Staining with Held's molybdic haematoxylin (1909) was strongly advocated by the classical authors because of the clarity of the images and the absence of any stain taken up by the celloidin. The techniques mentioned above probably supercede Held's technique, but its use for staining the vitreous body, the basement membranes and the mucins have led it to figure in a large number of publications and it seems to me useful to give the *modus operandi* for purposes of the record.

The molybdic lake of haematoxylin is prepared by dissolving 1 g of this substance in 100 ml of 70% alcohol and adding an excess of molybdic acid (about 2.5 g); the suspension is allowed to mature, being stirred from time to time. The fluid goes blue in the early stages of maturation, and then turns black in 4 to 5 weeks; it is from this moment onwards that it may be used. Nevertheless, the best results are only obtained with solutions which have aged for one to two years.

In use, several drops of the solution whose preparation has just been described are added to distilled water (in general allow 3 drops for 50 ml); the liquid is filtered and the sections remain in it for 24 hours, at laboratory temperatures; they are then rinsed in distilled water which should be renewed two or three times, dehydrated, cleared and mounted. The nuclei, the striated muscle fibres and the bony tissue stain intensely blue, the erythrocytes black, and the collagen tissue grey-blue, sometimes with a reddish tint, the elastic fibres are violet as are certain mucins; the epithelial fibrils, the basement membranes, the eye-lashes and the acidophilic secretory granules show up very clearly. I presume that it is the lengthy maturation period of the staining lake which is to a large extent responsible for the abandonment of this technique by the great majority of modern authors.

The retina is only preserved satisfactorily on eyeballs fixed as a whole if the fixation has been carried out using perfusion techniques; the immediate opening of the sphere with the dissection of the required fragments is the technique of choice when the study of the retina alone is the objective, all the more so as the fixations needed differ according to the constituents whose demonstration is desired. In the case where any given retina cannot be examined by several different techniques it is best to cut the eye into two halves, one anterior and one posterior, to remove carefully part of the vitreous body from it and to immerse it in the fixative.

A topographical study would involve fixation in Bouin's fluid, Halmi's fluid or Heidenhain's Susa, or mixtures of the "Kaformacet" type (p. 184) or in the so-called cytological fixatives. Inclusion may be undertaken in paraffin wax except when very hard parts (crystalline lens, etc.) exist in the same block of tissue. Among the stains, Heidenhain's azan, ferric haematoxylin, the allochrome technique of Lillie, or the method using luxol fast blue give very revealing preparations; as Kolmer and Lauber (1936) have very justly commented, a good topographical study of the retina requires not only the exploration of sections perpendicular to the surface of the membrane but also the study of sections taken parallel to its surface.

Rhodopsin may be preserved on paraffin wax sections, after fixation by 2.5% chloroplatinic acid; when the dissection is carried out on an eye adapted to darkness, the orange colour of the external segments of the rods may be sufficiently intense clearly to demonstrate these structures on sections which have been simply dewaxed and mounted in Canada balsam. Karli's method was discussed on p. 483; despite the uncertainties which still surround its chemical mechanism, the morphological value of the preparations obtained in this way is great. As Lillie (1952) has commented, three *lipid pigments* exist in the retina; the first, which is localised in the acromeres, is well preserved on paraffin wax sections and may be detected by the PAS technique; the second, which is also localised in the acromeres, is less resistant than the first but is preserved on paraffin wax sections after fixation in fluids with a potassium bichromate base; it gives the reaction using Schiff's reagent and performic (or peracetic) acid; the third lipid, which is detectable using lysochromes and by staining with ferric haematoxylin, but which does not react, either with PAS or with performic acid-Schiff, exists in the ellipsoids where it is associated with a basic protein. The demonstration of *glycogen* results in an intense stain of the myoids which constitute the essential site of this polysaccharide in the retinal cells.

The nervous and neuroglial structures of the retina may be shown up by the technique set out in Chapter 40. Ramon y Cajal (1894), in the course of his monumental study of the retina, sets out the optimal conditions for silver chromate impregnation; the working technique which follows is recommended.

Immerse the posterior half of the eye, after removal of the vitreous body, in the mixture,
 a 3% aqueous solution of potassium bichromate .... 20 ml
 a 1% aqueous solution of osmium tetroxide .... 5 to 6 ml
 and leave it there for from one to two days;
Wipe carefully with absorbent paper;
Immerse for 24 hours in a 0.75% aqueous solution of silver nitrate;

Transfer directly, for 24 to 36 hours, into the mixture
    a 3% aqueous solution of potassium bichromate .... 20 ml
    a 1% aqueous solution of osmium tetroxide .... 2 to 3 ml
Wipe carefully with absorbent paper;
Immerse for from 24 to 48 hours in a 0.75% aqueous solution of silver nitrate;
Continue to treat the piece of tissue as in the original working technique specified in the rapid Golgi method (p. 916).

When impregnation using silver chromate is practised on fragments of the retina, it is of the greatest utility to clad the piece in gelatine (see p. 916).

Impregnation of blocks of tissue following Ramon y Cajal's technique (p. 927) also gives good results in the case of the retina, but the ease with which the different types of nerve cells can be demonstrated varies according to the species. Table 32, which is arranged according to the data of Romeis (1948), shows subjects which are particularly favourable within each category.

The methylene blue technique, when applied to the retina, gives very beautiful preparations; the working technique was set out by Dogiel (in Krause, 1926). Fragments of the retina, which should be dissected out rapidly, are moistened with a 0.2% aqueous solution of methylene blue, and kept in a damp atmosphere at 37°C or at laboratory temperatures, according to whether we are dealing with the eyes of homeotherms or of poikilotherms, for about 30 minutes; examination under the microscope allows us to examine the condition of the piece of tissue. Stabilisation and mounting are carried out according to the instructions given on p. 912.

Table 32. — SUBJECTS FAVOURABLE FOR THE SILVER IMPREGNATION OF THE TYPES OF CELLS IN THE RETINA
(according to the data of ROMEIS, 1948)

Cell type	*Species*
Multipolar cells (ganglion cells)	Rabbit, Guinea pig, Cat, Dog, Fowl.
Amacrine cells	Rabbit, Fowl.
Horizontal cells	Rabbit, Guinea pig, Cat, Dog.
Bipolar cells	Guinea pig.

HISTOLOGICAL EXAMINATION OF THE STATO-ACOUSTIC APPARATUS

The majority of authors have examined the statocysts of the invertebrates using topographical techniques alone, the methylene blue technique, impregnation with gold following Ranvier's method and neurofibrillar impregnation using ammoniacal silver complexes and reduced silver serve to show up their innervation. It would certainly be premature to attempt to codify the histological examination of these organs in the present state of our knowledge. I should comment that the techniques which have been set out above would benefit from supplementation using cytological techniques, notably those which are useful for demonstrating ciliatures on the one hand, and on the other hand by histochemical tests for calcium in the statolith or the statocones and by the demonstration of carbohydrate and protein constituents of their matrix.

The histological study of the stato-acoustic apparatus of the vertebrates, at the level of the light microscope, uses no staining technique particularly conceived for this objective, but the techniques used for fixing and embedding the inner ear are peculiar to this objective and should be set out in detail.

The outer ear, the middle ear and the specialised cutaneous glands attached to the external auditory meatus should be studied by the techniques described in relation to the histological examination of the integument, of the connective tissue and of cartilage.

Special precautions are essential when fixing **the inner ear;** only perfusion through the blood vessels will ensure an impeccable preservation of the structures in animals whose size exceeds that of the guinea pig, and even when using small rodents, such as are customarily used in physiological studies, the making of a very large and very careful incision prior to immersion in the liquid fixative is only a makeshift arrangement.

As Werner (1936) has commented, it is essential to carry out the perfusion with the liquid fixative at the body temperature of the animal; he advises the use of Wittmaack's fluid, prepared immediately prior to use by mixing 85 volumes of a 5% aqueous solution of potassium bichromate, 10 volumes of commercial formalin, 5 volumes of acetic acid and 100 volumes of distilled water. The block of tissue which is dissected after perfusion should be immersed in the same liquid and kept there for 24 hours in an oven at 37°C; the fluid should be renewed and fixation continued for 48 hours at laboratory temperatures. A bath consisting of a 4% aqueous solution of lithium sulphate, which should be continued for 24 hours, should precede a careful washing (for 24 hours in running water); the pieces of tissue should then be dehydrated and embedded in celloidin, decalcification with nitric acid being applied to the celloidin blocks (p. 246).

Romeis (1948) recommends treatment with formalin *in situ*, applying a catheter to the eustachian tube in cases where dissection cannot be undertaken immediately. Wittmaack (1906) advises that material derived from human autopsies and taken as rapidly as possible after death should be fixed for 6 to 8 weeks, at 37°C, in a mixture of 85 ml of 5% aqueous potassium bichromate solution, 10 ml of commercial formalin and 3 ml of acetic acid; the liquid need not be renewed during fixation and the tissue block does not require opening. It is then washed for 24 hours in running water prior to being cut up with a metal saw; it is then refixed for 3 to 4 weeks in a mixture of 85 ml of distilled water, 5 ml of acetic acid and 10 ml of formalin, then decalcified with nitric acid, washed for 24 hours in running water and then dehydrated, one of the semicircular canals and the cochlea being bared after passing through 70% alcohol; embedding should be carried out in celloidin.

Bulk staining of Corti's organ is possible after cold dissection and fixation, but it demands advanced training of the manipulator. Only *general methods* can be applied to pieces of tissue fixed without perfusion; ferric haematoxylin, azan, the PAS technique and techniques for the study of the ciliatures give very good results when the fixation has been correctly carried out; I might remark that it is practically impossible to avoid detaching the *membrana tectoria*. With material fixed in formalin it is preferable to use neurofibrillar impregnations, particularly using procedures derived from Bielschowsky's technique. It may be adviseable to cut frozen sections of material so fixed and to decalcify them using nitric acid.

CHAPTER 42

TECHNIQUES FOR THE HISTOLOGICAL STUDY OF ENDOCRINE GLANDS

A histological examination, when conducted solely using topographical methods, can afford serious presumptions in favour of the endocrine nature of an organ; the glandular appearance of the cells which constitute the parenchyma, the richness of vascularisation or the closeness of the relationships with the general cavity, depending on whether the circulatory system of the animal studied is closed or not, and lastly the absence of any excretory duct, represent the morphological characteristics of any endocrine gland. Data of this kind allowed A. Prenant (1899) to affirm the endocrine nature of the corpora lutea of the ovary at a time when no physiological argument favoured this interpretation; at a later date the moulting gland of the malacostracan Crustacea was identified in the same way (Gabe, 1953). Laguesse (1892) was able to take into account the histological characteristics of the islets of Langerhans and so to give a correct histophysiological interpretation of these formations scarcely four years after the first cases of experimental diabetes through surgical pancreatectomy had been obtained (von Mehring and Minkowsky, 1889).

Certain of the endocrine glands, techniques for the histological study of which should be discussed here, are in effect neurohaemal organs in the sense of current nomenclature, that is to say places where the secretory products and the hormones formed in the neurosecretory pericaryones are accumulated and stored, the endings of the axons which stem from these neurosecretory pericaryones being one of the essential features of the organs in question. We should include in this category the neurohypophysis, the urophysis and the rostral zone of the median eminence of the hypothalamus, the corpora cardiaca of insects, the sinus gland of the Crustacea, the cerebral gland of the chilopods and diplopods as well as the homologous organs in the Arachnida, in addition to the neurohaemal organs described in representatives of the old and heteroclite assemblage of the worms and in a few molluscs (see Gabe, 1966 for the bibliography).

Other endocrine glands are less closely linked with the nervous system and if we take into account the purely morphological data we should be led to divide them into two categories.

It happens that the activity of some of these glands does not give rise to the accumulation of secretory products in the morphological sense of the term, such as can be discerned under the light microscope. This is the case with the moulting gland of all the arthropods studied to date, of the androgen gland of the malacostracan Crustacea, of the corpora allata of insects and of the parathyroid gland of the vertebrates.

On the other hand the functioning of the other endocrine glands results in the accumulation of particulate substances. Into this third category we should place all the endocrine glands of vertebrates with the sole exception of the parathyroid gland.

TECHNIQUES FOR THE HISTOLOGICAL STUDY OF THE NEUROHAEMAL ORGANS

The technical features which dominate the histological study of the neurohaemal organs, and the pathways by which neurosecretory products reach them, are essentially the same as those which have been set out in Chapter 40 in relation to the histological study of the pericaryones.

Fixation using an aqueous mixture is preferable in all cases where the demonstration of the secretory product is to be undertaken as compared with alcoholic mixtures or with acetone. In fact, we know of a large number of neurosecretory products extracted from tissues or insufficiently denatured by alcoholic fixation whereas good preservation by alcoholic fixatives compared with losses in the case of the use of aqueous fixatives has never been suggested in any publication to which I have had access. Bouin's fluid and its variants, that of Halmi, and Heidenhain's Susa, are suitable in most cases, but there are examples of neurohaemal organs which compel us to have recourse to what are, properly speaking, cytological fixatives for a clear demonstration of the neurosecretory product; that is to say we have recourse to mixtures based on potassium bichromate and formalin and devoid of acetic acid. Only the existence, in the blocks of tissue, of very hard material could render *embedding in celloidin* necessary; *embedding in paraffin wax* is suitable in all other cases.

When choosing ***stains*** we should bear in mind the two possibilities envisaged on p. 963 in relation to the secretory products, these possibilities being the persistance of acidophilia despite permanganate oxidation or, on the other hand, the appearace of a basophilia following such an oxidation.

When, as a result of permanganate oxidation in an acid medium, the secretory product acquires no basophilia the so-called general methods, in particular those which assure a good demonstration of acidophilic structures, are the only ones which can be used for such studies. Azan, one step trichrome, Masson's trichrome and its variations, the method of Mann using methyl blue-eosin and that of Mann-Dominici, and techniques which use eosinates of azur are suitable in the majority of cases; no less advantageous are staining using neutral gentian violet and staining using Altmann's fuchsin provided that the material has undergone fixation appropriate to the use of these techniques.

On the other hand, when the neurosecretory product becomes basophilic after permanganate oxidation in a medium acidified with sulphuric acid or after oxidation with performic or peracetic acid—a frequent but not constant result—methods using chromic-haematoxylin-phloxin, paraldehyde-fuchsin, paraldehyde-thionin, or alcian blue, etc..., whose working techniques are described on p. 965 to 969 are the methods to choose, not only for a study of the axon pathways but also for that of the endings.

Tests for autonomic glandular cells and for secretory products differing from those which arrive at the neurohaemal organs by travelling along the axonal route should be practised in all cases. In fact, a distinct glandular activity involving the accumulation of a second secretory product frequently occurs in the case of the neurohaemal organs of arthropods. In cases where the neurosecretory product becomes basophilic after permanganate oxidation, what are subsequently to be shown as glandular cells and their secretory products often take up the acid background stain utilised in association with chromic-haematoxylin or with paraldehyde-fuchsin, thus ensuring their identification, but this eventuality may not come to pass and it may be necessary to put into effect a whole series of stains and of histochemical reactions to discover either the various dyestuffs affinities of the individual secretory products or the histochemical characteristics which would permit us to distinguish one from the other.

The nervous and neuroglial constituents of the neurohaemal organs should be studied by the techniques described in Chapter 40, the connective constituents being studied by those set out in Chapter 33.

The neurohypophysis and the median eminence of the vertebrates deserve particular mention because of their physiological interest and the multitude of publications devoted to them.

Fixation should be carried out using the mixtures indicated at the beginning of this section when the essential preoccupation of the investigator is the detection of the neurosecretory product. Nevertheless, when the objective of the study is neurofibrillar impregnation or impregnation of the neuroglia, special liquids should be used. In all cases rapid dissection of the tissue should be practised and whenever the dissection is likely to be lengthy perfusion through the blood vessels is to be commended. Embedding in celloidin is necessary only for very large pieces of tissue, the manufacture of paraffin wax sections or cutting on a freezing microtome being indicated for other cases.

So-called general methods suffice for anatomical studies; *vascular injection* may be useful in detailed studies on the irrigation of the organs, this being particularly true for the median eminence; in the course of anatomical studies on the hypothalamo-hypophyseal complex it is useful to know the total volume of the neurohypophysis which is determined by sketching the serial sections and then weighing the relevant outlines after cutting them out or by means of planimetry.

The demonstration of the neurosecretory product may be undertaken using the techniques set out below; the methods of Gros-Schultze, of Bodian and of Palmgren are particularly suitable for neurofibrillar impregnation. The pituicytes should be impregnated by del Rio Hortega's technique using silver carbonate, especially using the procedure intended for the detection of oligodendroglia; it may be necessary to resort to Penfield's variation when the essential requirements for fixation in the original procedure have not been respected. Romeis (1940) advises the following working technique to distinguish the pituicytes from connective elements or nerve fibres.

> Sections in paraffin wax taken from material fixed in Carnoy's fluid or in Bouin's fluid;
> Practise either silver impregnation of the neurofibrils or that of the reticulin; Bodian's technique, its variation due to Fitzgerald or Palmgren's technique are suitable in the first case, whereas Gomori's technique is suitable in the second;
> Wash for 30 minutes in running water;
> Stain for 5 minutes with the mixture
>
> | | |
> |---|---|
> | distilled water | 100 ml |
> | acid fuchsin | 2 g |
> | acetic acid | 1 ml |
>
> Rinse in distilled water;
> Treat for 5 minutes with a 1% aqueous solution of phosphomolybdic acid;
> Rinse in distilled water;
> Rinse in 1% acetic acid;
> Blot with absorbent paper;
> Dehydrate in absolute alcohol, clear in benzene and mount in a synthetic resin or in Canada balsam.

The nerve fibres or the connective fibres appear black, the pituicytes and their prolongations appear intensely red.

The concomitant demonstration of the nerve fibres in black, the pituicytes in violet and the connective tissue in blue may be obtained using azan staining, employing the technical conditions which Romeis (1940) described for the histological examination of the adenehypophysis, on sections which have undergone preliminary neurofibrillar impregnation.

TECHNIQUES FOR THE HISTOLOGICAL STUDY OF ENDOCRINE GLANDS WHOSE ACTIVITY DOES NOT GIVE RISE TO THE ACCUMULATION OF PARTICULAR SUBSTANCES

The absence of any apparent secretory product, which would give us a clue to the stages of the secretory cycle of the cells which make up the parenchyma of the endocrine glands falling into this category, severely limits the possibilities of a histological diagnosis and reduces the possible methods open to the investigator to general cytological techniques. Experience shows that criteria such as the size of the cells, the size and the morphology of the nuclei, do allow us to a certain extent to comprehend the functional condition of the cells in question, but we have indeed to recognise that the images so obtained provide much less information than in the case of the endocrine glands discussed in the following section.

The fixation of the organs should be subjected to the same rules as apply to other tissues; where tests for specific secretory products are lacking, the analysis of the nuclear structures and the general appearance of the cytoplasm should be borne in mind from the moment of dissection; the use of what are, properly speaking, cytological fixatives is not strictly necessary but all the manipulation preparatory to the section cutting and the section cutting itself should be conducted with all necessary care.

Any **topographical stain** will give a good delimitation of the cells and a proper study of the nuclei is appropriate; the use of selective stains for the connective tissue is to be commended in cases where the supporting web of the parenchyme is developed to a certain extent, its modifications giving some clues as to its functonal state. It is often important to undertake the measurement of the cells and of the nuclei by sketching them, followed by cutting around the outline and weighing the included paper, or better by planimetry; the general rules for the caryometric examination of cells should evidently be respected, but it would be outside the scope of this work to discuss them here.

The strictly cytological and histochemical study of the organs in question falls within the framework of research histology in the present state of our knowledge; it is not possible to codify the practices nor to indicate any method particularly valuable for the diagnosis of the functional condition and further progress in this matter will have to come from future work.

The parathyroid gland of vertebrates should receive special mention, not only because of its physiological interest but more particularly because its histological examination gives rather poor returns. So far as the diagnosis of the functional condition of this organ is concerned all the hopes founded on light microscopic techniques have been shown to be vain and only very general methods can be recommended for its histophysiological study.

The dissection of parathyroid glands may be difficult, as there is not always a very marked difference of colour or of consistency as compared with the lobes of adipose tissue; I might, moreover, mention the variability of its situation and the possibility of confusing it with lymph nodes. The inferior parathyroids of certain mammals, in particular of the rat and mouse, are included right inside the thyroid parenchyme and are impossible to separate from it by dissection; those of the dog are closely adpressed against the thyroid gland but can be identified by macroscopic examination because of their whitish tint.

Among the *fixatives*, Bouin's fluid or Halmi's fluid or Heidenhain's Susa preserve the general morphology quite well; fixation by mixtures with a potassium bichromate and formalin base are only rarely needed to distinguish the cellular types. It is, moreover, useful to bear in mind fixation using Carnoy's fluid to demonstrate the presence of glycogen and also the use of saline formalin or formaldehyde-calcium prior to examination for individual lipids.

Among the topographical techniques, azan, one step trichrome and the variations on Masson's trichrome distinguish the cell types clearly; glycogen should be investigated by the PAS technique using a malt diastase control, the lipids being shown up by staining with a lysochrome on frozen sections. It is only rarely useful to use mitochondrial stains, but these show up the oxyphilic cells with the greatest clarity; so far as the connective web is concerned, information furnished by preparations stained using general methods may be supplemented by silver impregnation of the reticulin using Gomori's technique (p. 813), fixation with Carnoy's fluid being an excellent preparation for this technique. I might mention how useful a caryometric study may be in any cases where the appearance of the parathyroid cells has not been seriously modified by the given experimental conditions.

TECHNIQUES FOR THE HISTOLOGICAL STUDY OF ENDOCRINE GLANDS WHOSE FUNCTIONING IS ACCOMPANIED BY THE ACCUMULATION OF SECRETORY PRODUCTS

All the endocrine glands of vertebrates, except for the parathyroid gland mentioned above, are characterised from the morphological point of view by the accumulation of individual secretory products whose demonstration is of capital importance when we need to identify the different cell types or to understand the functional condition of the organ. "Special" techniques have been described in large numbers for demonstrating the cell types of the adenohypophysis and of the endocrine pancreas; histochemical techniques, in particular those for the detection of lipids, have an important place in the study of the adrenal cortex of mammals and of the interrenal tissue of other vertebrates; the demonstration of catecholamines is one of the essential stages of the examination of the adreno-medulla of mammals and of the adrenal tissue of other vertebrates; the study of the endocrine part of the genital glands also benefits from a demonstration of individual lipids. So-called general methods and the PAS reaction allow us, in most cases, to obtain all the useful information from a histophysiological examination of the thyroid gland. To these glands we should add the epiphysis whose endocrine significance has been established by recent physiological and biochemical research although the histological study in no way provides us with information which can be used during a practical examination for diagnostic purposes.

A. — THE DISTAL LOBE OF THE ADENOHYPOPHYSIS

ANATOMICAL STUDY

The anatomical study of the distal lobe of the adenohypophysis and the analysis of its relationships with other constituent parts of the hypothalamo-hypophysial complex necessitate only a few technical comments.

Fixation, whether undertaken by immersion or by vascular perfusion, brings into play the so-called topographic stain mixtures; dissection prior to fixation is easy in certain cases (the Muridae, insectivores, certain carnivores, batracians) and more laborious in other cases (birds, reptiles, teleosts); it is contra-indicated in any case where parts of the hypophysis are embedded in bony or cartilagineous tissue forming the base of the skull (selacians, certain teleosts, etc...). Decalcification should be undertaken with nitric acid or trichloracetic acid; it is, for all practical purposes, never useful to embed in celloidin before undertaking this manoeuvre, but I would strongly recommend that the pieces of tissue should not be immersed in *the decalcifying* fluid until they have been partially dehydrated through passage into 96% alcohol. *Paraffin wax embedding* is the method of choice except when the pieces of tissue are very large in size.

Topographical stains are evidently adequate to distinguish the different lobes of the hypophysis; Heidenhain's azan gives spectacular preparations, but the passage into an azocarmine solution, warmed to 60°C, entrains a serious risk of unsticking the sections, particularly when bony or cartilagineous tissue has been cut together with the hypophysis; it may be prudent to content oneself in the latter case with one step trichrome or with a variant of Masson's trichrome, with Mann's method or with that of Mann-Dominici. The relative volumes of the different lobes may be determined by sketching them, followed by cutting out around the outlines or by planimetry of the serial sections; the number of sections requiring to be sketched in the series obviously depends on the size of the organ and on its anatomical peculiarities; sagittal sections are the most favourable for this sort of work. *The vascularisation* of the hypophysis whose physiological importance is too well known to need mention here may be studied on stained sections simply by topographic methods, but vascular injection is very useful in doubtful cases.

IDENTIFICATION OF THE CELLULAR CATEGORIES

The identification of the cellular categories of the distal lobe, unlike the anatomical study, poses difficult technical problems; a reading of recent studies, in particular the reviews of Herlant (1963, 1965), and Purves (1961, 1965), and of the proceedings of an international colloquium of the C.N.R.S. devoted to this question (colloquium no. 128, 1963) clearly illustrates the confusion which reigns over the nomenclature of the adenohypophysial cells and the present author finds it all the easier to admit that the effort to standardize the nomenclature undertaken by an international committee was unsuccessful, because he himself formed part of the committee in question. We know from the report edited by its president, P.G.W.J. van Oordt (1965) that agreement was attained so far as the functional nomenclature was concerned; seven cellular types correspond to the seven hormones produced by the organ; six of these cellular types exist in the distal lobe of species whose pars intermedia persists in the adult, whereas all seven may be looked for in the pars distalis when the intermediate lobe is absent or vestigial. These cellular categories are known by the names of the hormones which they secrete. But to collate the functional nomenclature and the morphological types described in innumerable investigations from preparations made by techniques which it is almost impossible to reduce to a single common denominator would be a superhuman task, all the more so because only further experiments could lead to absolute certainty in the choice of a functional name, such experimentation being impracticable in a large number of cases. The incredible confusion which has marked—and still marks—the development of our knowledge of the human adenohypophysial cytology clearly illustrates the desperate nature of the situation and we may well ask ourselves to what extent the total abandonment of all older morphological nomenclatures would not represent the most reasonable attitude. Because the use of Greek letters was introduced into the morphological nomenclature of the adenohypophysial cells by Romeis (1940) a table of their equivalences with the functional nomenclature is presented here (Table 33), but it should be clearly understood, nevertheless, that this is only a very rough first approximation, one and the same Greek letter being liable to designate different cell types in successive works by any given author.

Table 33. — Approximate equivalents of the functional names and designation by greek letters in the cytology of the adenohypophysis

Functional name	Greek letter	Observations
Somatotropic	α	Classical acidophils
Lactotropic	η	The distinction between lactotropic and corticotropic
Corticotropic	ε	cells has only been made in recent publications
Gonadotropic FSH	β	Classical basophils
Gonadotropic LH	γ	Corresponding, according to circumstances, to basophils or acidophils of the old nomenclature.
Thyrotropic	δ	
Melanotropic	—	Localised either in the pars distalis, or in the pars intermedia; are represented, in the human hypophysis, by the β cells of Romeis (1940).

I should like to draw attention, in passing, to the opportunity which presents itself of finally abandoning the terms "acidophil" and "basophil" to designate the two groups of "chromophil" cells of the distal lobe of the adenohypophysis; much more appropriate would be the names "erythrophil" and "cyanophil" (see p. 335).

In *fixing* the adenohypophysis for the identification of the cellular types speed is essential, as it is for any glandular parenchyme; the secretory granules of the adenohypophysial cells are very sensitive to postmortem autolysis although they are not as fragile as the chondriosomes.

The choice of fixatives merits particular attention; in spite of the diversity of the mixtures which are used, there is agreement as to the suitability of fixation by liquids containing mercuric chloride, the principal advantage being not so much better preservation of the secretory granules but a better preparation for certain of the stains which play an essential part in this kind of research. Most Anglo-saxon authors use mixtures of corrosive sublimate and formalin; many European authors prefer Gérard's liquid (p. 181); Halmi's fluid and Heidenhain's Susa are equally very suitable; even material fixed in Bouin's fluid may give satisfactory preparations. Fixation in formalin is not to be recommended although fixation in mixtures of formalin and potassium bichromate can be very useful in certain instances. The harmful nature of acetic acid and more particularly of the acetyl ion has been taken up several times by Racadot, but the views of this author are not shared by the majority of specialists in adenohypophysial cytology and my personal experience, does not permit me to sustain them at least so far as the post-foetal stages of vertebrate life are concerned.

The total elimination of bony tissue at the time of the dissection of the hypophysis is not indispensable and experience shows that well fixed tissue will withstand *decalcification* by trichloracetic acid for a reasonable period without coming to any harm.

Embedding should be undertaken in paraffin wax; the *sections* should be fine (5 μ at the maximum); most authors advise that they should be frontally oriented in cases where the programme of study requires a description of the zones of the adenohypophysial parenchyme or of the predominance in certain zones of certain cellular categories.

Staining

Staining which is devoid of chemical significance, marker staining, and histochemical reactions can be used for the distinction of the cellular categories of the distal lobe of the adenohypophysis on sections. A complete list of the techniques suitable for use with each group would be very long and only the essential methods can be given space here. During this identification the general morphological characters of the cells must evidently be taken into consideration but we shall not try to describe this process here.

Among the *staining* techniques there are some which have been widely used by the classical investigators in the subject and which may still at the present time be of service for the histological study of the adenohypophysis; these techniques include in particular that of Mann using methyl blue-eosin, Heidenhain's azan, one step trichrome, and Masson's trichrome together with its variations. The working techniques were described in the second part of this work and obviously we do not need to repeat them. The older staining techniques of Kraus (1912) for the demonstration of erythrophil cells, the technique of Erdheim and Stumme (1909) for the demonstration of cyanophil cells together with the techniques of Severinghaus (1932), Berblinger and Burgdorf (1935), and Wallraff (1939) have all been rendered out of date by improved techniques and the reader is referred to the reviews of Romeis (1940, 1948) for their description. On the other hand, the methods of Cleveland, Rucker and Wolfe (1932), Romeis' cresazan (1940) and Herlant's tetrachrome (1960) are freely used by modern authors and it is essential to describe them.

*a) **The technique of Cleveland, Rucker and Wolfe**.* — In the original specification the technique was executed on paraffin wax sections taken from material fixed in Regaud's fluid and postchromated, but satisfactory results can be obtained after fixation in one of the fluids mentioned below and without passage through potassium bichromate. Among the different formulae which have been put forward for the execution of this technique I would recommend that of Herlant (1956).

Paraffin wax sections, taken from material fixed in Gerard's fluid, Halmi's fluid or Heidenhain's Susa or, if necessary, Bouin's fluid, dewaxed, treated with collodion and hydrated;

Stain the nuclei in Groat's haematoxylin, avoiding any overstaining (use fairly fresh solutions and adjust the time the sections remain in the staining bath appropriately);

Wash for from 2 to 5 minutes in running water;

Stain for from 5 to 10 minutes (the optimum time to be determined by trial and error) with a 1% aqueous solution of erythrosin;

Rinse in distilled water;

Treat for from 1 to 3 minutes (the optimum time to be determined by trial and error) with the mixture

distilled water	100 ml
orange G	2 g
phosphomolybdic acid	1 g

Rinse *rapidly* in distilled water (it is often advisable simply to blot with absorbent paper);

Stain for from 1 to 5 minutes with the mixture

distilled water	100 ml
acetic acid	1 ml
aniline blue	0.5 to 1 g

Rinse very rapidly in distilled water, dehydrate in absolute alcohol, clear in a benzenoid hydrocarbon and mount in a synthetic resin or in Canada balsam.

The results are set out in Table 34: among the factors which lead to successful staining we may in particular mention the freshness of the reagents, which should never be prepared in advance in too large quantities, the quality of the commercial sample of erythrosin (it may be advisable to replace erythrosin with phloxin which is of more consistent quality from one lot to another) and that of the phosphomolybdic acid.

b) Romeis' cresazan. — This technique affords truly spectacular preparations, but it includes a certain number of trivial stages and the interpretation of the results may be rendered difficult by the fact that affinity for fuchsin-resorcin does not correspond, as used to be believed, to an affinity for paraldehyde-fuchsin or paraldehyde-thionin, even though these three stains demonstrate the presence of elastic tissue in a highly selective fashion (I might remark that the terms fuchsin-resorcin, cresofuchsin and fuchselin are synonymous). The poor keeping qualities of solutions of fuchsin-resorcin and the impossibility of predicting exactly the duration required for staining also explains the relative lack of confidence now placed in this technique.

Paraffin wax sections, taken from material fixed under the same conditions as for the method of Cleveland and his collaborators, dewaxed (treatment with collodion is possible but one should pay the greatest care and attention to the thinness of the covering) and taken into 80% alcohol;

Stain with a freshly prepared solution of fuchsin-resorcin (p. 819) until the β cells are intensely stained blue-black or brown-black; after rapid rinsing in 80% alcohol the sections should be periodically examined under the low power of the microscope, the time taken to secure a stain running from one hour to one night;

Differentiate in 3 baths of 96% alcohol until the background is totally clarified, the β cells and the elastic fibres alone being coloured; the last alcoholic bath should be prolonged, whatever the duration of the first two may have been, for 15 minutes;
Treat for 15 minutes, at laboratory temperatures, using aniline in alcohol (0.1% or 1%, see p. 220);
Stain for 1 hour with azocarmine G, in an oven at 60°C, as in Heidenhain's technique (see p. 220);
Differentiate in a solution of aniline in alcohol until the α cells appear quite clearly;
Treat with acetic alcohol as in Heidenhain's technique (p. 220);
Rinse rapidly in distilled water;
Treat for about 5 minutes with a mixture of orange G-phosphomolybdic acid-distilled water as used by Cleveland and his collaborators;
Blot with absorbent paper;
Treat for from 20 to 40 minutes with the mixture
  distilled water .... 100 ml
  aniline blue .... 0.5 g
  boil, allow to cool, add 8 ml of acetic acid and dilute with 2 volumes of distilled water;
Rinse rapidly in distilled water;
Destain the background using 96% alcohol (this stage often serves no useful purpose)
Dehydrate in absolute alcohol, clear in a benzenoid hydrocarbon and mount in Canada balsam or in a synthetic resin.

The results are set out in Table 34. Examination of the magnificent pictures which illustrate Romeis' monograph (1940) shows that the nuclei, under the working conditions in which the author of the method carried it out, take on a colour which differs from that using Heidenhain's azan, the cresofuchsin participating in their staining. The passage of the sections, stained with cresofuchsin differentiated in alcohol, into a solution of aniline in alcohol has the objective of rendering the tissues alkaline and suppressing the unfortunate effects on the uptake of azocarmine which would result from a preliminary passage through a liquid of a pH as low as the solution of cresofuchsin.

Experience shows that this technique, carried out without the staining using cresofuchsin, and the differenciation of the stain in alcohol, furnishes preparations which are even more striking than those given by Heidenhain's azan, and I wonder whether this "Romeis' azan" should not replace the original working technique used by Heidenhain for most purposes, all the more so because the time for its execution is shorter. From my own experience, Romeis' azan is admirably suitable as a background stain after paraldehyde-fuchsin has been used, the significance of the uptake of this latter stain by certain categories of adenohypophysial cells evidently being different from that relating to the affinity for cresofuchsin.

c) Herlant's tetrachrome. — Though considered by its author as being a technique derived from that of Petersen (1924) this method is in fact a quite original procedure which gives not only excellent differentiation of the cellular categories of the distal lobe of the adenohypophysis but also magnificent topographical preparations which are very useful for the histological study of a large number of tissues and organs. Its adoption as a general method seems to me highly desirable; naturally, Herlant's tetrachrome has this in common with Heidenhain's azan, one step trichrome, Petersen's stain and the "quad" of Kornhauser, that it is extremely demanding so far as the quality of fixation is concerned. Only material which has been freshly dissected and properly fixed allows one to be sure of good results.

> Paraffin wax sections, fixed as for the two preceding techniques, dewaxed, treated with collodion and hydrated;
> Stain for 10 minutes with a 1% aqueous solution of erythrosine (Racadot advises the acidification of the solution with 1 or 2 drops of acetic acid for every 100 ml); from my personal experience, erythrosine may be replaced by phloxin;
> Rinse rapidly in distilled water;
> Stain for from 5 to 10 minutes with aniline blue-orange G-acetic acid, as used by Mallory
>
> | | |
> |---|---|
> | aniline blue | 0.5 g |
> | orange G | 2 g |
> | distilled water | 100 ml |
> | acetic acid | 2 ml |
>
> this stain may be replaced, as my personal observations show, with the customary but diluted solution of aniline blue-orange G of Heidenhain, especially when the experimenter opts for the longest periods in the staining baths;
> Rinse rapidly in distilled water;
> Stain for 10 minutes with the aluminium lake of acid alizarin blue, prepared according to the prescription of Petersen (p. 225);
> Rinse rapidly in distilled water;
> Treat for from 5 to 10 minutes (I would advise the adoption of the second period in preference to the first) with a 5% aqueous solution of phosphomolybdic acid;
> Rinse rapidly in distilled water;
> Where appropriate, extract the excess erythrosine by rapid passage of the sections into 70% alcohol (this stage is not always indispensable);
> Dehydrate with absolute alcohol, clear in a benzenoid hydrocarbon and mount in Canada balsam or in a synthetic resin.

The results are given in Table 34. As I noted on p. 225, treatment with phosphomolybdic acid has the effect of changing the colour obtained using the aluminium lake of acid alizarine blue into a bluish violet; treatment with phosphotungstic acid causes this colour to become red, and is not suitable for the purposes we have in mind here, so that the two acids are not interchangeable. I should like to remark that the use of a fresh solution of phosphomolybdic acid, prepared from a chemically pure sample which has not been hydrated in contact with air, is one of the essential factors for success and that acid alizarine blue is not synonymous with alizarine blue S.

Histochemical Reactions

Among the histochemical reactions the metachromatic reaction using toluidine blue has a certain historical interest because it provided the first histochemical arguments in favour of the secretion of gonadotropic hormones in the cyanophil cells of the adenohypophysis (Herlant, 1943); the appearance of the preparations is particularly clear after fixation using Regaud's fluid, otherwise the working technique does not present any special features (see p. 346);

Table 34. — An indication of the Tinctorial Affinities and the Histochemical Characteristics of the Cell Types of the Distal Lobe of the Adenohypophysis; All specific peculiarities are not considered
(After Gabe, 1962)

Techniques	Delta	Beta	Gamma	Alpha	Epsilon-eta
Mann biacid	Bright Blue	Deep Blue	Violet to Red	Red	Red
Azan (Heidenhain)	Bright Blue	Deep Blue	Mauve to Red	Red	Orange
Cleveland-Wolfe	Sky Blue	Deep Blue	Purple	Orange	Pink
Berblinger-Burgdorf	Blue	Dark Violet	Mauve	Orange	Orange
Kresazan (Romeis)	Cobalt Blue	Violet	Mauve to Red	Red	Orange
One-step trichrome (Gabe and Mme Martoja 1967)	Bright Green	Deep Green	Grey to Red	Red	Red
Herlant	Deep Blue	Blue	Violet	Orange	Red
PAS	+++	++	+++ to 0	0	0
PAS + acid dye (orange G, naphthol yellow)	Violet	Mauve or Red	Brick or Yellow	Yellow	Yellow
Metachromasia	+	+	0	0	0
PAF and One-step trichrome	+++ Violet	± or + Blue-Green	0 to +++ Pink to Violet	0 Red	0 Pink
Elftman (1959)	Violet	Red	Red to 0	0	0
Paget and Eccleston (1960)	Blue-Black	Violet	Violet to 0	Blue-Green	?
Adams and Sloper	+++	++	0	0	0
DDD Neotetrazolium	0	±	+++	++	++
Tetrazo reaction (Danielli)	0	+	0	+	?
Indole groups	0	++	0	+	?
Acylamidocarboxylic groups	0	0	0	+	?
Sudan Black B	0	0	0	+	?
Acid Haematin (Baker)	0	0	0	+	?
Luxol Fast Blue	0	0	0	+	?

PAS = Periodic acid-Schiff reaction; PAF—Paraldehyde-Fuchsin stain; Elftman = Fuchsin stain—paraldehyde—PAS: Paget and Eccleston = staining with thionine-paraldehyde—PAS—Luxol Fast Blue; Adams+Sloper = staining with Alcian blue at a low pH after performic oxidation: DDD neotetrazolium = reaction of sulphydrylated proteins after Barrnett & Seligman (1952) and after Gomori 1956; Indolic groups = reaction of indolic nuclei after Glenner & Lillie 1957; Acylamidocarboxylic groups = Barrnett & Seligman technique 1958: Herlant = staining with erythrosine—Heidenhain blue—alizarin acid blue—phosphomolybdic acid after Herlant (1960).

however, this way of discerning, on sections, those cells which secrete glycoproteinaceous hormones is distinctly less advantageous than the *PAS reaction* whose introduction into research on the adenohypophysial cytology (Catchpole, 1948; Pearse, 1949; Herlant, 1950) marked a veritable turning point in the development of our knowledge of this organ.

The practice of the PAS reaction itself calls for no special comment arising from its application to the hypophysis, but it may be associated with other histochemical reactions or with diagnostic stains. Among the simplest of these procedures, I would enthusiastically advise Herlant's technique (1950, 1956) which consists of associating the PAS reaction, a nuclear stain using Groat's haematoxylin and staining of the erythrophil cells using the orange G-phosphomolybdic acid of Cleveland and his collaborators; other and more complex variations are described in the following section; Herlant's working technique is described on p. 400; the results are set out in Table 34 under the heading PAS + acid stain.

Tests for protein-bound sulphydriles using the technique set out on p. 517 to 531 disclose erythrophilic cells in the distal lobe of the adenohypophysis; a strong reactivity of the γ cells exists in certain cases and even the β cells may react weakly. The only cellular category which is negative under all circumstances is represented by the δ cells. *Danielli's coupled tetrazonium reaction* causes the β cells to appear in a highly selective fashion; these elements are rich in indole groups; tests for acylamidocarboxyl groups (p. 493) result in the demonstration of the presence of "acidophil" cells as does Baker's method using acid haematin (p. 469).

Marker stains

Marker stains, in Lison's (1953) sense of the term, whether used alone or associated with other methods, have an essential part to play in modern research on adenohypophysial cytology.

a) **Staining with naphthol yellow S,** whose advantages were discussed in relation to the histochemical demonstration of acidophilia of the tissue constituents (p. 333), has been suggested as a replacement for that of orange G, in association with the PAS reaction; the results are better and the working technique is simple, naphthol yellow at a concentration of 1% replacing orange G in the stain used by Cleveland and his collaborators, as shown on p. 400 and 996.

b) **Staining with lead haematoxylin** using the technique of MacConaill (p. 910) has been applied to the staining of the adenohypophysial cells using the same techniques as were used to demonstrate nerve fibres (Stahl, 1958; Olivereau, 1964; Carlon, 1966, 1967). Erythrophil cells are shown up in a highly selective fashion in teleosts and Olivereau considers that these are corticotropic cells, however, in the dog, the gonadotropic LH cells are the only ones to stain by this technique (Carlon, 1966, 1967).

It is, however, methods which use paraldehyde-fuchsin, paraldehyde-thionin and alcian blue which are the most important.

c) **Paraldehyde-fuchsin** has been used for the staining of adenohypophysial cells using various working techniques and it is appropriate to emphasize, as did Purves (1961, 1965), that certain differences in the results obtained will necessarily follow. For the preparation of this stain certain authors use the original method of Gomori (p. 350), others use stabilisation by synthesis in an aqueous medium (Gabe, 1953); in the first case acidification is secured by the use of hydrochloric acid and in the second using acetic acid, and the proportion of dye used is also different in the two formulae. Moreover, pretreatment plays an essential part; some authors use oxidation of the sections with Lugol's fluid, such as Gomori (1950) recommended, whereas others use potassium permanganate in an acid medium, which represents a second source of disagreement between their results. It seems essential, to me, that the preparation of the paraldehyde-fuchsin and the technique used for oxidation should figure in the working technique of the variations given below, even at the risk of adding to the length of these descriptions.

The paraldehyde-fuchsin-trichrome of Gomori (Halmi, 1952):

Paraffin wax sections, taken from material fixed as for the techniques described above, dewaxed, treated with collodion and hydrated;
Oxidise for 1 minute with a mixture of equal parts of a 0.03% solution of potassium permanganate and sulphuric acid at the same concentration;
Rinse in tap water;
Bleach with a 2% aqueous solution of sodium metabisulphite;
Rinse in tap water;
Stain for 5 to 10 minutes with the original paraldehyde-fuchsin solution of Gomori, prepared more than 3 days and less than 5 days previously;
Rinse in 3 baths of 96% alcohol; leave the slides in the last bath for about 10 minutes;
Rinse in tap water;
Stain the nuclei with haemalum;
Wash for from 2 to 5 minutes in tap water;
Stain from 1 to 2 minutes using the mixture

light green	0.4 g
chromotrope 2R	0.5 g
orange G	1 g
phosphotungstic acid	0.5 g
distilled water	100 ml
acetic acid	1 ml

Rinse in 1% acetic acid;
Dehydrate using 96% alcohol and then absolute alcohol, clear in a benzenoid hydrocarbon and mount in a synthetic resin or in Canada balsam.

Under such technical conditions, the secretory granules of the cells described as β cells by Halmi (1952) but which in fact correspond to the thyreotrope (δ) cells are the only ones to be stained purple; the erythrophil stains become orange, the gonadotropic cells green, the nuclei become a brownish-red.

Oxidation using a very dilute permanganate solution, which figures in this formula, may be replaced by keeping the sections in Lugol's fluid for 1 to 2 hours, followed by destaining using sodium hyposulphite; I might remark in passing that rapid treatment with Lugol's fluid, which is an obligatory stage in the preparation for staining after any mercuric fixation, has no effect whatsoever on the affinity of the tissues for paraldehyde-fuchsin.

The paraldehyde-fuchsin-Groat's haematoxylin picro-indigocarmine (Gabe, 1953) or orange G (Herlant, 1956). — Oxidation is carried out using potassium permanganate in a sulphuric acid medium, the concentrations being the same as for the demonstration of the hypothalamic neurosecretory product; staining is carried out using the stable, diluted and acidified solution (p. 351). Under such conditions, the thyreotropic and gonadotropic FSH cells take on a violet colour, the gonadotropic LH cells being either unstained or stained according to the species. The working technique includes the following stages.

Paraffin wax sections, dewaxed, treated with collodion where appropriate and hydrated;
Oxidise using the potassium permanganate sulphuric acid mixture of Gomori, as for the preparation for staining using chromic-haematoxylin phloxin; the average time for the oxidation varies around about 1 minute; the sections should take on a rather deep tobacco colour;
Rinse in tap water;
Destain using a 2-5% aqueous solution of sodium bisulphite;
Rinse in tap water;
Stain for 2 to 5 minutes using the diluted and acetified stock solution of paraldehyde-fuchsin;
Rinse in tap water;
Where appropriate, clear the background using absolute alcohol to which 0.5% of concentrated hydrochloric acid has been added;
Wash in tap water;
Stain the nuclei using Groat's haematoxylin;
Wash for from 2 to 5 minutes in tap water;
Stain the background using picro-indigocarmine or a 1% aqueous solution of orange G;
Dehydrate in absolute alcohol, clear in a benzenoid hydrocarbon and mount in Canada balsam or in a synthetic resin.

The behaviour of the cyanophil cells has been noted above; the erythrophil cells take on a pale yellow colour with the picro-indigocarmine, the yellow being much clearer if orange G has been used as a background stain.

Paraldehyde-fuchsin-one step trichrome (Gabe and Mme Martoja, 1957). — The working technique has been described in relation to the demonstration of the hypothalamic neurosecretory product (p. 965), the results being given in Table 34. Permanganate oxidation should be conducted as in the preceding variation so that the thyreotropic cells, the gonadotropic FSH cells and, where appropriate, the gonadotropic LH cells stain with paraldehyde-fuchsin, but in the case of the gonadotropic FSH cells the affinity for light green overlays the paraldehyde-fuchsin stain so that there is a clearer contrast with the background as after haematoxylin background staining.

PAS-paraldehyde-fuchsin (Elftman, 1959). The original feature of this technique rests in its abandonment of any oxidation of the sections but fixation is carried out using a liquid which has chrome alum as its basis.

> Fix for 1 night (a period of 48 hours in the fixative has no ill-effects) using the mixture, which should be prepared immediately prior to use—
> a 5% aqueous solution of mercuric chloride .... 100 ml
> chrome alum .... 5 g
> commercial formalin .... 5 ml
> Dehydrate without any special washing, embed in paraffin wax and cut into thin sections;
> The dewaxed sections, treated with collodion and hydrated;
> Stain for 30 minutes to 1 hour with a paraldehyde-fuchsin solution prepared by mixing 100 ml of a 0.5% solution of basic fuchsin in 70% alcohol, 0.75 ml of paraldehyde and 1.25 ml of concentrated hydrochloric acid; the higher content of hydrochloric acid as compared with Gomori's formula is considered to be very important; it takes 3 days for the solution to mature, at laboratory temperatures, and 26 hours at 37°C; the stain does not keep for much beyond 1 week;
> Rinse in 95% alcohol, acidified where necessary to decolourise the background;
> Employ the PAS reaction and wash for a long time in running water;
> Stain the erythrophil cells with a 3% solution (?) of orange G, which should be brought to a pH of 2 using hydrochloric acid;
> Rinse rapidly in tap water, dehydrate, clear and mount in Canada balsam or in a synthetic resin.

Under these technical conditions, the thyreotropic cells stain violet-purple, the gonadotropic cells red (with colour differences corresponding to the two categories), and the erythrophil cells in yellow. It is appropriate to mention that Elftman recommended a "sensitised" Schiff's reagent for the PAS reaction, a reagent which is poorer in SO_2 than are samples freshly prepared according to the usual formulae; from my own experience, the method of preparation used by Graumann (p. 361) is entirely suitable. The concentration of orange G in the background stain is patently above the solubility of this compound; I would therefore advise using a saturated solution (about 2%).

d) Paraldehyde-thionin, a stain already mentioned on p. 354, has been applied to adenohypophysial cytology by Paget and Eccleston (1960), the working technique recommended by these authors including the association together of staining by paraldehyde-thionin, the PAS reaction and staining with luxol fast blue.

> Paraffin wax sections, taken from material fixed with formalin-corrosive sublimate, dewaxed and, where appropriate, treated with collodion (pay special attention to the thinness of the coating) and hydrated;
> Oxidise for 2 minutes with a mixture of equal parts of a 2% aqueous solution of potassium permanganate and a 0.5% solution of sulphuric acid;
> Destain using a 2% aqueous solution of potassium metabisulphite (avoid using oxalic acid for destaining the sections);
> Wash for several minutes in running water;
> Stain for 10 minutes using a well matured solution of paraldehyde thionin (p. 354);
> Rinse in tap water;
> Pass the slides first through 70% alcohol and then through 96% alcohol;
> Stain for 30 minutes, at 57°C, with a 0.1% solution of luxol fast blue in 96% alcohol, which has been acidified by the addition of 0.5 ml of acetic acid for every 100 ml of staining solution;
> Rinse in 96% alcohol and then in water;
> Differentiate with a 0.5% aqueous solution of lithium carbonate;
> Rinse 4 times with 70% alcohol;
> Rinse in tap water;
> Oxidise for 10 minutes using a 1% aqueous solution of periodic acid;
> Wash for 2 minutes in running water;
> Treat for 30 minutes with Schiff's reagent;
> Wash vigorously in distilled water;
> Wash for 10 minutes in running water;
> Dehydrate in absolute alcohol, clear in a benzenoid hydrocarbon and mount in a synthetic resin or in Canada balsam.

The results can be seen in Table 34. From my own experience, staining using paraldehyde-thionin can be replaced in this formula using paraldehyde-fuchsin.

Ezrin (1963) prefers to stain the erythrophil cells with orange G; the working technique recommended by this author includes the following stages.

> Paraffin wax sections, dewaxed, treated with collodion where appropriate and hydrated;
> Oxidise for 2 minutes with a mixture of equal parts of a 0.5% aqueous solution of potassium permanganate and a 0.5% solution of sulphuric acid;
> Destain for 1 minute with a 2% aqueous solution of potassium metabisulphite;
> Wash carefully in tap water and rinse in distilled water;
> Stain for 50 minutes with a well matured solution (3 to 7 days) of paraldehyde-thionin, prepared according to Paget's formula (p. 354);
> Rinse in distilled water;
> Oxidise for 5 minutes using a 0.5% aqueous solution of periodic acid;
> Rinse in distilled water;
> Treat for 15 minutes with Schiff's reagent;
> Wash in 3 baths of sulphur dioxide water (3 minutes in each bath);
> Wash for 15 to 30 minutes in running water;
> Stain for about 20 seconds using the solution
>   distilled water .... 100 ml
>   phosphotungstic acid .... 5 g
>   orange G .... 2 g
> Rinse in distilled water only when there is excessive staining;
> Dehydrate in absolute alcohol, clear in a benzenoid hydrocarbon and mount in Canada balsam or in a synthetic resin.

The results correspond to those obtained using Paget and Eccleston's technique, with the exception that the erythrophil cells are stained yellow.

*e) **Staining with alcian blue after vigorous oxidation*** was introduced into the cytological study of the adenohypophysis by Adams and Swettenham (1958), whose objective was to distinguish more readily the types of cyanophil cell (thyreotropic and gonadotropic). These authors used performic oxidation; their working technique was founded on the method used by Adams and Sloper (p. 524) for staining structures rich in cystine, but as a second stage of the process the sections undergo the PAS reaction and staining with orange G. The technique therefore includes the following stages.

Paraffin wax sections, dewaxed and treated where appropriate with collodion and then hydrated;
Oxidise for 5 minutes at laboratory temperatures using a freshly prepared solution of performic acid (p. 467);
Wash in distilled water (for about 5 minutes taking care not to cause the sections to come away from the slide);
Treat for 1 hour at laboratory temperatures with the following freshly prepared solution;

concentrated sulphuric acid .... 5.4 ml
distilled water .... 94.6 ml
alcian blue .... 1 g

pouring the sulphuric acid with the customary precautions into the water; the rise in temperature assists the solution of the alcian blue; it may be necessary to warm slightly;
Wash for 5 minutes in distilled water;
Oxidise for 5 minutes with a 0.5% aqueous solution of periodic acid;
Wash for 2 minutes in tap water;
Treat for 15 minutes with Schiff's reagent;
Wash very vigorously in distilled water;
Wash for 10 minutes in tap water;
Stain for about 1 minute with a 2% solution of orange G in 5% phosphotungstic acid;
Wash in tap water;
Dehydrate in absolute alcohol, clear in a benzenoid hydrocarbon and mount in Canada balsam or in a synthetic resin.

The results are set out in Table 34.

As I mentioned in relation to the discussion of Adams and Sloper's method (p. 524) the results of peracetic oxidation are strictly equivalent to those of performic oxidation and Lillie (1965) considers the latter as being better, since the oxidising solution can be kept whereas the solution of performic acid only keeps for a few hours. Moreover, experience shows that the results are strictly the same as those of performic oxidation even if the mixture of potassium permanganate and sulphuric acid is used as an oxidant. From the practical point of view, this oxidation, which is easier, is adopted by Herlant (1960) whose technique using PAS and alcian blue includes the following stages.

- Paraffin wax sections, dewaxed, treated with collodion where appropriate and hydrated;
- Oxidise with the potassium permanganate ,sulphuric acid mixture as for staining the hypothalamic neurosecretory product;
- Rinse in tap water;
- Destain using a 2% aqueous solution of potassium metabisulphite or sodium metabisulphite;
- Wash in tap water;
- Stain for from 15 to 30 minutes with a 1% solution of alcian blue, prepared either with 2 N sulphuric acid, as in Adams and Sloper's formula (pH = 0.2), or with 1% acetic acid (pH = 3);
- Wash for 5 to 10 minutes in running water;
- Oxidise for 5 minutes in a 1% aqueous solution of periodic acid;
- Wash for 2 minutes in tap water;
- Treat for from 6 to 30 minutes using Schiff's reagent (I would advise the adoption of the average time of 15 minutes);
- Wash very vigorously in distilled water;
- Wash for 10 minutes in tap water;
- Stain the nuclei where appropriate using Groat's haematoxylin;
- Wash for 2 to 5 minutes in tap water;
- Where appropriate, stain the erythrophil cells either using orange G-phosphomolybdic acid, as used by Cleveland and his collaborators (p. 996), or using a 1% solution of naphthol yellow in 1% acetic acid;
- Rinse rapidly in distilled water;
- Dehydrate in absolute alcohol, clear in a benzenoid hydrocarbon and mount in Canada balsam or in a synthetic resin.

The thyreotrope cells become intensely blue, the gonadotropic FSH cells become violet, the gonadotropic LH cells stain red, the erythrophil cells stain yellow if the staining by orange G or naphthol yellow has been used. Herlant (1960) remarks that the gonadotropic LH cells of the Reptilia and the Anamniota often take up alcian blue at pH 3, but that they do not stain at pH 0.2; in the mammals studied by Herlant even the higher of these two pH values suffices to distinguish the three categories of cyanophil cells of the adenohypophysis. Whether staining by orange G or naphthol yellow is appropriate or not depends on the PAS activity of the gonadotropic LH cells; when this reactivity is marked it is advantageous to employ such staining, but it is better not to use it in cases where the gonadotropic LH cells react only feebly towards PAS so as not to diminish the selectivity with which they can be distinguished from the erythrophil cells. Nuclear staining using Groat's haematoxylin is also optional; in my opinion it always improves the legibility of the preparations.

GENERAL HISTOCHEMICAL AND CYTOLOGICAL TECHNIQUES

All techniques used in general cytology, as well as all the histochemical reactions, can be applied as research methods for the study of the distal lobe of the adenohypophysis; I would in particular mention the attempts to identify the cellular categories according to their histo-enzymological nature (see Arvy, 1963 and 1971; Pearse and Van Noorden *in* Colloque international du C.N.R.S. no. 128).

B. — THE INTERMEDIATE LOBE OF THE ADENOHYPOPHYSIS

The anatomical study of the intermediate lobe, and in particular the evaluation of its relative volume, has been discussed in relation to the distal lobe (p. 992).

The techniques required for its *histological study* call for no special commentary. The methods of fixation and staining described in relation to the distal lobe permit the cells of the intermediate lobe to be shown up clearly, allowing us to recognise the types of cell and showing up the cells of the distal lobe includded within the parenchyme proper to the intermediate lobe. We may recall the particular interest which attaches, during histological studies of the intermediate lobe of the adenohypophysis, to the detection of the hypothalamic neurosecretory product which is present in a certain number of species in the nervous fibres which come from the neurohypophysis and are to be found between the cells belonging to the intermediate lobe.

The histological study of the *pars tuberalis* of the adenohypophysis calls for no special technique and the methods set out in relation to the other lobes will demonstrate all its morphological characters.

C. — THE ENDOCRINE PANCREAS

The histological examination of the endocrine pancreas, when carried out with diagnostic ends in view, should afford not only data about the different types of cell and their functional condition but, equally, numerical and volumetric data on this organ; in fact, that information which weighing, carried out before or after fixation, affords in the case of the other endocrine glands of the vertebrates can come only from a study of sectioned tissue in this instance because the endocrine pancreas is not sufficiently distinct anatomically. It is appropriate to mention at the outset that it is not always easy to reconcile the requirements of the techniques capable of furnishing these two types of information.

TECHNIQUES FOR THE QUANTITATIVE STUDY OF THE ENDOCRINE PANCREAS

Very numerous methods have been proposed to estimate the absolute or relative volume of the endocrine pancreas beginning with the first attempts of Heiberg (1906). There can be no question of making a complete list of these here; an abundant bibliography and very useful technical details are to be found in the reviews devoted to the endocrine pancreas (see in particular Bargmann,

1939; Ferner, 1952) as well as in the monograph of Tejning (*Acta med. Scand.*, suppl., 198, 1947) and in the publications of Hellman (*Acta Endocrinologica*, 1959). On the other hand, the difficulties which arise in this kind of work should feature in the present section.

Evaluation of the relative volume of the endocrine pancreas by techniques involving linear integration as set out in the first part of this book is made difficult by the fact that the distribution of the Langerhans' islets within the exocrine pancreas is far from random; there is always a distinct tendency for the endocrine tissue to be concentrated at the splenic pole of the organ and this may be carried so far that there is a complete absence of the islets in the juxta-duodenal part (head) of the pancreas. It is therefore necessary to carry out the examination on the various regions of the gland or to cut up the entire organ into serial sections. This requirement is very easy to satisfy in the case of animals of small size, in particular the mammals currently used in physiological research, but in the case of animals of a certain size it may result in the fixation of pieces of tissue whose dimensions are no longer compatible with cytological examination. Moreover, certain techniques involve the cutting of the organ into sections whose thickness is such that the study of the types of cell in the islets could not even be considered (celloidin sections of 30 μ in Tejning's technique). We may add to this that most of the techniques for the quantitative study of the Langerhans' islets leave out of account the isolated insular cells which are far from negligible in number. Moreover, methods aimed at evaluating the apparent surface of the Langerhansian tissue from sections and at deducing from these studies the real distribution of endocrine and exocrine tissue within the organ are founded on the mathematical studies of Wicksell (1925, 1926), carried out at the request of Hellman *sen.*; we know from such studies that the real distribution can be deduced from the apparent one in cases where the Langerhans' islets conform closely to spheres or to ellipsoids; such conformity may occur in the case of small mammals, but it may lead to gross errors for one type of islet in the birds, and for the islets of the reptiles and batracians.

It would, then, be dangerous to forget the sources of error in any of the methods set out below; their results represent an approximation to the truth and should never be treated in the same way as the results of gravimetric studies when working up the raw data of an experiment.

The enumeration of the islets as proposed by Heiberg (1906) does not of itself provide any valid indication of the extent of the endocrine pancreas; as Glaser (1926) has quite rightly commented the mass of Langerhansian tissue which corresponds to a small number of islets of large size may be greater than that corresponding to twice the number of small islets. From the technical point of view this manoeuvre evidently presents little enough difficulty; the exploration of the sections can be carried out using lens systems sufficiently powerful to ensure that even the small islets do not escape examination. Lucas (1947) suggests that an enumeration of the islets should be combined with an evaluation of their surface area.

Evaluation of the relative surface area of the insular parenchyme in a fixed number of microscope fields was put forward by Richardson and Young (1937) as a means of expressing the relative volume of the insular organ. From the technical standpoint, these authors use the classical method which consists of sketching a certain number of microscope fields in a camera lucida and evaluating the surface areas which correspond to the different tissues by cutting out the relevant parts and weighing them or by planimetry of the surface areas. Richardson and Young's ratio is calculated by dividing the surface area (or the weight of paper) corresponding to the islets by the value which corresponds to the exocrine parenchyme and then multiplying by 100. Naturally, this technique gives only relative values devoid of any significance so far as the real volume of the insular organ is concerned; moreover, the estimate should be made on an appreciable number of microscopic fields and the total amount of physical work is far from negligible. In fact, the ratio of insular tissue to exocrine tissue is much easier to determine by techniques which involve linear integration, as described in Chapter 7.

The measurement of the islets of Langerhans can be carried out either under the microscope, particularly in cases where their form approaches that of a sphere or of an ellipsoid, or by sketching them, followed by cutting up the sketch and weighing the relevant parts or by planimetry, the simplest way of expressing the result being the calculation of the radius of a circle whose surface is equivalent to that which has just in fact been measured; an approximation which is often adequate may be obtained according to Tejning (1947) and Hellman *jun.* (1959) by placing in the focal plane of the eyepiece a transparent plate inscribed with circles and ellipses of known surface, comparison with the islets being made by superposition. The investigations of the authors who have just been cited show how useful it is to classify, in categories of increasing size, the islets on which the measurements have been made.

Tejning's volumetric method consists of fixing the pancreas in formalin and, after fixation, removing the tissues other than the glandular parenchyme (lymph nodes, adipose tissue, peritoneum) by means of a careful dissection, carried out under the dissecting microscope. The organ is then dehydrated, care being taken to give it a form which will minimize the number of sections to be cut, and then embedded in celloidin. The sections are cut at 30 μ, one section out of every 10 or every 5 being kept for a numerical analysis. Staining is carried out using a commercial mixture, the composition of which has not been divulged (Kernechtrotkombination H, Hollborn, Leipzig), which stains the islets blue and the exocrine parenchyme red. In each of the sections which have been set aside the area occupied by the Langerhansian tissue is determined by projection and sketching, followed by cutting out of the relevant parts and weighing, or by planimetry, the total volume of the islets of Langerhans being subsequently calculated according to the formula

$$V = \frac{S \times T \times (I+1)}{M^2}$$

where V represents the volume in mm^3, S the surface in mm^2, T the thickness of the sections, I the interval between two sections which are being studied (these two values in mm), M the linear magnification used during projection. We know from Tejning's calculations that the study of one section out of every ten, under the technical conditions which have been defined, will suffice to estimate the volume with adequate precision, the gain in precision which results from the examination of one section out of every five being incommensurate with the additional work involved. Naturally, this way of proceeding makes it impossible to study the cellular composition of the islets, evaluation of the volume of the insular organ being the only outcome of a histological examination of the pancreas such as has just been considered

Tejning's numerical method depends on the distribution of the real and observed size of spherical or ellipsoidal solids as seen in the sections and included in a medium which differs from them. When we group the surfaces measured on sections into frequency classes, for the different islets of any given pancreas, we see that the curve representing the distribution is strongly asymmetrical, the number of islets increasing very rapidly for small dimensions, whereas the curve representing the volumetric distribution is symmetrical, indicating that the greater part of the insular parenchyme is represented by islets of average fize. By using Wicksell's equations we can calculate the total volume of the insular organ from the surface areas measured, this calculation being greatly sacilitated by the tables set out by Tejning, which are valid only for the rat.

The method used by Hellman jun. depends on the existence of a linear relationship between the logarithm of the number of islets and the diameter appropriate to each size class as defined by Tejning; this fact, taken together with Wicksell's data, obviously suggests that there may be a simple correlation between the number of islets and the real volume of the insular organ. A statistical study, carried out on the rat, does indeed show the existence of a linear correlation between the volume of the insular organ on the one hand, and, on the other hand, the number of islets whose surface area, measured on sections, is at least equal to that of a circle whose diameter is 109.4 μ; the analysis of a substantial number (75 rats) shows that a supplementary factor needs to be taken into account, that is to say the age of the animal. Graphs drawn up by Hellman thus allow us to read off directly the approximate volume of the insular organ if we know the number of islets whose surface area is at least equal to that of a circle of 109.4 μ in diameter. It goes without saying that the entire organ needs to be examined, the sections being taken at regular intervals; these ready-reckoners were set up for the case of a 300 μ gap between the optical sections, the use of any other gap involving the multiplication of the number of islets by 300/E, E being the separation of the optical planes adopted for the work. The validity of the regression equations on which Hellman's graphs depend is, evidently, established only for albino rats of the Wistar strain.

A considerable advantage of this latter method is its rapidity, circles and ellipses of the desired volume being inserted into the eyepiece to allow an immediate appreciation of the approximate surface area of the islets. Experience verifies a very satisfactory agreement as compared with the volumetric method. The sections examined may be thin and stained by techniques which show up the different types of cell, the only limitation to the use of these methods stemming from the size of the pieces of tissue, when the methods are applied to species other than the rat.

Counts of the cells belonging to the different types, when carried out by the application of the techniques described in the second part of this section, should also take into account various methodological features. Naturally, only those cells or fragments of cells whose nucleus is entirely or partly included in the section should be counted; any inequality of the nuclear diameters thus leads to an over estimation of the numbers of cells in a particular nuclear category whose nuclei are the most voluminous and a caryological study may be necessary to correct this error. The counting should include at least 2,000 cells since, in the rat, the errors only become slight for counts of 3,000 cells (Larsson, 1956). These errors increase in direct proportion to the thickness of the sections. Moreover, the distribution of the types of cells varies considerably according to the size of the islets, so that it is necessary to include in the examination islets belonging to all size classes.

TECHNIQUES FOR IDENTIFYING THE DIFFERENT TYPES OF CELL IN THE ENDOCRINE PANCREAS

The existence of several types of cell characterised by different secretory granules in the islets of Langerhans has been known since the beginning of the twentieth century, but the histophysiological interest of this multiplicity of cells in the organ was only siezed upon in 1940, an appreciation which was greatly stimulated by research on alloxan diabetes. At the present time, the identification of the types of cells, the study of their secretory granule content and the establishment of their percentages in any given animal has a greater part to play in the histological study of the organ than has the quantitative study set out in the preceding section.

We should not hide from ourselves that progress in our knowledge has led to a certain confusion in the definition of one of the classical types of cell, that is, the D cells; on the other hand, there is agreement about the B cells; which are responsible for the secretion of insulin. As for the cellular category designated by the name of A cells, and until recently considered as being responsible for the secretion of glucagon, its heteroclite nature is now established, researches by Hellman's school providing weighty arguments for the proposition that there are in fact two sub-categories.

Preparation of the material for the demonstration of the types of Langerhans' cells

Naturally, any cytological or histochemical technique can be used as a research tool during work which bears on the pancreatic islets, *fixation* taking place with an eye to the requirements of such techniques. But the methods used for the identification of the different types of cell, by showing up their secretory granules, all permit fixation by Bouin's fluid, Halmi's fluid, Heidenhain's Susa and mixtures of corrosive sublimate and formalin; I rather tend to consider the first two of these liquids as being the best and it seems to me permissible to advise their adoption as routine fixatives for the study of the islets of Langerhans. The preservation of the secretory granules is a little better when Halmi's liquid is used than after the use of Bouin's fluid, but this latter fluid prepares the material better for the silver impregnation which has become indispensable for a study of the Langerhans' cells as it is for the demonstration of indol groups which is also very useful.

Rapid fixation is absolutely imperative; it is rendered necessary by the presence, in the parenchyme, of proteolytic proenzymes whose activation, which is linked to the death of the cells, will bring about the destruction of all the structural details of the exocrine and endocrine cells; this possibility also explains the need to reduce one of the dimensions of the pieces of tissue to 5 ml or less. In practice, the pancreas of the small mammals used in physiological research may be fixed as a whole, their texture being soft enough for even the cytological fixatives to penetrate them rapidly, but the same is not at all true when we have to deal with an animal whose size is greater than that of the rabbit.

The preparation of the material for section cutting and this procedure itself require only a few comments. Prolonged immersion of the tissues in ethyl alcohol should be avoided, particularly if the alcoholic concentration of the liquid is slight; it is best to embed rapidly in paraffin wax, the necessity of cutting thin sections in fact rendering this type of embedding necessary. The thickness of the sections should not exceed 5μ.

The fact that there were several types of Langerhans' cells has been agreed since the beginning of this century, but it is only since 1940 that we have been able to link the cells of any given type with the secretion of either insulin or of glucagon. Currently, new types of cell have been identified in the islets of Langerhans; some of these can only be recognised on electron micrographs. Generally speaking, research over the last ten years abundantly illustrates the difficulty of collating the results obtained on preparations intended for light microscopy with those intended for electron microscopy. There are a certain number of inconsistencies in the terminology of the types of cell in the endocrine pancreas because many investigators see fit to pursue their researches without taking the slightest account of the results obtained by other workers; nevertheless, this terminology is not as confused as that of the cells of the distal lobe of the adenohypophysis. The definitions of the types of cell which we adopt here is that put forward by Falkmer and Patent (1971).

Techniques for the selective demonstration of B cells

The general morphological characteristics of the B cells will, obviously, allow their identification by an investigator trained in the histochemical examination of the endocrine pancreas of any given species, and even the site where they occur within the islets of Langerhans is, in the majority of cases, quite characteristic. Topographical techniques generally show up differences between the staining affinities of their secretory granules and those of the secretory product of the A cells. These latter are, for all practical purposes, always distinctly erythrophilic, whereas the secretion of the B cells is either more weakly erythrophilic or distinctly cyanophilic when stained with mixtures containing several acid dyestuffs. Mann's method using methyl blue-eosin (Dobell's variation) has been put forward by Grobety (1947) as a routine method for the study of the endocrine pancreas. When applied to material which has been fixed in Bouin's fluid it does indeed show up the A cells which become red and the other types of cell, including the B cells, which become a violet blue, but the contrast between the different types of cells are distinctly less marked than it is with some of the techniques described below.

Bensley's staining technique (p. 756) using neutral gentian violet, as well as the technique using ethyl violet-orange G, clearly stains the B cells violet, the other cell types becoming yellow. Both the techniques which have just been mentioned gave rise to Lillie's method (1954) which is simpler and quite as effective. It involves the use of a mixture containing eriocyanin A, an acid stain of the triphenylmethane group related to the acid violet of the classical authors, as well as of safranin, the selectivity of the uptake of stain by the A cells being ensured by the use of a solvent buffered to pH 3.75. The technique in question involves the following stages:

> Dewaxed sections, treated with collodion where appropriate and hydrated;
> Stain for a period which has to be determined by trial and error (see below) using the following mixture, prepared immediately prior to use from stock solutions which keep well
>
> | | |
> |---|---|
> | a 1% aqueous solution of eriocyanin A | 2 ml |
> | a 1% aqueous solution of safranin O | 2 ml |
> | an M/10 aqueous solution of citric acid | 1.3 ml |
> | an M/5 aqueous solution of disodium phosphate | 0.7 ml |
> | distilled water | 34 ml |
>
> Rinse in distilled water;
> Blot with absorbent paper;
> Dehydrate in acetone, clear in a benzenoid hydrocarbon, and mount in a synthetic resin or in Canada balsam.

Since a buffer of pH 3.75 has been used, staining by eriocyanin A is automatically limited to the A cells which become blue; the other types of cell, including the B cells, become red or violet; the ergastoplasm of the exocrine pancreatic cells and the nuclei become red and the erythrocytes blue; the contrast between the islets of Langerhans and the exocrine parenchyme is excellent. From my own personal experience, the solutions of citric acid and of sodium phosphate, prepared with distilled water and methyl alcohol as indicated in relation to the preparation of the McIlvaine-Lillie buffer (p. 667), can be substituted without the slightest ill-effect for the aqueous solutions indicated in the above formula. The optimal duration of staining is very variable and depends on the commercial samples of eriocyanin A; it may last as long as 24 hours. A personal and unpublished variation of this technique consists of replacing the eriocyanin A in the staining bath by cyanol (xylene-cyanol) FF, a dye which it is easier to obtain in samples whose properties are identical from one batch to another. In this case, the optimal time of staining is 30 minutes and the rinsing with distilled water should last for from 20 to 30 seconds. The A cells are stained intensely green.

The major objective of staining with eriocyanin A and its variations is to allow thorough delimitation of the islets and of the exocrine parenchyme; from the point of view of the identification of the B cells it is evidently less useful than the techniques described below.

The best techniques for demonstrating the B cells are those which depend on one of the essential characteristics of their secretory granules, namely the acquisition of an intense basophilia following strong permanganate oxidation in a sulphuric acid medium. It was in the course of studies on the endocrine pancreas that Gomori (1939, 1941) discovered this "shift" of the staining affinity of certain structures, a shift whose importance has been underlined in Chapter 29. It seems legitimate to explain this property of the secretory granules of the B cells in terms of their higher content of protein-bound sulphydryls, the cystine and cysteine being transformed into cysteic acid as a result of the oxidation, and so the cells become basophilic.

Any of the techniques described in relation to the selective staining of the hypothalamic neurosecretory product can, then, be employed for the demonstration of the B cells of the endocrine pancreas and indeed they are so used. The oldest of these methods is that using chromic haematoxylin-phloxin used as described on p. 759; it confers an intense blue colour, tending towards black, on the secretory granules of the B cells, the A cells being stained red by the phloxin. The absolute necessity for re-fixing the sections and the instability of the chromic lake of haematoxylin often makes it preferable to use paraldehyde-fuchsin; this confers an intense violet colour on the secretory product of the B cells. The variable results obtained by staining with paraldehyde-fuchsin according to the way in which it is prepared, as noted in relation to the study of the distal lobe of the adenohypophysis, do not seem to exist in the case of the endocrine pancreas; all investigators have used permanganate oxidation in a sulphuric acid medium as a pre-treatment (Gabe, 1953; Scott, 1953); the unstable solution prepared according to Gomori's formula (1950) and the stable solution, diluted and acidified (Gabe, 1953), give identical results. The colour assumed by the Langerhans' cells, other than the B cells, after staining with paraldehyde-fuchsin in the way described in the preceding chapters, obviously depends on the particular background stain used. With Groat's haematoxylin and picro-indigocarmine these other types of cells become yellow, the colour being sufficiently clear for their identification but insufficient for a study of their structural details. Nevertheless, the preparations so obtained are highly advantageous for black and white photography when the object of the work is the study of the B cells. When the background staining is carried out with one step trichrome the A cells become red, the D cells green; the A cells and all the insular cells other than the B cells may be stained red with acid fuchsin used in dilute and acidified solution; ponceau or phloxin may also be used for this purpose. This red background stain may assist the analysis of the preparations but not their photographic reproduction in black and white. The way in which paraldehyde-fuchsin should be used is shown on p. 761 and 965; I might comment that refixation of the sections is only useful in cases where the tissue from which they are taken has been poorly fixed; most authors do not use it.

The Mann-Dominici method, when applied to sections refixed in Bouin's fluid and oxidised by the addition of chrome alum to the fixative, as in the case of staining with chromic haematoxylin-phloxin, very clearly shows up the B cells of the endocrine pancreas which are stained blue; the A cells become red and the other types of cell pink (Gabe, 1950). Unlike staining with paraldehyde-fuchsin, this technique requires the sections to be refixed but the stability of the stains used is a considerable advantage compared with the chromic haematoxylin-phloxin method. The working technique is shown on p. 760 and at that point I commented on the need for the individual differentiation of the slides using 96% alcohol; this requirement is obviously a nuisance when large numbers of slides need to be handled.

Paraldehyde-thionin, as put forward by Paget (1959), gives preparations which are in all respects comparable to those given by paraldehyde-fuchsin; the preparation and use of the stain are described on p. 354; in my opinion the impossibility of stabilising the dye solutions is a serious disadvantage compared with the use of paraldehyde-fuchsin.

The strong affinity of the secretory granules of the B cells for a large number of basic dye stuffs, an affinity which appears after permanganate oxidation in a sulphuric acid medium, was expressly noted by Gomori (1941) and all those techniques which depend on this principle are in effect "Gomori's methods". In addition to the dye-stuffs which have just been mentioned many others can be used; Victoria blue in an alcoholic solution acidified with acetic acid has been recommended by Ivic (1959); a more complicated formula, due to Humberstone is mentioned on p. 969; Müller (1951) recommends a 5% aqueous solution of Bismarck brown (vesuvine) to which 0.5 g of zinc acetate has been added to every 100 ml of solution; a combination of this formula together with a stain selective for the A cells is to be commended when dealing with the latter type of cell. Alcian blue and astra blue can be used to good effect; experience shows (Gabe, 1969) that permanganate oxidation in a sulphuric acid medium confers a strong affinity for phthalocyanins on the secretory granules of the B cells, even when the pH of the dye bath is very low; it is at pH 2.6 or 3 that the intensity of the stain taken up by the B granules reaches its maximum whereas the background remains quite pale. The use of solutions of higher pH does not increase the intensity with which the B cells are stained and the greater intensity of the background stain results in less clearly marked contrasts. Very good results can be obtained using the following working technique.

Dewaxed sections, treated with collodion where appropriate, and hydrated;
Oxidise using potassium permanganate in a sulphuric acid medium following Gomori's recommendations (p. 1001);
Rinse rapidly in tap water;
Destain using a 2 to 5% aqueous solution of sodium metabisulphite;
Wash for 2 minutes in running water;
Stain for from 10 to 20 minutes (depending on the commercial sample of the dye) with the solution
Citric acid-disodium phosphate buffer
    of pH 2.6 (McIlvaine-Lillie) .... 4 ml
    distilled water .... 96 ml
    alcian blue or astra blue .... 0.2 g
Rinse in distilled water;
Stain the nuclei using the aluminium lake of nuclear fast red;
Wash for 2 minutes in running water;
Dehydrate in absolute alcohol, clear in a benzenoid hydrocarbon and mount in a synthetic resin or in Canada balsam.

The B cells become intensely blue-green, the other types of cell in the islets and in the exocrine parenchyme take up the background stain; the secretory granules of the exocrine cells are also stained with copper phthalocyanin when they have been preserved during fixation.

Performic or peracetic oxidation can be substituted for permanganate oxidation in a sulphuric acid medium. Contrary to the erroneous opinion which I expressed in the French edition of this work, such a substitution has considerable practical advantages. In fact, experience shows that oxidation by one or other of the two peracids is much more selective than that by potassium permanganate. Under such conditions, the sections may remain in the diluted and acetified solution of paraldehyde-fuchsin for a time which may be prolonged up to 15 minutes without there being the slightest need to extract an excess of the dye; the background stain is much less strong than after permanganate oxidation and I rather tend to consider peracetic oxidation followed by staining with paraldehyde-fuchsin-one step trichrome as the method of choice for routine work on the B cells of the endocrine pancreas. The working technique which follows has regularly given me very satisfactory results.

> Dewaxed sections, treated with collodion where appropriate, and hydrated;
> Refix where appropriate using Bouin's fluid to which chrome alum has been added as in the method using chromic haematoxylin-phloxin (p. 759); this stage is only rarely useful;
> Wash, where appropriate, in running water until the yellow colour disappears;
> Oxidise for from 20 to 30 minutes using performic or peracetic acid prepared according to the formula of Greenspan (p. 467);
> Wash for 1 minute in running water;
> Stain from 10 to 15 minutes in a diluted solution of paraldehyde-fuchsin acidified with acetic acid (p. 352);
> Rinse in tap water;
> Stain for 10 minutes with one step trichrome (p. 217);
> Wash for 30 seconds to 1 minute in distilled water;
> Dehydrate in absolute alcohol, clear in a benzenoid hydrocarbon and mount in a synthetic resin or in Canada balsam.

The B cells, whose secretory product takes on an intense violet tint, show up with the greatest clarity; the secretory granules of the A cells stain red, those of the D cells green.

We know from experience (Gabe, 1968, 1969) that oxidation by either of the two peracids confers on the secretory product of the B cells a strong metachromasia towards toluidine blue or azur A; this metachromasia, which is of the γ type, withstands dehydration by alcohol and in this way is distinguished from the fugitive metachromasia noted in the B cells of various mammals and in the frog (Fujita and Takaya, 1968). This fact illustrates a very clear distinction between the results of oxidation by the two peracids on the one hand, and that by permanganate oxidation using Gomori's technique on the other hand. In fact, this latter oxidation results in the orthochromatic basophilia mentioned above when the pH of the solution of toluidine blue or azur A is higher than 4.2, although when the thiazine used for staining is dissolved in a liquid whose pH is less than 4.2 there is a highly fugitive metachromasia which does not withstand treatment with alcohol (Fujita and Takaya, 1968). The stable metachromasia described here ensures that the B cells are very clearly shown up; mounting in synthetic resins is possible provided that the stains are stabilised using the classic ammonium molybdate treatment. The working technique involves the following stages.

Dewaxed sections, treated where appropriate with collodion, and hydrated;
Oxidise for about 20 minutes using performic or peracetic acid;
Wash for 5 minutes in running water;
Stain for about 5 minutes in a 0.2% solution of toluidine blue in Walpole's buffer using a 0.2 M solution of acetic acid-sodium acetate of pH 4.2;
Rinse in distilled water;
Mount in sorbitol F if one desires to avoid dehydration or
Treat for 5 minutes with a 5% solution of ammonium molybdate;
Wash for 2 minutes in running water;
Blot with absorbent paper, dehydrate in absolute alcohol, clear in a benzenoid hydrocarbon and mount in a synthetic resin or, where necessary, in Canada balsam.

The secretory product of the B cells becomes reddish violet; only the nuclei are stained in the other types of insular cell. The basophilia of the ergastoplasm of the exocrine parenchyme is not changed by performic or peracetic oxidation; the metachromasia of the mucins is also preserved. The effect of the pH of the dye bath on this metachromatic basophilia was noted during the discussion of Adams and Sloper's method (p. 524).

Performic and permanganate oxidation in a sulphuric acid medium confers on the secretory product of the B cells the same metachromasia, after staining with pseudo-isocyanins, as that noted in relation to the hypothalamic neurosecretory product (Schiebler, 1958; Schiebler and Schiessler, 1960). The yellow fluorescence described in relation to the study of the neurosecretory cells also exists and some authors consider this technique as particularly advantageous for the study of the B cells of the endocrine pancreas. In fact, the chemical significance of the method is the same as that of the other procedures which involve permanganate, performic or peracetic oxidation. The data of Schiebler and Schiessler strongly support the idea that this metachromasia towards pseudo-isocyanin is in fact due to the oxidation of the disulphide links of the insulin molecule, but it is in no way true that the reaction is "specific" in the chemical sense of the term since other anionic groupings can give rise to the same metachromasia and other compounds rich in protein-bound sulphydryls can acquire such a metachromasia following oxidation. The working technique has been described in relation to the demonstration of the hypothalamic neurosecretory product; it is taken up again in the course of Epple's (1967) account of the sequence of stains.

It is appropriate to mention that the technique due to Solcia and his collaborators (1968) confers an intense metachromasia on the secretory product of the B cells but this metachromasia arises solely when the sections are taken from material fixed with mixtures having a glutaraldehyde base.

Among **the histochemical techniques** which are capable of demonstrating the B cells, the principal one is the test for protein-bound sulphydryls. The high proportion of sulphur-containing amino acids in the insulin would fairly obviously have induced the pioneers of the histochemistry of these compounds to try out such tests in the endocrine pancreas; strongly positive results are obtained not only by the method using DDD (p. 518) but by that using tetrazolium salts (p. 331) or ferric ferricyanide (p. 323). The theoretical interest of these results is great but the optical quality of the preparations is not superior to that given by the stains described above. Tests for protein-bound sulphydryls should then be reserved for doubtful cases. This remark is, *a fortiori*, valid for the histochemical tests for zinc using the technique set out in Chapter 13. A selective demonstration of these cells may be obtained by such methods but the working conditions are much less advantageous than are those relating to the use of selective stains and the preservation of the preparations as well as their optical qualities are less good.

Techniques for the selective demonstration of the A cells

Many authors consider that all the Langerhans' cells other than the B cells form a homogeneous category whose selective detection rests either on an acidophilia which persists despite permanganate oxidation or on an argyrophilia and whose demonstration is in any case ensured "by difference" because of the staining of the secretory product of the B cells. Recent work, in particular that of Hellman's school, makes it necessary to revise this point of view. Cytometric criteria, the staining affinities, some of which have been known since the classical studies of Thomas (1937), differences of argyrophilia using certain techniques, and lastly the ultrastructural and histophysiological data prove that only some of the cells which keep their acidophilia after permanganate oxidation in an acid medium are responsible for the secretion of glucagon. Such elements which therefore correspond to the histophysiological definition of an A cell are designated by the Swedish school under the name of A_2 cells, whereas other cells which are also acidophilic after permanganate oxidation but which have no part in the secretion of glucagon are designated by the same authors under the name of A_1 cells. Only these cells, which in all probability correspond to the

D cells of Bloom (1931) and Thomas (1937, 1940, 1942), are argyrophilic under the technical conditions of Davenport's method as modified by the Swedish authors.

The A cells, whose secretory granules are characterised by their intense erythrophilia, may be identified in principle by any staining technique in which two acid dyes with sufficiently distinct diffusion coefficients play a part. Thus, we find that the elements in question take up azorubin S from the one step trichrome which is utilised as a background stain after paraldehyde-fuchsin. They also take up eosin in the Mann-Dominici technique, and acid fuchsin from Masson's trichrome etc. However, the use of more selective methods is particularly indicated when we need to obtain a vivid stain of the elements in question. Iron haematoxylin, phosphotungstic haematoxylin and azocarmine allow us to attain this result. In addition, silver impregnation and the histochemical reactions should be mentioned here.

Staining with iron haematoxylin, combined with the demonstration of the B cells by Bismarck brown (Müller, 1951), depends on the fact that the A cells keep their siderophilia (which in this case, as in others, constitutes an acidophilia) despite permanganate oxidation in an acid medium; this oxidation which restricts the siderophilia also serves as a preparation for the staining of the B cells using the zinc lake of Bismarck brown. It includes the following stages:

Sections taken from material fixed in Bouin's fluid, embedded in paraffin wax without prolonged immersion in ethyl alcohol, dewaxed, treated where appropriate with collodion and hydrated, the picric acid having been removed by careful washing in running water;

Oxidise for 2 minutes using a mixture of equal parts of a 0.25% aqueous solution of potassium permanganate and a 0.5% solution of sulphuric acid. The preparation of this mixture amounts to the dilution with 9 volumes of distilled water, instead of 6 to 8, of the mixture of stock solutions of these two compounds as recommended by other authors; evidently this minor modification has no important effect on the result of the staining;

Rinse in tap water;

Destain using 2% oxalic acid or with a 2 to 5% solution of sodium metabisulphite;

Wash carefully in running water (for at least 10 minutes);

Mordant for 24 hours at laboratory temperatures with a 5% aqueous solution, freshly prepared, of iron alum;

Wash in 3 or 4 baths of distilled water;

Stain for 24 hours at laboratory temperatures using Heidenhain's haematoxylin or that of Regaud;

Wash for 3 to 4 minutes in running water;

under microscopic examination, with the solution of iron alum which was used as a mordant; continue the destaining until the A cells are selectively demonstrated; the B cells should remain unstained;

Stain for 2 minutes with the solution

Bismarck brown (vesuvine)	0.5 g
zinc acetate	0.5 g
distilled water	100 ml

filter after standing for 24 hours at laboratory temperatures and add 1 ml of acetic acid;

Differentiate under microscopic examination using very dilute acetic acid (20 drops for every 100 ml of distilled water) to the point where the connective tissue is virtually completely decolourised;

Wash for 2 minutes in tap water;

Dehydrate in absolute alcohol, clear in a benzenoid hydrocarbon and mount in a synthetic resin or in Canada balsam.

The A cells are easy to identify because their secretory granules are black, the B cells appear red or orange according to the abundance of the secretory granules contained in their cytoplasm.

The staining of the A cells by phosphotungstic haematoxylin seems to have been put forward for the first time by Gomori (1941); a variation intended for frozen sections, which is due to Hultquist and Tegner (1949) is given below. From my own personal experience it is the working technique of Levene and Feng (1964) which gives the best results on paraffin wax sections.

The staining of frozen sections using Hultquist and Tenger's (1949) technique involves the following stages:

Frozen sections, taken from material treated with formalin and steeped in tap water;

Oxidise for from 60 to 90 seconds in a 0.5% solution of potassium permanganate (non-acidified);

Destain using a 0.5% solution of sodium bisulphite;

Pass through 2 baths of distilled water;

Mordant for 3 to 4 hours in a 2 or 5% solution of iron alum;

Pass through 3 baths of distilled water;

Stain for 6 to 20 hours (the optimum should be determined by microscopic examination) in phosphotungstic haematoxylin prepared according to the original formula of Mallory (p. 212);

Rinse rapidly in tap water;

Remove the excess stain using 95% alcohol, complete the dehydration with origanum essence, clear in a benzenoid hydrocarbon and mount in Canada balsam.

The staining technique due to Levene and Feng, which is more particularly intended for paraffin wax sections, involves the following stages:

Paraffin wax sections, taken from material fixed in Bouin's fluid, dewaxed and where appropriate treated with collodion and hydrated, and freed from any picric acid which remains in it by washing in running water;

Oxidise using potassium permanganate acidified with sulphuric acid following Gomori's technique (for about 30 to 40 seconds);

Rinse in tap water;

Decolourise in 2 or 5% sodium metabisulphite solution;

Wash for 3 minutes in running water;

Rinse in distilled water;

Mordant for about 2 hours in a freshly prepared 4% solution of iron alum;

Rinse in distilled water;

Stain for 16 hours using phosphotungstic haematoxylin prepared according to the formula of its originators (p. 212);
Rinse in 96% alcohol to extract the excess dye;
Dehydrate in absolute alcohol, clear in a benzenoid hydrocarbon and mount in a synthetic resin or, if necessary, in Canada balsam.

The A cells are stained, by both methods, a deep blue, the selectivity of their demonstration being perfect. From my own personal experience, the lake prepared according to the formula of Terner *et al.* (p. 823) which starts with haematin can be used in the place of that of Levene and Feng but the duration of the stages should be reduced. The other elements of the sections are stained as if phosphotungstic haematoxylin had been used without oxidation.

The staining of the A cells using azocarmine also has strong advantages. It was Heidenhain's original working technique (p. 220) which allowed Bloom (1931) to describe 3 categories of cells in the human pancreas, namely the A cells stained red, the B cells stained yellow or grey and the D cells stained blue, but these results are only obtained if the critical features of the fixing process are strictly observed (Helly's or Maximow's fluids, without osmium tetroxide, acting for not longer than 8 hours). A variation of this method, due to Gomori (1941), ensures success under any circumstances and dispenses with fixation by fluids with a potassium bichromate base. The working technique of a personal variation, which I have used since 1957 and whose satisfactory results have been mentioned several times (Beaumont, 1960; Agid *et al.*, 1962), is still simpler, the results being obtained in a practically automatic fashion.

Staining following Gomori's recommendations involves the following stages:

Sections taken from material fixed in Bouin's fluid, dewaxed, treated with collodion and hydrated;
Oxidise for about 1 minute with potassium permanganate in a sulphuric acid medium, as for the demonstration of the B cells;
Rinse in tap water;
Destain using a 2 or 5% aqueous solution of sodium metabisulphite;
Wash with great care (for at least 10 minutes) in running water;
The elimination of the last traces of sodium metabisulphite is an essential factor for success since the azocarmine does not take well on acid tissues;
Stain for about 16 hours in an oven at 60°C using a saturated aqueous solution of azocarmine G to which acetic acid has been added as in Heidenhain's formula; the prolongation of the staining time as compared with that in the original formula is due to the great reduction of the affinity of all the tissues for azocarmine, because of the permanganate oxidation in an acid medium;
Rinse in distilled water;
Differentiate, where necessary, in aniline-alcohol as in Heidenhain's formula; it is not necessary to carry out any differentiation in some cases, the B cells remaining unstained by the azocarmine; in any case, it is necessary to obtain the selective demonstration of the A cells, only the nuclei being coloured in the other insular cells;
Allow to stand for 1 minute in the acetic alcohol, as in the original formula; it is possible to set the preparation aside in this liquid;

> Rinse in distilled water;
> Treat for about 30 minutes with a 5% aqueous solution of phosphotungstic acid;
> Rinse in distilled water;
> Treat for about 30 minutes with a dilute solution of aniline blue-orange G following Heidenhain's recommendations (p. 220);
> Dehydrate directly in absolute alcohol, clear in a benzenoid hydrocarbon and mount in a synthetic resin or in Canada balsam (see p. 222 for a discussion of the circumstances in which it is useful to rinse in distilled water or in 96% alcohol).

The general appearance of the preparations is that given by Heidenhain's azan but the tendency of the B cells to cyanophilia is reinforced and the A cells appear with great selectivity because of the intense red colour of their secretory product.

Staining the A cells by a personal variation of the azan technique has been developed in order to shorten the time taken for the staining, which is long when Gomori's azan is used, and to avoid the prolonged incubation of the sections in an oven at 60°C with the consequent risk that the sections will come unstuck, as well as to suppress the subjective element which results from differentiation under the microscope. My own personal procedure is derived from a variation of the azan technique described by Schleicher (1948), which is more particularly intended for the demonstration of collagen tissue; the working technique involved is set out below. My own procedure does indeed attain the objective which was sought at the beginning, but the brilliance of the stain taken up by the other tissues is less than it is with the variations of the azan technique which employ hot staining. So far as the A cells of the endocrine pancreas are concerned results which are as satisfactory as those obtained using staining by phosphotungstic haematoxylin have been obtained with representatives of all the Gnathostome vertebrate classes. The stages involved in this technique are as follows:

> Sections in paraffin wax, dewaxed, treated with collodion where appropriate and hydrated;
> Oxidise for 1 minute using potassium permanganate in a sulphuric acid medium as for the demonstration of the neurosecretory product;
> Rinse in tap water;
> Destain using sodium metabisulphite as is employed with Gomori's azan;
> Wash for about 10 minutes in running water;
> Stain for 15 minutes at laboratory temperatures using a saturated aqueous solution (about 0.1%) of azocarmine B (*and not G*), acidified with 1 ml of acetic acid for every 100 ml of solution;
> Rinse rapidly in distilled water;
> Treat for 15 minutes at laboratory temperatures with a 5% aqueous solution of phosphotungstic acid;
> Rinse rapidly in distilled water;
> Treat for 15 minutes at laboratory temperatures with a dilute solution of aniline blue-orange G as used by Heidenhain (p. 220);
> Dehydrate directly with absolute alcohol, clear in a benzenoid hydrocarbon and mount in Canada balsam or in a synthetic resin.

So far as the secretory granules of the insular cells are concerned the results are rigorously comparable to those obtained using Gomori's variation; the staining of the other structures is satisfactory but the brilliance of the preparation is not as great as it is after staining with azocarmine G.

Numerous methods of silver impregnation can demonstrate the A cells, but none of them is rigorously selective and some cases where the D cells have shown up have been reported by some of the most careful workers using the techniques in question. The different variations of Bielschowsky's method, which were used following Ferner's suggestion (1939), are mentioned here only for completeness since they lead to the demonstration of a mixture of A and D cells. Grimelius' technique using silver proteinate, as described below, gives simultaneous impregnation of the A and D cells with certain commercial samples of this product, whereas with others a very selective impregnation of the cells is obtained. The best chance of success is offered by Grimelius' technique using silver nitrate (1968), described in the discussion of the demonstration of gastro-intestinal endocrine cells.

Among *the histochemical reactions* which allow us to identify the A cells the most important is the test for indol groups whose positive result agrees well with our knowledge of the chemical structure of glucagon. After fixation in Bouin's fluid, the techniques due to Glenner and Lillie (p. 514) and of Glenner (p. 515) give satisfactory results; but the preservation of the indol compounds is much better after fixing by the GPA as used by Solcia et al. (1968). When this latter fixative is used the xanthydrol reaction (p. 516) is superior to other methods for demonstrating indol groups, according to my own personal experience. It is indeed superior not only so far as the contrasts obtained with these preparations are concerned but also for their preservation. The plasmal reaction also gives positive results in the A cells (Wolter, 1950; Hellman et al., 1962), but naturally this is not a technique which we should advise for investigations in which the identification of the A cells is carried out with diagnostic or histophysiological ends in view.

Techniques for the selective demonstration of D cells

The D cells were discovered through the use of so-called general histological techniques (Bloom, 1931; Thomas, 1937, 1940, 1942); both stains and silver impregnations permit of very selective demonstration. Two negative histochemical characteristics should also be mentioned because they may be useful in doubtful cases, namely the absence from the cytoplasm of these elements of protein-bound sulphydryls characteristic of the B cells and the indol groups whose abundance is diagnostic of A cells.

Cyanophilia after staining with the usual trichromes is to a greater or lesser extent clear according to the species involved; it persists despite permanganate oxidation of the sections or their peracetic oxidation, so that techniques put forward for demonstrating the B cells cause the D cells to appear when trichromes are used for background staining. In the same way, the variations of the azan technique described in relation to the selective staining of the A cells render the D cells blue, but the cyanophilia of the B cells is also accentuated in these circumstances.

The metachromasia of the D cells, after fixation by Bouin's fluid and embedding in paraffin wax, was discovered by Manocchio (1960); and a variation of the staining technique initially used was suggested by the same author in 1964. The technique used by Solcia et al. (1968) represents a great advance on Manocchio's method whose working technique is described for completeness.

Test for "spontaneous" metachromasia using Manocchio's method (1960):

> Sections taken from pieces of tissue fixed in Bouin's fluid, dewaxed, treated where appropriate with collodion, hydrated and freed from any excess of picric acid;
> Stain for several minutes to 1 hour with a 0.01 or 0.005% aqueous solution of toluidine blue or azur A at a pH above 4.5; the duration of staining, the optimal concentration of the stain and the optimal pH should be determined for each animal species by trial and error;
> Rinse rapidly in distilled water or mount in the stain; mounting in sorbitol F or syrup of Apathy is possible, but all dehydration should be avoided.

Test for metachromasia after methylation and saponification using Manocchio's (1964) technique:

> Sections taken from pieces of tissue fixed in Bouin's fluid, dewaxed, treated with collodion and freed from all picric acid by washing in 96% or 70% alcohol;
> Treat for 1 hour in an oven at 60°C with the mixture
>
>   methanol .... 100 ml
>   hydrochloric acid .... 0.8 ml
>
> Rinse rapidly in 80% alcohol;
> Treat for 20 minutes, at laboratory temperatures, using the mixture
>
>   80% alcohol .... 100 ml
>   caustic potash .... 1 g
>
> Wash for 3 to 5 minutes in 80% alcohol;
> Hydrate the sections and carry out staining with toluidine blue as in the test for "spontaneous" metachromasia.

These two methods confer on the cytoplasm of the D cells a metachromasia which is clear but fugitive and it is essential to photograph the preparations immediately. It is appropriate to emphasize that the clarity of the appearance of the preparations varies a great deal from species to species.

The method of Solcia *et al.* (1968), described in relation to techniques for the study of secretory granules, represents a substantial advance on that used by Manocchio. After hydrochloric acid hydrolysis under the technical conditions defined by the authors who have just been quoted, the D cells of all the species of gnathostome vertebrates studied from this point of view take on an intense red metachromatic colour after staining with toluidine blue; the preservation of this colour after stabilisation with ammonium molybdate, dehydration, clearing and mounting in a synthetic resin is possible. The optical qualities of the preparations are evidently superior to those of the preparations given by Manocchio's method and their photographic reproduction poses no problems. The A cells, under the same technical conditions, take on an orthochromatic colour which is very different from that of the metachromasia of the D cells; the B cells remain unstained except when the tissue has been fixed in mixtures with a glutaraldehyde base in which case they are metachromatic like the D cells. We should, then, prefer fixation using liquids which do not contain glutaraldehyde when the object of the work is the certain detection of the D cells using the method of Solcia *et al.* It is relevant that the appearance of the metachromasia after hydrochloric acid hydrolysis goes hand in hand with that of a strong affinity for phthalocyanins of the alcian blue group, which should be dissolved for use in buffers of pH 5 or 5.5. In most cases the colour of the D cells is intense, that of the A cells moderately intense, and the B cells remain practically unstained.

Silver impregnation following Davenport's technique was applied for the first time to the study of the islets of Langerhans by Volk and his collaborators (1955); in the hands of the Swedish school (Hellman and Hellerström, 1960; Hellerström and Hellman, 1960) it has become the method of choice for distinguishing the D cells (A_1) which are argyrophilic and the A cells (A_2) which are not argyrophilic under the technical conditions defined below. We must stress the fact that the work of the authors who have just been mentioned marks a turning point in the development of our knowledge of the types of cell in the endocrine pancreas.

Impregnation using Hellerström and Hellman's technique involves the following stages:

Sections in paraffin wax taken from tissue fixed in Bouin's fluid (see below), dewaxed, treated where appropriate with collodion (a thin film) and hydrated;
Refix for 2 hours, at 37°C, using Bouin's fluid (without the addition of chrome alum);
Wash for 1 hour in running water;
Rinse in distilled water;
Dehydrate in 96% alcohol;
Impregnate for 18 to 24 hours, at 37°C, or 48 to 60 hours at laboratory temperatures using the solution
    silver nitrate .... 10 g
    distilled water .... 10 ml
    96% alcohol .... 90 ml
    N nitric acid .... 0.1 ml

the impregnation bath being prepared as in the original formula of Davenport by first of all dissolving the silver nitrate in the distilled water and then adding the other reagents; the content of nitric acid is 5 times less than in the original formula; moreover, the pH has been brought back to about 5 in cases where the impregnation is practised at 37°C by the addition of several drops of ammonia (3 to 4 drops per litre of bath); this adjustment serves no useful purpose when the impregnation is carried out at laboratory temperatures. Keep the solution in a brown bottle in which it keeps well whether or not ammonia is added and it will serve several times.

Wash rapidly (about 10 seconds) in 96% alcohol;

Reduce for 1 minute and keep the slides vertical and, if possible, in motion, using Davenport's mixture

> pyrogallol .... 5 g
> distilled water .... 100 ml
> commercial formalin .... 5 ml

Rinse in 3 baths of 96% alcohol (1 minute per bath);

Dehydrate in absolute alcohol, clear in a benzenoid hydrocarbon and mount in a synthetic resin or in Canada balsam.

The D cells appear with a striking selectivity because their secretory granules are impregnated with black; the cytoplasmic prolongations of these elements are very easy to follow. The background of the preparation is a clear yellow or brown; the A cells may take on a brown colour which is more intense than that of the B cells, but except in the cases of some of the Reptilia there is no likelihood of confusion so far as their distinction from the D cells is concerned. In most cases impregnation at laboratory temperatures is preferable.

Once examined and photographed, the preparation may be used for the demonstration of the different cell types and the detailed study of suitably chosen microscope fields obviously has a considerable value for teaching purposes. The following working technique is that advised by the originators of the method.

> Carry out silver impregnation of the D cells (A_1 cells) in conformity with the working technique set out above;
> Where appropriate, mount in a medium miscible with water after the sections have been hydrated and examine the preparation photographing suitably selected fields;
> Remove the preparation from the mount and, if necessary, hydrate it;
> Oxidise using the potassium permanganate-sulphuric acid of Gomori as if preparing for staining with paraldehyde-fuchsin and chromic haematoxylin; this procedure results in the total destaining of the impregnated tissues;
> Destain with sodium bisulphite;
> Stain using chromic haematoxylin-phloxin or with paraldehyde-fuchsin, using a background stain which will show up the A cells;
> Dehydrate, clear in a benzenoid hydrocarbon and mount in a synthetic resin or in Canada balsam;
> Rephotograph the same microscope fields as after the first mounting and compare the two sets of photographs.

As Fujita (1968) has quite rightly remarked, phloxin, under the technical conditions of this method, stains both the A cells *and* the D cells; the cells impregnated in the first stage of the method should thus correspond, if the technique has been properly employed, to the cells which are phloxinophil after the second stage of the staining technique, but the use of a background stain which at one and the same time includes a green or blue constituent as well as a red constituent shows that the impregnated cells are cyanophil, the A cells which are not impregnated during the first stage being erythrophil.

Preparations which are rather more synthetic, in which one can preserve the results of the two stages of the method, can be obtained, from my own personal experience, by toning with gold in the impregnation techniques which employ Davenport's method, thus allowing us to carry out, without destaining, the permanganate oxidation and staining using paraldehyde-fuchsin or, more particularly, that of my personal variation using azan, which was described in relation to the demonstration of the A cells. The method involves the following stages:

> Sections in paraffin wax, impregnated so as to demonstrate the D cells, using Hellerström and Hellman's technique;
> Verify the result of the impregnation by microscopic examination of the section mounted in 96% alcohol; photograph it where appropriate;
> Hydrate the section and rinse in distilled water;
> Treat for 5 to 10 minutes with a 0.2% aqueous solution of gold chloride (without any addition of acetic acid);
> Rinse in distilled water;
> Treat for 1 minute with a 5% aqueous solution of sodium thiosulphate (hyposulphite);
> Wash for 2 to 5 minutes in running water;
> Oxidise using potassium permanganate in a sulphuric acid medium, following Gomori's method, destain using sodium bisulphite and carry out azan staining (my personal variation p. 1023);
> Dehydrate in absolute alcohol, clear in a benzenoid hydrocarbon and mount in a synthetic resin or in Canada balsam.

The D cells are impregnated with black, the A cells are stained red by the azocarmine and the B cells, whose cyanophilia is much increased by the treatment as a whole, stained blue. Staining by paraldehyde-fuchsin can be practised in the place of azan but the contrast between the black of the impregnation and the violet stain of the B cells is less advantageous.

Impregnation using silver proteinate following Grimelius' technique (1964), which was carried out using German samples of protargol, has been put forward as a method for demonstrating the former assemblage of A cells, that is to say the D cells (A_1 cells) and the A cells (A_2 cells). The author of the method himself emphasizes the essential role of the particular commercial sample of silver proteinate in securing a successful impregnation and he notes in a more recent publication (1968) that no brands of protargol at his disposition permit him to reproduce the results which he published earlier. Experience proves that Grimelius' method using protargol carried out with samples of the product which are currently available on the French market ensure an excellent demonstration of the D cells, the selectivity and the optical qualities of the preparations equalling those of the best impregnations by the method of Hellerström and Hellman. This fact was noted during work on the endocrine pancreas of *Eliomys quercinus* (Gabe and Mme Martoja, 1969); results obtained since then allow me to state that the same is true in the islets of Langerhans of all the gnathostome vertebrates. Grimelius' technique using protargol should then be retained, with reservations made inevitable by the uncertainty as to the constitution of silver proteinate, as a method for the detection of D cells. According to the original description, which I would advise investigators to follow to the the letter, this method is practised in the following way.

Reagents:

Buffer	1.7% acetic acid		1.2 ml
	1.6% sodium acetate		0.3 ml
	distilled water to make up to		100 ml
Reducer	Hydroquinone		1 g
	Crystalline sodium sulphite		5 g
	Distilled water to make up to		100 ml

A 2% aqueous solution of oxalic acid.
A 5% aqueous solution of sodium thiosulphate (hyposulphite).

Working technique:

Paraffin wax sections, taken from material fixed in Bouin's fluid, dewaxed, and where appropriate treated with collodion (a thin film), hydrated and washed in distilled water renewed several times;
Impregnate for 48 hours, at about 45°C, in the solution
    buffer .... 100 ml
    silver proteinate .... 2 g
(this bath may be used once again);
Wash in 2 baths of distilled water;
Treat for 10 minutes at laboratory temperatures with the reducer;
Wash rapidly in distilled water;
Treat for 3 minutes with oxalic acid;
Rinse in distilled water;
Fix for 10 minutes in sodium thiosulphate;
Wash in running water (for about 5 minutes), dehydrate, clear and mount in Canada balsam or in a synthetic resin.

The D cells are impregnated with an intense black, with a striking selectivity, on a yellow or purple background. The nuclei are also very clearly shown up and the connective fibres may be impregnated. Other special features of this excellent method, whose use is unfortunately subject to factors outside the users control, have been discussed in relation to the calcitonine cells and the gastro-duodenal endocrine cells.

Staining sequences for demonstrating different types of cell in selected islets

The difficulties of selection which arise as soon as we have to confront the results obtained by various techniques of staining of adjacent sections of one and the same piece of tissue explain the usefulness of synthetic preparations which show several types of cell simultaneously on the one hand, and on the other sequences of stains carried out on one and the same slide with a photographic record of the results obtained at the successive stages in suitably chosen islets. One such sequence, as used by Hellerström and Hellman (1960), was described above and deals with the silver impregnation of D cells using a modification of Davenport's method. A more complicated sequence was put forward by Epple (1967) which includes the following stages.

Paraffin wax sections, taken from material fixed in Bouin's fluid;
Stain using toluidine blue following Manocchio's technique, *without methylation*, mount in the stain, and examine and photograph selected islets (for preference using colour photography);
Remove the coverslip and impregnate the section with silver following Hellerström and Hellman's technique; the stain due to toluidine blue disappears entirely; examine and rephotograph the selected islets;
Oxidise with potassium permanganate in a sulphuric acid medium following Gomori's technique;
Destain using a 3% aqueous solution of oxalic acid;
Wash for at least 10 minutes in running water;
Rinse in distilled water;
Stain for 10 minutes or longer (according to the species of animal) using the solution
  distilled water .... 100 ml
  NN'-diethylpseudoisocyanin chloride .... 0.020 g
(this mixture will keep in a refrigerator for several months; allow it to return to laboratory temperature before use);
Mount in distilled water and examine for the B cells either in white light, for colour photography, or in monochromatic light, at 578 mμ, or in ultraviolet light (using the UGI excitation filter, and the ultraviolet filter k430 of Leitz);
Wash the sections, re-oxidise using potassium permanganate in a sulphuric acid medium and stain with paraldehyde-fuchsin, staining the background with a combination of acid fuchsin, ponceau and light green approximating to the Masson-Goldner trichrome. This latter procedure will enable the A cells to be picked out.

Techniques for demonstrating other types of cell

In addition to the three fundamental types, whose existence in the endocrine pancreas of all the gnathostome vertebrates is agreed by the vast majority of modern authors, other types of cell have been noted; their presence has generally been remarked upon only for one or for a small number of species, so that a definitive statement on the matter will have to await further work.

The C cells of the endocrine pancreas of the guinea pig (Bensley, 1912) and of man (Bloom, 1931) are characterised by the absence of cytoplasmic granulations and by the diffuse affinity of the cytoplasm for the orange G in neutral gentian violet as well as for Heidenhain's azan; their absence from the islets of Langerhans in other mammals has been categorically stated by Thomas (1938). Brief fixation in Helly's fluid is the only method used by these authors and is in any case highly to be commended as a preparation for staining with neutral gentian violet. Examination at the level of ultrastructural cytology confirms the validity of this type of cell whose functional significance and relationship with other types of insular cells remains to be discovered.

The E cells of the islets of Langerhans in the opossum (Thomas, 1938) seem to exist only in this animal. They are characterised by their relatively peripheral position in the islets and by the magenta colour of their granulations after fixing in Helly's fluid and staining with Heidenhain's azan; the very widespread assertion that these granulations take up magenta (basic fuchsin) is erroneous. Electron microscopy confirms the validity of this type of cell (Caramia *et al.*, 1965) but, as in the case of the C cells, we do not know its functional significance.

The F cells of the processus uncinatus of the dog's pancreas resemble the A cells in their affinity for stains. Lazarus and Volk (1956) recognised them from their more general morphological characteristics and they have also been discovered on electron micrographs by Caramia *et al.* (1965). Their significance is unknown and there seems to be no way of staining them in a fully selective fashion.

The agranular hyaline cells, which are to be found particularly in the endocrine pancreas of teleosts, may correspond to the immature cells of other categories (Falkmer *et al.*, 1964).

D. — THE ADRENAL GLAND

The technical details which require mention for a histological examination of the adrenal gland are diverse and may be set out schematically in three groups. Some methods are particularly to be recommended for the anatomical study of this organ, for the demonstration of its constituent parts and in order to obtain certain information of a histophysiological order; others are intended for the examination of the adrenal cortex in mammals and of its equivalent in other vertebrates, that is to say, for a study of the interrenal tissue; yet others provide cytological and histochemical data on the medullo-adrenal of mammals and on its equivalent in the other vertebrates, the adrenal tissue.

TECHNIQUES FOR THE TOPOGRAPHICAL STUDY OF THE ADRENAL GLAND

The rapid postmortem autolysis of the adrenal gland is not the only feature to be taken into consideration during the dissection of this organ when a histological examination is to be undertaken; modern research on the general syndrome of adaptation abundantly illustrates the surprising speed with which morphological modifications take place in the adrenal tissue, and also in the interrenal tissue of animals subjected to stress, so that it is essential to avoid any rough treatment of animals whose adrenal gland is destined for histological examination.

Dissection should be rapid and the dimensions of the pieces of tissue to be fixed should be adapted to the requirement of a rapid penetration of the fixatives; slicing the tissue may be rendered awkward because of the soft consistency of the organ so that it is valuable to use an extremely sharp blade and to proceed with sawing movements avoiding any pressure, however slight, on the fragment being sectioned. Dicing the tissue is useful in cases where the dimensions of the gland are greater than those of the adrenal of the rabbit or the cat; even in smaller animals cutting into two halves may be useful when perfect preservation of the medullo-adrenal is required.

The choice of fixatives is a delicate one because of the need to use methods as diverse as topographical stains, tests for free lipids and the detection of catecholamines, and even certain histo-enzymological reactions. It is thus impossible to recover all the data required by a histological study from a single piece of tissue fixed in a single fluid, even though the objectives are diagnostic ones. Fixation in diluted formalin, whether saline or not, using calcium formaldehyde is indispensable during tests for free lipids, whereas fixing with a mixture based on potassium bichromate and which does not contain corrosive sublimate should be used for the histochemical localisation of catecholamines. Even though it is true that topographical techniques can be used on frozen sections and on paraffin wax sections taken from material so fixed, the use of a fixing bath such as Bouin's fluid or Halmi's fluid nevertheless remains desirable, even though it is not indispensable. Fixing in acetone chilled to about 4°C or, better, using saline formalin, chilled to the same temperature, is a suitable preparation for histo-enzymological research, and even sections taken from fresh tissue, cut up in a cryostat or in a microtome with a frozen blade, may be useful.

The preparation of the tissue for section cutting and the section cutting itself must inevitably take into account the requirements of the techniques for which they are a preparation. Some pieces of tissue should be sectioned in a freezing microtome, others after paraffin wax embedding; embedding in celloidin is useful only in those very rare cases where voluminous adrenals require to be sectioned as a whole.

Among **the topographical stains,** those which give a good demonstration of collagen fibres are particularly suitable; in addition to azan, one step trichrome and techniques using naphthol black B (Curtis' method and its variations) are particularly to be commended in the case of mammalian tissue; Masson's trichrome and its variations also give very good topographical preparations and, in addition, they show up the erythrophil cells of Vines. In addition to a clear delimitation of the zones of the gland, these techniques are remarkable for facilitating tests for the connective hyperplasia which, in cases of reduced activity of the adrenal, occurs at the edges of the glomerular and fasciculated zones on the one hand, and in the internal part of the reticulated zone on the other (the internal and external transformation fields of Tonutti, 1942). Silver impregnation of the reticulin will obviously give preparations which are particularly useful for the analysis of the connective web of this organ.

The delimitation of the cortex and of the medulla poses no problems in the case of the adrenal gland of mammals, but the distinction between interrenal and adrenal tissue may be more difficult in Anamniota and Sauropsida, in which the two tissues are often intermingled. In fact the high lipid content of the interrenal cells explains their "clear" aspect in preparations treated by topographical techniques and it makes this distinction more evident; it is nevertheless true that techniques for the demonstration of free fats on the one hand, and those techniques which enable us to detect catecholamines on the other, give preparations the contrast of which is much improved and it can only be helpful to use them even for the anatomical study of the organ.

The evaluation of the relative volume of the cortex and of the medulla should be conducted by the usual procedures (sketching followed by cutting out and weighing or by planimetry) in the case of the adrenal gland of mammals. When the form of the gland is well defined and constant, measurements on suitably oriented sections may give an order of magnitude which is sometimes sufficient for the comparison of the individual reactions of animals which form part of a single experimental lot. Techniques of linear integration should be applied for the evaluation of the proportions of interrenal and adrenal tissue in the adrenal gland of Sauropsida. In the Anamniota, the adrenal cells may be isolated, a fact which seriously complicates the quantitative analysis of the organ.

The vascularization of the adrenal gland may be studied by procedures described in Chapter 36; *the demonstration of the nerves* clearly forms a part of the neurofibrillar techniques; Gros-Schultze's method using frozen sections and the methods of Bodian, Holmes and Palmgren generally give good results. The introduction of the osmium-iodide technique may be useful in certain cases.

TECHNIQUES SPECIALLY RECOMMENDED FOR THE STUDY OF THE INTERRENAL TISSUE

Any cytological and histochemical technique may be applied for research purposes to the adrenal cortex of the mammals and to the interrenal tissue of other vertebrates; only methods which are useful when the examination is undertaken with diagnostic ends in view are set out below.

Among *the so-called general techniques,* those which ensure a clear demonstration of the collagen tissue are particularly useful in the case of the adrenal gland of mammals; the demonstration of connective hyperplasia in the "transformation fields" of Tonutti, already noted in the preceding section, is diagnostic of a reduced activity of this organ. Moreover, the analysis of the *nuclear structures* is useful whatever the zoological status of the animal studied; the caryometric studies of Sandritter and Hübotter (1954) which illustrate the valuable results obtainable from nuclear and nucleolar measurements during a histophysiological study of the adrenal cortex have been mentioned on p. 164. Even in the course of a qualitative analysis, the reduction of size and increase in density of the nuclei, the deformations of their outlines or, on the other hand, their clear and vesicular appearance have a definite diagnostic value. The *demonstration of the chondriomes,* which is fairly easy in the case of interrenal tissue, gives very spectacular preparations and may be combined with the pheochrome reaction, as practised during research on the adrenal tissue. Any of the techniques indicated in the preceding parts of this work are suitable for these purposes.

Among *the histochemical techniques,* tests for *free fats* represent an essential stage in the examination of the adrenal cortex and, more generally, of the interrenal tissue, fixation in dilute formalin, whether saline or not, using calcium formaldehyde, followed by frozen sectioning, being obligatory in all cases. The staining of free fats by lysochromes and their examination in polarised light, with the precautions described on p. 457 to distinguish the birefringence of crystalline lipids in the section from that produced by the presence of liquid crystals, is sufficient when the objectives of the work are diagnostic. I might mention again that it is impossible to detect the ketosteroids histochemically (see p. 371) and also of the necessity of a correct interpretation of the results afforded by lysochrome staining; hyperactivity of the interrenal cells is shown by a depletion of the fats and fats which do not take part in the genesis of the steroids may accumulate in large amounts within the interrenal cells when these are functionally at rest. Tests for sterols using Liebermann's reaction or Windaus' reaction may also be useful.

The detection of PAS-positive compounds completes the demonstration of the collagen fibres and affords information on the possible presence of glycogen, a polysaccharide which is abundant in the adrenal gland of certain Anamniota and Sauropsida and it ensures a clear demonstration of the adrenal "colloid" noted in mammals and in reptiles, but whose functional significance is not yet known.

Naturally *tests for chromolipoids* are essential, the preferred site of the oxidised derivatives of the lipids (lipofuscins) of the adrenal gland of mammals being the internal part of the reticulated zone; the techniques indicated on p. 483 will serve to identify them.

The demonstration of iron may assist the diagnosis of the functional condition of the interrenal tissue, the intracellular accumulation of iron-bearing inclusions being a sign of reduced activity; in the corticoadrenal of the mammals; the greatest frequency of such inclusions is to be found in the internal part of the zona reticularis.

The detection of ascorbic acid is of considerable theoretical interest, the fluctuations of this substance being closely linked to the functional condition, but quantitative estimations are evidently much superior to histochemical demonstrations.

Among *the histo-enzymological techniques,* tests for alkaline phosphomonoesterase activity and of unspecific esterase activity often give positive results in the interrenal cells, but tests for Δ^5-3-β-hydroxysteroido-dehydrogenase activities is much more important from the histophysiological point of view (see Arvy, 1963 who has set out the results in detail and has given a bibliography).

I might mention that *the histochemical tests for proteins and those for nucleic acids* give only poor returns when the interrenal tissue is examined for diagnostic purposes.

Special types of cell exist in the interrenal tissue of certain vertebrates; among these *the erythrophil cells of Vines* are quite selectively shown up by variations on Masson's trichrome and by those of Altmann's fuchsin; *the Stilling cells* (*summer cells*) of the adrenal gland of anuran batracians of the genus *Rana* are easy to identify because of their acidophilia; Mann's method using methyl blue-eosin, that of Mann-Dominici and stains which employ the eosinates of azur and azan give particularly striking preparations. Histochemical reactions also afford a very clear demonstration of the summer cells; the same is true of the PAS method (Verne and Delsol, 1956) and of tests for protein-bound sulphydryls (Gabe, 1956).

TECHNIQUES PARTICULARLY SUITABLE FOR THE STUDY OF THE ADRENAL TISSUE

As in the case of the interrenal tissue, any of the cytological and histochemical techniques may be used in the course of research work on the adrenal tissue and only those methods which are most useful during an examination carried out with diagnostic ends are mentioned here.

Fixation by fluids with a potassium bichromate and formalin base, which do not contain corrosive sublimate, is essential when the tissue is to be submitted to the pheochrome reaction; Helly's fluid or that of Maximow are quite suitable for studies using so-called general techniques; Bouin's fluid and its variants, that of Halmi and Heidenhain's Susa, as well as mixtures of corrosive sublimate and formalin, preserve the general morphological characteristics of the cells but the specific secretory granules are dissolved in most mammals; they may be preserved in the Anamniota and Sauropsida. Fixing in dilute formalin, whether saline or not, is imperative prior to examination for noradrenalin cells using Eränkö's method as is treatment of the pieces of tissue or of thick sections with potassium iodate prior to tests for the same cells using the method of Hillarp and Hökfelt. Fixation in dilute formalin, followed by frozen sections, is a suitable preparation for histochemical tests for lipids and for enzymatic activity. The time spent by the tissue in the fixative, which should be chilled prior to use, should be short.

Topographical stains permit us to study the general histological characteristics of the adrenal cells and, in certain cases, may disclose morphological differences between the noradrenal cells and the adrenal cells. It happens that the secretory granules of the noradrenal cells are often more voluminous than those of the other type of cells and their affinities for dyes may be slightly different. Moreover, the general methods give us a preliminary impression of the abundance of the secretory granules, but much more precise estimates may be obtained using histochemical techniques.

The certain distinction between the two types of cell in the adrenal tissue depends above all on **histochemical methods.** In addition, the pheochrome reaction furnishes the most informative pictures of the abundance of the secretory granules in any of the adrenal cells.

The classical pheochrome reaction should be carried out according to the directions given in Chapter 21 and will show up the secretory granules of any of the adrenal cells; this reaction serves, as well, for the demonstration of the pheochrome tissue which is anatomically independent of the adrenal gland and treatment of the tissue with a mixture of an aqueous solution of potassium bichromate (3 to 5%) and formalin is advisable as a preparatory stage to dissection (Watzka, 1943). The various ways of intensifying the contrasts given by the pheochrome reaction are also described in Chapter 21.

Hillarp and Hökfelt's technique, as well as *Eränkö's technique*, described in Chapter 21, show up the noradrenal cells selectively; in addition to these techniques, I would particularly recommend an excellent recent method, due to Tramezzani, Chiocchio and Wassermann (1964). The procedure set out by these authors depends on the fact that fixation using mixtures with a glutaraldehyde base confers a yellow colour on the noradrenal cells, the adrenal cells remaining uncoloured. The contrast between the two types of cell can be considerably reinforced by treating the frozen sections, taken from material so fixed, with an ammoniacal silver complex which causes the yellow colour to become black.

The technique of Tramezzani and his co-workers includes the following stages.

> Fix small pieces of tissue in a 6.5% solution of glutaraldehyde, dilution of the 25% commercial solution being carried out with the buffer proposed by Millonig for electron microscopy (7 ml of 0.2 M monosodium phosphate solution, 43 ml of 0.2 M disodium phosphate solution, 50 ml of 5.7% saccharose solution) and allow them to stand in the solution for 1 to several hours, at laboratory temperatures;
> Section on a freezing microtome, collecting the sections in the fixative;
> Rinse for about 30 seconds in distilled water;
> Treat for about 20 seconds with an ammoniacal silver complex (the preparation of which was not specified in the original description of the technique);
> Rinse in distilled water;
> Treat for several minutes with a 5% aqueous solution of sodium thiosulphate (hyposulphite);
> Wash for several minutes in tap water;
> Mount on slides, dehydrate in absolute alcohol, clear in a benzenoid hydrocarbon and mount in Canada balsam or in a synthetic resin.

The noradrenal cells, which are yellow before the treatment with the ammoniacal silver complex, take on a colour which varies from deep brown to black, the adrenal cells remaining uncoloured. From my personal experience, Gros-Schultze's ammoniacal silver complex, as well as that of Gomori for the impregnation of reticulin, and that of Del Rio Hortega employing the tanno-silver, and silver hexamethylene-tetramine variations of Gomori's preparation are all equally suitable; a background stain using the aluminium lake of nuclear fast red may be applied after the water bath which follows fixing and prior to mounting.

Tests for free lipids may to some extent help with the discrimination between the two types of cell; experience shows that the adrenal cells often contain a small amount of free lipid, whereas the noradrenal cells are generally devoid of it; I might also mention that the BZL blue method is a background stain which is highly advantageous for sections treated by Hillarp and Hökfelt's method, especially in the case of the Sauropsida where the interrenal and adrenal tissues are intermingled (Gabe and Martoja, 1961).

Tests for unspecific acid phosphomonesterase activity also serve as an element in the discrimination between the two types of cell; in fact, this activity is always less strong in the noradrenal cells which may be completely devoid of it, whereas the adrenal cells always react strongly.

E. — ENDOCRINE TISSUES OF VERTEBRATE GONADS

It is true that experimental results and the observation of different stages of the reproductive cycle provide evidence in favour of the secretion of "sex hormones" by the gonads of certain invertebrates but the fragmentary nature of our knowledge obviously prevents us from trying to codify the techniques to be used for a histological study of the structures in question. Methods for the examination of the interstitial tissue of the testis, of the internal theca of the ovarian follicles and of the *corpora lutea* of the ovary are on the other hand easy to codify. Because of the chemical relationship of the hormones secreted by these organs and by the interrenal tissue such methods correspond to those set out in relation to the study of the interrenal tissue.

INTERSTITIAL TISSUE OF THE TESTES

The anatomical study of the interstitial tissue of the testes of vertebrates uses the same techniques as for the examination of the seminiferous part of the same organ; it will be discussed in the following chapter. It is however appropriate to mention at this point that the evaluation of the relative volume of the interstitial tissue, carried out in the usual way (sketching, followed by cutting out and weighing or by planimetry and linear integration), gives results less important than those given by the analysis of the Leydig cells using cytological and histochemical techniques. As Hooker (1948) has quite correctly commented, the condition of the interstitial tissue is much more important than its amount.

Examination of the interstitial cells for general signs of activity or rest (extent of the cytoplasm, nuclear characteristics) may be undertaken on preparations stained by so-called general methods; techniques which are, strictly speaking, caryological are obviously more advantageous and the shrinkage, which is often difficult to avoid during fixation of small fragments of the testes using chromo-osmic fluids or mixtures such as that of Regaud, or of Maximow, in no way hinders this work.

Mitochondrial stains give spectacular preparations and it is to be regretted that they are used in only some of the studies devoted to the interstitial tissue of the testes. The absence of acidophilic secretory granules in the Leydig cells avoids any danger of confusion of these formations with the mitochondria and makes it unnecessary to resort to crystal violet staining. Altmann's fuchsin and the ferric or cupric lakes of haematoxylin will serve equally well.

Tests for free lipids represent an essential stage of the histophysiological study of the interstitial tissue of the testes. It is often advantageous to follow the fixing in diluted formalin, whether saline or not, using formaldehyde-calcium, by embedding in gelatin using Baker's technique (p. 92) as there is a rather substantial tendency for the sections to disintegrate during the subsequent handling. In addition to staining by lysochromes the outstandingly important technique is examination in polarised light with the precautions indicated on p. 457; staining with Nile blue may also help to distinguish the lipids which are implicated in the metabolism of androgenic hormones from those which have a different functional significance. As in the case of the interrenal tissue, the demonstration of the androgenic hormones themselves cannot be obtained by histochemical reactions and numerous discussions relating to the "battery" of reactions diagnostic of the presence of ketosteroids (see p. 475) are now only of historical interest. Tests for sterols using Liebermann's reaction or that of Windaus are as useful as they are in the case of interrenal tissue. It is also very helpful to test for the possible presence of chromolipids.

Among *the histo-enzymological techniques*, the detection of Δ^5-3-β-hydroxy-steroido-dehydrogenase activity yields the most direct information about the functional condition of the interstitial testicular tissue; the demonstration of unspecific esterase activity is also distinctly useful. The description of these techniques is given in Chapter 22.

INTERNAL THECA OF THE FOLLICLES

As in the case of the interstitial testicular tissue the anatomical study uses the techniques already recommended for the study of other parts of the ovary, techniques which are described in the following chapter.

An examination for the general signs of activity or of rest uses the same technical procedure as for the interstitial tissue of the testes; the examination of preparations treated by topographical techniques gives useful information in this respect, but caryological methods give the most distinct pictures. The usefulness of mitochondrial staining is less than in the case of the Leydig cells.

The detection of free lipids plays the same role as it does in the study of the other steroidogenic tissues (the interstitial testicular tissue, the corpora lutea and the interrenal tissue) and uses the same techniques. It is of course proper to take into account the birefringence of the collagen constituents of the external theca during the examination of preparations intended for tests for anisotropic lipids.

Technical details relating to *the histo-enzymological techniques* which were given in relation to the interstitial tissue of the testes are valid for the internal theca of the ovarian follicles.

CORPORA LUTEA

Topographical methods provide information about the general structure of these formations and bring to light the resemblance between the luteal cells and those of the adrenal cortex giving some indication of the amount of lipid material occluded within the cytoplasm. Fixing in Bouin's fluid, in Heidenhain's Susa or other topographical fixatives is quite suitable. As for the stains, azan, one step trichrome and variations on Masson's trichrome very clearly show up the organisation of the corpora lutea; the PAS reaction, followed by background staining with Groat's haematoxylin and picro-indigo-carmine or the allochrome method of Lillie (p. 400) also give very informative preparations. As in the case of the internal theca, the usefulness of *mitochondrial staining* is but slight.

Among **the histochemical techniques,** tests for free lipids and for chromolipoids are in the first rank, the technical details being the same as for the other steroidogenic tissues. Chromo-osmic fixation, of widespread use in the past, certainly shows up osmiophilic lipids, but staining by lysochromes and examination of frozen sections, taken from material fixed in formalin, under polarised light are much to be prefered; in fact, an accumulation of osmophilic lipids often occurs in the luteal cells during the first stages of involution so that osmic blackening frequently illustrates lipids which have no connection with steroidogenesis. The enzymatic equipment of the corpora lutea varies a great deal from one animal species to another; a strong Δ^5-3-β-hydroxysteroido-dehydrogenase activity exists in all cases studied to date; unspecific esterases may often be demonstrated (see Arvy, 1963 for an inventory of the results and for the bibliography).

F. — THYROID GLAND

The basic reasons motivating a histological examination of the thyroid gland, apart from what is, properly speaking, research into the microscopic anatomy, arise from the desire to obtain information about its functional state and to identify the epithelial cells other than the principal cells (calcitonin cells or macrothyrocytes, parafollicular cells, ovoid cells, etc., and the Langendorff cells or corridor cells).

The removal of the organ calls for no particular comment; fixation as a whole may be practised for small species, whereas in others slicing the organ may be necessary. I might mention the need to remove the region situated ventrally with respect to the branchial copuli as a single block, followed by the taking of serial sections during the histological study of the thyroid gland of most teleosts, this organ being diffuse and represented by isolated vesicles.

Fixing the thyroid gland when this has been dissected out for diagnostic purposes should be carried out using topographical mixtures; Bouin's fluid is perfectly suitable as are its variations or Heidenhain's Susa; mixtures with a potassium bichromate and formalin base will better preserve the colloid *in situ* but in fact the differences between the results so obtained and those given by fixatives containing acetic acid are not sufficiently great to render its systematic use necessary.

The preparation for section cutting and the section cutting itself call for only a few special comments. Embedding in paraffin wax is to be used in most cases; only very voluminous tissue, intended for the analysis of anatomical relationships, is worth embedding in celloidin. The thyroid colloid often shows a tendency to harden considerably during paraffin wax embedding so that it is helpful to soften the cut block by soaking it in water (p. 107).

In most cases *topographical stains* suffice to provide the evidence for a diagnosis of the functional condition; in addition to the disposition of the thyroid vesicles as a whole and of the general appearance of the epithelium, they show the height of the thyroid cells, the positioning of the nuclei, the homogeneous or vacuolised structure of the cytoplasm and the amount of colloid present. The techniques which make use of several acid stains (azan, Masson's trichrome, one step trichrome and Mann's technique using methyl blue-eosin) often cause erythrophil or cyanophil zones to appear within the colloid, this difference of staining affinity being considered by the classical authors as an index of the functional condition (cyanophilia corresponding to activity, erythrophilia to the resting condition); in fact, we now know that the differences of affinity for dyes correspond to differences of hydration and that histochemical techniques show up no significant differences between the two types of colloid so that these aspects are devoid of functional significance.

Techniques which are, properly speaking, cytological, especially those which show up the chondriome and the golgi apparatus, give very informative preparations so far as the activity or rest of the thyroid cells is concerned, but the results of the so-called general methods and of certain histochemical techniques are at the same time quite as clear and easier to obtain; the cytological tests therefore do not represent an obligatory step in the histological examination of the thyroid gland when this is undertaken for diagnostic purposes.

Among **the histochemical techniques,** the PAS reaction, followed by background staining as suggested on p. 400, is the technique of choice for the histological study of the thyroid gland; in fact, this method gives preparations of excellent quality in which the colloid and the secretory granules of the thyroid cells appear with the greatest clarity, the demonstration of the nuclei, of the basement membranes and of the general structure of the parenchyme being as good as it is with the best of the so-called general methods. It is, then, this technique which I would advise for adoption as a routine method during the histological examination of the thyroid gland, undertaken with a view to diagnosis. The ferric ferricyanide reaction also gives a very selective demonstration of the colloid, as does Danielli's coupled tetrazonium reaction.

The Langendorff cells (corridor cells) show up clearly on preparations treated with PAS or after staining with azan, the essential feature which allows us to identify them being the similarity of the affinity for dyes of their cytoplasm and of the colloid. Naturally, the nuclei of the cells in question are pycnotic.

The calcitonin cells (parafollicular cells, clear cells, macrothyrocytes, ovoid cells of the opossum etc...), whose autonomy as independent cell lineages has been recognised by virtue of the demonstration of the hormone which they secrete, are designated as C cells following Pearse. This name has the twofold inconvenience of not being descriptive and of utilising a name which was already used by Bensley (1912) for type of cell in the endocrine pancreas.

As Nonidez, to whom we owe the discovery of the argyrophilia of the elements in question has remarked (1932, p. 490), **the topographical staining techniques** give preparations in which the parafollicular cells are, because of their morphological peculiarities, not too difficult to identify, but naturally techniques for their selective detection greatly assist the study of such elements. Among the techniques in question we may mention silver impregnation, staining and histochemical reactions.

The fundamental investigations of Nonidez (1932, 1933, 1934) were undertaken using the second variation of the technique using reduced silver due to Ramon y Cajal and this method is an excellent technique for the impregnation of the cells in question in blocks of tissue, but we must insist on the fact that silver impregnation on sections is far and away preferable since its use can be combined with that of other techniques whereas impregnation in tissue blocks obviously prevents the piece of tissue from being used for any other purpose. Davenport's technique, carried out as for the demonstration of the D cells of the endocrine pancreas, gives very good results in most mammalian species (Solcia and Sampietro, 1965; Kameda, 1968; Gabe and Mme Martoja, 1969; Solcia et al., 1970). Grimelius' technique using silver proteinate (1964) which was described in relation to techniques for the study of the endocrine pancreas gives excellent impregnation of the calcitonin cells (Gabe and Mme. Martoja, 1969) when carried out using the samples of protargol currently available on the French market. Grimelius' technique using silver nitrate, which was described in relation to the study of the endocrine cells of the digestive tract, is much praised by Solcia et al. (1970) as a method for the silver impregnation of calcitonin cells. All these impregnations on sections give good results after fixing in Bouin's fluid, Halmi's fluid, the GPA of Solcia et al. (1968), formalin or glutaraldehyde, embedding being carried out in paraffin wax without any special precautions.

Among **the stains**, the selective affinity for phosphotungstic haematoxylin, which was discovered by Bensley (1914), seems to be limited to the calcitonin cells (ovoid cells) of the opossum. A strong cyanophilia of these elements has been noted in certain species, Mann's method using methyl blue-eosin, azan or one step trichrome giving preparations in which the calcitonin cells appear with the greatest clarity (Gabe, 1959). Permanganate oxidation in an acid medium, conducted as for the staining of the hypothalamic neurosecretory product, confers on the secretory granules of the calcitonin cells of certain species a strong affinity for paraldehyde-fuchsin (Gabe, 1959) and peracetic oxidation is even better as a preparation for this stain (Lietz and Zippel, 1969). The method used by Solcia et al. (1968) confers an intense metachromasia on the calcitonin cells; in some species a metachromatic stain of these elements can be obtained without hydrochloric acid hydrolysis simply by treating the sections with toluidine blue at pH 5.4, following the directions of the Italian authors. A strong affinity for copper phthalocyanins of the alcian blue group appears following hydrochloric acid hydrolysis. Staining with lead haematoxylin, following the formula of Vassallo and his collaborators, which was given in the section on the gastro-intestinal endocrine cells, selectively stains the calcitonin cells of an appreciable number of mammalian species.

Research work during the last fifteen years has resulted in considerable progress in our knowledge of the histochemistry of the calcitonin cells; most of the histochemical reactions requiring mention here are not indeed superior to the stains which have just been mentioned when the object of the work is the identification of the type of cell in question. The PAS reaction gives positive results in all cases (Kroon, 1958; Gabe, 1959, 1961; Idelman, 1962; Pearse, 1966), but the preparations obtained are not generally well contrasted; in the case of the rat the activity is sufficiently weak for Leblond's school (see Young 1968 for the bibliography) to have used the term "clear cells" to designate the calcitonin cells. The presence of protein-bound sulphydryls (Gabe, 1959, 1961; Lietz and Zippel, 1969) seems to be a constant characteristic; the reaction to DDD and that to ferric ferricyanide thus ensures the demonstration of calcitonin cells. We know from the methodical researches of Lietz and Zippel (1969) that the method using colloidal iron, when carried out following Müller's technique, but adjusting the pH to 5 by the addition of Michaelis' buffer in place of the acetic acid, gives positive results in the calcitonin cells of eight species of mammal including man; this capture of iron is greatly reinforced by preliminary hydrochloric acid hydrolysis as commended by Solcia and his co-workers (1968), whereas the classical reaction using colloidal iron, practised at pH 1.2, becomes entirely negative after this hydrolysis. The metachromasia after staining with 6,6-dichloro-N'N'-diethylpseudoisocyanin chloride is particularly clear, according to Lietz and Zippel (1969), in the calcitonin cells of the thyroid gland of the rat.

We may add to all this that the calcitonin cells show the histochemical characters of the APUD series; tests for α-glycerophosphate-dehydrogenase, when menadione (vitamin K_3) is added, following Wattenberg and Leong (1960), gives strongly positive results in these cells. Spectrographic study by electronprobe microanalysis discloses the presence of an important amount of calcium in the calcitonin cells of six mammalian species (Mme Martoja, 1971).

G. — EPIPHYSIS

As I remarked at the beginning of this chapter, recent progress in our knowledge of the epiphysis is due primarily to physiological and biochemical research, but the systematic study of the nervous connections of this organ, brought to fruition by Ariens Kappers (1965), has played an important part in the interpretation of the relationships of the pineal gland with the encephalon gland and with the other endocrine glands. Naturally, any cytological and histochemical technique can be recommended for work on the epiphysis forming a part of histological research; only methods which have proved their worth in demonstrating the normal constituents are set out below.

The dissection should take account of anatomical peculiarities, these being very variable according to the animal species involved. There are no problems in large animals; the closeness of the connections with the pia-mater, even the existance of adhesions with the dura-mater frequently leads the experimenter to remove the whole region instead of undertaking a true dissection. In smaller species the pineal gland can be removed together with the encephalon; adhesions to the skull may make it necessary to keep a sagittal band of bony tissue in position with subsequent decalcification.

The choice of fixatives depends closely on the object of the work. Bouin's fluid, Heidenhain's Susa, Zenker's fluid, Helly's fluid and that of Carnoy serve for topographical studies, saline formalin or formaldehyde calcium will prepare the tissue for tests for lipids on frozen sections, as does diluted formalin for neurofibrillar impregnations on frozen sections and brominated formalin for investigations on the neuroglia.

The subsequent treatment of the tissue also depends on the objective of the study. Material intended for topographical study should be embedded in paraffin wax, a short decalcification using nitric or trichloracetic acids often being necessary, especially when the epiphysis of older animals has been fixed in a fluid which does not decalcify it; embedding in celloidin should as usual be reserved for large pieces of tissue intended for anatomical study. Sectioning on a freezing microtome is essential for tests for lipids and for certain silver impregnations.

Among *the topographical stains*, Heidenhain's azan, one step trichrome and variations on Masson's trichrome give very good results; Bargmann (1943) recommends staining with iron haematoxylin-acid fuchsin-Mallory's blue, which was described for the study of the alveoli of the lung (p. 892). These techniques show up the connective constituents of the organ very clearly but it may be necessary to resort to silver impregnation of the reticulin (Chapter 33) in certain cases.

Histochemical techniques are also useful in the study of the epiphysis; the PAS method gives good topographical preparations and is a suitable preliminary for investigating the possible presence of carbohydrates; the frequency with which free lipids occur explains the appositeness of staining frozen sections taken from material treated with formalin by means of lysochromes, the other techniques for the histochemical detection of lipids being chosen in the light of the results obtained. It seems scarcely worth using the histochemical tests for proteins; I might in particular mention the negative results of tests for indole groups even though melatonine, which is itself an indole compound, is quite certainly present in the organ. Nevertheless, this negative result was obtained before it had been shown that glutaraldehyde had excellent qualities as a histochemical fixative for indole compounds. The pigments which so frequently occur in the epiphysis should be studied by the techniques described in the third part of this work in relation to the chromolipoids (p. 483) and the melanins (p. 580). Histochemical tests for calcium and micro-incineration may be appropriate, such tests obviously need to be carried out when the tissue has been fixed (see Chapter 13).

The nervous and neuroglial constituents of the pineal gland may be shown up by the techniques described in Chapter 40; Bodian's and Palmgren's methods are particularly suitable for neurofibrillar impregnation, Ramon y Cajal's technique using gold and corrosive sublimate being the method of choice for the impregnation of protoplasmic astrocytes. According to Bargmann (1943), and Romeis (1948) a technique due to del Rio Hortega (1923) shows up the pineal cells and their prolongations excellently. The technique, of which I have no personal experience, is described here, following to the letter the recommendations of the authors just cited.

Fix for at least 48 hours in dilute formalin (1 volume of formalin to 9 volumes of water);

Frozen sections;

Wash the sections with great care in several baths of distilled water;

Place the sections in a 2% aqueous solution of silver nitrate to which 3 drops of pyridine have been added for every 10 ml of solution; warm to about 50°C and maintain in an incubator at 37°C for several hours or at laboratory temperatures (in darkness) for 24 hours; the sections should take on an ochre tint;

Wash in distilled water to which 2 drops of pyridine have been added for every 10 ml;

Impregnate in the solution of silver carbonate intended for oligodendroglia (p. 959) the sections are placed in the solution which is warmed to about 50°C and the sections are kept in the impregnation bath until they have taken on a sepia tint;

Wash in distilled or tap water;

Reduce in 10% formalin for 1 to 2 minutes;

Rinse in distilled water;

Transfer to a 0.2% aqueous solution of gold chloride, warming it slightly where necessary to intensify the colour which should become violet;

Rinse in distilled water;

Fix for a short time (about 1 minute) in a 5% aqueous solution of sodium hyposulphite;

Wash for a long time in frequently renewed tap water;

Place the sections on slides, dehydrate, clear and mount as for neuroglial impregnation using ammoniacal silver carbonate (p. 958).

H. – HISTOLOGICAL STUDY OF HORMONAL TARGET ORGANS DURING HISTOPHYSIOLOGICAL STUDIES ON THE ENDOCRINE GLANDS

Experience shows that changes in the target organs for a hormonal secretion are, in many cases, a more sensitive reflection of the hormonal content of the blood than is the morphology of the gland where the hormones in question are secreted. Some of these changes are of a physiological or biochemical nature and would be out of place here. Other changes however may be followed by means of the morphological techniques described in this work. For this reason, it seems to me to be useful to stress the desirability of this histochemical examination of the target organs in any case where the histological study of an endocrine gland is carried out with diagnostic ends in view and to mention the special features in the form of a table. The working techniques do not need to be described because they are set out in other chapters of this work; an appreciation of the appropriate changes to be studied falls outside histochemical technique in the strict sense of the term.

Table 35. — Principal indications for the examination of hormonal receptors in histophysiological research on the endocrine glands of vertebrates

Endocrine gland examined	Hormonal receptors to be examined
Adenohypophysis	Skeleton (long bones). Thyroid gland Gonads Adrenal cortex and interrenal tissue Mammary gland (possibly)
Thyroid gland	Adenohypophysis Skeleton (young animals only) Liver Haemopoiesis Sub-maxillary gland (Muridae)
Parathyroid gland	Skeleton
Male gonads	Genital tract and auxiliary glands Sub-maxillary gland (Muridae) Kidney (Sauria and Ophidia). Digital callosity (Frog) Adenohypophysis
Female gonads	Genital tract Sub-parotid gland (Rat). Kidney (Sauria and Ophidia) Adenohypophysis
Adrenal cortex and interrenal tissue . . .	Lymphoid organs (lymph nodes, thymus, Peyer's patches).

CHAPTER 43

TECHNIQUES FOR THE HISTOLOGICAL STUDY OF THE REPRODUCTIVE SYSTEM

A great diversity of histological techniques may be used for the study of the reproductive system although there are no "special methods" restricted to this purpose, so that in this chapter we need only mention procedures which have already been described.

HISTOLOGICAL EXAMINATION OF THE MALE GENITAL SYSTEM

It is appropriate to consider, successively, the technical details of an anatomical study of the testes, particularly those of the vertebrates, then the cytological analysis of the various stages of spermatogenesis, and lastly consideration of the genital ducts and of the glands attached to them.

MICROSCOPIC ANATOMY OF THE VERTEBRATE TESTES

Research into the microscopic anatomy of the male gonad of vertebrates uses topographical techniques and calls for only a few special comments.

Although **dissection** should be carried out as rapidly as possible, the dangers arising from post-mortem autolysis are less for the testes than for other organs which normally secrete proteolytic enzymes; for this reason the removal of the testes should be carried out after that of the digestive apparatus, the kidney and the adrenal during a complete autopsy of an animal of small size, especially when it is only the anatomical study of the male gonad that we need to consider.

Fixation may be carried out as a whole for small blocks of tissue (testes not exceeding the dimensions of those of the mouse); many authors consider that fixing *in toto* reduces the risks of shrinkage and consider this procedure advisable even for tissue blocks of the size of a rat or guinea-pig testis. Bouin's or

Halmi's fluids, Heidenhain's Susa, or the fixatives of Helly, Maximow and Carnoy are entirely suitable.

The preparation of the tissue for section cutting requires certain precautions, especially in cases where shrinkage must be avoided at all costs. It is, indeed, the case that shrinkage takes place not at the time of fixation but during the dehydration and impregnation by a paraffin wax solvent. A technique of progressive dehydration was described by Allen (1918). This technique avoids any sudden change in the composition of the fluid by adding the new dehydration medium drop by drop to the old one. Allen even goes so far as to recommend that this procedure be adopted even for embedding in paraffin. Most modern authors rightly consider that such a long and complicated working technique is not justified by the results obtained. Romeis (1948) recommends the dehydration by suspension of the testes fixed as a whole in 96% alcohol, keeping the tissue blocks in this fluid, which is renewed two or three times, for two to three days. *Embedding* should be undertaken in paraffin wax. There is a serious risk of severe shrinkage when this method of embedding is applied to tissue fixed in dilute formalin, whether saline or not, or by formaldehyde calcium; it is desirable to allow the tissue to stand for two to three days in a 3% aqueous solution of potassium bichromate and then to wash it for 24 hours in running water before beginning the dehydration. Embedding in gelatin is useful for material from which frozen sections are to be cut.

The cutting of sections calls for no particular comment.

In addition to **topographical stains**, such as azan or Masson's trichrome and its variations, or one-step trichrome, the PAS technique, followed by background staining as described on pages 400–402, gives preparations which are very easy to study, which show clearly the basement membranes of the seminal ducts and on the one hand allow us to identify the various stages of spermatogenesis and on the other allow us to study the interstitial cells. The relative abundance of these latter cells may be evaluated on this kind of preparation by sketching the sections followed by cutting out and weighing or by planimetry; procedures using linear integration may also be applied.

THE MICROSCOPIC ANATOMY OF THE INVERTEBRATE TESTES

The technical details for the histological examination of the invertebrate testis are the same as those which have just been set out for the vertebrates; for most animals the testis may be fixed as a whole as in most cases its size will be less than that of the testes of small vertebrates.

The composition of the organ is usually more homogeneous than in the case of vertebrates and it is not always worthwhile to use techniques which ensure the easy detection of collagen fibres when choosing a topographical stain. The PAS method always give excellent preparations and, even for an anatomical study, it may be useful to employ techniques which allow the different affinities for dyestuffs of the various types of cytoplasm to be clearly shown up; Mann's technique using methyl blue-eosin and the Mann-Dominici technique, together with azan and one-step trichrome, are all equally suitable in this respect.

Special features of the anatomical structure may frequently necessitate the cutting of serial sections since the various regions of the male gonad may show substantial structural differences.

It is appropriate, moreover, to comment that the male gonad is not anatomically distinct in many invertebrates since the testicular tubules are buried in other tissue.

THE STUDY OF SPERMATOGENESIS

The various stages of spermatogenesis are usually quite easy to recognise even on sections stained by topographical techniques; no special precautions are required when sections of the testis are used for the summary estimation of the relative abundance of male gonocytes at different stages of maturation.

It is quite otherwise when the objective of the work is the cytological study of spermatogenesis, that is to say the detailed analysis of the transformations which take place between spermatogonia and the formation of spermatozoids ready to pass into the male genital ducts.

The study of smears is in itself sufficient for the analysis of spermatogenesis in cases where the maturation of the gonocytes takes place entirely or substantially in the internal medium of the animal (annelids, polychetes, sipunculids); it is indispensable in every case. Often the examination of sections gives less clear cut results than the examination of smears so far as the cytological details are concerned, but does give information about the situation of the different stages in the testicular tubes, and about their relationships, because of the grouping into bundles of the elements derived from the division of a single line of cells. The smears and sections should be studied concomitantly in all cases where the anatomical characteristics of the gonad permit one to make both types of preparation.

Smears may be made by techniques described for the study of the nucleus and of the chondriome (Chapters 24 and 26); their fixation should be undertaken using techniques described for this purpose. Among the stains, the variations on Flemming's triple stain, safranin-light green, variations on Altmann's fuchsin and staining using the regressive lakes of haematoxylin are all particularly to be commended; I might particularly mention the advantages of rapidity and simplicity when using iron haematoxylin staining after fixation using the vapour of osmium tetroxide (Grassé, 1926); the working technique was described on p. 790. Feulgen and Rossenbeck's nucleal reaction is also very useful and when Heidenhain's technique, described on p. 555, using aniline blue-orange G as a background stain, is brought into play most of the organelles are easy to identify on synthetic reparations. The PAS technique has the advantage of showing up the acrosome with complete selectivity in a large number of cases. Naturally, any other cytological and histochemical technique may be used so long as the fixation of the smears was carried out with the special requirements of the technique used in view.

In this context I might recollect how difficult it is to secure metallic impregnation of the Golgi bodies (dictyosomes) on smears whereas their staining by ferric haematoxylin is relatively easy to obtain. In cases where the investigator needs to study the structures by light microscopic techniques, metallic impregnation (osmic for preference) should be undertaken on tissue blocks and not on smears.

Sections intended for the cytological study of spermatogenesis should be taken from material fixed in a fashion suitable for general cytology; the fixation of the testis as a whole may only be undertaken for animals of very small size, the organ requiring to be sliced in all other cases. Chromic-osmic fluids which either do not contain acetic acid or only contain a small amount, as well as mixtures of potassium bichromate and formalin, with or without corrosive sublimate, are most suitable for a study of the structural details, followed by mitochondrial staining or Flemming's triple stain and the nucleal reaction of Feulgen and Rossenbeck as well as the PAS reaction all of which are standard options. Evidently any other cytological and histochemical technique may be required.

THE STUDY OF THE EXCRETORY DUCTS FOR SPERM AND OF THE GLANDS ATTACHED TO THE MALE GENITAL SYSTEM OF VERTEBRATES

The examination of the organs dealt with in this section has for a number of years become a routine in laboratories which undertake research into sexual endocrinology and most of the workers engaged in this task content themselves with using topographical techniques on the material in question. It is necessary to recognise that fluctuations in the amounts of androgen hormone in the internal medium entrain spectacular modifications of the morphology of the glands attached to the male genital system as well as of the excretory ducts for the sperm, so that there is indeed a partial justification for the attitude mentioned above. Nevertheless, cytological and histochemical techniques give such clear information that it seems to me desirable to mention them here.

The fixation of the epididymis, of the vas deferens, of the seminal vesicles and of the prostate or equivalent glands may be carried out as a whole in animals whose size does not exceed that of the rat, especially when only topographical techniques require to be used; even for a topographical study of larger animals cutting the organ into slices, whilst taking account of its particular anatomical features, may be useful; obviously it becomes essential even with the rat when mitochondrial techniques or the impregnation of the Golgi bodies need to be carried out. Bouin's or Halmi's fluid, or Heidenhain's Susa are quite suitable for topographical studies, those fluids with a potassium bichromate and formalin base should be used in preparation for mitochondrial techniques, the fixatives mentioned in Chapter 25 being obligatory for the metallic impregnation of the Golgi bodies (dictyosomes).

The preparation of the tissue for section cutting calls for only one comment, namely the desirability of embedding in celloidin when the complex formed by the prostate gland and the seminal vesicles of the animals of a certain size has been fixed as a whole with a view to a topographical study; we need hardly add that the use of fixatives containing picric acid is unsuitable in the latter case. Material fixed in cold formalin for the detection of enzymatic activity should be cut on a freezing microtome. The cutting of paraffin wax sections may be rendered difficult by the substantial amount of hardening of the secretory products accumulated in the lumen of glands attached to the male genital system; it is very useful to soften the tissue by soaking the cut blocks in water.

Among ***the topographical stains***, those which show up the collagen fibres are particularly to be recommended; I would recommend the use of azan, one-step trichrome, and the variations of Masson's trichrome; these techniques clearly show up the various secretory products whose erythrophilia or cyanophilia follow the rules set out in relation to the thyroid colloid at least in a certain number of cases.

Cytological techniques may be very useful for an appreciation of the functional condition of the organs discussed here. The extent of the changes in the chondriome of the excretory ducts for sperm, of the seminal vesicles and of the prostate gland as a function of changes in the androgen content of the blood is well known and renders apparent the desirability of calling mitochondrial techniques into play; the absence of accumulations of granules of a fuchsinophil secretion in the organs mentioned may lead one to confuse them with mitochondria and makes it pointless to use crystal violet, so that in fact variations on Altmann's fuchsin and the regressive staining by haematoxylin lakes applied as described in Chapter 26 are all quite suitable. Changes in the Golgi apparatus are no less important; techniques using silver impregnation succeed readily in these organs. The study of the nuclear structures is also of some importance since a sudden spurt of mitoses is one of the first manifestations of activity in the accessory glands when the androgen content of the blood rises; the clarity of the appearance is generally sufficient for an analysis using topographical techniques.

Among *the histochemical techniques* the PAS method, whether or not combined with alcian blue staining, ensures a very clear demonstration of the secretory products of the various auxiliary glands of the male genital system; it may be adopted as a routine staining technique. Methods for the histochemical study of proteins and lipids can be very useful in work which forms part of histological research but it is not necessary to have recourse to these in cases where the histological examination is undertaken for diagnostic purposes. Histo-enzymological techniques which are as easy to use as the detection of alkaline and acid phosphomonoesterase activity or of unspecific esterase activity are, on the other hand, of the greatest usefulness even when the organs discussed here are examined within the framework of a sexual endocrinological study.

STUDY OF THE MALE GENITAL TRACTS AND OF THEIR AUXILIARY GLANDS IN INVERTEBRATES

The anatomical and histological diversity of these structures makes it impossible to codify the techniques needed for their study; we can give only some general remarks at this point.

The anatomical study should be carried out using topographical methods; because of the generally small size of these organs fixation may be carried out as a whole, to be followed normally by embedding in paraffin wax. In addition to the usual trichrome stains, methods such as those of Mann using methyl blue-eosin and of Mann-Dominici are very useful for discriminating between the secretory products of different glands, the same remark holding good for stains based on the eosinates of azur.

Any *cytological or histochemical technique* may be used, the pretreatment of the tissue being carried out with the special requirements of these techniques in view. The special usefulness of the PAS technique combined with alcian blue staining is explained by the frequent occurrence of secretory products rich in carbohydrates in the auxiliary glands of the male genital system of invertebrates; the same is true for any histochemical reaction which serves to discriminate between different polysaccharides. In the same way techniques for the identification of proteins often give spectacular preparations, tests for ribonucleic acids being most valuable for the study of glandular cells.

The secretion of spermatophores occurs rather frequently in representatives of various invertebrate classes; the examination of the male genital system in such cases includes the histochemical study of the different layers of the spermatophore and tests for the compounds so identified in the male genital tracts in order to obtain information on the site and the mode of such secretion.

HISTOLOGICAL STUDY OF THE FEMALE GENITAL SYSTEM

As in the case of the male genital system the technical details differ according to whether the work involves the microscopic anatomy of the gonad, the cytology and histochemistry of ovogenesis or the histology of the genital tracts.

MICROSCOPIC ANATOMY OF THE VERTEBRATE OVARY

The technical problems posed by the histological examination of the vertebrate ovary vary according to the size of the animals and the structural details of the oocytes.

Fixation may be undertaken *in toto* in the case of small mammals; cutting into slices is required above a certain size. The less dense texture of the ovary of Anamniota and Sauropsida allows us to fix larger blocks of tissue *in toto* than in the case of mammals.

The choice of fixatives is determined by the size of the oocytes and whether they are full or empty of yolk. Bouin's or Maximow's fluids or Heidenhain's Susa or Stieve's fixative (p. 183) are entirely suitable for the mammalian ovary as is Carnoy's fluid. Fixing in Flemming's liquid is much to be recommended but blocks of tissue whose size exceeds that of the rat ovary are too voluminous to be fixed as a whole in this liquid. Acetic acid-corrosive sublimate and Carnoy's fluid are particularly to be commended in the case of the ovaries of the Anamniota. Naturally fixing in fluids with a picric acid base should be avoided in cases where celloidin embedding is made necessary either by the size of the tissue blocks or by their consistency.

The preparation of the tissue for section cutting should take account of the requirement just mentioned; embedding in paraffin wax is obviously the quickest method but passage through celloidin may be rendered necessary by the size of the tissue blocks, the presence of particularly voluminous oocytes which are rich in vitellus, or even by the abundance of connective tissue. During embedding in paraffin wax the use of methyl benzoate or salicylate as an intermediate between the dehydrating alcohol and the benzene is very much to be recommended; it is even better to embed by passing through butanol or through cedarwood oil.

The need to examine the various regions of the organ should be foreseen when the *sections are spread*; the procedure described on p. 115 is very suitable for small tissue blocks; for more voluminous ovaries the gap between the sections taken as samples from the ribbon may be greater (one section out of 50 or out of 100 when the ribbon is cut 5 or 10µ thick).

As for *the stains,* those which selectively demonstrate the collagen fibres are recommended for the mammalian ovary; one-step trichrome, variations on Masson's trichrome and azan additionally stain the vitellus of the oocytes of the ovaries of Anamniota and Sauropsida very clearly. Staining by safranin-light green is the method of choice when an important objective of the work is the clear demonstration of the nuclei in the yolk filled oocytes. Flemming's triple stain and the use of ferric haematoxylin are required when the material has been fixed in Flemming's fluid, and the nucleal reaction of Feulgen and Rossenbeck, followed by a background stain using picro-indigocarmine, or Heidenhain's aniline blue-orange G (p. 555) is suitable in any case where the fixation of the tissue is compatible with an adequate histochemical demonstration of deoxyribonucleic acid. Mann's method using methyl blue-eosin very clearly stains the vitelline platelets, as does the Mann-Dominici technique, this latter technique also providing information about the abundance of ribonucleins in the cytoplasm of the oocytes. Very good topographical preparations are obtained, in the case of ovaries which are poor in connective tissue and rich in immature oocytes, by staining with methyl green-pyronine provided that the material has been fixed in a liquid which prepares it suitably for this technique. The PAS reaction is also very advantageous for the study of the vertebrate ovary, its association with alcian blue staining being of no great usefulness in this particular case.

Counting of the ovarian follicles (of the *corpora lutea* etc...) may be required in studies of the ovarian cycle; topographical stains allow us to identify these structures and to classify them in stages. The quantitative study of the internal thecae necessitates sketching the serial sections, cutting out the sketches and weighing, or planimetry; this procedure is not used in the course of research on ovarian endocrinology as it is easier to obtain information about the oestrogen hormone content of the blood from a study of the hormonal receptors.

The connective web of the ovary, *its vascularisation and innervation* may be studied by techniques described in the appropriate chapters of this book.

MICROSCOPIC ANATOMY OF THE FEMALE GONADS OF INVERTEBRATES

The ovary of certain invertebrates is not anatomically distinct and it has to be dissected together with the neighbouring tissue (the digestive gland of gastropods for example). In most instances the size of the organ allows it to be fixed as a whole.

The fixative mixtures to be used are the same as for the vertebrate ovary, Flemming's, Carnoy's, Maximow's or Bouin's fluids being particularly useful.

The preparation of the tissue and the cutting of sections require only one special comment, namely the need for a rigorous orientation of the tissue blocks in all cases where the different stages of oogenesis are arranged in a definite order (insect ovarioles for example). Embedding in paraffin is the method of choice in most cases.

The choice of *stains* should be undertaken having regard to the extent to which connective tissue enters into the constitution of the organ; this is not generally very important so that it is unnecessary to use techniques such as van Gieson's stain or the picric acid-naphthol blue black stain whereas azan, Masson's trichrome, and one-step trichrome are to be recommended because they also clearly demonstrate the staining affinities of the cytoplasm. Safranin-light green, Flemming's triple stain, and regressive staining using the ferric and cupric lakes of haematoxylin will serve equally well as does the method of Mann using methyl blue-eosin and that of Mann-Dominici. The PAS method also gives very good results and shows up at the same time the vitellus and the basement membranes with the greatest clarity.

CYTOLOGICAL AND HISTOCHEMICAL STUDY OF OVOGENESIS

Because of the dimensions and the consistency of the oocytes of most Metazoa the preparation of smears plays only a minor part in the study of ovogenesis but it may be interesting to examine freshly dissected oocytes between a slide and coverslip; the technique of this examination, as well as that of vital staining call, for no special comment.

Fixation should be undertaken on cross sections of the body in the case of polychaete annelids whose oocytes complete their development within the coelom; the oocytes of Sipunculids leave the ovary at a very early stage of maturation so that the fixation of small individuals as a whole or the puncture of the general body cavity, followed by concentration by centrifugation, represent the practical means for obtaining working material from these animals.

Any cytological and histochemical fixative may be used according to the object of the study. Carnoy's fluid serves well for the analysis of the nuclear structures and for demonstrating cytoplasmic ribonucleins; preservation of cytoplasmic detail is ensured by chromo-osmic fluids; as a preparation for these reactions we should employ the fixatives recommended in relation to the various histochemical techniques. Bouin's fluid, Heidenhain's Susa and fixatives of the same kind generally preserve the vitelline platelets well.

The preparation of the tissue for section cutting in the vast majority of cases involves paraffin wax embedding carried out in such a way as to prepare for the use of histochemical and cytological techniques. It is only very rarely that celloidin embedding is made necessary by the consistency of the tissue. The histochemical study of lipids and of most enzymatic activity obviously requires the preparation of frozen sections; this latter procedure greatly benefits from preliminary embedding in gelatine, carried out according to Baker's technique (p. 92), for the study of lipids, and carried out according to Pearse's technique (p. 93) for the study of enzymatic activities.

Among *the stains* histochemical reactions and diagnostic stains, some are more particularly adapted for the study of nuclear structures; the nucleal reaction of Feulgen and Rossenbeck, the technique using methyl green-pyronine and staining with gallocyanine should be placed at the head of this group. The two last methods supply information simultaneously about the amounts of cytoplasmic ribonucleins, essential data in studies of the cytology of ovogenesis. The chondriomes may be studied by the techniques described in Chapter 26, the use of Benda's or Nassonov's techniques being rendered, perhaps, necessary by the difficulty of discriminating between mitochondria and vitelline platelets in the early stages of their formation. Any of the techniques recommended for the study of acidophilic secretory products show up the vitelline platelets whose histochemical study represents an essential stage in the histochemical examination of ovogenesis; the PAS technique, the general reactions of proteins and staining with lysochromes, these latter stains being applied to frozen sections taken from formalin-fixed material, serve as techniques for orientation and help us to choose reactions which may be employed at the later stages of the work. The yolk bodies are examined by the techniques described in Chapter 27.

HISTOLOGICAL STUDY OF THE FEMALE GENITAL TRACTS OF VERTEBRATES

Techniques which are, properly speaking, cytological play only a minor role in the histochemical examination of the genital tracts of mammals, when these are examined for diagnostic purposes; the modifications of these organs which result from fluctuations in the blood content of female sex hormones show up clearly on preparations stained by topographical methods, but certain histochemical techniques are of the greatest utility for their study. In the same way, the histological examination of the placenta calls for no "special" methods.

Fixation should be carried out using the so-called topographic mixtures for the purposes of general study and for the histochemical techniques to which I have just alluded, whereas for histoenzymological research we may use acetone or, better, dilute formalin, whether saline or not, chilled to the temperature of melting ice; tests for free lipids on frozen sections of formalin treated material are not necessary in diagnostic studies of the female genital tract. Naturally, the size of the block of tissue should be chosen having regard to the penetration of the fixatives and the usual precautions should be taken during the fixation of material such as the fallopian tube, the uterine horns or the oviducts in order to avoid deforming them during preparations for section cutting.

Material treated with formalin and intended for histo-enzymological studies should be cut on a freezing microtome; embedding of other tissue may be carried out using paraffin wax except when their size is too great.

Topographical stains which show up collagen tissue clearly are particularly to be commended for the study of blocks rich in muscular tissue; at the same time they show details of the structure which need to be taken into account for a diagnosis of the functional conditions based on the characteristics of the epithelial parts. The PAS method, combined with alcian blue staining, also gives very good topographical preparations.

Among **the histochemical reactions** the list is headed by those useful for the identification of carbohydrates; in addition to the PAS technique, which has already been mentioned, staining with toluidine blue, as set out in relation to the histochemical study of metachromasia (p. 346), is a great help in classifying the mucins secreted by the various segments of the female genital tract and the data so afforded may be supplemented by those derived from other techniques discussed in Chapter 17. The usefulness of the histochemical reactions of proteins is less in the study of the tube and of the uterus of mammals than in the case of the vagina and the female genital tracts of Sauropsida and Anamniota; it may be advantageous in the study of the vaginal cycle of mammals, although topographical stains and the PAS technique suffice for an analysis of this cycle. Tests for calcium are necessary in the study of the oviduct of oviparous vertebrates bearing eggs surrounded by a calcareous shell and any technique which gives positive results on the shell of the eggs should evidently be applied to the oviducts of birds, reptiles, teleosts and selacians.

Tests for many enzymatic activities can also be of diagnostic value in the study of female genital tracts; the monograph of Velardo and Rosa (*in* Graumann and Neumann, 1964) gives a fully documented review of the state of knowledge prior to that date.

The practice of **vaginal smears,** in work on female sex hormones, is sufficiently well known to make it unnecessary to emphasize this subject Sampling is carried out with a spatula, with a metallic strip or a glass stirring rod suitably calibrated; any lesion of the vaginal mucosa should be avoided with the greatest possible care. The smears are prepared by rapid spreading of material obtained by scraping the mucosa; they may be fixed in methyl alcohol, in acetone or in a mixture of equal parts of absolute alcohol and ether. Numerous stains derived from Masson's trichrome have been recommended in clinical gynaecology; in fact, a simple stain using toluidine blue suffices for the identification of mucous threads, of epithelial cells, granulocyte and corneal squamae, the presence or absence of which furnish the elements of a diagnosis of the stages of the vaginal cycle in Muridae; the use of a trichrome stain shows up more clearly the erythrophilia of the corneal plates characteristic of oestrus.

HISTOLOGICAL STUDY OF THE FEMALE GENITAL TRACTS OF INVERTEBRATES

As in the case of male genital tracts, the anatomical and functional diversity of these tracts according to the systematic position of the animals inhibits us from any true codification of the techniques useful for the histological examination of the female genital tracts of invertebrates and only a few very general comments can be given here.

Fixation should take account of the needs of topographical studies, but glands which secrete material rich in mucin on the one hand and proteins on the other are much better represented in the female genital tracts of a large number of invertebrates than in those of the vertebrates, so that techniques which are, properly speaking, cytological and histochemical have an interest in the second case which they do not have in the first.

In the great majority of cases **embedding** may be carried out in paraffin wax.

In addition to **topographical stains, histochemical methods** as indicated for the study of carbohydrates and proteins are particularly important in the cases which concern us here. Even tests for mineral substances may be of some interest.

In addition to the identification of the secretory products of the auxiliary glandular formations of the genital tracts, the determination of compounds which enter into the composition of the shells which surround the eggs, which link chains of eggs, or which constitute cocoons, etc... have an obvious interest and the comparisons of results so obtained with those stemming from an examination of the genital tracts give useful information on the sites of secretion of the sheaths which protect the genital products.

APPENDIX

THE MASS PRODUCTION OF HISTOLOGICAL PREPARATIONS FOR TEACHING PURPOSES

The need to stain a large number of slides in a rigorously identical fashion, each slide bearing a single section of the same tissue block, is practically never met with in histological research, even though it be diagnostic; it is, on the other hand, of common occurrence in the preparation of slides intended for teaching purposes and one can only express astonishment at the attitude of most teachers, who use the tricks of the trade indicated below but rarely, and consequently involve themselves in an expenditure of time as great as it is useless.

In fact, the basis of this problem is of the greatest simplicity. We need in effect to cause the sections to adhere to a support which simultaneously permits us to manipulate the whole together throughout the preparations for mounting and also to enable us to separate them one from another during this last stage of the technique. The manipulator has in fact several possibilities.

a) **Sticking the sections to plates of mica** is the oldest procedure of this kind. It consists of causing the slides to adhere to sheets of mica of suitable thickness (sheets of 0.1 mm in thickness which are industrially available are very easy to split into yet thinner platelets), then drying the sections and treating the sheets of mica as carrying slides, completing the staining in flat receptacles (photographic developing dishes or petri dishes) of the appropriate size. Once clearing in a benzenoid hydrocarbon has been obtained the mica sheet is cut with scissors into as many fragments as there are sections and each section is mounted on a slide with the section oriented upwards; it may be useful to press down on the sheet with a weight of about 20 g, in order to ensure the elimination of air bubbles.

b) **Obregia's technique,** described in relation to the sticking of celloidin sections, may be adapted to the treatment of paraffin wax sections. The procedure involves the following stages.

> Cover a perfectly clean glass plate with the mixture: —
> solution of dextrin-candy sugar (p. 122) and distilled water in equal parts
> and spread the sections on this mixture;

Dry in an embedding oven;
Dewax in 2 baths of a benzenoid hydrocarbon;
Flush out the benzenoid hydrocarbon with 2 baths of absolute alcohol;
Cover the glass plate with a 5% collodion solution and allow to drain so as to obtain as thin a coating as possible;
Harden the coating in a bath of 70% alcohol;
Cut the coating across 3 sides, 0.5 cm away from the edge of the glass plate, immerse in distilled water; the solution of the mixture of candy sugar and dextrin results in the coating coming loose but adhering along the uncut edge to the glass plate, thus facilitating subsequent manipulation;
Carry the sections on the glass plate from one staining bath to another;
Begin dehydration in 96% alcohol, finish it in phenolic benzene, clear in benzene and mount as in the technique using sheets of mica.

This second technique is less costly than that using mica sheets but the solidity of the support for the sections is less, so that it is necessary to fish for the sections as during the processing of frozen sections. As a result the manipulator necessarily inhales a far from negligeable amount of benzene vapour; this undesirable feature can be avoided by mounting on slides in 96% alcohol, only the completion of dehydration and the clearing necessitating the manipulation of the individual slides.

*c) **Varnishes*** whose composition has not been published but which are industrially available (Zyklonlack in the terminology of Swiss chemical industry, C-Lack, of I.G. Farben), suitably diluted with acetone (about 1 volume of varnish for 5–10 volumes of acetone), allow us to cover the stained slides after acetone dehydration with a coating which hardens very quickly and is easy to remove as a whole taking the sections with it. Mounting is then carried out in Canada balsam or in a commercial synthetic resin; sections so "wrapped up" in the coating of protective varnish may be preserved for a long time between two sheets of very smooth paper.

BY WAY OF A BIBLIOGRAPHY

The absence of a detailed bibliographical index at the end of this book cannot fail to shock certain readers and the three reasons for this state of affairs should be set out.

A list, however incomplete, of the publications consulted during the preparation of this work would have enormously increased its size. Naturally the authors of the publications which have formed the basis of this text have been directly mentioned or else indicated by referring the reader to recent reviews. Nevertheless, the transcription of the complete bibliographical details would have resulted in a disquieting increase in the number of pages in the book.

Moreover, some of the publications mentioned below, particularly those of Arvy (1957–58; 1963); Barka and Anderson (1963); Burstone (1962); Gray (1955); Lison (1960); Pearse (1960, 1968); and Romeis (1948, 1968) include bibliographical lists containing thousands of references. The preparation of a bibliography of histological techniques could be affected by cutting up and mounting on cards the indexes of which we have just spoken as well as the tables of contents of the principal periodicals devoted to histological technique which are also mentioned below. It would in fact be a heavy task and yet one the usefulness of which appears to be arguable since the texts and periodicals in question are easy to obtain.

Lastly but of the greatest importance, the present undertaking is the work of one who is irremediably inadapted to modern life, who attempts to carry out in person all the various tasks relating to his work; this work has benefited from no material aid whatsoever and the absence of any acknowledgements to scientific or technical colleagues is not an indication of ingratitude on the part of the author but of the solitary state in which the manuscript has been prepared. It was in fact the card index mentioned above, condemned in advance to be incomplete, which it was found necessary to sacrifice; and so it has been.

To aid the reader to consult the original sources the major periodicals substantially or wholly devoted to histological technique have been indicated below as have a certain number of books and treatises with the same orientation.

Journals of histological technique

Naturally there is a far from negligeable number of histological techniques published, together with the results obtained with their aid, in reports whose title would not even cause one to suspect that they had any technical relevance. When hidden in this way the techniques in question would certainly escape those who do not systematically consult the major histological journals the reading of which forms a part of the professional duties of any histologist.

Moreover, the journals whose names are listed below specialise to a greater or lesser extent in the publication of technical articles.

Acta histochemica, Jena.
American monthly microscopical Journal, Washington.
Annales d'Histochimie, Paris.
Bulletin d'Histologie appliquée, Lyon—Paris.
Bulletin de Microscopie appliquée, Paris (successor to the foregoing).
Bulletin de la Société belge de Microscopie, Brussels.
Folia histochemica et cytochemica, Warsaw.
Histochemie, Berlin.
Journal of Histochemistry and Cytochemistry, Baltimore.
Journal of the Royal microscopical Society, London.
Journal de Microscopie, Paris.
Mikroskopie, Vienna.
Rivista di Istochimica normale e patologica, Milan.
Stain Technology, Baltimore.
Transactions of the American microscopical Society, Lancaster.
Zeitschrift für wissenschaftliche Mikroskopie, Leipzig.

Books on histochemical technique

The list given here has no pretensions to completeness; omissions in no way imply judgements as to the value of the works which are not cited. Consultation of the books which are mentioned has been of the greatest utility during the preparation of this handbook and the author is fully aware of the debt that he owes to his predecessors.

ADAM (H.) & CZIHAK (G.). — *Arbeitsmethoden der makroskopischen und mikroskopischen Anatomie*, FISCHER (G.), Stuttgart, 1964.
APPELT (H.). — *Einführung in die mikroskopischen Untersuchungsmethoden*. Akadem. Verlagsgesellschaft, Leipzig, 1955.
ARVY (L.). — *Les techniques actuelles d'Histo-enzymologie. Biologie médicale*, 1957–1958.
ARVY (L.). — *Histo-enzymologie des glandes endocrines*. Gauthier-Villars, Paris, 1963.
ARVY (L.). — *Histoenzymology of the endocrine glands-* Pergamon Press, Oxford 1971.
BAKER (J. R.). — *Cytological technique*. 5th Edition. Methuen & Co., London, 1966.
BAKER (J. R.). — *Principles of biological microtechnique*. Methuen & Co., London, 1958.
BARKA (T.) & ANDERSON (P. S.) — *Histochemistry*. Hoeber, New York, 1963; 2nd Edition, 1965.
BENSLEY (R. R.) & BENSLEY (S. H.). — *Cytological technique*. Univ. Chicago Press, 1934.
BOURNE (G. H.) & DANIELLI (J. F.) (Eds.). — *International Review of Cytology* (a review series with annual publication; vol. 1–20). Academic Press, New York, 1952–1967.
BERTRAND (I.). — *Techniques histologiques de Neuropathologie*. Masson & Co., Paris, 1930.
BURSTONE (M. S.). — *Enzyme histochemistry and its application in the study of neoplasms* Academic Press, New York, 1962.
CASSELMAN (W. G. B.). — *Histochemical technique*. Methuen & Co., London, 1959.
CLAYDEN (E. C.). — *Practical section cutting and staining*. 4th Edition. Churchill, London, 1962.

COLOVICK (S. P.) & KAPLAN (N. O.). — *Methods in Enzymology.* Academic Press, New York, 1955–1967 (in course of publication).
"COLOUR INDEX". 2nd Edition. Society of Dyers and Colourists, Bradford, Yorkshire & American Association of Textile Chemists and Colorists, Lowell, Mass., 1956; supplement, 1963.
CONN (H. J.). — Biological stains, 7th Edition. Williams & Wilkins Co., Baltimore, 1961.
CONN (H. J.), DARROW (M. H.) & EMMEL (V. M.). — *Staining procedures used by the Biological Stain Commission.* 2nd Edition. Williams & Wilkins Co., Baltimore, 1960.
COWDRY (E. V.). — *Microscopic technique in Biology and Medicine.* Williams & Wilkins Co., Baltimore, 1948.
CULLING (C. F. A.). — *Handbook of histopathological technique.* 2nd Edition. Butterworth, London, 1963.
DANIELLI (J. F.). — *General cytochemical methods.* Academic Press, New York, 1958, 1961.
DAVENPORT (H. A.). — *Histological and histochemical technics.* Saunders, Philadelphia, 1960.
EHRLICH (P.) (Edit.). — *Encyclopädie der mikroskopischen Technik.* Urban & Schwarzenberg, Berlin, 1st Edition 1903; 2nd Edition published by R. KRAUSE, 1926–1927; 3rd Edition 1937.
ERÄNKÖ (O.). — *Quantitative methods in Histology and microscopic Histochemistry.* Karger, Basel, 1955.
GATENBY (J. B.) & BEAMS (H. W.). — *Bolles Lee's "The Microtomist's Vade Mecum".* Mc Graw-Hill Book Co., New York, 1950.
GOMORI (G.). — *Microscopic Histochemistry.* The University of Chicago Press, Chicago, 1952.
GRAUMANN (W.) & NEUMANN (K.). — *Handbuch der Histochemie.* G. Fischer, Stuttgart, 1958–1967 (in course of publication).
GRAY (P.). — *Handbook of basic Microtechnique.* The Blakiston Co., New York, 1952; 2nd Edition 1964.
GRAY (P.). — *The Microtomist Formulary and Guide.* The Blakiston Co., New York, 1954.
GURR (E.). — *Methods of analytical Histology and Histochemistry.* Hill, London, 1958.
GURR (E.). — *Encyclopaedia of microscopic Stains.* Hill, London, 1960.
GURR (E.). — *Staining animal tissues.* Hill, London, 1962.
HAITINGER (M.), EISENBRAND (J.) & WERTH (G.). — *Fluoreszenzmikroskopie.* Akademische Verlagsgesellschaft, Leipzig, 1959.
HARMS (H.). — *Handbuch der Farbstoffe für die Mikroskopie.* Staufen-Verlag, Kamp-Lintfort, 1965.
HAUG (H.). — *Leitfaden der mikroskopischen Technik.* G. Thieme, Stuttgart, 1959.
HUMASON (G.). — *Animal tissue techniques.* 2nd Edition. Freeman & Co., San Francisco, 1967.
JONES-MCCLUNG (R.). — *McClungs Handbook of Microscopical technique.* Hoeber, New York, 1950.
JONES-MCCLUNG (R.). — *Basic microscopic technics.* The University of Chicago Press, 1966.
KRAJIAN (A. A.) & GRADWOHL (R. B. H.). — *Histopathological technic.* 2nd Edition. The C. V. Mosby Co., St. Louis, 1952.
LANGERON (M.). — *Précis de Microscopie.* 5th Edition. Masson & Co., Paris, 1949.
LILLIE (R. D.). — *Histopathologic Technic and practical Histochemistry.* 3rd Edition. McGraw Hill, New York, 1965.
LIPP (W.). — *Histochemische Methoden.* Oldenbourg, München, 1954–1967 (in course of publication).
LISON (L.). — Histochimie et cytochimie animales. 3rd Edition. Gauthier-Villars, Paris, 1960.
MCMANUS (J. A. F.) & MOWRY (R. W.). — *Staining methods, histological and histochemical.* Hoeber, New York, 1960.
MAHONEY (R.). — *Laboratory techniques in Zoology.* Butterworth, London, 1966.
MALLORY (F. B.). — *Pathological Technic.* Saunders Co., Philadelphia, 1938.
MARTIN (L. C.) & JOHNSON (B. K.). — *Practical Microscopy.* Blackie, London, 1958.
MARTOJA (R.) & MARTOJA (M.). — *Initiation aux techniques de l'histologie animale.* Masson & Co., Paris, 1967.
MELLORS (R. C.) (Edit.). — *Analytical Cytology.* 2nd Edition. McGraw-Hill Book Co., New York, 1960.

OSTER (G.) & POLLISTER (A. W.) (Eds.). — *Physical techniques in biological Research.* 6 volumes. Academic Press, New York, 1955-1967 (in course of publication).

PANTIN (C. F. A.). — *Notes on microscopical technique for Zoologists.* Cambridge University Press. Cambridge, 1960.

PEARSE (A. G. E.). — *Histochemistry.* 2nd Edition. Churchill, London, 1960; 3rd edition 1968/72.

PETERFI (T.) (Edit.). — *Methoden der wissenschaftlichen Biologie.* 2 volumes. Urban & Schwarzenberg, Berlin, 1928-1929.

POLICARD (A.), BESSIS (M.) & LOCQUIN (M.). — *Traité de Microscopie.* Masson & Co., 1957.

RAMON Y CAJAL (S.) & DE CASTRO (F.). — *Elementos de técnica micrográfica del sistema nervioso.* Tipografia Artistica, Madrid, 1933.

ROMEIS (B.). — *Mikroskopische Technik.* Oldenbourg, München, 1968.

ROULET (F.). — *Methoden der pathologischen Histologie.* Springer, Wien, 1948.

SCHMORL (G.). — *Die pathologisch-histologischen Untersuchungsmethoden.* 15th Edition. Vogel, Leipzig, 1928.

SCHULZE (E.) & GRAUPNER (H.). — *Anleitung zum mikroskopisch-technischen Arbeiten in Biologie und Medizin.* Akademische Verlagsgesellschaft, Leipzig, 1960.

SPIELMEYER (W.). — *Technik der mikroskopischen Untersuchung des Nervensystems.* 4th Edition. Springer, Berlin, 1930.

STEEDMAN (H. F.). — *Section cutting in Microscopy.* Blackwell, Oxford, 1960.

VIALLI (M.). — *Introduzione alla Ricerca in Istochimica.* Industria Poligrafica Lombarda, Milan, 1953.

ZEIGER (K.). — *Physiko-chemische Grundlagen der histologischen Methodik.* Steinkopff, Dresden and Leipzig, 1938.

SUBJECT INDEX*

A

Acetate of 5 bromo-4-chloro-indoxyl, esterases, 631, 632
– – copper, cupric haematoxylin, 695, 696
– – p-N, N'-dimethylamino-phenylmercuric, detection of thiols, 520
– – – synthesis, 519
– – indoxyl, cholinesterases, 622
– – – esterases, 631, 632
– – manganese, oxidation of carbohydrates, 395
–, mercuric, chondriome mordanting, 724–725
– – naphthol AS, esterases, 628
–, α-Naphthyl, esterases, 628
–, β-Naphthyl, esterases, 628
–, naphthyl, cholinesterases, 623
Acetalphosphatides, definition, 449, 476
–, plasmal reaction, 477
Acid acetic, fixation, 50
– –, maceration, 770, 776
Acid, adenylic, phosphorylase, 641
–, alanine β-sulfonic, see cysteic acid
–, 8-amino-1-naphthol-3,6-disulfonic acid, see H acid
–, 8-amino-1-naphthol-5 sulfonic, see S acid
–, ascorbic, detection, 387
– –, after cryodesiccation, 387
– –, on cryostat sections, 387
– –, recommended tissue, 676
– –, at the cell scale, 388
– –, periodic oxidation, 391
– –, argentaffine reaction, 325
– –, ferric ferricyanide reaction, 322
– –, adrenal cortex and interrenal tissue, 1035
–, aurine tricarboxylic, aluminium detection, 311
–, boric, inhibition of oxidation by lead tetra-acetate, 416
–, carminic, 170
– –, see also carmalum
–, chloroplatinic, 46

–, p-chloranilido-phosphonic acid, phosphamidase, 619, 620
–, chloric, bleaching of melanin, 581
– –, see chlorine dioxide
–, chloroplatinic, fixation, 46, 58
– –, rhodopsine detection, 482, 982
–, chlorosulfonic acetic acid, esterification, 406
–, chromic and dichromates, decalcifying agent, 245
–, chromic, see chromium trioxide
–, citric, decalcifying agent (Lorch), 610
–, citric-ammonium citrate, decalcifying agent (Lillie), 611
–, cysteic, fuchsine-paraldehyde affinity, 353
– –, basophilia, 535
– –, fixation of metallic ions, 523
–, dehydro ascorbic, detection, 387
–, deoxyribonucleic, convenient tissues for detection, 677
– –, fixation, 565
– –, removal, by deoxyribonuclease, 563
– – – – nuclease, 563
–, deoxyribonucleic, see also nucleic acids, nuclear reactions
–, dimethylaminonaphthalene-5-sulfonic (chloride of), 276
–, formic, decalcification, 245
–, formic-sodium citrate (Greep) decalcification, 611
–, H, see amino-naphthol sulfonic acid, 511
– –, Morel and Sisley reaction, 511
–, 2,4-dinitrofluorobenzee reaction, 497
–, tetrazoreaction of Daninelli, 509–511
–, hydrochloric, decalcifying agent, 244–245, 840
– –, extraction of nucleic acids, 564–565
– –, fixation, 45
– –, normal solution, 672
– –, see also nuclear reactions, maceration, 771, 898
–, hydrochloric acid-sodium citrate, decalcifying agent (Lillie), 611

---

* For entries such as acetic acid, see acid, acetic.

Acid, adenylic *(cont.)*
 -, hyaluronic acid, depolymerisation, 418
 -, p-acetoximercurianiline, detection of thiols, 519
 -, p-hydrazino-benzene sulfonic, sulfonation, 432
 -, p-hydrazinobenzoic acid, carboxylation, 432
 -, o{2 – [α-(2-hydroxy-5-sulfophenylazo)-benzylidene] hydrazino} benzoic
 – – – – – – – –, see zincon
 -, 1,2-naphtholquinone-4-sulfonic, detection of steroids and their esters (Adam's reaction), 478
 -, nitrous, deamination, 503
 – –, diazotation, 498 511
 -, nitric, decalcification, 244 ú
 – –, fixation, 45
 – –, normal solutions, 663
 – –, ribonucleic acid removal, 564
 -, nucleic, 45, 47–48
 – –, basophilia, 339, 342, 540, 548
 – –, classification of detection methods, 539
 – –, definition, 538
 – –, differential basophilia, 545, 548
 – –, metachromasia, 348
 – –, methyl-green staining, 543–555
 – –, microspectrography in U.V., 539
 – –, pH of the staining solutions, 331–332
 – –, selective removal: by perchloric acid, 564
 – – – – –, trichloracetic acid, 563
 -, osmic, see osmium tetroxide
 -, oxalic, iron removal, 588
 -, peracetic, bleaching, of melanin, 582
 – –, preparation, 467
 – –, secretion products oxidation by, 468
 – –, thiols oxidation, 523–524
 – –, unsaturated lipid oxidation by, 468
 -, perchloric, extraction, for nucleic acids, 594
 -, performic, bleaching of melanins, 582
 – –, preparation, 467
 – –, secretion products, oxidation by, 758, 967, 1005
 – –, thiol oxidation, 523–524
 – –, unsaturated lipid oxidation by, 468
 – periodic, 391
 – –, alcoholic solution, for phosphorylase, 642
 – –, in Benson's method, 559
 – –, in Himes and Moriber's method, 558–559
 – –, starch detection, 430
 – –, substances oxidable by, 402–403

 – –, utilisation, first methods, 393; others, 399
 -, periodic-Schiff, see PAS
 -, phosphoric, tryptophane detection, 513
 – –, DNA hydrolysis, 553
 -, picric, 171
 – –, decalcification, 245
 – –, differentiation of Altmann fuchsine, 728–729, 731
 – – – –, ferric haematoxylin, 692
 – –, fixation, 46, 56, 59
 – –, removal of excess, 68
 -, ribonucleic, convenient tissues for research, 671
 – –, detection, 542, 551, 563–567
 – –, extraction by acid, 566–567
 – – –, by buffers, 567
 – – –, by ribonuclease, 547, 563–565
 – –, fixation, 567
 – –, lost during decalcification, 568
 – –, see also Nissl bodies, ergastoplasm, nucleolus
 -, rubanhydric, rubeanic acid, see dithioxamine
 -, S, Morel and Sysley reaction, 511
 -, sulphurated, affinity for fuchsin paraldehyde, 353
 – – – –, cupric phthalocyanines, 355, 523–524, 758
 -, sulphuric, normal solutions, 663
 -, sulphurous decalcification, 244–245
 – –, equivalent of the Schiff reagent, 362–364
 – –, fixation, 45
 – –, ribonucleic extraction, 567
 – –, Schiff reagent, 358–360
 -, sulphuric-acetic, esterification, 406
 – – –, anhydride, esterification, 406
 -, sulfuric-ether, esterification, 406
 -, thiacetic, thiocetic acid, see thiolacetic acid
 -, thiolacetic, carboxylic esterases, 626–627, 632
 – –, disulphide bonds reduction, 529
 -, thioglycolic, disulphide bonds reduction, 528
 -, thymic (apurinic), 557
 -, trichloracetic, decalcification, 244, 839–842
 – –, fixation by, 45, 58
 – –, nucleic acids extraction, 533, 563
 -, uric, argentaffine reaction, 326, 328, 592–593
 – –, basophilia, 339, 343
 – –, staining by carmin and methylene blue, 901–902

Acetic alcohol, azan, 220
– anhydride-acetic acid, -sulphuric acid, 504–505
– – – –, polysaccharides, 418–420
– – – –, vic-glycols, 419–420
Acetocarmin, caryotype, Belling, 702–703
– – –, Schneider, 703
Acetone, dehydration of sections, 148
– fixation, 44, 58, 597, 609, 615, 619, 624, 629, 633
p-acetoxymercurianiline, thiol detection, 519
n-acetyl-β-glucosaminidase, 635
Acetylation, principle, 419
–, working technique, 412
Acetylcholinesterase, cholinesterases, 622
Acidophily, definition, 134, 332
–, detection, 333
–, proteins, 532, 533
–, total, definition, 332
Acid resistance, chromolipoids, 484
Acriflavine, see trypaflavine
Acrolein, 52
Acylamino-carboxy-acids, detection, 493–494 (Barrnett and Seligman reaction)
Adenohypophysis, anatomical study, 992
–, identification of cellular categories, 993–1006
Adenosine-5-phosphate, 5-nucleotidase, 614–615
Adenosine-triphosphatase, detection, 612–613
–, suitable tissues, 678
Adenylic acid, phosphorylase, 641
Adrenal cortex, 11, 1031–7, 1047
Adrenaline, 575–579
Affinities, 50
Alanine β-sulfonic acid, paraldehyde fuchsine affinity, 365
Albumin, sticking the sections, 112
Alcohol, see ethanol
– celloidin, embedding, 88
–, -chloroform Auguste Prenant's method. for calcium, 307
–, diluted, maceration (Ranvier), 770
–, distillation, 71
–, formalin, Schaffer's fixative, 186
–, – for tanning, gelatin or albumin, 142
–, picric acid for haematoxylin differenciation, 693
–, sulfuric esterification, 406
Aldehydes, 54
–, affinity for fuchsine-paraldehyde, 353
–, argentaffine reaction, 328, 382
–, blocking reactions, 370
–, detection, 357, 370

–, distinction, with ketones, 371
–, ferric ferricyanide reaction, 325
–, peroxidase properties, 369
–, reactions of condensation, 496
Alizarine, 24–25
–, -cyanin, 168
–, -purpurine, see purpurine
–, -red S, 168
–, sodium sulfonate, 168
– – –, alkaline phosphatase detection, 299
– – –, bone staining (Lundwalle), 830
– – –, calcium detection, 299
– –, viridin, 168
Alkaloids, 46
Alkylamino-alcohols periodic oxidation, 391
Allochromasia, definition, 344
Alloxan, Romieu's reaction, 499
Alloxan-Schiff reaction, detection of α-amino-acids, 501–502
Alphazurine, see patent blue
Aluminium, detection with aurine-tricarboxilic acid (Lillie), 311
– – –, morin (pentahydroxyflavanol), 311
Amaranth, see azorubine S
Amines, 54
–, acetylation, 503–504
–, deamination, 503
–, detection (Lillie), 504
α-Amino-acids, detection, of terminal carboxyls, 493, 496
– – – –, by oxidative deamination, 499–502
– – – –, by azomethine formation, 496–497
– – –, fixation, 491
– – –, lead tetra-acetate oxidation, 394–395
– – –, periodic acid oxidation, 391–394
– – –, terephthalic aldehyde reaction (Danielli), 496
– – –, p-aminobenzaldehyde reaction (Danielli), 497
– – –, 2,4, dinitrofluorobenzene reaction (Tranzer and Pearse), 498
– – –, 3-hydroxy-2 naphthaldehyde reaction (Weiss and al.), 497
Amino-alcohols, periodic oxidation, 391
– – saponification after acetylation, 419
Aminonaphthol, 6-disulfonic acid, see H-acid, Morel and Sisley reaction, 511
4-amino-1-N, N'-dimethylnaphthylamine, cytochrome oxidase detection, 643–646
Aminopeptidase, see leucine-aminopeptidase
Ammonium acetate, 47–68
Amniotic fluid, 19
Amphophily, definition, 134
Amylase, glycogen lysis, 416, 423
α-amylase, phosphorylase detection, 641–642
β-amylase, phosphorylase detection, 642

SUBJECT INDEX

Amylo-1, 4, 1-6-transglucosidase detection, 640, 642
– –, suitable tissues for research, 678
Amyloid substance, 343
Amyl nitrite, 63
Angle of attack, razor, 99
Angle of the blade, 99
Angle of discharge, of sections, 99
Angle of facets, razor, 99
Anhydrides
–, acetic-acetic acid, or sulfuric acid, amines acetylation, 504–505
– –, pyridine, acetylation amines 504–505
– – – –, *vic*-glycols, 419–420
– – – –, polysaccharides, 418–424
–, phthalic, carboxylation, 432
–, succinic, carboxylation, 496–497
–, terephthalic, 496–497
Anilides 3-hydroxy-2-naphthoic, see naphthol A.S.
Aniline chlorhydrate, aldehyde blocking, 370
– –, dehydration of tissues, 74
Anilinic alcohol, azan, 233
Anthracogram, 291
Anthraquinone (chromophores), 133, 168
Anti-cholinesterases, 622–627
–, toxicity, 626
Apoferritin, detection by cadmium sulphate, 316
Apparatus of Kramer and Hill, 37
–, of Van de Kamer, 889
Aqueous humor, 19
Arginine, detection, 504–506
–, suitable tissues, 677
Argentaffin reaction, 328, 381–382
Argentaffinity, definition, 325
–, of aldehydes, 326
Argyrophilia, definition, 325
–, of secretions, 765
Arsenic, detection, 295
Artefacts, 10, 15, 19, 31–35, 46, 49, 53, 259, 264, 410, 596, 600, 682–683
Arthropod, 16, 210, 432
Arylsulphatases, see sulphatase
Arzac and Flores reaction, silver-piperazine, polysaccharides, 404–405
Ascite fluid, 19
Astrocytes, silver carbonate impregnation, 958
Astrocytes, see also neuroglia and neuroglia impregnation
Auramine 0, preparation of the Schiff equivalents, 170
Aurantia, 170, 867
–, Altmann's fuchsin, differentiation, 729–831, 736, 737

Autoradiography, 38, 282–287
Auxochromes and anti-auxochromes, 133
Azan of Heidenhain, 219–223
– – –, endocrine pancreas, 1022, 1023
Azan, novum (Geidees), 244
Azan, variants, azocarmine B, 223
– – –, endocrine pancreas, 1023
– –, Ziehl's fuchsine, 224
– –, nucleal reaction, 224
– –, nuclear fast-red, 234
Azine (chromophore group), 132
Azobordeaux, see Bordeaux R.
Azocarmine B, 168, 223, 1023
Azocarmine G, 168, 219–223, 997–998, 1022–1023
Azocarmine GX, see azocarmin
Azo-dyes, 132, 169–170
Azofuchsine 3 B, see sorbine red
Azomethine (chromophore group), 132
Azophloxine, 169, 214, 228
Azophloxine GA, see azophloxine
Azoreaction, 373–380
–, enterochromaffine cells, 584–585, 872–873
–, histamine detection, 586
–, histochemical interpretation, 380
–, noradrenaline, 577–578
Azorhodine 3 G, see sorbine red
Azorubine, see azorubine S
Azorubine S, see amaranth, 169, 217
Azur A, 172, 584
–, Schiff reagent equivalents, 362, 559–560
–, Lillie and Pasternak method, 235
Azur A, B, C, vital staining, 25
– – – –, metachromatic stains, 344–345
– – – –, contaminant of methylene blue, 345
– – – –, detection of basophilia, 339
Azur B, 172
Azur C, 172
Azurine-solochrome, beryllium (glucinium) detection, 308

B

Barium chlorate, to prepare chlorine dioxide, 581
–, chloride, biliary capillaries, 886
–, detection, 307
–, and strontium, contaminants of calcium deposits, 300
Basophily, misuse of term, 334–335, 756, 994
–, action of fixatives, 336
–, action of temperature, 336
–, chromolipoïds, 342

Basophily *(cont.)*
-, conditions of research, 334–335
-, definition, 130, 334
-, nucleic acids, 339, 342, 540–548
-, of acid polysaccharides, 339, 342, 434–439
-, purines, 593
-, tests for, on sections, 339–340, 540–548
-, urates, 339, 342, 591, 896
-, uric acid, 343, 592, 901
Basophiles in tissues, see mast cells
Basophily absolute, definition, 335
Basophily discrimination, nucleic acids, 545–548
Basophily relative, definition, 335
Basophily and characteristics of the staining solutions, 337–339
Basophily in cytoplasm and methylation, 421
Basophily in nucleus and methylation, 421
Basophily by oxidation, in secretions, 757, 962, 964, 1008
Balsam with gelatin, of Heringa and Ten Berge, 146
-, Canada, mounting media, 147, 148
-, oxidized (Masson), 148
Berberine, 170
Benzene, dehydration of pieces, 74
-, dehydration of sections, 146
-, dewaxing, sections, 141–142
-, impregnation of tissues, 74–77
-, recuperation, 75
Benzenic hydrocarbons, 38, 74–75–77
Benzidine, aldehydes staining, 366, 367
-, haemoglobin staining, 568–570
-, peroxidase detection, 648–649
-, blood vessels, staining, 858
Benzoate, benzyl, impregnation of tissues, 78
Benzoate, methyl, impregnation of tissues, 76–77
Benzopurpurine 4B, 169
3,4-benzopyrene, 453-454
6-benzoyl-2-naphthylsulfate of potassium, sulfatases, 634, 635
Benzoylation, tetrazoreaction block, 511
Benzoylation, polysaccharides, 419
Beryllium, detection, with azurine solochrome, 308
- -, quinalizarine, 308
- -, green naphthochrome B, 308
Bile pigments, 588–589, 591
Biliary capillaries demonstration with acid fuchsin, 886
- - -, haematoxylin, 886
- - -, indigo-carmine, 885
- - -, Scarlet R, 885
- - -, silver bichromate, 887

Bilirubine, see bile pigments
Bile salts, enzyme inhibitors, 622
- - -, activators, 622
Biogenic amines, detection, 571–580
Birefringence, 282
Bismuth, detection, 320
Bismuthate of sodium, glucides oxidation, 395–396
Bismuthate of sodium-Schiff, 403
Black Sudan B, for Golgi, 716
Bleaching of melanins, 581 (P. Mayer, method)
- bromine, 581
- chlorine, 581
- chloric acid, 581
- chlorine dioxide, 582
- chromium trioxide, 582
- peracetic acid, 582
- performic acid, 582
- potassium permanganate, 582
Blood cells, 16–17, 587, 718
- smears, 34, 44–45, 638, 704
- vessels, 587, 884
Blue, alizarin (acid), 168
- - - alum lake, 225
- - -Herlant tetrachrome, 998
- - - quad of Kornhauser, 818
- - - muscle (Neubert), 848
Blue, alcian, 172, 324, 355
- - adenohypophysis, 1005–1006
- - affinity for cysteic acid, 355, 523–524, 757–758
- - staining of acid mucosubstances, 412–413
- - staining after methylation, 421–422
- - mast cells, 825–826
- - -, Benson method, 559–560
- - -, Mowry method, 413
- - neurosecretion, 967–968
Blue alcian 8GS, 8GN 150, see Blue alcian
Blue alcian-yellow alcian, mucosubstances staining, (Ravetto), 436–437
Blue, alizarin RNB, see gallocyanine
Blue, aniline, 171
- -, azan of Gomori, 1016, 1022
- - -, Heidenhain, 219, 1022
- - -, Gabe, 1023
- - -, Romeis, 993
- -, allochromic method, Lillie, 400, 1013
- -, Cleveland and al., 996
- -, Gaussen method, 208
- -, Mallory, 212
- -, Masson, 213–214
Blue, aniline, see Lyon Blue
Blue, aniline, in alcohol, for lacuneous bone (Ranvier), 837

Blue, anthracene, SWR, 168
– –, SWX, see alizarin blue, acid
Blue astra, 172, 354–355
– –, mucosubstances, staining, 411, 412
Blue Benzo 3B, see blue trypan
Blue bromophenol protein staining, 533, 534
Blue BZL, 168
– –, staining technique, 452
Blue celestin, 171
– – B, see blue celestin
Blue, China, see blue aniline
Blue, chinoline, see cyanine
Blue, Congo 3B, see blue trypan
Blue cotton, see blue, aniline, methyl blue
Blue, cresyl brilliant, 171
– – –, vital staining, 25
– – –, Schiff equivalent, 362
– – –, reticulocytes, staining, 794
– – –, 2RN see blue, cresyl brilliant
Blue diamine BB, 170
– – –, Curtis method, 206–208
Blue 2B direct, see blue, diamine BB
Blue water, see blue, anilin
Blue water with orcein, Pasini method, 849–850
Blue, Evans, 170
Blue, gallamine, 171
– –, alum lake, 238
– –, bulk staining, 239
– –, muscular tissue, 847–848
– –, staining of sections, 238
Blue, gentian, see Lyon blue
Blue, Heidenhain, 219–223
Blue, Helvetia, see blue methyl
Blue, oil NA, 168
Blue, indophenol, 643–646
Blue, light, see blue, Lyon
Blue, luxol fast, 172 (see blue, methasol)
– – –, adenohypophysis, 1003–1004
– – –, lipids staining, 463
– – –, myelin staining, 950
Blue, Lyon, see spirit blue, gentian blue 6 B
– – –, rhodopsine staining, (Karli), 482–483
Blue, Mallory, 212
Blue, Meldola, see New blue R, 171
Blue, methasol, see luxol fast blue
Blue, methyl, collagen fibres staining (Dubreuil), 205
– –, Mann staining, 232–233
– –, allochromic method (Lillie), 400–401
Blue, methylene, 172
– –, basophily, detection, 339
– –, cartilage staining, 831–832
– –, hydrogen transport, 652
– –, isoelectric zone, estimation, 340–341

– –, neuroplasmic staining, 909, 911–912
– – – –, stabilisation, 912
– –, Nissl bodies, 909–910
– –, Schiff reagent equivalent, 362
– –, staining after sulfuric esterification, 406–407
– –, staining of reticulocytes, 794
– –, vital staining, 25
Blue, methylene polychrome, 345–346
Blue, naphthol R, see blue, Meldola
Blue, Niagara 3B, see trypan blue
Blue, Nile, 171
– – acid lipoids, staining, 461
– – chromolipoids staining, (Hueck), 484
– – vital staining, 25
Blue black B, 170
– – –, Curtis-Heidenhain method, 206–207
Blue black naphthol, 170, 206–208
Blue New R, see blue, Meldola
Blue New fast 3 R, see blue, Meldola
Blue, night, 172
Blue, patented V, VF, 172
– –, zinc-leuco-base, 569
Blue, Paris, see blue, Lyon
Blue polychrome, see polychrome blue
Blue pontacyl brilliant V, see patent blue
Blue, Prussian, 322
– –, vascular injection, 862–853
Blue, pyrrol, vital staining, 25
Blue, soluble 3 M, see aniline blue
Blue, Swiss, see methylene blue
Blue, tetrazolium, 330
– –, succino-dehydrogenase, 653–654
Blue, toluidine, 172
– –, basophily, detection, 339–340
– –, cartilage staining, 829
– –, Mann-Dominici method, 233–234
– –, metachromatic reaction, 344–349
– –, neurofibrils, detection, 919
– –, pheochrome reacion, 575
– –, Schiff reagent equivalent, 362–363
– –, staining of carboxylated sections, 432
– –, vital staining, 25
Blue, Unna, see polychrome blue
Blue trypan, 170
– –, athrocytosis, 825–826
– –, Curtis method, 206
– –, elimination by kidney, 902–903
– –, trachea of Arthropods, 894, 895
– –, vital staining, 25
Blue Victoria B, 172
Blue Victoria R, 172
Blue Victoria 4 R, 172
Blue Victoria, endocrine pancreas, 1016
– –, neuroglia staining, 954
– –, neurosecretion, 969

Bone, 25, 828–830
Bone cartilage, 11, 830–832
Bone marrow, 34–40, 804
Boracic carmin, 239
Borax solution, 607
Borax ferricyanide, Bensley, 695–696
– –, Loyez, 947
– –, Weigert, 469
Bordeaux R or B, 169
– –, background staining, 228
– –, preparation for ferric haematoxylin staining, 693
– –, trichohyalin staining, 781
Bordeaux SF, see azorubine S
Borders, brush, 752
–, striated, 752
Brain, 43, 688
Branchia, 16, 893–894
Branching enzyme, 641
Brasiline, brasilein, 170
Brenthol AS, see naphthol AS
Brilliant Dianil red, see Vital red
Bromine for melanin bleaching, 581
–, hydrolysis, nucleal reaction of Feulgen-Rossenbeck, 553
6-bromo-2-naphthyl-β-D-glucopyruronoside, β-glucuronidase, 635–636
Bromination, peracid oxidation, 468, 1018
Brown, Bismarck, 170
– –, endocrine pancreas, Müller, 1016, 1020–1021
– –, Schiff equivalent, 362–363
Brown excelsior, see brown, Bismarck
Brown, Manchester, see brown, Bismarck
Buccal cavity, 864–865
Buffers, 663–672
–, acetate, 616
–, citrate, 605, 611
–, glycine-hydrochloric acid, 668
–, maleic acid, 619
–, Sörensen, 667–668
–, "Tris", 608, 611, 656
–, Tris-hydrochloric acid, 646, 654, 656, 658, 659
–, Tris-maleate, 613
–, Veronal, 603, 618, 633, 657
–, Walpole, 618, 624, 625, 626, 634, 638, 639, 640, 641, 646, 666
–, Glycine-sodium hydroxide, 668
–, Gomori's tris-hydrochloric acid, 671
–, Gomori's tris maleate, 671
–, Holmes's borax-boric acid, 669
–, Hydrochloric acid-monosodium phosphate, 664
–, Hydrochloric acid-sodium citrate, 663

–, Laskey's N-maleic acid-0,1 N sodium hydroxide 665
– Mc Ilvaine's citric acid, dibasic sodium phosphate 667
–, Michaelis's hydrochloric acid-sodium veronal, 670
–, Michaelis's universal sodium veronal-sodium acetate 671
–, Oxalic acid-sodium oxalate, 669
–, Sodium oxalate-ferric chloride, 670
–, Walpole's acetic acid-sodium acetate 666
– Walpole's hydrochloric acid-sodium acetate 666
Bürker cell, for blood cells enumeration, 796
Butanol, dehydration of pieces, 71, 74
–, dehydration of sections, 335–336, 340, 544, 548
–, preservation of pieces, 78
Butyrates, enzyme substrate, 627
Butyrylcholine cholinesterases, 623

C

Cadmium chloride, 687, 713, 715
Calcitonin cells, 763, 1042–1044
Calcium, cartilaginous tissues, 830
–, detection, 298, 307, 676
–, distinction from urates, 594
–, formaldehyde fixation, 655, 656, 659
–, mineralogic forms, 282
–, osseous tissues, 838
–, phosphatases, 604
Capillaries, biliary, 885
–, vascular, blood, 857, 862
– –, lymphatic, 862–863
Carbohydrates, 43, 51
–, nomenclature, 674–675
Carbonates, detection by substitution, 303–304
Carbonate, silver (Arzac and Flores), 326, 327, 404
Carbonate, silver for quick impregnation, (Del Rio Hortega), 205–206
Carbonate, silver, see silver impregnation and tannosilver
Carbonate, lithium, indol reactivation, 513
– – –, solvent of uric deposits, 594
Carbonic anhydrase, 636–637
Carbonyl groups, 47, 49, 51
Carbonyls, lipidic, 472–475
Carboxyl, fuchsin paraldehyde affinity, 353
–, basophily, 339
–, metachromasia, 349
Carboxylation, neutral mucosubstances, 433
Carbowax, 93–94

Carmalum, bulk staining, 239–240
—, Fautrez and Lambert staining, 570
—, of Mayer, 570
—, preparation, 240
Carmin (carminic acid), 170
—, acetic, 702–703
—, alum, nuclear stain, 608, 632
—, purine staining, 593
—, uric acid staining, 901
—, vascular injection, 860–861
Carmin alum (Grenacher), 570
Carmin, Best's glycogen staining, 411
— —, nodal tissue in the heart, 853–854
— —, osmic haematoxylin (Schultze), 773
Carmine, lithium, athrocytosis, 826–827
— —, vital staining, 25
Carminate, ammonium, vital staining, 25
Carotenoids, 482–483
Cartilage, *in vivo* study, 828–829
—, histology, 830–833
Caryosomes, 705
Caryotype, acetocarmine, Belling, 703
— —, Schneider, 703
— 697, 699, 701–705
Catalase, 645
Catechol, polyphenoloxidase, substrate, 648
Catecholamines, detection, 573, 574–579, 678, 1037
—, periodic oxidation, 391
Causes of error, in enumeration of blood cells, 795–799
— — — —, leucocyte formula, 799
— — — —, microscopical measurements, 162
Celestin blue B, 171
Celloidin, embedding, 88–90
—, sections, 116–123
Celloidin, ese also nitrocellulose
Celloidin-congelation, (Petersen), 783
Celloidin-paraffin (Apathy), 96
— —, method of Millot, 76
— — — — Peterfi, 76
— — — —,, Pfuhl, 96
Cellular categories, adenohypophysis, 993–1006
— —, adrenal tissue, 1035
— —, endocrine pancreas, 1011–1031
— —, salivary glands, 879–881
Cells A, endocrine pancreas, argyrophilia, 1026–1029
— — — — other, methods, 1019–1024
— B, 1013–1019
— C, 1031
— D, 1024–1029
— E, 1031
Cells, adenohypophysial, functional nomenclature, 993–994

— —, morphological types, 993
Cells, adrenalinogen, adrenal tissue, 1037–1038
Cells, argentaffine, see enterochromaffin, Kultschitzky
Cells, chief, stomach, 858
Cells, chromo-argentaffin, see enterochromaffin
Cells, connectives, 825–827
Cells, enterochromaffin, 584–586, 875–877
Cells, gastrin, 877
Cells, glandular intestine, 871
Cells, hyaline, endocrine pancreas, 1031
Cells, in blood, morphological study, 787–799
Cells, Goblet, intestine, 871
Cells, neurosecretory, 961–967
Cells, noradrenalinogen, adrenal, 1037–1038
Cells, parietal, stomach, 868
Cells, round (dust cells) in lung, 892
Cells, thyroid, parafollicular, calcitonin cells, 1042
Cells, Kultschitzky, in stomach, 868
— — — —, intestine, 782
Cells, Kupffer, 884
—, Langendorff, 1042
—, Paneth, intestine 891
—, Rouget, see pericytes
—, Stilling (summer cells), 1035
—, Vines, erythrophil cells, 1035
Cellulose, detection, 429
Centrosome, 693, 700, 739, 747–50
Cerasine R, see Bordeaux R
Cetimine, 132
α-Cetols, periodic oxidation, 391
— —, lead tetra-acetate oxidation, 394–394
Chambers, Born, De Fontbrune, 19
—, desiccating chamber, 39
—, moist chamber, 17
—, oil chamber, 17
—, vacuum chamber, 38
—, Van Tieghem and Le Monnier chamber, 19
—, Vaseline chamber, 19
Chelation of cobalt, 654, 656, 658
—, of ferric ions, 689
—, with glyoxal, 301
Chitin, 11, 432–433
Chloramine T-Schiff, 502
Chloranilidophosphonic acid, for phosphamidase detection, 619–620
Chlorides, detection, after Leschke, 293
— — —, Lison, 293
— — —, Gersh, 293
— — —, Komnick, 293

Chlorine, for melanin bleaching, 581
– dioxide, 582
Chlorhydrate of L-leucyl-4-methoxy-2 naphthylamide, leucine aminopeptidase, 69
Chlorhydrate of tryptamine, mono-aminoxidase, 651
Chloroform, paraffin embedding (Apathy), 77
Chloroform, see Carnoy fixative
p-chloromercuribenzoate, as enzyme inhibitor, 613, 627
1,4-chloromercuriphenyl azo-2-naphthol, thiol detection (Bennett), 519
Chloropicrin, block for thiol, 530
Chlorophyll, 171
Chloride, cadmium, Aoyama fixative, 715
Chloride, ferric, bilirubin oxidation, 590
– –, Mallory haematoxylin, 692
– –, reaction with ferric-ferrocyanide, 322–325
– –, Weigert haematoxylin, 197–198
Chloride mercuric, see mercuric chloride
Cholinesterase, activities, detection, 522–527
–, myoneural synapse, 852
–, and iron, 605
–, tissues convenient for demonstration, 678
Chondriome, 717–742
–, definition, 717
–, fixations, 719–722
–, stainings, 722–741
–, vital observation, 717–718
–, – staining, 718–719
–, staining method of Altmann, 728, 729, 734
– – – –, Benda, 735
– – – –, Benoît, 729, 730
– – – –, Bensley-Cowdrey, 731–732
– – – –, Del Rio Hortega, 739–740
– – – –, Fernandez-Galiano, 741
– – – –, Gabe, 729
– – – –, Galeotti, 728
– – – –, Hollande, 729
– – – –, Kull, 729, 731
– – – –, Metzner, 728
– – – –, Nassonov, 735–737
– – – –, A. Prenant, 729
– – – –, Volkonsky, 729
Chondroblasts, 718
Chondrocytes, 31, 831
Chondrosulfatases, see sulfatases
Choroid, 980
Chromate, potassium, lead detection, 320
– –, cupric lake of haematoxylin, 695
– –, pheochrome reaction, 575

Chromate, silver, nervous cells impregnation, 910–919
Chromate, zinc-silver nitrate, neurones impregnation, 914–915
Chromatic, analysis, 134
Chromatin, 698–703
–, sexual, 704–705
Chromic oxidation, 716
Chromium trioxide, fixation, 48, 49, 57, 582, 684, 685, 980
– –, maceration, 770
– –, oxidation of carbohydrates, 396–397
– –, bleaching of melanin, 582, 980
Chromocenters, 705
Chromolipoïds, basophilia, 339–340
–, classification, 443
–, evolution, 484–485
–, histochemical characteristics, 483–484
–, in interrenal tissue, 1035
–, periodic oxidation, 391
–, tissues convenient for demonstration, 677
Chromo-osmic mixture, fixation, 684–685, 701, 704, 708, 748
Chromophore, definition, 132
–, principal groups, 132
–, list, 168–173
Chromotrope 2 R, 169
– – –, backgroup stain, 229
Chrysoïdin R, Schiff equivalent, 362
Chrysoïdin Y, 169
Chymotrypsine, 355
Ciliations, fixation, 747
–, staining, 753
Citric acid, for decalcification (Lorch), 610
Cleaning of glassware, 62–71
Closing bands, staining, 773
Coagulant, 43–44, 58–60
Cobalt, adsorption by mucosubstances, 306
–, detection, 317
–, substitution reaction (Stoelzner), 306
–, salts, for cytochromoxidase, 646
– – –, Golgi, 713
– – –, phosphatase, 603–604, 613
Coenzyme I, NAD, 655
Coenzyme II, NADP, 655
Collagen fibres, 811–812
– –, cartilage, 833
– –, selective staining, 201, 225
– –, enzymatic lysis, 825
– –, silver impregnation, 811
– –, in polarized light, 812
– –, staining, by competition between acid stains, 201–211
– – –, with phosphomolybdic (or -tungstic) acid, 211–227

Collagenase, 536
Collodion, see celloidin, nitrocellulose
Collodion, 76, 610
– directions for use, 142–143
Colloid in interrenal tissue, 1035
– – thyroid, 1041–1044
Compatibility, 56–59
Complexes of lipids, with chromium, 469–470
Complexes of silver, see silver impregnation (neurofibrils, neuroglia, connective fibres), argentaffin reaction
Compound fixatives, 56
– –, compatibility, 56–59
– –, incompatibility, 56–59
Compression of contrasts, 162
Concentration of dye, action on basophilia, 336
Condenser, 20
Congo red, 25
Connective fibres, 739, 774, 811–825
Conventions, 6
Cooling, 35
–, liquid air, 35
–, liquid nitrogen, 36
–, n-pentane, 36
–, isopentane, 36
–, propane-isopentane, 36
–, difluoromethane, 36
–, ethyl alcohol, 36
Coplin jars, 141
Copper, acetate, cupric hematoxylin, 696
– –, Holland's liquid, 181
–, detection, 317
–, sulphate, for cholinesterase detection, 624, 625
Coreine 2 R, see Celestin blue
Coriphosphine 0, 170
Cornea, 978
Corpora lutea, ovary, 1040
Cortex, adrenal, see also interrenal tissue, 1034
Cortex adrenal, 1031–1038
Cortex of hair, performic-Schiff reactivity, 524
Corticosterone, periodic oxidation, 392
Coupling, of diazonium salts, definition, 378–380
Cresazan, Romeis, 996–997
Creosote, 78
Cresofuchsine, see fuchsine resorcin
Cresyl Violet, 25
Cross, black, lipids (Ranvier), 945
Crystalline lens, histology, 980
Crystalloids, erythrophilous, 708
Crystals of mercury, removal, 143
Cryodesiccation, 33-40

–, for cytology, 683
–, for histochemistry, 261
–, for histoenzymology, 597
Cryostat, principle of, 261
–, improvements, 261
–, for histochemistry, 262
–, for histoenzymology, 597
Cupric lakes, 596
Cupric haematoxylin, 696
Curcumine, see brilliant yellow S
Cutting sections, 97–125
Cyano-acetylcoumarone, for cytochromoxidase, 645
Cyanine, chinoline blue
Cyanol FF, 172
–, haemoglobin detection (Fautrez and Lambert), 570
–, endocrine pancreas, 1014
–, see zinc-leucobase
Cyanosine, see phloxine
Cyanides, reducing agents, for disulphide detection, 528
Cyanol, 172, 884
Cysteine, 48
–, detection, 517–531
–, enzyme inhibitor, 604, 612
–, tetrazoreaction of Danielli, 511
Cystine, detection, 527–531
–, peracid oxidation, 523
–, reduction, 528–529
Cytoarchitectony, 944
Cytochemistry, definition, 253
Cytochrome C, 645, 718
Cytochrome oxidase, 643–646, 718, 726
– –, convenient tissues for detection, 678
Cytology, definition, 681–682

D

Dahlia violet, chondriome, 718
– –, vital staining, 25
Decalcifying, effects on tissues, 242–247
–, chromic acid and bichromates, 245
–, formic acid, 235
–, nitric acid, 244
–, organic buffers, 245
–, picric acid, 245
–, sodium ethylene tetracetate, 245
–, sulfurous acid, 244
–, trichloracetic acid, 244
–, acetic acid, 243
– – –, lanthanum acetate, 566
–, after celloidin embedding, 246
–, collagen fibres swelling, 243
–, dental tissue, 843–844
–, fixatives, 243

Decalcifying (cont.)
—, glycogen extraction, 839
—, histo-enzymological research, 610–611, 839
—, of sclerotic, 980
—, osseous tissues, 838–839
—, ribonucleic acid extraction, 565–566
—, vacuum, 243
—, verification, 243
—, versene, 242, 245
—, and ergastoplasm, 745
Decalin, 78
DDD, thiol detection, 518–523
Deformation, photographic, 162
Degeneration of myelin, Marchi, 950
– – –, Lillie, 951
Dehydration of pieces, 70–74
– – –, aniline, 74
– – –, benzene (toluene, xylene), 74
– – –, dioxane, 73
– – –, ethanol, 70–73
– – –, isopropanol, 74
– – –, time required, 71
– – –, stained sections, 147–149
– – – –, acetone, 148
– – – –, benzene (toluene xylene) phenolated, 147
– – – –, ethanol, 147–148
Dehydroepiandrosterone, substrate for Δ^5--3-β-hydroxysteroidodehydrogenase activity, 659–660
Dehydrocorticosterone, periodic oxidation, 392
Dehydrogenase aerobic, definition, 643
Dehydrogenase anaerobic, definition, 643
Denaturation, by fixatives, 34, 37, 38, 41, 43
DNP, DNPH, see NAD, NADH
Density of structures and staining, 137–138
Deoxyribonuclease, 639–640; deoxyribonucleic extraction, 563
Deoxyribonucleic acid, 640, 706
Depigmentation, iris (Kopsch), 980
—, of melanin, see bleaching
Deposits, silver, 318–319
Desmoenzymes, 598
Desmosomes, 751
Desiccation, 34, 37–40
Development, physical, (Liesegang) for iron, 316
Dewaxing sections, 141
– –, in benzenic hydrocarbons, 38
– – –, isopentane, 38
– – –, petroleum ether, 38
– –, for enzymes, 610
Dextrane detection, 430

o-diacetylbenzene, amino-acid detection, 499–500
Diamides of acids naphthol AS-phosphoric, phosphamidase, 619–620
Diamino-oxidases, detection, 651
o-dianisidine, aldehyde detection, 366
Dianthine B, see erythrosine B
Dianthine G, see erythrosine G
Diaphanol, see chlorine dioxide
Diaphorases, detection, 656–657
Diastase of malt, for glycogen removal, 417
Diazo, 4-amino-2, 5-dimethoxy-4-nitroazobenzene DDD reaction, 518–523
Diazo, acid S, indol detection, 514
– – –, preparation, 377
Diazo, benzidine, 509–510
Diazo, o-dianisidine, 367–368, 493, 497, 509–511, 521, 522, 608, 635–636, 651
Diazo, 5-nitroanisidine, DD reaction, 522
Diazo, pararosaniline, preparation, 377
Diazo, safranine, indol detection, 514
– – –, preparation, 377
– – – –, acetate of p-N, N'-dimethylaminophenylmercuric, 519–520
Diazotization, 2, 4-dinitrofluorobenzene reaction, 498
—, Morel and Sisley reaction, 511
2,4-dichloro-α-naphthol, arginine detection, Mc Leish, 506; Deitch, 506
2,6-dichloroquinone-chloro-imine, Gibbs reaction, 381
Dichotomous key for lipid analysis (Cain, Lison), 487–498
Diethyl-p-nitro-phenylphosphate, enzyme inhibitor, 627
Differentiation, definition, 131
—, theories, 136–137
Diffusion front, 45
Diformazan, 645, 660
Digestion of, collagen fibres, 824–825
– –, proteins, 534–535
Digitonine, α-hydroxysteroid detection, 479
Digestive gland in: Arachnida, 88
– – –, Crustacea, 888
– – –, Molluscs, 888
Digestive tract, 11, 864, 889
Dihydroxyphenylalanine, substrate of DOPA-oxidase, 646
Diisopropylfluoro-phosphate, 623, 626
Dimedone, aldehyde block, 370
—, APS glycogen detection (Bulmer), 427
Dimercaptopropanol, adenosine-triphosphatase inhibition, 612–613
—, reactivation of indolic compounds, 513
—, reducing agent, 529

Dimethylaminobenzaldehyde, indol detection, 514
p-Dimethylaminobenzylidene-rhodanine, silver detection, 1319
– – –, copper detection, 317
Dimethylformamide, as solvent, 606, 608, 618, 631, 638
Dimethylfuchsine, see magenta II
Dimethylnaphthylamine, for cytochrome oxidase, 644
Dimethylparaphenylene diamine, for acid mucoproteins, 435
– – –, cytochrome oxidase, 644
– – –, neutral mucoproteins, 431
– – –, peroxidase, 650
– – –, polyphenols (indoreaction), 380
Dimethylsulphoxide, 618, 631
Dinitrofluorobenzene, amino-acid detection, 497–499
–, tetrazoreaction (Danielli), 510
2,4-dinitrophenylhydrazine, carbonyles detection, 367–368
– – –, Albert and Leblond reaction, 368, 475
– – –, Monné and Slautterback method, 367, 401
– – –, nucleal reaction, 556–557
Dioxan, dehydration and impregnation, 73, 78
–, toxicity, 73
–, picric acid, fixation, 425
Dioxyhaematein of Hansen, 199–200
Dioxyphenylalanine, potassium iodate reaction, 578
Diphenylcarbazide, copper detection, 318
Diphenylthiocarbazide, see dithizone
Dipicrylamine, see aurantia
Diptera, salivary glands, 698
Distinction of cell organelles, 736
Disulfide of 2,2'-dihydroxy-6,6'-dinaphthyl, see DDD
Dithioxamide, calcareous deposits detection, 605
–, copper detection, 317
– silver detection, 319
Dithizone, zinc detection, 309
Dopamine, detection, 575
Dopa-oxidase, 646
Double coupling, 373–377
Double coupling, see also DDD-reaction, tetrazoreaction
Double-embedding, agar-paraffin, 95
– –, celloidin-paraffin, 96
Double-impregnation of Ramon y Cajal, Golgi method, 912, 916

Double impregnation, with silver nitrate, 874
Drops in a gram, 673

E

Echinoderm, 16
Elastase, 536
–, digestion of elastic fibres, 825
– – –, oxytalan fiblres, 824
Elastic fibers, 740, 816–821
Eleidin, 778
Embedding, 66
–, in agar, 14
–, in agar-paraffin 95
–, in alcohol-celloidin, 88
–, in celloidin-paraffin, 96
–, in gelatin, 14, 90–93
–, in glycerine-celloidin, 89
–, in methanol celloidin, 89
–, in nitrocellulose, 14, 37, 68, 85–88
–, in paraffin, 30, 34, 37, 50, 66–85
–, in polyethylene glycols, 93
–, in pyridine celloidin, 90
–, after picric acid fixation, 47
Emulsion, photographic, 285–286
– autoradiography, 283–286
Encephalon, phosphamidase, 620
Endocardium, 853
Endocrine pancreas, 757, 761, 763, 1011–1031
Endothelium, of vessels, nitration, 856
Enteramine, 584
Enteramine, see also 5-hydroxytryptamine
Enterochromaffine, cells, see argentaffin, basal granulated cells, Kultschitsky cells
– –, selective demonstration, 875
Enterocytes, 871–878
Eosin B, 173
Eosin 10 B, see phloxine B
Eosin G, J, Y, 172
Eosin in alcohol, see ethyleosin, methyleosin
Eosin in water, see eosin G, J, Y
Eosin, background stain, 228
–, Mann's method, 232
–, Pasini method, 850
–, for ferric haematoxylin, 693
–, for Gomori's trichrome, variant, 216–217
–, for orcein-water blue, 774
–, triple stain of A. Prenant, 693–694
Eosin azur, for blood smears, 791
– – –, topographical staining, 235
Enzymes, acid phosphomonoesterase, 615–618
– adenosine-5-phosphatase, 614–615
–, adenosine triphosphatases, 612–613
–, alcaline phosphomonoesterase, 602–611

SUBJECT INDEX

Enzymes *(cont.)*
–, carbonic anhydrase, 636–637
–, carboxylic esterases, 622–633
–, cholinesterases, 622–627
–, cytochrome-oxidase, 643–646
–, dehydrogenases, 650–660
–, deoxyribonuclease, 639–640
–, diaphorases, 655–656
–, esterases, 627–632
–, glucose-6-phosphatase, 620–631
–, glucosidases, 635
–, hydrolases, 601–640
–, hydroxysteroidodehydrogenase, 659–66
–, lipases, 632
–, oxidases, 643
–, oxido-reductases, 643
–, peptidases, 635
–, peroxidase, 648–650
–, phosphamidase, 619–620
–, phosphatases, 601–621
–, polyphenoloxidases, 647–648
–, succino-dehydrogenase, 653–655
–, sulfatases, 634–635
–, transferases, 640–642
–, tyrosinase, 646–647
Epidermal cells, 77–779
– –, histochemical reactions, 779–780
– –, fibrillar structures, 778
Epiphysis, 1044–1046
Epithelial fibrils, 739
– –, see also tonofibrils
Epithelioid pads, of arterio-veinous anastomosis, 855
Epithelium 16, 871
Equivalents: capacity, metric and weights, 674
Equivalents of Schiff's reagent, 362
– – – –, nuclear reaction, 557–560
Equivalents, thermometric scales, 672
Ergastoplasm, 47, 743–745
–, fixation, 744
–, staining, 745
–, vital staining, 744
Ergastoplasm, see also ribonucleic acid
Eriocyanin A, 171
–, endocrine pancreas, 1013
Eriorubin, see sorbine red
Errors, in microscopical measures, 162
Erythrocytes, enumeration, 794
Erythrophilous inclusions, in nucleus, 708, 756
Erythrosine B, 173
Erythrosine G, J, Y, 173
Erythrosine, background staining, 228
–, Cleveland's method for adenohypophysys, 995–996
–, Herlant's method, 997–998

Erythrosine-orange G, method of Mann-Dominici, 233–234
Eserine, enzyme inhibitor, 622, 627, 631
Essence of cedar, impregnation of pieces, 77
Esterases, carboxylic, 622–634
Esterification, detection of carbohydrates, 406–407
–, neutral mucosubstances, 430–433
Ester-wax, embedding, 94
Ester-phosphatides, 480
Ethanol, 6, 38, 44–46, 70–73
–, enzyme preservatian, 597
–, ergastoplasm preservation, 744
–, Nissl bodies fixation, 908, 928
Ethanol, maceration, by Ranvier's method, 770
Ether, 6, 54
Ethopropazine methylsulfate, cholinesterase inhibition, 623
Ethyl eosin, 173
Ethylene-diamine tetracetate of sodium, see versene
Ethylmaleilimide, block for thiol groups, 529
Euparal, 146
Examination, in polarised light, 282
– – – –, see also collagen fibres, muscular fibres, lipids
–, of sections, 13–14
–, vital, 15–21
– –, see also cells, organelles, organs
Extraction, 44
–, carbohydrate, 44
–, lipids, 44, 455–457
–, proteins, 44
–, of nucleic acids, 532, 563–565
–, by chloroform, methyl green, 543
–, by enzymes, 416, 534–537, 561, 563
–, by pyridine, 470

F

Factors of penetration, 27
Fahrenheit and centigrade degrees, 672
Fatty acids, 48
Ferric ferricyanide, reducing power, 322, 485, 576, 584
– –, thiol detection 316
Ferric salt, 707
Ferricyanide ferroso-ferric, 332
Ferritine, detection, 316, 589
Ferrocyanide, ferric, 322
Ferrous salt, 707
Fibres, collagen, 881
– –, enzymatic digestion, 825
– –, polarised light, 812
– –, selective staining, 200–227

Fibres *(cont.)*
- –, silver impregnation, 811
- –, staining by competition, 200–211
- –, staining with phosphomolybdic (or phosphotungstic) acid, 211–227
- – elastic, cartilage, 834
- –, enzymatic digestion, 825
- –, histochemical characteristics, 816–821
- –, silver impregnation, 739–740
- – muscle, 847
- – –, smooth, 851
- – –, striated, 848–850
- –, oxytalan, dyestuff affinities, 824
- –, of Purkinje, see heart
- –, reticuline, demonstration, 812–816

Fibrin, silver impregnation, 740
Fibrin, staining, 821–824
Fibrinoid, demonstration, 824
Fibroblast, 718
Fibroglia, gold-sublimate impregnation, 956–957
- –, silver carbonate impregnation, 958–959
- –, staining, 952–955

Fibrous proteins, 46
Filters, light, 282
Fixation, 11, 30–65
- –, by chemical agents, 15–34
- – – –, chloroplatinic acid, 46
- – – –, chromium trioxide, 48
- – – –, hydrochloric, nitric, sulfuric acids, 45
- – – –, mercuric chloride, 47
- – – –, methanol, ethanol, acetone, 44
- – – –, picric acid, 46
- – – –, potassium dichromate, 49
- – – –, trichloracetic acid,
- –, by physical agents, 33–42
- – – –, cryodesiccation, 33–35
- – – –, drying, 34
- – – –, freezing-substitution, 41
- –, by heat, 33
- – – –, drying, room temperature, 34
- – – –, low temperature, 34–35
- –, by vapours, 61
- –, by immersion, 61–61
- – – injection, 62
- – – perfusion, 62–63
- –, for autoradiography, 283
- –, under vacuum, 62

Fixatives, aqueous, 4, 48–51
- –, choice, 188
- –, duration, 59–60
- –, excess, 49
- –, ideal, 33
- –, indications and counter-indications, 42
- –, "indifferent", 43–44, 56
- –, "irrational" fixative, 57–59
- –, mixtures, 33, 42–45, 55–56, 60, 64–65, 70
- –, rate of penetration, 43
- –, universal, 42, 64
- –, Allen (Bouin-urea), 181
- – – B 15, caryological research, 701
- –, Altmann, 64, 684–685, 720
- –, Aoyama, 64, 688, 717
- –, Apathy (ethanol-mercuric chloride), 186
- –, Baker, 56–57, 60, 684
- –, Benda, 684, 699
- –, Benoît, 684–685, 730
- –, Bensley, 684–685, 699
- –, Bodian, 932
- –, Bouin, 10, 59–60, 180
- –, Brasil, 187
- –, Carnoy I, see Clarke's fixative
- –, Carnoy II, see Carnoy's fixative
- –, Carnoy, 186, 263, 425, 530, 544, 546, 701–702, 744, 807, 898, 908, 932
- –, Clarke, 186, 263, 425, 701–702, 744
- –, Champy, 57, 684–685, 711, 736
- –, Da Fano, 688, 713
- –, Danielli, 64
- –, Davidson, sex chromatin, 704
- –, Flemming, 684, 749, 830
- –, Gendre, 41, 71, 425
- –, Gérard, 181, 990, 994
- –, Gilson, 45, 247
- –, Halmi, 183, 688, 990, 994
- –, Heitz, 684, 701–702
- –, Helly, 55, 57, 60, 185, 686–687, 721, 806
- –, Henning, 247
- –, Hermann, 684
- –, Hirschler, 684
- –, Hollande, 181
- –, Kleineberg, 181
- –, Kolster, 686–687, 711, 734
- –, Kopsch, 57, 185, 382, 686–687, 710, 721
- –, Laguesse, 684
- –, Lang, 181–182
- –, Lindsay-Johnson, 684
- –, Mann, osmic impregnation 710
- –, Maximov, 55, 60, 64, 686, 687, 721, 800
- –, Mewes, 684–685
- –, Müller, 55
- –, Nassonov, 684–685
- –, Orth, 57, 382, 686–687, 721
- –, Rabl, 980
- –, Ramon y Cajal, formol uranyl-nitrate, 688, 713
- –, Regaud, 57, 185, 382, 686–687, 721
- –, Romeis, 183

Fixatives *(cont.)*
 -, Rossman, 425
 -, San Felice, 57, 183, 701
 -, Schaudinn, 187
 -, Slonimsky and Cunge, 858
 -, Slonimsky and Lapinsky, 858
 -, Stieve, 183
 -, Szent-Györgyi, 978
 -, v. Telliesniezky, 183
 -, Verhoeff, 978
 -, Wittmaack, 984
 -, Zenker, 55, 57, 184
Fixatives, choice, 188
 -, classifications, 33, 42–43
 -, coagulant, 43
 -, compound, see mixtures of fixatives
 -, cytological, 682–689
 -, decalcifying 242–243
 -, histo-enzymological, 597–598
 -, simple, 55
 -, topographical, 117
Flocculation, 27–43
Fluorescence, apparatus, 273
 -, definition, 272
 -, histamine, 586–587
 -, histochemistry, 275
 -, 5-hydroxytryptamine, 584–586
 -, immunochemistry, 275–277
 -, indol groups, 876
 -, morphology, 273
 -, noradrenaline, 577
 -, porphyrins, 591
Fluorochromes, 276
 -, dimethylaminonaphthalene-5-sulfonic chloride, 277
 -, fluorescein isocyanate, 276
 -, isothiocyanate of rhodamine B chloride, 277
  lissamine-rhodamine-sulfonic chloride, 277
Formaldehyde, fixative, 51, 55, 58–59, 61, 445, 578
 -, see also formalin
 -, calcium, 56, 179, 446–447, 609, 721
Formalin, 6, 32, 178–179, 446, 597, 721
 -, vapours (Lagounoff and al.), 586
Formalin-hydrochloric acid-sodium nitrite, (Voisenet-Furth reaction), 513
Formalin-lead-acetate (Lison), 568
Formalin-magnesium acetate (Schiller), 179
Formalin-mercuric chloride, Bouin, 182
 – – –, Dawson and Friedgood, 182
 – – –, Heidenhain, 182
Formalin-potassium ferricyanide, (Slonimsky and Lapinsky), 567, 858
Formalin-pyridine (Danielli), 64, 609

Formazan, 653, 659
Formic acid, for decalcification (Greep), 611
Free aldehydes, 357, 817
Free cells, 13, 16, 19
Freeze-drying, 33
Freezing microtome, 11
Freezing substitution, 33, 41
Freon, 38
Frozen sections, 29, 35, 124–127
Fuchseline, see resorcine fuchsine
Fuchsin, acid, 171
 – –, background staining, 229
 – –, biliary capillaries (Forsgren), 886
 – –, Cason, 213
 – –, Ehrlich triacid, 791
 – –, filling osseous cavities, 837
 – –, Goldner, 214
 – –, Mallory, 212
 – –, Masson, 213
 – –, phenolic (Seki), 727
 – –, Schiff equivalent, 362
 – –, van Gieson, 204
 – –, zinc-leucobase, 569
Fuchsin, acid, of Altmann, 726–732
 – – – –, Millot's triple staining, 229
 – – – –, pheochrome reaction, 576
 – – – –, preparation, 726
 – – – –, utilisation, 728
Fuchsin, basic, 171
 – –, chromolipoids, staining, 484
 – –, fuchsine paraldehyde, preparation, 350–352
 – –, Gaussen, 208
 – –, Schiff reagent, preparation, 358–362
 – –, Schiff reagent, regeneration, 358
Fuchsin, Gallago, elastic fibres, 820
Fuchsin paraldehyde, adenohypophysis, 1001–1003
 – –, anionic group affinity, 352
 – –, calcitonine cells, 1043
 – –, chemical constitution, 350
 – –, cysteic acid, affinity, 523
 – –, directions for use, 352
 – –, elastic fibres, 353, 821
 – –, endocrine pancreas, 1015–1016
 – –, epidermal keratin, 779
 – –, lipids, 475
 – –, mast cells, 825–826
 – –, maturation of solutions, 350
 – –, mucosubstances, 414
 – –, neurosecretion, 965–966
 – –, preparation, 350–352
 – –, secretions, 760–761
 – –, solutions, 351
 – –, stable samples, 351
 – –, tonofibrils, 751

Fuchsin paraldehyde *(cont.)*
— —, trachea, in Arthropods, 894–896
Fuchsin paraldehyde-haematoxylin picro-indigo-carmin, 760–761
Fuchsin paraldehyde-one step trichrome, 821, 965–966, 1002
Fuchsin-resorcine, adenohypophysis, see Cresazan, Romeis
— —, elastic fibres, 819
— —, preparation, 819
Fuchsin-resorcine-trichrome of Masson-Goldner, 820
Fuchsin RNF, see basic fuchsin
Fuchsin S, SN, SS, ST, S III, see acid fuchsin
Fuchsin phenolated, (Ziehl), 202
Fuchsin fast G, see chromotrope 2 R
Fumaric acid, 653
Fundamental organelles, see organelles
Fusorial apparatus, 688
— , spindle, 700, 739, 748

G

Galactosidases, 635
Gallamine blue, 603
Gallocyanin (Einarson), 541
—, basophilia, 705
—, caryology, 701
—, chromic lake, 541
—, directions for use, 542
—, ergastoplasm, 745
—, nucleic acids, 541–546
—, nucleolus, 706
Ganglia of Auerbach, 879
— —, Meissner, 879
Ganglion cells, 910–919
Gangliosides, chemical definition, 444
Gastric mucosa, 587, 865
Gastrin-cells, demonstration, 763, 872, 877–878
Gastropods, 65, 383, 428, 710, 747
Gastrula, fixation, 425
Gelatin, coating, Golgi method (Kallius), 917
—, embedding, 90–93
—, sections, 123
—, sticking sections, 113
—, vascular injections, 861–862
—, — — with carmine, 861
—, — — —, Prussian blue, 862
Gelose-paraffin embedding, Chatton, 95
— — —, Wigglesworth, 95
Geranine G, 170
Germ cells, in Annelids and Sipunculids, 17
Gills, 66, 893–894
Glands, adrenal, 1031–1038

—, cutaneous, 782
—, digestives, Invertebrates, 887–888
— —, secretory cycle, 889
—, of Brunner, duodenum, 882
Glands, gastric, fundic, 866
— —, neck, 866–867
— —, parietal, 866
— —, principal, 866–867
Glands, intestinal, 871–878
Glands, lacrymal, 979
Glands, parathyroid, 990–991
Glands, salivary, 879–882
Glands, thyroid, 1041–1044
Glisson's capsule, 884
Glucinium, see beryllium
Glucopyruronoside, for β-glucuronidase, 636
Glucose, convenient tissues for research, 676
—, demonstration, 384–385
—, fixation, 384
Glucose-6-phosphatase, 621
— — —, convenient tissues for research, 678
Glucose-1-phosphate of potassium, phosphorylase, 641
Glucose-6-phosphate of potassium, see glucose-6-phosphatase
Glucose-6-phospho-dehydrogenase, 657
Glucosidases, 635–636
—, convenient tissues for demonstration, 678
Glucosulfatase, 634
Glucuronidase, see glucosidases
Glucuronide of 8-hydroxyquinoleine, for β-glucuronidase, 635
Glutamate dehydrogenase, 657
Glutaraldehyde, fixation, 52–53, 585, 722
—, noradrenaline reaction (Tramezzani and al.), 1037
Glyceride, convenient tissues for demonstration, 677
—, definition, 443
—, histochemical characteristics, 480
Glycerin-albumine, sticking sections, 112
Glycerin-gelatin (Kaiser) mounting of sections, 145
Glycerin-gum (Farrants), 145
Glycerol, 38, 41
Glycerol-celloidin, embedding, 89–90
— iodated, for phosphorylase, 641
Glycerophosphate, labelled, for phosphatases, 603, 615
Glycogen, 41, 46, 48, 53, 54, 641, 881, 884
—, amylase, 416–417
—, evaluation, 428
—, fixation, 425–426, 428
—, metachromasia, 428
—, distribution in the cell, 425

Glycogen *(cont.)*
-, retina, 982
- -, staining, Best carmine, 411
- - -, Fischer, 410
- - -, Mancini iodine, 427
- - -, Mayer, 410
- - -, Takeuchi iodine, 641
- - -, Vastarini-Cresi, 410
-, sulfuric esterification, 406–407
-, tissue, Purkinje (heart), 854
Glycosidases, see glucosidases
Glycoproteins, see neutral mucosubstances
Glycyl (or alanyl)-naphthylamines, aminopeptidase, 637–639
Goblet cells, 871
Gold chloride, 706, 740
Gold orange, see orange II
Golgi apparatus, 12, 45, 55, 60, 64, 687, 707, 709–716
-, bodies, histochemical reactions, 716
- -, impregnation with osmium, 710–713
- - - -, silver, 713–715
- -, staining, 709–716
- -, vital observation, 310
Gonad, Invertebrates, male, 1049–1050
- -, female, 1054–1057
Gonocytes, 1050
Gossipymine, see safranine O
Gram solution, 641
Green acid, see light green, naphthol green B
- -, see also wool green, lissamine green B
- alcian, 172, 354–355
- -, mucosubstance staining, 412–415
- brilliant, 171
- diamant G, see brilliant green
- diazine, see Janus green B
- double SF, see methyl green
- emerald, see brilliant green
- fast acid N, see light green
- - FCF, acidophilia, 333
- - -, background stain, 230
- - -, Gomori's trichrome, 215
- - -, histone detection, 532
- - -, Masson's trichrome, 213
- - -, one-step trichrome, 217–218
- - JJO, 171
- - O, 171
- - -, see malachite green G
- Janus B, 169
- - -, chondriome, 718
- - -, myoneural-synapse stain, 852
- - -, vital stain, 25
- light, background stain, 228, 230, 555–556
- -, see methyl green
- - N, see malachite green

- - SF, 2G, S, 2GN, see light green
- lissamine, see wool green, Acid green S
- malachite G, 171
- - -, nucleic acids staining, 549
- - -, see brilliant green
- naphthochrome B, beryllium detection, 308
- - -, calcium detection, 300
- naphthol, see naphthol green B
- of Alsace, see naphthol green B
- - ethyl, 172
- - iodine, 607–608, 630
- - methyl, 543–549
- - -, cartilage staining, 829
- - -, differentiation of Altmann-fuchsin, 729
- - -, Pollister and Leuchtenberger technique, 544
- - -, purification, 543
- - - -pyronine, ergastoplasm, 745
- - - -, Nissl bodies, 908
- - - -, nucleic acids staining, 545–542
- - - -, nucleolus, 707
- - Prussian, see ferrosoferric ferricyanide
- PL, see naphthol green B
- Victoria B, see malachite green G
- wool S, 172
Ground substances, 31, 831–833
Groups, anionic, basophily, 334–340
-, carbonyls, detection, 357–371
- -, of oxidized hydrocarbons, blocking, 415–416
-, disulphur, convenient tissues for demonstration, 677
- -, reduction, 527–529
-, indol, detection, 513–517
-, phenol and naphthol, detection, 372–383
Guanidyl radical, 504–506
Guanine, 592, 594
-, convenient tissues for demonstration, 678
Guanidyl radical, 504–506

H

Haemalum, affinities and methylation, 421–422
-, bulk staining, 241–242
-, cartilage staining, 832
-, differentiation, 196
-, directions for use, 196
-, nuclear stain, 608, 618, 630
-, results, 197
Haemalum-eosin, 227–228
Haemalum-picro-indigo carmine, 201
Haematoidin, 589

Haematopoietic tissues, 800–808
– –, bone-marrow, 804–806
– –, lymph nodes, 807
– –, Peyer patches, 807
– –, spleen, 805
– –, tonsils, 807
Haematoporphyrin, 588
Haematoxylin, 690–695
Haematoxylin, alcoholic "mother-solution", 194
–, chemical and physical characteristics, 194–195
– fixation of stain, by chelation, 136–137
– – – –, by hydrogen bridge, 689
– myelin staining, 945–948
– progressive ferric lakes, 197–198
– – nuclear stain, 194, 197–198
– purine staining, 593
– regressive cupric lakes, 695–696
– – stainings, 136–137, 689–696
– – – of chondriome, 727–739
– ripening of solutions, by oxidation, 195, 691
– – – –, spontaneous, 691
Haematoxylin, acetic (Kultschitzky), 469, 886, 945–946
Haematoxylin, chromic (Gomori), 759, 965, 1015
– – (Hansen), 195, 199, 759
Haematoxylin chromic phloxine, granules of secretion, 759
– – endocrine pancreas, 1015
– – neurosecretion, 965
Haematoxylin, cupric (Bensley), 695, 696
– – (Cowdry), 695, 696
– – chondriome staining, 739
– – lipid staining (Fischler), 462–463
Haematoxylin, Dobell-Hirschler, 694–695
Haematoxylin, ferric, caryological research, 702
– – Heidenhain, 690–693 –
– – Heidenhain-Regaud, 691
– – mitochondrial staining, 734–739
– – phaeochrome reaction, 576
– – staining of wet smears (Grassé), 790
– – treatment of pieces, 690, 738
Haematoxylin, lead-lake (Mac Conaill), for nervous pericarya, 910–911
– – – for adenohypophysis, 1000–1001
Haematoxylin, lithium carbonate, Bacsich (for myelin), 948
– – – –, Weigert, 945–946
Haematoxylin molybdic, of Held, 981
– – – –, mucosubstance staining, 410
Haematoxylin, osmic (Schultze), 773
Haematoxylin, phosphotungstic, for endocrine pancreas, 1021
– – –, fibrin staining, 823
– – –, neuroglia, 954–955
– – –, preparation, Levene and Feng, 823
– – –, original formula, 823
– – –, Terner and al., 823
Haemofuscines, 487
Haemoglobin, 587, 884
– benzidine, detection, 568
– Dunn, staining, 569
– Fautrez and Lambert staining, 570
– fixation, 568
– histospectroscopy, 567
– iso-electric point, 570
– peroxidase activity, 567, 857
– zinc-leucobase (Lison), detection, 569
Haemosiderin, 567, 588, 591
– convenient tissues, for demonstration, 678
– organic substrate, 316
Halogen addition, lipids, 465–467
Hardening of pieces, fixation, 43–44, 53, 60
Heart, 853–854
– nodal tissue, 853
– Purkinje fibres, 854
Hedgehog quills, 866
Haematein, 171, 199
–, alum lakes, 195
–, chemical and physical characteristics, 194
–, chromic lakes, 199
–, ferric lake progressive, 197
–, – – regressive, 695
Haematein, acid (Baker) adenohypophysis, 1000
–, phospholipids staining, 469–470
Haematein I A (Apathy), bulk staining, 240–241
Hematology, 61, 787–799
Hematometers, Bürker, Levy-Hauser, Thoma, 796–797
Haematoxylin, 171
Hemocytes, Invertebrates, 799
Hemogram, 786
Heparinocytes, see mast cells
Hepatopancreas, see digestive glands, digestive caeca
Histamine, 586–587
–, see also mast cells
–, substrate for diamine-oxidase, 650–652
Histidine, detection, 507
–, tetrazoreaction (Danielli), 509–511
Histochemistry, definition, 252–254
–, evolution, 251–253
–, *extra-situm*, 253
–, *in situ*, 253

Histochemistry *(cont.)*
—, progress, 254–256
Histo-enzymology, 595–660
—, general considerations, 596–601
Histolipoids, see heterophasic lipids
Histological diagnostic, 9–10, 12
—, general principles, 13
—, limits, 6
—, possibilities, 6
—, research 9–10, 12
—, technique, 6
Histones, detection with fast green FCF (Alfert and Geschwind), 532
Histophotometry, definition, 267–268
—, errors, 270–271
—, gallocyanine staining, 541
—, limitations of the method, 270–271
—, methyl-green staining, 543
—, with two wavelengths, 270
Histo-polychrome of Gaussen, 208–209
Historadiography, 277–279
Histospectography, emission, 271–272
Histospodography, see micro-incineration
Honing, razor, 98
Hormonal receptors, 1047
Hormones, steroids, detection, 477–479
Hyaluronidase, hyaluronic acid depolymerisation, 418
Hydrate, barium, glucose detection, 384
—, iron, 409–410
—, piperazine, insolubility of guanine, 592
— —, solubility of uric acid, 592
Hydrazide 2-hydroxynaphthoic, carbonyls detection, 367–368
— — —, demonstration of terminal carboxyl groups, 493
— — —, mono-amine oxidase, 651
— — —, nucleal reaction, 557
Hydrocarbons, aromatic, dewaxing, 141–142
— —, clearing stained sections, 147–148
—, paraffin impregnation, 74–75
— — —, advantages, 74–77
— — —, toxicity, 75
Hydrogen peroxide and peroxidase, 648–650
— —, for bleaching excess of osmic impregnation, 712
— —, gold detection, (Elftman), 319
Hydrogen sulphide, bismuth detection, 320
— —, dehydro-ascorbic acid detection, 388
— —, mercury detection, 318
Hydrolases, definition, 601
Hydrolysis by bromine (Barka and Dallner), 553
— — hydrochloric acid, Feulgen and Rossenbeck reaction, 551–556
— — — — nucleal and cytoplasmal reaction (Turchini and al.), 549–550
— — — — nucleal reaction with fluorones (Blackler and Alexander), 550
Hydrolysis, perchloric, Feulgen and Rossenbeck reation, 553
—, phosphoric, nucleal reaction of Feulgen and Rossenbeck, 553
—, trichloracetic, nucleal reaction of Feulgen and Rossenbeck, 553
α-Hydroxyacids, lead tetra-acetate oxidation, 394
α-Hydroxyaldehyde, lead tetra-acetate oxidation, 394
Hydroquinone, for Golgi, 714–715
Hydroxyadipinic aldehyde, 52
Hydroxybutyrate-dehydrogenase, 657
Hydroxylamine, aldehyde blocks, 370
3-Hydroxy-2-naphthaldehyde, detection of α-amino-acids, 497
Hydroxy-naphthoic acid anilide (naphthol AS, brenthol AS), 606
1-Hydroxy-2-naphthyl-anilide, cytochromoxidase detection, 646
4-hydroxynapthyl-N-maleilimide, thiol detection, 520–521
8-Hydroxyquinolein (oxime), arginine detection, 505
— —, β-glucuronidase detection, 635
Δ^5-3β-hydroxysteroido-dehydrogenase, detection, 659–660
— — —, convenient tissues for demonstration, 679
Hydroxy-sulfophenylazobenzylidine, hydrazine, benzoic acid, see Zincon
5-Hydroxytryptamine, detection, 584
— —, argentaffine reaction, 325
— —, reaction with potassium iodate, 576
Hygroscopic substances, 36, 73
Hypobranchial gland, 65
Hypochlorite of calcium-chromium trioxide, iris bleaching, 980
Hypophysis, fixation, 668
—, staining, 757

I

Ice crystals, 35–36, 39–41
Ideal fixation, 31
"Images de fuite", shift of glycogen, in front of fixative, 426
Imidazol, detection, 507–508
Immuno-histochemistry, 275–277, 490, 596, 877
Impregnation, by gold, Carey, 920
— — —, Lowitt, 979
— — —, Ranvier, 916

Impregnation, *(cont.)*
– –, silver, of cell boundaries, 772
– – – –, chondriome, 739–741
– – –, nucleolonema, (Estable and Sotelo), 706
– – –, precautions, 927
– – – products of secretion, 765
– – –, reticuline, Gomori, 813
– – – –, Oliveira, 815
– – –, bichromate, biliary capillaries, 887
– – –, chromate, nervous pericaryons, (Golgi-Cajal), 916
– – – –, pericytes, 855–856
– – – –, retina, 982–983
– – – –, trachea of Arthropods, 896
– "en masse", 32, 131
–, neurofibrils, Agduhr, 925–926
– –, Bodian, 931–933
– –, Boeke, 926
– –, Davenport, 930–931
– –, De Castro, 844–945
– –, Favorsky, 930
– –, Fitzgerald, 932
– –, Foley, 929
– –, Gros-Schultze, 921–923
– –, Holmes, 933
– –, Palmgren, 935–937
– –, Ramon y Cajal, 928–929
– –, Schultze, 938–929
– –, Tinel, 923–924
–, neuroglia, Del Rio Hortega (astrocytes and fibroglia), 958
– –, Del Rio Hortega (Histiocytes and microglia), 961
– –, Del Rio Hortega (microglia and perivascular neuroglia), 959
– –, Del Rio Hortega (Oligodendroglia), 959
– –, Globus (Gold-sublimate), 957
– –, Penfield (microglia and oligodendroglia), 960
– –, Ramon y Cajal (Gold-sublimate), 956
– of Aoyama, Golgi bodies, 713, 715–716
– –, Da Fano, Golgi bodies, 713–714
– –, Del Rio Hortega, Pineal gland, 1046
– –, Elftman, Golgi bodies, 713
– –, nerve pericaryons, by mercury (Cox), 918
– – Ramon y Cajal, Golgi bodies, 713–714
–, tannin-silver Achucarro, 739
– – Del Rio Hortega, first variant, 739–740
– – – – –, 2nd variant, 813
– – – – –, 3rd variant, 811–812
– – – – –, 4th variant, 957–958
– – Fernandez-Galiano (chondriome), 741

– – Valmitjana-Rovira, 741
Impregnation of pieces, benzene, 84
– – –, benzyl benzoate, 78
– – –, butanol, 78, 85
– – –, celloidin-paraffin, 76
– – –, chlorofom, 77
– – –, decalin, 78
– – –, dioxane, 73
– – –, essence of Cedar, 77
– – –, hydrocarbons aromatic, 74–77
– – –, methyl benzoate, 84
– –, osmic, for Golgi apparatus, 710
Imprint, 698
Incidents, paraffin sections, 110–111
Incineration, 288
Inclusions of calcium, fixation, 307
– – iron, fixation, 315
– intranuclear, cristalloids, 708
– – non cristalloid, 708
– lipidic, 457–458
Incompatibility, 56
Indamine, 132
Indian ink, 25, 884
– –, see Chinese Ink
Indigo carmin, 171
– –, biliary capillaries, 885
Indolamines, 574
Indol, convenient tissues for demonstration, 677
–, detection, 513, 585
–, ferric ferricyanide reaction, 325
Indophenol blue, cytochrome oxidase, 644
Indoreaction, 380
Indoxyl acetate, carboxylic esterases, 631–632
– –, cholinesterase, 623
– –, halogenated, for carboxylic esterases, 632
–, esters, 599
Induline, 170
Inhibition, adenosine-triphosphatase, 612
–, amylo-1,4,1,6-transglucosidase, 642
–, carboxylic esterases, 622, 623, 628, 634
–, cytochromoxidase, 644
–, dehydrogenase, 644–646
–, glucose-6-phosphatase, 620
–, β-glucuronidase, 635
–, mono-aminoxidase, 651
–, phosphamidase, 620
–, phosphatases, acid, 615
–, phosphatases, alkaline, 604
–, phosphorylase, 642
–, polyphenoloxidase, 648
Inhibitors, carboxylic esterases, 623, 628
–, of cholinesterases: ethopropazine methylsulfate, 623

SUBJECT INDEX

Injections, of blood vessels, 859–862
—, lymphatic vessels, 862–863
Ink, Chinese, athrocytosis, 826
— —, vascular injection, 861
— —, vital staining, 25
Insect larvae, 60
Insolubilization, 48–51
Integration, endocrine pancreas, 1007–1011
—, linear and planimetry, errors, 165–167
—, measure of areas and volume
Integument, 775–785
Interdigital membrane, 16
Internal ear, 63
— —, fixation, 688
Interstitial cells of testis, 1038–1039
Intestinal crypts, 891
—, Golgi apparatus, 716
Intestine, 40
Intestine, diverticular, Arachnida, 888
—, Vertebrate, 869–871
Iodates, phaeochrome reaction, 382–383
Iodate, potassium, ripening of haematoxylin solutions, 195
— —, method of Cattaneo, 578
— — — —, Hillarp and Hökfelt, 576–577
— —, phaeochrome reaction, 382
— sera (Schultze), maceration, 770
Iodine, in thyroid, detection, 309
—, solution of mercury crystals, 143
—, oxidation of bilirubine, 590
—, reaction of Landing and Hall, 507
— — — Morel and Sisley, 511–512
—, staining of cellulose, 429
— — — galactogen, 428–429
— — — glycogen, 427
— — — starch, 430
—, thiol block, 529
Iodine green, nuclear stain, 607
Iodine-iodide solution (Gram's solution), for phosphorylase, 641
— — —, 700
— — —, for caryology, 750
Iodine research, 309
Iodonitrotetrazolium, 330
Ions, ferrous, melanin fixation (Lillie), 583
Ionic forces, staining solutions, 337
Iris, examination, 980
Iron and phosphatases, Arvy and Gabe, 605
—, unmasking, 314
Iron-alum for bilirubin oxidation, 590
— — —, centrosome, 693
— — —, haematoxylin differentiation, 690, 694
— — — —, mordanting, 689–690, 694
Islets of Langerhans, 1007–1031
Isocitrate dehydrogenase, 657

Isocyanate of fluorescein, 275–276
— —, rhodamine, 277
Isoelectric point, 44, 47, 50
Isoelectric zone, 338
Isonicotinic 2-isopropyl hydrazide, aminoxidases inhibitor, 651
Isopentane, 38
Isopropanol dehydration, 74
2-Isopropylhydrazide isonicotinic, see Marsilid
Isorubine, see fuchsine
Isothiocyanate of fluorescein, 277
— —, rhodamine, 277
Isotropic lipids, 458–459

J

Janus green, 24–25, 29, 169

K

Kaformacet, fixative, 184
Karion, mounting of sections, 146
Kava-kava, fixation of intestine, 870
Keratine, epidermic, 778
Keratohyalin, 778
Ketones, free 357
Ketosteroids, 371, 473, 475
Kidney, 40–43, 897, 903
—, of Amphibians, 747
Kodak, dektol, 466
Kultschitzky cells, see enterochromaffine cells
Kupffer cells, 884

L

Lactic dehydrogenase, 656
Lactose, detection, 385
Lakes, alizarin, 735
—, aluminium, 604
—, chromic, 210, 778
—, cupric 695
—, ferric, 689, 778
—, gallocyanin, 701
Lamellibranch, branchial epithelium, 747
Larynx, examination, 891
Latent structure, 31
Laurylcholine, cholinesterase, 623
Lead effect, 617
Lead nitrate, for cholinesterases, 626
— — —, deoxyribonuclease, 640
— — —, phosphatases, 616
Leather, strop, 100
Lecithins, definition, 444

Lepidoptera, spermatocytes, 747
Leucine-aminopeptidase, detection, 637
– –, convenient tissues for demonstration, 678
Leucocytes, 23, 799,
Leucoderivates, 648, 718
Leucyl-4-methoxy-2-naphthylamide chlorhydrate, for peptidase detection, 639
Leucyl β-naphthylamide, for peptidase detection, 638
Levy-Hauser, haematometer, 796
Light source, 20
Lipases, convenient tissues for demonstration, 678
–, detection, 636
–, eserino-resistance, 622, 632–633
–, pancreatic, 627, 633
Lipids, reactions by halogen addition, 465–466
–, anisotropy, 457–458
–, birefringence, 458–459
–, content of carbohydrates, 476–477
–, cross, in polarised light, 458
–, definition, 442
–, dichotomous key, 487–489
–, extraction, Ciaccio, 455
– –, Keilig, 456
–, formation of chromic complexes, 469–470
–, isotropy, 457–458
–, metachromasia, 349, 461–562
–, osmic blackening, 464–465
–, oxidation by peracids, 467–468
–, periodic acid oxidation, 391
–, solubility, 455
–, sphero-crystals, 458
Lipids, acidity, 459
–, fixation, 446–448
–, heterophasic, definition, 445
–, homophasic, definition, 445
–, unmasking, 448
Lipids, histogenic, see heterophasic lipids
Lipids "masked", see heterophasic lipids
–, staining, cupric haematoxylin, 462
– –, fuchsin paraldehyde, 475
– –, luxol fast blue, 463
– –, lysochromes, 449–454
– –, Nile blue, 460–461
Lipofuscines, 486, 583
–, distinction from melanins, 484–485, 580
–, histochemical characteristics, 486
–, reaction with ferric ferricyanide, 325
Liposolubility, 26
Liquid air, 37–39
Liquid fixation, 61
– –, by immersion, 61

– – –, injection, 61
– – –, perfusion, 61
–, nitrogen, 38
Lissamine-rhodamine-sulphonic chloride, 277
– brown B, 172
Lithium carbonate, 47, 68, 650, 727, 827
–, carmine, 884
Liver, 40–43, 883–987
Lugol, 68, 634, 650, 725, 740
Lung, 16, 891–892
Lutes, 150
Lymph nodes, 40
Lymphatic vessels, injection, 862–863
Lyo-enzymes, 598
Lysine tetrazoreaction, 511
Lysivane, see ethopropazine methylsulfate, cholinesterase inhibitor
Lysochromes, absorption, 589
–, chondriome, detection, 741
–, classification, 449
–, cutaneous free fats, 780
–, definition, 130, 449
–, fluorescent, 543–454
–, mode of utilisation, 449–454
–, nervous degeneration, 950
–, solubility, 598
Lysosomes, 640, 734, 765

M

Macerating agent, 70
Maceration, 769–774
–, nephron, 898–899
–, nodal tissue, of the heart, 854
–, olfactive cells, 976
–, osseous tissue, 835–836
Macrophages, in any tissue, 827
– –, the liver, 884
Macrothyreocytes, 1041–1044
Magenta acid, see acid fuchsin
–, see basic fuchsin
Magenta 1, 172
Magenta III, see new fuchsin
Magenta 9, 172
Magneson, magnesium detection, 309
Malassez, haematometer, 796
Malt diastase, for glycogen, 884
– –, in perfusion, 870
Mammary gland, 782
Mandarin G, see orange II
Manganese acetate, oxidation of carbohydrates, 396
Mannitane esters, for lipases, 633
Marsilid, mono-aminoxidase inhibitor, 651
Masked structure, 31

Mast-cells, 586–587
– –, in tonsillar tissue, 878
Masticatory structures, in Annelids, Arthropods, Molluscs, 865
Measures, errors, 162
–, of areas, 164
– –, length, 163
– –, volumes, 165
–, with histophotometer, validity, 269–270
Meissner's plexus, 879
Melanic pigments, in liver, 884
Melanins, 580–583
 –, convenient tissues for detection, 678
 –, bleaching of, 485, 980
 –, distinction from lipofuscines, 579
 –, methylation, 584
 –, oxidation, 579–581
 –, reaction, argentaffin, 582
 – –, with ferric ferricyanide, 582
 –, reducing power, 582–583
Melanophage-cells, definition, 580
Melanophorous-cells, definition, 580
Membranes, basal, 812
 –, dermal, 779
 –, spread, silver impregnation, 772
Mercaptides, 47, 519–520
Mercuric-acetate, mordanting for chondriome, 722, 724
 –, chloride, 45, 47, 52
 – – phosphorylase inhibition, 642
 – – transglucosidase inhibition, 642
Mercuric, crystals, 6
 –, fixative, 684, 686
 –, nitrate, urea detection, Leschke, 593
 –, plasmal reaction, 473
 –, thiol detection, 529
Mercury, detection, 318
 –, orange, see 1,4-chloromercuriphenylazo-2-naphthol
Metabisulfite, 759
Metachromasia, adenohypophysis, 999
 –, amyloid, 811
 –, cartilage, 832
 –, definition, 343
 –, effect of dehydration, 346
 –, lipids, 349
 –, mast-cells, 825
 –, mechanism, 345
 –, metaphosphates, 349
 –, mucosubstances, 348
 –, myelin, 949
 –, nucleic acids, 348
 –, sulfomucosubstances, 348
 –, theories, 345–346
 – and density of anionic groups, 346
 – –, pH, hydrocarbon detection, 405

– –, structural orientation, 346
–, see also reversible methylation
Metachromasia β, 340
Metachromasia γ, 340, 345
Metachromatic stains, 344
Metallic salts, 55
Methanol, fixative, 44, 55, 791
Methanol-celloidin, embedding (Seki), 89
Method, acid peracetic- (or performic-) Schiff, lipids, 467–468
 –, myelin, 949
 –, Adams and Tuquan, proteases, 639
 –, Alfert and Geschwind with methyl green FCF, 532
 –, allochrome (Lillie), 400–401
 –, α-naphthylphosphate of sodium, alkaline phosphatases (Gomori), 605–607
 – – – – –, acid phosphatases (Grogg and Pearse), 617–618
 –, Altmann-Gersch, 39, 40
 –, Apathy, 38
 –, AS-naphthol phosphates (Burstone), 608, 618
 –, Barger, 603
 –, Barrolier and Suchowsky, 466
 –, Benson, 559
 –, Cason, 213
 –, Chalkley, 166
 –, Cain, 460
 –, Curtis-Heidenhain, 207
 –, Daoust, 639
 –, Daoust and Amano, 639
 –, De Galantha, 591, 900
 –, Ehrlich-Biondi-Heidenhain, 231–232
 –, Eränkö, 578–579
 –, Everett, 478
 –, Friedenwald and Becker, 635
 –, Glenner, 515, 590
 –, Golgi-Cajal, 916
 –, Gomori-Takamatsu, 602–604
 –, Gram-Weigert, 430
 –, Hartig-Zacharias, 495–496
 –, Haug, 166–167
 –, Hennig, 167
 –, Hillarp and Hökfelt, 576, 577, 1037
 –, Himes and Moriber, 558–559
 –, Hueck, 488
 –, Kolatschev-Nassonov, 711
 –, Kopsch, 710, 712
 –, Kutlik, 590
 –, Landing and Hall, 507
 –, Leschke, 293, 592, 902
 –, Lillie and Pasternack, 235–236
 –, Lorrain and Smith, 460
 –, Mallory, 212–213
 – Mann, 232–233

Method *(cont.)*
–, Mann-Dominici, 233–235, 750, **965,** 1015
–, Mann-Kopsch, see Weigl method
–, Marchi, 950
–, Mazia and al., 533
–, Mendelson, 213
–, Menschik, 461
–, Mowry, 413
–, Norton and al., 466
–, Pappenheim 791–792, 801–802
–, Pappenheim-Unna, 544
–, Petersen, 225–226
–, Pollister and Leuchtenberger, 544
–, Saint-Hilaire, 393
–, Salazar, 496
–, Schultz, 433, 478
–, Smith-Dietrich, 469
–, Stein, 590
–, Tremblay, 639
–, Unna, 803
–, Van Gieson, 204–207
–, Weigl, 710
Methods, myelinic, Bacsich, 948
– –, Kultschitzky, 945
– –, Lillie, 951
– –, Loyez, 947
–, Nageotte, 946–947
– –, Pal, 946
– –, Weigert, 945
– –, Wolters, 946
Method of calculation of Tejning, for endocrine pancreas, 1010
Method, statistical of Hellman, for endocrine pancreas, 1010–1011
Methosulfate ethopropazine, see lysivane
Methyl eosin, 173
– violet, 25
Methylation, effect on lipofuscines, 486, 584
– – –, melanins, 584
– – –, siderophily, 136, 689
–, reversibility, 421–424
Methylene azur, 25
– blue, dehydrogenase, 643
– –, eosinate, 34
– – , hydrogen acceptor 652
– – –, transport, 653
– –, vital stain, 25–25, 29
Methylol group, 51
Microglia, impregnation, 959
Micro-incineration, 288, 292
Micrometers, 163
Microplanimeter (Caspersson), 164–165
Microradiography, 38
Microscopes, dark-field, 20
–, electron, 21, 31, 53–54, 717, 747

–, interference, 21, 31, 607, 718
–, light field, 20, 31, 705
–, phase contrast, 21, 31, 697
–, polarised light, 38
–, resolving power, 31, 40
–, ultra-violet, 573, 587, 591, 698, 764
Microtomes, 98–105
Mitosis, 697, 702
Mixture, chromic, chondriome fixation, 720
–, chromo-acetic, cytological fixation, **688**
–, chromo-osmic, cytological fixation, 684–685
– – –, chondriome fixation, 721
– –, cytological fixation, 686–687
– for buffers, 662
– of essential oils (Apathy), 96
– – fixatives, acidity, 57–59
– – –, adjuvant salts, 55–56
– – –, choice, 64–65
– – –, compatibilities, 56–57
– – –, definition, 55–56
– – –, incompatibilities, 57
– – –, penetration, 57
– – –, price, 64
– – –, time of action, 59
M-nadireaction for peroxidase, 649–650
Molluscs, 16, 66, 210, 314, 424, 475
–, digestive gland (zinc), 321
–, gastric cavity, cilia, 869
–, integument, 775, 784
–, salivary glands, 698
Monoamine oxidase, 650
– –, convenient tissues for demonstration, 679
Mordant, definition, 136
Mordanting with mercuric acetate, for chondriome, 724–725
– –, Müller fluid, 686
Morin (pentahydroxy-flavanol), aluminium detection, 311
Moulding blocks, 80
Mounting, 13–15, 17, 19
–, media, 19–20, 38
– –, balsam and gelatin (Heringa and Ten Berge), 146
– –, balsam, Canada, 147–148
– –, balsam, oxidized (Masson), 148
– –, euparal (Gilson), 146
– –, glycerol, 144
– – – and gum, arabic 145
– – – – gelatin (Kaiser), 145
– –, Karion F, 146
– –, resin, dammar, 147
– –, resin, synthetic, 147
– –, syrup of Apathy, 145
– – – – laevulose, 145

Mounting *(cont.)*
—, of sections, summary, 149–150
Mucins, 47, 604
 — see mucosubstances, mucopolysaccharides
Mucins, reduction of tetrazolium salts, 332
Mucoids, see neutral mucosubstances
Mucopolysaccharides, see mucosubstances, mucins
Mucoproteins, see neutral mucosubstances
Mucosa, fundic, 867–868
—, pituitary, 974–976
—, respiratory, 990–991
Mucosubstances, acid, histochemical characteristics, 434–439
— —, cartilage, 831–833
— —, discrimination, 434–435
— —, nomenclature (Spicer and al.), 424, 674–675
—, carboxylated, behaviour with PAS, 434
— —, metachromasia, 361, 434
—, neutral, 430–433
—, convenient tissues for demonstration, 676
Murexide reaction, uric acid, xanthine, guanine, 594
Muridae, stomach, 865
Muscle adenylic acid, for nucleotidase detection, 614
— — —, for phosphorylase detection, 641
Muscles, examination, 846–851
Myelin, haematoxylin lakes, 945, 951
 — diagnostic staining, 332, 949
—, see also lipids, myelinic methods
Myeloid tissue, 648
Myelotectonic, 944
Myocardium, 953
Myo-epithelial cells, 782
— — —, in salivary glands, 880
Myofibrils, staining, 848–849
— —, tanno-argentic impregnation 739–740
Myoneural synapse, 624
Myristoylcholine, cholinesterase, 623
Myrosulphatases, 634
NAD, NADH, 655–660
NAD-dehydrogenases, 657–659
— —, convenient tissues for demonstration, 679
NAD-diaphorases, 655–657
— —, convenient tissues for demonstration 679
G-nadi-reaction, see cytochromoxidase
M-nadireaction, 649–650

N

NADP, NADPH, 654–657
NADP-dehydrogenase, detection, 652, 657–659
NADP-diaphorases, 655–657
Naphthol α, for cytochrome oxidase, 644
— —, for peroxidase, 649–650
Naphthol AS acetate, carboxylic esterase, 629
— —, phosphate, alkaline phosphatase, 608
Naphthol green B, 171
Naphthyl acetates, carboxylic esterases, 624, 629
Naphthylamines, for peptidase detection, 637–639
Naphthyl phosphates, for phosphatases, 605–609, 617–618
Neotetrazolium, 330–331
Nervous system, 906–972
— —, neurofibrils, 707, 919–944
— —, Nissl bodies, 907–910
— —, pericaryons, 910–918
Neuroglia, 739, 952–961
Neurohypophysis, 988
Neuromelanin, 583
Neurosecretion, definition, 961–962
—, staining technique, 757, 963–969, 989
Neutral red, 24, 25, 29
Nickel, detection, 317
Nigrosine, 25, 170
Ninhydrin, oxidative deamination, 499–501
Ninhydrin-Schiff, amino-acid detection, 501–502
Nissl bodies, 541, 704, 744
— —, detection, 907–910
— —, gallocyanin staining, 541
— —, neurosecretory cells, 962
— —, gastro-intestinal tract, Auerbach ganglia, 879
Nitrate of cobalt, Golgi bodies fixation, 713–714
— — —, Stoelzner reaction, 305–306, 603
Nitrate of mercury (Leschke), 592
— — silver, ascorbic acid detection, 386–388
— — —, calcium detection, (von Kossa), 304–306
— — —, Golgi bodies fixation (Elftman), 713, 715
— — —, reduction by melanin, (Lillie), 583
— — —, see also argentaffine reaction, neurofibrils and neuroglia impregnation
— — uranyl, Golgi bodies fixation, 713–714
Nitro-blue of tetrazolium, 330, 652–659
Nitrocellulose, 37, 85–90
—, see also celloidin, collodion
Nitroprusside, 649

Nitroprusside *(cont.)*
—, thiol detection, 518
—, zinc detection, 309
Nomenclature azo-dyes, 169–170
—, hydrocarbons, 674–675
Nonane, 38
Noradrenaline, 575, 1037
Nothing dehydrogenase, 659
Nuclear fast red, 604
—, membrane, 49–51
—, reaction
— —, De Lamater, 557
— —, Feulgen and Rossenbeck, 551
— —, Himes and Moriber, 559
— —, Turchini and al., 549
Nucleolus, 705–708
Nucleoproteins 50, 538–566
—, definition, 538
5-nucleotidase, 614–615
— —, convenient tissues for demonstration, 678
Nucleotide of diphosphopyridine, see NAD and NADP
Nucleus, 50, 697–708

O

Observation chambers, 16–17
—, medium, 18
Oedematous ball (Ranvier), 825
—, reaction, 63
Oesophagus, 864–865
Oil of cloves Flemming triple stain, 749–750
— — —, neutral gentian violet, 757
— —, turpentine, bleaching of osmiated sections, 712
Oligodendroglia, silver carbonate impregnation, 959
Oogenesis, 1056–1057
Optic anisotropy, 282
Orange G, 169, 220, 228, 231, 233, 400, 995–996
— —, fuchsin of Altmann, differentiation, 729
— —, phosphomolybdic acid (Cleveland and al.), 995–996
— —, triple stain of Flemming, 750
Orange GG, GPM, see orange G
Orange II, 169
Orange, acridine, 170
— —, fluorochromy of the nucleus, 698
Orcein acetic, stain for chromosomes, 702–703
Orcein-water blue, Pasini-Walter, 849–850
— —, Unna, 774
Orcein, 171

—, chlorhydric (or nitric), elastic fibres, 817–819
—, stain for cilia, 753
Organ of Corti, 985
Organelles, in the cell, 45, 48, 49–51, 53, 57, 65, 234, 282, 640, 685, 705
Organs, hematopoietic, 803–808
—, neuro-hemal, 986–987
Osmic blackening, lipids, 464
Osmium iodide, 579–580, 943
—, tetroxide, 45, 53–54, 56, 59, 61–62, **64**, 579, 638, 683–684
Ovary, 1039–1040
Oven-microscope, 20
Oven, of Policard, micro-incineration, 290
— —, Schultz-Brauns, 290
— —, Scott, 290
Over-fixation, 46
Oxalic acid, 712, 733, 760
Oxazine, chromophore, 132
Oxidases, 643–648
Oxidation, adenohypophysis, 1001
— by iodide, 507
—, elastic fibres, 335, 818
—, endocrine pancreas, 1015
—, lipids, 469
—, Mann-Dominici staining, 233–234
—, neurosecretion, 967
—, peracetic, lipids, 469
— —, melanins, 582–583
— —, oxytalan fibres, 824
— —, secretions, 758
— —, sulphydrylated proteins, 523–526
—, performic, adenohypophysis, 1005
—, periodic, chitin, 432–433
— —, polysaccharides, 392–405
— —, specificity, 392–393
—, permanganate of potassium, Gomori (secretions), 757, 762, 964–966, 1001, 1020
— — — —, sulphydrylated proteins, 467
Oxido-reductases, 643–660

P

Panchrome of Pappenheim, 801
Pancreas, endocrine, 1011–1030
—, exocrine, 882–883
—, living, chondriome, 719
Paneth cells, 871
Paraffin, embedding, 68–85
—, sections, 105–116
Paraldehyde, 350–353
Paraminophenol, indoreaction, 380
Pararosaniline, preparation of paraldehyde fuchsine, 351–532

Pararosaniline, *(cont.)*
—, preparation of Schiff's reagent, 360–361
Parasites, 15
Parasomes, 743–744
Pars distalis, see adenohypophysis
PAS, adenohypophysis, 999
—, amyloid, 810
—, background staining, for contrast, 399–400
—, collagen fibres, 400, 811
—, connective cells, 825
—, Golgi apparatus, 713
—, interrenal tissue, 1034
—, lysosomes, 765
—, mast-cells, 825–826
—, polysaccharides, 440
—, reticulin fibres, 812–816
—, variants, 399
PAS-alcian blue, 413
PAS-argentaffine reaction, 415
PAS-dimedone, glycogen detection, 427
PAS-haematoxylin-orange G, 400
PAS-haematoxylin-picro-indigocarmin, 400
PAS-iron hydrate, 408
PAS-phaeochrome reaction, 575
PAS-reversible acetylation, 419–421
— —, methylation, 421
Paste, for razor, 101
Patent blue V, 172, 884
Penetration, of fixatives, 43–44
—, poor, 46
—, rapid, 45
—, slow, 46–48, 50–52, 54, 57, 59, 66
Pentahydroxyflavanol, (see Aluminium), 311
Pepsin, collagen and reticulin digestion, 825
Peptidases, detection, 637–639
Peracids, lipid oxidation, 467
—, see also peracetic and performic acids
Perfumed vaseline, 19
Pericardium, 853
Pericaryones, 31, 914–919
Pericytes, silver chromate impregnation, 855–856
Periodate oxidation, 716
Permanent preparations, 20, 31
Permanganate of potassium, bleaching, 712, 733, 852
— — —, oxidation of polysaccharides, 397
— — — — —, secretions, 758–762, 964–969, 1001–1002, 1030
— — — — —, thiols, 523–525
Peroxidases, blood vessel study, 857
—, convenient tissues for demonstration, 678
—, definition, 648
—, detection

Petroleum ether, 38
Peyer patches, 807
pH, basophilia, 337–338
—, diazo coupling, 378–379
—, fixatives, 49, 56, 59, 575
Pharynx, 864, 891
Phase contrast, 38
—, liquid, 35–36, 41
—, solid, 35–36, 41
Phenols and naphthols, detection, 372–383
Phenosafranine, 168
—, Schiff equivalent, 362
Phenylenediamine, cytochromoxidase, 645
p-phenylenediamine, detection of carboxyls (Scarselli), 369, 404
Phenylhydrazine, block for aldehydes, 370
—, coupling with diazo salt of *o*-dianisidine (Seligman), 367–368
Phenyliodoso-acetate, hydrocarbon oxidation, 396
N-phenyl-p-phenylene diamine (Burstone), 646
Phenylurethane as inhibitor, 644, 645
Phloxine, 173, 759, 965, 1015
— acid GR, see chromotrope 2 R
Phloxine B, see phloxine
Phosphamidase, convenient tissues for demonstration, 678
—, detection, 619–620
Phosphatases, 53, 64, 678, 752, 863, 870, 879
Phosphine 5 G, GN, Schiff's reagent equivalent, 362
Phosphine 3 R, fluorochromy of lipids, 454
Phosphogluconate dehydrogenase, 657
Phospholipids, 47
Phosphorylase, convenient tissues for demonstration, 678
—, detection, 640–641
Phthalaldehyde, histamine, detection 587
Phthalic anhydride, carboxylation, 432
Phthalocyanin dyes for acid mucopolysaccharide, 412–413
— — —, anion groups, 354–356
— — —, calcium, 300
— — —, lipids, 463
— — —, mucosubstances, 414
— — —, secretion, 758, 967, 1005
— — —, thiols, 523–524
Physostigmine, see eserine
Picrate-ammonium molybdate, stabilisation of methylene blue, 914
Picrate, methyl green, differentiation of Altmann's fuchsin, 729
Picro-blue black B (Heidenhain), 207
Picrofuchsine, Van Gieson's, 204–206
Picroindigocarmine, 201

Picro-methyl blue (Dubreuil), 205
Picroponceau, 205
Picro-scarlet, Biebrich's, 205
Picro-thiazine red (Domagk), 205
Pieces, softening of hard, 107
Pigments, biliary, convenient tissues for demonstration, 678
– – Glenner, 590–591
– – Kutlik, 590
– – Stein, 590
– ceroid, 486
– formalin, 52
– in retina, 982
Pinacyanol, 172
Pipette of Potain, 795
– – Thoma, 795
Pituicytes, in neurohypophysis, 988–989
– – –, azan, 989
– – –, silver impregnation, 989
Pituitary mucosa, 974–976
Planimetry, 162–163
Plasmal reaction (Hayes), 473–474
Platelets, in Mammals, 589, 798
Platinum trichloride, eye fixation, 482
Point, isoelectric, estimation, 337–338, 340–342
– –, in protides, 533–534
Polarised light, 38, 282, 603
Polonium, detection, 282
Polychaete, 17
Polychrome blue, 344–345, 803–804
– –, Nissl bodies, 909
Polyethylene-glycol, see carbowax
Polynucleotides, definition, 538
Polyphenols, silver salt reduction, 325, 328
–, tetrazolium salt reduction, 329–332
Polyphenoloxidase, convenient tissues for demonstration, 678
– detection, 647
Polysaccharides, acetylation, 419–421
–, basophily after chromic oxidation, 396–397
–, classification, 389
–, esterifications, 406–407
–, extraction, by enzymes, 416–418
–, fixation of metallic ions, 407–410
–, methylation, 421–423
–, oxidation reactions, 390–404
–, tests for, 439–441
Polyvinylpyrrolidone, 609, 656, 658
Ponceau, see sudan
–, B, see Biebrich scarlet
–, brilliant, see Ponceau 2R, RG, 4R
–, G, see Sudan III
–, R or LB, see Sudan IV
–, 2R, background stain, 228

–, –, detection of acidophily, 333
–, –, method of van Gieson, 204
–, –, polychrome method of Gaussen, 208–209
–, –, trichrome of Masson-Goldner, 213–214
–, S, 170
Porphyrins, 591
Postchromatisation, affinities for haematoxylin lakes, 738
–, after Elftman, 471–472
–, chondriome, 723–723
–, myelin, 945
–, phospholipids, 456
–, slides, 733, 737, 739
Potassium acetate, cytochromoxidase, 645
– alum, eye fixation (Karli), 483
– chromate, 695
– cyanide, enzyme activator, 638
– – – inhibitor, 604, 615, 646–648
–, detection, 297–298
– dichromate, 49, 55–56, 575, 583
– –, for erythrophilous crystalloids, 708
–, ferricyanide, 632, 707
–, ferrocyanide, 632
–, glucose-6-phosphate, 621
–, iodate, 577, 700
–, permanganate, for melanin bleaching, 582
– –, for bleaching excessive osmic impregnation, 711–713
Preen gland, of birds, 444
Preparation of sections, celloidin, 116–123
– – –, celloidin-paraffin (Apathy), 118, 120, 121
– – –, frozen, 124–127
– – –, gelatin, 123
– – –, paraffin-agar, 116
– – –, paraffin, 105–116
Preservation of blocks, celloidin, 89, 117
– – –, gelatin, 91
– – –, paraffin, 83
– – –, reagents for silver impregnation, 927
– – tissues, 30
Primary amine groups, acetylation, 503–504
– – –, deamination, 503
– – –, detection, 496
Propane, 38
Propylene glycol, for solution of naphthol AS acetate, 630
Proteolytic enzymes, 755
Protist, 17, 61
Purines, histochemical detection, Saint-Hilaire reaction, 592–594
–, in polarised light, 282
Purkinje fibres, in the heart, 854

Purple, ethyl 6B, see ethyl violet, 172
Purpurine, see alizarine
– brilliant R, in Curtis method, 208
Pyridine-celloidin, embedding, 90
–, extraction of lipids, 470–472
Pyrocatechol, see catechol
Pyrogallol, 707
Pyronine affinities for ribonucleic aids, 545
Pyronine B, 173
– –, equivalent of Schiff's reagent, 362
– –, reaction with α-naphthol, peroxidase, 649
– –, see erythrosine B
– G, J, Y, 173
– J, see erythrosine G
Pyrrol blue, 25
– ferric ferricyanide reaction, 325

Q

"Quad" of Kornhauser, 226
Quantitative study, blood, 795–804
– –, bone-marrow, 804
– –, endocrine cells, 1011
– –, endocrine pancreas, 1007–1011
– –, insular area, 1009
– –, islets enumeration, 1008, 1010
– –, Peyer patches, 878
– –, size of islets, 1009
– –, spleen, 805
– –, thymus, 806
– –, volume of langerhansian tissues, 1010
Quinalizarine, detection of beryllium, calcium and magnesium, 299
Quinones, 132, 647
Quinone-imines, 647

R

Radio-isotopes, for autoradiography, 283
Razor, 39
Razor-holder, 102
Reaction argentaffine, definition, 325–326
– –, detection of phenols and napthols, 381
– –, enterochromaffine cells, 584
– –, interpretation, 328
– –, lipofuscines, 583
– –, melanins, 580
– –, noradrenaline (Eränkö), 579
– –, principles, 329
– –, Arzac and Flores, 404
– –, Gomori, 403
– –, Lillie and Burtner, 328
– –, Masson, 328
– chromaffine, see phaeochrome reaction
– histochemical, direct and indirect, 257
– –, reliability, 259

– –, sensitivity, 258
– –, specificity, 256–257
– –, types, 263–265
– histo-enzymological, contradictory requirements, 598
– – –, validity, 600–601
– immuno-histochemical, 275–277
– metachromatic, considerations for use, 346–348
– –, hydrocarbon detection, 405–406
– –, interpretation, 348–349
– –, lipid detection, 349, 461–462
– –, mechanism, 345–346
– nucleal, 549, 560
– –, for caryology, 701–704, 707
– –, Blackler and Alexander, 552
– –, Danielli, 557
– –, De Lamater, 557–558
– –, Feulgen and Rossenbeck, 551–556
– – – – –, on chromatin, 701–706
– – – – –, on pieces, for bulk staining, 241
– –, Pearse, 557
– –, with alkaline complex of silver, 557
– – –, Schiff equivalents, 557–560
–, Adams (steroids), 478–479
–, Ashbel and Seligman, 368
–, Berg, 399
–, Bruckner, 476
–, Ehrlich, indol groups,
–, Gibbs, 381
–, Gram, 822
–, Grynfeltt, 383
–, Liebermann-Burchard, 477
–, Millon-Baker, 508
–, Millon-Polister and Ris, 509
–, Molisch, 476
–, Morel and Sisley, 511–512
–, Mulon, 383
–, Perls, 312
–, Quincke, 313
–, Roe and Rice, 476
–, Romieu, alloxan, 499
–, Romieu, phosphoric acid, 513
–, Sakaguchi (Carver et al., variant), 505
–, Sakaguchi (Deitch variant), 506
–, Sakaguchi (Mc Leish et al., variant), 506
–, Stoelzner, 305, 603, 611
–, Tirmann and Schmelzer, 313–314
–, Virchow, 383
–, Voisenet-Furth, 513
–, Von Kossa, 304, 603
–, Vulpian, 383
–, biuret, 493
–, gypsum, 307
–, murexide, 594

Reaction *(cont.)*
–, oxidation of polysaccharides, 390–405
–, precipitation, protides, 495
–, Prussian blue, 312
–, rosindole (Adams), 516
–, rosindole (Glenner), 515
–, Turnbull blue, 313
–, peroxydasic, myeloid tissue, 648–649, 788, 804
–, plasmal, Cain, 474
– –, Hayes, 473
–, phaeochrome, catecholamines, 50, 575–576
– –, definition, 382
– –, enterochromaffine cells, 584–585
– –, in adrenal tissue, 1036–1037
– –, mode of utilisation, 382–383
–, primary, in histo-enzymology, 599
–, pseudoperoxidasic, haemoglobin, 567–570, 805, 857
– pseudoplasmal, definition, 473
– –, myelin, 949
–, with acetate p, N, N'-dimethylamino-phenylmercuric (Lillie and Glenner), 519
– – alkalin thio-indoxyl (Pearse), 585
– – alloxan-Schiff, 501
– – benzidine, Gomori, 649
– – –, Lison, 568
– – –, Slonimsky and Lapinsky, 568
– – carbodiimides, 494
– – chloramine T-Schiff, 502
– – 1,4-chloromercuriphenylazo-2-naph-thol (Bennett), 519
– – DDD (Barrnett and Seligman), 520–522
– – digitonin (Lison), 479
– – dimethylbenzaldehyde-diazo of S acid, Glenner and Lillie, 514–515
– – dinitrofluorobenzene, 508
– – epoxyether, 494
– – ferric ferricyanide, detection of thiols, 518
– – – –, elastic fibres, 817
– – – –, enterochromaffine cells, 584
– – – –, interpretation, 328
– – – –, lipofuscines, 582
– – – –, melanin, 582
– – – –, phaeochrome reacton, 576
– – – –, principles, 322
– – – –, trachea of Arthropoda, 896
– – – –, Adams, 324
– – – –, Chèvremont and Frederic, 324
– – hydroxamate, 494
– – 4-hydroxynaphthyl-N-maleilimide, Barrnett and Seligman, 520–521

– – naphtholiodo-acetamide Barrnett and al., 520
– – neotetrazolium (Gomori), 330–331
– – ninhydrine-Schiff, 501
– – o-diacetylbenzene, 499
– – α-naphthol, 649
Reactivation of enzymes, 611
– – indol groups, 5134
Reagent, Léger, detection of bismuth, 320
–, Schiff, chemical constitution, 358
– –, elastic fibres staining, 817
– –, elimination of excess, 363
– –, equivalents, 360, 362–363
– –, preparation, 360
– –, regeneration of the stain, 358
– – and equivalents, histochemical interpretation, 364–465
– Sols, 492
Reconstruction, aim, 156
–, chamber of Born, 156
–, graphic, 158–160
–, plastic, 160–161
Red amidonaphthol G, see azophloxine
– B, see sudan B
– Bordeaux, see Bordeaux R
– cerasine, see sudan III
– Congo, 170
– – amyloïd, 810
– –, keratin, epidermic, 797
– –, osseous tissue, 842
– –, parietal cells (Romeis), 868
– –, vital staining, 25
– –, see vital red
– cotton 4B, see benzopurpurine 4B
– cotton B, C, see Congo red
– direct, see Congo red
– fast, see azorubine S
– neutral, 168
– –, vital stain, 25, 718, 788
– nucleal fast, 168, 299
– – –, alum lake, 203
– – –, picro-indigo-carmine, 203
–, acridine, 173
–, –, ribonucleic acid staining, 549
–, alizarine S, 168
–, diamide 4B, see benzopurpurine 4B
–, Magdala, 168
–, naphthalene, see Magdala red
–, naphthol S, see azorubine S
–, napthylamide, see Magdala red
–, Nile, stain for neutral lipids, 460
–, ruthenium, galactogen detection, 429
–, –, tendonous fibres, 852
–, sorbine, 169, 208
–, sudan, 452
–, thiazine, 169, 205, 849

Red *(cont.)*
-, toluylene, see neutral red
-, trypan, 170, 827
- oil 0, 4B, 170, 452, 564
- - IV, see sudan IV
- sulphydryl reagent, see 1,4-chloromercuriphenyl azo-2-naphthol
- vital, 170
- - brilliant, see vital red
- wool, see azorubine S
Reducing compounds, 321–332
- -, reduction of ferric ferricyanide, 322–325
- -, reduction of silver salts, 325–329
- -, reduction of tetrazolium salts, 329–332
Refractive index, 16, 21, 31, 698, 755
Rehydration, 35–37
Removal of blood, 63
- - excess fixatives, chromic, 68
- - - -, mercuric, 68
- - - -, osmic, 68
- - - -, picric, 68
- - lipid groups, 44
- - lipidic inclusions, 45
- - water molecules, cold trap, 37
- - - - by hygroscopic substances, 37
- - - - - mechanical pump, 36
- - - - - stream of dry gas, 37
Resins, as mounting medium, 148
Reticulation, as artefact, 35, 40, 45–46, 49
Reticuline fibres, 740, 812–816
Reticulocytes, 23, 793–794
Reversible acetylation, practice, 420
- -, principle, 419
- methylation, 421
Retina, 981–983
Rhodamine 3GO, equivalent of Schiff reagent, 362
Rhodizonate of sodium, calcium detection, 300–301
- - -, glycerophosphatase, 603
- - - -, lead detection, 320
Rhodopsine, 482
Ribbon of paraffin-wax, 109
- - -, handling, 109–112
Ribonuclease, (Brachet), 545, 561–563
Ribonucleic acid, 538–539, 705
Ring chamber, 19
Rodent, stomach, 866
Rosaniline chlorhydrate, see magenta I
Rosazine, see azocarmine G
Rose chlorazol Y, see thiazine red
Rosinduline GXF, see ozocarmine G
Rosophenine 10B, see thiazine red
Rubeanhydric acid, rubeanic acid, see dithioxamide

Rubin, basic, see basic fuchsine
- Victoria O, see azorubine S
Rubine S_i see acid fuchsin

S

Saccharate of iron, athrocytosis, 826–827
Saffron, 171
Safranine, equivalent of Schiff's reagent, 362
-, Fautrez and Lambert staining, 570
-, water-alcoholic solution, 230
-, nucleic acids staining, 543–544
-, orcein-water blue technique, 774
-, triple staining of Flemming, 749–750
- B, see phenosafranine
- light green, 230, 700, 712
- O, G, Y, A, 168
Salicylate of methyl for paraffin-wax impregnation, 76
Salivary glands, 879–882
- -, histo-enzymological study, 881
Salts biliary, lipases activators, 633
- brown R, see chrysoïdine R
- fast blue B, see diazo of *o*-dianisidine
- - - BB, alkaline phosphatases, 607–608
- - - RR, see carboxylic esterases
- fast corinth LB, see carboxylic esterases
- - garnet GBC, acid phosphatases,
- - - - - -, carboxylic esterases,
- - - - - -, leucine amino-peptidase,
- - red 3G, acid phosphatases,
- - - RC, alkaline phosphatase, carboxylic esterases,
- - - TR, alkaline phosphatase,
- - - violet LB, alkaline and acid phosphatases,
- - scarlet GG acid phosphatases,
- ferric, histochemical detection, 312–313
- ferrous, reduction, 313–314
- of diazonium, nomenclature, 374–375
- - -, purification, 378
- - -, staining of elastic fibre, 817
- - Reinecke, histamine detection, 586
- - tetrazolium, 329–332
- - -, elastic fibre staining, 817
- - -, see also detection of reducing compounds, dehydrogenases, diaphorases
- - vinyl, vascular injection, 860
Saponification of acetylated sections, 420
Sarcosomes, 850–851
Saturation pressure, 36–37
Scarlet B, see Biebrich's scarlet
- -, see sudan III
- of Biebrich, 169
- - -, method of van Gieson, 205
- - croceine, see Biebrich's scarlet

Scarlet B. *(cont.)*
- oil, see sudan II
- R, see sudan IV

Schiff reagent, aldehyde detection, 650
Schwarzschild-Villiger effect, 270
Scraping, 16
Secretory granules, 45–46, 754–765
Secretory granules, basophilia after oxidation, 758
- –, cyanophily, 756
- –, distinction from lysosomes, 765
- –, erythrophily, 756
- –, examination *in vivo*, 755
- –, fixation, 755
- –, techniques for cytology, 756
- – – –, topography, 755

Sections, after freezing, 124–127
- – – –, sticking, 126–127
- by grinding or polishing, dried bone, 836
- – – –, fresh bone, 835
- defects of ribbon, remedy, 110–111
- –, dehydration, clearing, 147
- of celloidin block, angle of attack, 118
- – – –, angle of cutting, 119
- – – –, sticking, 121–123
- – – –, under alcohol, 119
- – – – – terpineol, 120
- – – – paraffin blocks, 118–120
- – – – – –, angle of attack, 118
- – – – – –, angle of cutting, 119
- – – – – – –, sticking, 121–123
- – – gelatin blocks, 123
- – – – –, sticking, 123
- – – paraffin blocks, 105–112
- – – – –, angle of attack, 99, 118
- – – – –, draining, 115
- – – – –, dry sticking, 112
- – – – –, drying, 116
- – – – –, paraffin removal, 141–142
- – – – –, serial sections, spreading, 115
- – – – –, spreading, 114–115
- – – – –, sticking with glycerine albumin, 112
- – – – – – Ruyter's fluid, 113

Semicarbazide aldehyde block, 370
Sensitiveness of histochemical reactions, 258
Sepia officinalis, 56
Serotonine, 584–585
- –, see also enteramine and enterochromaffine cells
- –, substrate for mono-amine oxidase, 650
- –, see 5-hydroxytryptamine

Serum, iodated for maceration (Schultze), 770
Sex-chromatin, 704–705

Sheets of mica, for histological teaching, 1062
Shift, of glycogen, during fixation, 426
Shrinkage, 31, 37, 41, 43–44, 54, 58, 60, 74
Sialidase, sialomucines identification, 417–418
Sialomucines, 435–436
- –, convenient tissues for demonstration, 677

Siderophily and anionic groups, 689
Silica, removal from tissues, 242
Silicon, detection, 296
Silver, ammoniacal carbonate, 327
- –, carbonate, 404
- –, detection, by p-dimethylaminobenzylidene rhodamine, 319
- – – – dithioxamine, 319
- – – – hexamethylene tetramine, 326–328, 463, 593–594
- –, impregnation of chondriome, 739
- – – –, endocrine cells, 873
- – – –, lysosomes, 765
- – – –, nucleolonema, 706
- –, chromate, 713
- –, nitrate, Golgi, 715
- – –, ascorbic acid detection, 325
- piperazine, 327, 404
- proteinate (Grimelius), 875
- purines, detection, 592–593
- salts, reduction, 325

Sinusoids, 884
Skin, 781–785
- –, cutaneous glands, 782
- –, nail, horn, 781
- –, hair follicles, 781

Slides, cleaning and care, 114
Smears, definitions, 699
- –, desiccation at laboratory temperature, 683
- –, osmic fixation, 699–700, 788–789
- dry, Ehrlich triacid, 791
- – –, Giemsa, 791
- – –, May-Grunwald, 791
- – –, panoptic staining (Pappenheim), 792
- – –, preparation, 788–789
- – –, Wright, 793
- vaginal, 1059

- wet, fixation (Weidenreich), 789
- – –, gentian violet staining (Geitler), 700
- – –, haematoxylin staining (Grassé), 790
- – –, safranin-light green staining (Geitler), 700

Sodium alizarine sulphonate, see **alizarine**
- azide, cytochrome-oxidase **inhibitor**, 645
- bicarbonate, for carbonic anhydrase detection, 637

Sodium *(cont.)*
- bisulfite, 760
- chloride, 55–56
- citrate, for peptidase inhibition, 638
- – for swelling chromosomes, 702
- diethylmalonyl urea, see sodium veronal
- ethylene-diamine-tetra acetate, 608
- –, decalcification (Freiman), 611
- fluoride, maceration, 770
- –, inhibitor, 615–616, 622
- glycerophosphate, for phosphatases, 602–605
- hydrosulphite, reduction of nitro groups, 498
- – –, reduction of disulphide bridges, 528
- hypochlorite, 648
- – –, oxidative deamination, 500–501
- – –, Sakaguchi reaction, 506
- hyposulfite, 740
- iodacetate, thiol block, 529
- iodate, 577
- isocitrate, 657
- lactate, 656
- laurylsulphate, 608
- metabisulfite, 712, 733, 761
- nitroprusside, 309, 518, 649
- rhodizonate, 603
- succinate, 653
- sulfate, 46–66, 686
- sulfite, 714
- taurocholate, 627, 632
- tetraborate decahydrate, see borax
- thiosulfate, 68, 706, 714
- veronal, for phosphatases, 603, 612
- α-naphthylphosphate, 606
- β-naphthylphosphate, 606

Softening, of cuticle, 880–881
Solution, of mercury cristals, 143
Solution, Achard and Aynaud, 798
   –, Benson, 559
   –, Fontana, 326–327
   –, Himes and Moriber, 558
   –, Jores, 879
   –, Kaiserling, 879
   –, Locke, 18
   –, Lugol, 143
   –, Müller, 55
   –, Ranvier, 770
   –, Ringer, 18
   –, Ruyter, 113, 116
   –, Tyrode, 18
   –, von Albertini, 19
   –, Weigert, 945
Sorbine red, 169
Sorbitane esters, for lipase detection, 633
   – phosphate, enzyme inhibitor, 622

Soret line, haemoglobin, 567
Spectrography of fluorescence, 272–275
Spectrophotometry of absorption, 267–271
Spermatid, acroblast, 716
Spermatocytes, 747
Spermatogenesis, on sections, 1050–1051
Spermatozoa, 20
Spherocrystal, 458–459
Sphingolipids, characteristics, 481
   –, convenient tissues for demonstration, 670
   –, definition, 444
Spleen, 43, 719
Spodograms, definition, 288
   –, identification of ashes, 292
   –, mounting, 291
   –, see also micro-incineration
Spreading sections on albumin, 38
   – – – alcohol, 42
   – – – glycerine-albumin, 38
   – – – mercury, 38
   – – – mineral oil,
   – – – warmed slide, 38
Squash, 698, 702, 704
Stain, acid, definition, 133
   –, amphoteric, definition, 133
   –, anionic, definition, 133
   –, basic, definition, 133, 1016
   –, cationic, definition, 133
   –, choice, 129, 138–139
   –, classification, 131–133
   –, comparison, 129
   –, manufacturer, 129
   –, metachromatic, chromophores, 344–345
   –, neutral, definition, 133
   – –, endocrine pancreas, 1013–1014
   – –, secretory granules, 756–757
   –, Giemsa, 791–792
   –, Leishman, 791
   –, May Grunwald, 791–792
   –, Romanovsky, 11
   –, Wright, 792–793
   –, standardization, 129–131
   –, vital, 24–25
   – –, acid, 28
   – –, basic, 29
Staining, adjective, definition, 131
   – bulk, cell boundaries, 773
   – –, definition, 131
   – –, indications, 237
   – –, integument, 776
   – –, nucleal reaction (Feulgen and Rossenbeck), 55
   – by fluorochromes, definition, 272
   – – "montage" (Feyrter), 462

Staining *(cont.)*
 –, choice, autoradiography, 286
 –, combined, definition, 131
 – direct, definition, 131
 –, free sections, 855
 –, histological, aim, 129
 – –, definition, 129–130
 – –, nomenclature, 129
 – –, requirements, 130
 –, indirect, definition, 131
 –, mitochondrial, 726–742
 –, multiplicity, 128–129
 –, neuroglia, after Anderson, 953–954
 – – – Holzer, 952
 –, neurones with methylene blue, 911–194
 – panoptic (Pappenheim), sections, 801
 – – –, smears, 792
 – with phosphotungstic haematoxylin, 954–955
 –, Altmann, 726–734
 –, Altmann-methyl green picrate, 729–730
 –, Benda, 734–735
 –, Benoît, chondriome, 729–730
 –, –, osmic impregnation, 712
 –, Bensley-Cowdry chondriome, 729, 731
 –, Fautrez and Lambert, haemoglobin, 570
 –, Gerlach, with carmin, 910
 –, Heidenhain, with haematoxylin-Bordeaux R, 693
 –, Hollande, chondriome, 729, 730
 –, Klinger and Ludwig, sex-chromatin, 704
 –, Kull, chondriome, 729, 731
 –, –, osmic impregnation, 712
 –, Masson, with phosphotungstic haematoxylin, fibrin, 822–823
 –, Nassonov, chondriome, 736
 –, –, osmic impregnation, 710, 726
 –, Neubert, muscular tissue, 848
 –, Pasini, 849–850
 –, Schaeffer, osteoid tissues, 842
 –, Schmorl, phosphotungstic acid-thonine, 841
 –, –, thionine-picric acid, 840
 –, Taenzer-Unna, elastic tissue fibres, 817–818
 –, Volkonsky, 729
 –, Walter, muscular tissue, 850
 –, Weigert, with methyl violet, 822
 –, – – resorcine-fuchsin, elastic fibres, 819
 –, Wright, original technique, 793
 –, Ziehl-Neelsen, 484–485
 –, on sections, 131
 –, – slides, 140

 –, post-vital, 23
 –, progressive, definition, 131
 –, regressive, definition, 131
 –, "*signaletic*" (Lison), 258
 –, simple, definition, 131
 –, simultaneous, 131
 –, successives, 131
 –, theories, 134–137
 –, topographic, 192–193
 –, vital, aim, 24
 – –, advantages, 24
 – –, definition, 24
 – –, diffuse, 27
 – –, disadvantages, 24
 – –, granular, 27
 – with Altmann fuchsin-methyl green picrate, 729–730
 – –, cresyl violet-picrofuchsin, mast cells, 826
 – –, haemalum-Congo red keratin, 778–779
 – –, haematoxylin-thiazine red, 849
 – –, luxol fast blue, myelin, 949
 – –, orcein, mechanism, 137
 – –, performic acid-alcian blue (Adams and Sloper), 524–525, 967
 – –, pyrogallol-iron, nucleolonema, 707
 – –, "quad", of Kornhauser, elastic fibres, 818–819
 – –, sudan black B, myelin, 949
 – –, thiazine red-methylene blue (myofibrils), 849
Starch, 430, 641
Stato-acoustic apparatus, 983–985
 – – in Invertebrates, statocyst, 983
 – – – Vertebrates, 984–985
Stellar ganglion, 56
Steroido-dehydrogenase, 659
Steroidogenesis, 659
Steroids, 481
 –, convenient tissues for demonstrations, 677
Sticking sections, 97, 121–127
 – –, albumin (Apathy), 113
 – –, albumin-glycerine (Mayer), 112
 – –, albuminous-water (Henneguy), 113
 – –, by desiccation, paraffin sections, 116
 – –, gelatin, 113
Stomach, 866–869
Striated border, 748, 871
Strontium, detection, 307
Stylet, crystalline, in Molluscs, 869
Sublimation of water, 36
Substitution by cobalt, calcium detection, Stoelzner, 305
Substrates for enzymes, 598–599
Succinic anhydride, carboxylation, 432

Succinodehydrogenase, 53, 652
Sudan black B, 170
– – –, acetylated, Lillie and Burtner, 451
– – –, alcoholic solutions, 451–453
– – –, myelin, 949
Sulphocyanide-ammonium picrate, for methylene blue stabilisation, 907
Sulphomucosubstances, affinity for paraldehyde-fuchsin, 353
–, basophily, 342
–, convenient tissues for demonstration, 677
–, histochemical characteristics, 435–435
–, mast-cells, 825–826
–, metachromasia, 348
Sulphonation, p-hydrazine benzene sulfonic acid, 433
Sulphatases, detection, 634–635
–, suitable tissues, 678
Sulphate, detection, 295
– ferrous, melanine detection, 580
– of cadmium, apoferritine detection, 316
Sulphydrylated proteins, 526–530, 706
Susa, Heidenhain's, 182
Swelling, 35, 41, 43, 54
Swim bladder, 893
Sympathetic ganglional cells, Golgi, 716
Synapses, myo-neural, demonstration, 852
Syrup of Apathy, 145
– –, laevulose, 145
System, canalicular, in salivary glands, 882
– nervous, 969–972

T

Tactile corpuscles, 781, 973–974
Tannin-orange, of Unna, 728
Tanning, 48, 51, 647
Tannophilic protide, 495
Target organs for hormones, 1046–1047
Taste buds, 865, 976–977
Taurocholate of sodium, lipase activator, 622
Teasing, 16–17
Techniques, 10
–, automatic, 10
–, capricious, 10
–, choice, 2–3, 11–12
–, difficult, 10
–, easy, 10
–, general rules, 11
–, Ackerman, leucine-aminopeptidase, 638
–, Adams, indol groups, 517
– –, ferric ferricyanide, 325
– –, sterols, 478

– – and Sloper, neurosecretion, 967
– – and Swettenham, adenohypophysis, 1005
–, Altmann, chondriome, 728
–, Aronson, Vorbrodt, deoxyribonuclease, 640
–, Arvy, cholinesterase, 625
– –, – and phosphatase, on the same section, 605
– –, free lipids and mast-cells, red oil and toluidine blue, 462
– – and Gabe, cresyl violet–van Gieson picrofuschsin, for mast-cells, 827
– – – –, iron and phosphatase, on the same section, 605
– – and Rancurel, PAS-alcian blue, for mast-cells, 827
–, Bessis, blood reticulocytes, 794
–, Bethe, methylene blue stabilisation, 913
– –, neurofibrils, 919
–, Bielchowsky, neurofibrils, 921
– –, reticuline, 812
– – and Plien, Nissl bodies, 908
–, Bloom and Bloom, osseous tissues, 842
–, Bohm, biliary capillaries, 880
–, Bubenaite, silver chromate impregnation, 918
–, Burstone, acid phosphatases, 618
– –, alkaline phosphatases, 608
– –, carboxylic esterases, 631
– –, cytochromoxidase, 646
–, Chiquoine, glucose-6-phosphatase, 621
–, Chrzonszczewsky, biliary capillaries, 885
–, Clara, alveolar cells of lung, 892
–, Cleveland et al., adenohypophysis, 995
–, Coers, cholinesterase, 624
–, Cox, neuroplasm, 918
–, De Galantha, silver impregnation of urates, 593, 896
–, Dogiel, methylene blue stabilisation, 913
–, Donaggio, neurofibrils, 919
–, Elftman, adenohypophysis, 1003
– –, gold detection, 319
– –, Golgi bodies impregnation, 715
– –, postchromisation, 471–472
–, Eränkö, noradrenaline, 578–579
–, Ezrin, adenohypophysis, 1004
–, Farber and Louviere, succinodehydrogenase, 653
–, Forsgren, biliary capillaries, 886
–, Fox, neurone impregnation, 919
–, Galeotti, chondriome, 728
–, Gerebtzoff, cholinesterases, 625

Techniques (cont.)
 -, Gerota, lymphatic vessel injection, 862–863
 -, Glenner et al., mono-aminoxidase, 651
 -, Golgi-Cajal, silver chromate impregnation, 916
 -, Gomori acid phosphatases, 616
 - -, alkaline phosphatases, 602
 - -, carboxylic esterases, 630
 - -, DOPA-oxidase, 647
 - -, lipases, 533
 - - , 5-nucleotidase, 614
 - -, peroxidase, 649
 - -, phosphamidase, 619
 -, Gomori-Takamatsu, alkaline phosphatase, 604
 -, Grogg and Pearse, acid phosphatases, 618
 - Hagmann, Arthropod tracheae, 894–895
 -, Halmi, adenohypophysis, 1001
 -, Hellerström and Hellman, silver impregnation, endocrine pancreas, 1026–1027
 -, Hellman jun., size of Langerhans islets, 1010
 -, Hellman sen., lymphoid tissue in digestive tract, 878–879
 -, Herlant, alcian blue, adenohypophysis, 1006
 -, Hillarp and Hökfelt, adrenaline, 576, 1037
 - - - -, noradrenaline 576–1037
 -, Hitzeman, dehydrogenase, 658
 -, Holmer, biliary capillaries, 886
 -, Hultquist and Tenger, A cells, 1021
 -, Humberstone, neurosecretion, 969
 -, Koelle and Valk, mono-aminoxidase, 651
 -, Krompecher, fresh bone, 835
 -, Kurata, carbonic anhydratase, 637
 -, Laidlaw and Blackberg, DOPA-oxidase, 647
 -, Laskey, Nissl bodies, 908
 -, Levy et al., Δ^5-3-β-hydroxysteroidodehydrogenase, 660
 -, Lillie, amyloid, 810
 - -, dehydrogenases, 658
 - -, endocrine pancreas,1013
 -, Lundwall, bone and cartilage, 828–830
 -, Mc Conaill, lead haematoxylin, 910
 -, Marks and Drysdale, stomach, 867
 -, Metzner, chondriome, 728
 -, Meyer and Weinmann, phosphamidase 620
 -, Moog, cytochromoxidase, 645
 -, Müller, endocrine pancreas, 1020
 -, Nachlas et al., amino-peptidase, 639–640
 - - - -, cytochromoxidases, 645
 - - - -, diaphorases, 654
 - - - -, succinodehydrogenase, 656
 -, Obregia, sticking of celloidin sections, 122
 -, Oliver, urea, 592
 -, Oppenheimer, biliary capillaries, 885
 -, Oster and Schlossman mono-aminoxidase, 650
 -, Otami, biliary capillaries, 886
 -, Padykula and Herman, adenosine-triphosphatase, 612
 -, Paget and Eccleston, adenohypophysis, 1003–1004
 - Pappenheim reticulocytes 794
 -, Pearse, dehydrogenase, 653
 - -, succinodehydrogenase, 654
 -, Petersen, freezing-celloidin, 783
 -, Peute and van de Kamer, neurosecretion, 967
 -, Pischinger, Nissl bodies, 909
 -, A. Prenant, chondriome, 728
 -, Puchtler, amyloid, 810
 -, Ranvier, membranes, 772
 - -, neurofibrils, 920
 - -, nerves, 944
 - -, osseous tissue, 837
 -, Romeis, adenohypophysis, see cresazan
 - -, cartilage, 831–832
 - -, pituicytes, 989
 - -, stabilisation of methylene blue, 913
 -, Rutenburg et al., sulfatases, 634
 -, Sabrazes, reticulocytes, 794
 -, Scarpelli et al., diaphorases, 656
 -, Schabadash, methylene blue, 907
 -, Seligman et al., β-glucuronidase, 636
 -, Sterba, neurosecretion, 966
 -, Tramezzani et al., adrenal tissue, 1037
 -, Wachstein et al., esterases, 626–627
 - - and Meisel, adenosine-triphosphatase, 613
 - - - -, glucose-6-phosphatase, 621
 -, Wattenberg, Δ^5-3-β-hydroxysteroidsdehydrogenase, 659
 -, Weidenreich, bone, 841
 -, Weigert, fibrine, 821
 -, Wigglesworth, trachea of Arthropods, 895
 -, Wittmaak, internal ear, 984
 -, Zimmermann, stomach, 867
Technics for autoradiography, stripping, 285
Techniques, cytological, 681–688
 - histochemical, 251–252

Techniques *(cont.)*
- histo-enzymological, 595–596
- mitochondrial, 717–719
- neurofibrillar, 919
- neuroglial, 952

Teepol, 476
Tegument, 40
Tellurite of sodium, dehydrogenase, 653
Temperatures, 6, 20, 60
–, action on basophily, 336
–, fixation, chromic, 687
– –, chromo-osmic, 686
– –, drying of sections, 121
– –, for embedding, 79
Tendons, 852
Terephthalic aldehyde reaction, detection of α-amino-acid, 496–497
Terminal bars, 747, 751
Testicular interstitial cells, 11
Testis, 40, 1048
Tetra-acetate of lead, inhibition of oxidation, 416
– – – –, oxidation of polysaccharides, 394
Tetra-acetate of lead-Schiff, polysaccharide detection, 408
Tetrachrome, Herlant's, 226, 997
Tetrahydrofuran, as solvent of napthol AS, 608
Tetrahydropyridino-iminazol, condensation reaction, 587
Tetra-isopropylpyrophosphoramide, cholinesterase inhibitor, 623
Tetranitromethane, block for Morel and Sisley reaction 511–512
Tetrazolium salts, 643, 650, 652–653, 655–657
Tetrazoreaction of Danielli, 509–511
– – –, adenohypophysis, 999
Tetroxide of osmium, fixation, 54
– – –, impregnation, 710
– – –, maceration, 772
Theca of ovarian follicle, 1055
Thiazine, 132
–, caryology, 701–702
–, detection of nucleic acids, 540, 705
–, insolubilisation of ammonium molybdate, 339
–, Nissl bodies, 903
Thiocholinesterase, gastrin cells, 878
Thioflavine, S, T, 170
Thioglycerol, 528–529
Thiol, argentaffin reaction, 325
–, block, 529
–, convenient tissues for demonstration, 677
–, detection, 517–526
–, ferric ferricyanide reaction, 322
–, in tissues, lability, 526
–, tetrazolium salt reduction, 329
Thiolacetic acid, for cholinesterases, 623, 626
– –, for lipases, 633
Thionine, 172
–, detection of basophilia, 339
–, equivalent of Schiff's reagent, 362
–, lipid-stain, 462
–, metachromatic stain, 346
–, neurofibrils stain, 919
–, osseous tissue stain, 919
Thionine-paraldehyde, 354
– –, adenohypophysis, 1003–1004
– –, endocrine pancreas, 1016
– –, neurosecretory cells, 966
Thionine-paraldehyde PAS-naphthol yellow, 966
Thionine (or azur A)-SO_2, nucleal reaction, 557
Thionine-phenol (Nicolle), 840
Thiosemicarbazide, aldehyde block, 370
Thiosulfate of sodium, indol reactivation, 513
Thiovanol, see thioglycerol
Thoma, haematometer, 796
Thrombocytes, 798
Thymus, 806
Tissue, adipose, lipids, 825
–, adrenal, 1032, 1036
–, choice for detection, acid phosphatase, 678
– – – –, alkaline phosphatase, 678
– – – –, aminopeptidase, 678
– – – – –, amylotransferase, 678
– – – –, arginine, 677
– – – –, arylsulphatases, 678
– – – –, ascorbic acid, 676
– – – –, β-glucuronidase, 678
– – – –, bile pigments, 678
– – – –, calcium, 676
– – – –, catecholamines, 678
– – – –, cholinesterase, 678
– – – –, chromolipoids, 677
– – – –, cytochromoxidase, 678
– – – –, deoxyribonuclease, 677
– – – –, diaphorases, 679
– – – –, disulphur groups, 677
– – – –, DOPA-oxidase, 678
– – – –, galactogen, 676
– – – –, glucose, 676
– – – –, glucose-6-phosphatase, 678
– – – –, glycerides, 677
– – – –, glycogen, 676
– – – –, guanine, 678
– – – –, haemoglobin, 677
– – – –, haemosiderins, 678

Tissue *(cont.)*
– – – –, indolic compounds, 677
– – – –, ionic iron, 676
– – – –, lipases, 678
– – – –, melanin, 678
– – – –, monoamine-oxidase, 679
– – – –, peroxidase, 678
– – – –, phosphamidase, 678
– – – –, phospholipids, 677
– – – –, phosphorylase, 678
– – – –, polyphenoloxidase, 678
– – – –, polysaccharides, 440
– – – –, ribonucleic acid, 677
– – – –, sialomucines, 677
– – – –, sphingolipids, 677
– – – –, steroido-dehydrogenase, 679
– – – –, succinic dehydrogenase, 679
– – – –, sulfomucopolysaccharides, 677
– – – –, thiol groups, 677
– – – –, tunicin, 676
– – – –, tyrosinase, 678
– – – –, tyrosine, 677
– – – –, urates, 678
– – – –, zinc, 676
–, collagen, see collagen cells and fibres
–, connective, see ground substance and connective cells
–, cultures, 17, 698
–, dental, 843–845
–, interrenal, 1034
–, lymphoid, in digestive tract, 878
–, "nodal", of the heart, 854
–, osseous and osteoid, 842
Toluene, 74
p-toluenesulfonechloramide of sodium, see chloramine T
Toluidine blue, 24, 576
– –, after hydrochloric acid hydrolysis, 877
Tongue, 16
Tonofibrils, fixation, 751
–, staining, 751, 773
TPN and TPNH, see NADP and NADPH
Trachea, 891
–, in Arthropods, 894
Transferases, definition, 640–641
Transglucosidase, 640–641
Triacid, Ehrlich, fixation, 34, 231–232
Trichloride of platinum, rhodopsine fixation, 482
– – –, see also chloroplatinic acid
Trichloride of titanium, 498
Trichohyalin, 781
Trichoxanthin, 583
Trichrome, Gomori, 215–216
–, Masson, 213
–, Masson-Goldner, 213

–, Ramon y Cajal, 202
–, one-step, 217–218
–, variant of Gomori, 216–217
Triglycerides, 47
Trihydroxymethalaminomethane, 654
Trioxide of chromium, fixation, 48–49, 57, 694
– – –, maceration, 770
– – –, melanin bleaching, 582, 980
– – –, oxidation, 396–397
– – – see also chromic acid
Trioxyhaematein, Hansen, 198
Triphenylmethane, 132
Triphenyltetrazolium, 330–331
Triple staining, Flemming, De Winiwarter variant, 749
– –, for nuclear structure, 702
– –, Matthey variant, 750
– –, A. Prenant, 209
– –, Millot, 229
Tropeoline G, see metanil yellow
Trypan blue, 25–28
– red, 170
Trypsine, elastic fibre digestion, 825
–, direction for use, 525
Tryptamine chlorhydrate, for aminoxidase (Koelle and Valk), 651
Tryptophane, 48, 513–514, 584–586
–, tetrazoreaction of Danielli, 509–510
Tubes, Borrell, 141
–, Caullery and Chapelier, 73
–, Fairchild, 68–73
–, Jolly, 141
Tunicine, see cellulose
Turbellaria, gonocytes, 777
Turpentine, for bleaching, osmic impregnation excess, 711–712
Tween for lipase detection, 633
Tyramine, substrate for monoamine-oxidase, 650, 652
Tyrofusine KA, 19
Tyrosinase, 646
Tyrosine, 48
–, convenient tissues for demonstration, 677
–, in nucleolus, 706

U

Ultrafiltration, 26–27
Ultrastructural cytology, 31
Universal fixative, 42
Unmasking, iron, 314
–, lipoids, 448
Uranyl nitrate, fixative, 687
– –, for nucleolonema, 706, 713

Urates, basophilia, 339, 343
 –, convenient tissues for demonstration, 678
 –, detection, 593
 –, distinction from calcium, 594
 –, reactions, argentaffine, 325, 328, 593
 – –, ferric ferricyanide, 900
 –, solubility, 316, 594
Urea, 591
 –, detection, Leschke, 592
 –, – Oliver, 592

V

Vacuoles, 27
Vacuum, 34–35, 61, 610
Van de Kamer apparatus, for fixation, 893
Vapour, dehydration, dioxan, 73
 –, fixation, formaldehyde, 61
 – –, iodine, 61
 – –, osmium tetroxide, 61
Varnishes, 1062
Vaseline chamber, 19
 – iodated, glycogen detection,
Verdoperoxidase, 644, 648
Versene, for peptidase inhibition, 638
 –, see sodium ethylene-diamine tetra-acetate
Vessels, cutaneous, 780
 –, gastric and intestinal, 879
 –, in liver, 884
 –, lymphatic, 862–863
 –, staining, content, 857
Vesuvine, see Bismark brown
Vic-glycols, acetylation, 420
 – –, oxidation, 390–405
Violamine R, see violet-acid 4R
Violet, acid, see eriocyanine A
Violet acid, zinc leuco, 569
Violet, acid 4R, 171
 –, C, FB, C, see crystal violet
 –, crystal, chondriome, 734
 – –, fibrin, 822
 – –, neuroglia, 952
 – –, Schiff equivalent, 362
 – –, triple staining of Flemming-Matthey, 750
 – – -methyl violet, amyloid, 810
 – – -resorcin (Lillie), 820
 –, ethyl-orange (Bailey), 756
 –, hexamethylated, see crystal violet
 –, cresyl, 171
 – –, mast cells, 826
 – –, metachromasia of lipids, 462
 – –, Nissl bodies, 909
 – –, reaction, metachromatic, 347

– –, vital stain, 25
 –, ethyl, 172
 – – see ethyl purple 6B
 –, fast cresyl, see cresyl violet
 –, gentian, osseous tissue staining, 841
 – –, see methyl violet, violet crystal
 – –, smears, chromosome staining, 700
 – –, triple staining of Flemming, 749
 – – neutral, (Bensley), 756
 –, Hofmann, see dahlia
 –, iodine, see dahlia
 –, Lauth, see thionine
 –, methyl, Schiff equivalent, 362
 – –, staining of fibrin, 822
 – –, vital stain, 25
 – – 10B, 172
 – –, see crystal violet
 –, methylene, 172, 729, 802
 –, Paris, see methyl violet
 –, R, RR, 4RN, see dhalia
Visual apparatus, 977
 – Invertebrates, 977
 – Vertebrates, 977–983
Vital examination, 15–21
 – –, drawbacks, 15
 – –, limits, 15
 – stains, 22–29
 – –, acid, 29
 – –, advantages, 24
 – –, basic, 29
 – –, classification, 24–25
 – –, disadvantages, 24
 – –, for Golgi apparatus, 698
 – –, for nucleus, 698
 – –, objects, 24
 – –, post-vital, 23
 – –, supra-vital, 23
 – –, theories, 25–26
Vitamin A, demonstration, 482
Vitreous body, 981
Volume, appreciation, 6, 31, 36, 53, 61

W

Washing of pieces, 67–68, 711, 722, 724
Water, anilinic, Altmann fuchsin, 735
 –, sulfurous, washing, 363
Wax, definition, 444
Weights, 6
Wing, 16
Worms, 60

X

Xanthine, 594
 – oxidase, 650

Xanthydrol, indol groups, detection, 876
–, urea detection (Oliver), 592
Xylene-cyanol, see cyanol FF

Y

Yellow acid, see fast yellow (azo-dyes)
– – R, see metanil yellow
–, alcian, 172
– –, mucosubstances (Ravetto), 412–413
– –, neurosecretion (Peute and Van de Kamer), 967
–, brilliant, 169
–, butter 169
– –, see also yellow oil D, yellow oil III, yellow fast oil B
–, fast (azo-dye), 169
–, FY, G, S, see fast yellow (azo dye)
–, GG, (pyrazolone), 172
–, imperial, see aurantia
–, Manchester, see Martius yellow
–, of acridine, 170
– – –, fluorochrome, 274
– – –, Schiff equivalent, 362
– – Martius, 171
– – –, Millot staining, 229
– – –, one-step staining, 217–218
– – metanil, 169
– – naphthol, see Martius yellow
– – –, S, 171
– – – –, adenohypophysis, 1000, 1006
– – – –, Benson's method, 559
– – – –, Himes and Moriber's method, 558–559
– – – –, one step trichome, 217–218
– – – –, total acidophily, 332–333
–, thiazol, see yellow Titan G
–, titan, magnesium detection, 309
– – G, 170
Y-erythrosin, 173
Yolk nuclei in Araneid ovocytes, 746

Z

Zea mais, 49
Zinc-iodide (Maillet), 943
– -leucobases, 648
– chloride, detection of cellulose, 429
– – – chitin, 433
– – – haemoglobin, 569–570
– – – peroxidase, 648
Zincon, detection of zinc, 310
Zonation, in fixation, 40, 53, 59
Zone, iso-electric, 338

MASSON, Éditeur.
120, Bd St-Germain, Paris (VIe),
Dépôt légal: 1er trimestre 1976

Printed in Hungary